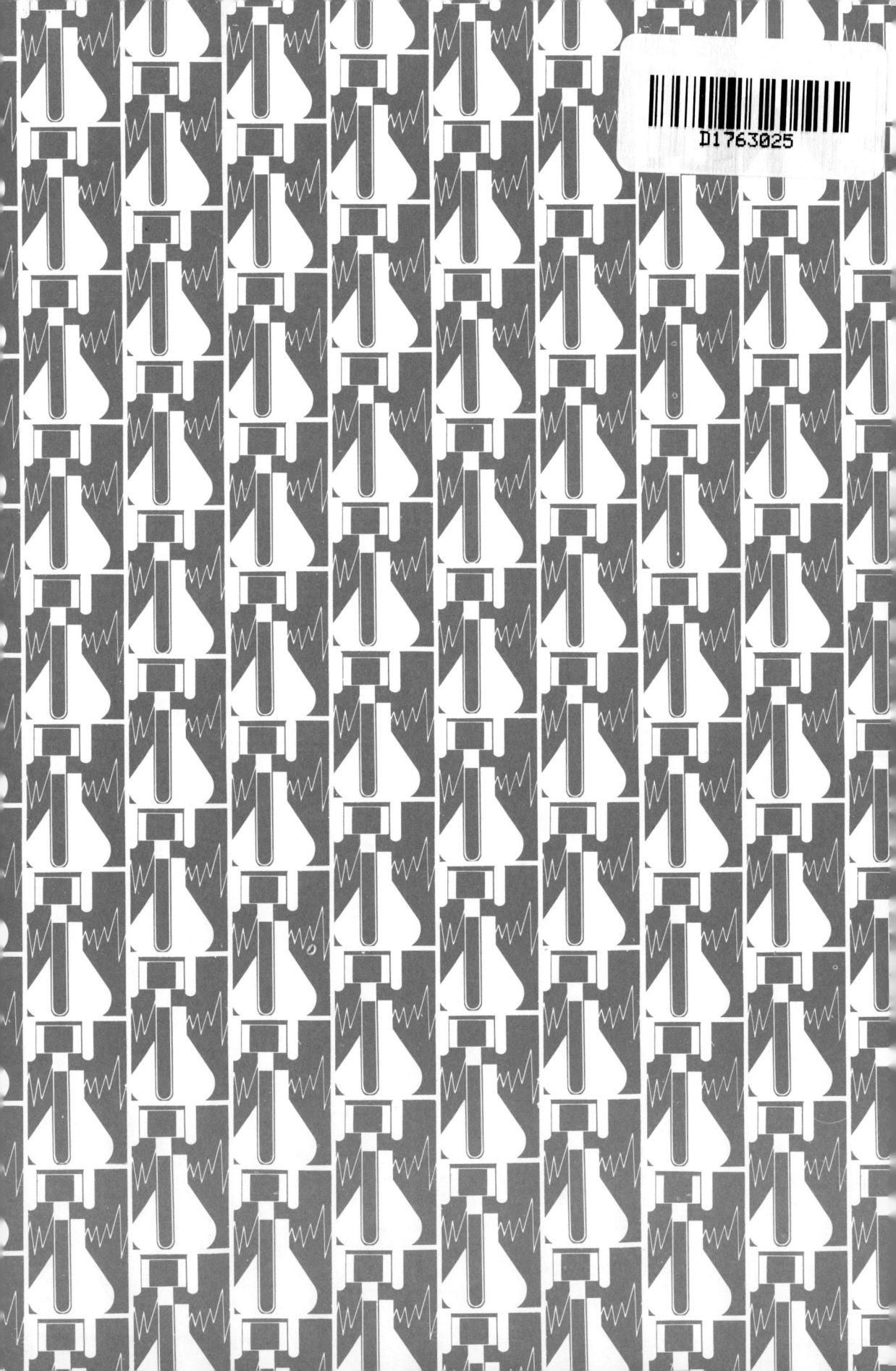

MODERN LEGAL MEDICINE, PSYCHIATRY, AND FORENSIC SCIENCE

MODERN LEGAL MEDICINE, PSYCHIATRY, AND FORENSIC SCIENCE

WILLIAM J. CURRAN, J.D., LL.M., S.M. Hyg.
FRANCES GLESSNER LEE PROFESSOR OF LEGAL MEDICINE
HARVARD MEDICAL SCHOOL AND SCHOOL OF PUBLIC HEALTH
CHAIRMAN, MASSACHUSETTS STATE MEDICOLEGAL INVESTIGATION COMMITTEE
BOSTON, MASSACHUSETTS

A. LOUIS McGARRY, M.D.
PROFESSOR OF CLINICAL PSYCHIATRY
STATE UNIVERSITY OF NEW YORK AT STONY BROOK
DIRECTOR, DIVISION OF FORENSIC SERVICES
NASSAU COUNTY MEDICAL CENTER
EAST MEADOW, NEW YORK

CHARLES S. PETTY, M.D.
DIRECTOR, SOUTHWESTERN INSTITUTE OF FORENSIC SCIENCES AT DALLAS
CHIEF MEDICAL EXAMINER, DALLAS COUNTY
PROFESSOR OF PATHOLOGY AND FORENSIC SCIENCES
UNIVERSITY OF TEXAS SOUTHWESTERN MEDICAL SCHOOL AT DALLAS
DALLAS, TEXAS

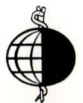 **F. A. DAVIS COMPANY • Philadelphia**

Copyright © 1980 by F. A. Davis Company

All rights reserved. This book is protected by copyright. No part of it may be reproduced, stored in a retrieval system, or transmitted in any form or by any means, electronic, mechanical, photocopying, recording, or otherwise, without written permission from the publisher.

Printed in the United States of America

Library of Congress Cataloging in Publication Data
Main entry under title:

Modern legal medicine.

   Includes bibliographies and index.
   1. Medical jurisprudence.   2. Forensic pathology.
3. Forensic psychiatry.   4. Criminal investigation.
I. Curran, William J.   II. McGarry, Armand Louis, 1929-   III. Petty, Charles S.
RA1051.M54   614'.19   79-19477
ISBN 0-8036-2292-9

PREFACE

The Russian word *troika* may best describe our role as editors of this book: three acting together with unity of purpose. We represent three different areas of specialization, but we are united in an effort to bring the knowledge and skills of the medicolegal fields and allied forensic sciences to bear upon the administration of the courts, penal systems, and law enforcement programs. We recognize the divergences in methodology in forensic medical areas, the forensic behavioral sciences, and the many related scientific fields examined in the book, but all of the contributing authors join us in our devotion to one goal: justice. These are years when the basic concept of justice has been assailed, when the administration of the courts and the management of law enforcement programs in North America and in other western nations have been under grave suspicion by many elements of their populations.

Medicolegal professionals and forensic scientists are dedicated to thorough investigation, impartial reporting to proper authorities, and scientific truth in the formulation of their findings and conclusions. Through these principles they seek the constant improvement of the relationship between science and justice in the interest of personal rights, responsibilities, and freedoms. It is our hope that the cooperative efforts that made this book possible will enhance public confidence in the courts and law enforcement programs in future years.

This book is intended as the first comprehensive, single-volume work covering the entire field of legal medicine and the allied forensic sciences. That it has been accomplished after over four years of interdisciplinary planning and production is a tribute primarily to our authors, selected from among the most authoritative and articulate spokespeople for their fields in the United States. We are indebted to all of them for their cooperation and dedication in making this ambitious undertaking a reality.

It may be helpful to readers to be apprised of the separate viewpoints and goals of the editors as well as our common objectives. In the following paragraphs we will try to summarize these views.

CHARLES S. PETTY

It has been my goal to provide physicians, scientists, attorneys, jurists, law enforcement personnel, and students in college programs and graduate professional schools with a readable book that is practical and usable. The sections of this book dealing with scientific, medicolegal investigation of death and scientific investigation of crime are intended as broad, general illuminations of the fields covered in each chapter. These sections are also intended to aid the consumers of this information—law-enforcement investigators, prosecutors, defense attorneys, and the courts—in dealing more intelligently and effectively with specialists in the various medicolegal and forensic scientific fields.

No earlier work of American origin has covered the interfaces of legal medicine, psychiatry, and the forensic sciences. Several excellent texts have been produced in recent years on various aspects of medicolegal death investigation, but even in this field the coverage has not generally been as broad as in this book. Our effort has been to emphasize not only the more traditional areas of trauma-related deaths and suicide investigation but modern medicolegal investigational aspects of automobile and airplane deaths, medical care-related deaths, and deaths related to public health hazards and neoplastic diseases. We have included not only chapters on scientific methods, but on the practical aspects of operating a public death investigation program, performing a medicolegal autopsy, investigating rape and other sexually related crimes, and managing a forensic crime laboratory.

The authors of these chapters have done their best to present their subspecialties in relation to the overall objectives of the book. It is they who have created and who should be praised. Technical interpretations are the authors' alone; the thrust of the book is ours as general editors.

In closing I wish to cite a second *troika:* the close cooperation of the editors, the authors, and the publisher. The latter should not be overlooked. Patience and help to the fullest were the watchwords of the publishing staff throughout the long months necessary to produce this book in an accurate and attractive form.

A. LOUIS McGARRY

Psychiatrists and psychologists specializing in fields related to the administration of justice have joined with other professional colleagues and forensic scientists to produce this comprehensive text. This is in keeping with the general movement of behavioral clinicians to work more directly with the mainstreams of medicine and science and with community agencies generally, including courts and law enforcement agencies. In recent years we have seen the decline of the large state mental institutions and the development of psychiatric wards, including forensic psychiatric and psychological units, in community general hospitals and university teaching hospitals. There has been a biological revolution in the practice of psychiatry with the introduction and widespread effectiveness of antipsychotic, antianxiety, and antidepressive drugs along with greater understanding, through promising and sophisticated research, of the neurophysiological and biochemical determinants of behavior. This text is intended to reflect these modern trends toward the greater application of clinical psychiatry and psychology in the legal and penal systems of this country.

I would also note that behavioral clinicians have not always been seen as working from as firm a scientific base as other physicians and forensic scientists contributing to this book. In all behaviorally related chapters, however, the editors have tried to present the most broadly authoritative, professionally accepted, and scientifically reliable findings and conclusions available for the consideration of readers.

No single-volume text can be totally exhaustive in every field covered. We have thus not dealt in depth with child custody, juvenile justice systems, or spousal abuse and other nonfatal, behavioral-legal issues in the family-law field. We have chosen to give primary attention in this section of the book to the most frequently encountered interfaces of forensic psychiatry and psychology with the administration of justice, including therein the most recent developments in psychological assessment for juvenile and adult courts, as well as the highly controversial subject of assessing, predicting, and treating dangerous, violent conduct.

I am grateful to the chapter contributors from many professions and disciplines whose efforts are contained in this section. Their writings are consistent with the highest traditions of the Hippocratic oath to instruct those who come after them in the best precepts of their chosen fields.

WILLIAM J. CURRAN

In this last section, I will attempt to explain the design of this book. As it is the first comprehensive, one-volume text dealing with all of the medicolegal and allied forensic science fields, our first concern was with coverage. We wanted to call attention to all areas of such specialization devoted to aiding the courts, correctional programs, and law enforcement. This may seem a clear-cut objective, but it was found to be quite novel in the field. The unifying source was the courts, the administration of justice, not the sciences themselves. We chose to make a contemporary survey and to include, if practicable in a text of manageable size, attention to each medicolegal and allied forensic science specialty currently seen in any appreciable degree of frequency in regular contact with courts, investigators, and correctional authorities. The subjects covered in this book represent these fields. We also sought to achieve cohesiveness in the relationship of the fields one with another. We identified important links among them in their voluntary association within respected organizations such as the American Academy of Forensic Sciences and in their groupings in official units or offices of medical examiners or forensic scientific investigation. We found keys also in the intraprofessional efforts to achieve national standards for accreditation as forensically related, evidence-producing experts. Our effort was therefore intended in this respect to establish the practical and operational boundaries of the medicolegal and allied forensic scientific fields in a way not previously described in a single reference book.

In the individual chapters, it is our intention to describe the current state of the art at the end of the 1970s with a view to application to modern problems of the respective fields into the 1980s and beyond. We asked authors to deal in practical terms with the basic skills and methodologies and with the important technological advances in their fields. Readers should not expect fresh, first-hand reports on research findings. This is a textbook of general applicability, not a collection of independent research results presented in professional journal style.

This last remark leads me into the next issue of design. Most of the authors selected were independent and well-established contributors from the various fields covered in the book; they could be expected to provide important contributions, but not necessarily related one to another, unless a plan of design addressed interrelationships and a comprehensive product. I attempted to address these requirements. Along with the other editors, I sought to have the various sections of the book follow a common pattern of development. The first chapters in each section should address operational, management problems for their broad areas and then should lay down requirements for education, advanced training, and accreditation. The next chapters should then deal with the basic methods and practices of diagnosis (or identification of the problem) in their fields. The other experts could then branch off into numerous specific applications, coming together again in concluding materials on the common core of methods and problems in the presentation of evidence in the courts of law.

With minor variations, this format has been followed throughout the completed book. The major section on medicolegal death investigation, under Dr. Petty's editorship, sets the tone. The first chapter in the section is a detailed and relatively long chapter on operational aspects pointing out the many interrelationships of a modern medicolegal office. There is next a chapter on qualifications and training followed by two chapters dealing with technical and practical aspects of the basic tool of the field, the medicolegal autopsy. There follows a chapter on another general conceptualization of the field, the definition and time of a death. Specialized chapters follow leading up to the concluding chapter on courtroom presentation in death cases.

In the large section on forensic psychiatry and psychology, Dr. McGarry follows the same structural pattern. The opening chapter deals with operational problems and also gives attention to qualification and training. Since the organizational and management issues are not as complex as in the death investigational systems, this shorter, combined coverage is warranted. However, a second chapter is given over entirely to a consideration of psychiatric professional relationships to the courts on substantive issues in the administration of justice. Next, Dr. McGarry's section moves on to two chapters on the basic diagnostic tools, psychiatric and psychological testing, and the reporting of findings and conclusions to the courts on mental status examinations, psychological assessment results, and special psycholegal reporting in legal areas such as capacity to stand criminal trial, criminal responsibility, and contractual and testamentary capacity. Specialized subjects are then dealt with in a series of chapters ending with two chapters relating to the trial process and evidence presentation.

The final major section on the allied forensic sciences follows a similar model of exposition. The first chapter deals with operations from the point of view of the term approach to investigation, gathering and preserving evidence, and reporting on findings and conclusions. Dr. Peterson's chapter introduces many of the forensic scientific specialties in relation to on-scene investigation. The next chapter deals with the organization and management of a forensic-crime laboratory, the focal point of the laboratory-based technical support systems. The following chapters deal with the major forensic science fields. Within the chapters, the basic format is followed. Thus they cover matters of qualifications and training, basic techniques of the field, and the scientific basis for the field itself. Two chapters are more general, dealing with matters of personal identification and the statistical foundations of many forensic scientific applications. The last chapter of the book returns to the basic theme, the all-important end product, the presentation of forensic scientific evidence in the courts of justice.

Two sections of the book do not follow the format indicated above. These are more general sections where the specialties are not grouped. The first section contains chapters on historical development and ethical standards. These subjects are intended to provide foundations for the field as a whole. The remaining section, covering special investigations, provides a bridge between major groupings in death investigation and behavioral science fields. It contains chapters on subjects which do not easily fit solely in one major section or another. We are particularly appreciative of the contributions regarding rape investigation. Much of this type of material has never before appeared in a medicolegal or forensic science text. The other chapters in this section are also quite novel in their scope and attention to community aspects of sensitive investigations.

Certain qualifications should also be stated concerning what this text does not attempt to accomplish. It is not a law book, though we hope to reach trial lawyers, judges, and students in forensic study programs. This is a book concerning scientific methods and scientific evidence. We hope that it will encourage more effective use of expert witnesses from medical, psychological, and other forensic science fields.

We have not examined directly certain aspects of police science and technology such as ballistics, fingerprinting, or the general aspects of witness interrogation. We have also not included a separate chapter on anthropology and personal identification, although two chapters deal with these subjects extensively. One is Dr. Petty's chapter on personal identification issues in forensic pathology. The other is Dr. Schwartz's chapter on forensic dentistry, in which the central issue of the entire chapter is accurate identification of human remains by anatomical means and personal dental characteristics. We also do not include attorneys and their practice as such, even though there is a section of lawyers (Jurisprudence) in the American Academy of Forensic Sciences. We view attorneys as essential to the presentation of understandable and relevant scientific evidence in the courts and as vital factors in the challenge to ineffective and improper evidence in their role as cross-examiners, but we do not classify them as forensic scientists per se. We have therefore distinguished the legal from the scientific role as a proper separation of powers and authority in the administration of justice. Again, readers may differ with our position, but we have tried to take it consistently throughout the book.

It is my strong belief that the medicolegal and forensic science fields will be among the most significant areas of professional work in this country over the remaining decades of this century. The United States must give high priority to the aims of the medicolegal and forensic science fields for the sake of its own social security. As contagious diseases are being conquered, and as greater attention and public expenditures have been allocated to chronic illnesses, the next decades must be concerned with social pathology, violence, accidental injuries and death, and more effective systems of justice. This trend in national emphasis is already becoming apparent in the greatly improved public support for forensic pathology service programs, scientific work in criminal and accident investigation, legal psychiatry programs, deviancy research, alcohol abuse and alcoholism rehabilitation programs, drug abuse and addiction programs, and for court and prison reform.

We wish again to thank the chapter authors whose wholehearted efforts have given this book a truly comprehensive scope. Their contributions, together with the encouragement and assistance of the editors and staff at the F.A. Davis Company, have helped us to realize our goals in presenting a thoroughgoing examination of modern legal medicine, psychiatry, and forensic science.

William J. Curran, J.D., LL.M., S.M. Hyg.
A. Louis McGarry, M.D.
Charles S. Petty, M.D.

CONTRIBUTORS

MARVIN E. ARONSON, M.D.
Medical Examiner, City of Philadelphia
Adjunct Associate Professor of
Pathology
University of Pennsylvania
School of Medicine
Philadelphia, Pennsylvania

CHARLES R. BAXTER, M.D.
Professor of Surgery and Medical
Director
Skin Transplant Center for Burns
University of Texas Southwestern
Medical School at Dallas
Dallas, Texas

JAMES A. BENZ, M.D.
Associate Professor of Pathology
Indiana University School of Medicine
Chief of Pathology Services
Wishard Memorial Hospital
Indianapolis, Indiana

JOSEPH P. BUCKLEY, M.S.
Director, John E. Reid and Associates
Laboratory
Chicago, Illinois
Lecturer in Polygraph Technology
Northwestern University School of Law
Chicago, Illinois

L. MAXIMILIAN BUJA, M.D.
Associate Professor of Pathology
University of Texas Southwestern
Medical School at Dallas
Dallas, Texas

MAUREEN CASEY, B.A.
Chief Document Examiner
Criminalistics Division
City of Chicago Department of Police
Chicago, Illinois

JOHN I. COE, M.D.
Medical Examiner, Hennepin County,
Minnesota
Chief of Pathology
Hennepin County Medical Center
Professor of Pathology
University of Minnesota
School of Medicine
Minneapolis, Minnesota

MURRAY L. COHEN, Ph.D.
Professor of Psychology
Director, Clinical Community
Psychology Program
Boston University
Boston, Massachusetts

JONATHAN O. COLE, M.D.
Staff Psychiatrist
McLean Hospital
Belmont, Massachusetts
Lecturer in Psychiatry
Harvard Medical School
Consultant in Research
Boston State Hospital
Boston, Massachusetts

WILLIAM J. CURRAN, J.D., LL.M., S.M. Hyg.
Frances Glessner Lee
Professor of Legal Medicine
Harvard Medical School and
School of Public Health
Chairman, Massachusetts State
Medicolegal Investigation
Committee
Boston, Massachusetts

JOSEPH H. DAVIS, M.D.
Chief Medical Examiner
Metropolitan Dade County, Florida
Professor of Legal Medicine
University of Miami School of Medicine
Miami, Florida

HAROLD W. DEMONE, JR., Ph.D.
Dean and Professor of Social Work
Graduate School of Social Work
Rutgers—the State University
New Brunswick, New Jersey

RISA G. DICKSTEIN, J.D.
Chief Counsel
New York State Commission on
Investigation
Formerly, Director of Planning
Heroin Research and Rehabilitation
Program
Vera Institute of Justice
New York, New York

VINCENT J. M. DI MAIO, M.D.
Medical Examiner, Dallas County
Associate Professor of Pathology
University of Texas Southwestern
Medical School of Dallas
Dallas, Texas

SIMON DINITZ, Ph.D.
Professor of Sociology
The Ohio State University
Columbus, Ohio

AMIRAM ELWORK, Ph.D.
Assistant Professor of Psychology
University of Nebraska—Lincoln
Lincoln, Nebraska

RUSSELL S. FISHER, M.D.
Chief Medical Examiner
State of Maryland
Professor of Forensic Pathology
University of Maryland
School of Medicine
College Park, Maryland

JAMES C. GARRIOTT, Ph.D.
Chief Toxicologist
Criminal Investigation Laboratory
Southwestern Institute of Forensic
Sciences at Dallas
Assistant Professor of Forensic Science
University of Texas Southwestern
Medical School at Dallas
Dallas, Texas

THOMAS P. HACKETT, M.D.
Eben S. Draper Professor of Psychiatry
Harvard Medical School
Chief of Psychiatry
Massachusetts General Hospital
Boston, Massachusetts

ELLEN L. HECK, B.S., M.T.
Faculty Associate
Department of Surgery
Director, Skin Transplant Center
for Burns
University of Texas Southwestern
Medical School at Dallas
Dallas, Texas

ELAINE HILBERMAN, M.D.
Associate Professor of Psychiatry
Assistant Director of Psychiatric
Residency Training
University of North Carolina
School of Medicine
Chapel Hill, North Carolina

CHARLES S. HIRSCH, M.D.
Director of Forensic Pathology
Hamilton County Institute of Forensic
Medicine, Toxicology, and
Criminalistics
Cincinnati, Ohio

LARRY B. HOWARD, Ph.D.
Director, Georgia State Crime
Laboratory
Atlanta, Georgia
Assistant Professor of Clinical Pathology
Emory University School of Medicine
Atlanta, Georgia

JULIAN KIVOWITZ, M.D.
Senior Psychiatrist and Director
Child Inpatient Ward
Neuropsychiatric Institute
University of California at Los Angeles
Los Angeles, California

ROBERT E. LITMAN, M.D.
Co-Director and Chief Psychiatrist
Suicide Prevention Center and
Institute for Studies of Destructive
Behaviors
Los Angeles, California
Adjunct Professor of Psychiatry
University of California at Los Angeles
Los Angeles, California

WILLIAM T. LOWRY, Ph.D.
Chief, Regulated Substances Section
Southwestern Institute of Forensic
Sciences at Dallas
Assistant Professor of Pathology
University of Texas Southwestern
Medical School at Dallas
Dallas, Texas

MORTON F. MASON, Ph.D.
Professor of Forensic Medicine
and Toxicology
University of Texas Southwestern
Medical School at Dallas
Dallas, Texas

A. LOUIS McGARRY, M.D.
Professor of Clinical Psychiatry
State University of New York
at Stony Brook
Director, Division of Forensic Services
Nassau County Medical Center
East Meadow, New York

WILLIAM A. MEISSNER, M.D.
Professor of Pathology
Harvard Medical School
Formerly, Chairman
Department of Pathology
New England Deaconess Hospital
Boston, Massachusetts

HERBERT C. MODLIN, M.D.
Professor of Community and Forensic
Psychiatry
The Menninger Foundation
Topeka, Kansas
Associate Clinical Professor of
Psychiatry
University of Kansas Medical Center
Kansas City, Kansas

CAROL C. NADELSON, M.D.
Associate Professor of Psychiatry
Harvard Medical School
Boston, Massachusetts

MALKAH T. NOTMAN, M.D.
Associate Clinical Professor of
Psychiatry
Harvard Medical School and
Beth Israel Hospital
Boston, Massachusetts

CHARLES P. O'BRIEN, M.D., Ph.D.
Professor of Psychiatry
University of Pennsylvania
School of Medicine
Director
Drug Treatment and Research Center
Veterans Administration Hospital
Philadelphia, Pennsylvania

GEORGE V.C. PARKER, Ph.D.
Clinical Psychologist
Austin, Texas
Formerly, Associate Professor of
Psychology
University of Texas
Austin, Texas

JOSEPH L. PETERSON, D.Crim.
Associate Professor and Director
Center for Research in Criminal Justice
University of Illinois, Circle Campus
Chicago, Illinois

CHARLES S. PETTY, M.D.
Director
Southwestern Institute of Forensic
Sciences at Dallas
Chief Medical Examiner, Dallas County
Professor of Pathology and Forensic
Sciences
University of Texas Southwestern
Medical School at Dallas
Dallas, Texas

SEYMOUR POLLACK, M.A., M.D.
Professor of Psychiatry and Director
Institute of Psychiatry, Law and
Behavioral Science
University of Southern California
Los Angeles, California

EARL F. ROSE, M.D., LL.B.
Professor of Pathology
University of Iowa School of Medicine
Iowa City, Iowa

LOREN H. ROTH, M.D., M.P.H.
Director, Law and Psychiatry Program
Western Psychiatric Institute and Clinic
University of Pittsburgh
Pittsburgh, Pennsylvania

JOSEPH C. RUPP, M.D., Ph.D.
Chief Medical Examiner
Nueces County (Corpus Christi), Texas

FAY A. SABER, J.D., M.P.H.
Assistant Professor of Medicine in Society
Wright State University
School of Medicine
Dayton, Ohio

BRUCE DENNIS SALES, Ph.D., J.D.
Associate Professor of Psychology and Law
Director, Law-Psychology Graduate Training Program
University of Nebraska—Lincoln
Lincoln, Nebraska

STANLEY M. SCHWARTZ, D.M.D.
Forensic Dental Examiner
Commonwealth of Massachusetts
Associate Professor of Oral Pathology
Head, Section on Oral Diagnosis
Tufts University
School of Dental Medicine
Boston, Massachusetts

R. KIRKLAND SCHWITZGEBEL, Ed.D., J.D.
Associate Professor of Psychology
California Lutheran College
Thousand Oaks, California

THEOHARIS K. SEGHORN, Ph.D.
Clinical Associate
Department of Psychology
Boston University
Boston, Massachusetts
Director of Clinical Services
Massachusetts Treatment Center
Bridgewater, Massachusetts

LAURENCE R. SIMSON, JR., M.D.
Associate Pathologist
Edward W. Sparrow Hospital
Lansing, Michigan
Associate Clinical Professor of Pathology
Adjunct Professor
School of Criminal Justice
Michigan State University
East Lansing, Michigan

IRVING C. STONE, JR., Ph.D.
Chief, Physical Evidence Analysis Section
Southwestern Institute of Forensic Sciences at Dallas
Assistant Professor of Forensic Sciences
University of Texas Southwestern Medical School at Dallas
Dallas, Texas

WILLIAM Q. STURNER, M.D.
Chief Medical Examiner
State of Rhode Island
Professor of Pathology and Laboratory Medicine
Director of Forensic Medicine
Brown University
Providence, Rhode Island

DONALD L. TASTO, Ph.D.
Clinical Psychologist
San Francisco, California
Formerly, Director
Center for Research on Stress and Health
SRI International
Menlo Park, California

OSCAR I. TOSI, Ph.D., Sc.D.
Director, Institute of Voice Identification
Director, Speech and Hearing Sciences Research Laboratory
Michigan State University
East Lansing, Michigan

CHARLES F. VORKOPER, M.S.S.W.
Psychotherapist
Dallas, Texas
Formerly, Clinical Director
Suicide Prevention Center of Dallas
Dallas, Texas

JAMES T. WESTON, M.D.
Chief Medical Investigator
State of New Mexico
Professor of Pathology
University of New Mexico
School of Medicine
Albuquerque, New Mexico

GEORGE E. WOODY, M.D.
Associate Clinical Professor of Psychiatry
University of Pennsylvania
School of Medicine
Assistant Director
Drug Treatment and Research Center
Veterans Administration Hospital
Philadelphia, Pennsylvania

RONALD K. WRIGHT, M.D.
Assistant Professor of Pathology
Associate Professor of Epidemiology
and Public Health
University of Miami School of Medicine
Miami, Florida
Deputy Chief Medical Examiner
Dade County, Florida

NORMAN E. ZINBERG, M.D.
Associate Professor of Psychiatry
Harvard Medical School
Staff Psychiatrist
Cambridge Hospital
Psychiatrist-in-Chief
Washingtonian Center for Addictions
Boston, Massachusetts

ROSS E. ZUMWALT, M.D.
Deputy Coroner
Cuyahoga County, Ohio
Assistant Professor of Forensic
Pathology
Case Western Reserve University
School of Medicine
Cleveland, Ohio

CONTENTS

PART 1   GENERAL CONSIDERATIONS

    1   HISTORY AND DEVELOPMENT   1

        William J. Curran, J.D., LL.M., S.M.Hyg.

        Ancient Origins   1
        The Amicus Curiae of Roman Law   2
        Developments in the Middle Ages   2
        The Seventeenth and Eighteenth Centuries   5
        Significant Dates in Medicolegal and Forensic Science History   5
        Methods of Proof   10
        Medicolegal Specialization   11
        The Emergence of Forensic Science   14
        Scientific Criminal Investigation and Forensic Science   21
        Contemporary Conditions: The State of the Art   22

    2   ETHICAL STANDARDS   29

        William J. Curran, J.D., LL.M., S.M.Hyg.

        The Scope of Ethical Inquiry   29
        Ethical Codes for Professions   30
        Monopoly and Legal Enforcement   31
        Ethical Codes in Forensic Science: Delayed Development   31
        Truth and Advocacy   36
        Impartiality in Public Agencies   37

Excessive Publicity 38
Investigational Procedures 39
Improperly Obtained Confessions 41
Psychiatric and Psychological Issues 42
Issues in Forensic Pathology 43
Unethical Advertising and Publicity 45
Enforcement of Ethical Codes 45

PART 2 MEDICOLEGAL DEATH INVESTIGATION

3 OPERATIONAL ASPECTS OF PUBLIC MEDICOLEGAL DEATH INVESTIGATION 51

Charles S. Petty, M.D., and
William J. Curran, J. D., LL.M., S.M.Hyg.

The Mores of Death 51
Legal Source for Programs 54
Government Support and Protection 56
Legal Liability Problems 59
Operational Interfaces 61
Forensic Medical Expert "Pool" Concept 75
Medicolegal Records and Confidentiality 76
The Death Certificate 78
Time of Death Problems 80
Relations with Organ Transplant Programs 82
Relations with the Press and Other Media 82
Support Facilities 83
Scene Examination and Body Removal 84
Appendix 87

4 QUALIFICATIONS AND TRAINING FOR FORENSIC PATHOLOGY 97

Russell S. Fisher, M.D., Ronald K. Wright, M.D., and
Charles S. Petty, M.D.

Anatomic Pathology 97
Clinical Pathology 97
Subspecialties of Pathology 98
Forensic Pathology 98

5 MEDICOLEGAL AUTOPSY: FUNDAMENTAL PROCEDURES 111

James T. Weston, M.D.

Clothing 111
External Examination 112
External Evidence of Injury 112
General Comments Concerning Injury 113

    External Evidence of Therapy   113
    Opening the Thorax and Abdomen   114
    Internal Examination   116
    Internal Evidence of Injury   117
    Internal Evidence of Therapy   117
    Systems Review   117
    Specimens   118
    Disposition of Evidence   118
    Photographs   119
    Diagnosis   119
    Summary of Protocol   119
    Specimens and Samples to be Recovered Before and During a Postmortem Examination   119
Special Problems Encountered in Medicolegal Autopsies   123
Common Mistakes Encountered During the Medicolegal Autopsy   124
Medicolegal Photography   125

6   MEDICOLEGAL AUTOPSY: PRACTICAL PERSPECTIVES   129

Charles S. Hirsch, M.D.

    Preservation of Evidence   130
    Other Evidence   131

7   DEFINITION AND TIME OF DEATH   141

John I. Coe, M.D., and
William J. Curran, J.D., LL.M., S.M.Hyg.

    Fundamental Concepts   141
    The Brain Death Concept   143
    Forensic Pathology Issues   150
    Early Postmortem Period   151
    Late Postmortem Changes   160
    Practical Problems   164

8   SUICIDE INVESTIGATION   171

Charles F. Vorkoper, M.S.S.W., and Charles S. Petty, M.D.

    The Physical Signs of Suicide   172
    The Psychological Signs of Suicide   176
    The Crisis of Suicide   180

9   HEART DISEASE, TRAUMA, AND DEATH   187

L. Maximilian Buja, M.D., and Charles S. Petty, M.D.

    Autopsy Procedures   187
    The Scene Investigation and Historical Data   195

10   **TRAUMA AND DEATH RELATED TO NEOPLASTIC DISEASES**   209

William A. Meissner, M.D.

    Significance of Trauma   209
    Relationship of Trauma to Tumors   210
    Trauma to Normal Tissue   211
    Effect of Trauma on Abnormal Tissue   213
    Repeated Minor Trauma and Chronic Irritation   213
    Role of the Medicolegal Investigator   214

11   **PEDIATRIC DEATHS**   219

William Q. Sturner, M.D.

    Abortion Cases   219
    Stillbirths   220
    Sudden Natural Deaths   220
    Sudden Infant Death Syndrome   224
    Asphyxia in Children   226
    Blunt Force Trauma   228
    Childhood Poisonings   233
    Child Abuse   236
    Childhood Drowning   241
    Childhood Suicides and Homicides   242

12   **ASPHYXIAL DEATHS**   249

Joseph H. Davis, M.D.

    Sudden Death Mechanisms   252
    Autopsy Findings   253
    Investigation and Reporting of Asphyxial Deaths   258
    Death Certification   261
    Drowning   262
    Scuba Deaths   264

13   **THERMAL DEATHS**   269

James A. Benz, M.D.

    Scope of Investigation   269
    Deaths Due to Fires   271
    Deaths Due to the Thermal Injury Caused by Hot Liquids, Steam, or Hot Objects   286
    Deaths Due to Heat Exhaustion and Heat Stroke   290
    Death Due to Cold Exposure   291
    Cases   295

14   **AUTOMOBILE DEATH INVESTIGATION AND PREVENTION PROGRAMS**   307

Joseph H. Davis, M.D.

    History   307

Problems   308
  The Cause of the Crash   309
  Pre-Crash Factors   310
  Crash Phase Investigation   320
  Motorcycle Deaths   323
  Pedestrian Fatalities   325
  "The Florida Accident"   328
  Post-Crash Fire Hazard   329
  Intentional Automobile Crashes   330
  Post-Crash Medical Care   331
  Tort Liability   333
  Prevention of Traffic Fatalities   334

15 AIRCRAFT DEATH INVESTIGATION: A COMPREHENSIVE REVIEW   339

Laurence R. Simson, Jr., M.D.

  Aircraft Crash Investigation: Developing Principles   339
  Magnitude of the Problem   342
  Investigative Authority   343
  Organization of Crash Site Investigations   344
  Aviation Accident Pathology   346

16 DEATH BY TRAUMA: BLUNT AND SHARP INSTRUMENTS AND FIREARMS   363

Charles S. Petty, M.D.

  Blunt-Force Trauma   364
  Head Injury   390
  Sharp Instrument Injury   405
  Firearms Injury   415
  Some Questions and Answers on Trauma   472
  Autopsy Records in Trauma Situations   479

17 COURTROOM PRESENTATION OF EVIDENCE IN DEATH CASES   491

William J. Curran, J.D., LL.M., S.M.Hyg.

  Distinguishing Characteristics of Death Cases   491
  Preparation for Trial   492
  The Story to be Told   493
  Pretrial Consultation   494
  Forensic Pathologists as Expert Witnesses   495
  Courtroom Testimony: Some General Situations   496
  Direct Examination: Qualifications   497
  Presentation of Findings: Demonstrative Evidence   498
  "Gruesome" Photography   499
  The Appearance of Nonpartisanship   500
  Range of Direct Interrogation   500
  Correcting the Examiner   500

Testimonial Style 501
Medical Certainty 501
Cross-Examination 502
Different Types of Judicial Proceedings 504

PART 3 SPECIAL INVESTIGATIONS

18 THE RAPE EXPERIENCE 509

Carol C. Nadelson, M.D., Malkah T. Notman, M.D., and Elaine Hilberman, M.D.

Definition of the Crime 509
The Rape Victim's Experience 510
The Mythology of Rape 510
Legal Considerations 513
Rape as Stress 516
Life Stage Considerations 519
Long-Term Consequences of Rape 520
Counseling Issues 521
Medicolegal Considerations 527

19 THE PSYCHOLOGY OF THE RAPE ASSAILANT 533

Theoharis K. Seghorn, Ph.D., and Murray L. Cohen, Ph.D.

Basic Assumptions 534
Psychological Functioning 534
Factors in Developmental History 538
The Dynamics of Rape 540
Prognosis and Treatment 548

20 COMMUNITY INVESTIGATION OF RAPE AND SEXUAL ASSAULT 553

Ross E. Zumwalt, M.D., and Charles S. Petty, M.D.

Medical Examination 555
Chain of Custody 558
Laboratory Analysis 558
Anal and Oral Intercourse 559
Victims of Sexual Assault Other Than Adult Females 560
Examination of the Suspected Rapist 560
The Prosecution of the Sexual Assault Suspect 560
Rape Crisis Center 561
Assessment of the Criminal Justice System 562
Instruction Sheet for Rape Examination 564
Medical Report: Suspected Rape 565
Sexual Assault Instruction Sheet (Male Patients) 569
Sexual Assault Examination (Male Patients) 570

21 SEX-RELATED DEATHS 575

Joseph C. Rupp, M.D., Ph.D.

Deaths During Sexual Activity 576
Trauma and Mutilation of the Genitals 577
Female Death Related to Sexual Activity 578
Simultaneous Sex-Related Deaths 580
Sex-Related Homicide 580
Child Molestation Deaths 581
Homosexually Related Deaths 582
Autoerotic Asphyxia 584

22 DEATHS RELATED TO MEDICAL CARE 589

Earl F. Rose, M.D., LL.B.

Approach and Analysis 589
Researching the Medical Literature 592
Adverse Drug Reactions and Drug-Related Deaths 593
Deaths Related to Surgical Care 599
Deaths Related to Anesthesia 600
Cardiac Arrest 601
Incidents in Intensive Care Unites 602
Diagnostic X-Ray Procedures 603
Transfusion Reactions and Serum Hepatitis 604
Cancer Deaths Related to Medical Care 605
Deaths Related to Hospital Care and Nosocomial Infections 607
Incidents Involving Institutionalized and Elderly Patients 609

23 PUBLIC HEALTH ASPECTS OF MEDICOLEGAL DEATH INVESTIGATION 615

Marvin E. Aronson, M.D.

Public Health Deaths 615
Health Departments and Death Investigations 616
Deaths in Hospitals and Nursing Homes 616
Health Department Location: Advantages and Disadvantages 617

24 TRANSPLANTATION PROGRAMS AND MEDICOLEGAL INVESTIGATION 621

Charles R. Baxter M.D., Ellen L. Heck, B.S., M.T., and Charles S. Petty, M.D.

25 MULTIPLE DEATH INVESTIGATIONS 629

Vincent J.M. Di Maio, M.D., and Charles S. Petty, M.D.

Multiple Natural Death 629
Multiple Accidental Death 631

Multiple Homicide   633
Police Investigation of Multiple Death   636
Proper Medicolegal Investigation of Scenes of Multiple Death   637
Common Grave Discovery   639

PART 4   FORENSIC PSYCHIATRY AND PSYCHOLOGY

26   OPERATIONAL ASPECTS, TRAINING, AND QUALIFICATIONS IN FORENSIC PSYCHIATRY   643

A. Louis McGarry, M.D.

Psychiatric Involvement in Legal Settings   643
Clearer Questions and More Relevant Answers   644
The Mental Status Examination   645
Probative Value   645
Structure and Operation   646
Security Facilities   647
Qualifications and Training   648
Statutory Attempts to Establish Forensically Qualified Psychiatrists   649
Toward a Standard for Forensic Psychiatry   650

27   PSYCHIATRY AND THE ADMINISTRATION OF JUSTICE   655

Seymour Pollack, M.A., M.D.

Forensic Psychiatry as Forensic Fact-Finding for Legal Purposes   658
Ethical Issues of Psychiatric Fact-Finding for Legal Purposes   659
Psychiatry in the Cause of Justice   664
Individualization in Law as Justice   664
The Humanistic Aspect of Law as Justice   666
Criticisms of Psychiatric Evidence   669
Cost-Benefits of Forensic Psychiatry for the Criminal Justice System   670
Conflict of Values in Psychiatry with Those of Law

28   CORRECTIONAL PSYCHIATRY   677

Loren H. Roth, M.D., M.P.H.

Definition of the Field   678
The Inmate Experience   683
Psychiatric Problems of Prisoners   687
The Role of the Correctional Psychiatrist   704

29   PSYCHIATRY AND THE CIVIL LAW   721

Herbert C. Modlin, M.D.

Personal Injury Suits   721

  Anxiety Neurosis 722
  Hysterical Neurosis (Conversion Type) 724
  Psychophysiologic Reaction 725
  Dependency Reaction 725
  Worker's Compensation Claims 727
  Secondary Gain 729
  Malingering 730
  Special Psychiatric-Legal Problems 730

30 PSYCHOLEGAL EXAMINATIONS AND REPORTS 739

 A. Louis McGarry, M.D.

  Testamentary Capacity 740
  Guardianship 745
  Examiner as Agent or Impartial Expert 749
  Competency to Stand Criminal Trial 750
  Criminal Responsibility 758
  Amnesia 759
  Malingering 759

31 PSYCHOLOGICAL TESTING IN LEGAL SETTINGS 763

 George V.C. Parker, Ph.D.

  Basic Concepts and Guidelines 763
  Psychological Tests Defined 764
  Test Scores 764
  Psychodiagnosis 764
  Major Areas of Psychological Testing 765

32 PREDICTION OF DANGEROUSNESS AND ITS IMPLICATIONS FOR TREATMENT 783

 R. Kirkland Schwitzgebel, Ed.D., J.D.

  Predictive Accuracy 783
  Approaches Toward Increasing Predictive Accuracy 786
  Treatment Implications 790

33 THE ANTISOCIAL PERSONALITY 799

 Simon Dinitz, Ph.D.

  Early Formulations 800
  Etiologic Perspectives 804
  Biological Substrates of Sociopathy 808
  Heterogeneity of Sociopathy 810

34 PEDOPHILIA

 Donald L. Tasto, Ph.D.

  The Crime of Pedophilia 815

Classification of Pedophiles 816
Preventive Factors 816
Sexual Arousal to Children 817
Heterosexual Pedophilia 818
Homosexual Pedophilia 821
Treatment 821

35 EXHIBITIONISM 827

Thomas P. Hackett, M.D., Fay A. Saber, J.D., M.P.H., and William J. Curran, J.D., LL.M., S.M.Hyg.

History 828
Treatment and Patient Management 829
Psycholegal Aspects 830
Case Studies 830

36 PSYCHOLEGAL ASPECTS OF SUICIDE 841

Robert E. Litman, M.D.

The Certification of Suicide 841
Psychological Autopsies 845
Accident versus Suicide 845
Drug Automatism 846
Insurance Aspects of Suicide 847
Worker's Compensation and Suicide 849
Suicide and Medical Malpractice 850
Suicide Assessment 852

37 MENTAL RETARDATION AND THE LAW 855

Julian Kivowitz, M.D.

Definitional Concepts 855
Legal Issues 856
Institutionalization of the Retarded 857
Right to Treatment or Habilitation 857
Other Human Rights 858
Guardianship 860
The Criminal Justice System and Retardation 861
Retardation and Dangerousness 862

38 ALCOHOLISM AND ALCOHOL ABUSE 865

Harold W. Demone, Jr., Ph.D.

Historical Perspective 865
The Criminal Law and Intoxication 866
Legal Rights of Alcoholics 868
Civil Commitment Procedures 868
Driving While Intoxicated 870
Enforcement of Drunk-Driving Laws 870
Alcohol Beverage Control Legislation 871

      Alcohol Education in the Public Schools   872
      Other Issues of Interest   873

39   DRUG ABUSE TREATMENT PROGRAMS   879

Charles P. O'Brien, M.D., Ph.D., and George E. Woody, M.D.

      Definitional Concepts   879
      Patterns of Drug Abuse   880
      Methods of Treatment   886
      Overview of Ancillary Services   891
      Confidentiality in Drug-Abuse Treatment   892
      Trends in Drug Abuse   893

40   PSYCHOACTIVE DRUGS   897

Jonathan O. Cole, M.D.

      Antipsychotic Drugs: Benefits and Risks   897
      Antidepressant Drugs   899
      Antianxiety Drugs   899
      Stimulants   900
      Drugs in Children   900
      Drugs for Impulse or Antisocial Disorders   900
      Drugs and Criminal Responsibility   902

41   PRESCRIBING CONTROLLED SUBSTANCES: PHYSICIANS' RIGHTS AND RESPONSIBILITIES   905

Norman E. Zinberg, M.D., and Risa G. Dickstein, J.D.

      The Legal Context: Regulating the Freedom of Physicians to Prescribe   906
      Separating Medical Use, Abuse, and Recreational Use: The Doctor's Role as Prescriber   915

42   THE JURY AND TRIAL PROCESS: PSYCHOLOGICAL PERSPECTIVES   927

Amiram Elwork, Ph.D., and
Bruce Dennis Sales, Ph.D., J.D.

      Alternative Approaches to Organizing Research   928
      Civil and Criminal Trial Proceedings   928
      Review of Research Findings   930
      Some Final Considerations   953

43   COURTROOM PRESENTATION OF PSYCHIATRIC AND PSYCHOLOGICAL EVIDENCE   963

A. Louis McGarry, M.D., and
William J. Curran, J.D., LL.M., S.M.Hyg.

      State of the Art Problems   963

Judicial and Legal Practices   964
General and Special Evaluations   966
Testimonial Presentation   996
Illustrative Testimony   975

PART 5   THE FORENSIC SCIENCES

44   THE TEAM APPROACH IN FORENSIC SCIENCE   991

Joseph L. Peterson, D.Crim.

Forensic Science Specialty Areas   992
The Adversary System of Justice   993
Forensic Science Involvement   995

45   ORGANIZATION OF A CRIME LABORATORY   1009

Larry B. Howard, Ph.D.

Definitions and Misconceptions   1009
Need for a Crime Laboratory   1010
Service Features   1010
Organizational Considerations   1012
Physical Facility   1015
Personnel   1029
Procedures   1031
Transportation   1036
Cost   1037
Appendix   1037

46   QUALIFICATIONS AND TRAINING FOR FORENSIC TOXICOLOGY   1041

Morton F. Mason, Ph.D.

General Qualifications   1041
Forensic Pathologists   1042
Technicians   1043
Academic Programs   1043
Supervisory Qualifications   1044
Board Certification   1045
Laboratory Quality Control Measures   1047
Expert Qualifications and Testimonial Issues   1048

47   FORENSIC TOXICOLOGY: GENERAL CONSIDERATIONS   1051

James C. Garriott, Ph.D.

Laboratory Considerations   1053
Interpretation of Toxicologic Results   1065

48 SPECIALTY AREAS OF FORENSIC TOXICOLOGY 1079

William T. Lowry, Ph.D.

- Toxic Substances 1079
- Toxicity and Hazard Ratings 1080
- Environmental Factors Affecting Toxicity 1080
- The Forensic Toxicologist and Evidentiary Responsibility 1082
- Speciality Areas of Forensic Toxicology 1083

49 THE ROLE OF THE PATHOLOGIST IN CHEMICALLY INDUCED DEATH CASES 1119

Charles S. Hirsch, M.D.

- Deaths Due to Natural Causes 1120
- Deaths Due to Mechanical Violence 1121
- Deaths Due to Drugs 1122

50 FORENSIC DENTISTRY 1133

Stanley M. Schwartz, D.M.D.

- Dental Identification: General Principles 1133
- Anthropology 1134
- Age Determination 1134
- Race Determination 1137
- Personal Habits 1138
- Sex Determination 1140
- Radiologic Evaluation 1141
- Examination of Sinuses 1144
- Child Abuse Investigations 1145
- Examination of Bite Marks 1146
- Other Issues of Dental Identification 1148

51 FUNDAMENTALS OF VOICE IDENTIFICATION 1151

Oscar I. Tosi, Ph.D., Sc.D.

- A Model of Voice Communication 1152
- Methods of Voice Identification 1153
- Theory of Speech Production 1154
- Subjective Methods of Speaker Recognition 1160
- Objective Methods of Speaker Recognition 1168
- Legal acceptance of Voice Identification 1172
- Field Procedures 1175
- Court Appearances 1181
- Training of Voice Identification Examiners 1182
- The Future of Voice Identification 1183

52 POLYGRAPH TECHNOLOGY 1187

Joseph P. Buckley, M.S.

- A Diagnostic Procedure 1187
- Historical Development 1187
- Control Question Technique 1188
- The Instrument 1188
- The Examination Room 1189
- Examiner Qualifications and Training 1189
- Test Procedure 1190
- Test Questions 1190
- Construction and Number of Tests 1192
- The Diagnosis 1193
- Supplementary Tests 1199
- The Accuracy of Examination Results 1200
- The Legal Status of the Polygraph Technique 1201
- Future Legal Status 1203
- The Testimony of the Polygraph Examiner 1203

53 IDENTIFICATION PROCEDURES IN DEATH INVESTIGATION 1207

Charles S. Petty, M.D.

- Fingerprints 1208
- Footprints 1211
- Palm Prints 1211
- Fingerprints on Skin 1211
- Dental Patterns and Restorations 1211
- Frontal Sinus Pattern 1213
- Skull Suture Pattern and Vascular Grooves 1213
- Normal and Abnormal Bone Comparisons 1213
- Other Fortuitous Comparisons 1216
- Less Positive Methods of Identification 1217
- Identification by Circumstances 1218
- Anthropologic Identification 1219
- "Positive" Identification 1219

54 QUESTIONED DOCUMENT EXAMINATION 1223

Maureen Casey, B.A.

- Scope of the Field 1223
- The Forensic Document Examiner 1224
- The Comparison of Handwriting 1225
- Signature Comparison 1235
- The Comparison of Mechanical Impressions 1240
- Alterations and Methods of Decipherment 1252
- Restoration of Burnt, Charred, and Water-Soluble Papers 1258
- Decipherment of Indented Writing 1259
- Paper Examinations and Comparisons 1260
- Dating of a Document 1260
- The Examination of Machine Copies 1263

Sequence of Writings   1265
Latent Fingerprints on Paper   1266
Preservation of Document Evidence   1266
The Document Examiner as an Expert Witness   1267

55 STATISTICAL ASPECTS OF FORENSIC SCIENTIFIC EVIDENCE   1271

Irving C. Stone, Jr., Ph.D.

Preparation and Organization of Data   1271
Common Pitfalls   1272
Statistics in Testimony   1273

56 COURTROOM PRESENTATION OF FORENSIC SCIENTIFIC EVIDENCE   1279

William J. Curran, J.D., LL.M., S.M.Hyg.

Forensic Scientists and the Courts   1279
Expert Opinion in the Common Law System   1279
Scientific Evidence: Rules of Admissibility   1280
Preliminary Matters on Admission   1280
The Weight of the Evidence   1283
Possibilities, Probabilities, and Proof   1284
Courtroom Appearances   1285

INDEX   1289

PART 1 GENERAL CONSIDERATIONS

CHAPTER 1

William J. Curran is Frances Glessner Lee Professor of Legal Medicine at Harvard University and Chairman of the State Medicolegal Investigation Committee of Massachusetts. Professor Curran writes regularly for the *New England Journal of Medicine* and teaches at the Medical School, Law School, and School of Public Health at Harvard. He was formerly Robert R. Utley Professor of Legal Medicine and Director of the Law-Medicine Institute of Boston University. He also served as Assistant Professor of Law and Government and Assistant Director of the Institute of Government at the University of North Carolina. Professor Curran is the author of several books in the medicolegal field including *Law, Medicine and Forensic Science* (with E. D. Shapiro); *Trauma and the Automobile; The Doctor as a Witness;* and *Medicolegal Proof in Litigation.* He is an Associate Editor of the *American Journal of Law and Medicine* and was formerly Medicolegal Editor of the *Massachusetts Law Quarterly.*

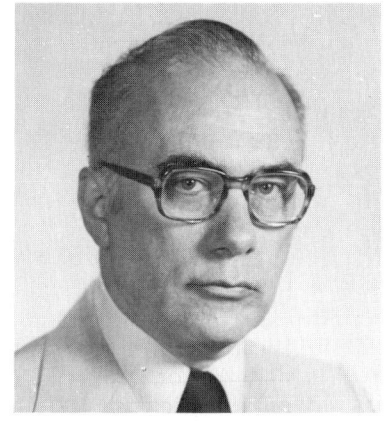

HISTORY AND DEVELOPMENT

William J. Curran, J.D., LL.M., S.M.Hyg.

ANCIENT ORIGINS

In the early history of man, only fragments of a scientific approach to judicially related inquiry can be found. The study of primitive cultures reveals an interrelationship of the magic of the sorcerer or medicine man with the development of science and law. Sir James Frazer traces the beginnings of the scientific method to the magician's association of ideas in their orderly incantations.[1] I believe that the same studies also indicate a relationship to the development of law. The magician's incantations were based upon precedence, or a cause and effect relationship, observed over time. The term "cause" is generally accepted as originating in the Greek and Roman legal usage of "cause of action," meaning the basic facts from which a right to justice has been derived. Only later was the theory of causation adopted into scientific terminology along with the concept of natural "laws" of science.[2]

Historians of the ancient Egyptian civilizations assert that experts were called in judicial inquiries and that post-mortem examinations of human bodies were required in some investigations.[3] Sydney Smith has called the Egyptian Imhotep (ca. 2980 B.C.–2900 B.C.) the first medicolegal expert because he was both the chief justice and the personal physician to Pharaoh Zoser.[4] The same Imhotep has also been claimed as the "God of Medicine," more entitled to acclaim as the founder of the healing arts than Hippocrates.[5] Personally, I find both claims rather romantic and lacking in historical support. Imhotep was essentially an architect and the Pharaoh's master builder. He was untrained in either medicine or law. He acquired responsibilities as a justice along with his duties as the head of civil affairs. As for his medical prowess, it seems to have been largely related to his deification in the centuries after his death.

Evidence of medicolegal relationships and the orderly collection of legal evidence can be found in early legal systems such as the Code of Hammurabi in Babylonia (ca. 1700 B.C.) and the Code of the Hittites of 1400 B.C. The Hammurabic Code is most noted for its provisions on the punishment of physicians for improper treatment. The Hittite Code contained a lengthy table of legal compensation for personal injuries. The most important of the pre-Christian legal codes, however, was the Roman law contained in the Twelve Tables of the decemvirs, which governed the Roman Empire for 900 years, beginning in 451 B.C. The Tables contained a number of provisions of medicolegal significance concerning such matters as the competency of the mentally ill and the gestation period for development of the human fetus.[6]

THE AMICUS CURIAE OF ROMAN LAW

The effective utilization of expert evidence in the judicial system had its origins in the Roman practice of appointing *amicus curiae,* friends of court, to advise the judges on matters requiring specialized knowledge or wisdom of any kind. These friends were nonpartisan advisers who took part in the hearing of the cases and in the deliberation of the justices. No rigid distinction was drawn between the evidence taken from the witnesses and the advice given by the experts; in fact, the Roman Codes dealt very little with what would be called evidence law under the Anglo-American common law system of today.[7] The Roman practice of court-appointed nonpartisan experts was contained under the civil law systems of Europe and South America. The practice was never adopted in England or in America for trial court matters. Its only appearance in the United States legal system can be found in the acceptance of *amicus curiae* briefs at the appellate court level. These briefs offer arguments on the law, not on matters of factual or scientific opinion, and usually come from special interest groups advocating their own views concerning the particular case. They are "friends of the court" only to the extent that they are not the paid representatives of the parties to the litigation. Otherwise, they are as partisan as all other parties in the American adversary system.

DEVELOPMENTS IN THE MIDDLE AGES

The Capitularies of the Emperor Charlemagne (768–814) contained express provisions concerning requirements for "proofs as clear as day" in cases of a serious nature, such as where a man's life was at stake. They required the courts of the realm to seek medical advice in all cases of physical injury, infanticide, rape, bestiality, and marital matters such as annulment and divorce.[8]

The lasting foundations of legal medicine and forensic science can be traced most clearly as a part of the rebirth of scholarly research and inquiry from the thirteenth to the sixteenth centuries (Fig. 1-1). Legal and medical professional cooperation became evident in Bologna about the middle of the thirteenth century. Rules concerning the appointment of medical consultants to the courts were formulated in Bologna at that time and were later adopted in other cities on the Italian peninsula. Medicolegal autopsies were first performed in Bologna in 1302. Singer has asserted that the modern science of anatomical dissection grew out of publicly ordered medicolegal postmortem examinations of homicide and suicide victims and of the bodies of executed criminals in Italy.[9] For many years,

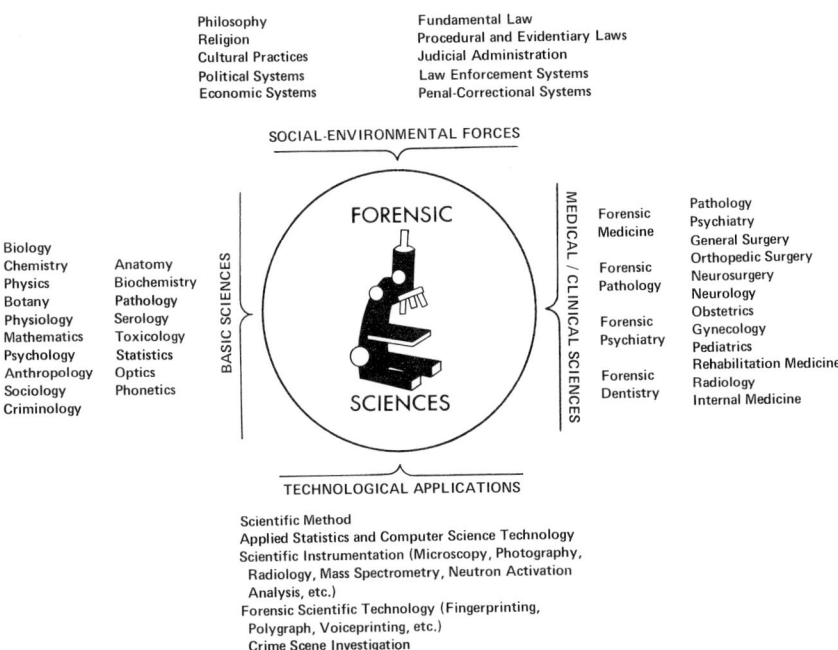

FIGURE 1-1. Schematic view of influences upon the development of the forensic sciences.

executed criminals were the chief source of anatomical materials for medical school instruction all over Europe, inasmuch as the Church forbade the dissection of persons dying in a state of grace.

In this same period a treatise appeared, evidencing similar developments in China. In 1924, a professor of Chinese at Cambridge University translated a work alleged to have been published in China between 1241 and 1253.[10] It is an instructional booklet concerning methods of public investigation of violent deaths and is attributed to a Commissioner of Justice named Sung Tz'u. Professor Giles gave its title as "Instructions to Coroners," a rather English terminology. In a footnote he suggested the literal meaning as "Record of the Washing Away of Wrongs." The translation itself seems questionable in its interpretations in many substantive areas. Giles admitted to having taken considerable liberties with the Chinese text in order to present a useful modern interpretation.

The first scholarly works in legal medicine in the West began to appear toward the end of the sixteenth century. The first is alleged to be that of a physician who was a teacher in Naples and Palermo, Giovanni Filippo Ingrassias (1520–1570). His work was called *Constitutiones et capitula necro uirisdictiones regii promedicatus officii* and is alleged to have first appeared in 1564. Another early work was a small treatise on mortal wounds by the famous French surgeon, Ambroise Paré (1510–1590), entitled *De rapports et des maijens d'embaumer les corps morts*. It was published in Paris about 1575.

The two leading texts of the period, however, were produced somewhat later. Both were encyclopedic in scope and were highly influential in the establishment of the field itself. One was the work of a Sicilian physician, Fortunatas Fidelis (1551–1630), bearing the title *De relationibus medicorum* and published in Palermo between 1598 and 1602. It collected not only a wide range of Italian and Greek materials, but also for the first time reflected the Arabic influence felt in Sicily in these years. Later editions were published in Venice and Leipzig. The other great product of this period was the massive, multivolume work by the physician to the Papal Court in Rome, Paulo Zacchias (1584–1659) (Fig. 1-2), entitled *Questiones medico-legales*. It was published in installments between 1621 and 1634. The text covered the spectrum of medically related issues which came before the *Sacra Rota Romana*, the most sophisticated court system of its time. Zacchias' work became the standard in the field for centuries and earned him the title of "the father of legal medicine."[11]

In the behavioral science field, the most outstanding medicolegal figure of the Middle Ages was Johann Weyer (1515–1588). As the personal physician to William, Duke of Cleves, Weyer opposed the cruel persecution of alleged witches by the clerical and secular judicial authorities. In his classic work, *De praestigiis daemonum,* Weyer refuted the claim that all persons alleged to be witches were dangerous to the public. He demanded

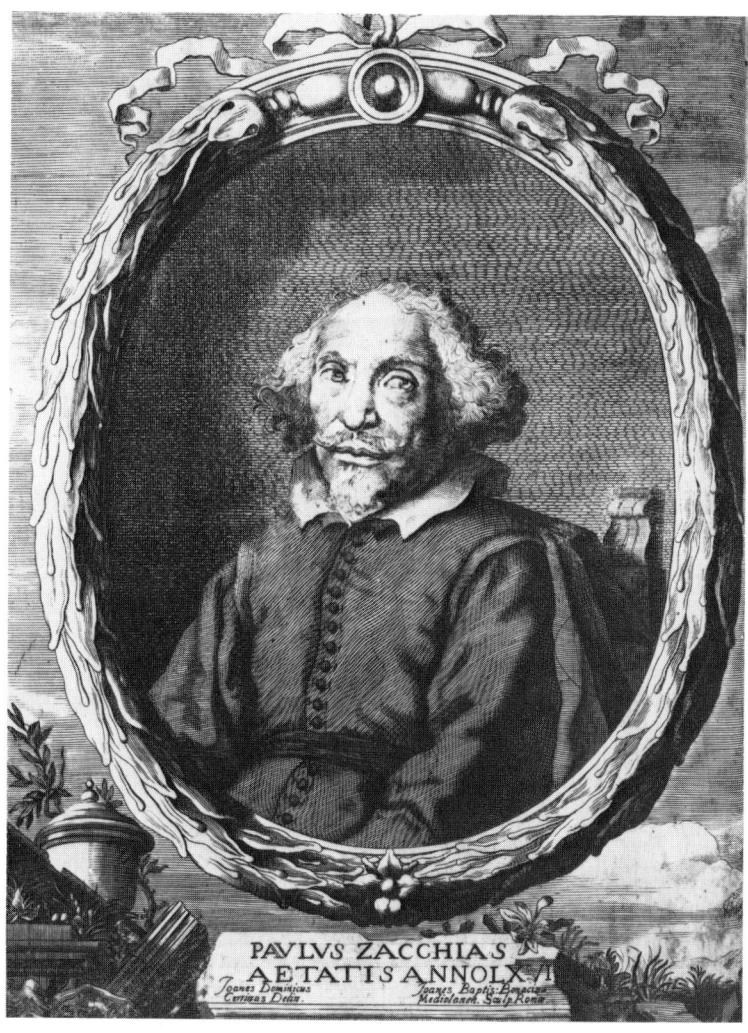

FIGURE 1-2. Paulo Zacchias at age 66.

that proof be produced in each case that the accused, usually a woman, had committed harmful acts or crimes against the state. Weyer advocated that a distinction be drawn between those who commit crimes due to a "corrupted will" and those who are shown merely to have a "troubled spirit." Zilboorg called Weyer the first scientific and humanistic medicolegal psychiatrist.[12] More recently, Szasz has also praised the medicolegal contributions of Weyer, but denies that Weyer found any significant number of the persecuted women to be mentally ill.[13]

THE SEVENTEENTH AND EIGHTEENTH CENTURIES

The next centuries were marked by substantial developments in medicolegal relations and by severe struggles to encourage the more effective use of scientific methods. Ackerknecht wrote of the "queer mixture of backwardness and progress" in the medicolegal texts produced in Europe through the middle of the eighteenth century.[14] The movement away from the superstitions of the Dark Ages can be found in the works of Weyer, Condronchi, Fodéré, and Bohn. An important departure is also found in a small treatise by the Portuguese physician, Rodrigo de Castro, who blended public health and public medicolegal investigational techniques in his unique work, *Medicus politicus*, published in 1614.

METHODS OF PROOF

In the court systems, progress was very slow, and proof of innocence in criminal cases was essentially based on superstition and physical endurance. The criminal defendant was expected to display his innocence under the various methods applied. Trial by ordeal was common in all countries. It traditionally included four tests: ordeal by fire, water, poison, and battle. In the test of fire, the defendant was required to carry hot coals or iron. If he was burned in any way, he was declared guilty. In the ordeal by water (Fig. 1-3), he was submerged for a period of time, and if he survived, he was set free. The poison test should not be difficult to imagine. All sorts of obviously toxic or deadly poisons were forced upon the accused and if even the slightest discomfort was displayed, he was condemned. These tests, the cruelest applications of trial by ordeal, were outlawed by the Church at the Lateran Council of 1215. Trial by battle survived much longer as a means of judicial proof. The parties or their substitutes engaged in physical combat with the question of guilt or the winner in a lawsuit determined by the outcome. Perhaps the most enduring and the simplest form of judicial proof in these religious times was that of sacred oath or compurgation. Parties in both criminal and civil cases could satisfy the demands of the court by swearing to the facts under Christian oath. In compurgation, the parties were allowed to produce oath-takers who would swear to the truth of their claims. The decision would often go to the party who produced the largest number of compurgators. These methods of proof still survive to a certain degree in both the civil law system and in common law.

During all of these centuries in both Europe and America there was a heavy reliance on confession by the accused as a means of disposing of criminal cases. Various forms of torture and somewhat milder methods of persuasion and intimidation were used. Incarceration without trial for long periods was common in many countries, especially for political prisoners and defendants thought highly dangerous. These methods have by

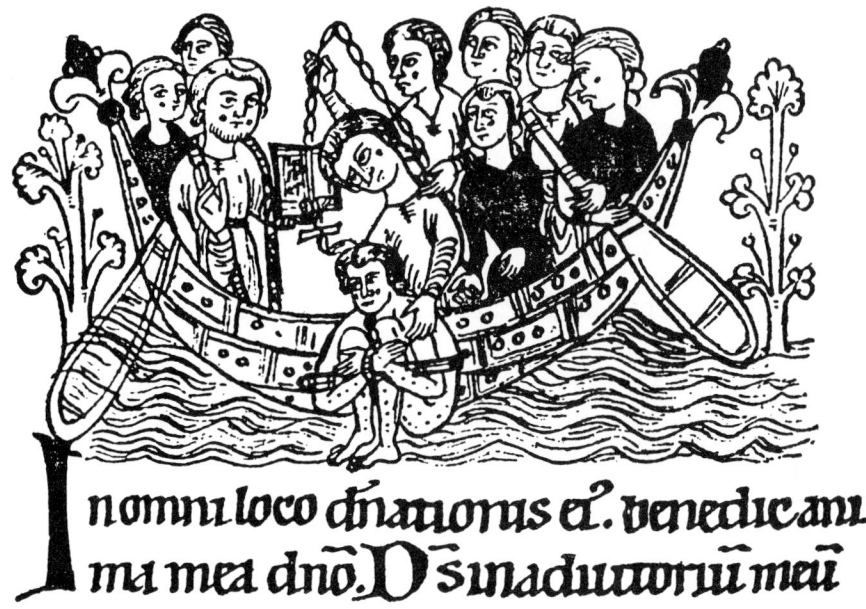

FIGURE 1-3. Medieval trial by water. (From Sayre, F.B.: *Cases on Criminal Law*. Lawyers Co-operative Publishing Co., Rochester, N.Y., 1927.)

no means disappeared in modern times. They have merely become more sophisticated and technical, with the aid, at times, of forensic scientists.

MEDICOLEGAL SPECIALIZATION

From its Italian beginnings the specialty of medicolegal work spread throughout continental Europe in the eighteenth and early nineteenth centuries. The German states were particularly responsive because of their excellent criminal codes which imposed substantial requirements for medical evidence to support criminal convictions. The most important early procedural law was the Code of Bamberg, adopted in 1507. It was the basis for the later Criminal Code of 1532, which was adopted widely in the German states under Kaiser Karl V. Another important criminal code which included medicolegal requirements was that of Austria-Hungary, promulgated in 1769.

The early university teaching in the field combined three areas: (1) the presentation of medical findings and opinions in court, especially in death cases; (2) public health regulation and control of infectious diseases; and (3) medical care of the poor. It was not until the later part of the nineteenth century that these areas split into separate specialty fields.

The first lectures in forensic medicine in Germany were given in the mid-seventeenth century and are generally attributed to Professor Johann Michaelis of the University of Leipzig. The successor to Michaelis at Leipzig was the famous Johann Bohn (1640–1719) who was the leading figure in the field in Europe at the time. In his influential textbook, published in 1704, Bohn referred to the field as "Official Medicine" or "State Medicine," indicating the wide scope of its coverage.

The first independent chair in the field was established at the University of Vienna in 1804. The occupant was Ferdinand Bernhard Vietz and the title given the post was "State Pharmacology," which combined forensic medicine and toxicology with public health regulation, the latter administered by "medical police." The developments at Vienna stimulated further academic progress throughout the Austro-Hungarian Empire. A chair was established in Cracow in 1805 and in Prague in 1807. Medicolegal instruction began in Russia in 1804 when it was combined in a new chair in medicine which also included anatomy and physiology.

In Scandinavia, the first chair in the field was established at the University of Copenhagen in 1819. It was combined with pharmacology as in Vienna. The first medicolegal instruction in Sweden was offered at the Karolinska Institute in Stockholm in 1841. It did not become a professorship until 1889. A professorship in State Medicine and Pathological Anatomy was begun at the University of Helsinki in 1857. The first independent professorship in forensic medicine on the Iberian peninsula was founded at the University of Coimbra in Portugal in 1836. A chair was established at the University of Madrid in 1843.

It is quite true that medicolegal scholarship and public service were much later in beginning in the British Isles and America than on the Continent. There is no evidence of medicolegal work earlier than the late eighteenth century. However, once the field was introduced, the establishment of independent professorships in the nineteenth century closely paralleled academic progress on the Continent—a historical fact rarely noticed by the commentators on medicolegal history.

The first medicolegal lectures given in a British medical school were offered at the University of Edinburgh in 1791 by Sir Andrew Duncan (1744–1828), who was then a professor of the institutes of medicine. Duncan adopted the term "Medical Jurisprudence" for his course of lectures. He included all of the forensic areas common to the field since the time of Zacchias as well as the German field of "medical police." The first chair in the field was established at Edinburgh in 1807. Its first occupant was Andrew Duncan, Jr., the son of Sir Andrew. The second Scottish professorship in medical jurisprudence was established at Glasgow in 1839. The first professorship in England was established at King's College, University of London, in 1831, though lectures were offered in the subject in earlier years.

In the United States the inaugural lectures in legal medicine were presented at Columbia College of Physicians and Surgeons in 1804 (the same year the famous chair was established at Vienna) by an Edinburgh medical graduate, Dr. James S. Stringham. In 1813, Stringham was named to the first American professorship in the field, but he died before he could lecture under the new title. The next professorship was established at Harvard University Medical School in 1815, where it was combined with Obstetrics until 1878. In Canada the first professorships were established at McGill University in Montreal in 1845 and at Laval University in Quebec City in 1856.

In most of the university programs, the coverage of subject matter was very broad, but the individual professors tended to have their own specialties for public service or research work. Most of them selected pathology, or at least bench laboratory scientific work. The technological discoveries of the late nineteenth century confirmed and strengthened these tendencies. However, efforts were also extended in areas of forensic psychiatry. The greatest obstacles to progress in forensic psychiatry were lingering superstitions about supernatural origins for strange and bizarre behavior and the lack of objective, laboratory-based proof of mental illness. The greatest pioneer work in forensic psychiatry was undoubtedly that done in Paris. Philippe Pinel (1745–1826) reformed the entire system of treatment for the mentally ill when he became head physician of the Bicêtre in 1798 (Fig. 1-4). He struck the chains from the patients, allowed them freedom of movement within the hospital, and gave them nourishing food. He ordered that the patients be treated humanely and with dignity rather than cruelly and with contempt. In a structured way he referred to this new method of patient care as "moral treatment." However, Pinel also strongly advocated the separation or alienation of the mentally ill from the cruelties and fears of the general population. He believed that the moral education of the insane could take place only in the isolated, closed mental hospital.

Pinel's greatest pupil was Jean Esquirol (1772–1840) who actually surpassed his master as a teacher and a scholar of mental illness. Esquirol was one of the great pioneers in the nosology of psychiatry, having provided the first descriptions of what he called hallucinations and delusions and having clearly distinguished mental deficiency (idiocy) from mental derangement. He was one of the first psychiatrists to take an interest in criminal conduct attributed to the insane. He described it as caused mainly by different forms of monomania and advocated treatment rather than punishment for the criminally insane. His classic text, published in 1838, was the bible of French psychiatry for over half a century. Alexander and Selesnick describe Esquirol as laying the foundations for the new

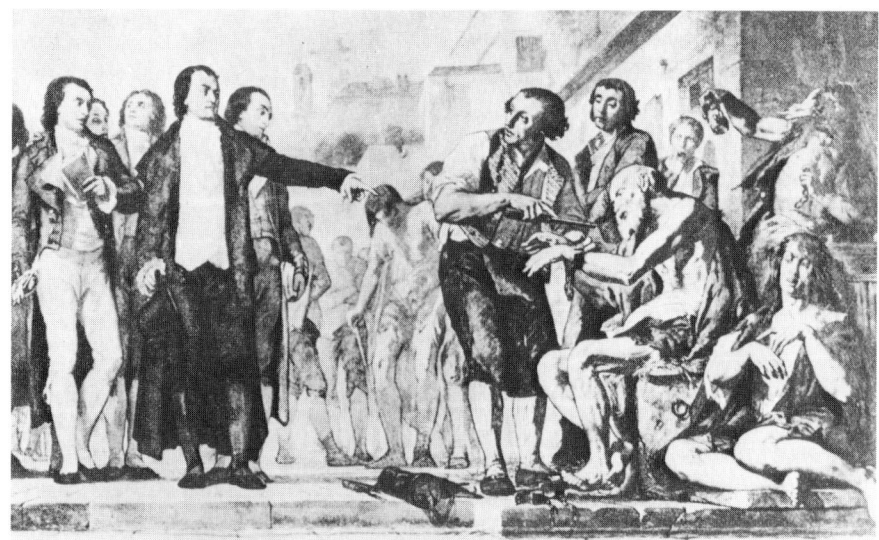

FIGURE 1-4. Philippe Pinel demanding the removal of chains from the insane at the Bicêtre Hospital in Paris. (Painting by Charles Muller.)

medical discipline of clinical psychiatry.[15] Overlooked, however, in most general historical commentaries is Esquirol's extraordinary contributions to legal psychiatry in both the strictly legal and the clinical areas. He was the chief psychiatric consultant in the drafting of the famous French mental health law of 1838, which is, incredible as it may seem, still the basic law of France. Esquirol's textbook was addressed very heavily to the medicolegal field, stressing the medical, public health, and forensic aspects of the subject. Its title was *Des maladies mentales considérées sous les rapports médicale, hygiénique et médico-légal*. In my own judgment, Jean Esquirol of Paris was the modern founder of legal psychiatry.

Followers of Esquirol, particularly Guillaume Ferrus (1784–1861) and

Francois Leuret (1797–1851), established the medicolegal specialty of forensic or legal psychiatry. Leuret was the first medical witness to testify in the courts concerning the defendant's irresistible impulse or psychological drive to commit a particular crime. The theory was derived from Esquirol's emphasis upon monomania as the causal link between the person's insanity and the commission of repeated criminal acts.

On the Continent, forensic psychiatry became associated with other fields of medicolegal work in the university departments of legal medicine. In later years, many of the chairs in legal medicine were occupied by professors whose main interest was in psychiatry. During the nineteenth century, the most influential of this group was the Italian, Cesaré Lombroso (1836–1909). Lombroso combined indefatigable energy and enthusiasm with painstaking scholarship. He has been called the father of criminology because of his demand that criminal law and penology be related to the character of the criminal rather than to the type of crime he has committed. Lombroso began his academic medicolegal career at the University of Turin in a traditional way; his first book was a treatise on postmortem examinations. He soon began to take an interest in studying the physical makeup of the inmates of a nearby prison. Under the influence of Darwin's theory of evolution and Morel's psychiatric theories of inherited mental disease, Lombroso espoused the idea that most criminals are examples of arrested physical and mental evolution, contemporary "throwbacks" to an earlier, more primitive, more aggressive period in man's development. Prison populations all over the world were examined during the latter half of the nineteenth century, and most of these studies seemed to confirm Lombroso's theories. The dominant explanation for criminal behavior became anthropological. The "typical criminal" was described as having a small brain and brain case, a sloping forehead, a broad nose and mouth, and a strong jaw. Lombroso's ideas remained strong in Europe and America into the early decades of the twentieth century.

Medicolegal service programs united with the teaching of medical students and law students in the institutes of legal medicine all across the Continent. Despite the advances made in forensic psychiatry, however, forensic pathology was the predominant specialty field for the leaders of the field from M.-G.-A. Devergie in Paris to Johann Ludwig Caspar in Berlin. The first European medical journal devoted solely to medicolegal and public health subjects is said by Nemec to have begun publication in 1782 in Stendal, Germany.[16] The first continuously published medicolegal journal, and still the most noted in the world, was begun at the University of Paris in 1829 under the title *Annales d'hygiène publique et de médecine légal.*

THE EMERGENCE OF FORENSIC SCIENCE

Prior to the nineteenth century, the only scientific work associated with law on any continuing basis was medicolegal in character. All other technical assistance tended to be drawn from the regular ranks of the professions and occupations of the time. The French courts developed a system of panels of "experts" drawn from a wide variety of fields to provide evaluations and opinions on a broad spectrum of subjects from the value of land and chattels to complex problems of engineering and medicine, but none of these panelists devoted full time to court activities.

It is difficult to draw the line between medical and nonmedical developments in forensic science. The medicolegal specialists were very prompt in embracing the new technological discoveries of the late eighteenth and early nineteenth centuries, including microscopy, photography, and radiology. In Europe the expanded fields of forensic science were very often incorporated into the activities of the university-based institutes of legal medicine. This, however, was not always the case. Some of the most famous programs, such as those of Hans Gross in Graz, Austria, and R. A. Reiss at the University of Lausanne, Switzerland, were independent efforts in forensic science and criminalistics from their very beginnings. In the common law countries, forensic scientific efforts have almost universally developed independently of medicolegal work. They have been supported by national or local law enforcement organizations such as the Home Office in England, the Royal Mounted Police and the Attorney General's Department in Canada, and the Federal Bureau of Investigation and the Chicago Police Department in the United States. It seems quite clear that for the English-speaking countries on both sides of the Atlantic, the "pedigree" of forensic science is, in the words of H. J. Walls of the Metropolitan Police Laboratory at Scotland Yard, "by forensic medicine out of police work" with, in my judgment, the nurture after birth coming very largely from the police agencies.[17]

Forensic Toxicology

The first forensic scientific field mentioned after pathology in the medicolegal areas has usually been forensic toxicology. In fact, an independent field of toxicology, the study of poisons, probably did not exist prior to concerns for its forensic applications. In more recent years, of course, general toxicology has been developed considerably, along with a number of subspecialty fields. There was material on poisons in most of the medicolegal texts published from the sixteenth through the eighteenth centuries. The most famous early figure in forensic toxicology was J. M. B. Orfila (1787–1853), a Spaniard by birth, educated in Valencia, Barcelona, and Madrid, who became Professor of Legal Medicine at the University of Paris. Unlike his predecessors and his contemporaries in other French medicolegal programs, Orfila devoted his major attention to chemistry and pharmacology rather than pathology. He is generally acknowledged as the father of toxicology for his classic text on the subject published in 1815. Another leading figure in medicolegal work in Scotland took a course similar to that of Orfila. This was Sir Robert Christison (1797–1882), who was the successor to Andrew Duncan, Jr., the first occupant of the chair in medical jurisprudence at the University of Edinburgh. Christison's text on toxicology was published in 1829. It should also be recalled that the first medicolegal chair at a university in Central Europe, that at Vienna, was originally entitled a professorship in "State Pharmacology," indicating the importance of investigations into the subject of poisons and other chemical compounds.

The most well-known poison in history has been arsenic. It was a favorite weapon of murderers in the Middle Ages since it was commonly available, undetectable in the human body, and gave symptoms similar to those of widespread diseases of the times, especially cholera. Orfila and others used various methods to detect the poison, but it remained for the English chemist, James Marsh, in 1836, to develop a highly accurate technique for discovering very small traces of arsenic in human tissue. Marsh's breakthrough led to much improvement in toxicolegal work over the next decades. There are many fascinating accounts of investigations and trials of murder cases involving arsenic poisoning. My own favorite is the trial of Marie La Farge in France in 1840, involving sensational testimony by Orfila.[18]

Identification and Criminalistics

The core issue in most of the forensic sciences is identification. Some trace of the criminal, or some verbal description, may be available, but how is this matched up with one human being out of hundreds or thousands? This problem has plagued police investigation for centuries and continues to do so. More effective and more accurate methods of personal identification are constantly being sought. The identity of materials is also a problem, from poisons to paint, from blood to bullets, from sperm to sand.

The initial exploratory efforts in applying orderly methods and classification to personal identification involved oral descriptions of suspects and criminals. It is claimed that the ancient Egyptians and some early Chinese civilizations applied painstaking approaches to describing the physical characteristics of wanted criminals and prisoners. The practice of branding some convicted criminal offenders was widespread in Europe, Asia, and the Americas in past centuries as a means of permanent identification and classification. (Readers of American classics will recall Hawthorne's *The Scarlet Letter*. The red "A" was sometimes used to brand adulterers in Colonial times.) The first scientific application of anthropological classification methods to criminal identification was developed by Alphonse Bertillon of the Paris Criminal Investigation Department in the 1880s (Fig. 1-5). A very elaborate system of physical description and clas-

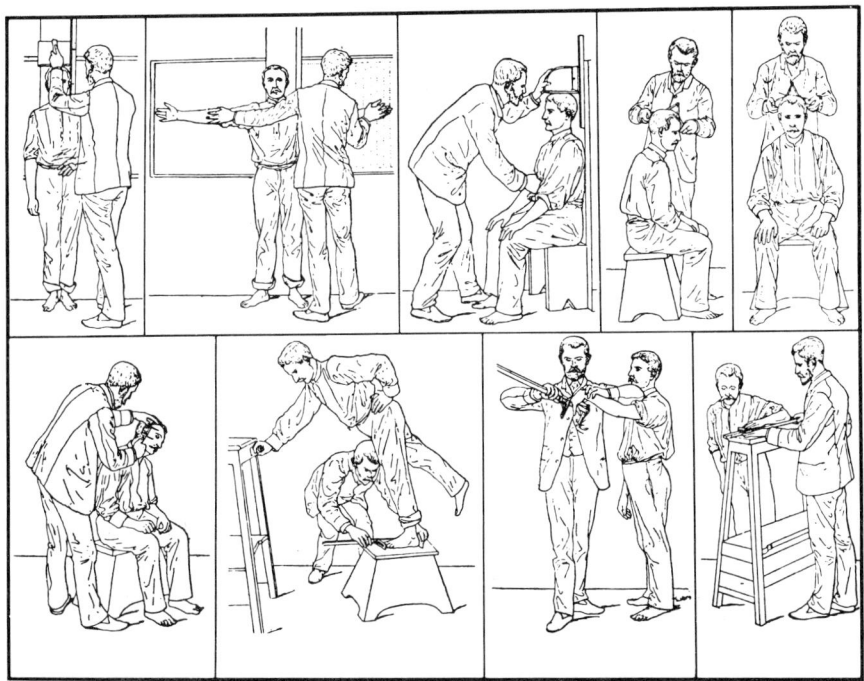

FIGURE 1-5. Sketches illustrating the main parts of the anthropometric system of Alphonse Bertillon.

sification was devised and huge files were kept of these *portraits parle,* or word pictures, of thousands of persons arrested or convicted by the law enforcement agencies. Line drawings and later black and white photographs supplemented the system. The method was very expensive in personnel, time, and space, and had clear limitations as an investigatory technique. Though it remains today, largely in photographic files, it has been substantially replaced by the much more effective method of fingerprinting. The individuality of finger-end markings was originally proposed by J. E. Parkinje, a Czech physiologist, in 1823. It is said to have been first applied to identification by Sir William Herschel, who used it in the 1870s in India as a means of registering documents for illiterates. The technique was developed for police work by Sir Francis Galton in England, whose treatise on the subject appeared in 1892. The first country in the world to adopt fingerprinting as the foundation of a national system of criminal identification, however, was not England but Argentina, prompted by the great early leader in the field, Juan Vucetich. In most parts of the world, fingerprinting is still limited to criminal classification, and noncriminals are rarely fingerprinted. In the United States, however, the Federal Bureau of Investigation has long conducted a campaign for universal fingerprinting, and it has been highly successful. Fingerprinting has proved its value in the United States in matters of identification considerably beyond the criminal field.

The broad use of scientific techniques in criminal investigation and law enforcement generally has developed rapidly since the later 1800s. The major pioneers in Europe were Hans Gross of Austria and R. A. Reiss of Switzerland, who were mentioned earlier. Gross was a lawyer and police-court magistrate who advocated the use of all available technologies in crime detection. He later became the head of a university-based Institute of Criminology in Prague before he returned to his birthplace, Graz, in Austria, to direct a similar university program which served the law enforcement agencies all over Austria. Reiss' earliest work was in photography, but he soon moved on to develop a highly systematic approach, with characteristic Swiss precision, all across the field of criminal investigation which he called "criminalistics." His Institute of Police Science at the University of Lausanne began offering such courses just after the turn of the century. Police and judicial officials came from all over Europe to take instruction at Lausanne under Professor Reiss. Another of the great early leaders was Edmond Locard, who headed an Institute of Criminalistics at the University of Lyon in France. His encyclopedic work was published in 1923.

The product of criminal investigation depends heavily upon what is found at the scene of an alleged crime. It was Professor Locard, mentioned above, who coined the *theory of interchange* at the scene: that the person or persons at the scene when the crime is committed will almost always leave something and take something away. It is the task of the trained investigator to examine the scene thoroughly enough to find the traces left behind, from fingerprints to blood to bits of cloth, and to locate materials on or about a suspect which were picked up at the scene, from dust to paint to the victim's blood or clothing. The connection of the suspect with the scene may not provide totally adequate evidence to sustain a conviction, but it will provide *objective proof* that he or she was at the scene, thus refuting alibis and lending support to other adequate evidence.

The use of the terms "criminalistics" and "police science" has the obvious result of limiting the field to its applications to criminal investigation on the side of the police and court prosecutors. In practice, this is an accurate description in most cases, since the laboratories and institutes of the field have been, almost without exception, supported and operated by and for police agencies. However, many of the techniques developed in the laboratories have uses in other civil areas of the law, as well as in non-legally related fields. Blood identifications have been used extensively for paternity claims in noncriminal cases. Questioned document examinations have been utilized in will cases and in many situations where the authenticity of documents and signatures has come into question. For this reason, the term "forensic science" is preferable for describing all uses of science in systematic reporting and evaluation for all types of courts and law enforcement and penal agencies.

American Beginnings

Efforts to install medicolegal and other forensic scientific methods on the American continent suffered from the same restrictions found in the British Isles. The common law has not been receptive to scientific proofs, and American lawyers have rarely been trained in science or its uses. If there is a single principle that the history of forensic science has taught us, it is that there must be a cooperative relationship between the basic legal system of proof and the development of scientific work related to the law. Without a fertile soil in the law, forensic science cannot grow. The fertilizing of the legal foundation has taken a very long time in this country, and it cannot be said, even today, that the American courts are readily willing to allow science a legitimate place in the everyday administration of justice.

It was noted earlier that the first formal medicolegal lectures in an American medical school were presented in 1804 by Dr. James S. Stringham at Columbia College of Physicians and Surgeons in New York. Stringham had studied at Edinburgh, the leading British medical school in medicolegal work. Another Edinburgh graduate, Benjamin Rush, also included the subject of "medical jurisprudence" in his famous series of lectures on medicine at the new College of Medicine in Philadelphia in 1810. Unlike his Edinburgh teachers, however, Rush placed his primary stress upon forensic psychiatry. He was to go on to become primarily a psychiatrist, though not limiting himself to the forensic area, and he is generally acknowledged as the father of American psychiatry.[19]

The first great leader in legal medicine in America was Dr. Theodoric Romeyn Beck (1791–1855) (Fig. 1-6), who taught the subject at the College of Physicians and Surgeons of Western New York and at Albany Medical College in New York. His two-volume treatise, published in 1823, was the pioneer work in this field by an American and was considered the authoritative source on all medicolegal subjects for decades.[20] Dr. Beck's scholarship was not limited to the medicolegal field. He also taught materia medica at Albany and was the editor of the *American Journal of Insanity*, the official publication of the American Psychiatric Association, from 1850 to 1855.

The most controversial early figure in American medicolegal relations was the psychiatrist Isaac Ray (1807–1881). Dr. Ray was the superintendent of a mental hospital in Augusta, Maine, and was one of the founders of the American Psychiatric Association. It was actually while he was still in private practice in Eastport, Maine, two years before he became superintendent at Augusta, that Ray wrote his polemical medicolegal text, *The Medical Jurisprudence of Insanity*. In his work, published in 1838, Ray reviewed the contributions of the French and English forensic psychiatrists and advocated the establishment of a much broader rule of criminal irresponsibility for the mentally ill than was then being applied in America or in England. He pleaded that any mentally ill person should be found innocent of any criminal act related to his mental condition. A New Hampshire judge, Charles Doe, read Dr. Ray's book shortly after it was published and corresponded with him. The judge informed Dr. Ray that he agreed with his views and said that he had applied a similar rule in a case of testamentary capacity. Later Judge Doe was influential in having the Supreme Court of New Hampshire adopt a rule of criminal responsibility similar to that advocated in the Ray treatise.

Other American courts did not follow the New Hampshire law, and Ray's thesis was also rejected in England when the House of Lords adopted the *M'Naghten Rules*. The so-called "product test" of criminal irresponsibility seemed destined to become only a nineteenth-century anachronism of New Hampshire, not even cited often in its home jurisdiction, when it was adopted in the District of Columbia in 1954 in a famous decision by Judge David Bazelon.[21] The *Durham* case provoked a national reexamination of the law of insanity. The State of Maine enacted the "product test" by statute in 1963.[22] In later years, however, the enthusiasm for the Ray-inspired rule has cooled substantially. The District of Columbia has now virtually abandoned the *Durham* decision and returned to a more traditional test. No other American jurisdiction has adopted the "product test" in recent years.

MEDICOLEGAL DECLINE

Little progress seems to have been made in the United States in the medicolegal field during the middle decades of the nineteenth century. In 1876, as a part of a series of papers on the history of the various specialty fields of medicine during America's first century as a nation, Sanford Chaillé reported that accomplishment in legal medicine had been dismal and bleak to the point of being disgraceful.[23] The author, who was not a medicolegal specialist himself, did not name a single major scholarly contributor or practitioner in the field since Theodoric Beck. Chaillé blamed this sorry state of affairs almost entirely on the unreceptive nature of the common law system. Before we become too provincial in our medicolegal criticism, however, we should note that Nemec, in his *Highlights in Medicolegal Relations*, which deals much more with Europe than with the Americas, calls attention to a "famous speech" in 1888 by Emil Ungar, Professor of Pediatrics and Legal Medicine at the University of Bonn, wherein Ungar deplored the low status of legal medicine and its teaching in Germany, a country usually considered to have maintained the best of standards in the field.[24]

THE SECOND CENTURY: AUSPICIOUS BEGINNINGS

Dr. Chaillé was particularly emphatic in his criticism of the coroner system in America, and he seemed to hold out no hope for its reform in the near future. Yet it was only a year later that Massachusetts became the first state to abolish the system totally and to replace it with physicians who would report upon suspicious deaths in their respective districts of

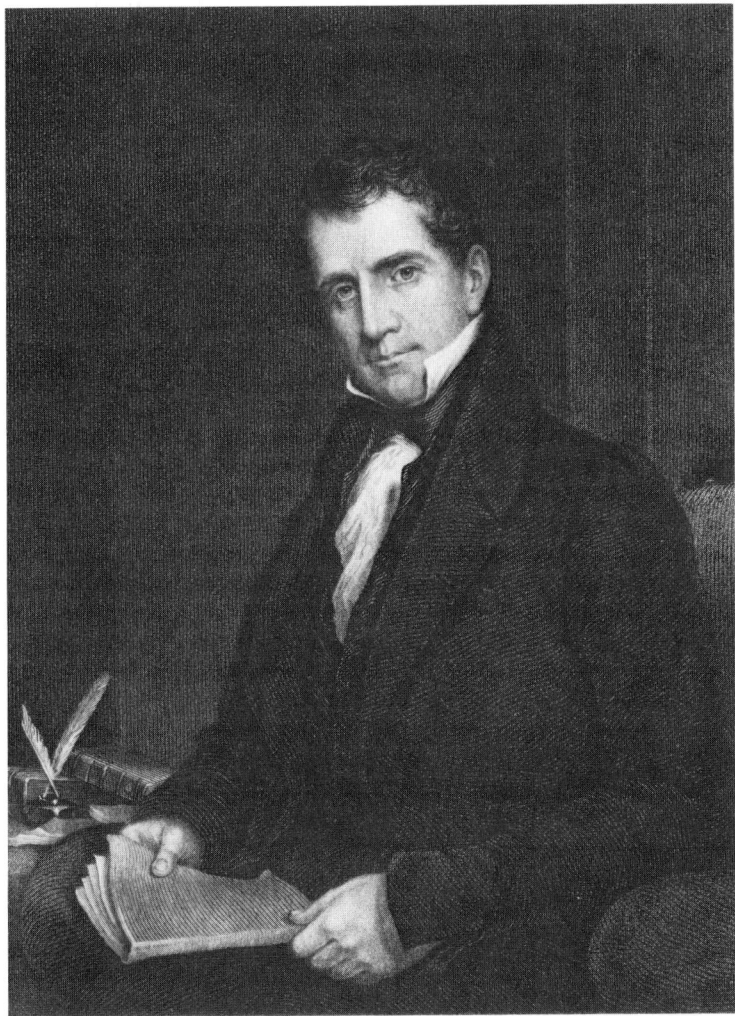

FIGURE 1-6. T.R. Beck.

the state. The new group was given the simple title of "medical examiners." They carried no legal or judicial authority, but functioned as the nation's first appointive impartial medical consultants to the law enforcement and court systems. Properly famous as this reform was in Massachusetts, it caused no quick stampede away from the politically strong coroner systems in other states. Only the nearby New England states of Connecticut and Rhode Island adopted medical examiners during the remainder of the nineteenth century, and neither of these states totally abandoned the coroner system.

There was evidence of growing interest in medicolegal affairs in the United States in the late decades of the century when one examines the proceedings of the International Medico-Legal Congress held in New York in 1895.[25] European and American leaders in the field attended and read important papers on a wide range of medical and legal subjects. The President of the Congress and its primary organizer was Clark Bell (1832–1918), a New York attorney, who was also editor of the *Medico-Legal Journal*, the official organ of the Medico-Legal Society of New York. The *Journal* had begun publication in 1883 and was the first general periodical in the medicolegal field in the United States. It was continuously published on a quarterly basis until 1933. The New York Medico-Legal Society was particularly significant in the history of American medicolegal relations because of its early adoption of a very broad scope for the field. The core membership was the huge group of elected coroners in the state, but the organization also contained physicians and lawyers active in other aspects of the subject including personal injury litigation.

After the turn of the century, the most significant medicolegal reform in the United States was the adoption all across the country of workmen's compensation laws which replaced the highly inequitable common law of torts as a means of compensating employees for personal injuries sustained "out of or in the course of" their work. In 1910, New York was the first state to adopt the new no-fault system of recovery united with a simplified administrative method of handling claims against employers. As important as the legal reform was, the growth of liability insurance was equally important since it enabled industry to make injury compensation a regular cost of doing business. It was the existence of this insurance which later encouraged the courts to liberalize the entire law of personal injury recovery in many fields from automobile accidents to medical malpractice claims. Currently, however, the liberality of the courts in allowing extensive recoveries is blamed for the inability of the private insurance companies to provide liability insurance coverage at reasonable rates.

MEDICAL EXAMINERS AND CORONERS

In the first two decades of the twentieth century, the only jurisdiction which joined Massachusetts in abolishing the coroner system was the City of New York in 1915. Again it was not physicians who led the reform. It was not lawyers either. The step was based upon a devastating report on the corruption and expense of the old system by the City's Commissioner of Accounts, Leonard W. Wallstein. Like the reform in New England, however, the change in New York City provoked no rush of converts to the medical examiner system. In the next ten years, only the City of Newark, contiguous to New York City, followed suit.

In an effort to stimulate further medicolegal reform, the National Research Council in 1925 commissioned a study and report on coroner and medical examiner systems across the country. The project was under the direction of a Committee on Medicolegal Problems headed by Dr. Ludwig Hektoen of Chicago. The Report of the study, published in 1928, strongly supported the establishment of medical examiner programs throughout the country and the abolition of all coroner systems. It also suggested that in large urban centers the medical examiner's offices should offer a wide range of expert medical assistance at all stages of criminal investigation, prosecution, and disposition. Lastly, it was recommended that in large urban areas "medicolegal institutes" should be established under the direction of the medical examiner and "affiliated as far as practicable with public hospitals, medical schools and universities."[26]

In 1932, the National Research Council published a supportive study to the last recommendation cited above. It was entitled *Possibilities and Need for Development of Legal Medicine in the United States*.[27] The Report was prepared by Oscar T. Schultz, who had been medical director of the survey of death investigation systems. Like Dr. Chaillé in 1876, Dr. Schultz was of the opinion that the legal system was to blame for the lack of development of legal medicine in America. He asserted that the failure to establish medicolegal institutes was the "severest criticism which can be made against the coroner system. . . ."[28]

Useful as the NRC Reports were at the time, they were not successful in stimulating any of their objectives. Much of the reason for the failure can probably be related to the fact that they were published in the late 1920s and early 1930s, at a time of economic decline all across the country followed by a decade of economic depression.

SCIENTIFIC CRIMINAL INVESTIGATION AND FORENSIC SCIENCE

In ballistics, the European pioneers were again forensic physicians as was the case in so many other areas of forensic science. Comprehensive efforts at classification were American, however, and were initiated by Charles E. Waite, an investigator in the Office of the District Attorney in New York City. Waite was joined by John Fisher, Calvin Goddard, and Philip Gravelle. It was Gravelle who developed the comparison microscope for ballistics work. Together the group established and operated the first Bureau of Forensic Ballistics in America in New York City in 1924. On Waite's death, Goddard, who was a physician, took over the leadership of the program and became the foremost figure in forensic ballistics in the world. After being involved in many famous cases, Goddard was called to Chicago in 1929 to aid in the investigation of the St. Valentine's Day Massacre, a gangland killing which was the climax of the reign of organized crime in the Middle West in the 1920s. Goddard's investigations of the machine gun bullets and shells left at the scene and in the dead gangsters' bodies led to the arrest and conviction of a member of the Al Capone gang. After the successful work on the case was completed, Dr. Goddard was persuaded to stay on to set up a comprehensive program of scientific criminal investigation. He was sent on a tour of European medicolegal institutes and criminology programs and returned to become the head of the privately endowed Scientific Crime Detection Laboratory located on the campus of Northwestern University in Evanston, Illinois. The entire field of scientific criminal investigation, known in Europe as criminalistics, was developed at the Evanston Laboratory. It was the model for the national laboratory established by J. Edgar Hoover for the FBI in 1932. It also stimulated the establishment of the *American Journal of Criminology and Police Science* at Northwestern University in 1930. The Laboratory became the focal point for the development of many of the modern techniques in forensic science. In 1938, the Laboratory could no longer continue under private support. In a quite logical move, it became a part of the Chicago Police Department. Some of the scientific work continued to be based in Northwestern University as did the *Journal*, which continues to be published today by the Northwestern University Law School.

Forensic scientific work has continued to be supported in the United States primarily by law enforcement agencies with the continued stimulation and encouragement of the Federal Bureau of Investigation in the Department of Justice. In 1950, the American Academy of Forensic Sciences was established under its first President, Dr. Richard Hayes Gradwohl (1877–1959), who was Director of the Police Crime Laboratory for the City of St. Louis. The *Journal of Forensic Sciences,* official organ of the Academy, began publication in 1956.

CONTEMPORARY CONDITIONS: THE STATE OF THE ART

It can probably be said that conditions are improving for the forensic sciences, including legal medicine, in this country. This observation depends, however, on an agreement that it is a relative assessment: conditions were far worse in the past.

Dr. Chaillé, whose evaluation of legal medicine in the United States one hundred years ago was so dismal, would at least be pleased that elected lay coroners are now very uncommon with only a small handful of states still relying on them. Organized, statewide medicolegal death investigation systems under a chief medical examiner have been created in many states, while large metropolitan centers such as Dallas, Miami, Philadelphia, Los Angeles, and Washington, D.C., have recently established comprehensive medicolegal death investigational programs. Many of these agencies also include excellent laboratories which have capabilities in a wide range of criminalistic fields as well as in biologically related forensic sciences.

Most of the medical schools and a large majority of the law schools in the United States currently offer at least one medicolegal course, and many medical schools offer forensic clinical placements. There are a number of accredited residency programs in forensic pathology located in medical examiner and coroner programs across the country. University training in forensic toxicology has been improving steadily to the point where over 25 programs now exist for advanced degrees in the field. In the other forensic sciences, the practitioners are nearly all people who have gained their forensic knowledge and skills on the job, even though they may have had professional or scientific degrees when they began their forensic science careers.

Academic programs in various aspects of the forensic sciences, police science, and criminalistics have been developed in a scattering of universities, community colleges, and junior colleges, most of them state schools, over the past ten or fifteen years. Most of the courses are quite elementary so that on the job training continues to be essential for most specialty fields.

A national survey of the state of the art of the forensic sciences was conducted by the Forensic Sciences Foundation, an affiliate of the American Academy of Forensic Science, and was published in 1975.[29] The study produced both encouraging and discouraging results. A questionnaire survey of judges and practicing lawyers in the criminal law field indicated that a substantial majority (85%) believed that scientific evidence had more credibility than lay witness testimony. Among the same respondent groups, an even larger majority (92%) indicated that they thought scientific evidence should be used more frequently in criminal cases. A large majority (78%) reported that they would like to see forensic psychiatric services more readily available to the courts in their jurisdictions. Lastly, some two-thirds of these judges and lawyers thought changes in the law were essential to allow the forensic sciences to be used more effectively in American courtrooms.[30]

Among the general public, however, the study found that the forensic science profession was essentially unknown. Even important public agencies in the criminal justice field, such as the Federal Law Enforcement Assistance Program, were found to give very little attention to the field.

The study indicated that there was very little research going on in any of the forensic sciences. There was also no data base from which a reliable assessment could be drawn of the contribution being made by any of the forensic sciences to law enforcement or to the administration of justice.

More will be said in specific chapters of this text on the results of this survey regarding qualifications and training of professional practitioners in the various specialty fields in forensic science. It is enough to say at this point that the report indicated in an overall way that degree-oriented educational programs in the forensic sciences were "extremely limited."[31] At the time of the survey, only one of the specialties, forensic pathology, had a formal accreditation requirement. Since that time, however, a number of other specialties have set up accreditation boards, including anthropology, document examination, forensic psychiatry, forensic odontology, and forensic toxicology.

Our concluding evaluation must be related to the legal system, the environment within which most forensic scientists work. Trust and confidence in the forensic sciences have undoubtedly improved over the past century, as the forensic sciences themselves have progressed in reliability and effectiveness.[32] Law enforcement agencies rely on scientific investigation to a constantly growing extent, but budgetary constraints have limited the growth of comprehensive programs and have all but prohibited research. The trial courts are probably more receptive to scientific expert opinion and objective technological devices and tests than can be judged by reviewing appellate court cases. There are some very progressive and scientifically sophisticated appellate opinions by thoughtful judges,[33] but there are also many rather discouraging decisions displaying scientific ignorance and prejudice and a blind resistance to any invasion of the traditional powers of the common law judges and juries.[34] The greatest resistance is still displayed toward any scientific method of measuring the credibility of witnesses, that primary bulwark of the lay juror's functions. Thus the polygraph continues to have a stormy time of it in the appellate courts. Yet there are excellent opinions, even in this field, stressing the areas where the polygraph is most highly reliable and pointing out the absolute need for competent, trained polygraph operators working under proper conditions.[35] The newer methods of personal identification, such as the voiceprint, are still experiencing their ups and downs of judicial recognition,[36] while the battle of conflicting experts on scientific subjects continues to baffle the trial and appellate courts alike.[37] Except in regard to death investigation and some forensic psychiatric examinations, the common law jurisdictions continue to resist establishing impartial medical or scientific expert systems.

We would have preferred our concluding remarks to be more broadly hopeful. However, the analysis must be offered as we see it. Nothing less can be expected if our evaluation is itself to maintain the proper standards of objectivity, reliability, and completeness which must be the hallmark of the forensic sciences.

SIGNIFICANT DATES IN MEDICOLEGAL AND FORENSIC SCIENCE HISTORY

3000 B.C.   Imhotep, chief architect and builder to Pharaoh Zoser,

	also court justice and perhaps medical consultant. Later worshiped in Egypt as "God of Medicine."
1700 B.C.	Code of Hammurabi.
449 B.C.	Roman Code (Twelve Tables).
400 B.C.	Oath of Hippocrates.
44 B.C.	Public medical examination of the body of Julius Caesar.
130 A.D.	Testimony of Gaius Manicuis Valerianus, oldest known written medicolegal opinion, Greece.
200 A.D.	Claudius Galen's *Quomodo morbum simulantes suit deprehensi,* a treatise on malingering, perhaps the earliest text on a legally related medical subject.
475 A.D.	Code of the Visigoths.
600 A.D.	Hsu Chich-Ts'i, *Ming Yuang Shih Lu,* early Chinese medicolegal text.
800 A.D.	Capitularies of Charlemagne.
925 A.D.	Office of Coroner established in England.
1241–1253	Sung Tz'u, *Record of Washing Away of Wrongs,* early Chinese instruction booklet for public investigation of suspicious deaths.
1302	First medicolegal autopsy, Bologna.
1533	Code of Carolina.
1563	Johann Weyer, *De praestigiis daemonum et incantationibus ac veneficiis libri quinque,* a treatise refuting the public condemnation and execution of witches.
1564	G. P. Ingrassias, *Constitutiones et capitula necro uirisdictiones regii promedicatus officii,* Naples, earliest comprehensive medicolegal treatise in Europe.
1598–1602	Fortunatas Fidelis, *De relationibus medicorum,* Sicily.
1634	Paulo Zacchias, *Questiones medico-legales,* Rome, the most famous early medicolegal text.
1636	Election of the first Coroner in an English colony in America, by the General Court of Plymouth Colony, Massachusetts.
1650	First medicolegal lectures in Germany by Johann Michaelis at the University of Leipzig.
1663	Bartholin's discovery of hydrostatic test for determining whether infant breathed before death (also announced by Swammerdam in 1667).
1725–1736	Michael Alberti, *Systema jurisprudential medical,* multivolume German treatise, influential in introducing term "medical jurisprudence."

1769	Criminal Code of Empress Maria Theresa of Austria-Hungary, made medical evidence obligatory in certain cases, laying foundation for development of university medicolegal programs throughout Central Europe.
1779–1817	Johann Peter Frank, *System einer vollständigen medizinischen Polizei*, a comprehensive treatise on "medical police" published in Germany.
1791	The first medicolegal lectures in English language, at University of Edinburgh, by Andrew Duncan, Sr.
1794	French national decree reorganized medical education including mandatory courses in legal medicine.
	Thomas Percival, *Code of Ethics*, highly influential principles of medical ethics, originally titled, *Medical Jurisprudence, or A Code of Ethics and Institutes, Adapted to the Profession of Physics and Surgery*, Manchester, England.
1796	Pinel struck the chains from the mentally ill at Bicêtre Hospital, Paris.
1804	Independent chair in State Pharmacology established at Universities of Vienna and Salzburg, by Emperor Franz II of Austria-Hungary.
	Independent chair in Legal Medicine and Medical Police established at University of Cracow, under same decree of Emperor Franz II.
	First lectures on medical jurisprudence in America, at Columbia College of Physicians and Surgeons, by Dr. James S. Stringham.
	Combined chair in Legal Medicine (with Anatomy and Physiology) established at Moscow University.
1810	Medical lectures by Dr. Benjamin Rush at University of Pennsylvania, including lecture on "Medical Jurisprudence," with emphasis on forensic psychiatry.
1815	M. J. B. Orfila, *Traité des poisons*, Paris.
1823	T. R. Beck, *Elements of Medical Jurisprudence*, first American medicolegal text.
	First use of fingerprints for identification proposed by J. E. Parkinje.
1829	Robert Christison, *A Treatise on Poisons*, Scotland.
1836	Toxicological test for presence of arsenic in the human body, by James Marsh, English chemist.
1838	J. E. D. Esquirol, *Des maladies mentales considérées sous les rapports médicale, hygiénique et médico-légal*, Paris.
	Isaac Ray, *Treatise on Medical Jurisprudence of Insanity*, Boston.

1843		M'Naghten's Case, England (rules of insanity).
1847		Code of Ethics, American Medical Association.
1855		F. Wharton and M. Stillé, *A Treatise on Medical Jurisprudence,* Philadelphia.
1857		J. L. Caspar, *Praktisches Handbuch der gerichtlichen Medizin,* Berlin.
1859		J. J. Elwell, *A Medicolegal Treatise on Malpractice and Medical Evidence,* New York.
1860		Mrs. E. P. W. Packard's national campaign in U.S.A. for civil rights for mental patients.
1869		*State v. Pike,* 49 N.H. 399. (First adoption of "product test" for criminal irresponsibility.)
		John Ordroneaux, *Jurisprudence of Medicine,* New York.
1876		Cesaré Lombroso, *The Delinquent Man,* Milan.
		Sanford Chaillé's speech on Medical Jurisprudence at the Philadelphia Centennial Congress.
1877		Medical examiner system established in Massachusetts.
1879		Bertillon introduces system of personal identification for criminal investigation, Paris.
1881		Trial of C. J. Guiteau for assassination of President Garfield.
1883		Hans Gross, *Handbuch für Untersuchungsrichter,* Graz, the pioneer textbook in criminalistics.
1892		Sir Frances Galton, *Finger Prints,* London.
1908		Hugo Munsterberg, *On the Witness Stand,* New York.
1909		Psychiatric Court Clinic, Juvenile Court, Cook County, Chicago.
1910		Workmen's Compensation Law, New York.
1913		C. B. Goring, *The English Convict: A Statistical Study,* London. (First application of modern statistics to criminology, refuting Lombroso's theories.)
1915–1918		Chief Medical Examiner's Office, New York City.
1917		Psychiatric Court Clinic, Supreme Bench, Baltimore.
1920		Institute of Police Science, University of Lausanne.
		School of Criminology and Scientific Police, Lyon.
1921		Development of combined instrument for physiological measurement of detecting deception (blood pressure, pulse, and respiration) by John A. Larson, Berkeley, California.

1923	Edmond Locard, *Manual of Police Technique*, Lyon.
	Frye v. U.S., 203 F. 1013. (Leading case on acceptance of scientific tests in evidence.)
	Development of the comparison microscope for forensic ballistics by Philip O. Gravelle, New York.
1924	Identification Division, Bureau of Investigation, Department of Justice, Washington, D.C.
	Bureau of Forensic Ballistics, New York.
1925–1932	Medicolegal Reports, National Research Council, Washington, D.C.
1926	Development of polygraph instrument for detection of deception by Leonarde Keeler, Chicago.
1927	*Buck v. Bell*, 274 U.S. 200 (upholding compulsory sterilization).
1929–1930	Scientific Crime Detection Laboratory, Evanston, Illinois. (First comprehensive forensic science laboratory in America.)
1930	*American Journal of Police Science.*
1932	Federal Bureau of Investigation Laboratory, Department of Justice, Washington, D.C.
	Scientific Institute of Forensic Medicine, Soviet Union. (Highest authority in legal medicine in U.S.S.R.)
1934	Home Office Forensic Science Laboratory, England. (Foremost criminalistics laboratory in Great Britain.)
1938	International Academy of Legal and Social Medicine.
	Institute of Criminology, University of California, Berkeley.
1939	First statewide medical examiner system, under a chief medical examiner, Maryland.
1947	Code of Nuremberg, war crimes trials, Germany. (Code on human experimentation.)
1948	*International Digest of Health Legislation*, World Health Organization, Geneva, Switzerland.
1950	American Academy of Forensic Sciences.
1952	Law-Medicine Center, Case Western Reserve University, Cleveland.
	Law-Medicine Institute, University of Texas Law School, Austin.
1958	Subspecialty in Forensic Pathology, American Board of Pathology. (First recognized specialty in medicolegal field in United States.)

	National Interprofessional Code for Physicians and Attorneys.
	Law-Medicine Research Institute, Boston University.
1961	Development of voiceprint spectrograph by Lawrence Kersta, Bell Laboratories, New Jersey.
1962	Model Penal Code, American Law Institute.
	Vera Institute of Justice, New York.
1963	Trial of Jack Ruby for murder of alleged assassin of President Kennedy.
1968	Report on Medical and Legal Definition of Brain Death, Harvard Ad Hoc Committee.
	Trial of Sirhan Sirhan for assassination of Robert Kennedy.
1969	National Commission on Causes and Prevention of Violence, Washington, D.C.
	Southwestern Institute of Forensic Sciences, University of Texas, Dallas.
1973	National Commission on Criminal Justice Standards and Goals, Washington, D.C.
1973–1975	National Assessment of Personnel of the Forensic Science Profession, Forensic Sciences Foundation, Bethesda, Maryland.

REFERENCES

1. Frazer, J.G.: *The Golden Bough, A Study in Magic and Religion.* Macmillan, New York, 1958.
2. Nagel, E.: Types of Causal Explanation in Science, in Lerner, D. (ed.): *Cause and Effect.* The Free Press, New York, 1965.
3. Rawlinson, G.: *History and Ancient Egypt.* Scribner & Welford, New York, 1881.
4. Smith, S.: History and Development of Legal Medicine, in Gradwohl, R.B.H. (ed.): *Legal Medicine.* C.V. Mosby, St. Louis, 1954.
5. Hurry, J.B.: *Imhotep.* Oxford University Press, London, 1926.
6. Brittain, R.P.: Origins of Legal Medicine: Roman Law, Lex Duodecim Tabularum. *Medico-Legal Journal* 35:71–72, 1969.
7. Radin, M.: *Handbook of Roman Laws.* West Publishing Co., St. Paul, Minn., 1927.
8. Brittain, R.P.: The Origins of Legal Medicine: Charlemagne. *Medico-Legal Journal* 34:121–123, 1969.
9. Singer, C.: *A Short History of Medicine.* Oxford University Press, New York, 1928, p. 71.
10. Giles, H.A.: The Hsi Yuan Lu, or Instructions to Coroners. *Proc. R. Soc. Med.* 17:59–107, 1924.
11. Ackerknecht, E.H.: Early History of Legal Medicine. *Ciba Symposium* 2:1286–1289, 1950–1951.
12. Zilboorg, G., with Henry, G.W.: *History of Medical Psychology.* W. W. Norton, New York, 1941, p. 226.
13. Szasz, T.S.: *The Manufacture of Madness.* Dell, New York, 1970, p. 76.
14. Ackerknecht, op. cit., p. 1297.

15. Alexander, F.G., and Selesnick, S.T.: *The History of Psychiatry*. Harper & Row, New York, 1966, p. 138.
16. Nemec, J.: *International Bibliography of Medicolegal Serials, 1736–1967*. National Library of Medicine, Bethesda, Maryland, 1969.
17. Walls, H.J.: *Forensic Science*. ed. 2. Sweet & Maxwell, London, 1974, p. 1.
18. Sanders, E.: *The Mystery of Marie La Farge*. Crerke & Cockeran, London, 1951.
19. Deutsch, A.: *The Mentally Ill in America*. Columbia University Press, New York, 1949.
20. Ordronaux, J.: *The Jurisprudence of Medicine*. T. & J. W. Johnson and Co., Philadelphia, 1869, p. 6.
21. *Durham v. United States*, 214 F. 2d 862 (D.C. cir., 1954).
22. Maine Code, Chapter 311, Section 3.
23. Chaillé, S.E.: Origin and Progress of Medical Jurisprudence, 1776–1876. *Transactions of the International Medical Congress of Philadelphia*, Collins, Philadelphia, 1877.
24. Nemec, J.: *Highlights in Medicolegal Relations*. rev. ed. National Library of Medicine, DHEW Publication (NIH) 76-1109, Bethesda, Md., 1976, p. 95.
25. *Bulletin of the International Medico-Legal Congress* (1895). Medico-Legal Society of New York, 1898.
26. Schultz, O.T., and Morgan, E.M.: The Coroner and the Medical Examiner. Bulletin No. 64, National Research Council, Washington, D.C., 1928, p. 89.
27. Schultz, O.T.: Possibilities and Need for Development of Legal Medicine in the United States. Bulletin No. 87, National Research Council, Washington, D.C., 1932.
28. Schultz and Morgan, op. cit., p. 84.
29. Field, K.S., et al.: *Assessment of the Personnel of the Forensic Science Professions*. Forensic Sciences Foundation, Inc., Rockville, Md., June 1975.
30. Schroeder, O., Jr.: *The Forensic Sciences in American Criminal Justice, A Legal Study Concerning the Forensic Sciences Personnel*. Forensic Sciences Foundation, Inc., Rockville, Md., June 1975, pp. 13–21.
31. Field, K.S., Lipskin, B.A., and Reich, M.A.: *A Survey of Educational Offerings in the Forensic Sciences*. Forensic Sciences Foundation, Inc., Rockville, Md., June 1975, p. 4.
32. Curran, W.J., and Shapiro, E.D.: *Law, Medicine and Forensic Science*. ed. 2. Little, Brown, Boston, 1970.

ADDITIONAL READING

Ackerknecht, E.H.: Legal Medicine Becomes a Modern Science. *Ciba Symposium* 2:1299–1304, 1950–1951.
Brittain, R.P.: *Bibliography of Medico-Legal Works in English*. Rothman, South Hackensack, N.J., 1962.
Burns, C.R. (ed.): *Legacies in Law and Medicine*. Science History Publications, New York, 1977.
Cuthbert, C.R.M.: *Science and the Detection of Crime*. John Wiley & Sons, London, 1960.
Foucault, M.: *Madness and Civilization*. Random House, New York, 1965.
Gray, J.C.: *The Nature and Sources of the Law*. Columbia University Press, New York, 1909.
Havard, J.D.J.: *The Detection of Secret Homicide*. Macmillan, London, 1960.
Kind, S., and Overman, M.: *Science Against Crime*. Aldus Books, London, 1972.
Kozelka, F.L.: Legal Medicine in the United States. *Ciba Symposium* 2:1305–1311, 1950–1951.
Maine, H.S.: *Ancient Law*. Oxford University Press, New York, 1931.
Mannheim, H.: *Pioneers in Criminology*. Quadrangle Books, Chicago, 1960.
Moreland, N.: *An Outline of Scientific Criminology*. Butterworth, London, 1958.
Nemec, J.: *International Bibliography of the History of Legal Medicine*. National Library of Medicine, DHEW Publication (NIH) 73-535, Bethesda, Md.

Smith, S.A.: The History and Development of Legal Medicine. *Br. Med. J.* 24:599–606, 1951.

Thorwald, J.: *The Century of the Detective.* Harcourt, Brace & World, New York, 1965.

Walker, N.: *Crime and Insanity in England.* Vol. 1. Historical Perspective. University Press, Edinburgh, 1968.

CHAPTER 2

William J. Curran is Frances Glessner Lee Professor of Legal Medicine at Harvard University and Chairman of the State Medicolegal Investigation Committee of Massachusetts. Professor Curran writes regularly for the *New England Journal of Medicine* and teaches at the Medical School, Law School, and School of Public Health at Harvard. He was formerly Robert R. Utley Professor of Legal Medicine and Director of the Law-Medicine Institute of Boston University. He also served as Assistant Professor of Law and Government and Assistant Director of the Institute of Government at the University of North Carolina. Professor Curran is the author of several books in the medicolegal field including *Law, Medicine and Forensic Science* (with E. D. Shapiro); *Trauma and the Automobile; The Doctor as a Witness;* and *Medicolegal Proof in Litigation.* He is an Associate Editor of the *American Journal of Law and Medicine* and was formerly Medicolegal Editor of the *Massachusetts Law Quarterly.*

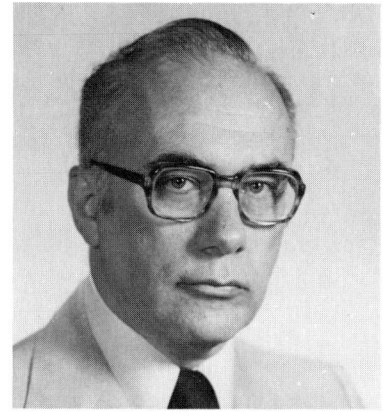

ETHICAL STANDARDS

William J. Curran, J.D., LL.M., S.M. Hyg.

THE SCOPE OF ETHICAL INQUIRY

A review of ethical standards in the forensic sciences was considered by the editors of this text an essential part of the development of a comprehensive presentation of the state of the art in the field. There were two approaches which could have been taken: (1) each author of a particular chapter could have been left to review or not review ethical matters as that author saw fit; or (2) a separate chapter could be prepared covering the subject of ethical standards. We chose the second approach. However, we have also encouraged chapter authors to include discussions of ethical considerations relevant to their own coverage. Discussions of ethical issues, even though not always identified as such, appear in the chapters on operational and administrative aspects of the subject, in some chapters on examination standards and techniques, and in some of the chapters which cover the broad scope of the specialty field as such.

The rationale for including a general chapter on ethical standards is based on the position that there are fundamental ethical issues which cut across the various specialties of the forensic sciences. We also believe that an examination of the general principles of ethical conduct in professional practice is necessary to an understanding of particular applications of ethical rules to any given field.

Frankena describes ethics as a part of the field of philosophy or more specifically moral philosophy.[1] It is the study of morality, moral problems, and moral judgments. We find the equating of "morals" with "ethics" to be quite common in the writings of general ethicists and philosophers. For example, the title of a currently popular book on ethics is *Morality: An Introduction to Ethics*.[2] The study of morals or ethics is essentially an examination of what is right and what is wrong, what is virtuous and what is evil, in the human conduct of individuals and groups of individuals.

ETHICAL CODES FOR PROFESSIONS

The practice of issuing sets or codes of ethical principles for professional groups is of long standing and is generally identified as one of the essential attributes of a profession.[3] These codes are not limited to expressions of proper moral conduct. They generally contain admonitions concerning loyalty to the group itself and to the maintenance of standards of practice traditional among the group. The inclusion of such provisions has been disparagingly referred to as making the principles matters of "etiquette" rather than "ethics."[4] This should not be taken as a criticism. It is entirely proper to broaden statements of group conduct to include matters of importance to the group itself and its self-preservation. Thus the Hippocratic Oath required the physicians of that Greek minority of doctors to honor and protect their teachers and to preserve their learning and traditions. Without the solidarity of the group, there would be no way of identifying or enforcing the moral aspects of the code. The Hippocratic Oath also contained a provision prohibiting Hippocratic physicians from going beyond their calling into other fields, since it required that the group not engage in any cutting (surgery) of their patients. This prohibition preserved the identity of the group as physicians and discouraged association with other practitioners following different principles.

The ethical codes of professional groups are also necessary to express the independence of individual practitioners to offer their services as they see fit in accordance with their ethical standards, even in defiance of the request or demand of their patients, clients, or employers. The Hippocratic Oath contained more promises *not* to do certain things than it did affirmative expressions. The Hippocratic physicians promised *not* to give deadly potions, even if their patients asked for them; *not* to perform abortions (a common practice at the time by other physicians), even if requested; and *not* to cut their patients, even if it seemed needed for the patient's good. They also promised *not* to disclose confidences of patients, even if demanded by authorities.

These promises of "I shall not" are essential to the protection of the character of the professional person. They make it clear that he or she is not the unthinking instrument of the client, available to do anything that the client wants, willing to make the knowledge and skills of the professional calling work for the client's interest irrespective of the inherent wrongness or group corruption of the action itself. This incorruptibility of professional action is not related solely to moral wrongness. It is also intended to prevent lowering of the standards of the profession, even at the request of the client or employer who wants short-cuts in methods, a cheaper price, or a flattering result. These admonitions have often been attributed solely to the altruism of the professions and to the requirement of acting always on behalf of the public good. I disagree. They are also related to group identity and pride in one's work. The artist who paints pictures which are not popular paints for his own perfection and satisfaction. The architect who refuses to design an ugly and tasteless building is following his own and his group's concept of proper standards, even if the building meets utilitarian needs and a low budget. The scientist who publishes the results of his experiments whether successful or not does so in the interest of truth and knowledge, even though no particular public good may be achieved. The scientist takes pride in following lines of inquiry no matter where they may lead. The search for knowledge is very personal in science. The group of scientists protects the individual scientist in his personal search, often against the outcry of employers and government agencies who may see no immediate public good being achieved in the scientist's work.

The need for independence of professional judgment has led many to doubt whether a profession can be maintained on a salaried basis, especially where all or nearly all members are salaried. Those who argue that professions can be salaried are even more dependent upon the support of strong ethical standards to hold members of the group to proper principles in the face of employer demands.

MONOPOLY AND LEGAL ENFORCEMENT

At the present time criticism can be heard against many of the larger and more powerful professional organizations, especially from consumer groups and consumer advocates. Much of the criticism is due to the monopolistic position achieved by some professional societies, often with the help of federal and state legislation. Licensing laws have been used by lawyers, for example, to integrate admission to the bar with membership in the state bar association. Nearly all of the professions which are licensed have been able to convince the legislatures to provide for revocation of licenses on the basis of vaguely worded "unethical conduct," or "violations of professional standards," and even to list in the law particular bases for revocation such as advertising and fee-splitting.

In recent years, the legislatures and regulatory bodies have taken it upon themselves to enact provisions imposing requirements in areas formerly left solely to ethical standards within the professions. Thus the Federal government has become active in establishing laws and regulations (often called "guidelines," but promulgated and enforced as regulations) in animal and human experimentation.[5] The courts have also imposed their own interpretation of professional requirements with or without statutory grounds in areas such as informed consent of patients[6] and experimental subjects[7] and confidentiality of client relationships.[8] Lastly, the courts have struck down some statutorily imposed ethical standards, such as the prohibition of professional advertising, as unconstitutional deprivations of free speech.[9] A large part of the rationale for the decisions has been the monopolistic position of many of the professions today.

ETHICAL CODES IN FORENSIC SCIENCE: DELAYED DEVELOPMENT

Even though the American Academy of Forensic Sciences was formed in 1950, it was not until 1976 that a proposal for the development of an ethical code was openly discussed at the organization's annual meeting. At that time, only one of the specialties represented in the Academy, the questioned documents examiners, had adopted their own national code.[10] One state association in criminalistics, that in California, had adopted a code.[11] In 1977, the Academy adopted its first general ethical principles.[12]

The long absence of an ethical code in the forensic sciences can be explained on various grounds. First, some of the professional groups in the Academy already had their own general professional codes (medicine, dentistry, and law) or their own specialty code (questioned document examiners). Next, the promulgation of a code was not as common among scientists who were not licensed as among legally registered and licensed professional groups who offer their services largely on a fee for service

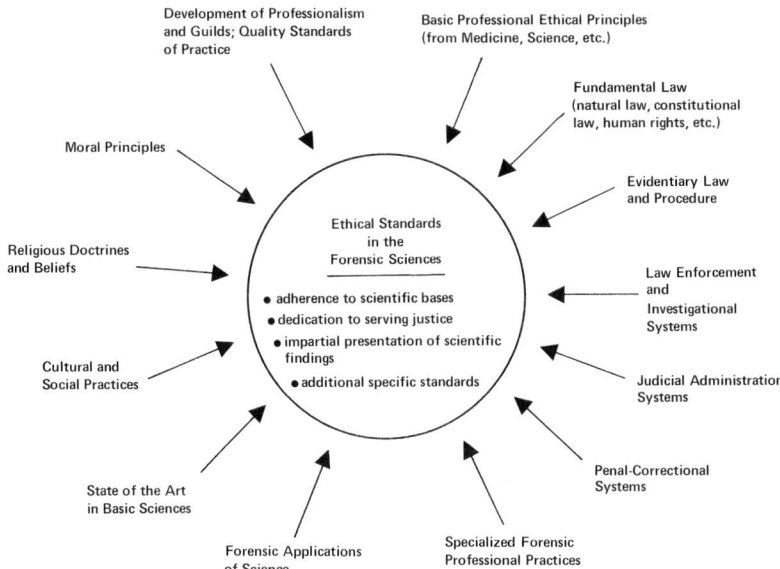

FIGURE 2-1. Contributions to ethical standards.

basis. The Academy then saw itself more as an interdisciplinary scientific group than as a new, integrated profession. Also, many of the specialties in the Academy were too recent in development and too loosely constructed in identity and qualifications to be primarily concerned about codes of ethics.

In this chapter, we will examine both general principles of ethical conduct applicable to all forensic scientists and specific standards developed for particular groups. We will discuss ethical issues and dilemmas presented by the environment in which forensic scientists work within the courts, the penal system, and the law enforcement agencies of this country. Figures 2-1 and 2-2 are offered as schematic presentations of the multidisciplinary contributions to the development of codes of ethics in forensic science.

A General Interprofessional Code

The first generalized code to which attention should be called is that jointly developed and promulgated by the American Medical Association and the American Bar Association in 1958.[13] It applies to medical litigation and is called a National Interprofessional Code for Physicians and Attor-

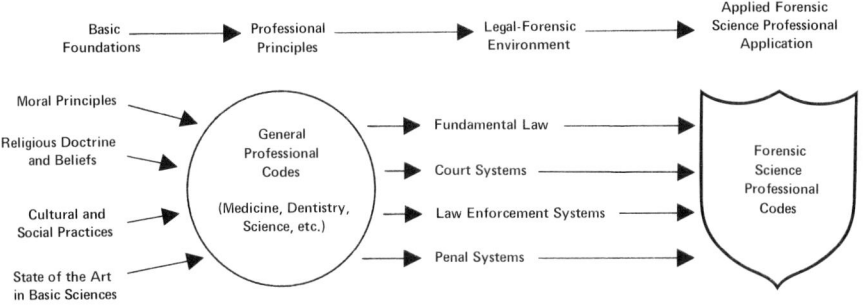

FIGURE 2-2. Ethical development in the forensic sciences.

neys. The Code covers matters concerned with litigation such as the making of reports, testimony, and the payment of fees to doctors for services in litigation. Most of the principles in this Code could properly be found to apply to any other forensic scientist or expert witness. For example, the expert medical witness is admonished never to become an advocate in his testimony and is encouraged to enlighten the court and jury rather than to try to impress them with his status or to prejudice their judgment. Pretrial conferences concerning testimony are encouraged to avoid inadequate preparation. The Code provides that the expert witness is entitled to reasonable compensation for all time spent on preparation, pretrial conferences, and for court and other appearances as a witness. The amount of the witness' fee is prohibited from being contingent on the outcome of the case or the amount of money damages received by the party calling the witness. The Interprofessional Code places responsibilities upon lawyers as well as physicians. For example, it prohibits harassment and abuse of medical witnesses and attempts to influence a medical opinion.

The approach of an interprofessional code has much in its favor. It must be admitted that it would be difficult for any of the forensic sciences to make an ethical code work effectively without the cooperation of the courts and the judges and lawyers who function in them. As will be pointed out, many of the ethical problems for forensic scientists are intimately connected with court practices and attorney behavior.

A Specific Code: Questioned Documents Examiners

An examination of an ethical code currently in force for a national specialty group in forensic sciences is appropriate at this point. The American Society of Questioned Documents Examiners first adopted a Code of Ethics in the late 1940s. It was later amended in the 1950s and was last amended in 1972. It begins with a preamble on aims and purposes of the document. Mentioned first is the promotion of justice through the discovery and proof of facts relating to questioned documents. Next (and last) the Code is said to be intended to maintain and advance the technical as well as the ethical standards of the profession. The preamble thus relates the profession exclusively to forensic applications and dedicates the group to serving justice, not merely a client's interests. The preamble also accepts the importance of relating high-quality standards of practice with proper ethical standards, as was suggested for professional codes earlier in this chapter.

The first specific principle in the QDE Code can be considered a first commandment for all of the forensic sciences: It pledges members to apply the principles of science and logic to their field and to follow the truth courageously no matter where it may lead. A later provision supplements this principle by admonishing members to act at all times, in and out of court, in an "absolutely impartial manner." Caution and modesty in presenting opinions are also pledged. Conclusions should be offered only to the extent justified by the findings, and the examiner should admit that some questions cannot be answered because of the nature of the problem (i.e., the limits of the science), inadequate material available to examine, or insufficient opportunity to examine.

The second principle in the Code pledges members to keep well informed about developments in their field so as to remain competent to carry out their professional responsibilities.

There are important provisions concerning charges for consultation services. It is stipulated that services should not be undertaken on a contingent fee basis. As for the amount of the fee, the Code allows consideration of three elements: (1) extent and character of the service rendered; (2) the importance of the matter in litigation; and (3) the relationship of the problem submitted to the controversy as a whole. This provision endorses the practice of most QD professionals in basing their fees in particular cases not only on the time and effort spent, but also on the circumstances of the case itself. In civil law matters, the circumstances are essentially related to the money involved, such as the value of a disputed contract or the amount of an estate passing on a contested will. In criminal cases, the importance of the matter could relate to the gravamen of the charge or the severity of the potential sentence of the defendant. The commission or percentage nature of the fee is common to many professions, occupations, and undertakings from the salvaging of a sunken ship to taking out a rich man's appendix. Care must be taken, however, in applying this practice to fields heavily dependent upon opinions as to genuineness or relative value. The amount of the fee could well depend on the outcome (genuine or forgery; high value or very low value) such as to make the fee essentially contigent in nature. There is another provision in the QDE Code which requires that the "best possible service" be given in all cases irrespective of the importance of the matter. Thus the amount of the fee may differ, but not the degree of effort and standard of quality rendered. The law of malpractice for all professional work imposes the same rule, even if the practitioner is paid nothing for the services. The legal standard of "ordinary and accepted practice" applies in all cases except where an even higher standard may be imposed or agreed to by the professional and the client.[14]

The Code also contains a provision on confidentiality and conflict of interest, both of which relate to loyalty to the client. The practitioner is required to keep information given by the client strictly confidential. It also provides that the examiner must refuse to perform services for any other person whose interests oppose those of the client, except by permission of the client or as required by established administrative procedure or law.

In the most recent amendments in 1972, the Code was expanded to cover examiners who are fully salaried as well as fee for service consultants.[15] Specifically, Provision 7 was clarified in regard to charges for services. Members are now authorized to serve on an annual salary or employment contract basis. Conditions of payment may be controlled by the policies of the employing organization. The provision on conflict of interest noted earlier also applies differently to employed examiners who generally do not choose their own clients. An impartial public agency may properly conduct investigations involving parties with conflicting interests. Such conduct on the part of an independent document examiner would, under the Code, be considered unethical.

A General Ethical Code

The two codes reviewed above provide the background for the examination of the Code of Ethics adopted by the American Academy of Forensic Sciences in 1977.

The Code is in two parts. The first part contains the only officially binding portion of the principles adopted by the Academy. It contains two principles as follows:

1. Every member of the American Academy of Forensic Sciences shall avoid any material misrepresentation of training, experience or area of expertise.
2. Every member of the American Academy of Forensic Sciences shall avoid any material misrepresentation of data upon which an expert opinion or conclusion is based.

The rather studied language of the two provisions indicated that the Academy was being quite careful to limit the scope of the Code and that some conservative lawyers were involved in the drafting. The document does not display the broad and sweeping style of most ethical pronouncements. Essentially, the two principles express a single ethical demand, namely, truthfulness. They are worded, like many professional codes, in the negative, thus requiring members not to issue "material misrepresentations." Apparently, small inaccuracies are allowed. It should be noted also that the second principle does not cover an untruthful opinion or conclusion. It covers only material misrepresentations of data on which the opinion is based. This is rather strange. It is entirely possible for people to tell the truth about data (which can be checked), but to lie or misrepresent their opinion. Admittedly, it is difficult to prove that an opinion is not genuinely held by an expert. Nevertheless, this should not deter an admonition in an *ethical* code against lying about opinions. Again we see the fine hand of the lawyers at work. Lawyers (and police officials as well) are uncomfortable with laws that are difficult or virtually impossible to enforce. But this Code is not law; it is a set of group principles, an ideal of proper conduct. It certainly should not hedge on the fundamental standard of truth in all professional and scientific work. We should also point out that it is not impossible to prove that an opinion is untruthful. In fact an American court has convicted a physician of perjury for what was found to be an untrue medical opinion. The conviction was upheld on appeal.[16] Personally, I believe the case of *State v. Sullivan* so significant that it is the first decision included in my own casebook in the section of expert medical testimony.[17] It seems to me that all expert forensic science witnesses should be aware of this decision before they undertake any courtroom testimony.

The second part of the ethical standards adopted in 1977 are described as "guiding principles" which are voluntarily subscribed to by all forensic scientists. They would seem to go sufficiently beyond the careful wording of the official Code as to require separate treatment. Apparently, members of the Academy can be subject to censure, suspension, or expulsion from membership only for violation of the official Code. The three guiding principles are as follows:

1. The forensic scientist should maintain his professional competency through existing programs of continuing education.
2. The forensic scientist should render technically correct statements in all written or oral reports, testimony, public addresses, or publications and should avoid any misleading or inaccurate claims.
3. The forensic scientist should act in an impartial manner and do nothing which would imply partisanship or any interest in a case except proof of the facts and their correct interpretation.

These three guidelines are closer in style and content to traditional ethical principles than the official AAFS Code. The first guideline refers to professional competence. As noted earlier, a principle of this type is common in professional codes. This statement is rather more specific than most in referring directly to continuing education programs. The licensing laws and certification requirements for some of the professions are moving toward specific requirements for periodic relicensure and recertification based upon certain required hours of continuing education.

The second guideline seems in part a commentary or extension of the two official and binding principles. It deals with truthfulness in a more expansive way than the Code. The forensic scientist is admonished ("should") to render "technically correct" statements and to avoid misleading or inaccurate "claims." It is not clear whether or not the guideline covers expert opinions.

In the last guideline, the forensic scientist is cautioned to maintain impartiality in all cases. This is a very important provision. It does not seem to be worded as cautiously as the other guidelines or the official Code.

It should be clear that the Academy's ethical standards are intended to cover members (under the Code) and forensic scientists generally (under the guidelines), but not lawyer members who are acting professionally as lawyers. Lawyers in practice do not offer expert scientific opinions and certainly cannot be expected to be impartial in the cases they handle. The forensic scientist who also has a law degree (not uncommon among Academy members) would be covered by the Code and guidelines when acting as a forensic scientist. General principles of truthfulness should, of course, apply to all members of the Academy.

TRUTH AND ADVOCACY

Certain general themes can be seen to be supported in the ethical codes reviewed above. The primary functions of forensic science personnel in every specialty are investigation, examination, and evaluation. The courts and law enforcement agencies receive their reports and must rely on their findings and expert judgments. Therefore, the first principle in the ethical codes of the field relate to truth in reporting and testimony. From this one standard many applications and refinements can be made. Reports should be complete as well as accurate. Conclusions should not go beyond the findings to the point that they cannot be supported, and expert opinions should reflect truthfully the viewpoint of the expert. Of the available ethical codes, the most detailed on all aspects of truthful testimony and reporting is the Code of the California Association of Criminalists, referred to earlier. The Code has separate sections on ethical aspects of court presentation (with 13 subsections), ethics relating to opinions and conclusions (with 10 subsections), and ethical aspects of the use of the scientific method (with 6 subsections).

The greatest danger to truth for a forensic scientist is in becoming an advocate. The temptations to advocacy are severe. The strongest of all is the court system itself. Truth is not the objective of most contested cases. The objective is the peaceful settlement of disputes with reliance upon the burden of proof to resolve issues of fact.[18] The attorneys for the parties are admittedly advocates of the causes they represent and are allowed substantial leeway in fighting for their clients' legal interests. The forensic scientist is cast into the midst of this battle. The pressure is greatest upon the independent expert evaluator. The attorneys seek out forensic scientific consultants and pay them for their services. Though interested in the truth, the lawyers are essentially seeking support for their client's cause. They may go from expert to expert seeking one who is able and willing to offer conclusions favorable to their side of the case. Currently, the standards of legal ethics do not condemn such practices as long as the lawyers do not knowingly produce false or misleading testimony in court. They are not required to call to the witness stand or to produce the reports of each of the experts they consulted but determined not to use because their conclusions were adverse to their client's interests. Thus the independent experts who appear in court for the parties in the common law system are the screened-out results of the lawyers' advocacy methods. The lawyers expect the expert to support the cause of the client. If a forensic science consultant wishes to continue in the field and to be paid to appear in court, it is said that he must "play the game" according to the court's rules and in compliance with the advocacy system.

Despite pressures and temptations, the ethical forensic scientist must resist acceptance of an advocate's role. He must present his findings and conclusions truthfully and fully without unjustified overreaching to favor the client who called him. Nevertheless, the expert witness must be able to defend his position on cross-examination. He should not allow the cross examining attorney to destroy the value of his findings and conclusions by trick questions or misleading statements. Avoiding the role of advocate does not mean that the witness should become a straw in the wind blown from side to side by whatever lawyer is questioning him. At times the badgering of a cross-examiner can cause the opposite to occur. The expert witness who was not entirely certain of various parts of his examination or report may stiffen under personal attack and defend the weak parts much more forcefully than they deserve. Extremes on either side should be avoided, and the forensic scientist should adhere to the accuracy of the findings and conclusions with dignity and firmness.

IMPARTIALITY IN PUBLIC AGENCIES

Moving into a salaried position in a public agency such as a police laboratory or a medical examiner's office does not eliminate all of the problems of truth, advocacy, and impartiality. The pressures will be different but can often be just as severe as in private consultation. The client of the forensic scientist in a public setting should be the public. However, in reality, it may be a politically elected or appointed administrator who does not understand or respect the science that the forensic specialist practices.

The strongest pressures on the public employee may be related to inadequate scientific equipment and facilities and inadequate time to carry out investigations and evaluations properly. The Report of the Forensic Sciences Foundation on conditions in the forensic sciences in the 1970s indicated that virtually all public laboratory facilities in the criminal justice field were operating in inadequate space and were understaffed and overworked.[19] Ethically, the forensic scientist should have the freedom in a public agency to refuse to offer an opinion or a conclusion based on inadequate grounds.

The temptation for the forensic scientist in a law enforcement agency or the medical examiner's office is to become a servant of the police and the criminal prosecutor's office to the extent that truth is sacrificed to arrest, disposition of cases, and a good prosecution record. In such conditions, evidence is rarely evaluated to find a suspect innocent. At best it is found "inconclusive." Such forensic scientists improperly join in the chase for a likely suspect and resolve doubts in support of their colleagues in the police department.

Ethical impartiality demands another approach for forensic scientists. Administratively, it is advisable for forensic science laboratories and their personnel to be separated from the investigative arm of a law enforcement agency.[20] A coroner or medical examiner should not be responsible to a law enforcement agency and should not be dependent upon the permission of a prosecuting attorney to conduct an investigation or to order an autopsy.[21]

The urging of civil service status and job security or tenure for medical examiners and other forensic scientists in public employment is directly related to the need for impartiality of judgment. At least after a period of probation, forensic scientists should be assured of job security.

A controversial subject in this area is the proper relationship of publicly supported forensic science programs to the defense in criminal cases. In the early stages of an investigation, a confidential attitude may be necessary in order to avoid damage to reputations. Personnel in medicolegal agencies and forensic science laboratories should generally refrain from premature public statements or from releasing information to anyone except those in charge of the investigation. At later stages, however, cooperation with attorneys and with other forensic scientists retained by an accused person may be ethically advisable because the agency or laboratory may be in total control of the evidence in the case. Court cases and statutes have authorized medical examiners to furnish copies of autopsy protocols and other evidence to the defense. Oliver Schroeder, in his report for the Forensic Sciences Foundation study referred to earlier, points to a number of statutory authorizations to furnish evidentiary materials to the defense for their own analysis.[22]

In a useful paper on ethical problems for criminalistics laboratories, Bradford urges greatly improved practices in these programs to preserve evidentiary material and to make and preserve complete notes and records on all cases handled.[23] He describes graphically the weaknesses of many current laboratories. Such laboratories cannot substantiate the accuracy of their reports and certainly cannot aid in a later re-examination of the findings and conclusions in a case, either by the defense, an independent review board, or their own agency administrators.

EXCESSIVE PUBLICITY

The ethical demand for an attitude of impartiality does not apply only to the courtroom. It applies also in the investigative and pretrial periods when the news media may be exerting strong pressures for interviews and statements. Due process of law and fundamental fairness require the use of restraint in dealing with the press and with other persons who may release information to the press.

In recent years, the American Bar Association, with the aid of a committee of outstanding judges and lawyers, has issued important statements on the problems of maintaining a free press and also assuring fair trial for criminal defendants.[24] In amendments to the Canons of Professional Ethics, the Bar Association has provided that from the time of arrest or indictment until trial, no attorney for the prosecution or the defense shall release any extrajudicial statement relating to a number of prejudicial areas including (1) the performance of any examinations or tests on the accused, or the refusal of the accused to submit to any examinations or tests; and (2) the existence or contents of any statement, admission, or confession of the accused, or the refusal or failure of the accused to make any statement.

As a matter of professional ethics, these same standards should apply to forensic scientists involved in criminal investigations. It should be noted that the rules deal with disclosures of refusals to submit to examinations or tests as well as to disclosures of results. A reading of some of the leading American cases on excessive publicity in criminal matters reveals that forensic science personnel were involved in some of the practices and procedures which were alleged to have resulted in violations of due process of law and the right to a fair trial.[25]

The justification for the early release of information in some criminal investigations has been to assure the public that the person who committed the offense or offenses is no longer at large. The pressure for such public assurance can be very great, especially in multiple crimes committed over a period of time and creating substantial public fear and disturbance. News media coverage usually becomes more intensive and more sensational as additional crimes are committed. Are lawyers, police, and forensic scientists ethically justified in releasing information in such matters where their motives are solely to quiet public fears? No exception to the ethical demand for impartiality has been adopted or seriously proposed in any of the professions in such circumstances. In his report for the Forensic Sciences Foundation noted earlier, Professor Schroeder comments favorably on the forensic scientist's role in allaying the fears of citizens.[26] Commenting on a case of mass murder, Schroeder asserts that the work of the laboratory represented "a valuable contribution of the forensic sciences to allay the fear of citizens when an apparent criminal situation creates an atmosphere of fear in any neighborhood."[27] In this case, the laboratory investigation indicated that one of four members of a family found dead in a house had murdered three of them and then killed himself. The quoted report on the case ends with the statement: "Although shocked by the incident, the neighbors were relieved to know that it was not a fifth party who might still be free."[28] It was not indicated how the neighbors were reassured. Release of the information by the forensic scientists would not be ethically proper. However, if the investigation were closed as a result of their work and an official report were released to the public, the head of the laboratory, or the head of the agency, could comment further on the case to provide public assurance, as long as the rights of persons involved were not prejudiced thereby.

INVESTIGATIONAL PROCEDURES

Ethical codes related to the forensic sciences have not considered issues of questionable participation in investigational procedures against persons accused of crime or under suspicion. To what extent can physicians and other forensic science professionals become involved in forcible actions against an accused without consent? Such actions can become so aggravated that they can be described as "cruel or inhuman treatment," or "torture." The Declaration of Tokyo, an ethical statement adopted by the World Medical Association in 1975, admonishes physicians not to engage in any such practices upon prisoners under penal sentence or in detention under criminal charges. Included as "cruel or inhuman treatment" are forcible treatment with drugs to aid in obtaining a confession and forcible feeding of prisoners on a hunger strike. The Declaration of Tokyo and another statement of principles by the World Health Organization on the same subject would allow medical involvement in such procedures only with the free consent of a mentally competent, adult prisoner or detainee.[29] Obviously, the "free consent" of a detained person to any painful or dangerous procedure would be highly suspect.

Medicolegal and forensic science personnel would probably correctly deny involvement in outright "torture" of suspects or convicted prisoners, but cases can be suggested of questionable conduct which is not uncommon on the American scene and which can raise serious ethical issues. Consider the following examples: Blood samples have been taken from unwilling arrestees. Persons suspected of swallowing illegal drugs or other substances have had their stomachs pumped out in order to produce the evidence. Surgical operations have been performed without consent to remove bullets from suspects for ballistics examination. Persons have been forced to talk into a recording device, or have had their voices recorded without their knowledge while in custody, in order to have the recordings available for identification by a witness, or to be analyzed by a voiceprint technician. Which of these practices, if any, are ethically unjustified?

The primary guidance on the propriety of the above examples comes from decisions of the American courts on the violation of constitutional rights of accused persons subjected to such practices. Space limitations allow only a summary of the conclusions in the most important cases.

The taking of blood samples against the strong protest of persons arrested for drunken driving has been upheld by the U.S. Supreme Court as proper so long as it is done by competent physicians under sterile, clinical conditions.[30] The forcible use of a stomach pump in a case which also involved illegal entry and some other "strong-arm tactics" on the part of the police was held, in a famous opinion passed down in 1952 by Justice Frankfurter, to be brutal conduct that "shocks the conscience" and violates due process of law.[31] In other later cases, however, lower courts have sanctioned the use of stomach pumps and other body-cavity searches by physicians to aid the police.[32] In a recent case, however, the California Supreme Court returned to the ruling of 1952 and found the forcible use of a stomach pump on a protesting woman to be an unreasonable and improper search.[33] In this case, police had a warrant to inspect the house and the "person" of the suspect. She was seen to swallow two bags which the narcotics agents believed contained heroin. The suspect was arrested and taken to a hospital where the agents showed a doctor the warrant and requested him to pump the woman's stomach. The doctor denied any medical necessity to pump her stomach, even if she had swallowed heroin. He indicated that the only reason he did so was because of the warrant. After the procedure, the subject regurgitated seven bags of heroin. The Court held that the warrant did not extend to forcible entry into the body. Under the Declaration of Tokyo, the physician's actions, in the absence of any medical reason for the use of the stomach pump or drugs to induce vomiting, would be unethical.[34]

The use of surgical procedures to remove bullets from unconsenting suspects has been allowed by a few courts where it has been alleged that the risk was minimal and local anesthetic was used.[35] The Indiana Supreme Court has declared that any use of surgery to remove bullets, even under local anesthetic, is an unreasonable search and a violation of due process.[36] Two other courts have outlawed risky procedures involving general anesthetics, but have indicated that they might approve minor invasions of the body to remove bullets where no anesthetic or a local anesthetic was appropriate.[37] Interestingly enough, in the most risky of these cases, where the bullet was lodged in the defendant's lower back in the spinal canal, the surgeons involved recommended that the procedure be performed, even though they admitted that it was "major surgery" and involved "at least" the risks associated with general anesthesia.[38]

Where no risk of physical harm to the defendant is involved, such as in breathing into an analyzing device or blowing up a balloon, the courts have sanctioned the procedure.[39] These procedures have been held not covered by the prohibitions against self-incrimination because they do not involve oral or written statements. Somewhat more difficult have been the cases in which the suspect was forced to speak in a line-up or had his voice recorded secretly and without his consent. The courts have allowed both practices, as long as the statements were used only for identification purposes.[40]

Some of these situations could involve forensic scientists. Two types of involvement may be reviewed: (1) the active participation of the forensic scientists in improperly producing the evidence; and (2) the passive reception and testing of evidence (such as a blood sample) which was obtained improperly by other personnel such as the police. The violation of ethical standards may be more aggravated in the first situation, but it would also be ethically improper to cooperate in the latter situation if the circumstances of the use of improper coercion were known.

Cases such as those described above raise the issue of what ethical justification the professional may have for pleading that he was acting under the orders of a superior. In many situations of doubt as to whether the act was unethical per se, or where the professional was unaware of significant facts which made the action unethical, such as not knowing or having reason to know that a piece of evidence or a blood sample was obtained illegally or through use of unwarranted force, the professional would be justified in obeying his superiors. If the action was clearly unethical, however, and the professional was in possession of the necessary facts to show that it was, it would be improper to follow the order. The Nazi crimes against humanity as exposed at Nuremberg clearly laid to rest any doubt about the invalidity of such a defense by professional personnel dealing inhumanely with prisoners or detainees. The Code of Nuremberg concerning improper medical experimentation on prisoners was essentially a restatement of accepted ethical principles.[41] It was enforced against physicians and nurses who claimed they were only obeying orders. The Declaration of Tokyo clearly requires physicians to refuse to obey superiors or to cooperate with other personnel in any treatment of prisoners or accused persons under detention which is deemed cruel or inhuman.

IMPROPERLY OBTAINED CONFESSIONS

It can be unethical conduct for a physician or forensic scientist to use improperly the skills of his or her profession to obtain or to aid in the obtaining of a confession from an accused. The use of deception, coercion, or the administration of drugs without the person's consent would be examples of improper conduct. In a landmark case, the United States

Supreme Court severely criticized the conduct of a psychiatrist in using subtle, persuasive techniques to extract a confession from a youthful suspect.[42] The Court appended to the opinion a transcript of the psychiatrist's interview with the accused to demonstrate its impropriety and coercive nature. The psychiatrist said, among other things, the following:

> I want you to recollect and tell me everything . . . It's entirely to your benefit to recollect them because, you see, you're a nervous boy . . . Tell me, I'm here to help you.
>
> I am going to put my hand on your forehead, and as I put my hand on your forehead, you are going to bring back all these thoughts that are coming into your mind. . . .
>
> If you tell us the details and come across like a good man, then we can help you. We know that morally you were just in anger. Morally, you are not to be condemned. Right?[43]

This questioning was considered improper, particularly because it was used by a physician who had misled the accused into assuming he was there to help him. Also, as a psychiatrist, he was said to be using skilled psychological techniques in a corrupt manner. The case occurred in the early 1950s, before the Supreme Court imposed the *Miranda* warning requirements before interrogation.[44]

The form and substance of the questions above are not uncommon in police interrogation where gentle persuasion is used in place of, or in alternating fashion with, more aggressive confrontation. This type of questioning by police has been recommended as quite successful by authorities on interrogation and truth-seeking.[45]

Forensic scientists such as polygraph and voiceprint technicians are frequently involved in situations where suspects are encouraged to confess or make admissions prior or subsequent to scientific tests. Care must be taken by forensic scientists not to engage in coercive or deceptive actions (such as telling a suspect he had "failed" a polygraph test when the results were inconclusive or negative) when such deception is intended to provoke a confession.

PSYCHIATRIC AND PSYCHOLOGICAL ISSUES

The view has been held by some psychiatrists that members of their profession should not participate in criminal trials because of their belief that the courts distort psychiatric testimony and impose psychiatrically unsound laws of personal responsibility. Among the proponents of this view are Dr. Gregory Zilboorg,[46] who has received the Isaac Ray Award of the American Psychiatric Association for his contributions to legal psychiatry, and Dr. Thomas Szasz, who has written extensively on psychiatric-legal subjects.[47] The same view has also been expressed by Dr. Karl Menninger.[48] No ethical issues are raised by the testimony of psychiatrists in most legal matters where, like any other experts, they merely report on their own clinical findings or observations, expressing themselves in terms applicable to the situation, whether or not they are in court. The only time that psychiatrists have objected on scientific and ethical grounds has been where the courts have imposed their own behavioral standards upon the issues at hand, such as in criminal responsibility. It would seem ethically proper for a psychiatrist to decline to evaluate a case or to appear in court as an expert in criminal responsibility if he sincerely holds the belief that he could not agree with the applicable law and could not report within his own professional competence and skills. This is not to say that other psychiatrists could not hold opposite views on involvement in criminal responsibility evaluations.

In most clinical situations, psychiatrists (and clinical psychologists) are alleged to exercise their doubts about a patient's condition in favor of offering treatment, if the patient desires it. This tendency may be ethically proper (though I have my own doubts about it) in clinical practice, but it has serious consequences when applied to patients who are evaluated in criminal matters or commitment proceedings, or when the patient's potential for dangerous conduct is in question. Various chapters in this book will be found to deal with these issues substantively. At this point, we would only say that clinicians, especially those untrained in forensic psychiatry or psychology, must be cautioned not to exercise their judgment improperly in this regard. Often the untrained clinician has a great fear of what will happen to his patient if the latter is "turned over to the law." Therefore, he answers the key questions the "right way" to get the patient committed to his clinical care, or to prolong the commitment indefinitely. At other times, the clinician exercises his judgment conservatively, as on questions of "dangerousness," in order to avoid public or professional attack if the patient gets into difficulty after release. This type of conduct on the part of clinicians is ethically reprehensible and should be condemned strongly. Yet we must realize the great difficulty for even the most experienced of forensic psychiatrists and psychologists in making predictions of future conduct by their patients. Statutory immunity from civil damage actions for clinicians who act in good faith in such situations is commendable as encouraging objective evaluations. The difficulties of prediction and the vulnerability of clinicians to damage suits have been graphically presented in the *Tarasoff* case[49] in California. The Court therein held the clinicians of a university health service liable in damages to the family of a person murdered by a patient of the health service. The decision has been severely criticized by psychiatrists.[50] It has been praised by most legal commentators,[51] but not by all.[52]

One of the most difficult ethical situations for legal psychiatrists and psychologists is found in prison settings where clinical services are provided.[53] The inmates sometimes tell clinicians about incidents of their own behavior or that of other inmates which are violations of prison rules, or tell them about future plans for violent action, protest movements, or prison breaks. Distinctions are generally drawn by experienced prison therapists between information about past conduct, where confidences are kept, and information about serious future dangers to the inmate, fellow inmates, prison personnel, or the entire prison community, where the therapist may deem it necessary for the patient's welfare and that of others to reveal the information. This ethical standard is essentially the same as in private practice. The prison clinicians should clarify the limits of confidentiality before therapeutic sessions begin. The prison authorities should also be apprised of the ethical standards to be applied so that misunderstandings can be avoided and unreasonable demands are not placed on clinicians to cooperate in investigations of prison problems.

ISSUES IN FORENSIC PATHOLOGY

Matters discussed earlier concerning ethical standards in making reports and in testimony apply to forensic pathologists as well as to all other forensic scientists. There are, however, some special issues in this field which should be examined.

It is a universal rule that medicolegal autopsies performed under the jurisdiction of a coroner or medical examiner do not require the consent of next of kin. The constitutionality of this law has rarely been tested. In a recent challenge to the law in Maryland by an Orthodox Jewish family on grounds of violation of rights to freedom of religion, the highest court of the State held the law constitutionally valid.[54]

Medical examiners and coroner's physicians should, however, use their power to order autopsies with proper discretion and prudence. They should not allow a hospital, for example, to procure an autopsy against the wishes of the family by "taking medicolegal jurisdiction" in a situation where it is clearly not justified by the circumstances of the case.

Forensic pathologists, like all physicians and scientists, have an ethical obligation to contribute to further knowledge, research, and education in their field. This obligation means that forensic pathologists should keep accurate and complete records and should contribute to research and general education in medicine, not merely to its forensic aspects. Most forensic pathology programs are very busy with service obligations, but cooperation with research efforts should be encouraged. For example, the Medical Examiner-Coroner of Los Angeles County contributed substantially to suicide research by making available to behavioral scientists his collection of suicide notes left by deceased persons in closed cases.[55] Another area of cooperation is making certain anatomical materials available to medical and dental schools for anatomical instruction. Often the medical examiner's office is the only source of such materials. The supplying of tissues and organs is ethically justified if not prohibited by law, if it does not compromise the investigation in any way, if it does not cause unnecessary delays in making the body available to a funeral director for burial or cremation, and as long as the family is not caused distress by visible disfigurations.

The same rules would apply to donations of minor tissues for research or for transplant procedures, at least where the tissues, such as skin or bone or small glands, are very difficult to obtain otherwise and where no objection of next of kin can normally be expected. In cases of doubt about propriety, the consent of next of kin should be obtained.

In the donation of major organs, however, such as the kidney, heart, or liver, consent of next of kin should always be obtained, unless the law allows donations in such cases by the medical examiner or coroner, or where the deceased has consented and signed a valid document for such a donation (as currently provided by law in all 50 states) or has consented to such donations under the recent amendments to the motor vehicle license laws in many states.

Medical examiners called in to investigate deaths in hospitals or other medical settings sometimes feel that they, as a part of the medical care community, should avoid exposure of a medical professional colleague's mistakes which could have contributed to the death. This is an ethically and legally improper interpretation of the public responsibility of a medical examiner or any physician retained by a coroner. The physician in these situations is obliged to report fully on the circumstances and manner of the death. The facts should be described objectively, however, without unwarranted speculation about what could have been done medically to prevent the death or to "save" the person after the difficulties had occurred. It is no simple matter to lay down exact rules about these situations. Primarily, the forensic physician should avoid special efforts to "cover up" medical negligence or intentional wrongdoing. The same standards would apply to any investigation where the facts are "embarrassing" to police actions in the case, or to the work of other forensic scientists.

UNETHICAL ADVERTISING AND PUBLICITY

As pointed out earlier, ethical admonitions against professional advertising have been struck down recently by the courts. Antitrust and restraint of trade actions have also been brought against professional organizations attempting concerted actions to enforce bans on advertising. In the forensic science field, some institutional advertising has been fairly common for consultant and laboratory services, except where ethically prohibited by their own professional societies. Discretion should be used in the format of such advertising, and the claims for the technology should be modestly stated.

Despite the actions of the courts in advertising cases, forensic scientists should continue to act with professional dignity and should avoid professional actions designed solely for publicity purposes or personal adulation. The only ethical code for forensic scientists containing provisions on publicity is that of the California criminalists group. Two subsections are of interest:

> *Section 5(C).* In the interests of the profession, the individual criminalist should refrain from seeking publicity for himself or his accomplishments on specific cases. The preparation of papers for publication in appropriate media, however, is considered proper.
>
> *Section 5(D).* The criminalist shall discourage the association of his name with developments, publications, or organizations in which he has played no significant part, merely as a means of gaining personal publicity or prestige.

These are not easy standards to follow, especially when forensic scientists become involved in sensational cases with heavy news media coverage. Some practitioners may, in fact, disagree entirely with the position taken here. We do not mean to discourage necessary cooperation with the press. However, we do believe that devotion to the truth and resistance to the many pressures to compromise ethical standards call for an attitude of restraint regarding self-advertising and publicity.

ENFORCEMENT OF ETHICAL CODES

Enforcement of ethical standards is essentially a matter for the professional organizations, except where, as noted earlier, the ethical rules are enacted into licensure laws. The American Academy of Forensic Sciences has provided a detailed procedure for enforcement of its new Ethical Code. The procedure is intended to work equitably and fairly in the interest of the profession and the general public. Members of specialty groups within the Academy are also subject to enforcement of ethical standards in their respective professions. In the medicolegal field, the Interprofessional Code reviewed earlier contains provisions for joint investigation of complaints with censure and loss of membership left up to the respective professional organizations.

The forensic sciences have a unique relationship to a controlling body which is not common to other scientific undertakings; this is their relationship to the courts. Since all forensic scientists fundamentally serve the courts and the administration of justice, an enforcement method for serious ethical violations which compromise the forensic scientist's functions within the courts and administrative legal tribunals could be developed. Forensic scientists could be made "officers of the court" similar to attorneys and could be made subject to investigation and censure by the courts. At least this is an area of exploration for the future in the continuing relationship between law and the forensic sciences.

REFERENCES

1. Frankena, W. K.: *Ethics.* ed. 2. Prentice-Hall, Englewood Cliffs, N.J., 1973.
2. Williams, B.: *Morality, An Introduction to Ethics.* Harper Torchbooks, New York, 1972.
3. Bradford, L. W.: Problems of Ethics and Behavior in the Forensic Sciences. *J. Forensic Sci.,* 21:750–756, 1976.
4. Leake, C.: Theories of Ethics and Medical Practice. *J.A.M.A.* 208:842–847, 1969.
5. Curran, W. J.: Government Regulation of the Human Subjects in Research: The Approach of Two Federal Agencies. *Daedalus* 98:542–594, 1969.
6. Plant, M.: An Analysis of Informed Consent. *Fordham Law Rev.* 36:639–650, 1968.
7. Freid, C.: *Medical Experimentation, Personal Integrity and Social Policy.* North Holland Publishing Co., Amsterdam.
8. Zenoff, E.: Confidentiality and Privileged Communications. *J.A.M.A.* 182:656–663, 1962.
9. *Goldfarb v. Virginia State Bar,* 421 U.S. 773 (1974); *Bates v. State Bar of Arizona,* 97 S. Ct. 2691 (1977).
10. Code of Ethics of the American Society of Questioned Documents Examiners. *Am. Bar Assoc.* 40:690–691, 1954. (The amended Code was published recently in *J. Forensic Sci.* 21:782, 1976.)
11. California Association of Criminalists: Code of Ethics, 1974. (Personal communication from President, John I. Thornton, Berkeley, California, October 1, 1974.)
12. *Newsletter,* American Academy of Forensic Sciences, 1977, No. 3, pp. 1–2.
13. National Interprofessional Code for Physicians and Attorneys. *Am. Bar Assoc. J.* 45:650–653, 1958.
14. Curran, W. J.: Professional Negligence: Some Comments. *Vanderbilt Law Rev.* 12:535–545, 1959.
15. Hilton, O.: Ethics and the Document Examiner Under the Adversary System. *J. Forensic Sci.* 21:779–782, 1976.
16. *State v. Sullivan,* 24 N.J. 18, 130 A 2d 610 (1957), cert. denied, 355 U.S. 840 (1957).
17. Curran, W. J., and Shapiro, A. D. (eds.): *Law, Medicine and Forensic Science.* ed. 2., Little, Brown, Boston, 1970, pp. 338–342.
18. Frank J.: *Courts on Trial.* Princeton University Press, Princeton, N.J., 1949; Cardozo, B. N.: *The Nature of the Judicial Process.* Yale University Press, New Haven, 1921.
19. Field, K. S., et al.: *Assessment of the Personnel of the Forensic Science Profession.* Forensic Sciences Foundation, Inc., Rockville, Md., June 1975.
20. *Report on Police.* National Advisory Commission on Criminal Justice Standards and Goals, Washington, D.C., January 1973, Standard 12.1, pp. 3–4.
21. Curran, W. J.: The Medicolegal Autopsy and Medicolegal Investigation. *Bull. N.Y. Acad. Med.* 47:766–772, 1971.
22. Schroeder, O., Jr.: *The Forensic Sciences in American Criminal Justice: A Legal*

Study Concerning the Forensic Sciences Personnel. Forensic Sciences Foundation, Inc., Bethesda, Md., June 1975, pp. 33–37; Schroeder, O., Jr.: Old Ethics for New Sciences—What Confronts Justice. *J. Forensic Sci.* 21:748–758, 1976.
23. Bradford, op. cit.
24. Report, Committee on the Operation of the Jury System. *Federal Rules Decisions* 45:381, 1969; 51:135, 1971.
25. *Sheppard v. Maxwell,* 384 U.S. 333 (1966); *State v. Van Duyne,* 43 N.J. 369, 204 A. 2d 841 (1964). See accounts of the Sheppard case in Pollack, J. H.: *Dr. Sam, An American Tragedy.* Henry Regnery, Chicago, 1972; Holmes, P.: *The Sheppard Murder Case,* McKay, New York, 1961. See also *Hampton v. Chicago,* 484 F. 2d 602 (7th Cir. 1973).
26. Schroeder, op. cit., pp. 89–91.
27. Ibid., p. 90.
28. Loc. cit.
29. *Health Aspects of Avoidable Maltreatment of Prisoners and Detainees.* World Health Organization, Geneva, Switzerland, Document A/Conf. 56/9 (1975).
30. *Schmerber v. California,* 384 U.S. 757 (1966).
31. *Rochin v. California,* 342 U.S. 165 (1952).
32. Constitutionality of Stomach Searches. *U. San Francisco Law Rev.* 10:93–95, 1975.
33. *People v. Bracamonte,* 15 Cal. 3d 394, 124 Cal. Rptr. 528 (1975).
34. Curran, W. J.: Ethical and Legal Problems in Medical Participation in Criminal Investigations. *N. Eng. J. Med.* 294:764–765, 1976.
35. *Creamer v. State,* 229 Ga. 511, 192 S.E. 2d 340 (1942); *Allison v. State,* 129 Ga. App. 364, 199 S.E. 2d 587 (1973); *U.S. v. Crowder,* No. 73-1635 (D.C. Cir., July 12, 1976); Surgery and the Search for Evidence. *U. Pittsburgh Law Rev.* 37:429–431, 1975.
36. *Adams v. State,* 299 N.E. 2d 834 (Ind., 1973), cert. denied, 415 U.S. 935 (1974).
37. *Bowen v. State,* 510 S.W. 2d 879 (Ark. 1974); *People v. Smith,* 80 Misc. 2d 210, 215 N.Y.S. 2d 909 (1974).
38. *Bowen v. State,* 510 S.W. 2d at 881.
39. *State v. Berg,* 76 Ariz. 96, 259 P. 2d 261 (1953).
40. *People v. King,* 266 Cal. App. 2d 437, 72 Cal. Rptr. 478 (1968); *Foster v. California,* 394 U.S. 440 (1969).
41. Nuremberg Medical Tribunal, Medical Cases, *U.S. v. Brant,* U.S.G.P.O., Washington, D.C., 1947; Beecher, H. K.: "Experimentation in Man." *J.A.M.A.* 169:461–473, 1959.
42. *Leyra v. Denno,* 347 U.S. 556 (1953).
43. *Leyra v. Denno,* 347 U.S. at 580–585.
44. *Miranda v. Arizona,* 384 U.S. 436 (1966).
45. Inbau, F. E., and Reid, J. E.: *Criminal Interrogation and Confessions.* Williams & Wilkins, Baltimore, 1962.
46. Zilboorg, G.: *Psychology of the Criminal Act and Punishment.* Harcourt Brace, New York, 1954.
47. Szasz, T.: *The Myth of Mental Illness.* Harper & Row, New York, 1961.
48. Menninger, K.: *The Crime of Punishment.* Viking Press, New York, 1966.
49. *Tarasoff v. Regents of University of California,* 108 Cal. Rptr. 878 (1973); 13 Cal. 3d 177 (1974); 131 Cal. Rptr. 14 (1976).
50. Stone, A. A.: The Tarasoff Decisions, Suing Psychiatrists to Safeguard Society. *Harvard Law Rev.* 90:358–378, 1976.
51. Fleming, J., and Maximov, S.: The Patient or His Victim: The Therapist's Dilemma. *Cal. Law Rev.* 62:1025–1068, 1974; Duty to Act for Protection of Another. *Vanderbilt Law Rev.* 28:631–640, 1975.
52. Curran, W. J.: Confidentiality and the Prediction of Dangerousness in Psychiatry. *N. Engl. J. Med.* 293:285–286, 1975.
53. Halleck, S. L.: *Psychiatry and the Dilemmas of Crime, A Study of Causes, Punishment, and Treatment.* Harper & Row, New York, 1967.
54. *Snyder v. Holy Cross Hospital,* 30 Md. App. 317 (1976); Curran, W. J.: Religious Objection to a Medicolegal Autopsy: A Case and a Statute. *N. Engl. J. Med.* 297:260–261, 1977.

55. Curphey, T. J.; Role of the Forensic Pathologist in the Medicolegal Certification of Modes of Death. *J. Forensic Sci.* 13:163–171, 1968; Litman, R. E.: Psychological-Psychiatric Aspects of Certifying Modes of Death. *J. Forensic Sci.* 10:263–273, 1969.

ADDITIONAL READING

Dyck, A. J.: *On Human Care, An Introduction to Ethics.* Abington Press, Nashville, 1977.
Edelstein, L.: Professional Ethics of the Greek Physician. *Bull. Hist. Med.* 30:391–419, 1956.
Fletcher, J.: *Situational Ethics.* Westminster Press, Philadelphia, 1966.
Fox, M. (ed.): *Modern Jewish Ethics.* Ohio State University Press, Columbus, 1975.
Jones, W. H. S.: *The Doctor's Oath.* University Press, Cambridge, 1924.
Ramsey, P.: *Basic Christian Ethics.* Charles Scribner's Sons, New York, 1950.
Rawls, J.: *A Theory of Justice.* Belnap Press of Harvard University Press, Cambridge, Mass., 1971.
Reiser, S. J., Dyck, A. J., and Curran, W. J. (eds.): *Ethics in Medicine, Historical Perspective and Contemporary Concerns.* M.I.T. Press, Cambridge, Mass., 1977.

PART 2 MEDICOLEGAL DEATH INVESTIGATION

CHAPTER 3

Charles S. Petty is Director of the Southwestern Institute of Forensic Sciences at Dallas, Chief Medical Examiner of Dallas County, Director of the Dallas County Criminal Investigation Laboratory, and Professor of Pathology and Forensic Sciences at the University of Texas Southwestern Medical School at Dallas. Dr. Petty holds degrees in pharmacy and physiology from the University of Washington and received his medical education at Harvard Medical School. He is a diplomate of the American Board of Pathology in pathologic anatomy, clinical pathology, and forensic pathology. Dr. Petty is former President of the American Academy of Forensic Sciences and is a Fellow of the American Association for the Advancement of Science, the American College of Physicians, the American Society of Clinical Pathologists, and the British Academy of Forensic Sciences.

William J. Curran is Frances Glessner Lee Professor of Legal Medicine at Harvard University and Chairman of the State Medicolegal Investigation Committee of Massachusetts. Professor Curran writes regularly for the *New England Journal of Medicine* and teaches at the Medical School, Law School, and School of Public Health at Harvard. He was formerly Robert R. Utley Professor of Legal Medicine and Director of the Law-Medicine Institute of Boston University. He also served as Assistant Professor of Law and Government and Assistant Director of the Institute of Government at the University of North Carolina. Professor Curran is the author of several books in the medicolegal field including *Law, Medicine and Forensic Science* (with E. D. Shapiro); *Trauma and the Automobile; The Doctor as a Witness;* and *Medicolegal Proof in Litigation.* He is an Associate Editor of the *American Journal of Law and Medicine* and was formerly Medicolegal Editor of the *Massachusetts Law Quarterly.*

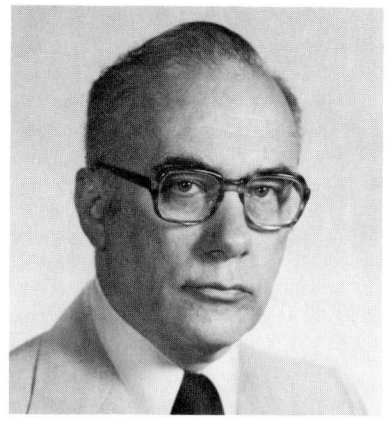

OPERATIONAL ASPECTS OF PUBLIC MEDICOLEGAL DEATH INVESTIGATION

Charles S. Petty, M.D., and
William J. Curran, J.D., LL.M., S.M.Hyg.

Medicolegal death investigative systems represent one arm of the governmental structure of a nation, state, province, county, or municipality. Their operational life springs from the law of the nation or political subdivision charged with the investigation of death for public rather than private reasons.

Operational problems experienced by medicolegal investigative agencies may range from an ineffectual law to conflicting interrelationships with other public or private agencies. This chapter is devoted to examining those operational problems most frequently affecting medicolegal investigative systems.

THE MORES OF DEATH

Although, according to some religions, death is considered to be the moment of rebirth, as far as the individual is concerned, death represents the end of life, at least on this planet. Perhaps because of the fear of death, the dead body is accorded a special place in many cultures. Customs and cults concerning death and the disposal of the dead body have developed. Some of these influence the medicolegal investigative system.

The sanctity accorded the dead body is, in various forms, used as an argument to prevent autopsy or even a simple postmortem examination,* and

---

*The term "postmortem examination" is used herein to refer to an external examination of a dead body without incisions being made, although blood and other body fluids may be collected for examination. The term "autopsy" indicates that, in addition to an external examination, the body is opened and an internal examination is conducted. The full procedure and documentation of a medicolegal autopsy are described in Chapter 5.

thus to hamper the medicolegal investigational system in the fulfillment of its legal obligations. Funeral practices, emotional reactions of the surviving family members, religious concepts, desires of transplantation surgeons, and many other beliefs and practices contribute vectors of force, some pushing the body toward a rapid interment, others serving as counter forces to delay the ultimate disposal of the lifeless form.

For more than a century the most commonly used technical funeral practice in the United States has been that of embalming. It has been said that this practice began to increase in popularity during the American Civil War. The desire to return the bodies of dead soldiers to their homes was strong, but transportation was not yet rapid. Cooling of the body with ice, when it could be procured, was not very effective for prolonged periods of time. Embalming was an available technique for preserving bodies on their homeward journey. Now worthy only of a historical note, the early embalming fluids frequently contained large quantities of arsenic. This caused an operational problem that foreshadowed a modern but similar one: arsenic poisoning obviously could not be proven by analysis of specimens procured during the autopsy of a body embalmed with an arsenic-containing fluid. The modern counterpart has many forms; one is the impossibility of proving poisoning by any substance that is also contained in the fluid used for embalming (e.g., methyl alcohol).

The provision of embalming by all funeral establishments in the United States has gradually brought about the practice of keeping the body in an unburied state for several days during which time it is kept or displayed in a ritualized fashion.

Embalming is carried out by two entirely different procedures, both of which are frequently applied to a single body. *Arterial embalming* is accomplished by replacing the blood in the blood vessels with a suitable embalming fluid. The fluid of choice usually contains formaldehyde and a variety of other substances including coloring matter. The exact composition of embalming fluids is a well-kept commercial secret. *Trochar embalming* is performed by introducing a large trochar (or needle) through the abdominal wall. By means of this trochar the fluids contained within the viscera and cavities of the chest and abdomen are removed and replaced with a kind of embalming fluid.

The interfaces of the medicolegal investigative system with the funeral establishment are many: most are negative; a few are positive when viewed by the medicolegal officer. The following are major objectives of funeral directors and embalmers:

1. The embalmer would prefer to work with a very recently dead body. The longer the body has been dead, the more the blood will settle and eventually cause discoloration of the dependent (downside) parts of the body which is difficult to erase.
2. The embalmer would prefer to work with an intact body, not one on which an autopsy has been performed. In the autopsy process, many of the blood vessels are necessarily cut. The vascular integrity is lost, and poor evacuation of blood and leakage of embalming fluid contribute to poor embalming and localized islands of insufficiently preserved tissues. Premature decomposition, discoloration, odor, swelling, and much less than "lifelike" appearance may result.
3. The funeral director would prefer to obtain the body immediately after death so as the better to plan for embalming and the subsequent funeral services. He may be much pressured by the family to prepare the body at once and to have the body ready for viewing.

These three objectives are probably the major reasons that the funeral establishment prefers little if any medicolegal investigation, for such requires time and may require autopsy. These objectives may conflict with the operational goals of medicolegal investigators, as follows:

1. The pathologist or medicolegal officer would prefer time in which to conduct an investigation into the circumstances of the death. Considerable time, sometimes many hours, may be required. This is particularly true when several agencies are concerned, especially when there are overlapping jurisdictions.
2. The pathologist or medicolegal officer would prefer an unembalmed body. There are many reasons for this preference: embalming alters the appearance of the body, tissues, and organs, making interpretation of any injury or disease process difficult; the toxicologic examination of fluids and tissues removed from embalmed bodies is difficult, and toxic substances may be masked, altered, destroyed, or sequestered by the embalming process. Some pathologists, perhaps not as concerned with medicolegal events, seem to prefer working on embalmed bodies. Permitting the embalmer at least to carry out arterial embalming makes him less apt to object to autopsy. The use of the trochar may remove accumulations of blood or fluids most necessary in the proper interpretation of wounds and disease. Moreover, the trochar makes tracks and these markedly alter the tissues.
3. On the positive side regarding the issues of embalming is that the practice provides for long retention of the body in an unburied state and thus longer availability to the medicolegal officers should it be discovered that investigation and autopsy are necessary. This is of particular importance if cremation, the ultimate in body destruction, is planned.
4. The funeral director provides a most valuable service for the medicolegal officer and the vital statistical arm of the state by providing much of the information needed to complete the death certificate.
5. The funeral director and his embalmer may be of great aid to the medicolegal officer by notifying him of instances where the examination of the body in the funeral parlor reveals evidence of trauma or inconsistency with the medical certification of death, as carried out by the practitioner of medicine.
6. Funeral practices and customs make the funeral parlor (or funeral home) the center of activity of the surviving relatives and provide a place of contact between the family and the medicolegal officer. A line of communication is thus possible, and the funeral director frequently is willing to serve as an intermediary in dealing with matters of sensitivity to the family.

Other mores of death are concerned in the interface between the medicolegal officer and the surviving family. After the death of any individual, the surviving family members (and sometimes even friends) have varied emotional outbursts. A feeling of guilt may pervade if the survivors feel that they might have done more to save the life—or that they somehow were responsible for the death. Grief is expressed in many ways, including hysteria, hostility, hate, and fear, among others. Any or all of these emotions may well cause the family members and friends to become irrational and to object to the medicolegal officer's interference with what they consider to be a very private matter. The idea of an autopsy may be abhorrent. Even the most circumspectly placed question may provoke an intense emotional outburst. The concept that the public interest must be served by a medicolegal investigation is understood only in the context that privacy will be violated, even though the investigation may prove eventually to be of great use and consolation to the same family. This is a true operational problem and one which must be contended with by means of tact, personal sensitivity, and sympathy. It is an easy matter to convince the family when their suspicions have been aroused that a homicidal attack was responsible for the death of their family member. It is quite a different matter to try to educate a hostile family to the benefits that may arise from a medicolegal investigation, particularly if it must be admitted that the investigation and autopsy might show that no insurance or other benefits should accrue to the family.

It must be remembered that the family members are part of the public at large, and that it is these people who are the taxpayers and who ultimately support the medicolegal investigative system. Although the medicolegal officer may be well within the operational law to perform an autopsy in a given case, he may have to convince the family that it is proper or necessary to do so. In some instances when a homicidal death is not suspected and the family is uncompromisingly opposed to autopsy, it may be in the best public interest not to proceed with the autopsy examination. However, should this latter course be adopted, the medicolegal officer must be certain to explain the medicolegal ramifications to the family. It may be well to put the facts of the case in writing and have the guiding family member attest by signature that he understands the entire problem.

LEGAL SOURCE FOR PROGRAMS

A public medicolegal investigative program (including both coroner and medical examiner systems) can be no more effective than the law providing for the establishment of the system. There will always be problems concerning the interpretation of the law, the constitutionality of the law, the applicability of the law, and finally the interdigitation of the fingers of law relating to the needs of the state versus the rights of the individual.

There will also continue to be arguments within and without the forensic science professions about the relative merits of the coroner and medical examiner systems. There is general agreement that the least effective system was the ancient English form of the coroner's office wherein the coroner was a layman performing only the quasijudicial functions of holding hearings, or inquests, with a coroner's jury and having no power to retain expert medical and scientific assistance in his work. This system disappeared long ago in England and is continued in only a few American jurisdictions. In England the coroners are either lawyers or physicians and all have medicolegal experience. Expert forensic science consultation is provided for all English coroners nationally by the Home Office.

In the United States, reforms in the lay coroner systems have taken many directions. Most of the reforms have two objectives: (1) to divorce the system from political control and influence, and (2) to provide expert forensic pathology and laboratory services to the system. The most direct way chosen to achieve both objectives in one reorganization has been the abolition of the coroner's office and substitution of a medical examiner system. The medical examiner is a physician who is appointed to the position by the government authority on a nonpartisan basis. He carries out only the forensic medical aspects of the public investigation, not the quasijudicial functions which are handled by the courts. This method was first installed in Massachusetts in 1877 and is operational currently on a statewide basis in approximately 20 states. It is also functioning in a number of other states for certain metropolitan areas or counties on the basis of local option laws. The first metropolitan area to adopt the medical examiner system was New York City which adopted its Chief Medical Examiner Law in 1915. The first fully organized medical examiner system for an entire state was that of Maryland, enacted in 1939.

Some states, counties, and municipalities have reformed their medicolegal systems without abolishing the office of the coroner. In many of these the coroner is a physician who is either a qualified forensic pathologist himself or is empowered to retain forensic pathologists as his assistants, along with other forensic specialties. The inability to abolish the office of coroner can often be attributed to the fact that the post was earlier made a required political office, and usually elected popularly, under the state constitution. It is generally very difficult to amend a state constitution to eliminate one political office; it is more practical in these jurisdictions to provide for medicolegal assistance to the elected coroner.

Thus, at the present time, an effective medicolegal system may be fully organized under a chief medical examiner on a statewide basis (as in Virginia, Maryland, Oregon, and Connecticut); or on a permissive basis allowing for local option to adopt a medical examiner system (as in Alaska, California, Florida, Georgia, New York, and Texas); or as combinations of elected coroners on the local level with a state-level chief medical examiner (as in Kentucky, North Carolina, and Tennessee). Many other variations have been adopted and maintained because of local conditions. There have been attempts at compiling these laws. The National Municipal League has conducted a campaign for improved medicolegal investigational systems and has published state by state reviews on a periodic basis.[1] There have been other recent compilations of value.[2,3]

In the appendix to this chapter, we have reprinted in their entirety the laws of two jurisdictions: one is an example of a statewide system (Maryland), and the other is an example of a permissive county-option system (Texas). These were chosen because of the personal experience of one of the authors under the two systems for a total of 17 years. The laws were found to operate quite effectively. The Maryland law in particular has been used as a model for legislation in other states. It was also the basis for the Model Law prepared by the National Municipal League in 1951.

Most laws provide for the intervention of the medicolegal officer in the usual orderly process of the disposal of the dead body. It should be realized that this is an interjection of the state into what would usually be considered a private matter. Most laws delineate the types of death situations that call for medicolegal investigation. There are usually three or four general types of cases where the law makes a specific requirement of the medicolegal officer to investigate the death:

1. Deaths due, or suspected to be due, to violence, including accidental, suicidal, and homicidal situations.
2. Deaths that occur in specific locations, such as jails or prisons, or in hospitals where admission has been quite recent (usually less than 24 hours).
3. Deaths that occur outside of a physician's care, or where no cause of death is apparent. Included herein are those instances where the death is sudden, unexpected, and with the deceased having presumably been in good health.
4. Deaths that occur as a result of a suspected communicable disease or other hazard to the public health.

The medicolegal officer should realize that the original death investigation laws were often established primarily to uncover murder. Although there are many other reasons for a medicolegal investigation, the investigation of homicide or suspected homicide clearly has the cloak of tradition and custom. The opinions of some courts and attorneys general are still to be found among the citations which would make it appear that homicide is the only reason for a medicolegal investigation. Any medicolegal officer who has been long in office has usually been challenged concerning the legality of investigating other than homicidal deaths.

The first decision to be made by the medicolegal officer in considering a case proferred to him is whether or not the case fits into one (sometimes more than one) of the case categories previously outlined. This is the prime decision; indeed it is an actual operational problem to be surmounted.[4] If the death situation does fit readily into a case category included in the law of the jurisdiction in which the death occurred, then the medicolegal officer is not only within his legal rights to accept the case, but he actually has a legal *obligation* to accept it.

The law usually will provide that if an autopsy is deemed necessary, the medicolegal officer should perform it or arrange for its performance by a qualified physician. Stated or implied is the reason for the performance of an autopsy: to determine the cause of death. The law does not require or permit the medicolegal officer to perform an autopsy merely for his curiosity or to improve his confidence in the certificate of death, but only to determine the cause of death. It should be noted that a paradox exists here, since rarely if ever is an objection made to the autopsy of a victim of homicide, even though the cause of death may be quite apparent without autopsy examination. Again, the traditional concept of the medicolegal investigative system existing for the detection of homicide is apparent even in the modern operational interpretation of the office. We should note, however, that the autopsy in a homicide case is also desired in order to have a thorough documenting of the cause, mechanism, and manner of the death and in order to insure the availability of expert testimony for the court trial which may follow from the homicide investigation. (These issues are further discussed later in this chapter in the sections on legal support, immunity, and legal liability of medical examiners and coroners.)

The law itself may be defective and may not provide a reasonable basis for proper medicolegal investigation. The interpretation of the law by the attorney general of the state or by the courts may prevent the medicolegal officer from operating with a reasonable degree of security. In one such instance[5] the medical examiner resigned after the law was narrowly interpreted by the state Supreme Court.[6]

GOVERNMENT SUPPORT AND PROTECTION

Medicolegal investigative agencies need at least two kinds of public or governmental support: financial and political. In regard to the former, medicolegal investigative agencies have frequently been undersupported. The central role of modern medicolegal investigation is frequently not understood by the budget- and decision-making officials of the governmental jurisdiction involved. Perhaps part of the failure to understand fully the medicolegal investigative system is the fear of death and all its ramifications by those very individuals who find themselves responsible for supporting the death investigative system. It has been said that "the dead are no one's constituents."

If the medicolegal investigative system is of the traditional coroner's type, the office may well be among the lowest ranking of all the political segments of the party and government. Other departments and segments of government such as welfare, security, and education have many spokesmen and frequently are more vociferous. When the medical examiners office has replaced the coroner system, a gap may exist between the physician-pathologist appointed to head the death investigative system and the lay persons with budget-making authority. The two are not likely to communicate effectively and cooperatively.

Good, modern, in-depth death investigation is expensive. The per capita cost of such a system, whether it be of the coroner or medical examiner type, may well range from 30 to 60 cents per resident per year, assuming a population base of at least one million. Few death investigative organizations find themselves that well supported. Lack of proper facilities, necessary equipment, and competent personnel results. Such a situation is common, unrecognized by the citizens until, too late, the immediate survivors of the deceased find that they have been afforded less than competent death investigation with resulting improper and unjust settlement of estate, insurance, and survivors' benefits. But who is to speak for them? Who is there to plan and conduct death investigation and to place it in proper perspective for the public?

The second type of support of a public or governmental nature necessary for good medicolegal investigation is the provision of an apolitical environment in which to work. No governmental controlling body would dream of telling a surgeon working in a public hospital how to remove a cancerous bowel from a patient. On the other hand, the budget makers of the hospital may fail to provide satisfactory financial support and thereby deny adequate nursing care for the patient after the surgical procedure. Nevertheless the operative act itself is a medical (or surgical) technical procedure and outside of direct governmental control. Is not the medicolegal investigation of a death just as medical and therefore should it not be held just as inviolate? Yet the temptation to interfere with the medicolegal death investigator in the performance of his duties as defined by law seems always to be present. Medicolegal officers have been subjected to various political pressures because of dissatisfaction on the part of a single citizen, usually in a quarrel over a death certificate. Most frequently, this complaint takes the form of a request (sometimes an order) by an elected politician to change the death certificate to reclassify a suicidal death as one due to accident. Medical examiners, subjected to this political pressure, have been known to resign in protest against such undue interference. In some way, the medical nature of the death certification is not seen to be as clear-cut as the surgical removal of the bowel from the patient with cancer.

To provide effective medicolegal investigation of death, the responsible official must not be subjected to such pressures. Indeed, he must be protected from them. It may well be that the coroner, who is elected and, in a sense, is a self-contained political entity, is not subjected to the same pressures as is the appointed medical examiner whose tenure in office depends upon those who may exert pressure to alter the work products of his legal duties.

It is essential, then, that the medicolegal officer be supported with an adequate fiscal policy and be provided with protection from undue pressure to alter his opinions. Ideally, he should stand as a person of integrity whose actions are not subject to pressure, favor, or bribe.

To accomplish the objectives pointed out above, we suggest that the medicolegal investigational law include the following provisions:

1. The medicolegal officer should be afforded job security under the civil service systems, or by special statute, to assure independence from political pressures. The officer should be removable, after a probationary period, only for good cause proved, such as incompetency or unethical conduct in carrying out his or her duties.
2. The actions of the medicolegal officer in ordering or carrying out an autopsy or other medicolegal investigation under the applicable law should be personally protected from legal action by any party for unauthorized touching or cutting of the body, or invasion of privacy, or for the exercise of judgment in his report as long as the action was taken within the officer's jurisdictional powers and in "good faith" reliance on the law and the statements of police, physicians, and others concerning the particular case.

The office of medical examiner or coroner, or physician to the coroner, should be viewed as a quasijudicial function. As such it requires legal protection so that it can operate free of political and other pressures to influence decisions of the office. The two areas suggested above are the keys to this independence.

In addition to the job security noted above, the salary of the medicolegal officer should be high enough to encourage full devotion to the duties of the office. A university faculty appointment is further inducement to full devotion to duties because of its professional recognition of the importance of the function in the medical and academic community. The medicolegal officer can also achieve academic tenure within the university under certain conditions, thus adding academic security to job security.

As regards personal immunity, this type of protection is common for other types of public officials who must make difficult decisions involving licenses or certifications, or relating to legal liability. These include judges, administrators, and inspectors. An immunity law in the County of Los Angeles covering public employees in the exercise of their duties and in making reports was interpreted to cover the county coroner in a suit for negligently performing and reporting the cause of death following an autopsy. A second autopsy by the plaintiff was claimed to have shown the coroner's earlier determination to have been erroneous. Nevertheless, the action was dismissed on the basis of the immunity. The decision of the trial court was upheld on appeal.[7]

In this day of suit-consciousness and growing numbers of medical malpractice cases, we suggest a special immunity law for medical examiners, coroners, and forensic pathologists performing official medicolegal autopsies.

In a recent case, the vulnerability of a State Chief Medical Examiner to personal suit was dramatically presented.[8] The Chief Medical Examiner of Oklahoma was refusing to conduct certain autopsies because of a lack of adequate facilities. In a particular case where homicide was suspected, the District Attorney of Oklahoma City sought and obtained a writ of mandamus from the Supreme Court of Oklahoma ordering the Chief Medical Examiner to perform the autopsy. The CME, Dr. A. Jay Chapman, complied with the order by performing the autopsy out of doors, though in a protected area, behind screens, in the rear of the Oklahoma National

Guard Armory. The daughter of the deceased brought an action against Dr. Chapman in his official capacity and also on a personal basis. The damages claimed were $150,000 for mental anguish because of the delay in performing the autopsy, another $150,000 for mental anguish due to the autopsy itself, and an added $200,000 in *punitive damages* against Dr. Chapman for his conduct in the case. The CME was forced to defend the case personally. The Supreme Court of Oklahoma found that the CME had acted properly in following the letter of the order. It also found nothing improper in performing the autopsy out of doors under the circumstances of the case. Having so ruled, the Court declined to answer the question of the personal immunity of the CME from suit. It is unfortunate that the Court did not see fit to make this ruling, since it would have provided important guidance for the future.[9]

LEGAL LIABILITY PROBLEMS

The medical examiner or coroner should be aware of the areas of his or her personal vulnerability to suit.[10] Based on experience in American courts, the most important areas of vulnerability are the following:

1. Negligently performing or negligently drawing erroneous conclusions on a medicolegal autopsy.
2. Intentionally exceeding his or her authority or jurisdiction in performing or ordering a postmortem examination or medicolegal autopsy.
3. Intentionally performing or ordering an unnecessary medicolegal autopsy.
4. Removing and disposing of organs or parts of the body of a deceased without proper authorization.
5. Making public statements of a defamatory nature about persons, whether or not under legal charges, where the statements were not a part of official duties, or were not made in "good faith."

Medicolegal officials have at one time or another been sued personally under each of the above categories, though the number of actions has not been large. Malpractice insurance generally available to physicians covers only the first-named category.

An immunity statute, such as applied in the California case noted earlier, may cover negligence in performing or reporting an official medicolegal investigation. Also, if the report of the investigation were filed in a court of law, it would have received a common law immunity as a statement of a witness. This form of immunity covers good-faith judgments or conclusions made by the witness or reporting official. There may be some weaknesses in the coverage of this immunity where the pathologist fails to perform expected and necessary procedures, where he or she falsely and knowingly reports on procedures not performed, or where the report is so without supporting evidence as to be found arbitrary or capricious.[11]

The second and third categories of vulnerability are currently presenting the most serious problems for medical examiners and coroners. The second category concerns a direct exceeding of authority or jurisdiction, i.e., performing or ordering a postmortem examination or autopsy not covered under the law. Special care must be taken in systems which have narrow grounds for coroner or medical examiner jurisdiction without the permission of next of kin. Poorly drafted laws tend to cover only suspicion of homicide. Where there is doubt, the medicolegal official should seek legal interpretation from the official legal counsel (attorney general, corporation counsel, or city solicitor) and should act only under that legal advice. The legal counsel may even wish to seek court interpretation through a declaratory judgment. Some laws require that the medical examiner obtain the permission of a county prosecutor or district attorney before performing an autopsy. A Florida Supreme Court decision enforced provisions of this type against an associate county medical examiner in very strict fashion.[12] Two Florida statutes were applied in the case. One required permission of the prosecutor. Such permission was not sought or received. The medical examiner was relying on the broader general law which authorized medicolegal autopsies without next-of-kin permission and without prosecutor's permission when the death was determined by the medical examiner to have taken place in "suspicious" circumstances. The Court refused to apply this statute to a case where there was doubt about the cause of death and where the hospital physicians would not certify the death without a medicolegal autopsy. The Court ruled that "suspicious" circumstances covered only deaths where there was "an inference of foul play."

Other courts have found medicolegal autopsies unauthorized where the cause of death, even if due to negligent or criminal conduct, was sufficiently clear to make an autopsy "unnecessary." A recent New York case[13] applied a very strict test of necessity for the autopsy in an injunction case where the family of the deceased, who were Orthodox Jews, sought to prevent the procedure. The Court found that the religious objections "outweighed" the authority to conduct the autopsy where the "cause" seemed apparent in a road accident. It seems clear that the Court was unwilling to allow an autopsy to investigate underlying causes, such as pre-existing illness, and unwilling to allow detailed medicolegal investigation of the manner and mechanism of the death.

Understandably, prosecutors and courts are most lenient in allowing or ordering medicolegal autopsies in homicide investigations, even though, to the forensic pathologist, these may be the type of cases where the *cause* of the death is most readily apparent. (See the discussion by Dr. Hirsch in Chapter 6.) These are, after all, cases where the interests of the prosecutors and the courts are most clearly being served.

In a case where the medical examiner is sued only after the autopsy was performed and the allegation is that it was "unnecessary," the pathologist has available the findings as a means of pointing out what was determined beyond the apparent cause and manner of death prior to the procedure. On the contrary, if the autopsy was unproductive and added little or nothing, it will tend to strengthen the charges against the pathologist. In such situations, the pathologist must rely on two points: (1) that the type of case involved *was covered* by the law authorizing medicolegal investigations, and (2) that the cause of death was *not apparent* within *reasonable medical certainty* prior to the performance of the autopsy.

Lawsuits under these two categories can be avoided in large part if the medicolegal investigational law is properly worded in the public interest. The categories of investigation should be adequately broad to assure protection of the public and of the medical examiner acting in good faith under the law. (See the Maryland and Texas law appended to this chapter for models of adequate medicolegal coverage.) Medicolegal autopsies covered by the investigational provisions should *never* be subject to the prior authorization of a criminal prosecutor, or district attorney, or any other public official outside the coroner or medical examiner system. These officials are often popularly elected and subject to political and personal pressures to prevent autopsies which may embarrass important local people or result in legal action or loss of insurance benefits. Moreover, these officials are often interested only in homicide investigations which may be significant to only a small part of the legitimate jurisdiction of the medical examiner or coroner system. Lastly, these officials may not want to incur the public expense of a full medicolegal investigation and autopsy.

The fourth category is discussed in other chapters in this text. It is clear that some body tissues must be removed in any adequate postmortem examination and autopsy for purposes of further evaluation and for preservation in the interests of the official investigation. Also, the medical examiner or coroner may wish to cooperate with an anatomical education program or a tissue bank, or with an organ transplant program. Some lawsuits have been brought charging unauthorized removal and/or disposition of organs or parts. Most of these cases were brought some years ago before the use of tissues and organs had become so widespread and clearly beneficial to the living. Suggestions are made in Chapter 24 for proper legal procedures in donating organs and tissues to transplant programs.

The last category of vulnerability, the making of statements charged to be defamatory, is also covered by public-official immunity in most instances, as long as the statements were made as part of the official duties of the medicolegal officer. However, the immunity protects the officer only if the defamatory statements were made in "good faith" reliance on the evidence, even if negligently determined. The immunity would not cover a statement which was *knowingly false* and intended with malice to damage the reputation of the person or cause him or her to be charged with a crime.

OPERATIONAL INTERFACES

It has been said the medicolegal investigative system, if it is active and well-supported, is in the mainstream of the community. By this is meant that the system has many operational interfaces with public agencies, the private sector, and the surviving relatives of the deceased. A partial list of those groups and individuals with which interaction is necessary would include law enforcement agencies (police and sheriffs); fire departments; emergency medical services; public health agencies; professional medical societies and bar associations; individual practitioners of medicine, dentistry, and law; insurance company investigators and claims adjusters; medical schools; jails and prisons; courts of all jurisdictions and levels; district attorneys and attorneys general; government officials of all types and on all levels; service and civic organizations; funeral directors and embalmers; hospitals (including medical-record librarians, administrators, medical staff, and nursing staff); and the relatives and friends of the deceased.

Each of these individuals and groups has a prime objective in dealing with the death investigator. These objectives differ and some of them may conflict with one another. In the first section of this chapter we detailed some of the conflicts encountered in relation to the funeral director and embalmer. It was pointed out that the embalmer would like to embalm first and only then allow the body to be subjected to autopsy, whereas the pathologist would like to perform autopsy and only later permit the embalmer to alter the body for his own purposes. It would be an exercise in futility to detail all of the operational interfaces, conflicts, and problems which can occur. The discussion below will be confined largely to a listing of the major objectives of some of the groups or individuals with which the medicolegal officer must deal, frequently on a daily operational basis.

Law Enforcement Groups and Individuals

Since the underlying reason for the existence of law enforcement agencies is crime, death investigation in its broad aspects is not a prime interest of such agencies. Thus it is that police officers and sheriffs tend to become disinterested in any death case after the possibility of homicide has been eliminated. Yet the medicolegal investigator may need to depend upon the investigative talents of such persons to resolve the questions presented by the dead body—after these officers no longer consider the case of any real significance! This day-to-day operational interface may well cause problems. Premature dispatch of the body from the scene, failure to search the scene thoroughly for leads as to why death occurred at a particular time and place, lack of sufficient medical knowledge to make judgments as to disease present, and many other shortcomings may be noted when the law enforcement agent carries out the investigatory phase for the medicolegal official. Yet this is the standard in many jurisdictions. The office of sheriff-coroner seems to be more popular than ever in California, despite drawbacks such as those noted above.

A source of friction between the law enforcement agency and the medicolegal officer may develop over the determination of the manner of death assigned to an occasional case. In practice, the law enforcement agency may be called on to investigate into the circumstances of death, as may the medicolegal officer. Both offices properly conduct an investigation but arrive at different conclusions as to the manner of death. In most jurisdictions it is the medicolegal officer who, by law, is responsible for that determination. But the investigating law enforcement officers unofficially arrive at a conclusion and make note of that conclusion on the official written report. Ordinarily, because of the facts surrounding the death, both agencies arrive at the same impression of the manner of death, or it is mutually agreed that the determination of the manner of death must await the results of autopsy andNor toxicologic examination. Rarely, however, there is a disparity. Usually this occurs when the medicolegal investigator determines suicide, while the investigating law enforcement officers maintain that the death occurred as the result of an accident. A second type of situation finds the law enforcement officers maintaining accident or suicide, while the medicolegal investigator determines the manner of death to be homicide. Still other combinations are found.

When the investigating authorities include their determination of the manner of death in their report, and when the direction and intensity of investigation become outwardly dependent on this "determination," the unofficial act may rapidly become known to the relatives and friends of the deceased, as well as to the media, the funeral director, and others. Only later the medicolegal officer may arrive at his *official* position regarding the manner of death, only to find great opposition to his ruling. The newspapers may print stories noting that "authorities differ," television groups may want interviews, and radio stations may make repeated calls to representatives of both agencies, recording and playing later the "off the cuff" answers to questions. Occasionally, the apparent difference in "rulings" is carried into the political arena, or to other interested groups, all to the detriment of good working relationships between the law enforcement agencies and the medicolegal investigation agency.

To prevent this type of disparity, each investigation should carry only the title of a "death inquiry" and not a case of homicidal, suicidal, or accidental death. Such labels should be applied only later, when all facets of the case have been developed. Good working relationships are thus engendered and the public image of both organizations is enhanced.

Fire Department

The prime interest of firefighters is to extinguish and prevent fires. It is the former objective that often overlaps with the duties of the death investigator. To fight the fire properly may result in exposing the body to further damage by fire or by the materials used for extinguishment of the flames. It may be important to move the body prematurely and to disturb the scene. All of these actions may be carried out in the interests of good firefighting technique, but to the detriment of good death investigation. The use of fire to cover homicide or the deliberate setting of a fire (arson) to accomplish various objectives may not be considered by the company-level firefighters, and telltales may be destroyed by them if care is not taken. Moreover, it is not an uncommon observation that the fire department (collectively speaking) is frequently very guarded in its operation, and the obtaining of opinions and reports from the department may be difficult and time-consuming.

Emergency Medical Technicians

Emergency medical technicians (EMTs) are individuals with special paramedical training and operational organizations devoted to the administration of medical care and transportation in emergencies. Many communities now have well-trained and highly capable emergency medical care technicians, frequently operating as an arm of the city fire department. Their primary mission is to save lives. Thus it is that the potential homicide victim is quickly and efficiently moved to a hospital environment for prompt resuscitation or care. In so doing, the scene of what may be declared a homicide is disrupted and the chain of custody of the body, the clothing, and other items of great importance to the apprehension of the murderer and his eventual course through the criminal justice system is disturbed. This occurs over and over again in relationship to all manner of already dead and dying individuals. But who can quarrel with the prompt movement of the victim to accomplish preservation of life? Thus the prime objectives of emergency medical care and death investigation are at cross-purposes.

Public Health Departments

Chapter 23 examines the interrelationship with public health agencies. Further discussion is not warranted here.

Professional Medical Societies

Medical societies embody what is sometimes called organized medicine. With the rise in medical negligence litigation, individual physicians and their medical societies have become highly sensitive to possible malpractice suits. The medical society may challenge the medicolegal officer in his investigation of deaths where the question of medical negligence may arise. Since the medical examiner (and often, the coroner) is a physician and may even be a member of the challenging medical society, that group may exert a subtle pressure upon the death investigator. Obviously, the development of truth is the prime objective of both, but the pathways to attain that objective may be quite different.

Individual Practitioners of Medicine

The preceding comments regarding the medical negligence problem may be encountered by the medicolegal officer in attempting to investigate cases where a medical practitioner has knowledge of the treatment of the deceased. If the physician fears that the medicolegal officer will be aligned with surviving family members and will directly or indirectly help in the development of a medical negligence suit, he may be reluctant to open his records for inspection. He may even be unwilling to speak with the medicolegal officer himself and by his unavailability may hamper the death investigation.

Insurance Companies

Insurance companies are among the most avid consumers of information generated by the medicolegal official. The official reports of the agency, death certificates, proof of death forms, and autopsy and investigational reports are all used to help settle the insurance ramifications of the estate of the deceased person. Many specifics regarding each individual death are needed as promptly as possible. Life insurance policies (some with double and sometimes triple indemnity clauses) are not the only issues which may need to be settled. In the instance of long-dead bodies (decomposing or skeletonized), the date of death is important from the insurance carrier's point of view to establish if the policy was in force on the day of actual death. The manner of death (accident, suicide, homicide, natural disease) is most important to determine. Clauses in life insurance policies often exclude payment if the death is due to a deliberately self-inflicted wound. Such exclusionary clauses most frequently become null two or three years after the policy has been in force, another reason that the insurance company depends so heavily upon the determination of the exact date (and time) of death by the medicolegal officer.

Thus it is that the medicolegal certification of death is of great importance to the everyday operational existence of life insurance companies. The determination of the date, time, and manner of death is of particular importance from the insuring carrier's point of view. Other types of insurance may also be dependent upon the proper medicolegal certification of death. This is especially true in the instance of workmen's compensation insurance. Most "accidents" in industry occur suddenly and without warning, converting the healthy employee into an injured or dead person. Two other ramifications of compensation law must be considered. The first is the effect of a culminating series of "minor traumas" which may cause death. The so-called occupational diseases are examples of this phenomenon. Prolonged occupational exposure to particulate material in the inhaled air is not infrequently encountered. "Black lung disease" in coal miners is the cause of many workmen's compensation claims, and the ultimate extension of this disease, death, must be certified properly if surviving family members are to be compensated. It should be noted that although this type of "minor trauma" initially affects the lungs, the ultimate and fatal effect may be on the cardiovascular system.

The second major ramification of compensation law involves a much less easily defined series of events. This concerns the relationship of disease, not induced by labor or work, but pre-existing or coexisting, to death on the job. Such a relationship can be a real conundrum. By far the most frequently encountered case of this type is the relationship of the work to heart disease.

As an example, a 50-year-old man was employed as a delivery truck driver by a wholesale hardware company. He had an assistant who helped him unload goods from the truck and place them on the loading docks where deliveries were made. On the day of the driver's death, it was extremely hot and humid. The driver's assistant was sick and did not report to work. The driver unloaded the truck himself, working extremely hard and at a faster than normal pace, trying to make the same delivery schedule outlined for both him and his assistant. He collapsed on a loading dock and died there despite resuscitative measures given by the emergency medical crew who were nearby and responded quickly to the call for help. The autopsy revealed severe and long-standing arteriosclerotic heart disease. The question raised by the workmen's compensation insurance carrier is easily stated: Did the work impose such stress and strain on the already diseased heart as to precipitate the death? In this instance the answer would appear to be in the affirmative. There was an easily authenticated history of greater than normal stress and strain imposed on the worker by the nature of the work and the environmental conditions. In such an instance, the medicolegal officer, if he is properly apprised of the circumstances of the death, can opine that there was a reasonable relationship between the work and the death from heart disease. Such would not appear on the death certificate, where the cause of death would be indicated as "arteriosclerotic heart disease." However, the medicolegal officer would have the duty to complete properly item 25e on the death certificate form (see Fig. 3–1), indicating that the deceased person was at work at the time of death. This entry would make the initiation of a workmen's compensation claim by the next of kin much easier.

In the preceding example, the association of the unusual stress and strain of employment and the pre-existing heart disease is rather clear. In some instances an association may be much less apparent, perhaps even occult. There are two major situations that may obscure the relationship between occupation, coexisting or pre-existing disease, and death:

1. The death is delayed until after the workman leaves the job.

Example: A stevedore experiences some twinges of chest pain while on the job. At the end of the working day the worker leaves and goes home. Upon arrival at home he relaxes by watching television. He is found dead sitting in his chair when his wife comes to call him for dinner. The onset of the heart attack during work is not recognized, and a potential workmen's compensation claim is never filed. Indeed, the cause of death may never be determined with any certainty because no adequate medicolegal investigation is undertaken. The death may appear to be due simply to "natural causes."

Example: Assume the facts to be the same as in the above example, but the longshoreman's heart attack, which had its onset while he was at work, does not become manifest until the next day when he collapses and dies while mowing his lawn.

Example: Assume the same situation as above, but also assume that on the job on the day in question the temperature in the hold of a ship where the worker was employed was 105° with a relative humidity of 85 percent. The ventilation in the hold was poor because one of the two main blowers failed to work properly. There was an accumulation of some carbon monoxide due to the forklift truck used in the hold. By the time of the death, 24 hours later, the carbon monoxide, present in the blood as carboxyhemoglobin, will have disappeared. The combination of excessive heat and humidity with the load for body cooling thrown upon the heart may have been forgotten, or at the least not documented. If the circumstances of the last job undertaken by the worker are not properly investigated, then the work/death relationship may never even be suspected.

2. The possibility of an occupation-related death is not considered until long after death has occurred. Documentation of the circumstances of the death has also been precluded by the passage of time (witnesses scattered, records no longer available, etc.), and the "the trail is cold." A hint of this situation has been given in the preceding examples. As time passes, investigation becomes more and more difficult. The death certificates, original investigation reports, and the autopsy report with its stated conclusions all begin to assume more important and apparent permanence with the passage of time.

The importance of the medicolegal investigator to the insurance carrier may not be apparent until late in the investigative stage as carried out by the insurance company. It may appear as if the medicolegal officer were overlooked by the carrier. The opinion of the medicolegal officer may not be sought by either the insurance carrier or the claimant's counsel until the case has nearly reached the courtroom. The trail will grow ever more cold as further time elapses.

The above situation is reason for the medicolegal officer to build a good working relationship with insurance company investigators so that cases that may be questioned by the carrier will come early to the attention of the medicolegal death investigator. It should be remembered that many insurance carriers, both large and small, employ firms or individuals to carry out investigations for them. Just because the investigator identifies himself as being from Equifax does not mean that the probe has nothing to do with an insurance problem. Indeed, a good working relationship between the medicolegal officer and private investigators may prove to be of great value to both. Information of use to both may be officially exchanged. This may prove true of the relationship with the claimant's counsel or investigator as well. The medicolegal officer must be a gatherer of information, and some of the data necessary to certify properly the cause and manner of death may originate from other than "official" sources.

Medical Schools

Most physicians subscribe to the Hippocratic Oath or a more recent version of it. Part of the Oath deals with passing on of skills and information to beginning physicians and students of medicine. When the medicolegal officer is a physician, he may have a strong desire to participate in the teaching of medical students and younger physicians. Many physician medicolegal officers seek a relationship with a medical school or teaching hospital where physicians are in training as house officers.

The medicolegal officer offers his services and the medical school may well respond by offering a faculty appointment. Frequently this takes the form of a so-called clinical faculty position, and the medicolegal official is expected to give of his time to lecture and demonstrate his particular specialty to the medical students and possibly also the house officers. He may be expected to demonstrate autopsy techniques and findings to the students in the autopsy room.

Some problems can occur relative to such activity. The medical school may offer to provide payment to the medicolegal officer for his teaching services. An annual stipend, a fee for each lecture, or other financial arrangements may be employed. Such income may or may not be permitted, depending upon the rules and regulations of the governmental subdivision that employs the medicolegal officer. Even if a source of income from a medical school is permitted, the ultimate effect may be to stifle the more orderly growth of income from the principal (governmental) employer. To avoid this salary problem, an arrangement to participate as a paid faculty member of a medical school should be completed with the political representatives of the state, county, or city long before faculty membership is anticipated.

When the medicolegal officer does become a faculty member, he will appear primarily in that role to the remainder of the faculty, with those members tending to overlook his primary medicolegal commitments. Multiple operational problems may result. One is more apparent than real, but difficulties may ensue. There may be an apparent conflict of interest in that the medicolegal officer may be expected to be less rigorous in his investigation of deaths that may be associated with therapeutic or diagnostic procedures that occur at the medical school's teaching hospitals. This sort of inculpation may originate with the plaintiff's attorney in instances where medical negligence is alleged. Presumably a faculty appointment would not affect the judgment or persuasion of the medicolegal officer. However, individual faculty members who are also members of the teaching staff at the medical school's teaching hospitals have been known to apply not so subtle pressure in such circumstances.

Another result of faculty appointment is the discovery of the lack of understanding by other faculty members of the duties imposed by law on the medicolegal investigator. This is usually evidenced in three ways: (1) the belief that the medicolegal officer can (and should) carry out autopsy examination in any instance when an individual medical school faculty member is interested in obtaining it; (2) the expected provision of organs, tissues, and sometimes even entire bodies for use at the medical school; and (3) the anticipation that the bodies under the jurisdiction of the medicolegal officer can (and should) be used by young physicians to practice diagnostic and therapeutic procedures. All three of these misconceptions probably stem from the lack of formal exposure of most students in medical school to a program devoted to forensic medicine. Many medical schools offer no such teaching; some offer only a modicum of instruction in forensic medicine. In only a minority of medical schools is a basic background of teaching provided in the specialty. The Committee on Medicolegal Problems of the American Medical Association has outlined a 19-hour didactic course suggesting, as a reasonable compromise between ideal and practical, a curriculum divided into two main components: medical law and forensic aspects of medical specialties.[14] Some schools of medicine, including Harvard University, have adopted this approach.

Another problem which may be of practical importance is the necessary rigidity of any teaching schedule. It is not inconceivable that the medicolegal officer, who must frequently appear in court as an expert witness, sometimes on very short notice, may not be able to meet a long-scheduled teaching assignment. Some of his fellow faculty members may not understand this failure to appear to instruct, and misinterpretation may well result with some deformity of the medicolegal officer's image.

Jails and Prisons

Deaths in jails and prisons frequently result in charges of police brutality, insufficient surveillance to prevent suicide, and lack of adequate medical care for prisoners. Any or all of these accusations may be true in given instances. However, most deaths in custody, when adequately investigated, prove to have been free of these complications. Nevertheless, custodial care imposes a barrier to the free and open investigation of deaths occurring in such institutions simply by near-total control of the environment, witnesses, and others who are present as guards or nurses, prisoners or patients. This poses an operational problem and sometimes an actual barrier to the usual actions of the medicolegal investigator.

The Courts

There are several potential problems here. The first is concerned with the medicolegal officer's true role in the court. Most medicolegal officers feel that it is their responsibility to present the medical technical facts of the case at hand to the court, in language understood by all, and then to offer their opinion as to the cause of death, the manner of death, and other related questions regarding time of death, duration of life after fatal wounding, and identification. To most medicolegal officers it is of little moment whether they are subpoenaed at the request of the prosecution or the defendant's counsel. What does concern them is that there be a contact with the attorneys prior to the courtroom appearance and that they not be required to wait many long hours in a witness room prior to testifying. When the medicolegal officer is expected to wait with all of the other witnesses with no apparent regard for his other pressing duties, he may feel misused, and the quality of his courtroom work may well suffer. The medicolegal officer must of necessity spend a percentage of his time in the courtroom. He may find that he is expected in more than one court at the same time, and at least sometimes feels more or less like a "professional witness." It is difficult for him to understand sudden, apparently capricious orders to appear in court, followed by prolonged waiting to testify, being kept in the witness room, not being released after he has given his testimony, and sudden, often unannounced, continuances of cases. The medicolegal officer should recall that each court is a separate, independent entity. However, when he has many case folders stacked on his desk, each with its attached subpoena, he cannot help but view them as a group. He knows that in many instances the case will be continued, that in others his testimony will not be required because of stipulation, and that in still other instances he may never know without making an inquiry why he was never actually called upon to appear. From the point of view of the court, the subpoena is unique to that particular case; from the medicolegal officer's viewpoint the orders to appear all blend together.

Another phase of court activity is bothersome to the medicolegal officer: it is obviously necessary for him to have some vacation and time for professional development. The latter frequently is attempted by attending professional meetings and continuing education seminars, workshops, and courses. Indeed, some states and medical specialty boards are now requiring physicians to attend a stipulated minimum of continuing education activities each year or a multiple of years to maintain licensure or certification as a specialist. It would seem quite natural that the courts should recognize the needs of the medicolegal officer to carry out the necessary functions of rest, relaxation, and professional development. Yet each court, operating independently, views its own requirements as paramount. This is a disturbing problem and one perhaps not possible of solution. In at least one medicolegal investigative agency (Dallas County, Texas), all medical examiners review each autopsy record and subscribe to an opinion which is worded to be acceptable to all. This has been accepted by the courts as a reasonable device to insure the presence in the courtroom of a medical examiner with knowledge of the case. In some other medicolegal investigative areas, at least two medical examiners view each autopsy or postmortem examination so that more than one person has knowledge of each case and "cross-testifying" is possible.

District Attorneys

Since the medicolegal officer is charged by law with the investigation of homicidal or suspected homicidal deaths, he must work closely with prosecuting attorneys. The point at which the duties of the two begin to coincide will vary greatly. In some jurisdictions the district attorney is very active in the investigation of the homicide from the moment the victim is discovered. In such instances both the district attorney and the medicolegal officer or their investigators may work the scene with the law enforcement officers. Indeed, the district attorney or the coroner may actually be the senior law enforcement officer of the county. During the preparation of the case for presentation to the grand jury or later for presentation of the case in court, the district attorney and the medicolegal officer will of necessity work together.

One problem that may be encountered is the desire of the district attorney to view the medicolegal officer as an extension of his office and to consider him an advocate. Most medicolegal officers consider themselves to be nonbiased and truly feel that the work product of their office is for the use of all, not just the district attorney. This difference in outlook may cause much tension between the two. If the other legal advocate, the defendant's counsel, also applies pressure to the medicolegal officer, the latter may well find himself in a most unenviable position. To prevent such from occurring, the medicolegal officer must work out with the district attorney a *modus operandi* so that all will be truly understanding of the evidentiary needs of both offices.

Frequently the district attorney's office is understaffed and little time is available for prolonged study of individual cases prior to the presentation of the case in the courtroom. Thus it is that a pretrial conference, considered to be most desirable, between the district attorney and the medicolegal officer may be held just before the former takes the witness stand or may be eliminated altogether. Limitation of time for a conference does not help to build good relationships between the two officials. The medicolegal officer may well feel subordinated because he is more or less at the beck and call of the district attorney. This may further modify the relationship between the two who should, in a very real sense, be on the same operational level. Great must be the understanding between these officials to prevent schism between them.

Perhaps basic to the differences in the points of view between the district attorney and the medicolegal officer is that the former is an elected official, while the latter may be appointed, either as a medical examiner or as a coroner's physician. This difference of position does seem to be a point of departure of views and philosophies and may serve to exaggerate minor grievances. It may make operational differences appear to be greater than they really are. This is not a unique phenomenon. The elected sheriff and the appointed medical examiner may find themselves similarly afflicted.

Defense Counsel and Other Private Attorneys

Lawyers not attached to the district attorney's office are outside of the establishment. They sometimes feel that the medicolegal officer, like some other officials, is an advocate. Considerable unnecessary pressure may be generated by defense counsel to force the medicolegal officer to reveal the results of his investigation. The deposition for the purpose of discovery is a tool frequently employed to obtain the work product of the medicolegal official. In some jurisdictions *habeas corpus* hearings are used for similar reasons. Both techniques are time-consuming and may be unnecessary: the medicolegal officer may well be anxious to provide a copy of his investigation and autopsy findings to the defense counsel. The medicolegal officer may truly feel that the results of his work must stand very much like the results of the analysis of physical evidence, available for all to use as they see fit. In addition, the medicolegal officer may find himself in the center of an argument between the district attorney and the defendant's counsel or between the counsel for the defendant and the plaintiff. This situation may embitter him somewhat as he may feel that the search for the evidence has turned into a perversion of the facts.

The use of the conference of all parties involved may help to prevent the impasse described above. Though expensive in time, it spares the emotional involvement of all and preserves the value of fact and opinion developed at its own price in time and energy.

City, County, and State Government

Here the concern is not with support for the medicolegal investigative system, but with other relationships. The governmental controlling group (city council, county fathers, etc.) may not really understand the central role the medicolegal officer must assume if he is to carry out his duties with efficiency. Those composing the governmental structure may not realize the need for maintaining in a confidential state many of the medical and some of the medicolegal ramifications of individual cases subject to investigation.

The medicolegal officer, if he is a physician, may feel very strongly regarding the confidential nature of a case at hand. Representatives of the government may not understand this point of view and may insist upon release of information that may damage the physician information source of the medicolegal official. In a very real sense this may be similar to the desire of some elements of government to reveal the identity of the police informant.

Since the true role of the medicolegal official may not be apparent to the members of the governmental authority, it may result that medical (and sometimes legal) duties far removed from the usual are added to his workload. He may suddenly, perhaps without consultation, find himself in charge of the medical care of the jail population or responsible for the examination of apparent victims of child abuse. Another form of misunderstanding may occur, that of being appointed to committees or boards dealing with matters only very remotely associated with medicolegal investigative objectives. Perhaps such assignments could be avoided by an educational program aimed at the members of the governmental power structure and provided by the medicolegal officer. Such a program would be a time-consuming task to say the very least, and not necessarily a productive one. A pretty paradox indeed!

Service and Civic Organizations

Community service groups are active in nearly every city and town. They not infrequently invite medical-technical individuals to speak at their meetings, often scheduled as luncheons. The medicolegal official is not exempted from such invitations, and he is expected to respond. It does present an opportunity to meet with interested and perhaps influential citizens. However, speaking engagements pose a time problem and sometimes a scheduling problem: although courtroom appearances usually do not take place during the noon hour (the judge himself may be a member of one or more such service clubs), the need to remain close to the court may cause cancellation of the intended appearance. The organization may feel that it was let down, and the image of the medicolegal official may suffer. No doubt each medicolegal officer will have to work out his own escape route to the courthouse! In the long run, the opportunity to give some good exposure to the usually low-profiled system of death investigation will outweigh the stress and strain imposed on both the medicolegal officer and the civic clubs.

Funeral Directors

Close liaison with funeral directors is an essential for smooth operation of the medicolegal investigative system. Some of the necessary interactions with the funeral director have been detailed in the first part of this chapter. Both the funeral director and the medicolegal official must help to construct the final, completed death certificate. The former provides the basic data dealing with the identification of the deceased such as complete name, date of birth, address, etc. The funeral director is also concerned with that portion of the death certificate dealing with the ultimate disposal of the body. The medicolegal officer, on the other hand, is responsible for the more medical-technical portion of the death certificate, including the cause and manner of death; and how, where, and when the accident occurred. It might be wise for the two to work together and to share the burden of preparing this most vital of the vital statistical papers.

The funeral director is always under the pressure of the family. He must get the body in time to meet the scheduled funeral service. He must get the death certificate as completed by the medicolegal officer in time to have it copied and ready for the use of the family of the deceased. Such copies are necessary for the settlement of estate problems, payment of insurance benefits, claiming death benefits from the Social Security

Administration or the Veterans Administration, and numerous other purposes. Not to be forgotten is the need of the death certificate copy to allow the funeral director himself to claim burial insurance benefits. The funeral director may have to apply for a certificate to permit cremation in those jurisdictions where such is the law. The medicolegal official should help to provide prompt viewing of the body (if required) and preparation of the necessary certificates. Delay on these matters will injure the image of that particular funeral director.

It is absolutely necessary that smooth channels be established to allow the rapid and expeditious processing of items of mutual interest to the funeral director and the medicolegal officer. The latter must realize that the public view of the medicolegal investigative officer depends to a large extent upon the picture the public is provided by the funeral directors of the community. If the funeral directors are frustrated, the medicolegal official will eventually find his own image tarnished, and he in turn will be frustrated.

Another area is of great importance today. The cooperative, forward-looking, well-informed funeral director can be of great help in seeking permission from the family of the deceased to use organs and tissues for transplantation. Here the two, funeral director and medicolegal official, can join hands to benefit the living.

Since the funeral director and medicolegal official see two different sides of the entire processing of the body after death, they may find each other's assistance most useful in aiding the passage of bills of mutual interest through the legislature. Each may find an ally in dealing with matters difficult to explain to legislators and others not usually involved in death situations. It should not be forgotten that funeral directors frequently have a very powerful lobby group in the state legislature.

One service that the medicolegal official may offer the funeral director is the investigation and preparation of the death certificate in those instances where the physician charged with the proper certification of death is out of town, ill, or expired before his certification task was completed. Upon default of the physician, the medicolegal official may step into the breach.

Hospitals

Numerous are the points of contact of the medicolegal officer and the hospitals in his jurisdiction. An expanding role of the hospital is its use as a place to die. Furthermore, with the advent of effective resuscitative methods and rapid transportation, a great many individuals arrive at hospitals in the "dead on arrival" state. Thus the modern hospital provides the point of entry of many bodies into the medicolegal death investigative system. The types of cases which have their initiation at the hospital are these:

1. Dead on arrival cases. The hospital personnel may know little, if anything, of the circumstances of the death, and medicolegal death investigation is usually necessary.
2. All homicidal, suicidal, and accidental death cases.
3. Deaths following a hospital stay of less than 24 hours if the so-called 24-hour rule obtains.
4. Deaths related to therapeutic or diagnostic procedures.
5. Deaths where the cause is unknown to hospital medical personnel.

It is the responsibility of the medicolegal officer to establish a smooth working arrangement with each hospital in his jurisdiction so as to insure prompt reporting of those deaths that are required by law to be investigated. Not only is reporting necessary, but there also must be established a free flow of the necessary information. Provision must be made to obtain the hospital charts in all instances where the death is reported by the hospital. There may be constraints upon the proferring of the original hospital chart, either in its entirety or those parts that seem important to the medicolegal officer. If the former is received, then a good receipting system needs to be established, so that receipts will be exchanged between the hospital and the medicolegal investigator each time the chart changes hands. This helps greatly to keep track of the chart and to establish responsibility for its custody. It follows that the hospital chart, when received by the medicolegal officer, should be put to prompt use and that its return be timely so the hospital will have the use of it. As received with the body, the chart will still ordinarily be incomplete. The medicolegal officer should be aware of this, as the key notations and results of laboratory examinations may not at that point be incorporated into the hospital record.

The death may have occurred outside of the hospital where the deceased had been previously treated. Yet, in the course of investigation, access to the hospital records may be necessary to review the health history of the deceased person. Such provides a second type of case where the hospital is called upon to provide records. From the hospital point of view, the relationship between the prior hospitalization (which may have been days, months, or even years before) and the recent death may be quite obscure. Patient and tactful dealing with personnel in the hospital record room is absolutely necessary, and again prompt return of the chart (if borrowed in its original form) is essential. Another essential is the arrangement with the hospital administration for the prompt reporting of cases and the rapid procurement of written material in individual cases under investigation.

Interfaces with the hospital are not concerned simply with hospital chart procurement. The need for x-ray films, electrocardiograms, and the like may arise suddenly. Another associated requirement of the medicolegal death investigator is receiving the body in the same condition as at the time of death. This implies that all of the apparatus (tubes, clamps, etc.) so much a part of modern intensive medical care be left in place in the body so that the position of these tubes can be noted at the time the body is examined. For example, the wrong placement of the endotracheal tube may have been responsible for, or at least contributed to, death. Although the removal of many catheters and tubes might seem to be a proper part of preparation of the body for its next stopping point prior to the final disposal, this will only serve to make adequate death investigation more difficult, if not impossible.

When the medicolegal officer investigates a death that originates in the hospital and performs an autopsy examination of the deceased individual, he is engaged thereby in a mutually interesting situation. Such activity may well help to improve relationships with the medical staff of the hospital and may be of great value to the medicolegal officer in the establishment of his medical image among all manner of hospital personnel. This type of activity, not delineated by law, is of utmost importance to the proper functioning of the medicolegal office.

One rather far-reaching side issue of importance to teaching hospitals, but not realized by some medical educators, is that a well functioning medicolegal investigative system drains away from the teaching hospitals all cases in which death is due to trauma. This leaves no opportunity for physicians in training, especially pathologists, to see instances of trauma in the autopsy room. Thus the efficiency of the one organization actually causes a lack of medical instructional opportunity in the teaching hospitals. Two ways of circumventing this are easy to effect. The first is to take the resident physicians into the medicolegal investigative system for short periods to permit them to see instances of trauma causing or contributing to death. Here they may assist the forensic pathologist in the autopsy room and become acquainted with the various ramifications of trauma. The second method might be for the medicolegal officer to release certain well-defined cases of traumatic death to the teaching hospital, thereby allowing the resident pathologists to undertake the necessary autopsy examinations. Problems are undoubtedly associated with both courses of action. There may be other options that could be employed.

Relatives and Friends of the Deceased

Few families are completely aware of the many ramifications of death. As Thomas Mann so aptly put it, "A man's dying is more the survivors' affair than his own." Only rarely do the members of a given family experience more than one death that must be investigated by the medicolegal investigative system. Thus, in a very real sense, the medicolegal investigator of most deaths must involve families that not only do not understand the forensic aspects of the death, but are not even aware of the existence of the medicolegal official. As previously noted, the reaction of family members may be greatly varied. The intrusion of the medicolegal officer into the grief of the family may well be met with great resistance. Protestations regarding questioning, or the performance of an autopsy, may be firm or may become hysterical. "He has suffered too much already, don't cut him up" is a thought often expressed.

Organized resistance to the medicolegal investigation may take many forms. Threats on the part of family members may be made by telephone, or all the mobile family members may descend *en masse* on the offices of the medicolegal investigator. Calls from ministers, priests, and attorneys retained by the family may follow. Judges may be prevailed upon to issue restraining orders preventing the planned autopsy. The mayor, governor's office, or state representatives may all be asked to exert pressure upon the medicolegal official who is seeking only to follow the laws regulating his conduct.

Rarely, however, does the objection of the family to medicolegal investigation reach such levels of resistance. In the majority of instances, when the family raises questions regarding the investigative procedure, calm, sympathetic, and firm explanation prevails, and in many instances the medicolegal officer may be able to use the opportunity to educate the family to the value of the medicolegal investigation.

Friends of the deceased sometimes pose a greater problem to the medicolegal officer than do the family members themselves. This might be because the friends want very much to prevent the family further grief and tend to interpose themselves almost as buffers between the family and the medicolegal investigative office.

Obviously, there are many other operational interfaces that might be detailed and discussed. But these are the principal ones. Neglected in the foregoing discussion is the relationship of the entire federal bureaucracy to the death investigative system. Many interfaces are possible here. Certification of the laboratory phase of medicolegal systems is not yet in effect; the inspection and accreditation program of the National Association of Medical Examiners is a recent accomplishment.[15] This latter is the first effort that is aimed at the standardization of work output of medicolegal investigative systems. (See Chapters 48 and 49 concerning forensic toxicology for further details regarding Federal agencies with which medicolegal officers are required to deal.)

FORENSIC MEDICAL EXPERT "POOL" CONCEPT

As a medicolegal investigative system develops, it should gradually attract more capable, well-educated, and trained specialists to it. It should be obvious that there is provision for only one medicolegal office in each jurisdiction. This is determined by the legal source that provides for the establishment and existence of the system. Private laboratories devoted to the forensic sciences including forensic pathology and medicine, although few in number, have had an impact in the field. However, in the usual situation, there is only one medicolegal investigative system, and, if it is well established and well supported, it will represent the only such collection of experts and expert experience in the area. Thus it becomes a "pool" of forensic medical expert capability.

Again, it must be emphasized that the traditional reasons for the establishment of medicolegal investigative systems are the detection of homicidal deaths, the provision of means of documenting the investigational and autopsy findings, and finally, the provision of expert testimony in the criminal courts. This has previously been pointed out in this chapter. Most medical examiners, and pathologists who carry out autopsy examinations for other types of medicolegal officials (coroners, justices of the peace), try to maintain complete impartiality in their courtroom appearances. Indeed, many of them feel that they serve in the capacity of *amicus curiae*. It should also be noted that the number of cases of homicidal death investigated is small when compared to the other types of death where medicolegal investigation is required by law. There is great variation in the types and numbers of deaths investigated by the medicolegal officer, but only 5 to 12 percent will be classified as "homicidal," even in a large urban system.

What, then, is our responsibility in regard to those cases where death was not due to homicidal means? Is not the medicolegal officer involved *ex officio* in civil suits? Such does occur, particularly in instances of accidental deaths. Not only is there a need for his forensic medical abilities in the courtroom, but also in consultation and in deposition form. This activity can be challenging and may well gradually expose the medicolegal officer to many forensic problems that he would otherwise never face. However, such activity is very time-consuming and in one sense takes the medicolegal investigator away from his primary task, that of watchdog for the community.

Because the well-developed medicolegal investigative system harbors within it the single concentration of forensic medical and scientific expertise in the community, great may be the desire of medicolegal officers of other jurisdictions to submit bodies for autopsy and individual attorneys to submit cases for review and to seek consultation, opinion, and deposition and/or courtroom testimony as an expert witness. If uncontrolled, the time demands of this "outside" activity may be considerable.

In many medicolegal jurisdictions this problem is dealt with by allowing the medicolegal officer to undertake a modest amount of this type of activity and to make a charge for such service. This accomplishes several objectives: it controls to a degree what might otherwise amount to a free service which might be exploited to the detriment of the medicolegal investigative system; it augments the income of the involved individuals; and, finally, it makes available the forensic "pool" of experts and their capabilities to a wider community. In a real sense, this permits the governmental "monopoly" to be utilized for other than direct governmental purposes. This is an important consideration and should be kept in mind in the design and implementation of medicolegal investigative systems.

MEDICOLEGAL RECORDS AND CONFIDENTIALITY

One of the long-standing points of contention between the individual and the state is the right of the individual to have access to records compiled by the state and the desire of the state to maintain some degree of confidentiality in the performance of state functions, also presumably in the interest of the citizens. In a parallel manner, the various media claim the right of access to records in the interest of the public, while the state may prefer to carry out certain tasks while maintaining silence and confidentiality. Moreover, when dealing with medicolegal death investigation, some of the facts and allegations which are developed in the course of the investigation are of a medical confidential nature. In some states medical privilege has long been recognized by law. That there are two distinct viewpoints regarding the degree of confidentiality to be afforded the records and work product of the medicolegal investigative system is a fact that must be dealt with on a day to day basis in any medicolegal investigative agency.

To further complicate an already difficult subject, the plethora of "open record" laws poses another problem. Even the sanctity of the reports compiled by law enforcement agencies (ranging from local police and sheriff's departments to the Federal Bureau of Investigation) is being challenged. The compilation of the dossier with all of the attendant good points and faults is now very nearly proscribed.

With the greater availability and accessibility of records, the medicolegal investigative agency experiences various difficulties such as the following:

1. Requests (sometimes demands) by attorneys that a given record be delivered for examination. This may be followed by an insistence that the individuals within the medicolegal investigative system be available for questioning of an informal nature, or sometimes appear to depose in a more formal atmosphere.
2. Requests by relatives that any and all records be open for inspection.
3. Court orders to produce records in their entirety.
4. Requests by members of the media that, since the records are "open" or "public," all records dealing with one type of death (most frequently drug deaths or suicidal deaths) be delivered so that a "story" can be constructed.
5. Demands by various medical school or university faculty members that the records in their entirety be open for use in various research projects.
6. Demands or requests from the suicide prevention agency for monthly access to all suicide case records, or from the welfare department for periodic review of all cases dealing with child abuse.

These and many other requests, sometimes demands, for access to copies of records are common and must be dealt with in a reasonable manner, recalling that the privacy of the relatives of the dead person must be respected and that there are medical-confidential matters that necessarily need to be kept from all except those with a definite "need to know."

Little consideration is afforded in these numerous requests for the nature of the records involved. These may be greatly varied. Some of the types of records are listed below. Those not initiated or prepared by the medicolegal investigative officer are designated by an asterisk (*).

1. Death investigation reports.
2. Autopsy reports.
3. Clothing lists and descriptions.
4. Working diagrams and worksheets prepared in the autopsy room.
5. Internal memoranda (intradepartmental) including requests for toxicologic analyses, toxicology reports, and requests for and reports of other types of analytical work such as firearms residue analysis, pacemaker examination, etc.
6. Ancillary pathology reports prepared by persons other than the autopsy surgeon, such as neuropathologic or cardiovascular pathologic examination.*
7. Notations of telephone conversations with all manner of people, including relatives of the deceased, friends of the deceased, employers, and insurance adjusters.
8. Police reports, including traffic accident reports, investigating officer reports, statements made by witnesses, and "rap" sheets.*
9. Polygraph examination reports.*
10. Hospital record copies.*
11. Letters from relatives, friends, and employers of the deceased.*
12. Photographs of the death scene, of the autopsy, and of weapons, clothing, etc.
13. Letters requesting autopsy and investigation reports from various attorneys, public agencies, etc.
14. Copies of transcripts of depositions or trials.

Surely there are other records that find their way into the master file in each case investigated by the medicolegal officer. Some of the records are memoranda that are really of an "internal" nature. Some, such as the autopsy report and death investigation report, represent the work product of the medicolegal office.

If the cooperation of the law enforcement departments is to be assured so that there is a continuous flow of information from those agencies to the medicolegal investigative official, then it would follow that copies of these reports be held confidential. The same would obtain in regard to the hospital medical records. One way to destroy effective cooperation with physicians, hospitals, law enforcement agencies, and other groups and individuals is to release the written reports, charts, and memoranda prepared by them.

There is a particular problem relating to the death investigation reports. These usually are prepared by the coroner's or medical examiner's investigators. More rarely they will be prepared by the coroner or the medical examiner himself. In the former instance, release of the report may eventuate in the necessity for the investigator to testify in court or to depose before a court reporter when being questioned by attorneys. It was once the custom for the coroner or medical examiner to testify or depose regarding not only the autopsy findings, but also the investigatory aspects of the case at hand. However, this approach in a sense admits hearsay evidence and prevents the cross examination in the courtroom of the collector of the information. More and more the lay investigator is required to testify from his report as to his findings, actions, and, sometimes, opinions. This requirement is costly in time and tends to dilute the personnel available on duty at a given time in the medicolegal investigative agency. The photographer is not immune: he may have to appear in court to testify that he did, in fact, take the photographs relating to the particular case.

If the investigative report is to be admitted in evidence in the courtroom, and if the individual who prepared the report is to testify regarding it, the composition of the report should meet certain standards and be legible. One of the frequently encountered failures in the preparation of the report is the inability of the investigator to differentiate between fact (observation) and opinion. The two become so hopelessly entangled in many reports that, after the passage of time, not even the person who prepared the report can determine the difference. Indeed, even the source of much of the "statement" type of inclusion in the report may be questionable. Certainly the medicolegal investigators should be required to adhere to the same standards as any law enforcement officer in making reports.

THE DEATH CERTIFICATE

The medicolegal official is required to complete a death certificate (or at least the basic vital statistics and so-called medical certification) in each instance of death that he investigates. Indeed, the body may not be committed to its final resting place without it. The estate of the dead person with its many potential complications cannot be settled without copies (sometimes 10 to 20 copies) of this final document relating to the individual. There are great pressures exerted by many individuals and groups to push the medicolegal officer into promptly completing a death certificate every time he accepts jurisdiction of a body. The medicolegal officer is required by law to determine both the cause and the manner of death, and the death certificate form provides room for these to be recorded. But it must be recognized that these are *opinions,* not facts. The opinion of one medicolegal officer can differ from another. The opinion of a given medicolegal official could change if more facts regarding the death were available at the time of death certification.

Example: A 60-year-old man was found dead, lying on his bed at his residence. No injury was noted. Severe heart disease was found at the time of autopsy. The death was certified as being due to heart disease, and the manner of death was indicated as "natural" (natural disease process). However, analysis of blood removed at the time of autopsy revealed the presence of a lethal amount of a fast-acting barbiturate. The analysis was not completed and the report was not received by the medicolegal officer until seven days following his prompt issuance of the death certificate. Clearly the death was miscertified. To further complicate matters, armed with this new piece of information regarding the cause of death, the wife of the deceased person stated that she was aware that her husband was contemplating suicide, and she considered him to be quite capable of taking his own life. It is now apparent that not only was the cause of death as indicated on the death certificate in error, but so also was the manner of death. The medicolegal officer must now alter the original certificate. The vital statistical laws of the individual states provide mechanisms for this procedure. In some states a "supplemental form" must be completed by the medicolegal officer; alteration of the original certificates or substitution of a second certificate may be the designated method. The problem of miscertification is one that affects every medicolegal officer.

Another problem that frequently must be faced is the failure to determine the cause (and probably also the manner) of death before the body leaves the morgue and the medicolegal officer faces the requirement to complete a death certificate. The determination of the cause and manner of death may well depend upon studies which may take days or weeks to complete. The longer time is particularly apt to be the case when the materials to be analyzed must be sent out to another agency or laboratory for examination. There are several methods in use to avoid the problems caused by a necessary delay in the determination of the cause and manner of death. A frequently employed technique is to issue the death certificate with the word "pending" written in the medical certification (cause of death) section. (See Figure 3-1 for the U.S. Standard Medical Examiner or Coroner Death Certificate form.) By reference to this figure it may be seen that items 23 and 25a may be temporarily completed as "pending." When the cause and manner of death have finally been determined to the satisfaction of the medicolegal officer, the registrar of vital statistics can be notified, and items 23 and 25a may then be completed. In some states there is a time period specified by law within which the death certificate must be completed in all particulars; in others no period is delineated. Certain states require that an "amendment" form be completed and signed by the certifier; this form serves to notify the registrar of vital statistics of the completion of the

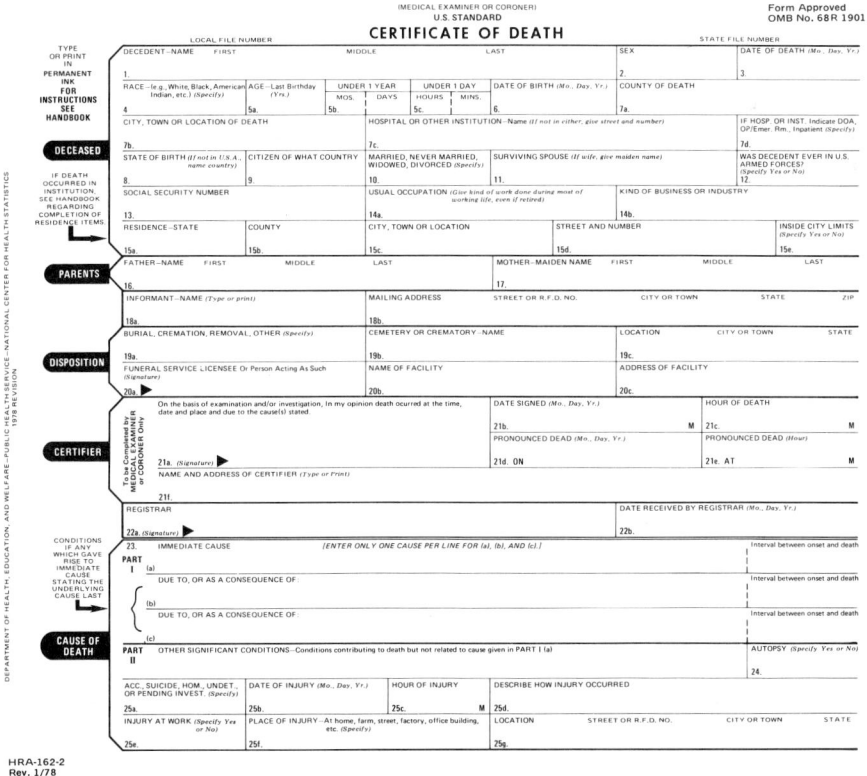

FIGURE 3-1. U.S. Standard Certificate of Death.

death certificate. With this *modus operandi* both the death certificate and the supplemental form are then issued by the vital statistics bureau when a copy of the death certificate is requested.

Reference to item 25a on the model death certificate will reveal that the manner of death is to be indicated as "accident," "suicide," "homicide," or "undetermined." Many medicolegal officials prefer to add (in pertinent instances) "natural disease." Such is a useful maneuver to make absolutely clear the manner of death; this may well forestall telephone or letter requests for further definition of the manner of death, a time-saving measure to be sure.

Again, with reference to Figure 3-1, it seems that many medicolegal officers avoid completing that portion of item 23 dealing with the approximate interval between onset and death. Perhaps this is because such an approximation is difficult or impossible to judge with reasonable certainty, particularly in those types of deaths coming to the attention of the medicolegal officer. In many such cases death occurs without witness, and the death certifier may not want to approximate this interval because such a degree of potential error exists that he may regard the request as calling for only a guess.

One other operational difficulty regarding the death certificate should be noted. How should the death certificate be completed when no cause and manner of death have been ascertained? The certifier should state on the death certificate form the following:

Item 23: cause of death not ascertained upon investigation, autopsy, and toxicology examination
Item 25a: undetermined

There are two general types of cases where the cause and manner of death are not determined. In the first of these the body is so decomposed (perhaps only a skeleton remains) that autopsy and toxicologic examination are markedly hampered and the cause of death (and usually the associated opinion as to the manner of death) is not apparent. In the second type of case, the most determined investigation and the most modern techniques of autopsy and toxicologic examination applied in the best way yield no clue as to the cause and manner of death. There is no injury; there is no significant natural disease process; there is no drug and no poison. With the techniques available to him, the death investigator has failed to define why that individual chose to die at that time and under those circumstances. Any medicolegal investigative agency will occasionally encounter a death of this type.

Although little has been written about this aspect of death certification, the National Center for Health Statistics has compiled a *Handbook* dealing with the coroners' and medical examiners' role in properly certifying death.[16] This text was prepared to aid medicolegal officers in properly certifying death and was issued in time to accompany the 1968 revision of the model death certificates.

TIME OF DEATH PROBLEMS

Many of the forensic pathology complexities relating to the determination of time of death are discussed in detail in Chapter 6. It is not our intent herein to review these areas. There is a practical side to the time of death conundrum, however, and this should be discussed. In each instance of the extinguishment of life there must be a point at which the whole person is, to all intents and purposes, dead. That point, from the practical point of view, is usually the time at which the cardiac and respiratory action ceases; that is, when heartbeat and breathing are no longer detectable. The individual may be resuscitatable, but without help from some other person, the death state will remain inflexible.

If the individual is watched while in his agonal state, the point of death (provided resuscitative measures are not imposed) is easy to determine. But a large percentage of those individuals whose deaths are investigated by the medicolegal officer die alone and unwatched. It is in such circumstances that an operational problem for the medicolegal investigator appears: just when did death occur? As pointed out in Chapter 6, determining after the fact the exact time of death is not easy, is rarely accomplished with precision, and is often no more than an educated estimate. Because of this, the usual device employed by medicolegal officers and encouraged by vital statisticians and others is to indicate the "time of death" as the time at which the person was "pronounced dead." There are some rather obvious complications inherent in this practice.

The time of pronouncement of death depends in full measure upon when the body was discovered and when the body is then viewed by someone empowered by law to make the pronouncement. The statutes of various states vary greatly in their wording and as to who can or cannot pronounce an individual dead. This person in many states must be a physician or health officer; in other states directors of hospitals are added to the list of those with the prerogative to pronounce death. In still other instances, anyone can apparently make the pronouncement of death. If the medicolegal officer is in an area where a physician (a holder of the degree of Doctor of Medicine or Doctor of Osteopathy) is required to view the body and pronounce death, quite a different "time of pronouncement" will result than when any person can legally say that death has taken place. In the former instance the body may have to be taken to a place where the physician can actually view the body, issue the pronouncement, and record the time of pronouncement. As hospitals frequently have physicians present at all hours, the body may well be removed, as a routine measure, to the hospital where it may be pronounced "dead on arrival." Some medicolegal officers feel comfortable in pronouncing death themselves or deputizing others to carry out this function. Others, perhaps fearing that a given body might be resuscitatable or that the question of resuscitatability might be raised, prefer to have all bodies first seen in a hospital accident room where treatment may be undertaken if it seems indicated. Local problems probably dictate the solution to be applied.

The death certificate form in some states is designed to allow for the time of "pronouncement" of death to be indicated. In other states, the death certificate, following the last revision (1978) of the model certificate designed under the auspices of the National Center for Health Statistics, allows for the recording of two different times: the time of pronouncement of death and the time that the medicolegal officer estimates death actually to have taken place.

As has been pointed out previously, much hinges upon the time of death. If the insurance policy were paid until midnight, and the body was found in the morning, both the insurance carrier and the family of the deceased person are most anxious for the medicolegal officer to indicate the actual time of death.

One way that the medicolegal officer can beg the issue is to indicate, instead of the time of death, the time the body was found dead. This practice may be necessary in instances where the body has been long dead and where a badly decomposed body or a skeleton is recovered. However, if this practice is resorted to in most instances, simply because the death was not witnessed, the medicolegal officer is clearly abrogating his responsibility in properly completing the death certificate.

RELATIONS WITH ORGAN TRANSPLANT PROGRAMS

The medicolegal investigative office is probably the best source for organs and tissues for transplantation to patients. So-called cadaver transplants have proven most useful. In particular, eyes, skin, and kidneys have been procured from the dead and transplanted to the living. A working relationship between the physicians in a medicolegal investigative office can be beneficial. Many of the people who die and come under the jurisdiction of a medicolegal officer have signed organ donation cards during their lives. Also many relatives of persons whose bodies are under the jurisdiction of medical examiners will wish to donate organs of the deceased, if they are asked. Technical aspects of this subject are discussed in Chapter 24. The ethical aspects of organ transplantation programs and their relationship to medicolegal programs are discussed in Chapter 2.

RELATIONS WITH THE PRESS AND OTHER MEDIA

Ordinarily, death is a rather private matter. But when death is of a homicidal nature, or occurs in plain view of all, or is of a spectacular type, or when the victim is well known or a public figure, then the representatives of the press and other mass media will be seeking details concerning the circumstances of the death, the appearance of the body, the ultimate disposition of the body, etc. With excellent communication systems available, newspapermen, television cameramen, and others may even be at the scene of death before the medicolegal officer or his representative arrives. Experience would indicate that the representatives of the media are most apt to interact with the medicolegal investigative system at the scene, at the time of the autopsy examination, and after the latter, particularly if the issuance of the death certificate is deferred for any reason.

Requests may be made by the representatives of the media to photograph the body and its removal, and the scene of the death, to be present at the time of the autopsy, to be allowed access to all records and details concerning the investigation of the death, and to interview any and all members of the medicolegal investigative system staff who were involved in the death investigation.

Such requests are routinely handled in the death investigation agency. The requirement of strict adherence to operating policies precluding photography of the body, presence at the death scene until all information and evidence are collected, and witnessing of the autopsy may obviate operational frictions.

Other requests may be more difficult to resolve. The press and the other mass media do have a right to information in the name of and as representatives of the public.[17] But there is no one spokesman for all of the various television channels, newspapers, radio stations, and magazines. In the instance of the death of a well-known public figure, the small medicolegal investigative office may be overwhelmed by large numbers of individual requests for information regarding the death. Two devices may be employed to help control such a situation. The first is the issuance of a "press release" or prepared statement which can be read in identical fashion to answer any and all requests for information. Because a release of this type cannot be expected to answer all questions, it may very well temporarily frustrate members of the media. A second device, sometimes of great use, is to hold a press conference where much more interaction is possible than with the "press release" technique. The press conference is, of course, costly in the time required and may not satisfy all.

Experience has shown that there must be available a member of the medicolegal investigative staff who can be contacted at any time and who can give the basic details concerning the case at hand to the requesting members of the media. Many of the questions asked deal not with individual, designated deaths, but more generally with recent deaths and the circumstances involved. The medicolegal officer should be certain not to release the names of those whose next of kin have not been informed of the death.

Another form of request sometimes presents difficulty. It is somewhat similar to a class-action suit since it involves the request for information concerning "all persons who have died as a result of narcotic or drug abuse" or "the names and addresses of all citizens who died while in jail." The medicolegal officer is being asked to use his data-recovery system (computerized data or a simple card file) to select those files which have a common denominator of interest. The parameter of dates of death is also often included here, such as "all suicidal deaths where handguns were employed for the year 1971." Even though the medicolegal investigative system records are often declared to be public (see Texas and Maryland Medical Examiner Laws in the appendix to this chapter), there is considerable doubt that such exposure of records was intended by the law makers. This type of request almost implies that the requester be allowed in the file room to peruse the files with complete freedom of action. Requests of this nature most often are an expression of intense, well-meaning interest on the part of the investigative reporter. Indeed, a public service may result: a hazard to life can be pointed out, or an interesting feature of modern living may be detailed in the newspaper or on radio or television. It is important that the medicolegal officer consider each request carefully, evaluate the possible public benefits to be obtained, and weigh these benefits against the time required of the office staff to search the files and the possible exposure to the public gaze of quite private details of the deaths being scrutinized under the request.

One other relationship of the medicolegal officer to the media should be noted. There is always the rather flattering aspect of personal exposure by the newspapers, radio, and television. The possibility exists that the medicolegal officer himself, or members of his staff, will become so enamored with the publicity thus gained as to seek out and exploit it. In so doing, perspective may well be lost, and the involved persons may find that they have demeaned their agency as well as themselves.

SUPPORT FACILITIES

Ideally, the medicolegal investigative system should be provided with all the supporting services that are necessary to its efficient functioning. In the main, these are:

1. investigatory capability;
2. autopsy facility;
3. histology service;
4. photographic support;
5. toxicology laboratory.

These five areas embrace the principal activities of the medicolegal investigative system. Adequate clerical support is presupposed, and some minor ancillary phases of the activity of a good medicolegal investigative system have not been listed.

Since the medicolegal officer is in charge of his office and organization, these activities should be centered in his office, where he can supervise them. In large organizations, these five major functions are usually in one location. However, in smaller medicolegal investigative offices, and occasionally in larger ones, there is a tendency for one or more of these major divisions to be split away and to be conducted out-of-house, at a different location and away from the immediate availability and supervision of the medicolegal official. Thus it is that the medicolegal office is at one location and the autopsy examinations are conducted at an entirely different place. Or, perhaps, the law enforcement agency conducts the investigatory phase and the medicolegal officer rarely if ever has direct contact with these investigators, and certainly has little if any control over the nature and quality of their work. Perhaps the most frequently employed out-of-house gambit is to send body fluids and tissues for toxicologic analysis to a distant laboratory. Often this laboratory is not even in the same city or community as the medicolegal office where the specimens were collected. There are instances where the physician who performed the actual autopsy has been obliged to send samples of tissues to an outside laboratory for their preparation for microscopic examination. The actual histologic study may even be made by an individual who never saw the body and may have no access to the preliminary autopsy report.

Some of this division of functions stems from the misconception that the medicolegal officer is only interested in and capable of conducting the autopsy phase of the total investigation. Part of the reason may originate from the desire of the officials of the community to save money by utilizing the law enforcement officers as the death investigators for the medicolegal investigative system. Undoubtedly, and with particular reference to toxicology services, the out-of-house arrangement results from the paucity of toxicologists combined with the expense of creating a new in-house supporting toxicology laboratory.

Such splitting of support services causes operational problems that hamper the proper, efficient, and prompt investigation of deaths in the interests of the public. Criminal, civil, and social justice have been thwarted over and over again by inadequate death investigation primarily resulting from the splitting of the major functions away from the medicolegal officer, making it impossible for him to perform properly those duties mandated by law.

SCENE EXAMINATION AND BODY REMOVAL

It has been pointed out elsewhere in this chapter dealing with operational problems that the existence of a modern, well-trained, and well-equipped emergency medical service will result in an increased flow of bodies to hospitals. Most such dead persons are of the resuscitatable or near-resuscitatable type. Some will not be, but are moved due to pressures developed at the place where the body was found. At every scene of death the next of kin, friends of the deceased, and the well-meaning (to all of whom the lifeless body is an unfamiliar object) often insist upon rushing the body to the hospital, hoping or expecting for revival of life.

This insistence upon action is understandable. The response of the ambulance crew or the paramedical group is straightforward and easy to comprehend. But the end results are predictable and necessarily counterproductive to ideal death investigation:

1. The body is removed from the scene and its relationship to the scene is thereby irrevocably damaged or destroyed.
2. Some of the physical evidence associated with the body may be lost, altered, concealed, or destroyed.
3. The scene of the death will be cluttered with the inevitable discarded wrappers of disposable EMT paraphernalia and other, sometimes difficult to identify materials.

The traditional response of the coroner or the medical examiner to the discovery of the body has been to proceed to the scene and there to aid in initial investigation of the death. The death investigation expertise possessed by the coroner, or the medical knowledge of the medical examiner, has always been regarded as being of great help in the early assessment of the cause and manner of death. Moreover, the study of the body in relationship to the scene has proven to be useful in the interpretation of injuries and marks observed at the time of the autopsy or postmortem examination.

The advent of rapid response by the emergency medical care team and the removal of the body for resuscitative purposes have caused a marked drop in the number of bodies that remain at the scene. Indeed, although the body may remain at the scene, the paramedical team may well have responded to the call for help and probably will have at least examined the body, altering its position and appearance, and may even have attempted resuscitation. In doing this, many things of importance are altered so that the death investigator will find many difficulties in performing his task. Thus it is that the standard, rule, or dictum once applicable to the medicolegal investigation no longer really applies. As most homicide victims are marked by easily observable injuries, these bodies are among those most apt to be promptly removed by the paramedical team. This is most often because of the bleeding associated with the wounds. The blood renders quick evaluation of the wounds difficult, and the wounds themselves seem to trigger a response on the part of the paramedics which culminates in transportation of the person to the nearest hospital.

Because of this situation the medicolegal officer may no longer be expected to carry a major scene investigation load. Lay investigators, trained by the medical examiner or coroner, are becoming more commonly employed. The medicolegal official is thus freed for more selective scene examination and for other pressing duties. This would appear to be a reasonable solution to the rapid increase in urban and suburban population with the attendant increase in deaths that require investigation in addition to the establishment of swiftly responding emergency medical technical groups.

It should be emphasized that retrospective scene investigation (after the body has been removed) may be of great help in understanding the death. If such an investigation appears indicated, the medicolegal officer or his trained representative should undertake it. This may be a most useful procedure during or after the postmortem examination or autopsy. Indeed, the use of the postmortem examination as a device to raise questions regarding the scene of death may well be a proper approach to the puzzle posed by the death, rather than vice versa.

An associated operational problem is that of the removal of the body from the scene to the point where it is to be examined. To accomplish this properly, the body removal must be carried out with these objectives:

1. The custody of the body must be complete at all times, and with a provable chain of custody.
2. The body and all of the items associated with it (clothing, stains, fibers, etc.) must be protected so that no item is lost.
3. The body must be protected from contamination so that unexpected and confusing items will not appear *de novo*.
4. Valuables and personal objects must be protected from theft.
5. The body must not be exposed to the gaze of the curious, and it must be protected from excessive heat, cold, wetting, and other hazards.

To accomplish these objectives, much more than just an ambulance or a funeral coach is needed. An entire system of body handling and removal is necessary. Without this, the operational problems may be insurmountable.

The medicolegal official may operate vehicles for body removal as part of the death investigative system. An alternative method is to contract with a private company for body hauling. It is probably best to avoid contractual relationships with a funeral home so as to prevent a conflict of interest from developing. Unethical individuals have been known to utilize the early notification of death and attendant immediate access to the family of the dead person to enhance their own interests as funeral directors. This is a situation which has every potential to damage the reputation of the medicolegal official and to build resentment among the public that he serves. It bears re-emphasis that the medicolegal officer has a difficult task at hand: that of investigation of death from an unbiased viewpoint. He must depend upon the family of the deceased person for aid and cooperative support. He cannot afford to jeopardize his neutral community standing by any alliance, real or imagined, with a funeral business interest.

The foregoing discussion has outlined twelve major areas in which operational problems can be expected in any medicolegal investigative system. No doubt there are many other sources of problems. Although remedies are not proposed here for all encountered problems, none is beyond correction. Any medicolegal officer will find himself sorely tried by one or more of these operationally difficult areas from time to time. In planning a medicolegal investigative agency, awareness of the points of friction, difficult interfaces, and frank problem areas may permit some of them to be eliminated before they cause difficulties.

REFERENCES

1. *Coroners, A State by State Symposium of Legal Bases and Actual Practices.* National Municipal League, New York, 1975.
2. *Death Investigation: An Analysis of Laws and Policies of the United States, Each State and Jurisdiction.* DHEW Publication (HSA) 78-5252, Rockville, Md., 1978.
3. Wecht, C. H.: *The Medico-legal Autopsy Laws of the Fifty States, the Canal Zone, Guam, Puerto Rico, and the Virgin Islands.* rev. ed. American Registry of Pathology, Armed Forces Institute of Pathology, Washington, D.C., 1971.
4. Petty, C. S.: Decisions, Decisions, Decisions! The Medical Examiners' Duty to Decide. *Forensic Sci. Gazette* 6:1–2, 1975.
5. Rupp, J. C.: Death of a Medical Examiner's System. *J. Forensic Sci.* 16:420–437, 1971.
6. Davis, J. H., Sevier, F. A. C., and Feegel, J. R.: Investigative Powers of the Medical Examiner in the Light of Rupp versus Jackson. *J. Forensic Sci.* 17:181–188, 1972.

7. *Stearus v. County of Los Angeles,* 79 Cal. Rptr. 757 (Ct. of App. 1969).
8. *Dean v. Chapman,* 556 P.2d 257, 1977.
9. Curran, W. J.: Damage Suits Against Medical Examiners for Authorized Autopsies. *N. Engl. J. Med.* 297:1220–1221, 1977.
10. Annotation, Liability for Performing in Autopsy. *Am. Law Reports 2d,* 83:953 et seq., 1962.
11. *Vanderpool v. Rabideau,* 557 P.2d 21, 16 Wash. App. 496, 1976.
12. *Rupp v. Jackson,* 238 So. 2d 86 (Fla. 1970).
13. *Weberman v. Zugibe,* 91 Misc. 2d 254, 394 N.Y.S. 2d 371, 1977.
14. Fisher, R. S.: Teaching Medical Law. *J.A.M.A.* 204:245–246, 1968.
15. *Standards for Inspection and Accreditation of a Modern Medicolegal Investigative System.* National Association of Medical Examiners, Wilmington, 1974.
16. *Medical Examiners' and Coroners' Handbook on Death and Fetal Death Reporting.* U.S. Department of Health, Education and Welfare, Publ. No. 78–1110, G.P.O., Washington, D.C., 1978.
17. Curran, W. J.: Medicine, Medicolegal Programs and the Press: A Reassessment. *N. Engl. J. Med.* 297:483–484, 1977.

APPENDIX

Maryland Post Mortem Examiners Law

1. The Department of Post Mortem Examiners is hereby created and established. The head of said Department shall be a Commission, consisting of the Professor of Pathology of the University of Maryland, the Professor of Pathology of the Johns Hopkins University, a representative of the State Department of Health selected by the Board of Health, the Commissioner of Health of Baltimore City and the Superintendent of Maryland State Police. The members of said Commission shall serve without compensation and shall select one of its members as Chairman, and one as Vice-Chairman, who shall act as Chairman in the absence or inability of the Chairman.

2. The said Commission is hereby authorized and directed to appoint six medical examiners, one to be known as Chief Medical Examiner, one as Deputy Chief Medical Examiner, and the other four as Assistant Medical Examiners, a toxicologist, two assistant toxicologists, a serologist, four residents training in Forensic Pathology and a Chief Traffic Investigator. The Commission with the approval of the Secretary of Personnel, shall fix their compensation which shall be paid by the Comptroller of the State of Maryland out of that portion of the funds collected by the Racing Commission allocated and paid to the several Counties of the State and Baltimore City. The Chief Medical Examiner and the Assistant Medical Examiners shall be licensed Doctors of Medicine and shall have had at least two years post-graduate training in pathology. The said Commission shall appoint, to such extent as may be authorized by the Board of Estimates of Baltimore City, such other professional or technical personnel, clerks and other employees as may be necessary for the proper administration of the Department and at such compensation as may be provided for by said Board of Estimates in the Ordinance of Estimates of Baltimore City. Such other professional or technical personnel and the clerks and employees shall be appointed in accordance with the provisions of Sections 142 to 156, inclusive, of Baltimore City Charter (1949 Edition), known as the Merit System.

Nothing in this section shall be construed to prevent the Commission from employing the services of physicians on a contract basis for part-time services, as may be authorized by the Board of Estimates of Baltimore City.

3. The said Commission is hereby authorized to appoint a deputy medical examiner, who shall be a licensed doctor of medicine, for each county in the State; provided, however, that an additional deputy medical examiner or examiners may be appointed for any county whenever, in its discretion, the said Commission shall deem it necessary or desirable to do so. The deputy medical examiners shall be appointed from a list containing the names of not less than two qualified persons submitted by the medical societies of the respective counties; provided, however, that if there be no medical society in any county, or if the medical society of any county fails or refuses to submit such list of names, the said Commission shall proceed to appoint a deputy medical examiner, or examiners, for said county. Each deputy medical examiner shall receive as compensation not less than twenty-five ($25.00) and not more than fifty dollars ($50.00) for each death he investigates, in accordance with the provisions of this article; such deputy medical examiner, when it becomes necessary, shall have the power to deputize any other physician in the county to act as deputy medical examiner in his place and stead. In addition to the foregoing services, whenever any such deputy medical examiner shall be called as a witness in any proceedings before the Grand Jury or in any criminal case, he shall receive as compensation for his services as such a fee which shall be determined by the court before which such proceedings are conducted.

4. The said Commission is hereby authorized to adopt and promulgate such rules and regulations not inconsistent with law as it may deem necessary to make effective the provisions of this Article.

5. It shall be the duty of the Chief Medical Examiner, the Assistant Medical Examiners and the Deputy Medical Examiners to attend to all the medical functions now devolving upon the coroners or Justices of the Peace, acting as Coroners, in the several counties of the State, and to perform all the duties imposed upon them by the provisions of this Article.

The office of said Chief Medical Examiner, and the Assistant Medical Examiners, shall be maintained in such building in Baltimore City as may be provided by the City of Baltimore, and the said Commission shall see that proper equipment is provided for the use of said Chief Medical Examiner and Assistant Medical Examiners, or arrange for the use of the Laboratory and other equipment of the State Department of Health, the Health Department of Baltimore City, the State Police Department, and the Police Department of Baltimore City. It shall be the duty of the Chief Medical Examiner, or an Assistant Medical Examiner, to be on call at all times for the performance of the duties set forth in this Article.

6. When any person shall die in Baltimore City, or in any county of the State, as a result of violence, or by suicide, or by casualty, or suddenly when in apparent health or when unattended by a physician, or in any suspicious or unusual manner, it shall be the duty of the police or sheriff immediately to notify the Chief Medical Examiner and Assistant Medical Examiner, or a Deputy Medical Examiner, as the case may be, and the State's Attorney of Baltimore City, or of the county, as the case may be, of the known facts concerning the time, place, manner and circumstances of such death. Immediately upon receipt of such notification, the said Medical Examiner shall go to the dead body and take charge of the same. Such Medical Examiner shall fully investigate the essential facts concerning the medical causes of death and may take the names and addresses of as many witnesses thereto as may be

practicable to obtain, and, before leaving the premises shall reduce such facts, as he may deem necessary to writing and file the same in his office. The Police Officer or Sheriff present at such investigation, or if no officer be present, then the Medical Examiner shall, in the absence of the next kin of the deceased person, take possession of all property of value found on such person, make an exact inventory thereof on his report and deliver such property to the Police Department in Baltimore City or Sheriff of the county, as the case may be, which shall surrender the same to the person entitled to its custody or possession; such Medical Examiner shall take possession of any object or article which, in his opinion, may be useful in establishing the cause of death, and deliver them to the State's Attorney.

7. (A) If the cause of a death described in Section 6 of this article is established beyond a reasonable doubt, the Medical Examiner shall so report and file in his office within 30 days after his notification of the death. If, however, in the opinion of the Medical Examiner, an autopsy is necessary, the same shall be performed by the Chief Medical Examiner, an Assistant Medical Examiner or by any competent pathologist as may be authorized by the Chief Medical Examiner, except those cases as provided in Subsection (B). A detailed description of the findings written during the progress of the autopsy, and the conclusions drawn from the findings, shall be filed in the Office of the Chief Medical Examiner, or in the office of the Deputy Medical Examiner in the county where the death occurred. A copy of the findings and conclusions as to the autopsies performed in the several counties shall also be filed in the Office of the Chief Medical Examiner. Provided, however, a Deputy Medical Examiner may call upon the Chief Medical Examiner or an Assistant Medical Examiner, or other person authorized and designated by the Chief Medical Examiner, to make an examination or perform an autopsy whenever he deems it necessary or desirable, and it shall be the duty of the Chief Medical Examiner or Assistant Medical Examiner to perform the examination, except in those cases as a competent pathologist is so authorized by the Chief Medical Examiner to perform the autopsy. The necessary expenses for transportation of a body for autopsy by the Chief or an Assistant Medical Examiner or an authorized pathologist and any reasonable fee payable to the authorized pathologist as has been approved by the Chief Medical Examiner for each autopsy the authorized pathologist may perform, shall be paid by the Comptroller of the State of Maryland out of the revenues of the Racing Commission, pursuant to the provisions of Section 19 of Article 78B of this Code.

It shall be the duty of the Governor to provide for these payments in the budget for the fiscal year 1957 and every year after that, and the expenses may not be paid by the Comptroller unless provision for it has been made in the budget.

(B) If the family of the deceased objects to the autopsy on religious grounds, the autopsy may not be performed unless authorized by the Chief Medical Examiner or his duly authorized agent.

8. It shall be the duty of the Chief Medical Examiner, and the Deputy Medical Examiners, to keep full and complete records in their respective offices, properly indexed, giving the name, if known, of every such persons, the place where the body was found, date and cause of death, and all other available information relating thereto. The original report of the Chief Medical Examiner, Assistant Medical Examiners, or Deputy Medical Examiners, and the detailed findings of the autopsy, if any, shall be attached to the record of

each case. The Chief Medical Examiner, or in case of his absence or inability, an Assistant Medical Examiner, and the Deputy Medical Examiners, shall promptly deliver to the State's Attorney of Baltimore City, or the State's Attorney of the county, as the case may be, copies of all records relating to every death in which, in the judgment of such Medical Examiner, further investigation may be deemed advisable. The State's Attorney of Baltimore City, or the State's Attorney of any county, may obtain from the office of the Chief Medical Examiner, or of the Deputy Medical Examiners, as the case may be, copies of such records or other information which he may deem necessary. The records of the office of the Chief Medical Examiner, and of the several Deputy Medical Examiners, made by themselves or by any one under their direction or supervision, or transcripts thereof certified by such Medical Examiner, shall be received as competent evidence in any Court in this State of the matters and facts therein contained. A reasonable fee shall be charged for filing insurance blanks, etc., and all such fees collected by the Chief Medical Examiner and Assistant Medical Examiners shall be paid into the City Treasury of Baltimore City on or before the tenth day of each month, but the Deputy Medical Examiners of the respective counties shall be permitted to retain the fees collected by them. The records which shall be admissible as evidence under this section shall be records of the results of views and examinations of or autopsies upon the bodies of deceased persons by such Medical Examiner, or by any one under his direct supervision or control, and shall not include statements made by witnesses or other persons.

9. The Chief Medical Examiner, the Assistant Medical Examiners and the Deputy Medical Examiners, shall have the power to administer oaths and affirmations, and take affidavits and make examinations as to any matter within the jurisdiction of their respective offices, but said Chief Medical Examiner, Assistant Medical Examiners and Deputy Medical Examiners shall not have the power or be required to summon a Jury of Inquisition.

Texas Medical Examiner Law (Optional)

Office Authorized

Section 1. Subject to the provisions of this Act, the Commissioners Court of any county having a population of more than 500,000 and not having a reputable medical school as defined in Articles 4501 and 4503, Revised Civil Statutes of Texas, shall establish and maintain the office of medical examiner, and the Commissioners Court of any county may establish and provide for the maintenance of the office of medical examiner. Population shall be according to the last preceding federal census.

Multicounty District; Joint Office

Sec. 1–a. (a) The commissioners courts of two or more counties may enter into an agreement to create a medical examiners district and to jointly operate and maintain the office of medical examiner of the district. The district must include the entire area of all counties involved. The counties within the district must, when taken together, form a continuous area.

(b) There may be only one medical examiner in a medical examiners district, although he may employ, within the district, necessary staff personnel. When a county becomes a part of a medical examiners district, the effect is the same within the county as if the office of medical examiner had been established in that county alone. The district medical examiner has all the powers and duties within the district that a medical examiner who serves in a single county has within that county.

(c) The commissioners court of any county which has become a part of a medical examiners district may withdraw the county from the district, but twelve months' notice of withdrawal must be given to the commissioners courts of all other counties in the district.

Appointments and Qualifications

Sec. 2. The commissioners court shall appoint the medical examiner, who shall serve at the pleasure of the commissioners court. No person shall be appointed medical examiner unless he is a physician licensed by the State Board of Medical Examiners. To the greatest extent possible, the medical examiner shall be appointed from persons having training and experience in pathology, toxicology, histology and other medico-legal sciences. The medical examiner shall devote so much of his time and energy as is necessary in the performance of the duties conferred by this Article.

Assistants

Sec. 3. The medical examiner may, subject to the approval of the commissioners court, employ such deputy examiners, scientific experts, trained technicians, officers and employees as may be necessary to the proper performance of the duties imposed by this Article upon the medical examiner.

Salaries

Sec. 4. The commissioners court shall establish and pay the salaries and compensations of the medical examiner and his staff.

Offices

Sec. 5. The commissioners court shall provide the medical examiner and his staff with adequate office space and shall provide laboratory facilities or make arrangements for the use of existing laboratory facilities in the county, if so requested by the medical examiner.

Death Investigations

Sec. 6. Any medical examiner, or his duly authorized deputy, shall be authorized, and it shall be his duty, to hold inquests with or without a jury within his county, in the following cases:

1. When a person shall die within twenty-four hours after admission to a hospital or institution or in prison or in jail;
2. When any person is killed; or from any cause dies an unnatural death, except under sentence of the law; or dies in the absence of one or more good witnesses;
3. When the body of a human being is found, and the circumstances of his death are unknown;
4. When the circumstances of the death of any person are such as to lead to suspicion that he came to his death by unlawful means;

5. When any person commits suicide, or the circumstances of his death are such as to lead to suspicion that he committed suicide;

6. When a person dies without having been attended by a duly licensed and practicing physician, and the local health officer or registrar required to report the cause of death under Rule 41a, Sanitary Code of Texas, Article 4477, Revised Civil Statutes, General Laws, 46th Legislature, 1939, page 343, does not know the cause of death. When the local health officer or registrar of vital statistics whose duty it is to certify the cause of death does not know the cause of death, he shall so notify the medical examiner of the county in which the death occurred and request an inquest; and

7. When a person dies who has been attended immediately preceding his death by a duly licensed and practicing physician or physicians, and such physician or physicians are not certain as to the cause of death and are unable to certify with certainty the cause of death as required by Rule 40a, Sanitary Code of Texas, Article 4477, Revised Civil Statutes, Chapter 41, Acts, First Called Session, 40th Legislature, 1927. In case of such uncertainty the attending physician or physicians, or the superintendent or general manager of the hospital or institution in which the deceased shall have died, shall so report to the medical examiner of the county in which the death occurred, and request an inquest.

The inquests authorized and required by this Article shall be held by the medical examiner of the county in which the death occurred.

In making such investigations and holding such inquests, the medical examiner or an authorized deputy may administer oaths and take affidavits. In the absence of next of kin or legal representatives of the deceased, the medical examiner or authorized deputy shall take charge of the body and all property found with it.

Sec. 6a. (a) When death occurs to an individual designated a prospective organ donor for transplantation by a licensed physician under circumstances requiring the medical examiner of the county in which death occurred, or his duly authorized deputy, to hold an inquest, the medical examiner, or a member of his staff will be so notified by the administrative head of the facility in which the transplantation is to be performed.

(b) When notified pursuant to Subsection (a) of this Section, the medical examiner or his duly authorized deputy shall immediately go to the transplant facility, perform an inquest on the deceased prospective organ donor, and determine if an autopsy is required.

(c) If an autopsy is required, the medical examiner or his duly authorized deputy will examine the organ to be transplanted in its whole state and will examine any other clinical evidence on the condition of the organ.

(d) The organ to be transplanted will then be released to the transplant team for removal and transplantation.

(e) Thereafter, the remainder of the body will be removed to some convenient and suitable area designated by the administrative head of the transplant facility for completion of the autopsy.

Reports of Death

Sec. 7. Any police officer, superintendent of institution, physician, or private citizen who shall become aware of a death under any of the circumstances set out in Section 6 of this Article, shall immediately report such death to the office of the medical examiner or to the city or county police departments; any such report to a city or county police department shall be immediately transmitted to the office of medical examiner.

Removal of Bodies

Sec. 8. When any death under circumstances set out in Section 6 shall have occurred, the body shall not be disturbed or removed from the position in which it is found by any person without authorization from the medical examiner or authorized deputy, except for the purpose of preserving such body from loss or destruction or maintaining the flow of traffic on a highway, railroad or airport.

Autopsy

Sec. 9. If the cause of death shall be determined beyond a reasonable doubt as a result of the investigation, the medical examiner shall file a report thereof setting forth specifically the cause of death with the district attorney or criminal district attorney, or in a county in which there is no district attorney or criminal district attorney with the county attorney, of the county in which the death occurred. If in the opinion of the medical examiner an autopsy is necessary, or if such is requested by the district attorney or criminal district attorney, or county attorney where there is no district attorney or criminal district attorney, the autopsy shall be immediately performed by the medical examiner or a duly authorized deputy. In those cases where a complete autopsy is deemed unnecessary by the medical examiner to ascertain the cause of death, the medical examiner may perform a limited autopsy involving the taking of blood samples or any other samples of body fluids, tissues or organs, in order to ascertain the cause of death or whether a crime has been committed. In the case of a body of a human being whose identity is unknown, the medical examiner may authorize such investigative and laboratory tests and processes as are required to determine its identity as well as the cause of death. In performing an autopsy the medical examiner or authorized deputy may use the facilities of any city or county hospital within the county or such other facilities as are made available. Upon completion of the autopsy, the medical examiner shall file a report setting forth the findings in detail with the office of the district attorney or criminal district attorney of the county, or if there is no district attorney or criminal district attorney, with the county attorney of the county.

Disinterments and Cremations

Sec. 10. When a body upon which an inquest ought to have been held has been interred, the medical examiner may cause it to be disinterred for the purpose of holding such inquest.

Before any body, upon which an inquest is authorized by the provisions of this Article, can be lawfully cremated, an autopsy shall be performed thereon as provided in this Article, or a certificate that no autopsy was necessary shall be furnished by the medical examiner. Before any dead body can be lawfully cremated, the owner or operator of the crematory shall demand and be furnished with a certificate, signed by the medical examiner of the county in which the death occurred showing that an autopsy was performed on said body or that no autopsy thereon was necessary. It shall be the duty of the medical examiner to determine whether or not, from all the circumstances surrounding the death, an autopsy is necessary prior to issuing a certificate under the provisions of this section. No autopsy shall be required by the medical examiner as a prerequisite to cremation in case death is caused by the pestilential diseases of Asiatic cholera, bubonic plague, typhus fever, or smallpox, named in Rule 77, Sanitary Code of Texas, Article 4477, Revised Civil Statutes of Texas, 1925. All certificates furnished to the owner or operator of a crematory by any medical examiner, under the terms of this Article, shall be preserved by such owner or operator of such crematory for a period of two years from the date of the cremation of said body.

Waiting Period Between Death and Cremation

Sec. 10a. The body of a deceased person shall not be cremated within forty-eight hours after the time of death as indicated on the regular death certificate, unless the death certificate indicates death was caused by the pestilential diseases of Asiatic cholera, bubonic plague, typhus fever, or smallpox, or unless the time requirement is waived in writing by the county medical examiner or, in counties not having a county medical examiner, a justice of the peace.

Records

Sec. 11. The medical examiner shall keep full and complete records properly indexed, giving the name if known of every person whose death is investigated, the place where the body was found, the date, the cause and manner of death, and shall issue a death certificate. The full report and detailed findings of the autopsy, if any, shall be a part of the record. Copies of all records shall promptly be delivered to the proper district, county, or criminal district attorney in any case where further investigation is advisable. Such records shall be public records.

Transfer of Duties of Justice of Peace

Sec. 12. When the commissioners court of any county shall establish the office of medical examiner, all powers and duties of justices of the peace in such county relating to the investigation of deaths and inquests shall vest in the office of the medical examiner. Any subsequent General Law pertaining to the duties of justices of the peace in death investigations and inquests shall apply to the medical examiner in such counties as to the extent not inconsistent with this Article, and all laws or parts of laws otherwise in conflict herewith are hereby declared to be inapplicable to this Article.

CHAPTER 4

Russell S. Fisher is Chief Medical Examiner of the State of Maryland and Professor of Forensic Pathology at the University of Maryland School of Medicine. He holds two additional posts at Johns Hopkins University, those of Lecturer in Forensic Pathology in the School of Medicine, and Associate in Forensic Pathology in the School of Hygiene and Public Health. After receiving his undergraduate degree in chemical engineering, Dr. Fisher attended the Medical College of Virginia, graduating in 1942. He became Maryland's second Chief Medical Examiner in 1949. An active member of the Council of Medical Education of the American Medical Association, Dr. Fisher also served as Chairman of the AMA's Liaison Committee on Graduate Medical Education during 1977–78.

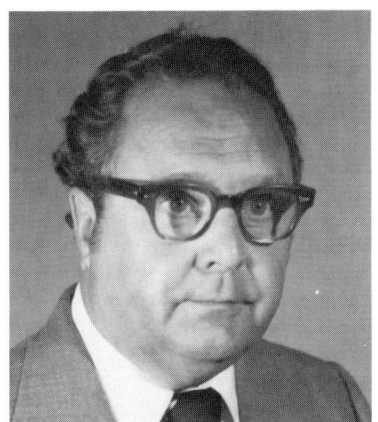

Ronald K. Wright is Assistant Professor of Pathology and Associate Professor of Epidemiology and Public Health in the University of Miami School of Medicine. He is also Deputy Chief Medical Examiner for Dade County, Florida. Dr. Wright holds his medical degree from Saint Louis University and recently completed studies at the University of Miami School of Law. He is a diplomate of the National Board of Medical Examiners and of the American Board of Pathology. The author of numerous articles, Dr. Wright is on the Board of Directors of the National Association of Medical Examiners, and is a member of the Council on Forensic Pathology of the American Society of Clinical Pathologists.

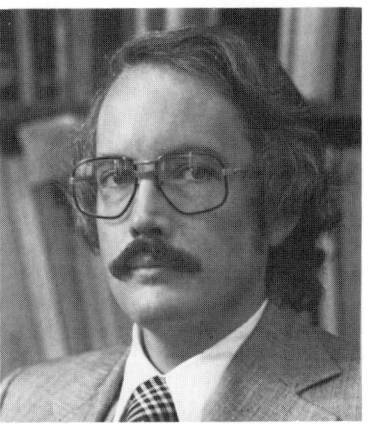

Charles S. Petty—See biographical sketch on page 50.

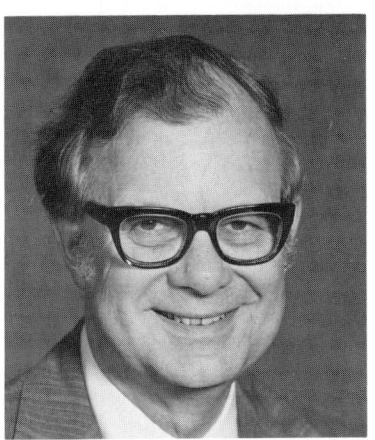

QUALIFICATIONS AND TRAINING FOR FORENSIC PATHOLOGY

Russell S. Fisher, M.D., Ronald K. Wright, M.D., and Charles S. Petty, M.D.

Pathology may be defined as the study of the reaction of the body to disease. Disease is defined in a very broad sense to include any departure from a state of health. So it is that pathology is that specialty of medicine which deals with the study of the reaction of the body to pneumonia, to cancer, to a gunshot wound, or to being struck by a motor vehicle. Pathology can be said to include two major divisions: anatomic pathology and clinical pathology.

ANATOMIC PATHOLOGY

The anatomic pathologist studies the tissues and organs of the body to determine changes from normal as a reaction of the body to disease. This is done by either gross examination of the body, or a part of it, or by the examination by microscope of small, specially prepared fragments of tissues. After death the entire body may be examined grossly and by microscopic techniques in an autopsy, sometimes termed necropsy. Also, a portion of the body removed during surgery may be examined by a variety of techniques.

CLINICAL PATHOLOGY

The clinical pathologist is concerned with the examination of blood, urine, sputum, and other body fluids and substances to determine the reaction of the body to disease. The causative agents of disease are also studied. This branch of medicine is frequently termed "laboratory medicine," and ordinarily the hospital laboratory is under the direction of a clinical pathologist. The specialty of clinical pathology involves the use of a variety of disciplines including chemistry, bacteriology, immunology, and hematology.

SUBSPECIALTIES OF PATHOLOGY

A number of subspecialties have been recognized by the American Board of Pathology, the national qualifying board established to examine and certify those pathologists who meet the educational and clinical requirements. These subspecialties include the following:

   Relating to clinical pathology:
     blood banking;
     chemical pathology;
     hematology;
     medical microbiology;
     radioisotopic pathology.
   Relating to anatomic pathology:
     forensic pathology;
     dermatopathology;
     neuropathology.

Special requirements have been established by the American Board of Pathology for qualification and certification in each of the above subspecialties. Certification by the American Board of Pathology in one or the other or both major divisions of pathology is required prior to subspecialty certification.

FORENSIC PATHOLOGY

Forensic pathology deals with the application of the science and methods of pathology to the resolution of problems at law. The borders of the specialty are hazy and at least partially include and overlap the fields termed legal medicine, forensic medicine, and medical jurisprudence.

The Forensic Pathologist

Most of the forensic pathologists in the United States who are active in that subspecialty are involved in either a direct or indirect manner with a government agency or with a political subdivision. The usual position occupied is that of medical examiner or pathologist to a coroner. In the former instance, the forensic pathologist serves as the medicolegal officer by appointment of the governing body of the state or county; in the latter, he serves indirectly, not as the medicolegal official, but rather as the pathologist responsible for the conduct of autopsies for the coroner who is generally an elected public official. Forensic pathologists may also engage in practice by carrying out autopsies at the request of families of the deceased, or upon request of an attorney. Cases of importance where a review of autopsy and pathologic findings is necessary to courtroom presentation may also be a subject of a forensic pathologist's activity.

Professional Education

The professional education of a forensic pathologist begins with his college or university studies. To examine the university career of forensic pathologists is revealing in that there is little uniformity of course choice; indeed, the converse appears true. Perhaps it is variety of university information and experience that is most sought by those who eventually choose forensic pathology as a career. Also, a wide range of summer employment is to be expected. It may be true that variety of educational and job experience is a factor in preselection of those who eventually become forensic pathologists. As far as the authors are aware, no studies or surveys of this background have been undertaken and brought to completion.

The medical school education of a forensic pathologist is much the same as that undertaken by all other physicians. Indeed, until recent years, only a very rigid curriculum was available to any medical student. The trend of medical education is now away from the unvarying curriculum, and in the third year and even more in the fourth year of medical school, opportunities for elective courses are now to be found.

Only a few medical schools have departments (or subdepartments) devoted to forensic pathology. In most medical schools, forensic pathology is offered in the form of a group of several lectures as part of the general pathology course, or perhaps dealing more in the jurisprudence area when offered in the third or fourth years. As a consequence, few graduating medical students have any true concept of forensic medicine or pathology, legal medicine, or medical jurisprudence. This is probably a major reason that only a few medical school graduates evidence interest in the forensic aspects of medicine.

Postdoctoral education is available in the form of residency training in forensic pathology in a variety of institutions, each with a formal arrangement with an operational medicolegal death investigative system.[1] Approved training programs are listed each year in the *Directory of Residency Training Programs*.[2]

Certification

Certification of forensic pathologists is the responsibility of the American Board of Pathology. The applicant must satisfy the requirements of the Board and successfully pass an examination in the field of forensic pathology. The American Board of Pathology was formed in 1936. One need not be a diplomate of the American Board of Pathology to practice anatomic pathology, clinical pathology, or any of the subspecialties of pathology. Most practicing pathologists, however, are certified by the American Board of Pathology.

Study of Figure 4-1 will show that a basic certificate in anatomic and clinical pathology, or anatomic pathology only (or, in special instances, clinical pathology only) is a prerequisite to taking a year-long period of supervised training in forensic pathology. Moreover, it is possible to combine training in anatomic pathology and forensic pathology (two years of each), leading to a combined certificate. Under some circumstances diplomates in anatomic pathology (but rarely in clinical pathology) can substitute full-time experience for formal training in forensic pathology.

Regardless of the route chosen to meet the requirements of the American Board of Pathology, the candidate must sit for an examination and pass it. This examination involves a written segment, the examination of gross specimens, microscope slides, and photographs of tissues, organs, wounds, etc. The examination in forensic pathology usually consumes an entire day and is given annually.

Originally, some qualified pathologists were awarded certificates under a so-called grandfather clause. Such is no longer the case with forensic pathology certificates; all individuals seeking certification in forensic pa-

FIGURE 4-1. Qualifications for examination by the American Board of Pathology for subspecialty in forensic pathology.

All applications to take the examination are considered by the Credentials Committee of The American Board of Pathology and the following items are evaluated in this process.

I. General

1. The candidate must hold a currently valid, full and unrestricted license to practice medicine, or osteopathy.
2. The candidate must devote professional time principally and primarily to pathology.

II. Professional Education

1. Graduation from a medical school in the United States approved by the Liaison Committee on Graduate Medical Education, graduation from an osteopathic college of medicine, or graduation from medical schools in other countries acceptable to the ABP.

2. For those who have not graduated from an approved medical school in the United States or Canada, certification by the Educational Council for Foreign Medical Graduates is required or successful completion of the "fifth pathway" as described and approved by the Council on Medical Education of the American Medical Association.

III. Qualifications

The American Board of Pathology recognizes several pathways to qualification for examination and certification, including training, experience, or a combination of training and experience. To acknowledge the diverse activities in the practice of pathology and to accommodate the interests of individuals wishing to enter the field, The American Board of Pathology offers certification through one of three routes (combined anatomic and clinical pathology, anatomic pathology only, or clinical pathology only) and a variety of special competence examinations. It is intended that the basic certifying examination is to establish competence to practice whereas the special competence examinations are utilized to indicate expertise in one segment of anatomic or clinical pathology.

A. Basic certificate

1. Training—the candidate must complete satisfactorily pathology training in a program approved by the Liaison Committee for Graduate Medical Education:

   a. combined anatomic and clinical pathology — four years of training—two full years in anatomic pathology and two full years in clinical pathology.

   b. Anatomic pathology only—
   (1) Three years of anatomic pathology, and
   (2) an additional year which may be spent either in further training, research, or practice of anatomic pathology. The additional year may also be in

FIGURE 4-1. *Continued.*

approved graduate education in internal medicine, surgery, pediatrics, or family practice.
   c. Clinical pathology only—
      (1) Three years of clinical pathology, and
      (2) an additional year which may be spent either in further training, research, or practice of clinical pathology. The additional year may also be in approved graduate education in approved internal medicine, surgery, pediatrics, or family practice.
2. Experience — candidates may be considered as being qualified to take the examination by acceptable experience in the specialty rather than by training. Under certain circumstances the candidate may receive one year's credit for each two years of experience. Thus, for a basic certificate, at least eight years of experience acceptable to the Board is necessary.
3. Other credit mechanisms—such credits are evaluated on an individual basis as being acceptable to the Board. To avoid misunderstandings, potential applicants should communicate with the Office of The American Board of Pathology early in the training period in order to ascertain if credit will be granted.
   a. Training time during medical school in an approved pathology training program (which was not part of the requirements to graduate from medical school) may be accepted upon satisfactory documentation by the program director. The maximum credit which may be granted is 12 months.
   b. A fellowship or instructorship in a preclinical department of a medical school if, in the opinion of the ABP, the experience was applicable to pathology. The maximum credit which may be granted is 12 months.
   c. Candidates holding a master's degree or a doctor's degree in a special discipline of pathology or a basic science may obtain credit for not more than 12 months regardless of whether it was received before or after the medical degree. The evaluation and approval of the amount of time credit will depend on an assessment by the Board regarding relevance of the subjects covered.

FIGURE 4-1. *Continued.*

d. Research with a direct application to the practice of anatomic and/or clinical pathology may be considered for credit not to exceed one-third of the training time requirement. The ABP encourages research and believes that all candidates should carry on investigation, teaching, and the publication of scientific papers during training. The ABP also allows up to one-third of training time to be spent in a related clinical activity, or a combination of the two.

The ABP will allow full credit for the first year of graduate medical education (internship) approved as a categorical program in pathology. The ABP will also accept for credit that portion of an approved diversified (flexible) first year program which is spent in pathology.

e. Credit for military service — Training or experience, or both, of reserve officers in the military service is evaluated on an individual basis. Credit depends upon the assignment the applicant has had, e.g., in a military institution approved for training in pathology by the LCGME as compared with an assignment to an unapproved location. For evaluation of credit for military service, write to the ABP Office.

B. Special Competence Certificates

1. Forensic Pathology

    a. For those applicants holding a certificate in anatomic and clinical pathology, or anatomic pathology only, or in special instances, clinical pathology only—one year of supervised training in forensic pathology in institutions approved by the LCGME, or by the ABP.

    b. For certification in anatomic pathology and forensic pathology — two years of approved training in anatomic pathology and two years of approved training in forensic pathology.

    c. In addition, candidates holding a certificate in anatomic pathology only, or in special instances, clinical pathology only—two years of full-time experience in forensic pathology in a situation comparable to that of an institution approved for training in forensic pathology.

thology must meet all requirements of the American Board of Pathology. It has been estimated that fewer than one-third of these diplomates practice forensic pathology as a full-time activity. More often than not, the diplomate devotes only a modest amount of his professional time to forensic pathology. Perhaps as many as 100 diplomates do not make any regular use of their forensic pathology background and certification.

The effect of the American Board of Pathology in recognizing forensic pathology as a subspecialty of pathology has been marked. The first examinations were held in 1959. Since that time, approximately 400 pathologists have been certified by the Board. A second and equally important effect has been the establishment of many more residency training programs for pathologists in this field. Thirty centers are now approved and offer about 60 residency positions annually in the subspecialty of forensic pathology.

The definition and approval of training centers has formalized training in forensic pathology to such an extent that much less "on the job" training has been utilized. This has permitted much more structuring of educational efforts and has stimulated research activities in these centers. Some of the trainees have undertaken research projects, and the result has been that the development of new knowledge, techniques, and concepts has been much more rapid than ever before.

With approved training programs and the development of research potential and capabilities, some medical schools which traditionally overlooked forensic pathology as a distinct discipline are now beginning to accord recognition to the subspecialty. Indeed, a few medical schools have entered into close relationships with operational medicolegal investigative systems to the enhancement of medical education, organ transplantation services, and the training of residents in anatomic as well as forensic pathology.*

The four objectives of the American Board of Pathology in the special field of forensic pathology (i.e., identification and recognition of competent individuals, definition of adequate training centers, encouragement of research, and insertion of the specialty into medical schools) have all been met in whole or in substantial part. In general, then, the effect of establishing forensic pathology as a recognized field or specialty of medicine has been to encourage the growth and recognition of the field. One interesting byproduct of these clearer definitions of the subspecialty of forensic pathology has been the recognition of the need for forensic pathology expertise in the wording of statutes authorizing medicolegal investigative systems. For the first time, some recently enacted statutes have required certification in forensic pathology as a requirement for employment as medical examiners.†

---

*Two examples may be cited: the University of New Mexico, where the Office of the Chief Medical Investigator (Medical Examiner) is actually a part of the medical school organization and campus, and the University of Texas Southwestern Medical School at Dallas, where the Dallas County Medical Examiner's Office is geographically situated immediately adjacent to (and physically connected with) the medical school, and where all professional members of the Office and the affiliated Criminal Investigation Laboratory are faculty members of the Department of Pathology and (in some instances) have joint appointments in the Department of Pharmacology.

†Recent examples are the State Chief Medical Examiner Law in Massachusetts and the Cook County (Illinois) Medical Examiner Law.

Part of the professional competence of a specialist in any field is founded upon his opportunity to associate with his peers. Forensic pathologists need this opportunity which is offered in large degree by professional societies devoted entirely or in part to forensic pathology and its closely allied fields. There are two national societies specifically organized for this purpose. The American Academy of Forensic Sciences, founded in 1950, numbers among the members of the Section on Pathology and Biology most of the certified forensic pathologists in the United States. It provides a forum for the exchange of ideas and for the presentation of research results. The National Association of Medical Examiners offers the same opportunities and in addition is active in the inspection and accreditation of medicolegal investigative systems.* In the United Kingdom, the Forensic Science Society and the British Academy of Forensic Sciences are active professional bodies. A Canadian Society of Forensic Sciences has also been established. All of these organizations are interested in the promotion of forensic *sciences*. A greater or lesser amount of emphasis is devoted to forensic *pathology*. Another society, the International Association of Coroners and Medical Examiners, has traditionally supported the activities of coroners and has undertaken extensive educational efforts for elected medicolegal investigative officials.

There are some societies that exist for the benefit of pathologists and the specialty of pathology generally, but have some special interest in forensic pathology. The American Society of Clinical Pathologists, within its Commission on Continuing Education, has maintained for many years a Council on Forensic Pathology. The Council is charged with continuing education efforts in the special field of forensic pathology. This has been effected by means of check sample programs, educational seminars, and workshops. Some of the latter have been week-long efforts and have been designed for basic, intermediate, or advanced training in the specialty. Teaching television cassettes have also been produced, dealing with subjects of forensic scientific importance.

The College of American Pathologists has long had a standing Committee on Forensic Pathology. By way of this Committee, a Federal Law Enforcement Assistance Administration (LEAA) grant for the training of a modest number of forensic pathologists has been effected. Another such LEAA grant was accepted to provide forensic pathology training (given in seminar form) for anatomic pathologists. This resulted in the publication of *Forensic Pathology, A Handbook for Pathologists*.[3] The College of American Pathologists, through its Committee on Forensic Pathology, has conducted seminars and panel discussions with special emphasis on such topics as battered children and rape, subjects with many community interfaces with the practicing pathologist.

Another organization which for many years has offered educational programs in the specialty of forensic pathology (and some closely associated subjects such as forensic toxicology and forensic dentistry) is the Armed Forces Institute of Pathology. Indeed, for some years, the week-long course in forensic pathology offered annually was the only didactic course given in the United States. One advantage of attending this course has been the opportunity for the students to meet experienced and nationally recognized forensic pathologists.

---

*A rigorous on-site inspection and an extensive questionnaire must be completed before accreditation is conferred upon a medicolegal investigative system. Reinspection must be effected at periodic intervals to maintain accreditation.

The American Medical Association maintained for many years a Committee on Medical-Legal Problems. During a major reorganization of the AMA, the functions of the committee were transferred to the Committee on Transplantation and Transfusion, and the former committee was abolished.

A special offshoot of the American Academy of Forensic Sciences should also be noted. This is the Forensic Sciences Foundation, funded specifically to provide a vehicle for research and education. The Forensic Sciences Foundation has been involved in the presentation of forensic science educational programs to attorneys and law enforcement officers as well as to forensic pathologists.

Specialized periodicals may be expected to continue to provide information exchange in the field. Early in its existence, the American Academy of Forensic Sciences recognized this and undertook the publication of the *Journal of Forensic Sciences*. This journal publishes scientific papers all across the forensic medical and forensic science fields. Other forensic science journals are also available, including the *Canadian Journal of Forensic Sciences;* the *Journal of the Forensic Science Society; Medicine, Science and the Law;* and the *Legal Medicine Annual*. Some well-established medicolegal investigative systems publish "house organs," some of which are widely distributed. It should also be noted that articles of forensic scientific interest are very apt to be published in nonforensic scientific journals such as the *Journal of Trauma,* the *Journal of the American Medical Association,* and the *New England Journal of Medicine*.

It should be realized that much forensic pathology practice in the United States is undertaken by pathologists who do not have special certification in forensic pathology. It is probably still true that more medicolegal investigations are undertaken in the United States each year by nonforensic pathologists than by those holding special certification in the subspecialty. It should also be admitted that the certification of an individual as qualified in forensic pathology by the American Board of Pathology does not always insure that the individual will carry out forensic tasks in a fully-competent and thorough manner.

Subdisciplines

The field covered by the term forensic pathology is very broad and involves many subareas or subdisciplines. Those practicing forensic pathology have found it difficult to define all of these precisely. Three areas seem to be especially important. These are clinical medicine, special areas of trauma, and certain crime-laboratory related areas.

CLINICAL MEDICINE

A physician is a physician, and although the curriculum may vary somewhat from one medical school to another, basic medical education is much the same regardless of where it is obtained. The curriculum offered at osteopathic colleges of medicine has become, in recent years, very similar to that offered by medical schools. The general rule of evidence law is that physicians may testify as experts in medicine and that expertise may include areas ordinarily embraced by medical specialists. There does not appear to be any standard guide available to indicate where general physicians should stop testifying and medical specialists begin. Moreover, there is no rule to apply to indicate when one specialist should stop his testimony and turn over his responsibility to a specialist in another field.

Perhaps the forensic pathologist, as much as any specialist, feels the lack of defined perimeters of his speciality. Pathology as a segment of medicine pervades all specialties (except possibly certain subareas of psychiatry), and there is a natural urge of the pathologist to apply his knowledge and experience to surgery, internal medicine, obstetrics, and so forth. However, the pathologist must realize that he does not treat the patient, even though he may well understand the disease involved and the fundamentals of therapy. It may be difficult for the pathologist to answer the question frequently put to him in medical negligence cases: Is this the standard of the practice of medicine in the community?

SPECIAL AREAS OF TRAUMA

Although the forensic pathologist is not an electrical engineer, for example, he may have a good working knowledge of electricity as applied to cases of electrocution. He may not be a scuba diver, but may well understand the problems associated with underwater breathing apparatus. He may not be a hunter, or a gunner, but he may have an excellent knowledge of firearms as applied to wound ballistics. Furthermore, he may never have fought a fire, but he is usually very knowledgeable about conflagrations, fire extinguishment, and the effects of carbon monoxide on the body, as well as the pathology of burns. Because of his special knowledge in areas not ordinarily considered to be part of the medical specialty of pathology, it may appear as if he is overwilling to testify in court as an expert in areas that appear not to be part of his background training and experience. This is generally not the case; these areas are a part of his regular environment if he is in full-time forensic pathology work.

CRIME-LABORATORY RELATED AREAS

The establishment of the range of fire in a gunshot wound case may involve the examination of the body for evidence of firearms residues. This is ordinarily considered to be a normal function of the forensic pathologist. However, if the firearms residue is found on the clothing of the victim, the forensic pathologist may not be considered by some courts to be within his field of expertise to testify in the matter of range of fire. There are many other extensions of the forensic pathologist into what is ordinarily considered the area of expertise usually reserved for those who work in the crime laboratory. The interpretation of blood-alcohol levels, effects of drugs on the ability of the individual to drive, and the definition of toxic levels of drugs in the blood are some of these areas.

Presumably, the forensic pathologist will use good judgment in deciding what limits there should be to his own expertise. Lack of challenge in the courtroom in case after case may well result in an unjustified expansion of his confidence and his area of expertise, perhaps with disastrous results. The forensic pathologist should take care to delineate sharply his personal area of solid knowledge, experience, and skill, be certain to recognize his limits, and be certain to recommend specialists in those areas of medicine and other sciences when they are needed.

Nonmedically educated persons are usually not aware that there is often very limited, if any, teaching of students in medical schools in forensic pathology and the other forensic sciences. Indeed, very little of the forensic aspect of pathology is taught in residency training programs in anatomic and clinical pathology. If there is a good medicolegal system in the community, then it tends to drain away from the ordinary pathology residency training systems those cases of trauma and those of forensic importance so that the training of residents in anatomic and/or clinical pathology suffers. So it is that the average physician, indeed nearly all physicians, in the United States have no basic body of knowledge in the fields of forensic medicine, forensic pathology, or forensic science. It is this void of knowledge, experience, and skill that points to the following needs:

1. It should be obvious from the foregoing reference to the small number of forensic pathologists certified by the American Board of Pathology that even if the qualified forensic pathologists were geographically distributed efficiently throughout the United States in a scientific manner based upon population, there would still be too few to fulfill the needs of the country. This situation is improving, but only slowly.
2. To fill the current need for forensic pathology expertise, pathologists without certification in forensic pathology must be utilized to resolve many forensic problems.
3. These nonforensic pathologists sometimes acquire some forensic expertise by experience and by voluntary attendance at seminars, workshops, and short courses. (Some general pathologists have little if any forensic capability, but profess such, and fail to attempt to acquire some knowledge and expertise.)
4. Most medical schools have failed to recognize the growing need in the United States for forensic medical specialists. These schools need to be encouraged to establish some modicum of exposure of their medical students to forensic medical matters.
5. Pathology residency training programs should also be encouraged to include forensic pathology as part of their basic education and training plan, joining with and utilizing strong existing medicolegal investigative systems. There is little chance that any pathologist completing his residency training in the future will not be involved in cases of forensic importance; he or she should have received at least an introduction to this type of work before being expected to perform adequately. The administration of justice in this country deserves at least a modestly competent pathologist in every forensic medical case where pathological investigation, evaluation, and testimony are required.

When forensic pathology investigation and expert opinion testimony are sought, the qualifications of the individual candidate should be evaluated as follows:

1. Certification in the subspecialty of forensic pathology by the American Board of Pathology in addition to adequate practical experience in the field of forensic pathology investigation.
2. Certification in, or eligibility for certification in, pathological anatomy and/or clinical pathology by the American Board of Pathology, in addition to practical experience in handling forensic pathology cases and an exposure to formal postgraduate courses, workshops, or seminars in basic, intermediate, or advanced forensic pathology. The candidate could have received education in special courses conducted by medical examiner's offices of recognized competence directed by certified forensic pathologists.
3. Education and training in pathology (anatomical or clinical areas, or both) with practical experience, probably in hospital-based pathol-

ogy, for a number of years, in addition to some experience in handling forensic cases (trauma-related, of different types, depending on the case at hand) and, hopefully, some exposure to formal postgraduate courses, seminars, or workshops in forensic pathology.
4. The same basic qualifications as given in background 3, with some experience in handling forensic pathology cases (trauma-related, of different types, depending on the case at hand), but without exposure to any formal postgraduate courses in forensic pathology.

Obviously, the choice of qualified candidates should be in descending order of the backgrounds above. It is best to select an individual who is fully qualified as a forensic pathologist (background 1 above). At a minimum, an interest in forensic medical matters and adequate pathology education, training, and experience should be expected of any physician presenting himself or herself as an expert, or expecting to serve as an expert, in the field. Just any pathologist or physician will not do.

Personal Characteristics

Perhaps something should be said about the personality of the ideal forensic pathologist. This is a very demanding specialty of medicine. The successful practitioner must be active and energetic. Since he is a seeker of facts, he should be a good observer. He must carry out his activity with some basic routine procedures, and thus he should be something of a routinist. The forensic pathologist deals with all manner of nonmedically trained individuals; he must be able to communicate with them easily and with the use of understandable nonmedical terms. Since he must testify as both an ordinary and an expert witness, he should be articulate. Such character traits might well describe a forensic pathologist of the type most in demand.

Forensic pathology, then, may be described as a relatively new arrival into the group of medical specialties. It is a subspecialty which cannot be sharply delineated, one which tends to encompass general areas of medicine and also most of the specialties of medicine. Forensic pathology has not yet been fully accepted by those who arrange the curricula of medical schools, despite the growing impingement of law upon all aspects of medical practice. Perhaps the very relationship of forensic pathology to law and law enforcement—to courts, police, and crime—has in the past clouded this subspecialty's professional medical image. This cannot be allowed to continue as the active cooperation of medicine with the administration of justice assumes a role of ever-increasing importance.

REFERENCES

1. *The American Board of Pathology Booklet of Information.* American Board of Pathology, Tampa, Florida, 1978.
2. *Directory of Residency Training Programs, 1977–78.* Liaison Committee on Graduate Medical Education, American Medical Association, Chicago, 1977.
3. Fisher, R. S., and Petty, C. S. (eds.): *Forensic Pathology, A Handbook for Pathologists.* National Institute of Law Enforcement and Criminal Justice, Government Printing Office, Washington, D.C., 1977.

CHAPTER 5

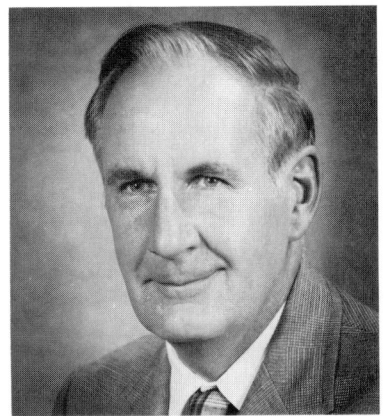

James T. Weston is Chief Medical Investigator of the State of New Mexico and Professor of Pathology at the University of New Mexico. He is Past President of the American Academy of Forensic Sciences and a member of the Board of Trustees of the Forensic Sciences Foundation, Inc. Dr. Weston was formerly Chief Medical Examiner of the State of Utah, and has worked as a forensic pathologist in Philadelphia and in San Diego, California. He has taught courses in forensic pathology at the Armed Forces Institute of Pathology in Washington, D.C.

MEDICOLEGAL AUTOPSY: FUNDAMENTAL PROCEDURES*

James T. Weston, M.D.

Forensic pathology is the study of the effects of violence or unnatural disease in its various forms in or on the human body. The external examination conducted before the autopsy is of paramount importance in determining cause, manner, and circumstances of death. Before conducting internal examinations, the pathologist should insure, if possible, that the body is removed from the scene of death in the same condition as it was found. Prior to beginning the dissection, the pathologist should advise the associated law enforcement agencies, morticians, and other involved parties of his need to review the physical evidence associated with the scene and the body. The information to be ascertained from a medicolegal autopsy and subsequent use of the information in the public interest dictate to a great degree the routine methodology that should be employed.

CLOTHING

While it is the primary responsibility of the forensic physical scientist or laboratory technician to conduct the expert examination of the clothing, the pathologist should remove and submit these articles to the laboratory. This type of evidence can, and usually does, provide important information in cases of doubtful identity and assault (i.e., rape, shooting, stabbing, stomping, or striking with a blunt object which may leave a pattern mark). The pathologist should describe briefly all clothing and jewelry left on the body, noting their position and any disarray. The description of the clothing position should note presence or absence of any buttons,

---

* This chapter was adapted by the author from material first appearing in Weston, J. T. (ed.): *Medicolegal Investigation of Death in New Mexico*, Chief Medical Examiner's Office and University of New Mexico, Albuquerque, 1977.

degree of dressing or undressing (i.e., whether the buttons are undone or torn from the garment, zippers zipped or unzipped, shoe laces tied or untied, and belt buckles buckled or unbuckled). Clothing should be removed from the body without cutting or tearing, and garments must not be allowed to fall to the floor. If cutting is unavoidable, the cuts should not extend through any important evidentiary tears, stains, bullet holes, or other types of external evidence. If the clothing is blood-soaked or otherwise wet at the time of removal, it can be transferred to a clean place to be air-dried. No attempt should be made to clean the clothing.

After drying, each significant article of clothing or jewelry should be carefully placed in a separate plastic bag. These bags, along with remaining articles of clothing, should be placed in a larger plastic bag and then labeled and sealed. Any significant external evidence on the clothing should be photographed; evidence such as bullet holes and stabbing defects should be described and measured in inches from clothing landmarks (i.e., collar, hem, etc.).

EXTERNAL EXAMINATION

After removing the clothing, the body weight is ascertained, if possible. If not possible, the weight is estimated and noted on the report as such. The following is an example of a general appraisal of the state of nutrition, development, and preservation of a deceased for use in the introductory sentence of the autopsy report. "This well-developed, well-nourished, Caucasian male weighs an estimated 175 pounds, measures 69 inches in length, and appears to be of stated age of 33." (See the section on external examination for a description of the external findings.) The use of verbally taped descriptions allows for considerably more detail in recording the external evidence of injury. Scars, however well healed, which appear to be a part of a pattern leading to the terminal episode (i.e., battered children) are included in the body of the protocol.

EXTERNAL EVIDENCE OF INJURY

This portion of the medicolegal autopsy, perhaps more than any other, describes the most important portion of the examination. The detailed observation of injuries, such as their location in relationship to landmarks on the body and to each other, in addition to body stature (i.e., the length of the wound above the gluteal fold in order to assist in reconstructing injuries inflicted to a sitting individual or the length of the injury above the heel in an erect individual), often preclude adequate description by note-taking. The very nature of note-taking and its constant repetition by an individual expending a significant portion of his time in forensic pathology will ultimately lead to short cuts, which will often result in a less than adequate postmortem report. This is particularly lamentable in instances when detail becomes of paramount importance. Therefore, while a standard form may be used for much of the note-taking on the external and internal portions of the body (i.e., body weights), the pathologist is strongly urged to procure a relatively inexpensive recording device so that he may record the external injuries as he actually views, measures, and locates them. The description should commence with the uppermost portion of the body, extend over the head, face, anterior surface of the trunk, and posterior surface of the trunk, and then proceed to the upper and lower extremities, respectively. In making this type of description, it is important that the pathologist recognize pattern marks or any marks giving a clue to the nature of the object which inflicted the injury. In cases where there are either singular or several injuries of major significance and, possibly, several minor injuries, the pathologist may prefer to delineate in the first paragraph of "External Evidence of Injury" those injuries he considers to be the most significant or those he may have to correlate with internal injuries in a subsequent paragraph.

When there are several significant injuries, list them individually in numerical paragraph form. This technique allows for subsequent correlation with the internal findings resulting from any given external injury. When many wounds are present, the wounds of a similar nature may be grouped, the number approximated, and the maximum and minimum diameters and color variations recorded. The pathologist should also record the external injuries in considerably more detail than he would during the course of a similar routine hospital examination.

GENERAL COMMENTS CONCERNING INJURIES

Numerous clues can be identified in the pattern of minor injuries which will indicate the nature of the assailant. These clues are often subtle defense wounds which can be readily missed if not searched for carefully. Often considerably more information is available, such as the direction of force in blunt injuries, than the pathologist might initially expect. During the first 24-hour period after death, recent hemorrhages, particularly in the nondependent portions of the body, become obvious as the blood settles from the superficial tissues. Later, hemorrhages may become even more evident after the postmortem examination has allowed much of the blood to drain, or after embalming procedures have removed livor mortis from the dependent portions of the body.

Drying of denuded skin allows for better delineation of recent abrasions. The position of the heaped-up epidermis often indicates the direction of the injuring force and assists in distinguishing abrasions from broken or dried blisters. The imprint outline on the skin surface often indicates the shape and dimension of the injuring object.

Sometimes it is most difficult to distinguish between cuts and lacerations of the skin, particularly on the head. Lacerations occur more commonly in the scalp or on the face; their edges tend to be ragged with some blunt force contusion of the adjacent skin. Strands of connective tissue or dermal skin elastic fibers may bridge the defects. On the other hand, incisions or cuts, except those caused by glass, usually have sharp edges and little or no evidence of adjacent contusion.

EXTERNAL EVIDENCE OF THERAPY

When a survival interim follows injury and surgical or other therapeutic measures are taken in attempting to save life, these measures should be categorically enumerated in order to avoid confusion in the minds of those subsequently reviewing the report. This portion of the report should include all of the surgical procedures, applied dressings, and other diagnostic and therapeutic measures evident from the external examination (i.e., an airway in the nose or mouth, indwelling catheters, plastic catheters through surgical incisions into the veins, needle puncture marks on the various parts of the body, bruises on the anterior thorax and abdomen incident to resuscitative attempts, etc.). Sometimes it is impossible to distinguish between injury and therapeutic effect on the exterior of the body as a result of either inadequate information prior to the autopsy or an inability to communicate with the surgeon prior to commencement of the autopsy. Under these circumstances, the wise pathologist should objectively describe the external findings grouped as "External Evidence of Injury and Therapy."

OPENING THE THORAX AND ABDOMEN

The usual Y-shaped primary incision is generally suitable, but sometimes it may have to be modified to extend the lateral ramifications high into the tip of the shoulder to completely expose the neck in those cases where exposure is necessary. The incision should not pass through injuries caused by either stab or bullet wounds, although it may pass through or be concurrent with post-injury surgical incisions.

Whenever pneumothorax is suspected, the pleural cavities are punctured under water contained in a trough between the subcutaneous tissues and the chest wall.

As the peritoneal cavity is exposed, it should be inspected for the presence of free blood, fluid, or exudate. If indicated, the amounts of fluid or blood are measured and swabs of exudate taken for culture.

In cases of pregnancy, the pathologist should examine the large abdominal veins for the presence of air by gently moving aside the bowel before the thoracic cavity is opened and the internal mammary vessels are incised.

The chest is opened by cutting through the rib cartilages near the costochondral junction in instances when the spinal cord is not examined in situ. If the latter is contemplated in order to allow the parallel vertical sagittal electric saw cuts in the vertebral column, it is suggested that the thoracic cage be opened by additional lateral cuts in approximately the anterior axillary line. The pleural cavity should be examined before complete removal of the sternum to prevent leakage of blood from the subclavian and jugular veins into the pleural cavity before inspection.

In a medicolegal autopsy, before any of the organs are removed by the technician, it is imperative that the forensic pathologist completely inspect all of the organs in situ after all of the internal blood and/or fluid is removed and measured. Care must be exercised during removal of blood and other fluid, particularly if there is a suspicion of gunshot wound or introduction of another type of foreign object which a suction device might remove. The correlation of external and internal injury and tracing bullet pathways through the body are more readily accomplished with the organs in situ than after the initial dissection by either removing the individual organs, the organ systems, or the organs *en bloc*.

Generally, it is better to commence dissection of the thorax by removing the larynx and esophagus in the neck after ligation and transection of the great vessels. Before removal of the thoracic organs, in situ inspection should include:

1. observation of the lumen of the main pulmonary vessels;
2. observation of the right atrium and ventricle for air embolism; and, thereafter,
3. incision into the right atrium for collecting a blood sample for toxicologic examination.

This procedure should be preceded by puncture for blood culture if deemed necessary.

Whether or not strangulation is initially suspected, the pathologist should carefully inspect the organs of the neck in situ, prior to removal by a technician, in order to rule out the possibility of:

1. artifactual hemorrhage into the soft tissues or neck muscle; and
2. fracture of one of the cartilages or bones of the larynx during the process of removal.

The natural disease process must be described in detail since questions frequently arise in court concerning the role of disease in:

1. predisposition to accidents;
2. aggravation of the effects of injury; or
3. hastening the demise of the deceased.

Pathologists should also remember that the time of the postmortem examination is usually the single opportunity he will have for obtaining any type of specimen, be it for toxicology, histopathology, serology, or other tissues. One should avoid the dilemma of placing oneself in a situation where additional evidence may be desired at a time when the collection of this material is virtually impossible. The detailed *step by step* procedure is as follows:

Neck: In the dissection of the neck, avoid squeezing and forcible pulling since pressure may produce excessive artifactual hemorrhage or dislodge foreign bodies from the pharynx or larynx. The presence of food or gastric contents in the upper respiratory passages should be noted. Keep in mind the possibility of postmortem spillage. Inspect the great vessels of the neck and cervical vertebrae after removal of the neck organs.

Thorax: Inspect pleural cavities before removing the sternum. Examine the superior vena cava and its main tributaries, the aorta and its branches. After opening the pericardium, take blood cultures. This is readily accomplished by puncturing the right atrium. At this time, blood samples for chemical analysis should also be taken from the right atrium. Open and examine the main pulmonary artery prior to removal of the heart. During removal of the heart, the prosector should watch for air or gas bubbles in the blood. Following removal of the thoracic viscera, inspect the pleural surfaces, ribs, thoracic spine, and diaphragm. The esophagus should be clamped or ligated and divided proximal to the diaphragm.

Abdomen: Inspect the entire gastrointestinal tract. Note if the appendix is present. Place a double ligature around the bowel in the region of the duodenojejunal junction with division between the ligatures. Inspect the rectum to detect possible objects concealed therein (i.e., drugs, money, etc.). Take urine samples, either directly from the bladder by syringe or from the external urethral meatus while applying steady pressure to the bladder. After removal of the abdominal and pelvic viscera, examine the lumbar spine, the pelvic walls, pubic rami, and symphysis. Accomplish this examination by dissecting the iliopsoas muscles laterally from their attachment along the spine. If sufficient blood for chemical analysis was not obtained during removal of the heart, obtain additional samples from the inferior vena cava, exercising care that there is no contamination from the gastrointestinal contents. In cases of suspected poisoning, toxicologic specimens should be collected as subsequently described.

Head: In reflecting the scalp, note and describe in detail any bruising on its deep surface. Often this inspection becomes extremely important in determining the number and direction of blows to the head or the nature of the weapon or weapons causing the blows. Not only should the description include an enumeration of the size of these bruises, but also their relationship to each other and the distance separating them. In removing the skull cap, avoid a hammer and chisel as much as possible since these devices may produce fractures. If possible, measure accumulations of extradural or subdural hemorrhage. In the event that the latter are solid, express in terms of grams of weight or area covered over the superior portion of the brain. Describe variation in thickness if the material is semiliquid and not readily gathered. Samples of these accumulations should be submitted for blood alcohol analysis. In instances when a detailed examination of the brain is of considerable importance, it is best to preserve the brain from 10 days to two weeks before sectioning, if time and facilities permit. In cases when an examination of the brain is conducted simply to rule out the possibility of some other pre-existing or coexisting condition, the brain may be cut in the fresh state in a manner similar to that in which the pathologist usually examines the fixed brain. In the fixed brain, cortical contusions and hemorrhages are much more distinct; however, in this condition it is usually extremely difficult or virtually impossible to dissect out ruptured berry aneurysms or small hemangiomas. Ruptured berry aneurysms may be more easily dissected under a flow of cool running water, pursuing a careful blunt dissection from the origin of the greater intracerebral vessels, around the circle of Willis, to the major branches of the circle. Often the degree of the hemorrhage in any one location within the subarachnoid space belies the location of the ruptured aneurysm. Strip the dura from the entire internal surface of the skull in order to visualize fractures. Since they often indicate the nature of the object or the direction of force which caused them, record the dimensions, course, contours, and degree of depression of fractures with some precision. The mobility of the atlanto-occipital joint should be tested.

Spinal Cord: Usually it is not necessary to remove and examine the spinal cord except in cases where injuries to the vertebral column are suspected or evident.

INTERNAL EXAMINATION

The internal examination should follow external evidence of injury on the description report. It does not, of necessity, have to describe the autopsy incisions on the body but should note the general situs of the organs and the appearance of the serosal surfaces. Note should be made of the presence or absence of old or recent adhesions, or other material found on initial internal inspection. This paragraph should also indicate the degree of muscular development as noted in the thoracic and abdominal walls and the degree of adiposity in the thorax and/or abdominal panniculus.

INTERNAL EVIDENCE OF INJURY

It is suggested that all non-natural conditions be individually listed in a subsequent section entitled "Internal Evidence of Injury." Specific external findings may be numerically correlated.

Since it is suggested that the numbering of these internal lesions coincide with the external lesions, the description would proceed from the head toward the lower extremities. When one lesion appears to be causally related to another, the primary lesion is designated with a number, and the causally related lesion associated with it is subdesignated by letter. The description of a gunshot wound, for example, would ordinarily include the angle of pathway and the general dimension of the track created. The underlying subparagraphs would enumerate in respective order those structures and organs the bullet track traversed, indicating in some detail the nature of the injury associated with penetration or perforation.

Similarly, when force to the thorax is associated with multiple rib fractures and compression of the chest, this should be enumerated as a major subheading under Internal Evidence of Injury. Multiple lacerations of the visceral, parietal pleural, retropleural, or intermuscular hemorrhage are designated as subheadings beneath the major lesions.

The orderly presentation of the injuries from above to below in the body allows the prosector to refer to the paragraph by number where he describes a particular lesion in the event that he is queried concerning that lesion. It is also for his guidance so that he can easily and rapidly refer to the location where the lesion is most likely to be described. The presentation within the body of the protocol of pertinent external and internal findings in close proximity to each other, in addition to the co-numbering of similar lesions, external and internal, allows the prosector and either the prosecuting or cross-examining attorney to more readily understand the cause and effect relationship involved.

The orderly description of the injuries prior to subsequent examination of other organs requires that the prosector set aside injured organs or tissues in a group until he has completed this section of his description prior to a more careful dissection in search of underlying or natural disease conditions.

INTERNAL EVIDENCE OF THERAPY

After the detailed internal examination and description of injury, the pathologist should inspect for, and carefully note, the internal findings consistent with surgical intervention during the surviving interval. The examination should carefully note the extent of such treatment. When heroic measures were taken during a very short time interval, it is sometimes impossible to discern the difference between injuries inflicted by an assailant and those associated with drastic therapeutic measures (i.e., blunt force to the abdomen associated with surgical manipulation during the perimortal injury). Under similar circumstances the pathologist should regroup these findings under a single heading entitled "Internal Evidence of Injury and Therapy."

SYSTEMS REVIEW

Following the detailed description of internal injury and therapy, the pathologist should proceed to careful dissection of internal organs with the customary inspection of external and cut surfaces and lumina of hollow viscera, and the weighing of parenchymal organs.

Again, for the convenience of the prosector and the individual preparing the report, and since so many of the medicolegal autopsies are conducted on young, otherwise healthy individuals, much of the remaining portion of the report may be systemized, depending upon the wish of the prosector. For this reason, it is important that the prosector does not incorporate into his protocol a statement in which he discusses a variety of organs in a single sentence. For example, "the heart, lungs, spleen, kidneys, adrenal, pancreas, etc., are otherwise normal." The implication of such a statement is that the pathologist has examined these organs carefully and rendered a gross judgment that these structures presented no significant abnormality. As a result, he has precluded some other individual subsequently reading his report from reaching an independent judgment based on his findings.

A description of the organ systems does not have to be lengthy or verbose. It should be limited to a clear, concise, objective description of shape, color, and consistency, as well as the presence or absence of any discrete lesions other than those systematically described under trauma.

SPECIMENS

In the section on specimens, all samples recovered from the body are listed together with the purpose for which they were retained. An example of this kind of information is as follows:

> Samples of all organs are preserved in 10 percent formaldehyde for histopathologic examination. Samples of blood, urine, and bile are submitted for toxicologic analysis. Blood is withheld for ABO, MN, and RH groupings.

A detailed description of the specimens to be collected and the method of preferred handling appears in an upcoming section of this chapter.

DISPOSITION OF EVIDENCE

All of the evidence collected from the body together with how it was packaged and its ultimate disposition must be carefully enumerated in the paragraph on disposition of evidence. A receipt should always be obtained for any transmitted evidence. The original copy of the receipt should contain detailed enumeration of all evidence transmitted and should be retained by the pathologist. A carbon copy should be sent with the specimen to the individual listed first in the chain of evidence for transmission of this material to the laboratory. A sample of the type of information included within this paragraph is given below:

> The two approximately .22 caliber bullets recovered, one from the posterior aspect of the left upper arm and the other from the left intrathoracic cavity, are placed in yellow paper envelopes, appropriately labeled, sealed, and personally delivered to Detective Sergeant Wood of the Bernalillo County Sheriff's Office, together with the clothing. The receipt is retained within the case folder. . . .

PHOTOGRAPHS

The photographic report should enumerate the photographs taken in the presence of, or by, the pathologist and his assistant during the course of the examination. An example of this type of information is as follows:

> In addition to the routine identification photo, Kodachrome photographs depict the pertinent bullet perforations of the anterior portion of the shirt, the entrance wound on the anterior aspect of the thorax, the exit wound on the posterior aspect of the thorax and, after dissection, the bullet pathways through the lung and heart.

DIAGNOSIS

Immediately following the conclusion of his examination and the preparation of the objective portion of his protocol, the pathologist should clearly organize the anatomic diagnosis. The list should proceed from the most significant injury or disease to the least significant, followed by the remote surgical procedures and the underlying or pre-existing natural disease which coexisted with injury at the time of death. Again, if there is more than one significant injury, each injury should be afforded individual numerical designation. The lesions considered secondary to those already designated are listed as separate subparagraphs beneath the primary, numerically designated diagnosis.

Within the comments portion of the report, the pathologist may desire to add additional information concerning the nature of the injury which may be of benefit either to the law enforcement officer or to the prosecutor but which may not otherwise be included within the body of the report (i.e., a plain language interpretation of the findings denoted in the pathological diagnosis).

SUMMARY OF PROTOCOL

The various sections of the medicolegal autopsy protocol may be summarized as follows:

External Examination
Identifying Marks and Scars
External Evidence of Injury
External Evidence of Therapy
Internal Examination
Internal Evidence of Injury
Internal Evidence of Therapy
Systems Examination
Specimens
Disposition of Evidence
Photographs

SPECIMENS AND SAMPLES TO BE RECOVERED BEFORE AND DURING A POSTMORTEM EXAMINATION

Many specimens and samples are of routine nature and are obtained in virtually all instances where a postmortem examination is conducted. However, often there are special specimens to be obtained when the investigation or the initial findings of the prosector indicate that subsequent examination or investigation should be pursued. In general, the samples and specimens recovered may be designated for several distinct purposes which are discussed below.

Crime Laboratory Examination

The examination conducted within a criminalistics laboratory is undertaken by an evidence technician or a specifically trained criminalist and may include highly trained physicists, engineers, and others (see Chapter 45). The evidence collected from the exterior or occasionally the interior of the body for subsequent examination by the crime laboratory would be subjected to comparison microscopy or photography, comparison ballistics, spectroscopic examination, flame emission or other biologic examination, or a vast array of other increasingly complex and sophisticated methodologies including scanning electron microscopy. Evidence collected for this category should include the following:

1. Dried, carefully and individually packaged clothing that has been delicately handled when the identity of the assailant in a known or suspected criminal attack is unknown.
2. Samples of hair from the head, axilla, and pubic region in those instances where the identity of the perpetrator of a criminal attack is unknown.
3. Clippings of the fingernails when the identity of the perpetrator of a known or suspected attack is unknown. The nails of each hand are packed separately.
4. Samples of foreign material recovered from the outside of the body, but not a part of the clothing, when a criminal act is known or suspected. This includes hit and run cases as well as cases in which the identity of the perpetrator is unknown.
5. Combings of the pubic hair, together with the new comb utilized for these combings when there is a known or suspected sexual assault.
6. Tracings of pattern injuries on the outside of the body when there is a distinct pattern which might aid in the identification of a subsequent weapon or assailant (i.e., heel imprints on the thorax, abdomen, or scalp).

The material should be placed in a dry container, labeled properly, indicating the nature of the evidence, the source of the evidence on the body, the name of the deceased person, the name of the individual gathering this evidence, and the date it was collected.

Serologic or Biologic Examination

Materials intended for serologic or biologic testing are subject to prescribed methods of collection and examination.

In known or suspected sexual attack, either homosexual or heterosexual, the following routine preparations are suggested:

1. Two swabs of the contents of the mouth are immediately smeared onto glass microscopic slides, dabbed onto filter paper or a square of a new clean paper towel, and then placed in a screw-top test tube;

two similar swabs of the vaginal contents are similarly smeared onto glass slides, dabbed onto a 4-inch square of filter paper or a square of a new paper towel, outlined in pencil, labeled, air-dried, and sealed in an envelope.
2. In addition to the swabs prepared of the vaginal contents, the examiner may wish to place 5 to 10 ml of normal saline solution in the vagina with a disposable syringe. The fluid is then removed and placed in a sealed, refrigerated test tube for subsequent enzyme examination.

If the pathologist desires to conduct an examination for spermatozoa in his laboratory, smears may be stained by Papanicolaou technique and read. He should insure that the slides are ultimately cover-glassed and labeled with the name of the deceased and the date. The slide should also be etched with a glass marking pencil to insure that there is no subsequent error in identification. For purposes of standardization, the glass tubes containing the swabs from the various body orifices should be labeled, indicating the nature of the examination desired. The filter paper or paper towel containing the dabs of dried vaginal contents should be carefully folded, sealed in a paper envelope, and labeled. The latter samples are used in absorption serology in the event that the assailant is a secretor (as is the case with approximately 85 to 90 percent of the population) to determine the ABO and RH blood grouping of the spermatozoa from within the vagina. The diminished number of spermatozoa within the oral and rectal cavities, together with their rapid rate of deterioration, usually precludes this type of examination from these orifices.

From individuals who died a violent death with external bleeding or following a sexual attack with or without external bleeding, a sample of clotted blood should be preserved. Subsequent ABO, MN, and RH agglutination studies can be done to determine the specific blood group of the decedent in the event some of his blood was transferred to a weapon and/or clothing or to some other source on the assailant. It is also useful in determining the blood group of the victim in sexual assault cases. Samples of blood similarly preserved are useful in known or suspected hit and run vehicular fatalities and from abandoned babies. These samples should be refrigerated, but *not* frozen.

Toxicologic Examination

Some samples for toxicologic examination are virtually mandatory. The principal one is blood alcohol determination on adult drivers and pedestrians expiring of injuries within 24 hours after a vehicular accident. A blood sample is submitted in all such cases in a tube containing fluoride preservative, sealed and identified with a label. The identification should include the name of the decedent and the source of the blood (e.g., heart), as well as the name of the individual sealing the container or collecting the specimen. Appropriate samples of the vitreous humor (fluid from the anterior chamber of the eye) should also be routinely collected in any such accidental vehicular death, in suspected diabetics, or in early decomposing remains. For epidemiologic and/or evidential purposes similar specimens are submitted for alcohol determination when death occurs at or shortly after any other type of accident. This procedure pertains to all individuals expiring during or immediately after an industrial accident, suicides (regardless of the mode of death), and all individuals dying as a result of violence inflicted by another person or persons.

In summary, insofar as possible, a flouride tube container of blood and, if indicated or necessary, vitreous humor are to be submitted in all unnatural deaths. This submission is in addition to specimens which might otherwise be called for.

In addition to the alcohol specimens, in the following types of cases additional toxicologic samples should be submitted according to the following guidelines (Table 5-1).

TABLE 5-1. GUIDELINES FOR TOXICOLOGY SPECIMEN COLLECTION

Drug	Blood	Urine	Liver/Brain	Gastric	Bile
Alcohol (flouride only)	10 ml	10 ml	–	–	–
Carbon monoxide	10 ml	–	–	–	–
Aspirin	20 ml	50 ml	*	total	–
Antihistamines	20 ml	50 ml	*	total	–
Barbiturates	20 ml	50 ml	*	total	–
Stimulants	–	100 ml	*	total	–
Tranquilizers	20 ml	50 ml	*	total	–
Narcotics	–	100 ml	*	–	total
Other	20 ml	100 ml	*	total	total

*100 grams of liver/brain tissue may be submitted for more complete analysis and particularly should be submitted in cases where the toxic agent is unknown.

In cases where an individual expires during anesthesia, in addition to the toxicologic specimens outlined above, the pathologist, in the event of inhaled anesthesia, should submit:

one lung in a sealed quart container;
approximately 2 grams of fat from the mesentery;
approximately 10 grams of skeletal muscle;
approximately 100 grams of brain from the cerebral hemispheres;
100 grams of liver; and
100 grams of kidney, and all the urine available.

Histopathology

During the course of the dissection, the pathologist should place in a 10 percent formaldehyde solution samples of all organs as well as the portions of organs in which there is either a bullet perforation or samples of the skin and subcutaneous tissue depicting significant external findings on which he desires to do microscopic examination. This examination should be conducted:

1. To confirm gross impressions or the presence or absence of antemortem or postmortem lesions.
2. To assist in dating the incidence of unusual, unnatural lesions resulting from trauma and/or other physical or chemical injury.
3. To confirm the gross impressions the pathologist gained at his initial examination.

It is quite possible that in a young male who expired as a result of an automobile accident, the order of magnitude of trauma and the complete absence of any evident gross natural disease process may entirely preclude the necessity for a microscopic examination. Conversely, it should be remembered that the diagnosis of sudden, unexpected infant death may be made only after exhaustive gross microscopic examinations. Similarly, the conclusion that an infant died as a result of parental neglect can be reached only after microscopic examination has ruled out the possibility that pre-existing natural disease may have caused the death.

This is generally the only occasion on which the pathologist has an opportunity to collect any samples. It is wise to obtain these samples in as much detail as possible, whether or not microscopic examination is immediately contemplated. Whether or not a microscopic examination contributes significantly to his information, an experienced pathologist always conducts such an examination in instances where he may be called upon to present evidence in a matter of civil litigation, particularly when such litigation either derives from the coexistence of natural and unnatural disease or requires testimony concerning the ultimate life span of the individual involved.

The microscopic description may be limited to the positive findings. The pathologist should indicate those tissues he has examined and the number of sections he has noted in any one tissue. This may seem like a trivial, routine procedure, but often a pathologist may describe in detail an important lesion which is only documented in one section. When requested by counsel for either party or perhaps ordered to render his microscopic sections for subsequent review by another expert, the pathologist may find he has inadvertently set this important section aside. As a result, the diagnosis and conclusions reached by an opposing expert may not be the same as those reached by the initially examining pathologist, and with good reason.

SPECIAL PROBLEMS ENCOUNTERED IN MEDICOLEGAL AUTOPSIES

The forensic pathologist should be aware of unique problems which might be encountered in medicolegal autopsies. Examples of such problems are given below.

1. Are the remains of animal or human origin?
    a. availability of precipitin test
    b. x-ray and anthropologic examination may be necessary
    c. examination of hairs
2. What is the identity of the corpse?
    a. photography
    b. fingerprinting
    c. physical features, size, scars, etc.
    d. dental examination
    e. internal findings—operative, stomach contents, etc.
    f. personal effects
    g. availability of prospective identification in some instances
3. What was the time of death, not the time of injury, and what was the relationship of the two?
    a. witnesses
    b. changing process (temperature, rigor and livor mortis, decomposition)

c. physical evidence and associated events
4. Was the place of injury the same as the place of death?
5. Is reconstruction of probable circumstances pertaining to fatal injury possible by examination of scene and of death?
6. Is there evidence of special predisposition of the deceased to accident, suicide, or assault?
   a. chemical examination
   b. medical and psychiatric history
7. Is there objective evidence relating to time elapsed between injury and death?
8. If there are multiple injuries, in what sequence were they received? Are they all equally responsible for death?
9. Is there evidence that more than one assailant participated in the attack? If so, what injuries can be attributed to each?
10. Were the injuries immediately incapacitating? If not, to what extent and for how long was the deceased capable of movement?
11. Did the assailant leave anything in or on the body of the victim that might be of assistance for identification purposes?
    a. residues, traces, bullets
    b. pattern wounds—location
    c. evidence of struggle, rape, sexual attack
12. Is it likely that recognizable traces of the victim were carried away in or on the person of the assailant?
13. Are there any other unusual features about the crime which point to the nature or identity of the assailant?

COMMON MISTAKES ENCOUNTERED DURING THE MEDICOLEGAL AUTOPSY*

Among the most commonly seen mistakes by pathologists contributing to improperly or incompletely prepared medicolegal autopsies are the following:

1. Not being aware of the objective of the medicolegal autopsy:
   a. identification;
   b. time of death;
   c. circumstances of fatal injury.
   d. kind of weapon or agent responsible;
   e. predisposing or modifying effects on the injury, alcoholism, etc.;
   f. identity of assailant.
2. Errors and omissions due to an incomplete autopsy.
3. Problems created by embalming prior to autopsy.
4. The error of regarding a multilated or decomposed body as unproductive of useful evidence.
5. Failure to recognize postmortem artifacts as such.
6. Inadequate description of clothing and external marks of violence.

*This list of common errors is adapted from the well-known paper on this subject by Dr. Alan Moritz, Classic Mistakes in Forensic Pathology, *Am. J. Clin. Pathol.* 26:1383–1397, 1956.

7. Confusion of objective and subjective phases of the descriptive reports.
8. Failure to see the body at the scene.
9. Failure to photograph all of the injuries.
10. Failure to collect samples for toxicology.
11. Failure to gain custody of the body in appropriate instances.
12. Minor errors and omissions within the autopsy report which jeopardize the value of the entire account.

MEDICOLEGAL PHOTOGRAPHY

Increasingly, the medical investigator and the forensic pathologist will be challenged by expert witnesses available to the defendant at the time of subsequent litigation. The expert witness may very well request examination of all reports, documents, and/or other evidential matter in preparation for testimony in court. A completely prepared medicolegal investigation should allow, whenever economically feasible, the gathering of as much documentary evidence as possible in the course of the investigation and subsequent examination. Color photography which may be used not only for reconstruction, recollection and evidence, but also for illustration in court and subsequent teaching is one of the best tools to document evidence. Photographs should be taken as delineated within the prescribed protocol if the ultimate objective to reconstruct and recollect evidence is to be effectively achieved. Ideally, photographs should be taken in those cases in which criminal or civil litigation might be contemplated.

Additional Hints About Medicolegal Photography

Owing to the importance of photography to medicolegal investigation, certain practical points need to be remembered:

1. Whenever possible, color photographs should be taken and, if the shade of the color is extremely important in making the presentation in court (i.e., various ages of bruises in battered children), some type of color comparison chart should be included within the photo. The comparison chart can be used in court to indicate that color aberrations were not present.
2. Aberration lenses should be avoided in taking photographs to be subsequently introduced into court. This type of lens can be excellent in bringing a whole body or scene into the photograph for purposes of recollection or teaching. Frequently, however, considerable distortion is caused which may make it impossible to indicate to the jury that the photograph is a true representation of what was seen at the time the investigation or examination was conducted.
3. Sufficient photographs should be taken to insure that adequate documentation is obtained. If there is some question concerning the exposure of the light source, several photographs can be taken of the same area with different exposure times or light sources. If photographs are included, the report should contain information concerning who took the photographs, on what date, and at what time. Also, it is wise to put a footnote in the body of the autopsy report indicating what photographs were taken so that counsel for the prosecution and/or defense might know that photos are available.
4. Formerly, in taking photographs for evidentiary purposes in court,

it was often necessary to advise the judge and counsel for either plaintiff or defendant of the technical considerations involved in taking such photographs. The attorney for whom one is testifying should be advised so that he can avoid such cross-examination by simply querying along this line: "Does this photograph reasonably represent what you actually saw?" This is the basis of the entire cross-examination process with respect to photographic technique. If answered in the affirmative, other questions are usually unnecessary. Moreover, when attempting to introduce photographs into evidence, one should be prepared to state not only that the photos are a reasonable representation of what was actually seen, but also a necessity because the photos represent the best way, perhaps the only clear way, to present the evidence. It is extremely important to have photographs in which the body has been cleansed and inflammatory evidence such as blood has been removed from the exterior of the body. Owing to jury prejudice, the use of either messy, bloody photographs or photographs in which there are artifacts may preclude the utilization of this valuable form of evidence in court.

CONCLUSION

The foregoing has not been intended as an all-inclusive guide to the performance and recording of a medicolegal autopsy. We have dealt primarily with the basic essentials for the procedure as conducted by one experienced medicolegal office in the United States. We should note, moreover, that there are many styles and conventions encountered among written reports. This chapter should be highly useful to attorneys and law enforcement personnel in arriving at a better judgment of what an adequate medicolegal autopsy should contain.

ADDITIONAL READING

Adelson, L.: *The Pathology of Homicide.* Charles C Thomas, Springfield, Ill., 1974.

Camps, F. E. (ed.): *Gradwohl's Legal Medicine.* ed. 3. Year Book Medical Publishers, Chicago, 1976.

Gantner, G. E.: The Autopsy and the Law. *Am. J. Clin. Pathol.* 69:235-238, 1978.

Gresham, G. A.: *Color Atlas of Forensic Pathology.* Year Book Medical Publishers, Chicago, 1975.

Moenssens, A. A., Moses, R. E., and Inbau, F. E.: *Scientific Evidence in Criminal Cases.* Foundation Press, Mineola, N.Y., 1973.

Rezek, P. R., and Millard, M. (eds.): *Autopsy Pathology: A Guide for Pathologists and Clinicians.* Charles C Thomas, Springfield, Ill., 1963.

Saphir, O.: *Autopsy, Diagnosis and Technique.* ed. 4. Hoeber-Harper, New York, 1961.

Spitz, W. U., and Fisher, R. S. (eds.): *The Medicolegal Investigation of Death.* ed. 2. Charles C Thomas, Springfield, Ill., 1977.

Tedeschi, C. G., Tedeschi, L. G., and Eckert, W. G. (eds.): *Forensic Medicine.* (3 vols.) W. B. Saunders, Philadelphia, 1977.

Weston, J. T.: *The Medicolegal Investigation of Death in New Mexico: Handbook for Representatives of the Office of the Medical Investigator, State of New Mexico.* University of New Mexico Press, Albuquerque, 1976.

CHAPTER 6

Charles S. Hirsch is Director of Forensic Pathology at the Hamilton County Institute of Forensic Medicine, Toxicology, and Criminalistics in Cincinnati. Prior to assuming his present position, he was Associate Pathologist and Deputy Coroner for Cuyahoga County, Ohio, and Associate Professor of Forensic Pathology at Case Western Reserve University in Cleveland. Dr. Hirsch is Past President of the Cleveland Society of Pathologists and is a member of the Board of Editors of the *American Journal of Clinical Pathology*. He is a diplomate of the American Board of Pathology in anatomic and forensic pathology.

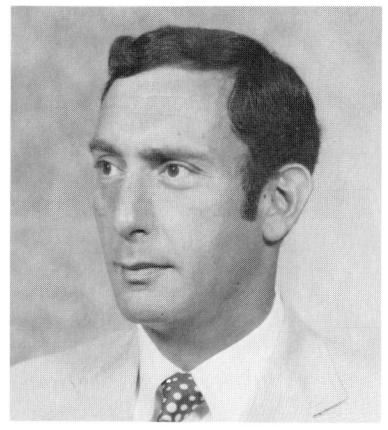

MEDICOLEGAL AUTOPSY: PRACTICAL PERSPECTIVES

Charles S. Hirsch, M.D.

This chapter is intended to provide insight into the objectives of the medicolegal autopsy, especially as it relates to homicide victims. We will also explain some of the cardinal differences between medicolegal autopsies and hospital autopsies done strictly for clinical-scientific purposes. We will offer some practical observations on medicolegal decision-making, the preservation of evidence, and courtroom testimony by forensic pathologists concerning the findings of a medicolegal autopsy. In particular, we emphasize that determining the cause of death is not the "be all and end all" of medicolegal investigation. In fact, determining the cause of the death is often the simplest, least controversial part of the investigation. The work of the forensic pathologist is but one part of a team effort in complete, effective medicolegal investigation of suspicious or violent deaths.

It might well be said: "An autopsy is *not* an autopsy is *not* an autopsy." It is somewhat misleading to use the word "autopsy" as a synonym for both the postmortem examination done in typical hospital deaths and in medicolegal situations. Both examinations begin with an inspection of the external surface of the body and then, using the same techniques, proceed to an evisceration and dissection of the organs. Appropriate samples are retained for indicated chemical and microscopic studies, and finally the observations are reduced to writing in the forms of an autopsy protocol and a report of laboratory findings. Superficially, the similarities between hospital and medicolegal postmortem examinations would seem to make the two procedures identical twins; actually they are no more than cousins that happen to look alike.

The two procedures are performed under different authorizations for different reasons. Some important medicolegal questions, such as identity of the decedent, time and place of death, and postinjury incapacitation and survival interval, never arise in hospital autopsies. Beyond these obvious differences, however, there is a conspicuous dissimilarity in the procedural and intellectual focus of the person performing the autopsy. In the typical hospital postmortem, external examination of the body is a perfunctory prelude to "getting on" with the primary business of determining the cause and mechanism of death and of evaluating medical, surgical, and radiologic diagnosis and treatment. The pertinent changes almost invariably reside internally, and an emphasis on the internal examination is entirely appropriate.

In contrast, the crucial objective observations in a medicolegal evaluation of violent death often are related to the victim's skin and clothing. The golden opportunity to observe and preserve important evidence usually is past history when the cadaver is incised. More often than not, the competent medicolegal autopsy could be conceptualized as an exercise in recognition, interpretation, and preservation of evidence which rests on or in the external surface of the body. This is not intended to denigrate the internal examination as an essential component of the medicolegal autopsy or to advocate that victims of mechanical violence be evaluated by inspection alone in lieu of a complete autopsy. An internal examination is necessary for many compelling reasons, but the forensic autopsy is concerned with a great deal more than dissecting viscera.

Lastly, all of us should recognize that the hospital pathologist who performs an occasional medicolegal autopsy is placed in a demanding, difficult, and frequently unfair position. He must be aware of the many differences between the two types of postmortem so that he can virtually shift perceptual gears when functioning as a forensic pathologist. Furthermore, he must perform the autopsy without the elaborate equipment and numerous support personnel found in sophisticated, modern, medicolegal institutes. Full-time forensic pathologists should be mindful that a substantial measure of our success is attributable to the environment in which we work and to the assistance which we receive from investigators, criminalistics technicians, toxicologists, and photographers. Our effectiveness would be greatly diminished if we had to work alone and received bodies for autopsy without clothing or a knowledge of the circumstances surrounding death.

PRESERVATION OF EVIDENCE

Photography

With the recognition that external findings commonly are the most important part of the medicolegal autopsy, it becomes immediately obvious that such evidence is perishable and frequently distorted by the examination. In fact, the dead body is the only "piece of evidence" in a homicide investigation which is intentionally altered. Consequently, we cannot overemphasize the necessity to preserve the appearance of external injuries prior to the addition of autopsy artifacts.

The only acceptable means to accomplish this goal is the use of color photography. There is absolutely no substitute for a good color photograph to preserve the appearance of a wound or injury. If the pathologist feels that blood spots or smears on the skin are important, the area in question should be photographed before and after the skin is cleansed. For example, when fouling by powder residue from a close-range gunshot wound is associated intimately with blood smears, a photograph of the bloody wound preserves evidence which might easily wash away. A second photograph after washing reveals the characteristics of the wound which were obscured by blood.

Regardless of whether a given court accepts color photographs as evidence, in the interests of the state and the defendant, they must be taken. Should questions arise as to the interpretation (or misinterpretation) of injuries by the pathologist who performed the autopsy, it is very much in the defendant's best interest to have color photographs available for independent evaluation by another expert. Acceptable black and white photographic prints can be made from color negatives for use in court in those jurisdictions where color prints are deemed inadmissible. Finally, it is not the pathologist's responsibility to decide whether or not photographs of the victim are admissible as evidence. The pathologist must be able to say (1) either that the photographs were taken by him or that they were taken under his direction, control, and supervision, and (2) that the photographs fairly and accurately portray what they purport to show. It is the judge's responsibility to rule on the admissibility of the evidence. In most jurisdictions, a bloody body and background greatly enhance the likelihood that photographs will be ruled inflammatory and inadmissible.

Other Evidence

If the pathologist fails to appropriately preserve and transmit evidence, whether it be foreign pubic hair and vaginal swabs from the victim of a rape-homicide, or a bullet, he might as well not observe it. The responsibility for initiating an unbreakable chain of custody rests with the pathologist. Careful attention to a few simple details is all that is required. The pathologist must be able to state what he removed or recovered from the body, what he did with it, when it left his possession, and to whom he gave it. The shorter the chain the better.

Usually, the pathologist has nothing to do with the evidence after it leaves his personal control, but he can do a good deal to simplify the evidentiary escort in his own institution. For example, it is asking for trouble if the pathologist recovers a bullet and then hands it to an autopsy room assistant, who places it in an envelope. The assistant gives the envelope to a secretary, who gives it to an orderly, who takes it to the office of the nursing supervisor. The secretary in the nursing office gives it to the supervisor on duty, who recognizes that it shouldn't have come to her in the first place. So she takes it to the office of the hospital administrator, whose secretary carries it to the security guard. None of these transactions is recorded. It would have been safer and a lot simpler if the police laboratory officer obtained the evidence directly from the pathologist and gave him an appropriate receipt.

The evidentiary chain doesn't have to be as tortuous as the foregoing, contrived example in order to cause the monumental headaches exemplified by the following actual case. Two colleagues performed autopsies on a man and a woman who had been shot to death and then partially incinerated in their home in an attempt to conceal the murders. One pathologist assumed primary responsibility for both examinations, composed the autopsy protocols, and testified about his findings in court. The second pathologist served as an assistant at the autopsies. When the first pathologist recovered bullets from both victims, he handed them to an autopsy diener. The diener placed them in containers which he had labeled. The first pathologist took custody of the bullets following completion of the autopsies and placed them in a locked cabinet in his office. He was not at work the next day, so the second pathologist gave the evidence to a police officer who came to the hospital. The bullets became vitally important when investigators ultimately found the weapon which had fired them and linked the gun to the suspect. Consequently, the assisting pathologist and the diener both had to testify in court to establish and maintain the chain of custody.

Had the trial been a local affair, this would not have imposed an undue hardship on anyone. However, a change of venue was granted because of excessive pretrial publicity. Counting travel time and waiting, the assisting pathologist and diener lost a day and a half to testify about their roles in the evidentiary escort. Insult was added to injury when a subsequent witness made grossly improper remarks which resulted in the declaration of a mistrial. This evoked more publicity, so the second trial was conducted at the other end of the state. The assisting pathologist and diener paid further with a tedious drive and another lost day. All of this inconvenience and wasted time could have been avoided if the pathologist who performed the autopsies had marked the bullet containers and personally handed them to the officer.

To summarize, "shorter is better" when forging custodial chains.

"Show It to Me Cold"

Totally objective study of gross and microscopic pathologic specimens is an instructive educational technique for students and practitioners of pathology. This is done in formally organized conferences and as an informal part of the professional relationship with one's colleagues in pathology. Whichever setting applies, the pathologist usually is given a microscopic slide containing X tissue. He examines it "cold" (i.e., without even being told whether or not the specimen is from a plant or animal, human or otherwise). The object is for the pathologist to deduce the origin of the tissue and the nature of the disease solely on the basis of objective examination. Some pathologists are more skillful than others at this exercise, and sometimes a bit of "gamesmanship" can make it seem as if a pathologic rabbit has been pulled out of the microscope. For example, after studying a tissue sample which he recognizes as a leaflet of the mitral valve showing a peculiar myxomatous degeneration and thickening, the experienced pathologist might amaze you by stating correctly that "This section is from a young woman with red hair who died suddenly and whose family history includes similar occurrences."

This is all fine and good. It's the way most of us learned pathology in the first place, and we continue to hone our diagnostic skills in the same fashion. It is an ongoing, serious, education "game" played with relish by most pathologists. "Show it to me cold" is an expression of our scientific "machismo." But in serious situations, it isn't the last word. One would not send a consultant a microscopic slide for diagnosis without accompanying historical and clinical information. Nor would one render a diagnosis of malignancy on a surgical pathology report without some knowledge of the clinical findings, particularly if such a diagnosis indicates the need for radical surgery, radiotherapy, or life-threatening chemotherapy. There is nothing wrong with objective evaluation of microscopic slides, but prudent pathologists consider all of the available information before rendering a final opinion.

Strangely enough, some highly competent pathologists fail to apply the same reasoning to evaluation of medicolegal autopsies. There sometimes is a reluctance to form opinions based upon anything which they cannot observe at the autopsy table or see under the microscope. Carried to their logical conclusions, such constraints deny reality in the name of objectivity. For example, consider the following situation. A previously vigorous, robust young man is found dead in wet grass on a construction site. An electric saw which he had been using is adjacent to his right hand. A complete autopsy shows no structurally demonstrable disease to explain his death; repeated, meticulous examination of the skin shows nothing which might be construed as an electrical burn, and chemical and toxicologic studies are negative. The saw's electrical cord has a faulty splice and its ground prong is missing. An electrical engineer who examined the saw reports that anybody operating the appliance would be at risk to receive an electric shock. Do you conclude that the victim was electrocuted despite the absence of cutaneous electrical burns, or do you steadfastly and unrealistically maintain that you cannot determine the cause of death?

Such an example is not at all far-fetched, and the forensic pathologist is attuned to considering historical, circumstantial, and other nonanatomic (nonobjective) data in evaluating cause and manner of death. If restricted to the practical and intellectual vacuum of the autopsy room and laboratory, we would be ineffective or make less of a contribution in many cases.

Drowning is a classic example of our reliance on information which we cannot observe personally. In many instances, there are no anatomic or chemical findings which prove or disprove that a person whose body is recovered from water has drowned. In these situations, a determination of death by drowning or from other causes rests as much upon an evaluation of the circumstances as it does on anatomic and chemical data. Consider the following example. The fully clothed body of a man is recovered from water at the foot of a fishing pier. Autopsy discloses severe arteriosclerotic heart disease and pulmonary edema. Did he drown or did he submerge in water following a fatal heart attack? This question cannot be satisfactorily resolved without additional historical information. The pathologist could spend all day in the autopsy room and study hundreds of microscopic slides, but the likelihood of resolving the issue by these activities is virtually nil. The history could indicate that the victim stepped on a slippery fish, tumbled off the pier, and submerged after thrashing about in the chilly water for a minute or two. On the other hand, the history might indicate that the victim was sitting quietly when he clutched his chest as his head rolled back, made a gurgling noise, slid off the pier, and submerged without a struggle. The objective anatomic findings are perfectly consistent with either history. In the absence of an eyewitness, one would have to attempt to resolve the issue on the basis of anatomic and chemical findings, physical evidence, common sense, and sound judgment. It isn't easy, and it's no place for rigid dogmatism.

Criminal prosecutions as well as civil controversies can hinge upon nonanatomic evidence which the pathologist is uniquely qualified to interpret in light of his own findings. A case in point concerned the disappearance of an 18-year-old woman. She left home as usual one October morning to go to work and vanished. Investigation disclosed that she never arrived at a bus stop three blocks from her home on that morning. She had been an emotionally stable, industrious person and had lived a quiet, sheltered life. Five months later, her skeleton was found in a wooded area approximately 10 miles from her home. There was no trace of clothing on, under, or near the body. Skeletonization had resulted primarily from animal feeding, and some of her bones were never found. Those that remained showed no fractures, and a cause of death was not demonstrable in the skeletal remains.

The history, circumstances of her disappearance, location of the body, and total absence of clothing indicated beyond reasonable doubt that her death was not the result of natural causes, an accident, or suicide. This left only homicide, and our inability to demonstrate the cause of death in her remaining bones did not deter us in the least from concluding that someone had killed her. In this instance, we chose to state that the cause of death was homicidal violence of undetermined type (i.e., the cause of death was undetermined, but the manner of death was homicide). A reliance solely upon gross and microscopic pathology would have produced no conclusion as to the cause or manner of death in defiance of the obvious truth that the girl was abducted, killed, and deposited nude at the scene of discovery.

Such cases are the antithesis of the "show it to me cold" attitude. In fact, the more a forensic pathologist knows about the total investigation, the more he can contribute from his autopsy. Conversely, the less the pathologist knows about the history and circumstances surrounding death, the greater is his likelihood of overlooking useful findings. Nobody sees everything all of the time, and there is nothing like a heightened index of suspicion to sharpen the focus of an autopsy.

The following example typifies coordination of medical findings and police investigation in the reconstruction of a violent death, a common nonanatomic goal of the forensic autopsy. An adult man was shot in the abdomen during a struggle over control of a revolver. He and his assailant walked to the assailant's car and drove off together, ostensibly en route to a nearby hospital. Instead, the assailant claimed that the victim grabbed the gun, forced him to drive to a park, and ordered him out of the car. Allegedly, they struggled again and the victim was shot twice in the head. One bullet entered his forehead and caused perforations of the skull and brain. The second bullet entered the left side of the face, perforated both eyes, and exited from the lateral aspect of the right eyebrow. When examined in the park, the dead man was prone with the right side of his face down. The police recovered a ⅜ inch bone fragment from the snow and ice beneath his face. The bone's configuration indicated that it came from the supraorbital rim.

At the ensuing trial the key issue was a reconstruction of the events in the park. The defendant admitted shooting the victim, and nobody doubted that death resulted from the gunshot wounds. The pathologist was the only one in a position to say that the gunshot wound which entered the skull and perforated the brain would have caused immediate incapacitation, and that the location of the bone chip beneath the exit wound further indicated that the victim's face was on the ground when he was shot through the eyes. Along with other evidence, the image of a shot fired at a motionless, helpless head on the ground proved fatal to the defendant's contention that he had acted in self-defense. The moral of this story is that a totally objective evaluation, restricting the pathologist to autopsy observations, would have added very little to an adjudication of the contested issue. "Show it to me cold" is all right so long as the attitude does not freeze one's perception of reality.

The importance of historical and other nonanatomic data in evaluation of sudden deaths due to natural causes is discussed in Chapter 49, Role of the Pathologist in Chemically Induced Death Cases.

"What's It All About?"

An understanding of the objectives of the medicolegal autopsy in homicide victims is enhanced if one is cognizant of the ultimate use made of medicolegal testimony at trials. To begin with, one element of an indictment for any degree of homicide deals with the unlawful death of a person. The pathologist's testimony must establish that the person is, indeed, dead and should include an opinion about the cause of death. Actually, in more than 95 percent of homicide trials, the defense has no quarrel with the pathologist related to these facts. Therefore, we ordinarily are not cross-examined concerning identity of the decedent or the cause of death. However, there are occasional instances in which the forensic pathologist enters controversial waters on the witness stand. His conclusions in such situations will be contested by cross-examination, and it is possible that a qualified expert with a contrary point of view will appear for the opposing side. He too will be cross-examined. The conflict of experts may prove sufficiently newsworthy to be highly publicized. This helps to create and maintain the mistaken notion that medical testimony in homicide trials is an emotionally charged, competitive experience in which the pathologist "wins" or "loses" the case. This is a gross distortion of common experience.

In the large majority of homicide trials, there is nothing controversial in the pathologist's testimony. This is not to say that the testimony is unimportant. It is just that in and of itself the medical evidence usually does not establish the guilt or innocence of the defendant, nor does it independently establish a degree of guilt. What it really is all about in the majority of instances is to provide expert opinions based upon objective, indisputable facts which help to evaluate the reliability and credibility of other witnesses. The pathologist is a "middle man" between the truth of the cadaver and the testimony of persons whose version of the fatal episode is at issue.

The following examples are intended to place in perspective the unusual and the usual in medicolegal testimony.

Case 1 (unusual). An apparently distraught man called the police at 3 a.m., requesting assistance for his wife whom he had just mistakenly shot. Allegedly, he thought that she was a burglar. They had been out together earlier in the evening, but he returned home first and went to bed. He was awakened by footsteps in the hallway outside his bedroom, grabbed the loaded shotgun which habitually was kept next to the head of his bed, called out to the person to leave his house, and fired. His wife was dead when the police arrived.

Examination of the victim and her clothing disclosed a contact-range shotgun wound of the lower presternal region and epigastrium, which had passed through her blouse, and a contact-range shotgun wound involving the back of her skirt and blouse, which did not injure her skin. The latter defects in the clothing could only have been produced by a shot fired when the skirt and blouse were held away from her body with the shotgun muzzle pressed against the garments. A third shot had perforated the bedroom door without injuring the victim. Furthermore, the interior of the shotgun muzzle contained dry blood and tissue, indicating unequivocally that the shot which entered her trunk was the last one fired. Had an additional shot been fired after the blood and tissues were deposited in the muzzle, the material would have been blasted out of the barrel by the shotgun charge and wads.

The objective observations, independent of other considerations, rendered the husband's claim of accidental shooting unbelievable. This case exemplifies the value of sound, scientific homicide investigation, and probably is suitable for a television drama or inclusion in a popular book for lay persons. Unfortunately, by publicizing such cases, one creates a false impression of the usual contribution of the forensic pathologist. Such cases account for less than 1 percent of all homicides investigated by our office. The assailant-husband was found guilty of manslaughter.

Case 2 (usual). A money-order salesman was robbed and killed as he left a delicatessen on his business rounds. Autopsy disclosed extensive, peculiar burns of his face and left eye, having the configuration of droplets and rivulets at their margins. The burned skin reacted in a strongly acidic fashion when touched with pH paper. It was concluded that an acid liquid had been thrown in the victim's face, and the police were requested to seek a likely container at the scene of the killing. They found a wax-lined paper cup which contained a residue of sulfuric acid. The victim also had a linear abraded laceration of his right retroauricular scalp and a faint, linear contusion in the same area oriented almost perpendicular to the former injury. He had been killed by two contact-range gunshot wounds of the left anterior chest.

Medical testimony at the separate trials of three defendants established that acid had been thrown in the victim's face, that he had been struck twice in the right occiput with a blunt object, and that he had been shot twice in the chest at contact range. This testimony was incontestable and noncontroversial. There was nothing in it which linked the victim to his assailants. In contrast, the crucial, bitterly contested testimony was that of a 12-year-old boy. He claimed that he saw two young men waiting in the doorway of the delicatessen and a third in a parked car, all of whom he recognized from the neighborhood. The eyewitness testified as follows. One of the men standing in the doorway held a paper cup from which he pretended to drink. When the salesman emerged from the store, the man with the paper cup threw its contents into the victim's face. As the salesman raised his hands to his face, the second assailant pulled a piece of pipe from his coat and struck the victim twice in the back of the head. The salesman fell to the pavement, and the man who formerly held the cup pulled a gun, bent over the victim, and shot him twice.

The problem faced by three juries was to decide whether to trust the eyewitness identification. All three defendants claimed that they were not there, and the defense theory in each trial rested upon mistaken identification. The medical testimony carried weight because it corroborated exactly the eyewitness account. It had no direct bearing on the witness' personal recognition of the defendants, but it indicated beyond doubt that his observation of the crime was precisely accurate. Each defendant was found guilty and sentenced to die in the electric chair.

In contrast to the rarity of the shotgun case described previously, medical testimony about the salesman typifies the day-in, day-out contribution of the forensic pathologist in court. Admittedly, the salesman's case is a more dramatic example than most, but the principle is the same in countless situations. How many times was the victim shot? At what range? Was he facing his assailant? Was the victim under the influence of alcohol, narcotics, stimulants, or other drugs? Did the victim have injuries indicative of a struggle or fight preceding infliction of the lethal wound? Did the ultimately lethal trauma cause immediate incapacitation? How long did it take the victim to die? Answers to these and similarly straightforward questions are the mainstay of medicolegal testimony in criminal trials and provide a sound factual basis for juries to use in evaluating the testimony of other witnesses. Also there are numerous analogous situations in civil litigation stemming from common occurrences such as traffic and industrial accidents. In actual trial experience, the pathologist frequently has a little good news and a little bad news for both sides. The prudent pathologist "tells it as it is" and doesn't choose sides.

"The Best Case"

"Which was your most memorable case?" Forensic pathologists hear this question, or something similar to it, with regularity. It's an invitation to tell entertaining "war stories," which usually have a common denominator. They generally end when the jury finds the suspect guilty of murder.

Perhaps a more thoughtful answer to the "best case" query would be a response referring to a class of cases rather than an isolated instance. There are many "best" cases, but their names and dates fade from memory. None of them is concerned with the detection of occult homicide because each of them hinges upon the recognition of "nonhomicide." And for most of us, the latter is a more rewarding and challenging pursuit than the former.

Complete autopsies on victims of apparent violence, whose deaths were surrounded by seemingly suspicious circumstances, commonly disclose that the fatalities resulted from natural causes. In some of these instances, the police arrest suspects prior to the autopsy on the basis of reasonable inferences drawn from their observations at the scene of death and from the external appearance of the decedent. "Medicolegal masquerades" of this nature often are spawned by the clumsiness, carelessness, fragility, and convoluted domestic relations of alcoholic persons. The classic example is that of a dead alcoholic woman with multiple bruises whose spouse admits that he occasionally "whacked her around." At the scene, the police find blood stains in several rooms. Their presumption of homicide and their willingness to accept the husband-assailant's admission of responsibility for her injuries are perfectly understandable.

The usual autopsy findings in such instances consist of multiple bruises of multiple ages on the extremities and trunk with a distribution suggesting that they probably were caused by stumbling into objects or falling. Facial contusions, consistent with spouse-abuse, complete the mistaken external appearance of a homicidal assault. None of us can evaluate such a death without a complete autopsy.

The presence or absence of lethal internal injury usually cannot be predicted accurately from an external examination of the cadaver. Sometimes internal injuries confirm the initial impression of a violent death, but in many cases the only visceral injury is chemical, induced by long-standing, abusive consumption of ethanol. Bleeding esophageal varices or peptic ulcers with hematemesis explain the widespread distribution of blood stains at the house and on the decedent's skin and clothing. At this point, the pathologist telephones the police to inform them that the decedent's injuries neither caused nor contributed to her death. They release her husband from jail.

One point in the above narrative warrants emphasis: Reference was made to a *complete* autopsy. The medicolegal autopsy should include appropriate chemical studies and examinations of the brain and neck as well as the thoracic and abdominal viscera. In medicolegal circumstances, partial autopsies are undesirable and are mentioned here only for the purpose of condemnation; they leave reasonable questions unanswered and erect an unwarranted facade of scientific validity.

Finally, and probably most importantly, pseudoviolent deaths demand the best of us; they test our independence and open-mindedness. As explained previously in this chapter, we need investigative information in advance of the autopsy if our examination is to achieve its potential, but we are not bound by the bias of first impressions. Our autoptic attitude can help to exonerate the innocent—a rare privilege and an exhilarating experience. There can be no greater stimulus to perform competent medicolegal autopsies.

CHAPTER 7

John I. Coe is Medical Examiner of Hennepin County (Minneapolis), Minnesota. He is also Chief of Pathology at Hennepin County Medical Center and Professor of Pathology at the University of Minnesota. Dr. Coe is currently President of the National Association of Medical Examiners and is a Fellow of the American Academy of Forensic Science. He has served on the Council of Forensic Pathology of the American Society of Clinical Pathology, and is Past President of the Minnesota Society of Clinical Pathology, the Minnesota Pathological Society, and the Minnesota Academy of Medicine.

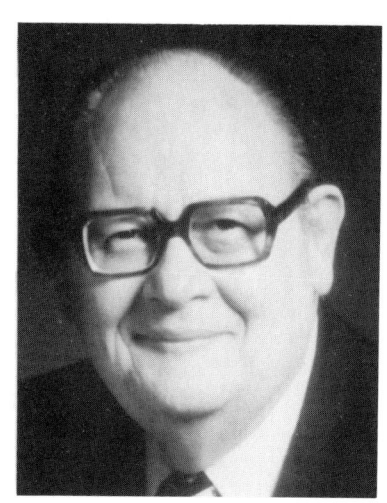

William J. Curran is Frances Glessner Lee Professor of Legal Medicine at Harvard University and Chairman of the State Medicolegal Investigation Committee of Massachusetts. Professor Curran writes regularly for the *New England Journal of Medicine* and teaches at the Medical School, Law School, and School of Public Health at Harvard. He was formerly Robert R. Utley Professor of Legal Medicine and Director of the Law-Medicine Institute of Boston University. He also served as Assistant Professor of Law and Government and Assistant Director of the Institute of Government at the University of North Carolina. Professor Curran is the author of several books in the medicolegal field including *Law, Medicine and Forensic Science* (with E. D. Shapiro); *Trauma and the Automobile; The Doctor as a Witness;* and *Medicolegal Proof in Litigation.* He is an Associate Editor of the *American Journal of Law and Medicine* and was formerly Medicolegal Editor of the *Massachusetts Law Quarterly.*

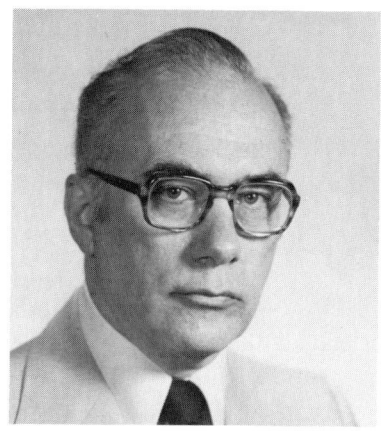

DEFINITION AND TIME OF DEATH

John I. Coe, M.D., and
William J. Curran, J.D., LL.M., S.M. Hyg.

FUNDAMENTAL CONCEPTS

Interrelated Issues of Definition and Time

Issues of the definition of death and determinations as to when death has occurred are conceptually interrelated. Traditionally, both law and medicine have held to the position that death is a single event in time, not a continuous process or series of phenomena.[1] This position is the key to the interlinking of the *definition* of human death and the establishment of a single *moment* when a person is said to have died. The selection of a specific time of a death is a practical necessity in family, social, and business affairs. Inheritance of property and control over a business often depends upon when a person died. It is said that "the law requires certainty." One of the most important applications of this rule is in death determination. In most primitive societies, all types of authority were personal and mortal. When the head of a family, a tribe, or a nation died, the power, usually absolute, passed to a designated successor. Uncertainty over the death of the leader was intolerable. Legal systems usually contain provisions for binding *presumptions* of a death when a person is lost in hazardous conditions where survival is essentially impossible (e.g., shipwreck, battlefield casualties, airplane disappearances, etc.). The time allowed for discovery in such situations is usually short, depending upon the evidence available. A recent famous application of this rule was the disappearance of the Prime Minister of Australia while swimming on a rocky, very deep seacoast near his home. Only a few days passed before he was presumed legally dead and his successor allowed to assume power over the nation. In more unusual circumstances, where there is no obvious explanation for a disappearance, these factually based presumptions do not apply. A period of uncertainty will exist with the hope that the person will return. For business and other purposes, temporary replacements of authority are usually installed, according to established rules such as corporate bylaws. Legal systems commonly provide for an arbitrary presumption of "death" after the passage of an established period of time. The traditional period has been seven years, especially when applied to marriage and inheritance.[2]

Legal controversies have also arisen over the question of which of two people died first in a common accident when both were found dead, or where both bodies were not recovered. If examination of the available bodies and the opinion of experts (such as the forensic pathologic evaluations discussed later in this chapter) do not provide factual support for a determination, the issue will remain unresolved. However, if the two were husband and wife, or other relatives such as siblings, testamentary documents may establish a rule of inheritance or succession by providing that property will pass in a certain way in the case of "simultaneous deaths" or common tragedies where the order of death cannot be resolved. Many states and foreign governments have enacted simultaneous death statutes which also help to resolve disputes over inheritance and passage of property in such cases, particularly where no will has been left by the parties.

Pronouncement and Certification of Death

In earlier years, the interlinking of the time of death and the definition of death presented no serious dilemmas. Death was associated with cessation of fairly easily observable signs of movement, breathing, and heartbeat. The soul was believed to leave the body when the heart stopped. Departure of the soul was clearly a single event in time; consequently, death was equally certain and marked by a point in time. This does not mean that no "mistakes" were made about determinations of death. Persons apparently dead did recover. Certain illnesses and physical shock could "mock death." As late as the nineteenth century there was widespread fear of incorrect pronouncement of death and premature burial.[3] Coffins could be obtained which contained bells and other ingenious devices which could be manipulated by the "corpse" if he or she should recover.

By the latter part of the last century, methods of determination of death had improved, especially where physicians involved in caring for the last illnesses also "pronounced" the death. Certification of death became largely a medical professional action. It was seized upon by the legal system as a method of removing uncertainty about the fact of death. The greatly increased number of deaths in hospitals, including the loosely defined "dead on arrival" cases, tended to make "pronouncements," and thus determinations of death, an accepted medical professional responsibility. Nevertheless, errors have continued. A patient's death has been pronounced by medical personnel and the person has later been revived, to the embarrassment of the pronouncer. These have often been "death on arrival" cases where the cause of the person's condition was unknown. The term "apparent death" appears in some medical dictionaries to cover these cases.

The Unified Concept of Death

Until recently, medical dictionaries defined death as the cessation of life (i.e., the ending of all vital functions and systems). Emphasis was placed on the cessation of respiration and cardiovascular function, but it was expected that all systems would fail quickly after one of the "vital functions" had stopped. Nervous system and brain function were considered particularly fragile and dependent upon the other systems.

This unified or interdependent concept of death remained unchallenged until quite recent times when medical care advances have made it possible to maintain some of the "vital functions" of a patient, but not all. Well-equipped hospitals can now resuscitate nearly all patients, and they can be maintained for long periods or essentially indefinitely on heart-lung machines or, in some cases, even under their own capacity in regard to heart and respiratory functions. The tragedy is that irreversible damage to the brain often occurs during the short period or periods when breathing and heartbeat have been suspended. Serious permanent impairment can occur with only four to six minutes of oxygen deprivation, and total loss of function is common when deprivation exceeds 15 minutes.

THE BRAIN DEATH CONCEPT

Development of the Concept

The first proposal to determine brain death by permanent loss of consciousness is generally attributed to Mollaret and Goulon in France in 1959. It remained, however, for an interdisciplinary group of faculty at Harvard University in 1968, under the chairmanship of Henry K. Beecher, M.D., to produce a complete set of medical criteria for determining brain death and a medicolegal procedure for pronouncing death.[4] The group, known as the Ad Hoc Committee of Harvard Medical School to Examine the Definition of Brain Death, was composed of 13 members. Ten were physicians representing the specialties of anesthesiology, neurology, pathology, psychiatry, neurosurgery, general surgery, internal medicine, electroencephalography, and nephrology. Some of the medical members were particularly interested in organ transplant medicine and surgery. The three nonphysicians were a lawyer, a theologian, and a historian of science. One of the authors of this chapter (W.J.C.) was the lawyer on the Ad Hoc Committee.

The Report of the Ad Hoc Committee, in 1968, set forth three criteria for determining the permanent nonfunction of the brain in a patient in deep coma. A fourth criterion was proposed as confirmatory. The three obligatory criteria were as follows:

> 1. *Unreceptivity and unresponsivity.* The patient must be totally unresponsive to applied stimuli. Even the most intensive effort to cause pain should evoke no vocal or other response and no movement or respiration.
>
> 2. *No movements or breathing.* Observation by physicians for at least an hour is required, during which no spontaneous muscular movement or breathing takes place, as well as no spontaneous response to touch, sound, or light. After a patient is on a respirator, the total lack of spontaneous breathing may be established by turning off the machine and observing the patient for three minutes. At the start of such a trial period of the respirator, the patient's carbon dioxide level should be within normal limits, and he or she should be breathing room air for at least 10 minutes.
>
> 3. *No reflexes.* The pupils of the eyes should be fixed, dilated, and unresponsive to bright light. Ocular movement and blinking should be absent. Swallowing, yawning, and vocalization should be in abeyance. Corneal and pharyngeal reflexes should also be unobtainable. Tendon reflexes

should not be elicited by tapping at biceps, triceps, pronator muscles, or quadriceps. Plantar or noxious stimulation should produce no response in the patient.

The added *confirmatory* test is, of course, a "flat" or *isoelectric electroencephalogram*. Details were provided for proper operation of the EEG. The reason for making the flat EEG only confirmatory of brain death was the realization that the machine will not always be available or that the patient's skull may be so crushed by trauma that there may be no way to affix the electrodes to the brain. Where it is available, however, the Ad Hoc Committee suggested that the EEG "should be utilized."

The Committee went on to provide that "all of the above tests" must be repeated *at least* 24 hours later with no observable change in results. At the time of the work of the Committee, most centers (even the Massachusetts General Hospital, where both Dr. Beecher, the chairman, and Dr. Schwab, the EEG specialist, practiced) were more conservative and repeated the tests every 24 hours over a 3-day period. After examining the world literature on survivorship, the Committee decided to reduce the repeat-test period to one observation at 24 hours.

The medicolegal discussion followed. It was provided that the determination of the above conditions should be the responsibility of a physician. After the determination, the physician in charge should inform other colleagues, including nurses, of the determination of a brain death. The family of the patient, if they are in attendance, should also be informed. The death of the patient should be declared by the physician in charge after consultation with at least one other physician involved directly in the case, and the declaration should always occur *before* the heart-lung apparatus is turned off. The Report specifically counseled the physician against placing the decision to turn off the machine in the hands of the family. Moreover, the Committee recommended that the physician declaring the death should not be among those later participating in any efforts to transplant organs from the deceased.

The criteria of the Harvard Ad Hoc Committee have since been generally accepted throughout the world. Two actions on the international level during 1968 greatly encouraged universal acceptance. These were the adoption of the brain death concept and the Harvard criteria by the World Medical Association in its *Declaration of Sydney* and the endorsement of the criteria by the Council of International Organizations of Medical Sciences.

During the years that have passed since the Report was first published, the basic criteria have survived essentially intact. It can be said, however, that the flat EEG is generally included as a criterion in most cases, rather than being merely confirmatory. The fact that the EEG is an *objective test,* while all of the others require subjective clinical judgments by physicians, adds to the strength of the EEG criterion.

The parts of the total procedure which have changed or been subject to disagreement have concerned the 24-hour waiting period before the retest and the medicolegal procedures. The Ad Hoc Committee fully expected these parts of the systems to change. The 24-hour waiting period was the shortest period which seemed acceptable at the time, but it was admittedly arbitrary. Currently, many groups favor a shortening of the period to 12 hours, or the removal of any fixed period with determination of a later confirmatory observation as needed in each case, depending on the circumstances and anatomic damage to the brain. In conducting the clinical tests, greater attention is now paid to the absence of brain-stem responses in many cases. Moreover, greater conservatism is now being shown in the handling of young children under 5 years of age and patients whose brain function has been depressed by drugs.

There has also been controversy over the terms brain death and irreversible coma. Some commentators have preferred the former term since it defines a status, while rejecting the latter as only a prediction or prognosis. Another form of status definition would be to describe the condition as permanent rather than irreversible.

Medicolegal Aspects of Brain Death

The Harvard Committee, in its legal commentary, described the definition of death as a question of fact rather than a law under then current American practice. The Committee did not suggest adoption of a statutory definition, at least until the medical community had accepted and was following the brain death concept. The very rapid acceptance of the concept was clearly unexpected by most of the Committee members. The first statutory definition of brain death was adopted by the Kansas Legislature in 1970.[5] It reads as follows:

> A person will be considered medically and legally dead if, in the opinion of a physician, based on ordinary standards of medical practice, there is the absence of spontaneous respiratory and cardiac function and, because of the disease or condition which caused, directly or indirectly, these functions to cease, or because of the passage of time since these functions ceased, attempts at resuscitation are considered hopeless; and, in this event, death will have occurred at the time these functions ceased; or
>
> A person will be considered medically and legally dead if, in the opinion of a physician, based on ordinary standards of medical practice, there is the absence of spontaneous brain function; and if based on ordinary standards of medical practice, during reasonable attempts to either maintain or restore spontaneous circulatory or respiratory function in the absence of aforesaid brain function, it appears that further attempts at resuscitation or supportive maintenance will not succeed, death will have occurred at the time when these conditions first coincide. Death is to be pronounced before artificial means of supporting respiratory and circulatory function are terminated and before any vital organ is removed for purposes of transplantation.
>
> These alternative definitions of death are to be utilized for all purposes in this state, including the trials of civil and criminal cases, any laws to the contrary notwithstanding.

The statute was well prepared. It should be noted that it includes no actual medical criteria. It leaves these matters open to determination and to change within "ordinary standards of medical practice." Furthermore, the definition provides an alternative, allowing the common definition to apply to most cases and the newer brain death concept to the special situations to which it is applicable. The statute also specifically deals with the issue of turning off the respirator after the pronouncement of brain death and adds that organs should not be removed until after the declaration. The statute thus recognized the interrelationship between transplant and brain death cases, a matter which many earlier commentators had tried to avoid.

It is also important to note what the statute does *not* contain. It does not complicate the pronouncement of death with strict requirements. Other suggested procedures would require two physicians to concur in the pronouncement and would also bar any physician who pronounces the death of a donor from "participating" in a transplantation. There is much to be said for this latter position. It deals with the concern for a possible conflict of interest between a transplant team and the patient's best interests. The Harvard Committee itself suggested this position, but did not recommend that it be adopted by statute. It would seem best left as a suggested precaution on ethical grounds, but allowable when involvement cannot be avoided. The trouble with the rule as law is that it would be impossible to enforce after the fact. It would seem inconceivable that an otherwise correct and uncontroverted pronouncement of a brain death would be voided because the physician who pronounced it later helped to prepare the dead patient for a transplant, or merely called a transplant group and helped to transport the body or organ. The law, as noted earlier, demands certainty in the declaration of death. If enacted into law, this rule would add uncertainty and make some pronouncements questionable where, when the death itself was pronounced, the physician was not a part of a transplant team and only afterward helped in the transplant. The Kansas Legislature wisely rejected inclusion of this prohibition, and later statutory definitions have followed this model. However, the original Uniform Anatomical Gift Act did adopt this position, and the Act as passed in many states includes this prohibition regarding transplantation. Not all states have included it. We caution readers that the state law on *both* brain death and anatomic gifts must be examined to clarify these medicolegal procedures in any one jurisdiction.

Since 1970, over 20 states have adopted statutory definitions of brain death. (Many of the statutes actually cover all types of death, not merely brain death.) None of the statutes is contradictory of the Harvard criteria or procedures. There are now three types of statutes on the subject: (1) those that follow the Kansas approach of allowing an *alternative* definition of death; (2) those *mandating* the application of brain death criteria whenever the person sustains loss of consciousness but retains heartbeat and respiration; and (3) an abbreviated definition suggested by the American Bar Association and applicable only to brain death.

In 1978, the National Conference of Commissioners on Uniform State Laws adopted a Uniform Brain Death Act. The Act has been suggested for passage to all 50 state legislatures. These Commissioners had earlier proposed the Uniform Anatomical Gift Act, which is now law in every state. It can be expected that the new bill will be influential, particularly in states having no legislation on brain death. Moreover, many states may elect to amend current legislation in order to achieve uniformity or at least substantial conformity in this area. Legislative uniformity has the advantages of minimizing confusion and encouraging interstate cooperation. The Uniform Brain Death Act is very similar in substance and length to the American Bar Association draft noted above. It reads as follows:

> For legal and medical purposes, an individual who has sustained irreversible cessation of all functioning of the brain, including the brain stem, is dead. A determination under this section must be made in accordance with reasonable medical standards.

The American Medical Association recently withdrew its opposition to a statutory definition of brain death. The AMA has prepared a model act on the subject which is substantively similar to the Uniform Act and has suggested a statutory immunity from lawsuits for physicians acting properly under the brain death law.

Some states have adopted a brain death concept by case law. Most of the litigation has involved homicide charges in which the defense has attempted to show that the death was improperly "caused" by the physicians in turning off the respirator after pronouncing the victim dead under a brain death definition. In all such cases in the U.S. and in foreign countries, this maneuver has failed. Nevertheless, attorneys keep asserting this defense in states where brain death statutes have not been adopted. In one of the most important cases, *Commonwealth v. Golston*,[6] the Supreme Judicial Court of Massachusetts limited the acceptance of the definition of brain death to a conviction for homicide. The Court thus left it to the State Legislature to adopt a statute for broader application of the brain death concept.

Constitutionality of Brain Death Laws

It was not until the late 1970s that the basic constitutionality of the brain death statutes was challenged in the courts of the United States. It is fitting that the first and currently the only case involving a constitutional challenge should have occurred in Kansas, the state passing the first brain death law.

In *State v. Shaffer*,[7] the defendant in a homicide case questioned the constitutional foundation of the law on the ground that it was "void for vagueness," or, that the statute was so unclear in its provisions as to be impossible of interpretation in criminal litigation. No criminal law can be so loose in its language as to require readers to guess at its meaning. The two areas of vagueness claimed by the defendant were as follows:

1. that the statute allowed alternative definitions of death, and
2. that the statute did not spell out the necessary criteria for the application of the brain death definition but left these criteria to be determined by "ordinary standards of medical practice."

Both of these challenges were dismissed by the Supreme Court of Kansas. On the first point, the Court found that the alternative method of determining death was supported by modern medical science and practice. It was held by the Court that the State Constitution did not require a single standard to be applied to all human deaths. On the second point, the Court held that the language was sufficiently clear for medical determinations where medical science is subject to change and progress. There are many areas of law where similar phraseology is used. It remains for individual situations to fill in the particulars. It should also be noted that this statute does not require the degree of specificity of a law which makes certain conduct a crime. This statute is intended to be applied by physicians in making declarations of death. Physicians can be expected to understand and apply "ordinary standards of medical practice."

The Shaffer case is also important in having recognized the interrelationship of the declaration of death and the appropriateness of organ transplants from the deceased. The Court expressly recognized the need to keep the heart-lung apparatus functioning and otherwise to prepare the body for the harvest of useful organs for transplantation. For the Court, Justice McGarland observed,

The increasing number of organ transplant operations complicates the situation further as organs such as kidneys may become too damaged for transplant within 5 minutes after the respiration ceases. So for kidney transplants, respiration must continue almost uninterrupted until the kidney is removed.

This part of the Kansas opinion is of great significance for transplant programs since it deals directly with a hidden or "closet" question of this field. Many transplant surgeons were greatly apprehensive about the legality of their procedures for preparing the body and for removing the organs while the donor was still maintained on the respirator. The Shaffer case legitimized this procedure as long as the donor is declared dead under the applicable law of the jurisdiction before any surgery is performed for the removal of the organs for transplantation. After these procedures are completed, the respirator can be turned off and the body can be released. A medical examiner or coroner should find nothing improper in the case if these steps are followed.

Time of Death: Problems of Legal Interpretation

An unresolved issue under the Harvard criteria and under many statutory definitions of brain death is when the death of the person actually occurs. It can be said that the Harvard group expected that the time of death and the pronouncement of the death by the attending physician would coincide. This belief was based on the fact that the Committee had required that the retest of the criteria be made at least 24 hours after the first application of the criteria. The retest was not considered merely confirmatory of the first examination; it was regarded as necessary to establish the irreversibility or permanence of the cessation of brain function. Moreover, selection of the time of pronouncement of death as the time of death is consistent with general medical practice and with death certificate and vital statistics practice, as is pointed out in Chapter 3. However, as the years have passed since 1968, and as pressure has grown to make the retest confirmatory only (or to eliminate it entirely), the tendency has grown to select the time of the first observation of cessation of brain function as the official *time* of death, no matter when the death is pronounced. If brain function is found on a retest, it means either that the patient has regained function or that the earlier observations were incorrect at the time they were taken.

Confusion can also arise if the physicians in attendance allow factors other than the application of the criteria for brain death to come into play before making a pronouncement of death. It is reported that some physicians ask the family or next of kin for their permission or for their concurrence in the pronouncement of the death and the turning off of the respirator. This procedure was specifically condemned by the Harvard Committee, but it is followed by some doctors and hospitals as a means of avoidance of family disputes and litigation. It is also reported that some physicians delay the pronouncement in order to allow a transplant decision to be made, or to permit arrangements to be made for the transplant. In all of these cases, an undetermined amount of time is allowed to pass from the time that the reevaluation is done (or from the time the original observation is made without a reevaluation) and a pronouncement is made. In such a situation, the lack of coordination of time of death and the pronouncement is obvious.

Under the Kansas statute, it is required that time of death occur when "these conditions first coincide." The conditions are that brain death occurs *and* that further attempts at resuscitation or supportive maintenance are found not to succeed. This seems to imply that further application of the respirator is expected, as under the Harvard procedure. Only after the reevaluation gives confirmatory evidence of death would the conditions "coincide." Thus death would occur only after some retesting, though a 24-hour period is not statutorily required.

Under the statutes of certain other states where the Kansas language above is not used, the question may be more difficult to answer. Under the New Mexico statute, which is otherwise similar to the Kansas law, it is provided that death has occurred "when the absence of spontaneous brain function first occurred."[7] It is argued that this takes place when the first observation of all the criteria is made and not at any reevaluation, as long as the reevaluation reaches the same result of no brain function. The retesting is merely confirmatory of the first observation. Thus, if the *time* of death is asked, the answer would be when the first complete observation was made, not when the death is pronounced, if this is at a later time.

Some of the case law has also applied a similar rule, at least where the official pronouncement of the death has been further delayed. In the *Golston* case noted earlier, there was a particularly confused situation. The homicide victim suffered a severe crushing blow to the skull. On August 26, he was examined under the criteria, and no brain function was found. The respirator was turned off for two minutes (according to the Court), and he failed to breath. On August 28, he was again taken off the respirator, and the criteria were applied with no change. After consultation with the family, the respirator was removed on August 31, and the patient's heartbeat and respiration stopped. In the trial court, the attending physician testified that in his opinion the patient was dead on August 26, when the remaining brain-stem functions disappeared and never again appeared. The local medical examiner, however, testified that in his opinion "the victim had been dead since August 28." The medical examiner's opinion would seem to be based upon the confirmatory observations taken on that day. Note that this was 48 hours after the first observations, not 24 hours as in the Harvard criteria. Several other physicians called as expert witnesses on "brain death" indicated that the Harvard criteria were the accepted tests of brain death, and based on these criteria and "observation over a 24-hour period," the victim was dead "by August 28." None of the experts chose to select as the time of death the date when it was officially pronounced, on August 31.

The opinion of the Supreme Judicial Court did not chose between the experts and the attending physician. The only significant point to the Court and to the jury below was that death occurred before the respirator was turned off.

In conclusion, it is apparent that the issue of time of death in brain death cases has not been settled, either in medical practice or in law. Readers are cautioned to examine closely the applicable statutory and case law of the particular state and to observe the practice of the local medical community.

FORENSIC PATHOLOGY ISSUES

Estimation of Time of Death

In any kind of case, no matter what the definition of death, forensic pathologists are often asked to give an opinion on the time of death of a body delivered into their jurisdiction. In most cases, the definitional concepts are not in issue, except as pointed out above. In all situations where a body is examined and the full circumstances of the death are not known and closely observed, it cannot be emphasized too strongly that there is *no accurate method* of making such a determination in our present state of scientific knowledge.

This is well documented by a number of review articles concerned with the problem and the different approaches used to solve it.[8-13] Experience has demonstrated the fallibility of all the methods and dictates that a wide range of latitude be allowed for any of the methods, whether considered individually or in concert. Fortunately, for most practical purposes, establishing a relatively broad time range to encompass the moment of death is all that is needed. Occasionally a more precise determination of the time of death becomes necessary, as illustrated in the following examples from the experience of one of the authors.

Case 1. An elderly gentleman with heart disease was last known to be alive at 9 p.m. and was found dead by the housekeeper of his apartment at 10 o'clock the following morning. The body was cool with appropriate dependent livor mortis, complete rigor mortis, and a vitreous potassium of 7.2 mEq/L.

It developed that the deceased had carried a term life insurance policy for which the last premium had not been paid and in which the grace period for payment expired at midnight on the day of his death. It thus became important for surviving relatives and the insurance company to determine whether death occurred before or after midnight. Both parties were surprised to learn that the author was not able to establish a precise time of death and, in fact, could not even narrow the range of time during which death occurred to a sufficiently small interval to resolve the problem.

Case 2. An elderly couple who had not been seen for over a day were found on investigation by police to be dead from violence. The woman's head was badly battered with massive depressed skull fractures and extruding brain. It appeared from the presence of a bloody trail that she had crawled a distance of approximately 20 feet after receiving these injuries. The man was found dead in an adjoining room from a self-inflicted shotgun wound to the head which would have been instantly fatal. The investigation supported the concept that this was a murder-suicide. Postmortem physical changes in each body were similar, and vitreous potassiums from the two were identical in value.

This was a second marriage for both individuals and each had surviving children from their first marriages. Their wills each directed that in the event of death the estate would be left to the spouse, and it thus became important to the two groups of surviving children to determine who died first. The attorneys for each group of survivors independently sought expert testimony from all over the world to resolve this problem before finally accepting the opinion of the author that for practical purposes the death of the two individuals should be considered to have occurred simultaneously since there was no way in which priority of demise could be legitimately established.

The methods of estimating time of death will be discussed for both the early and late postmortem period. The early postmortem interval is not defined on a time basis, but rather as the period between death and the visible onset of putrefactive changes. The methods commonly used to determine a range of time in which death occurred for this early period includes the classic triad of rigor mortis, livor mortis, and algor mortis, plus other physical factors and certain biochemical determinations. The later postmortem period includes putrefaction, mummification, adipocere formation, and possible timing of the postmortem interval by larvae, botanic specimens, etc.

EARLY POSTMORTEM PERIOD

Rigor Mortis

Following death the muscles of the body pass through three phases. There is an initial flaccidity which occurs immediately after somatic death with the muscles of the body and eyes relaxed but able to respond to electrical or chemical stimuli. The second stage is the onset of rigidity in the muscles, known as rigor mortis, during which there is no longer any response to electrical or chemical stimuli. Finally there is a phase of secondary flaccidity when the rigor mortis passes away that coincides with the onset of putrefaction. The onset of rigor mortis represents a complicated biochemical reaction which is not completely understood. It is recognized that during the development of rigor there is a firm combination of the myocin and actin filaments of the muscle which results in a decrease of extensibility. The linkage between myocin and actin filaments is inhibited by adenosine triphosphate (ATP), and rigor will occur with the disappearance of ATP from the muscle. Simultaneously, there will be a rise in lactic acid and a fall in hydrogen ion concentration due to glycolysis.

The body normally begins to stiffen 2 to 3 hours after death. Since the same postmortem biochemical reaction is presumably going on in all muscles simultaneously, rigor usually becomes apparent in the small muscle groups first and later progresses to larger muscle groups in order of increasing mass. Complete stiffness of the body usually develops in six to eight hours and will commonly remain from 12 to 36 hours before receding in approximately the same sequence in which the initial stiffness occurred.

Unfortunately, both external and internal factors may produce marked changes in the onset and duration of rigor mortis. Cold delays the onset of stiffening and then prolongs the period in which complete rigor exists before flaccidity of the muscle returns (see Case 4). In the frigid climates of a Minnesota winter it is not uncommon for an individual to show complete body stiffness due to freezing before rigor even sets in. In such cases, upon thawing of the body, the onset of rigor mortis will ensue. In contrast to the delaying effect of cold, a hot environment will hasten the onset of rigor.

Several internal factors are significant. The onset of rigor may be delayed in some emaciated individuals and, according to Burton,[11] may even be totally absent in those who are extremely obese. Conversely, infants routinely have a rapid onset of rigor. One of the authors is acquainted with many cases of sudden infant death syndrome where the child has been found in complete rigor less than 2 hours after being placed in the crib, apparently well. Strenuous exercise or terminal convulsions in muscular individuals may cause rigor to develop within a few minutes after death.

The duration of rigor is also variable and is reported to remain over 60 hours after death in some subjects. Such prolonged rigor is well illustrated in Case 4.

Problems connected with the use of rigor mortis for evaluating the time of death are best illustrated by the following examples:

Case 3. An 18-year-old lad was fleeing the scene of a robbery on foot with the police in hot pursuit when he was shot by one of the policemen after running approximately five blocks. The youth died in a matter of seconds. Medical investigative personnel arrived at the scene less than 15 minutes after the shooting, only to find the deceased in complete rigor mortis.

Case 4. During October a 15-year-old lad was found in a wooded area, partially covered by leaves. His hands were bound behind his back and he had been shot six times. The body was remarkably well preserved in all respects. Both the deputy medical examiner at the scene and the pathologist several hours later noticed the presence of rigor mortis involving all large muscle groups. Daytime temperatures during the week preceding the finding of the body varied from 40 to 60°F. The excellent state of preservation, the presence of rigor, and the relatively high daytime temperatures caused the pathologist to inform police that the deceased had probably been dead less than 72 hours. When asked his opinion, the present author fortunately expressed great reluctance to set any time limits. Vitreous potassium was determined to be 26 mEq/L, which was more consistent with the deceased having been dead for over 4 days. Ultimately, investigation established that the youth had been missing for 8 days prior to discovery of the body. Contents of the stomach at autopsy matched exactly the meal given to him by his mother only two hours prior to his disappearance.

In this case, cool earth, with the leaves covering the superior portions of the torso, effectively formed an "ice box" to prevent the onset of putrefaction and thus preserved the state of rigor mortis for a period of at least 7 days following death.

A phenomenon to be considered under the subject of rigor mortis is cadaveric spasm. This has been defined as complete rigor mortis occurring at the moment of death frequently involving only a portion of the body such as an arm. Its existence, at best, is very rare. Polson[14] admits to having seen only two examples in his extensive practice, but gives references to other reported cases. The majority of such reports concern people who are firmly grasping an object when the body is found, and the significance of this presumably is the fact that any injuries caused by the clutched agent (knife, gun, etc.) must have been self-inflicted.

The present author has never seen an example of truly instantaneous rigor mortis, nor has he been able to collect an acceptable example from a large number of professional colleagues in this country with whom he has been in contact. The closest approximation was supplied by Dr. Charles S. Petty, in which a young lady was seen, soon after death from an epileptiform seizure, with a fork firmly gripped in her teeth (Fig. 7-1). However, investigation revealed that this was inserted *after death* while

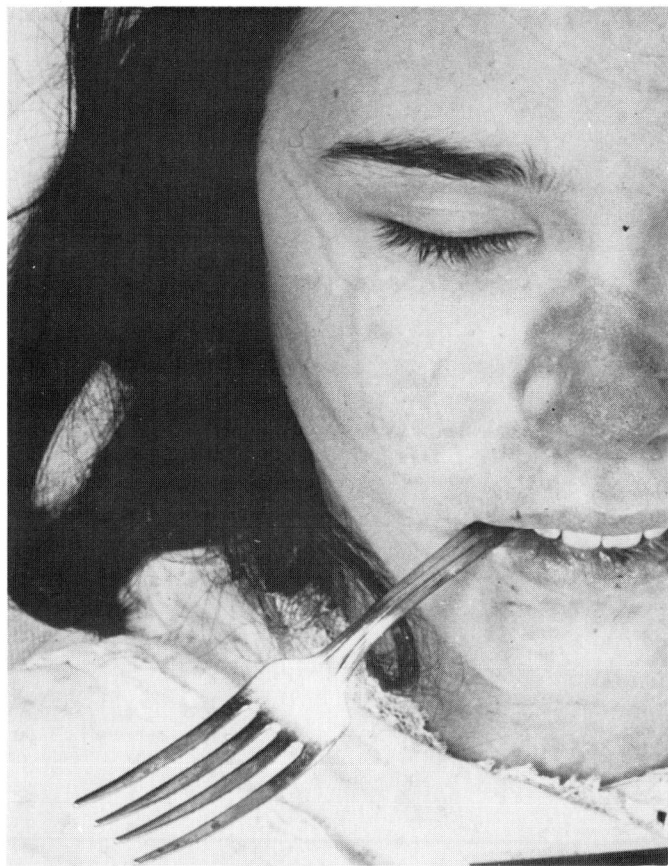

FIGURE 7-1. Fork handle firmly gripped in the mouth of a young woman who had expired only a few minutes earlier during an epileptiform seizure. This was initially thought to represent a case of cadaveric spasm, but investigation revealed that the fork had been inserted between the teeth *after death* while resuscitation was being attempted.

resuscitation was being attempted. It thus represents only an example of very rapid onset of rigor mortis similar to that described in Case 3.

Livor Mortis

After death the blood settles in the capillaries of the dependent parts of the body where it produces a reddish-purple discoloration of the skin called postmortem hypostasis or lividity. Pressure will cause gravitation of the blood into compressed points so that the body will have pale areas wherever the skin is touching an underlying surface or where bound by tight clothing. Thus a supine female dressed in normal attire will usually show blanched areas over the shoulder blades, buttocks and calves, as well as under such constricting garments as a brassiere (see Fig. 7-7B and D).

The postmortem discoloration will usually begin to manifest itself by purplish blotches appearing less than an hour after death. These blotches become increasingly intense and coalesce during the next few hours. The phenomenon is usually complete in 6 to 12 hours and is then said to be "fixed" (i.e., the lividity will not blanch on finger pressure and will not disappear upon changing of the body).

As with all postmortem changes, there is great individual variation so that use of the phenomenon is an unreliable guide to the postmortem interval. Livor may begin before death in severely debilitated patients having a lingering death or in individuals with prolonged terminal hypotension. Its onset frequently appears delayed in the presence of anemia and may never be visible in dark-skinned people. Completion of the process is equally uncertain. Fixation of livor has been observed in a man dead for less than 1 hour in a case discussed by Camps.[8] Conversely, Burton[11] has found shifting livor frequently in bodies moved 24 hours after death. However, once hypostasis has occurred, changing the postion of the body will not completely displace the blood so that evidence of its initial distribution will remain.

For the investigator the principal value in observing livor mortis is to ascertain whether a body has been moved from the position in which it originally lay when life ceased. Further helpful clues may be apparent from the color of the livor since a pink or red discoloration may replace the usual purple color in the presence of carbon monoxide or cyanide poisoning or when the body temperature is near freezing.

Algor Mortis

For many years observers have attempted to use cooling of the body as a means of determining the postmortem interval. Rather extensive scientific work has been carried out on temperature changes involving various areas of the body, and a number of different formulae for determining the postmortem interval have been developed as a result of these studies. In 1958, Fiddes and Patten[15] worked out a formula based on repeated observations of the difference between the rectal temperature and the surroundings in which the assumption was made that the rate of cooling of a dead body would follow Newton's law. However, Marshall,[16-20] in an extended series of studies with several different coworkers, established that a dead body does not obey Newton's law of cooling, but rather that the curve of cooling as measured by rectal temperature has a sigmoid shape with an initial plateau of slow cooling lasting up to 5 hours, followed by a straight portion of varying length and slope corresponding to the period of quickest cooling, and finally a slow falling curve of gradually decreasing gradient similar to that usually associated with the cooling expressed by Newton's law. Under ideal conditions, Marshall was able to develop the following double exponential formula from which a good representation of postmortem body cooling was possible when the height, weight, and external temperatures were known.

$$O = B \cdot e^{-Zt} + \frac{C}{Z-p} \cdot e^{-pt}$$

where O = the temperature excess of the rectum over the environment at time t; and B, C, Z, and p = constants for the corpse under observation.

As Marshall explained, this formula expresses the cooling of a naked corpse lying extended on his back in still air. Its use demands the knowledge of the constants B, C, Z, and p. While these would vary from case to case according to specific circumstances of cooling, sufficient data were available in his controlled experiments for their determination.

Unfortunately, as Marshall himself pointed out, there are a number of factors that make his formula impractical for routine use. First the formula must assume a constant environmental temperature which rarely exists. A change in the ambient temperature of only 5°F during the first 12 hours can introduce an error of ±2 hours when calculations are carried out on rectal temperatures taken 12 hours after death. Secondly, the effect of air movement can distort the values, or the body may well have been moved, clothing disturbed, and the scene generally changed prior to the time that the first rectal temperature could be taken. Finally, there is no way to know what the actual rectal temperature was initially. While it is usually assumed to be 99°F, there can be considerable variation.

Other investigators have felt that cooling formulae obtained from a different portion of the body would give more reliable results. In 1956, Lyle and Cleveland[21] reported that when simultaneous measurements were made on brain, rectum, liver, muscles, and skin, the falling temperature of the brain showed the least scattering and the steepest decrease in the beginning. However, their experiments were also carried out under uniform external conditions. In 1977, Simonsen and associates[22] substantiated the findings of Lyle and Cleveland that the measurements of brain temperatures gave the greatest accuracy in determining the time of death when compared with the fall in temperature of liver, axilla, calf, or rectum. Nevertheless, the technique seemed to be appropriate only for the first 20 hours after death, and Simonsen's group stressed that one factor which could not be calculated was the temperature at the moment of death. Their investigation revealed this to vary enormously. Such variation will make for inaccuracies that far exceed those inherent in the actual measurement of brain temperatures. For this reason Simonsen felt that the determination of the time of death must always be encumbered with uncertainty.

Besides the inherent inaccuracies of the various cooling formulae discussed, there is the very real problem of their practicality. Determination of the time of death using any of the above techniques requires multiple or continuous temperature observations over a period of time. This may be totally impossible because of the situation in which the body is found or the necessity of moving the body before a series of temperature readings can be obtained. Obviously none of the formulae will work where the ambient temperature equals or exceeds the body temperature (see Case 5). Furthermore, one of the authors is acquainted with a number of cases in which terminal temperatures of dying individuals exceeded the extremes given in the articles discussed above. Among these cases are several dying of heat stroke, in one of which the postmortem rectal temperature was observed to rise for over half an hour after death, reaching a high of 110°F rectally before cooling began. Conversely, numerous individuals have been brought into the Hennepin County Medical Center during winter suffering from extreme exposure, in which their temperatures upon entering the hospital were very subnormal. One woman entered the emergency room with a rectal temperature of 65°F and was revived only to die the following day of shock lung. Another patient entered the hospital with a rectal temperature of 67°F and survived to leave the hospital the following week. If either of these individuals had expired with their bodies discovered immediately after death, the temperature readings would have indicated that they had been dead for hours.

As Burton[12] has suggested, it is probable that the observation of heat that can be determined by feeling the body in exposed and unexposed portions, in conjunction with information obtained from the scene, gives as accurate an estimate as should be attempted from algor mortis.

Other Physical Observations

EYE

Observations of the eye reveal that a film will appear over the external surface of the exposed globe in a relatively short time. Cloudiness of the cornea will appear in a few hours to a day, depending upon the position of the eyelids, the temperature, humidity, and air currents. Intraocular pressure falls rapidly in the postmortem period, and attempts have been made to utilize this as an indicator of the postmortem interval. Finally, ophthalmoscopic observation will show segmentation in the retinal vessels and color changes of the different structures. Kevorkian[23] worked out a time table of postmortem color changes by which he felt he could judge the postmortem interval for periods up to 15 hours. However, his observations have not been confirmed by other experienced investigators. Wroblewski and Ellis[24] studied the eyes of 300 dead individuals admitted to a casualty department and were able to examine the fundi in 204 of the subjects. Segmentation was present in one or both eyes in 115, but absent in another 89. Clouding or haziness of the cornea was observed by them at 2 hours in three quarters of the subjects. They concluded that static segmentation was a postmortem change, but that any movement in the columns might be due to persistence of circulation. They felt static segmentation and clouding of the cornea were each indicative of death within the previous 2 hours.

Review of the literature would indicate that the study of the eye is more valuable in determining the presence of death rather than the postmortem interval, and, when used in the latter context, has a very limited time period in which it can be of value.

SUPRAVITAL REACTIONS

Schleyer[9] published, in 1963, an excellent review article discussing the postmortem excitability of muscles by faradic current and pupillary reactions to pilocarpine and homatrophine. The excitability of the smaller muscles of the eye, the mouth, and the hand was measured and gave reasonably constant information about the hour of death, but this was limited to the very early postmortem period and, of course, requires special equipment on the part of the investigator. The pupillary response to drugs requires injection of the compounds in the anterior chamber of the eye, followed by accurate measurements of the dilatation and constriction of the pupil. This procedure also has a very limited postmortem interval in which reactions would be of value, requires equipment at the scene, and contaminates the intraocular fluid from which more valuable data can be obtained by performing other tests.

STOMACH CONTENTS

Stomach contents may be of value in estimating the time of death if it can be compared with a known meal the deceased had eaten. Use of such data depends on the fact that a normal individual will usually empty the stomach in 2 to 3 hours after the last meal. However, experience in living individuals has shown that this time is not constant, and prolonged delays in emptying the stomach may be caused not only by organic disease in the intestinal tract, but also by psychologic factors or physical trauma, particularly to the head.[44] Nevertheless, observations concerning the stomach contents may on occasion be of great value, as illustrated in Case 4 above and Case 6 to follow.

Biochemical Reactions

SERUM AND CEREBROSPINAL FLUID

Mason and associates,[25] Naumann,[26] Fraschini and associates,[27] and Murray and Hordynsky[28] have all reported on the rise of potassium levels in the cerebrospinal fluid with increasing postmortem time. It was viewed as a possible means of determining the postmortem interval, but the results were found to be too erratic for accurate prediction, even in the very early postmortem period. Schleyer[9] found it to be completely unreliable beyond the twentieth hour after death.

Schleyer, in his excellent review article, discusses in detail the chemical determinations in serum and cerebrospinal fluid that have been tested for possible use as a postmortem clock. He has shown that values for aminonitrogen, nonprotein nitrogen, creatine, ammonia, and inorganic phosphorus all have some prognostic value. However, the range of error for each individual test is large. This can be obviated to some extent by combinations of chemical determinations, as shown in Table 7-1. The figures for this table are an update of those originally given and represent Professor Schleyer's opinion at the present time.[29]

TABLE 7-1.

	Time since Death (hours)	
	Maximum	Minimum

Amino nitrogen
  not exceeding 14 mg/100 ml
    (plasma and cisternal fluid)
	10	

Nonprotein nitrogen
  not exceeding 40 mg/100 ml
    (plasma)
  not exceeding 70–80 mg/100 ml
    (cisternal fluid)
	10
	
	24	

Creatine
  not exceeding 6 mg/100 ml
    (cisternal fluid)
  not exceeding 11 mg/100 ml
    (plasma)
	30
	
	28	

Ammonia
  not exceeding 3 mg/100 ml
    (plasma)
  not exceeding 2 mg/100 ml
    (cisternal fluid)
	10
	
	10	

Inorganic phosphorus
  exceeding 15 mg/100 ml
    (plasma and cisternal fluid)
		10

*Data from Schleyer, F.: Fehlerkritisch Betrachtungen über die Todeszeitberechnung anhand biochemischer Komponenten im zisternen Liquor und Serum. *Arch. Klin. Med.* 214:20–23, 1967.

VITREOUS HUMOR

Following Jaffe's[30] recognition that the levels of vitreous potassium would go up with increasing time after death, a number of studies were made verifying the relationship and pointing out the use of such tests in determining the postmortem interval. All of the investigators substantiated that the mean rise in any large group of individuals was arithmetic with time and appeared to be essentially independent of external factors. Sturner[31] and Lie[32] both found such a close correlation between the vitreous potassium concentrations and the postmortem interval that they believed the method could be used with a confidence limit of ±5 hours. They further felt that the standard error did not increase as the death interval lengthened. However, Adelson and associates,[33] Hughes,[34] Hanson and associates,[35] and Coe[36] all found the individual variation was greater than that reported by Sturner and Hughes, being in the neighborhood of ±10 hours in the first day after death. Hanson and associates, and Coe further showed that the standard error then continued to increase with longer postmortem intervals (Fig. 7-2).

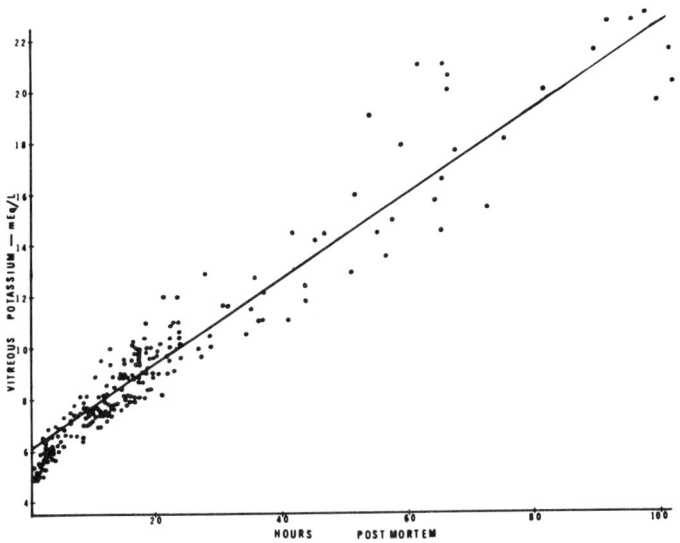

FIGURE 7-2. Vitreous potassium values of normal individuals plotted against the time after death with the line of least squares regression for all values having a postmortem interval of more than 6 hours. The slope is 0.1625 mEq/hr, and the intercept is 6.19 mEq/L. (Coe, J.I.: Postmortem Chemistries on Human Vitreous Humor. *Am. J. Clin. Pathol.* 51:741-750, 1969.)

It is interesting to note that all of the members of the seven original groups reporting resided in cool, temperate climates. This may have accounted for the feeling that individual variations were primarily a manifestation of internal factors within the body rather than the result of environment. In contrast, a recent study by Adjutantis and Coutselinis[37] indicates that the linear increase of vitreous potassium held for only a brief period of 12 hours in the less temperate climate of Greece. Three cases reported by Coe[38] substantiate that markedly elevated environmental temperatures do severely distort the vitreous potassium. The most striking example was the following:

Case 5. A 70-year-old white female went to the sauna in her apartment and was found between 2 and 4 hours later by the engineer of the building when he noticed that her clothing had remained on the outside of the sauna for an unusually long period. When viewed by medical investigative personnel, the body had fallen backward over a bench as shown in Figure 7-3. The temperature in the sauna was approximately 140°F, and the body was hot to the touch, darkly discolored, and showed extensive intravascular hemolysis. Skin bullae were noted

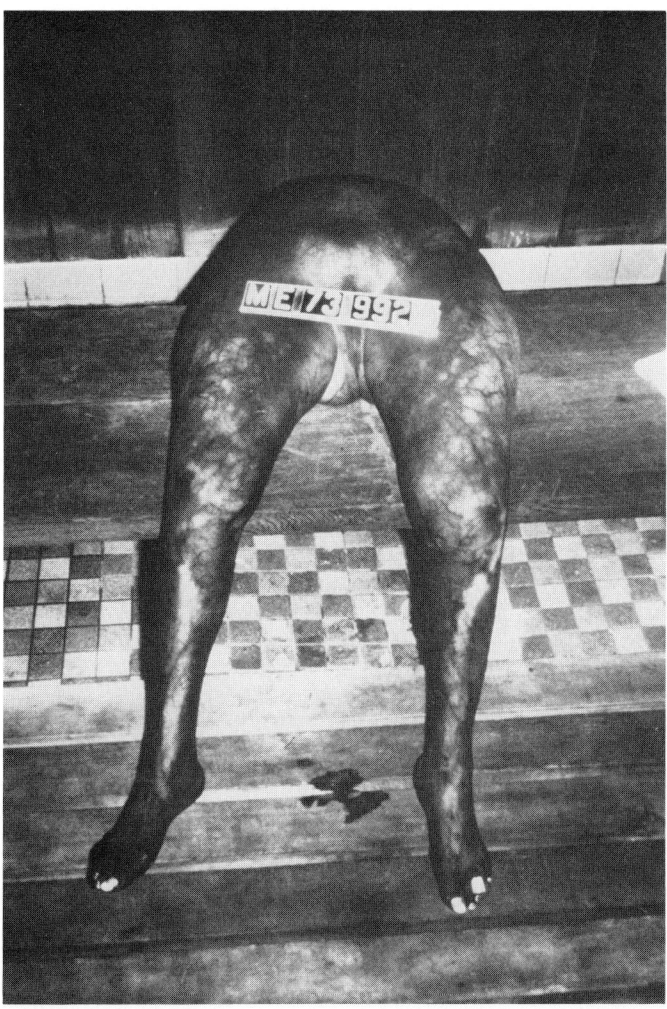

FIGURE 7-3. Body of an elderly female who died of a heart attack in a sauna where the body remained between 2 and 4 hours after death at a temperature of 140°F. Despite the relatively short time between death and the discovery of the body, there were skin bullae, blood-tinged purge coming from the nose and mouth, and extensive intravascular hemolysis. Vitreous potassium was 25.1 mEq/L. This case demonstrates the great rapidity with which all types of postmortem changes can develop in the presence of a high humid temperature.

and there was extensive skin slippage in many areas. Blood-tinged purge was coming from the nose and mouth. The body had the appearance of someone who had been dead for several days. Autopsy revealed severe coronary artery sclerosis and generalized autolysis but no evidence of gas formation. Vitreous chemistries showed a classic decomposition pattern[43] with low sodium and chloride values, while the potassium was 25.1 mEq/L. The vitreous potassium in this case would suggest that death had occurred at least 4 days previously, while it was known that the maximum time between death and obtaining the specimen was less than 7 hours.

While the margin of error is large with the use of vitreous potassium, it appears to be as reliable as the battery of tests suggested by Schleyer. Obtaining the specimens does not delay investigation, as would multiple tests of body temperature, and such specimens are much less likely to be contaminated by postmortem bacterial growth, perimortal injuries to the body, or by trauma in obtaining the specimen. For these reasons, despite the acknowledged limitations of the test, it has become a routine procedure in Hennepin County. In the cool climate of Minnesota there has been a surprisingly good correlation between the level of vitreous potassium and the postmortem interval in adults when unusual circumstances such as those described above have been excluded. The value of the procedure is attested in both Cases 4 and 6, where physical signs indicated a relatively short postmortem interval, while the vitreous potassium correctly indicated that death had occurred much earlier.

LATE POSTMORTEM CHANGES

Putrefaction

Putrefaction represents the process of destruction of body tissues caused primarily by anaerobic bacteria derived from the gastrointestinal tract in which coliform bacilli and *Clostridium welchii* are the principal agents. Other bacteria, molds, fungi, and cellular enzymes may all contribute to the final dissolution of the body's soft tissue.

Putrefaction is usually first evident as a greenish discoloration in the skin of the lower abdominal wall. This spreads to involve the whole of the abdominal wall and ultimately the skin of the entire body. Intravascular hemolysis with decomposition of the blood pigments causes staining of the vessel walls and makes the veins of the skin stand out prominently (Figs. 7-3 and 7-4). Blisters form and there is "skin slippage" in which the superficial layers of the epidermis become loose so that they can be pushed from the underlying tissues with minimal pressure while the hair of the scalp can be peeled off like a wig.

Gas formation causes the body to swell, and the rising internal pressure will cause blood-stained fluid to come from the nose and mouth (Fig. 7-4). This "postmortem purge" is frequently mistaken by the uninitiated for evidence of traumatic injury or gastrointestinal hemorrhage. Ultimately the whole body becomes so swollen and bloated that it is impossible to recognize the features. The tissues then slowly liquify and there is ultimately complete dissolution of all soft tissues.

The speed at which this entire process occurs depends on a number of factors including the condition of the body (state of nutrition, presence of

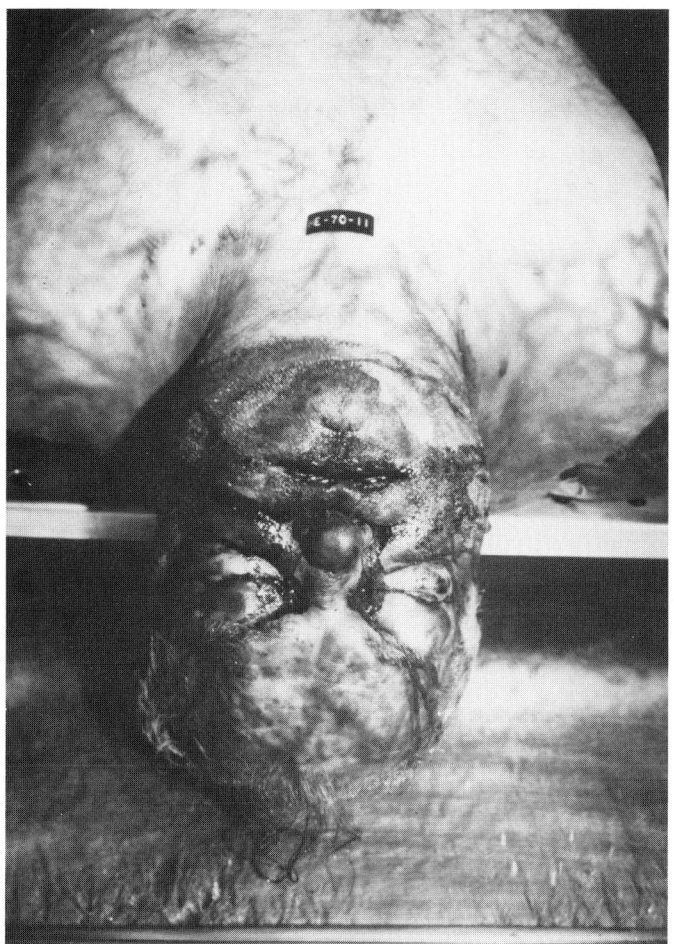

FIGURE 7-4. This body reveals the effects of advanced putrefaction with severe bloating of the trunk, intravascular hemolysis (marbling) in the skin over the shoulders and chest, marked distortion of the facial features by swelling, and the extrusion of blood-tinged material from the nose and mouth (purge). Such postmortem purge may be mistaken for evidence of traumatic injury or gastrointestinal hemorrhage.

terminal septicemia), presence or absence of bacteria, presence or absence of moisture in the air, the medium in which the body lies, and the temperature of the environment. Both Corbin[10] and Polson[14] state that the general discoloration of the skin takes approximately 7 days and the severe bloating that follows several weeks. Unfortunately, as with all previous generalizations concerning the postmortem interval, the factors just listed cause tremendous variation in the speed with which ordinary putrefaction occurs and even determine different forms of postmortem degeneration that may develop (e.g., mummification and adipocere).

The most common factor in distorting the time clock of postmortem change is that of environmental temperature. As putrefactive changes are the result of bacterial growth and biochemical reaction, it is not surprising that a very cool environment will slow down the entire process. This was apparent in Case 4, where there was excellent preservation of the body and maintenance of rigor mortis 8 days after death. It is not uncommon in the bitter Minnesota winters for stranded persons to die of exposure and be frozen. This gives excellent preservation of the body for prolonged periods of weeks or months.

Conversely, when the temperature climbs into the 90s, the author has frequently seen advanced putrefactive changes develop in less than 48 hours. The extreme speed with which changes can occur has already been attested in Case 5, where the high temperatures of a sauna caused extensive postmortem degeneration with marked staining of the vascular system, skin slippage, and bloody purge, all in a period of less than 7 hours from the time of death.

Differences in temperature can cause varying areas in the same body to show different rates of deterioration as shown in Figure 7-5. Here pillows put over and under the deceased's head prevented any circulation of air and caused much more putrefactive change in the face than was present in the skin of the remainder of the body.

The medium in which the body resides after death is also very important in determining the rate of decomposition and to some extent the character of the predominant degenerative process. In general, bodies deteriorate most rapidly in air and remain preserved the longest when buried in the ground. It is commonly stated that 1 week's exposure in air is equivalent to 2 weeks in water and 8 weeks underground. Obviously, such ratios hold only when other factors are constant. We have many examples of bodies deteriorating more rapidly in warm water than corresponding corpses exposed to cool air. Moreover, it is important to know that the body has remained in any single medium during the entire postmortem interval. The confusion that can arise in estimating the time of death under other circumstances is well illustrated in the case report of Majoska and Hololulu,[39] where submersion of a body in lye prior to throwing it into the ocean completely misled the investigators initially.

Mummification

On occasion, in the presence of a dry environment, the usual putrefactive changes will be inhibited and replaced by drying and shriveling of the tissues. This process is called mummification and is rarely seen in the bodies of adults, except in areas where the climate tends to be constantly dry and warm, as in the desert country of Africa or the southwestern United States. It can occur in more humid climates under unusual circumstances and the author is familiar with a case of mummification occurring in an adult who was shot to death and then thrown into a large van that remained unattended for the entire winter period. In this case the body was frozen and putrefactive changes were inhibited by the cold while general desiccation occurred. When the body was discovered in the spring, the extremities showed shrinkage of their normal size, and they were covered by dark brown, leathery epidermis. The skin of the trunk showed less change, but had a parchment-like character. The internal organs were decreased in volume and size, being largely autolyzed, but showed no putrefactive changes.

Such mummification is far more common in newborn infants who have no internal bacterial flora to produce the usual degenerative processes.

The time required for complete mummification of a body cannot be stated. It obviously is influenced by size, atmospheric conditions, and the place of disposal. However, peripheral mummification is a fairly common phenomenon with the trunk showing the usual putrefactive changes,

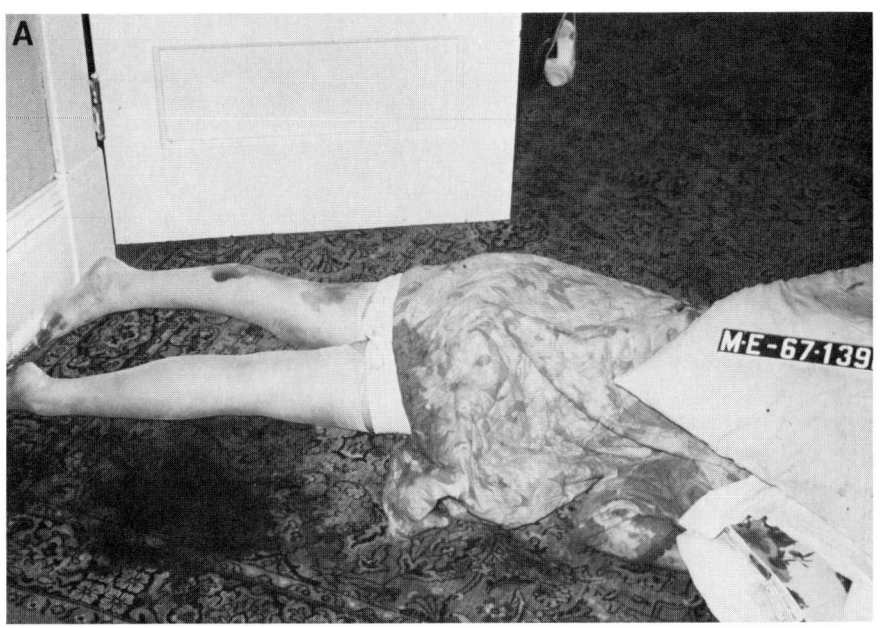

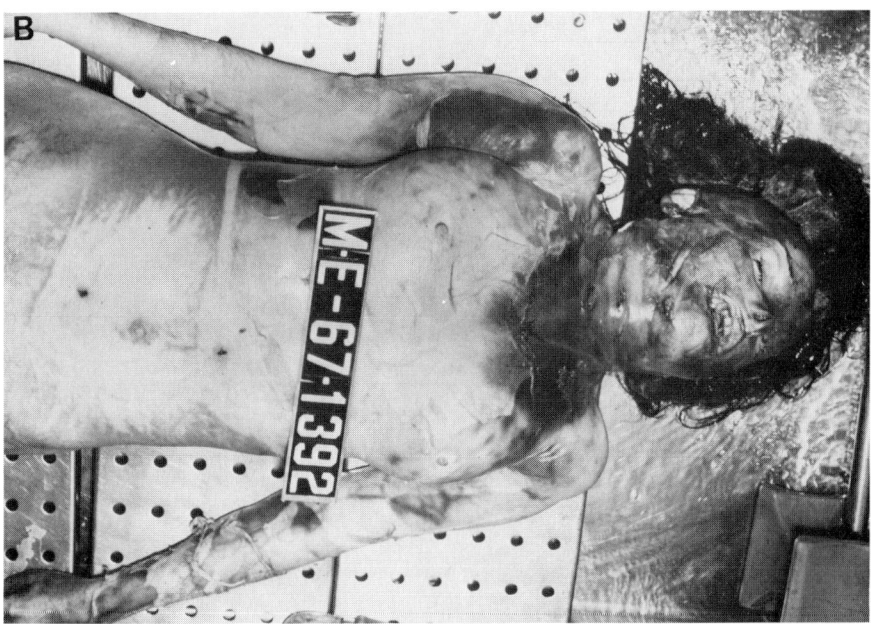

FIGURE 7-5. *A.* The position of a woman as initially seen several days after her death from manual strangulation. It will be noted that the head and upper torso were covered by pillows, and another pillow is extended under the face. *B.* The unequal rate of postmortem degeneration produced by the increased warmth of the portion insulated by the pillows contrasts with the remainder of the body where air currents caused a more rapid cooling of the tissues.

while the distal extremities, in particular the fingers and toes, show the desiccation and leathery changes of an essential drying process. This change involving the hands and feet may be found in people dead only 2 or 3 days.

Adipocere

Adipocere is a variant of putrefaction in which there is hydrogenation of unsaturated body fat into a peculiar, hard, yellowish-white, waxy substance consisting of saturated higher fatty acids. The optimum conditions for the formation of adipocere are apparently a damp, warm environment and the bacterial activity of *Clostridium welchii*. For those interested in the biochemical changes associated with this phenomenon attention is directed to the studies of Evans[40] and Mant.[41]

Although fat hydrolysis may begin within a few days of death, adipocere that can be recognized by the naked eye takes several months to be formed. An example of advanced adipocere is shown in Figure 7-6A. In this particular case the deceased was observed to go into the Mississippi River on May 1, and was recovered downstream on October 22 of the same year. The body had broken apart so that the upper torso and head were missing while the portions shown in the illustration were found as two separate pieces. Identification was established through material in the billfold that the deceased had in his rear trousers pocket, and the syndactylism of the second and third toes of the foot, as demonstrated in Figure 7-6B.

Biology

During warm weather in bodies exposed to various insects, a variety of flies may deposit eggs on the decaying flesh. These will pass through various larval and pupal stages to finally hatch into adult flies. Identification of the species involved and a knowledge of their life cycle will enable the pathologist to establish a minimum period of time which has elapsed since death.

No attempt will be made to take up the identification of the various insects or their life cycles, but the medical practitioner should appreciate their significance and collect specimens for examination by a competent entomologist. For those interested in more detail, an excellent discussion of all the sarcosaprophagous insects has been written by Nvorteva.[42]

In bodies lying in the outdoors during the growing season, information concerning the length of time a body has lain in a particular spot may be apparent from the restriction of growth underneath the body in relation to immediately adjacent plant life. As is true with the use of entomologic data, the use of plant growth to determine a minimal postmortem interval requires a specialist in botany or horticulture, but the investigator is reminded to consider always the possibility that such an expert may be able to give help so that the appropriate person will be called when conditions warrant.

PRACTICAL PROBLEMS

It has been the purpose of this discussion to point out the various physical and chemical techniques that are utilized to determine the postmortem interval and to demonstrate the marked deficiencies of each. Neverthe-

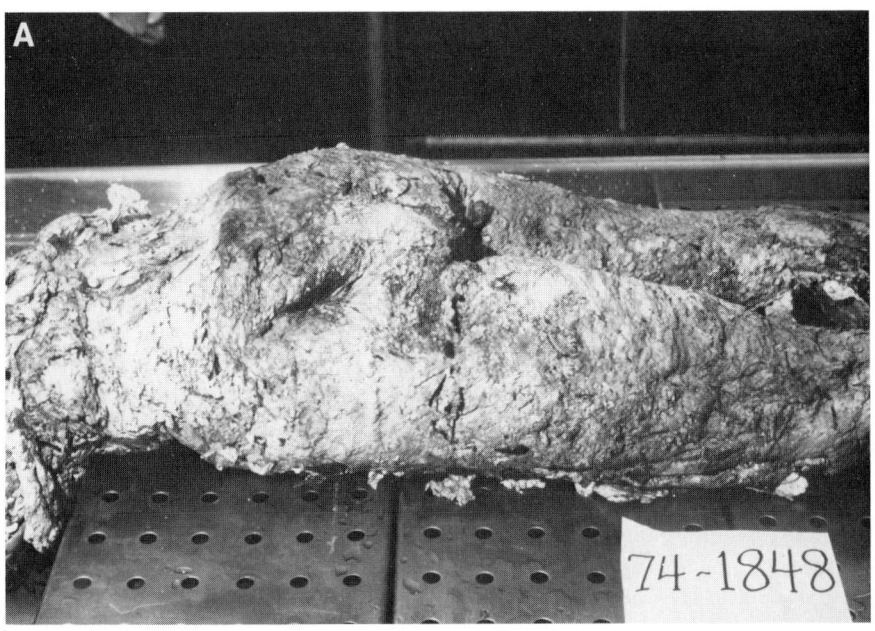

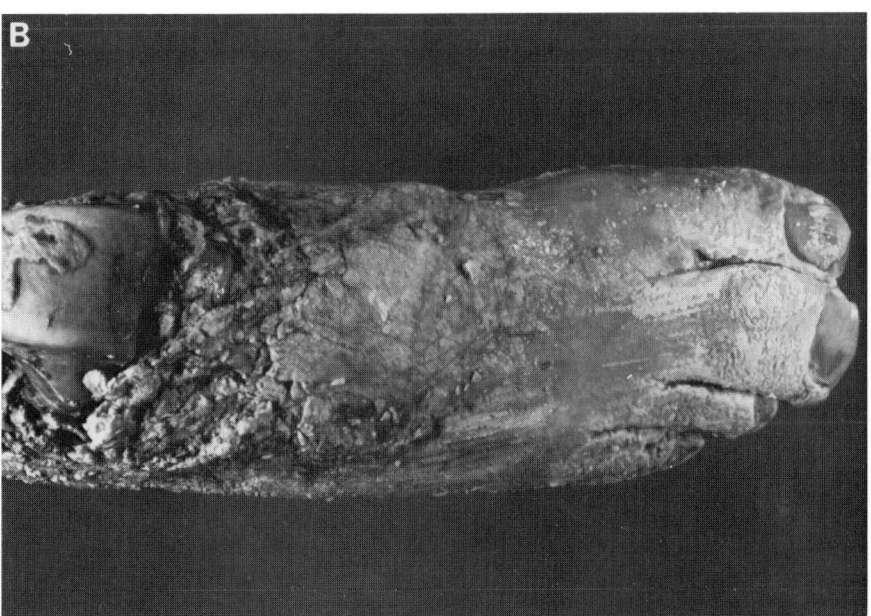

FIGURE 7-6. Advanced adipocere. This man was observed to go into the Mississippi River in early May and was recovered downstream in late October. The body had broken into several pieces with the portions photographed being the only parts recovered. Identification was established through the syndactylism of the second and third toes of the right foot. All fatty tissue of the body had a firm, flaky, white, waxy character.

less, it is frequently desirable for the forensic pathologist to aid police in their investigation by giving at least a range of time which they feel will encompass the moment that death occurred. The investigating officer should always be warned that the range of time provided is at best an educated guess and subject to error. He should thus not limit his investigation based on such an estimate, but utilize it only as it fits into other data that he is obtaining independently.

In providing his estimate, the pathologist is well advised to utilize all the available techniques for each particular case and to consider in his evaluation any factors from the scene investigation that may alter the usual result. Commonly the results from a multiplicity of tests will support each other, but if they are in conflict, an even greater time interval to encompass the projected postmortem interval should be proposed.

The way in which the pathologist can help is illustrated in the following case where several different techniques of estimating the postmortem interval were utilized.

Case 6. The body of a young woman was found by a passing teenager on November 25, as he was walking along the shores of one of the local lakes. When seen by medical investigative personnel, the deceased was lying face down in shallow water, as shown in Figure 7-7A. The deceased was clad in panty hose, a green wool skirt, white panties, a brassiere, and a heavy, long-sleeved, green sweater. The panty hose and panties were in normal position, but the brassiere had been pulled up in back and lifted in front to expose the breasts, as shown in Figure 7-7B. Tissues were excellently preserved, showing no evidence of putrefaction or destruction by aquatic life. The body was at ambient temperature with the water, and rigor had passed away. Livor mortis was fixed posteriorly. Postmortem vitreous chemistries revealed a classic decomposition pattern[43] with low sodium and chloride values and a potassium of 33 mEq/L. Autopsy revealed that the deceased had been manually strangled. The stomach was full of undigested food, as shown in Figure 7-7D.

Recognizing that the cold water would delay the onset and passing of rigor mortis, it was felt that the deceased had been dead for several days. The very high vitreous potassium supported this assumption and was consistent with death 5 to 6 days prior to discovery of the body. This estimate of the postmortem interval was given to police along with three other assumptions based on observation of the body. The first of these was that the deceased had lain for a prolonged period of time (over 12 hours) on her back immediately after death which would account for the fixed lividity apparent in the posterior portions of the body (Fig. 7-7B and C). A second assumption was that the brassiere had been removed from the breasts at a much later period as evidenced by the pattern of livor shown in Figure 7-7B. The last assumption was that death had probably occurred within a few hours after the deceased ate her last meal (Fig. 7-7D).

The police first questioned the young lad who had found the body and got him to admit that he had examined the deceased as she lay in the water, pulling up her sweater and brassiere, before he ever reported finding the body to the local officers. Further investigation on the part of the police established that the deceased had been with a boyfriend 8 days prior to discovery of the body. The boyfriend initially stated that they had gone out to eat, following which he had delivered the

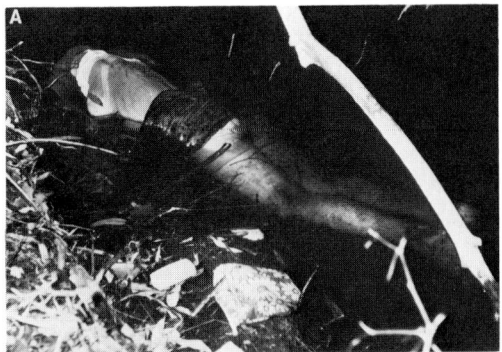
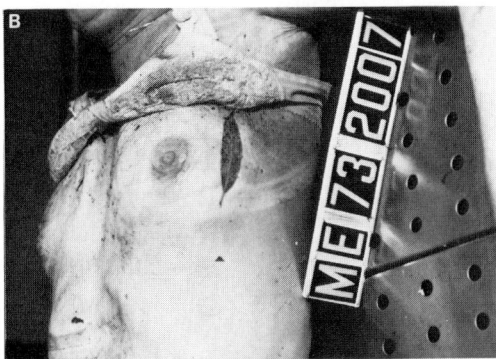
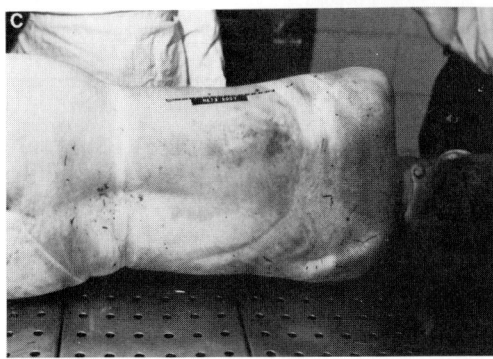
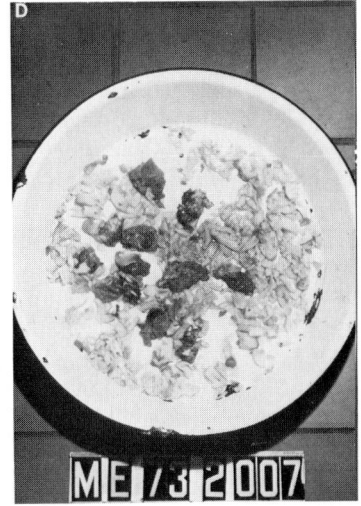

FIGURE 7-7. This young woman had been strangled and the body dumped in a lake, as shown in *A*. The pattern of livor and the intact food removed from the stomach were instrumental in resolving several problems concerning the death.

young woman to her home, and that he subsequently talked with her on the telephone approximately 10 hours later. The meal which he described her having eaten was identical in content to the food found in the stomach. When police confronted the boyfriend with the fact that the deceased had died within a few hours of eating the last meal and thus could not have answered the telephone 10 hours later, he broke down and confessed to having strangled the deceased while they were riding around in his automobile, following the meal. He had left her lying on her back in the rear of his car all that night and the following day. The next night he had taken her to the lake where he dumped the body into the water.

REFERENCES

1. Foster, H. H.: Time of Death. *N.Y. Med. J.* 35:2187–2197, 1976.
2. Madden, J. W.: *Handbook of the Law of Persons and Domestic Relations.* West Publishing Company, St. Paul, 1931.
3. Polson, C. J., and Marshall, T. K.: *The Disposal of the Dead* ed. 3. English University Press, 1975.
4. Beecher, H. K., et al.: "A Definition of Irreversible Coma. *J.A.M.A.* 205:337–340, 1968.
5. Laws of Kansas, Chap. 379, 1970; Revised Statutes of Kansas, Chap. 77, Article 202.
6. *Comm. v. Golston,* Mass. 366 N.E. 2d 744, 1977.
7. *State v. Shaffer,* 574 P. 2d 205, 1977.
8. Camps, F. E.: Establishment of the Time of Death—A Critical Assessment. *J. Forensic Sci.* 4:73–82, 1959.
9. Schleyer, F.: Determination of the Time of Death in the Early Postmortem Interval, in *Methods of Forensic Science.* Vol. 2 Wiley-Interscience, New York, 1963, pp. 253–293.
10. Corby, C.: Estimation of the Time Which Has Elapsed Since Death. *Current Med. Drugs* 3:3–15, 1963.
11. Burton, J. F.: Fallacies in the Signs of Death. *J. Forensic Sci.* 19:529–534, 1974.
12. Burton, J. F.: The Estimated Time of Death, in Wecht C. H. (ed.): *Legal Medicine Annual: 1976.* Appleton-Century-Crofts, New York, pp. 31–35.
13. Van den Oever, R.: A Review of the Literature as to the Present Possibilities and Limitations in Estimating the Time of Death. *Med. Sci. Law* 16:269–276, 1976.
14. Polson, C. J., and Gee, D. J. (eds.): *The Essentials of Forensic Medicine.* ed. 3 (rev.). Pergamon Press, Elmsford, N.Y., 1973.
15. Fiddes, F. S., and Patten, T. D.: A Percentage Method for Representing the Fall in Body Temperature after Death. *J. Forensic Med.* 5:2–15, 1958.
16. Marshall, T. K., and Hoare, F. E.: Estimating the Time of Death. The Rectal Cooling after Death and its Mathematical Expression. *J. Forensic Sci.* 7:56–81, 1962.
17. Marshall, T. K.: Estimating the Time of Death. The Use of the Cooling Formula in the Study of Postmortem Body Cooling. *J. Forensic Sci.* 7:189–210, 1962.
18. Marshall, T. K.: Estimating the Time of Death. The Use of Body Temperature in Estimating the Time of Death. *J. Forensic Sci.* 7:211–221, 1962.
19. Marshall, T. K.: The Use of Body Temperature in Estimating the Time of Death and its Limitations. *Med. Sci. Law* 9:178–182, 1969.
20. Brown, A., and Marshall, T. K.: Body Temperature as a Means of Estimating the Time of Death. *Forensic Sci.* 4:125–133, 1974.
21. Lyle, H. P., and Cleveland, F. P.: Determination of the Time of Death by Body Heat Loss. *J. Forensic Sci.* 1(4):11–24, 1956.
22. Simonsen, J., Voigt, J., and Jeppesen, N.: Determination of the Time of Death by Continuous Postmortem Temperature Measurements. *Med. Sci. Law* 17:112–122, 1977.
23. Kervorkian, J.: The Fundus Oculi as a Postmortem Clock. *J. Forensic Sci.* 6:261–272, 1961.
24. Wroblewski, B., and Ellis, M.: Eye Changes after Death. *Br. J. Surg.* 57:69–71, 1970.
25. Mason, J. K., Klyne, W., and Lennox, B.: Potassium Levels in the Cerebrospinal Fluid after Death. *J. Clin. Pathol.* 4:231–233, 1951.
26. Naumann, H. N.: Cerebrospinal Fluid Electrolytes After Death. *Proc. Soc. Exp. Biol. Med.* 98:16–18, 1958.
27. Fraschini, F., Muller, E., and Zanoboni, A.: Postmortem Increase of Potassium in Human Cerebrospinal Fluid. *Nature* 98:1208, 1963.
28. Murray, E., and Hordynsky, W.: Potassium Levels in Cerebrospinal Fluid and Their Relation to Duration of Death. *J. Forensic Sci.* 3:480–485, 1958.

29. Schleyer, F.: Fehlerkritische Betrachtungen über die Todeszeitberechnungan-hand biochemischer Komponenten im zisternen Liquor und Serum. *Arch. Klin. Med.* 214:20–33, 1967.
30. Jaffe, F.: Chemical Postmortem Changes in the Intraocular Fluid. *J. Forensic Sci.* 7:231–237, 1962.
31. Sturner, W. Q., and Gantner, G. E.: The Postmortem Interval: A Study of Potassium in the Vitreous Humor. *Am. J. Clin. Pathol.* 42:137–144, 1964.
32. Lie, J. T.: Changes of Potassium Concentration in the Vitreous Humor After Death. *Am. J. Med. Sci.* 254:136–143, 1967.
33. Adelson, L., Sunshine, I., Rushforth, N. B., and Mankoff, M.: Vitreous Potassium Concentration as an Indicator of the Postmortem Interval. *J. Forensic Sci.* 8:503–514, 1963.
34. Hughes, W.: Levels of Potassium in the Vitreous Humour after Death. *Med. Sci. Law* 5:150–156, 1965.
35. Hanson, L., Votila, V., Lindfors, R., and Laiho, K.: Potassium Content of the Vitreous Body as an Aid in Determining the Time of Death. *J. Forensic Sci.* 11:390–394, 1966.
36. Coe, J. I.: Postmortem Chemistries on Human Vitreous Humor. *Am. J. Clin. Pathol.* 51:741–750, 1969.
37. Adjutantis, G., and Coutselinis, A.: Estimation of the Time of Death by Potassium Levels in the Vitreous Humor. *Forensic Sci.* 1:55–60, 1972.
38. Coe, J. I.: Further Thoughts and Observations on Postmortem Chemistry. *Forensic Sci. Gazette* 5(5):2–6, 1973.
39. Majoska, A., and Hololulu, T. H.: The Determination of Time of Death in a Case of Suspected Infanticide. *J. Forensic Sci.* 5:33–38, 1960.
40. Evans, W. E. D.: *The Chemistry of Death.* Charles C Thomas, Springfield, Ill., 1963.
41. Mant, A. K.: Recent Work on Post-Mortem Changes and Timing Death. In Simpson, K. (ed.): *Modern Trends in Forensic Medicine: 2.* Appleton-Century-Crofts, New York, 1967, pp. 147–162.
42. Nvorteva, P.: Sarcosaprophagous Insects as Forensic Indicators, in Tedeschi, C. G., et al. (eds.): *Forensic Medicine.* Vol. 2, W. B. Saunders, Philadelphia 1977, pp. 1072–1095.
43. Coe, J. I.: Postmortem Chemistry of Blood, Cerebrospinal Fluid and Vitreous Humor, in Wecht, C. (ed.): *Legal Medicine Annual: 1976.* Appleton-Century-Crofts, New York, 1976, pp. 55–92.
44. Rose, E. F.: Factors Influencing Gastric Emptying. *J. Forensic Sci.* 24:200–206, 1979.

ADDITIONAL READING

Black, P. McL.: Brain Death. Part 1. *N. Engl. J. Med.* 299:338–344, 1978; Part 2. *N. Engl. J. Med.* 299:393–401, 1978.
Capron, A. M., and Kass, L. R.: A Statutory Definition for Determining Death. *U. Pa. Law Rev.* 121:87–109, 1972.
Curran, W. J.: Settling the Medicolegal Issues Concerning Brain Death Statutes: Matters of Legal Ethics and Judicial Precedent. *N. Engl. J. Med.* 299:31–32, 1978.
Hyland, W. F., and Baime, D. S.: In Re Quinlan: A Synthesis of Law and Medical Technology. *Rutgers-Camden Law J.* 8:37–64, 1976.
Sanders, D., and Dukemenier, J.: Medical Advance and Legal Lag: Hemodialysis and Kidney Transplants. *UCLA Law J.* 15:357–407, 1968.
Skegg, P. D. G.: The Case for a Statutory Definition of Death. *J. Med. Ethics* 2:190–192, 1976.
Veatch, R. M.: The Whole-Brain Oriented Concept of Death: An Outmoded Philosophical Formulation. *J. Thanatol.* 3:10–30, 1975.
Wassmer, T. A.: Between Life and Death: Ethical and Moral Issues Involved in Recent Medical Advances. *Villanova Law Rev.* 13:759–770, 1968.

CHAPTER 8

Charles F. Vorkoper is the former Clinical Director of the Suicide Prevention Center of Dallas, Inc. He is a graduate of the Central Lutheran Theological Institute and holds a master's degree in social work from the University of Texas. Mr. Vorkoper is a Past President of the Dallas Chapter of the Association of Humanist Psychology. He is currently engaged in the practice of psychotherapy in Dallas.

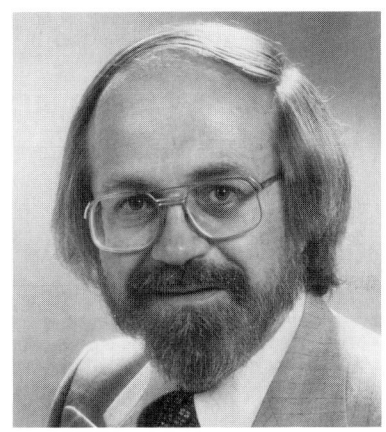

Charles S. Petty is Director of the Southwestern Institute of Forensic Sciences at Dallas, Chief Medical Examiner of Dallas County, Director of the Dallas County Criminal Investigation Laboratory, and Professor of Pathology and Forensic Sciences at the University of Texas Southwestern Medical School at Dallas. Dr. Petty holds degrees in pharmacy and physiology from the University of Washington and received his medical education at Harvard Medical School. He is a diplomate of the American Board of Pathology in pathologic anatomy, clinical pathology, and forensic pathology. Dr. Petty is former President of the American Academy of Forensic Sciences and is a Fellow of the American Association for the Advancement of Science, the American College of Physicians, the American Society of Clinical Pathologists, and the British Academy of Forensic Sciences.

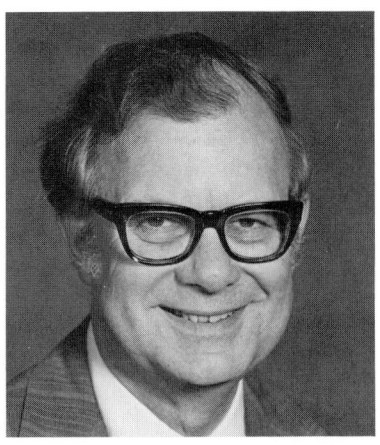

SUICIDE INVESTIGATION

Charles F. Vorkoper, M.S.S.W., and
Charles S. Petty, M.D.

From the point of view of the investigating officer, either law enforcement or medicolegal, each death should be approached as an unexplained death and no more. Much damage has been done to death investigation goals by premature labeling of the manner of death by the first official who views the scene of the death. Instances of snap judgment with actual guessing as to the manner of death are probably responsible for unwarranted and unjust estate settlements in more cases than are caused in any other way. This is particularly true when dealing with situations where suicidal death may be involved.

Off-the-cuff opinion or snap judgment as to whether or not the death is due to suicidal or other means has no place in good death investigative practice. Only after the investigation has taken into account all details should the case be assigned a presumptive or even tentative manner of death. There are many death situations that appear to be of suicidal type but are not. There are also death scenes where the body and the surrounding evidence point to a manner of death that is anything but suicidal, concealing what is in fact an occult suicide.

Numerous commentators have pointed out the risk factors or conditions predisposing to suicide. Since deaths due to suicidal activity are legion (death by suicide ranks among the "top ten killers"), any medicolegal officer dealing with the cause and manner (mode) of death must always be alert to these risk factors or predisposing conditions. Miles[1] estimates that the following percentages of individuals in major disturbance categories will die suicidal deaths:

Primary (endogenous) depression	15%
Reactive (neurotic) depression	15%
Schizophrenia	10%

Opiate addiction   10%
Psychopathic personality   5%

Miles further estimates that some 26,500 individuals with the foregoing conditions might die each year in the United States.

Risk factors have been put in tabular form and each factor assigned a risk potential so as to help physicians, nurses, and others to detect those individuals with the greatest suicidal thrust.[2]

Reference to Figure 8-1, the suicide target clock, shows that at different points from early to late life different suicide risk factors are expected. The teenager cannot compete; the oldster feels his existence is unordered or useless. The death investigator must consider all such factors.

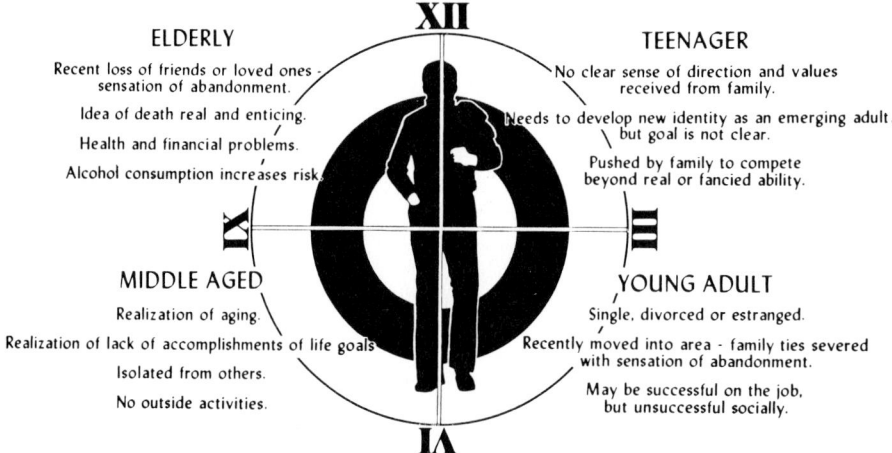

FIGURE 8-1. The suicide target clock. As the individual ages, his reasons for self-destruction may change. Loneliness and sensation of abandonment stemming from inability to make, or cutting off of relationships with others appear to be the common denominator.

THE PHYSICAL SIGNS OF SUICIDE

The death scene examiner finds himself working backward from the fact of death to the cause and manner of death. He no longer has the living person to interview and examine. He has only secondary sources to turn to for information. Some of these secondary sources may already be, or rapidly become, very unreliable. The medicolegal officer has available to him the following:

1. The dead body:
    cause of death
    placement of the fatal wound
    presence (if any) of disease
2. The scene:
    suicide note, record or tape
    position of the locks and access or egress routes
    suicidal apparatus
3. The witness:
    actual, "eyeball"
    telephone
    ear

4. The physician and hospital records:
   medical
   psychiatric
   suicide prevention center
5. Other records:
   school
   employer
   church
6. Relatives or friends

All of these mute or voluble witnesses are subject to misinterpretation by the medicolegal officer and may be a source of deliberate obfuscation on the part of individuals.

There are some guides as to the confidence which may be placed in the information developed as a result of the medicolegal officer's investigation. Suicide may be inferred in the following situations:

1. Suicide note—in victim's handwriting.
2. Suicide tape recording—in victim's voice, recognizable with a voice-print analysis.
3. Body found in room—with dead bolt or chain (not snap lock).
4. Suicide death witness—unbiased, neutral, eyewitness; telephone conversation; or overheard conversation.
5. Firearms discharge—contact wound or soot deposit on body; test for firearms residues on hands yields positive results.

In our experience, however, one of these five telltales of suicide is present in not more than 30 percent of cases where suicide appears to be the manner of death. Only one of those listed should be sufficient to "prove" that a death is suicidal. Sometimes more than one of the proof factors are found upon investigating a single death.

There are certain signs that point to suicide as a manner of death, but do not carry with them the degree of confidence that would enable the medicolegal investigator to come early to the conclusion that the death is suicidal in nature.

1. Wound character (with weapon still at hand):
   position
   "hesitation marks"
   contact gunshot wound
2. Drugs:
   Distribution consistent with apparent ingestion; intravenous, intramuscular, or intraperitoneal administration, complete with marks indicating the route of administration.
   Breakdown products of the drug consistent with recent large dose and not a series of small doses of a cumulative nature.

The distribution of the drug within the body may help to indicate its manner of administration. As an example, the presence of a large amount of unabsorbed drug in the gastrointestinal tract (usually stomach) indicates oral ingestion in large amount. This would point to a suicidal manner of death. The presence of marks due to the administration of drugs via needle (into vein, muscle, or peritoneal cavity), coupled with a very small quantity of the drug in the gastrointestinal tract, would indicate deliberate administration of the drug by parenteral means. If the injection apparatus is still present near the body, the suicidal nature of the death may be inferred.

There is no reasonable basis for the supposition that the fatal wound must have been in a position where the deceased himself could have inflicted it. The mere fact that the wound was located where it could have been self-inflicted does not constitute reasonable proof that the death was suicidal. It should also be noted that contact gunshot wounds are seen on the bodies of homicide victims and that "hesitation marks"* may be part of the wound complex in those dead at the hands of others.

In regard to drug-induced deaths, the distribution of the responsible agent may point to ingestion by mouth or an intravenous administration. Thus it is that when a very large amount of the drug is ingested, death may occur before all of the drug is absorbed from the gastrointestinal tract. A large amount may be expected to be recovered from the stomach, and the concentration of the drug in the liver would be expected to be high in comparison to the concentration in the blood. Similarly, intravenous injection may result in a high concentration of the drug in the lung.

The recent, spectacular advances in the field of forensic toxicology have provided useful tools for the study of drug overdoses. Of special interest is the ability to detect and quantitate certain of the breakdown products of drug metabolism. Since the metabolism of drugs is not an instantaneous matter, knowledge of this process for any given drug may eventually permit an assessment of the time from ingestion needed to degrade that drug and to appearance of breakdown products. The half-life of drugs varies widely from one substance to another. The capability of the laboratory to detect and quantitate the drug and its breakdown products is also most variable. But presupposing a good, well-equipped laboratory with high-level technical ability, the interpretation of the drug-breakdown product(s) (or ratios) may be of great aid in the resolution of a drug-related death. The time from ingestion to death may then be estimated and compared with investigational facets. Thus the old concept of "lethal level" of a drug may be expanded into a much more useful measuring device.

Suspicions of Suicide

Certain types of background information about a subject, brought to light in the course of a death investigation, may raise suspicions of suicide. These include:

1. Recent purchase of weapon employed in death.
2. Previous suicide attempt(s):
    documented history
    indicative scars
3. History of depression:
    change of habits

---

*These are marks which are part of the wound complex that indicate more than one cut, or more than one blow with a chopping instrument, or (occasionally) more than one shot. They are frequently found in instances of suicidal death. The subject may not know precisely where to place the wound to effect death, or may hesitate to cut too deeply because of initial pain; then summoning more courage, the subject makes a deeper cut or changes to a different method.

major recent upset such as divorce, death of close relative, emotional illness and treatment thereof.

Of course, the purchase of a revolver the day before the purchaser is found shot to death with his own brand-new and never before used handgun does not necessarily mean that he is dead of a self-inflicted wound. But it is suspicious. Just because the dead person has multiple, parallel scars on her forearm in the wrist area which seem to be the "hesitation cuts" of a suicide attempt does not prove that she died from a deliberate ingestion of the drug found in her blood stream. But it is suspicious. It is the weight accorded the many small, individual details that eventually tips the balance of the evidence to indicate either a suicidal or nonsuicidal death.

Scene Alteration

One possibility must not be neglected in the investigation of any death which may be of a suicidal nature. This is the alteration of the suicidal death scene inadvertently or deliberately, which may be accomplished by any of the following individuals or groups:

1. Emergency medical personnel
2. Investigatory personnel:
   law enforcement
   fire department
   medicolegal
   insurance
3. News media personnel
4. Relatives of deceased
5. Friends, neighbors, acquaintances
6. Passersby

Inadvertent alteration of the scene is generally one of two types. The first is the result of the emergency precipitated by the finding of a "sick person" or a body. In either instance the emergency personnel are obliged to take action, to provide care for the ill and resuscitation for the dead. Many emergency medical personnel are reluctant to consider the subject dead, not knowing if resuscitative procedures are apt to be effective. Physical evidence at the scene and on the body may be altered, destroyed, removed, or hidden by the actions of the emergency personnel. This is to be expected and perhaps there is little that can be done to anticipate and prevent such changes. The other type of inadvertent alteration is by all manner of persons whose presence at the scene may tamper with evidentiary material there. Here the major cause is lack of sufficient control by the law enforcement officer (or other official) in charge. As an example, the firearm present may be unloaded "to prevent it from injuring someone," thus obliterating fingerprints on the weapon. The ways in which the scene may be altered are clearly too numerous to bear listing here.

Deliberate alteration of the scene in instances of apparent suicidal death is not uncommon. Frequently the relatives of the dead person alter the scene in such a manner as to make the death appear to be something other than suicidal in nature. Many are the reasons for this, but most often these are of five major types:

For insurance purposes: "Suicide clauses," part of most life insurance policies during the first 2 or 3 years of the policy life, may be the reason to alter the scene so as to conceal the suicidal nature of the death. Accidental death or worker's compensation objectives may also motivate the family to alter the scene.

Because of feelings of guilt: Intense guilt feelings of family members may cause them to alter the scene to make the death appear to be of a nonsuicidal nature. Such feelings of guilt may stem from supposedly failing to help or understand the victim better prior to his fatal action, from failing to provide medical aid, or even (in the case of distraught parents) from having conceived the child.

Because of real or imagined social stigma: Among some groups and classes of society, suicide is viewed as an unacceptable act. This may motivate the family to conceal the suicidal nature of the death. The appearance of the word "suicide" on the death certificate may be abhorrent to some individuals.

For religious reasons: Among members of some religious groups, burial in consecrated ground has been denied to victims of suicide. The act of taking one's own life is proscribed in many religious teachings.

Because of wills: Instances have been recorded where the pattern of inheritance depends upon the nonsuicidal death of the person who prepared the will. In such an instance one or another family member may stand to gain or lose to such a degree that concealment of the act of suicide may be desirable.

The methods of concealing a suicidal death are many, but usually one or more of three different techniques are employed:

1. Altering the body:
    concealing the wound
    washing the body to remove blood or vomitus
    taking down the hanging body
2. Removal of items:
    note
    drug containers
    weapon
3. Confusing the scene:
    planting gun cleaning kit
    emphasizing illness of deceased
    not volunteering the actual story

These techniques of concealment and others have been encountered by every experienced death scene investigator. Sometimes they are detected by assiduous death investigations. In other instances the suicidal nature of the death has been stumbled upon. In many cases it undoubtedly remains unsuspected, and the manner of death is improperly determined.

THE PSYCHOLOGICAL SIGNS OF SUICIDE

Suicide is a total act. To develop an understanding of the suicidal act of any person it is important to begin with a clear perspective of the nature of suicide as a psychosocial event. While every aspect of what we will describe does not fit every person who commits suicide, this description has been widely used in suicide prevention centers.

A recent conceptual framework for categorizing suicide was presented by Shneidman.[3] He describes three kinds of suicidal acts. First is the impulsive act. The person responds to a hazardous event by impulsively using any available means to destroy himself. There are many individuals within this group who attempt to commit suicide but who are unsuccessful. The lethality of the means employed probably determines the difference between an attempt and death in many instances.

The second group includes those in whom the idea of suicide comes more slowly. The suicidal act is the high point of the drama. The greatest number of suicidal deaths are in this category. Suicide prevention centers have the greatest success in intervention with such persons. This group will be the focus of our description of suicide as a crisis.

The third group is made up of people who live for years, obsessed with the idea of suicide; theirs is virtually a suicidal career.[4] These people write, think, call crisis centers—in all cases about their suicides. In their eyes suicidal death is commonly perceived as the end of a last poem—the last scene in their personal drama.

Individuals who are subjected to the suicidal impulse, those who have a slowly unfolding suicidal idea or who live their lives on the brink of committing suicide, have certain characteristics which are common to all. These have been well summarized by Shneidman:[5]

1. The period during which the person is very lethal is a relatively short one (usually between 3 hours and 2 weeks). We will describe this in more detail when we discuss suicide as a crisis.
2. Most suicide events are dyadic. Even if the events prior to suicide are in isolation, the tension between two people continues to exist in one person's head. Frequently the tension is in the person's social relations: husband-wife, parent-child, lover-lover, employer-employee, etc. Danto has said that some suicides are "the last word in an argument."[6]
3. The person is ambivalent. He or she experiences strong wishes to die, even making plans to die, while at the same time having fantasies of being rescued. People frequently call suicide prevention centers immediately after they have taken dangerous drugs, an expression of this ambivalence.
4. During a suicidal crisis, a person will express heightened self-hate. This may or may not be the climax of long-term self-destructive experiences. What is significant is the sudden increase of self-hate.
5. The person will also experience an increased "constriction of intellectual focus."[7] While everyone wears intellectual blinders to some degree, in suicidal crisis people narrow their usual focus to only one or two ideas. A common experience encountered during crisis telephone calls is to hear people saying that suicide is the *only* option available to them.
6. The final event prior to a suicide is the idea, firmly implanted in the person's mind, that pain, abandonment, fear, and anger can be ended by terminating life. The person thinks that negative experiences can be stopped by his own action.

With the above lethality scale as a description of the internal world of a person in a suicidal crisis, there are some indicators which point to the greater or lesser possibility that a person will finish a suicidal crisis in death. Table 8-1 gives the lethality scale used by the Suicide Prevention

TABLE 8-1. LETHALITY SCALE*

Assess the lethality of your client as high, medium, or low in each of the 9 categories listed below. Translate the assessment into numbers (1) low, (2) medium, or (3) high and enter the numbers on the client sheet.

	Low	Medium	High
I. Stress	No significant stress	Moderate reaction to loss (loved person, money, status) Sickness (serious illness, surgery, permanent disability) Other significant environmental changes (success, increased responsibility, accident, etc.)	Severe reaction to loss (loved person, money, status, bodily functioning)
II. Communications Aspects	Direct and verbal—to one or more specific persons Direct, open and genuine with staff aides	Have interpersonalized suicidal goal (to cause guilt or force changes in others) directed toward world and people in general	Very indirect and nonverbal (acting out behavior) Have internalized suicidal goal Guilt
III. Age and Sex	Female 15 to 40 years old Male 15 to 34 years old	Female 41+ years old Male 35 to 44 years old	Male 45+ years old
IV. Resources	Help available	Family and friends available but unwilling to help Financial problems	Resources (family, professionals, clergy, employment) not available, hostile, or exhausted
V. Reactions of Significant Others	Ambivalence: responsibility and helpfulness outweigh anger and rejection	Indecisiveness and feelings of helplessness Little feeling of concern or understanding for client	Attitudes injurious to client (e.g., defensive, rejecting, punishing, withdrawn)

Sympathy	Ambivalence: anger and rejection outweigh responsibility and helpfulness	
VI. Life Style		
Consistent work history Stable peer and family relationships Stable personality (no history of prior suicidal behavior, acute onset of symptoms)	Acute suicidal behavior in stable personality Recent increase in long-standing disabling personality traits Recurrent outbreak of moderate symptoms	Suicidal behavior in unstable personality Recurrent outbreak of severe symptoms Severe character disorder, or borderline psychotic Repeated difficulty in peer, family and job relationships
VII. Symptoms		
No significant symptoms	(Moderate degree of "severe" characteristics listed on right) Alcoholism, drug addiction, homosexuality Prior suicidal attempts of low lethality; history of repeated threats and depression	Depression (sleep disorder, withdrawal, anorexia, weight loss, despondency, apathy, feelings of helplessness and exhaustion) Compulsive gambler Prior suicidal attempt(s) of high lethality Severe agitation (tension and anxiety, guilt and shame, hostile and vengeful feelings) Severe impairment of impulse control and judgment Severe frustration of dependency needs
VIII. Medical Status		
Psychosomatic illness (e.g., asthma, ulcers, etc.) Hypochondria (chronic minor illness complaints)	Pattern of failure in previous therapy Repeated unsuccessful experiences with doctors	Chronic, debilitating illness
IX. Plan		
No plan	Bizarre plans Moderately lethal attempt or specific plan	Specific plan and date Method very lethal and available

*Modified from the lethality scale used by the Los Angeles County Suicide Prevention Center.

Center of Dallas. This scale is adapted from forms which were developed in the Los Angeles Suicide Prevention Center in the middle 1960s.

This lethality scale is used by volunteers at the Suicide Prevention Center of Dallas when responding to callers. Each caller is rated as low or high on each item and assigned an overall subjective rating. This aids the volunteer in deciding on a response pattern to the caller. In using the scale it is important to weight the various items according to certain conventions in assessing apparent lethality. In the clinical experience at the Suicide Prevention Center of Dallas, age, sex, marital status, plan, and resources are weighted heavily, the remaining indicators less so.

A clinical observation about time of lethality is important. When a "lethal" person is deeply depressed, he is less likely to act on a suicidal idea than when his depression is "lifting" and his energy level is raised. A common experience is for people to be less concerned when a friend or family member becomes more alert and less depressed. These same people are later shocked to find that person dead. This observation is important in intervention tactics and in assessing statements of survivors of an apparent suicidal death.

THE CRISIS OF SUICIDE

Contemporary suicide prevention and intervention are based on the crisis theory and method which grew out of the studies of Lindemann after the Coconut Grove fire in Boston in 1943,[8] and, following Lindemann, the work of Caplan.[9] It is common clinical practice to assess suicidal lethality in all crisis situations in crisis intervention work. In reverse, the act of suicide is done in response to a crisis. This is particularly true of suicide as an impulsive and transient act.

In working with an apparent suicidal situation an understanding of the nature of crisis is important to assess the behavior of the participants. Crisis is a human event that is time-limited (extending from a few hours to a few months) in nonextraordinary situations. It is started by a hazardous event (defined as hazardous by the person in crisis). Immediately after the hazardous event the person's personal equilibrium is upset. Frightening and numbing sensations will be experienced. Persons cannot solve problems in their usual way (beginning of a narrowing of intellectual focus in suicidal crisis). People perceive a loss or threatened loss of something important (person or object). The resolution of a crisis can be useful or destructive, depending on the means and resources used by the person. It is important that people learn crisis skills so that they will use their resources when crises develop and thus learn to cope with possible future crises. What is critical is that people learn to pull toward interpersonal relationships in time of crisis, not away from these relationships.

Phases of Crisis

The crisis experience follows a broad pattern in the lives of most people. The *initial* phase is one of shock—with physical collapse, outbursts, dazed withdrawal, and denial as common experiences. The person's body (mind) is reacting to the hazardous event by shielding the person from its full impact.

The *second* phase is an extended cyclic period of intense release of feelings, regain of control, problem-solving, and then feelings released with loss of control. The pattern of behavior during this period is probably related to certain patterns learned very early in childhood. Most people depend on coping methods that they used in childhood to manage this period.

The *last* phase is the renewal phase in which the person renews social links to the outer world, rebuilds an inner world, and regains usual skills in problem-solving.

Handling the Family

Understanding this crisis process is critical in dealing with the families of suicide or suspected suicide victims. If a medical examiner is attempting to glean information from a family member after a suicidal death, the phase of crisis must be assessed: if the person is in the first phase of crisis, information gathered must be only tentatively relied upon. Reliable information and certainly a response to the request to assess the situation cannot be expected until the second phase has developed (usually initiated by an intense release of feelings). Understanding is also important in realizing that sensitivity and wisdom are the keys to making a powerful positive impact on the person in crisis. Frequently, sensitivity and wisdom are as important as education and technical knowledge (if not more so) in dealing with people in crisis. As has been stated earlier, if suicide is clearly indicated or evidence points to suicide, there are some important things to know and essential directions to follow. While every family is different, there are some general guidelines that grow out of our knowledge of the dynamics of crisis, grief, and mental health.

GENERAL GUIDELINES

When you begin your investigation with the family, explain what you are doing in simple terms. If there is the appearance of a suicide and the family appears willing to accept this fact, tell them calmly and professionally what you know the facts to be and what your conclusions are. Suggest that they may get help in this crisis from appropriate agencies, friends, clergy, or therapists.

If there is the suspicion of suicide and the family seems hostile, angry, or blank, you should first collect evidence. Ask questions about the past lethality of deceased. Ask how other people (friends and relatives) have reacted. Such people tend sometimes to absent themselves (emotionally, intellectually, or literally) in the case of a suicidal death or what appears to be such a death. Indicate to the families what you know about grief and crisis, and reassure them that what they are experiencing is natural and not uncommon. Suggest that they seek counseling if they seem open to the idea.

The family of a suicide experiences a double crisis. On top of the grief process that accompanies all of the reactions to loss is the added burden of the response to suicide. Families frequently are anxious about their possible role in the suicide. They want to know: "Is there something I could have done?" Conversely, some families and individuals respond by telling you that they are glad the deceased finally did it. They may be stung with the experience of the suicidal death as the "last word" in an argument and thus feel defeated. Families of those who commit suicide frequently are isolated from family friends, churches, and neighbors, and this experience generates a heightening of normal responses to grief. In addition to such factors, these people have lived with a person who has acted in the ways described above, and now they feel abandoned. It is essential to understand this reaction because such people are very vulnerable to committing suicide themselves. There is a strong possibility that their resources, both internal and community, are depleted. Knowing this will help you to respond to a family in a way that will be more likely to enlist their cooperation rather than their opposition.

DEALING WITH DENIAL

Any investigator of a suicidal or potentially suicidal death who must relate to the family should have a general idea of the process of grief because it must affect the investigation. The grief process begins with denial. People will block feeling, thoughts, and opinions from their consciousness. Some people experience numbness internally, and others experience a strange kind of unreality in their behavior.

There is no good way for an investigator looking for facts on which to base a decision to break through this shock mechanism. It may last from a few minutes to several days. Awareness of this process will help sensitize the investigator to the possibility that these people have literally blocked from their awareness something the investigator knows and wants to confirm or something that is suspected. It will not help to pursue or attack individuals experiencing the denial phase of the grief reaction. If there is something needed from a person in shock that he has not already reported, the only options are to wait until the shock phase is finished or to help that person enter the next phase.

EMOTIONAL RELEASE PHASE

When a grieving person finishes the denial phase, emotional release is experienced. It is a time when feelings are again accepted and reactions to those feelings are experienced in a full way. The person may express a wide range of emotions, including deep sorrow, anger, and fear.

Except during emotional outbursts, information can be obtained during this phase. A sensitive, caring approach to the persons grieving will produce the best results. It must be remembered that such people are now in a volatile emotional state. As previously noted, the grief process consists of general stages. The first period is one of shock-denial (the period of numbness). The second, acute stage lasts from 3 to 6 months. It is here that the worst anguish is experienced and the healing process gradually begins. This renewal stage follows an up and down pattern which is very individual. There will be unusual physical symptoms such as insomnia, indeterminate pains, and dietary changes. The third stage, beginning approximately 6 to 12 months after the suicidal death, is a time of reorientation and renewed stability.[10,11]

SIZING UP THE FAMILY

Short of a psychological autopsy, which Robert Litman describes in Chapter 36, it is important to evaluate the family to assess their reactions to the suicidal death and their involvement with the victim. There are some specific issues to keep in mind. The first is to notice how tightly this family lives together. It will be useful to know how tightly or loosely related this family is when there is no crisis. If the family is close-knit and tightly related to one another, working with the whole family in concert during the investigation will be productive. With the tightly related family, the possibility of a "family secret" structure will block responses of individuals confronted separately for fear that they will violate the family secret code. If the relatedness is loose, investigation with individual family members can be most productive.

The second issue is to notice the degree to which the family is being isolated. Families having experienced the suicidal death of a member will frequently be isolated from friends and resources such as church, family, and usual social contacts. Isolated persons from such families are unusually vulnerable to suicide themselves.

Families will frequently blame anyone who enters their door for the death of the family member. The families of adolescents who commit suicidal deaths are frequently especially hostile to police, medical examiners, and others who must undertake the investigation.[12] The process is one in which their frustration and self-blame is transferred to any figure of authority. The issue is not to respond personally to this blaming, but to respond to the awareness that this is a projection of the family member's self-blame and guilt.

If one experiences great difficulty in getting past the shock experience and tears, it would be useful to ask about former losses in the family. When people have had little previous experience they will probably demonstrate a higher degree of shock, but when there is unresolved grief from past losses, there may be exaggerated responses.

The circumstances surrounding the suicidal death are another variable in the response of the family. This will be very individual, ranging from someone dying alone to someone leaving an argument and committing suicide in full view of the family so as to have the last word.

FAMILY AMBIVALENCES

Just as a person thinking seriously about suicide experiences heightened ambivalent feelings, so a family member who survives a suicidal experience has conflicting thoughts. Both sadness about the loss and anger because the family member committed suicide will be experienced. Such persons are frightened about their own future and feel hopeless about any efforts to help the dead person. This ambivalence is a normal part of the grief process.

It is a good plan to inquire about earlier suicidal deaths in the same family. While suicide is not genetically determined, a suicidal death in a family will sensitize the whole family to suicide. What seems to happen is that the dead person gives a kind of permission for others to use suicide in that family as a way to act when life gets too difficult to endure.

FAMILY ASSESSMENTS: GENERAL CRITERIA

In a study which sought to describe and identify the healthy family, Lewis and coworkers[13] developed a scale to rank families. There are indicators which can be used to develop a picture of the health and/or pathology of any family to be studied. These are applicable to assessment of the family of a potential suicide victim. There is a range of behavior between the two statements made after each item.

1. *Power structure:* In healthy families leadership is shared between parents. In pathologic families there is absolute, dominant rule or chaos.

2. *Closeness:* In healthy families there is a high degree of closeness with each person demonstrating a separate identity. Pathologic families are "too close." There are indistinct boundaries between each member. In the middle of this spectrum are families whose members tend to stand apart from each other.
3. *Goal-directed negotiation:* Healthy families have devised efficient problem-solving processes. Pathologic families are inefficient problem-solvers.
4. *Communication of self-concept:* In healthy families, people communicate their feelings and thoughts clearly. In pathologic families, such communications are unclear and poorly expressed.
5. *Permeability:* Healthy families are open and receptive to each other. Pathologic families are unreceptive and closed to others.
6. *Expression of feeling:* Healthy families openly and directly express and verbalize their feelings. Pathologic families do not express their feelings unless they explode or become emotionally incapacitated.
7. *Mood and tone:* Healthy families are warm, affectionate, humorous, and optimistic. Pathologic families tend to be cynical, hopeless, and pessimistic.
8. *Conflict:* In healthy families there is conflict, but it is quickly resolved. In pathologic families, conflict leads to severe impairment of group functions.

For additional assistance we suggest that families get in touch with their local crisis telephone service, suicide prevention center, or crisis agency. Some of these centers have programs for the relatives of those who have committed suicide. They work with these "survivors" in groups, individually, in the home, or by telephone. They are trained to help persons and families work through their grief and feelings surrounding the suicidal death. Most of these centers operate with volunteer staffs, and it would be useful for medicolegal investigators to build a relationship with such centers so that the cooperation of volunteers can be secured.

HOMICIDE-SUICIDE PACTS

It might appear that the reaction of family and friends to homicide-suicide pacts would be quite different than that following a sole-victim suicide. Such is not the case. Any differences are probably more connected to the loss of two or more relatives or friends and the more involved investigation and greater publicity accorded the multiple deaths. In some instances the suicide victim, by his homicidal act, provides in himself a scapegoat for the use of the surviving family members.

There is an extensive literature dealing with various phases of suicide, including methods, prevention, and vital statistics, and with suicide as related to the young, the old, the middle aged, and to disease, stress, death certification, etc. No attempt will be made here to examine this extensive bibliography. This chapter deals with what the investigator of suspicious deaths should be aware of, in order to be able to carry out his charge.

REFERENCES

1. Miles, C. P.: Conditions Predisposing to Suicide. A Review. *J. Nerv. Ment. Dis.* 164:231, 1977.

2. Horoshak, I.: How to Spot and Handle High-Risk Patients. *RN* 40:58, 1977.
3. Shneidman, E.: A New Conceptualization of the Basic Components of the Suicidal Act. Presented at the May 1977 meeting of the American Association of Suicidology, Boston.
4. Alvarez, A.: *The Savage God, A Study of Suicide.* Random House, New York, 1972.
5. Shneidman, E.: An Overview of Suicide. *Psychiatric Ann.* 6:13, 1976.
6. Danto, B.: Post-Suicide Survivors: Bereavement. Workshop presented at the May 1977 meeting of the American Association of Suicidology, Boston.
7. Shneidman, E.: Psychological Theory of Suicide. *Psychiatric Ann.* 6:51, 1976.
8. Lindeman, E.: Symptomatology and Management of Acute Grief. *Am. J. Psychiatry* 101:141, 1944.
9. Caplan, G.: *Principles of Preventative Psychiatry.* Basic Books, New York, 1964.
10. Freese, A.: *Help for Your Grief.* Schocken Books, New York, 1977.
11. Westberg, G. E.: *Good Grief.* Fortress Press, Philadelphia, 1962.
12. Hatton, C. L., Valente, S. M., and Rink, A.: *Suicide Assessment and Intervention.* Appleton-Century-Crofts, New York, 1977.
13. Lewis, J. M., et al.: *No Single Thread.* Brunner-Mazel, New York, 1976.

CHAPTER 9

L. Maximilian Buja is Associate Professor of Pathology at the Southwestern Medical School of the University of Texas Health Science Center in Dallas. After graduating from Loyola University in New Orleans, Dr. Buja entered Tulane University, taking his medical degree in 1967, and a master's degree in anatomy the following year. Between 1972 and 1974, Dr. Buja was a senior investigator at the National Heart and Lung Institute in Bethesda, Maryland. He was also a surgeon in the Commissioned Corps of the U.S. Public Health Service between 1968 and 1974. In 1972, Dr. Buja became a diplomate of the American Board of Pathology.

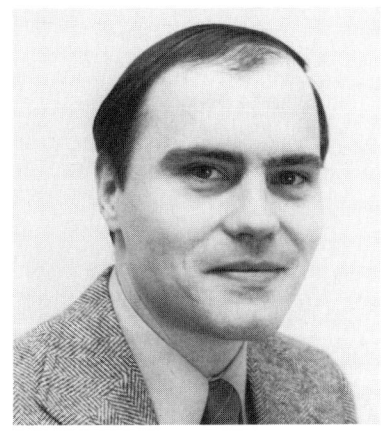

Charles S. Petty is Director of the Southwestern Institute of Forensic Sciences at Dallas, Chief Medical Examiner of Dallas County, Director of the Dallas County Criminal Investigation Laboratory, and Professor of Pathology and Forensic Sciences at the University of Texas Southwestern Medical School at Dallas. Dr. Petty holds degrees in pharmacy and physiology from the University of Washington and received his medical education at Harvard Medical School. He is a diplomate of the American Board of Pathology in pathologic anatomy, clinical pathology, and forensic pathology. Dr. Petty is former President of the American Academy of Forensic Sciences and is a Fellow of the American Association for the Advancement of Science, the American College of Physicians, the American Society of Clinical Pathologists, and the British Academy of Forensic Sciences.

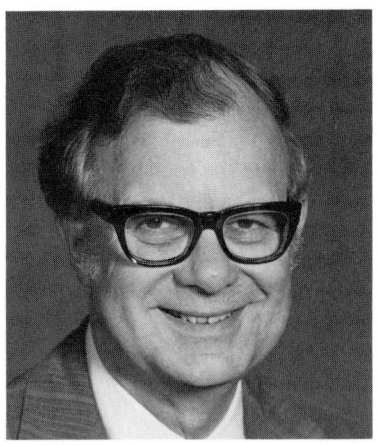

HEART DISEASE, TRAUMA, AND DEATH

L. Maximilian Buja, M.D., and
Charles S. Petty, M.D.

The forensic pathologist is frequently confronted with cases of fatal trauma in which autopsy reveals significant cardiovascular disease. In these situations, difficulty frequently is encountered in determining whether death was due to trauma and not immediately related to heart disease or whether cardiac disease was the primary factor causing death and initiating the accident. This chapter presents an analysis of the problem and an approach for determining the cause of death in cases of concurrent trauma and heart disease.

AUTOPSY PROCEDURES

Objective documentation of findings at autopsy is essential for determination of the role of heart disease in fatal trauma. The autopsy must include meticulous documentation of traumatic lesions and an appropriate toxicologic evaluation. These aspects of the forensic autopsy are discussed in detail in other chapters of this book. In this chapter, emphasis will be placed on the cardiovascular examination as it relates to the forensic autopsy.

Autopsy data should be gathered so as to exclude the presence of significant cardiovascular disease or to arrive at a diagnosis of a specific type of cardiovascular disease, which may be classified as shown in Table 9-1.

Much has been written about appropriate methods for autopsy examination of the cardiovascular system.[1-3] It is not our purpose to argue the pros and cons of specific autopsy methodology or to establish any rigid criteria for the cardiovascular examination. Nevertheless, we believe that the cardiovascular examination should provide information regarding certain essential points. These include documentation of the following: (1) any extracardiac vascular lesions, such as ruptured berry aneurysm or

TABLE 9-1. ETIOLOGIC CLASSIFICATION OF CARDIOVASCULAR DISEASE

Arteriosclerotic
Hypertensive
Valvular
Pulmonary (cor pulmonale)
Congenital
Degenerative:
   cystic medial necrosis (with or without dissecting hematoma)
   other
Inflammatory or Infectious:
  infective endocarditis
  myocarditis
  other
Traumatic
Neoplastic
Cardiomyopathy:
  idiopathic (primary)
    congestive
    hypertrophic
  secondary (associated with other cardiac lesions or systemic disease)

acute dissecting aneurysm or hematoma of the aorta; (2) cardiomegaly (dilatation and/or hypertrophy); (3) extent of coronary artery disease, primarily coronary arteriosclerosis; (4) extent of myocardial necrosis, fibrosis, or other lesions; (5) valvular or congenital cardiac lesions; (6) degree of generalized arteriosclerosis; and (7) extent of arteriolonephrosclerosis in excess of age-related change as an indicator of the duration and severity of systemic hypertension.

Examination of the Coronary Arteries

Since coronary artery disease is a leading cause of sudden death, the autopsy examination must provide an accurate evaluation of the coronary arteries. Recommended techniques for postmortem documentation of coronary artery disease range from classic and simple methods of coronary examination to relatively elaborate methods involving postmortem angiography and special dissection techniques.[1-5] Coronary examination has been further complicated by the advent of coronary bypass surgery, which has become one of the most frequently performed operations in this country.[6] Although the more elaborate postmortem techniques can provide much valuable information, especially for research purposes, we believe that many of these procedures are impractical for a busy general or forensic pathology service and that sufficient information can be gained by careful application of classic techniques.

The autopsy report should include a description of any significant variations in cardiac anatomy, such as anomalous origin of a coronary artery from the pulmonary trunk or major anatomic variants such as single coronary artery or left coronary preponderance.[7] The autopsy report also should contain descriptions of the presence or absence of acute coronary lesions, which may include various combinations of plaque rupture, plaque hemorrhage, and thrombosis[8] as well as an evaluation of the extent and severity of old arteriosclerotic disease. The severity of coronary disease is best categorized by grading the maximal degree of luminal narrowing of each of the major coronary arteries, including the left main, left anterior descending, major left diagonal and marginal branches, and the left circumflex and right coronary artery and its major branches. Although the exact point at which coronary luminal narrowing becomes clinically important has not been established definitively, available experimental evidence indicates that significant coronary blood flow reduction generally requires a narrowing of the vascular luminal area of at least 75 percent, which is equivalent to concentric narrowing of the luminal diameter by at least 50 percent, according to the formula $A=\pi(d^2/4)$.[9-12] Nevertheless, coexistent cardiovascular lesions, such as severe anemia, cardiomegaly, hypertension or valvular stenosis, may increase the functional significance of a given obstructive coronary lesion. Examination of the myocardium for evidence of fibrosis or necrosis can provide useful information in determining the functional significance of coronary arterial lesions, although the absence of grossly obvious myocardial lesions does not necessarily exclude the presence of significant coronary artery disease.

Of the two standard methods of coronary examination—namely, opening the coronary arteries in a longitudinal manner, versus cutting the coronaries in cross section at multiple levels and at intervals of 2 to 5 mm—the latter method in our experience is a much better approach for the estimation of the extent of luminal narrowing. Cross-sectioning of the coronary arteries, however, becomes increasingly more difficult according to the severity of coronary calcification, a phenomenon which is a frequent complication of coronary arteriosclerosis that increases progressively with age. In the face of extensive coronary calcification, coronary cross sections usually have to be cut at wider intervals, and this technique may then be combined with longitudinal dissection. In this circumstance, coronary examination can be aided by careful exploration with a small-bore probe prior to dissection of each segment. It must be stressed that the extent and severity of coronary arteriosclerosis can be easily over- or underestimated unless classic dissection methods are employed with meticulous attention to technique. In addition, the prosector should not fail to make a careful examination of the coronary ostia, since ostial stenosis may represent the most severe or only site of significant coronary disease in some cases.

Comprehensive examination of the coronary arteries is best achieved by combining gross study with microscopic study of appropriate histologic sections. Histologic examination is particularly helpful in documenting the nature of acute coronary lesions and, specifically, in determining whether an obstructive or occlusive lesion is due to plaque rupture, plaque hemorrhage, and/or thrombosis. In the absence of acute lesions, histologic sections can provide permanent documentation of sites of maximal coronary luminal narrowing by old arteriosclerotic plaques. Segments for histologic examination, especially those containing acute lesions, should not be repetitively sectioned at gross examination. Instead, these segments should be removed from the heart, fixed in formalin, and *decalcified* prior to histologic processing.

Characterization of Cardiomegaly

The autopsy report should include the following information: (1) a statement as to whether the heart is normal in size and shape, dilated and/or hypertrophied; (2) a designation of which cardiac chambers are dilated or hypertrophied; and (3) a description of any grossly visible areas of patchy myocardial fibrosis or necrosis or of discrete, subendocardial or transmural, old or recent infarcts.

One of the most useful pieces of information to be gathered at autopsy is an accurate heart weight obtained after extraneous debris has been dissected from the heart and blood removed from its chambers. Considerable data have been obtained regarding total heart weight and weights of individual ventricles.[1-3,13] Some controversy exists, however, regarding the exact criteria to be used for normal heart weight and cardiac hypertrophy. Some authors have proposed that the diagnosis of cardiac hypertrophy should be based on various ratios, including heart weight to body length or heart weight to body weight.[1-3,13] In our experience, cardiac hypertrophy in individuals of relatively normal size can be considered to be present with heart weights of 300 gm or greater in adult females, and 350 gm or greater in adult males. It is clear, however, that cardiac hypertrophy can exist at lower heart weights, especially in small, malnourished, or emaciated individuals. Furthermore, some evidence indicates that a mild "physiologic" hypertrophy, resulting in increased heart weights up to 500 gm, can occur in athletes and other individuals engaged in chronic strenuous physical activity.[13-16] For more detailed information, the cardiac weight tables in the standard texts should be consulted.*

Once an evaluation of cardiac size and coronary disease is made, further dissection of the heart is performed. Again, no one method of cardiac dissection is required; however, the two most commonly used approaches involve opening the heart according to direction of blood flow or cutting the heart into multiple transverse sections, the so-called bread-loafing technique. The latter method has the advantage of allowing a more thorough examination of ventricular myocardium for areas of scarring or necrosis. Although measurement of the circumference of the valve rings is a time-honored procedure, the information obtained has been shown to be of little value in assessing valvular insufficiency or chamber dilatation.[17] Measurement of wall thickness is a more useful procedure when combined with an overall assessment of the pattern of cardiomegaly. Upper limits of normal are usually taken to be 12 to 15 mm for left ventricle, and 5 mm for right ventricle.

We believe that accurate assessment of the pattern of cardiomegaly is extremely helpful in arriving at a specific cardiac diagnosis (Table 9-2 and Fig. 9-1). Selective or predominant right-sided cardiac dilatation without hypertrophy is indicative of acute cor pulmonale, usually secondary to acute pulmonary thromboembolism.[18] Right-sided cardiac hypertrophy usually occurs with variable dilatation and is characteristic of chronic or chronic and acute cor pulmonale. Cardiac dilatation with left-sided involvement in the absence of hypertrophy is indicative of acute cardiac failure and is characterized by a normal heart weight, chamber enlargement, and reduced thickness of the wall, and may be accompanied by a distinct softness and flabbiness of the myocardium.[14] This pattern of cardiomegaly is frequently caused by acute or subacute myocarditis, infective

---

*A good guide to "normal" heart weights, and "allowable" variations from the expected weights, may be found in the tables by Reiner and associates and Zeek for adults, and by Schulz and Giordano, Gruenwald, Naeye and Letts, Roessle and Roulet, and Keen for infants and children. To conserve space, the tables are not reprinted here, and the interested reader is directed to the original papers. The texts by Gould and by Pomerance and Davies reproduce the most useful tables.

TABLE 9-2. CLASSIFICATION OF HEART DISEASE ACCORDING TO THE PATTERN OF CARDIOMEGALY

No cardiomegaly:
  normal heart
  coronary artery disease
Cardiac dilatation without hypertrophy:
  coronary artery disease
  acute or subacute myocarditis
  infective endocarditis
  acute valvular incompetence
  acute cor pulmonale (selective or predominant right-sided involvement)
  other causes of acute cardiac failure
Cardiac hypertrophy without dilatation:
  hypertension (with or without coronary artery disease)
  valvular stenosis
  hypertrophic cardiomyopathy
Cardiac hypertrophy and dilatation:
  coronary artery disease
  hypertension (end-stage)
  chronic valvular incompetence
  congestive cardiomyopathy
  cor pulmonale (selective or predominant right-sided involvement)

endocarditis, or cardiac failure secondary to acute valvular insufficiency or coronary artery disease.

Concentric hypertrophy represents a distinctive pattern of cardiomegaly which is characterized by a relative or absolute increase in cardiac weight, a small cardiac chamber, and a symmetrical, excessively thickened chamber wall. This type of cardiomegaly is caused by processes which impose a chronic pressure load (afterload) on the involved ventricle. Concentric hypertrophy may be caused by valvular stenosis and, most commonly in forensic practice, by systemic hypertension. Cardiac

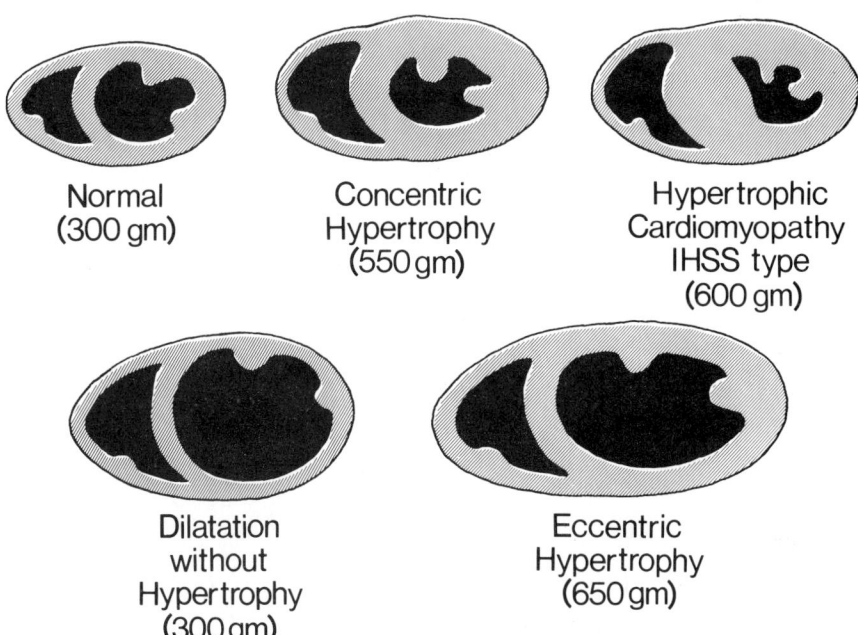

FIGURE 9-1. Patterns of cardiomegaly shown in transverse sections through the cardiac ventricles. Values in parentheses represent corresponding heart weights.

hypertrophy of the concentric type represents one of the earliest responses to systemic hypertension and may be found without other hypertensive lesions, such as arteriolonephrosclerosis.[19]

Another category of cardiomegaly, sometimes referred to as eccentric hypertrophy, is characterized by a combination of increased cardiac weight and generalized cardiac dilatation or specific chamber dilatation.[14] Even though the heart weight is increased, the involved chamber wall has a normal or decreased thickness because of the dilatation. Myocardial scarring, of variable degree and usually patchy in nature, frequently occurs in hypertrophied, dilated hearts, even in the absence of coronary arteriosclerosis, especially if the heart weight exceeds 500 to 600 gm. The causes of eccentric hypertrophy are multiple. This type of cardiomegaly may be due to chronic valvular insufficiency secondary to chronic rheumatic valvulitis or other causes. Cardiac failure superimposed on chronic coronary heart disease or hypertensive heart disease also can produce eccentric hypertrophy.[19,20] Finally, cardiomegaly with eccentric hypertrophy is the typical finding in cases of congestive cardiomyopathy or primary myocardial disease.[22-44] Although a specific etiologic diagnosis usually cannot be made, the two factors most frequently implicated as causes of idiopathic congestive cardiomyopathy are alcohol (alcoholic cardiomyopathy) and viral infection. It has been our experience that cases of hypertrophied, dilated hearts frequently are diagnosed as hypertensive heart disease on the basis of insufficient evidence, and we believe that such cases are best designated as congestive cardiomyopathy in the absence of definitive evidence of hypertension or significant coronary artery disease.

Additional comment is warranted regarding two other types of heart disease which have not received sufficient recognition as causes of sudden death. The first of these has been variously designated as floppy mitral valve disease or myxomatous (mucoid) degeneration of the mitral valve.[25-28] The gross morphologic changes are characterized by thickening and elongation of the chordae tendineae and mitral valve leaflets, particularly the posterior leaflet (Fig. 9-2). Histologically, the process is characterized by accumulation of loose, myxoid connective tissue and, in late stages, dense fibrous tissue, and by primary involvement of the fibrosa of the valves. In contrast to chronic rheumatic valvulitis, general valvular architecture remains intact.[25,26] The usual clinical findings in a patient with a floppy mitral valve consist of a midsystolic click and late systolic murmur (Barlow's syndrome). Patients with this syndrome are subject to arrhythmias and sudden death.[28] Sudden death also has been documented in individuals with hypertrophic cardiomyopathy.[23,24,29,30] The hypertrophic cardiomyopathies include idiopathic hypertrophic subaortic stenosis (IHSS) and less well categorized entities.[23,24,29] Classic IHSS is characterized grossly by disproportional ventricular septal thickening without chamber dilatation (see Fig. 9-1), and microscopically by a bizarre, disorganized arrangement of hypertrophied muscle fibers in the ventricular system.[23,24,29,31] Other cases of hypertrophic cardiomyopathy may lack the classic gross findings of IHSS and may exhibit a more generalized distribution of the disorganized muscle fibers (Fig. 9-3). The hypertrophic cardiomyopathies usually have a familial occurrence.[29,32]

Examination of the Myocardium

In cases of suspected heart disease, it is useful to supplement careful gross inspection by light microscopic examination of representative histologic

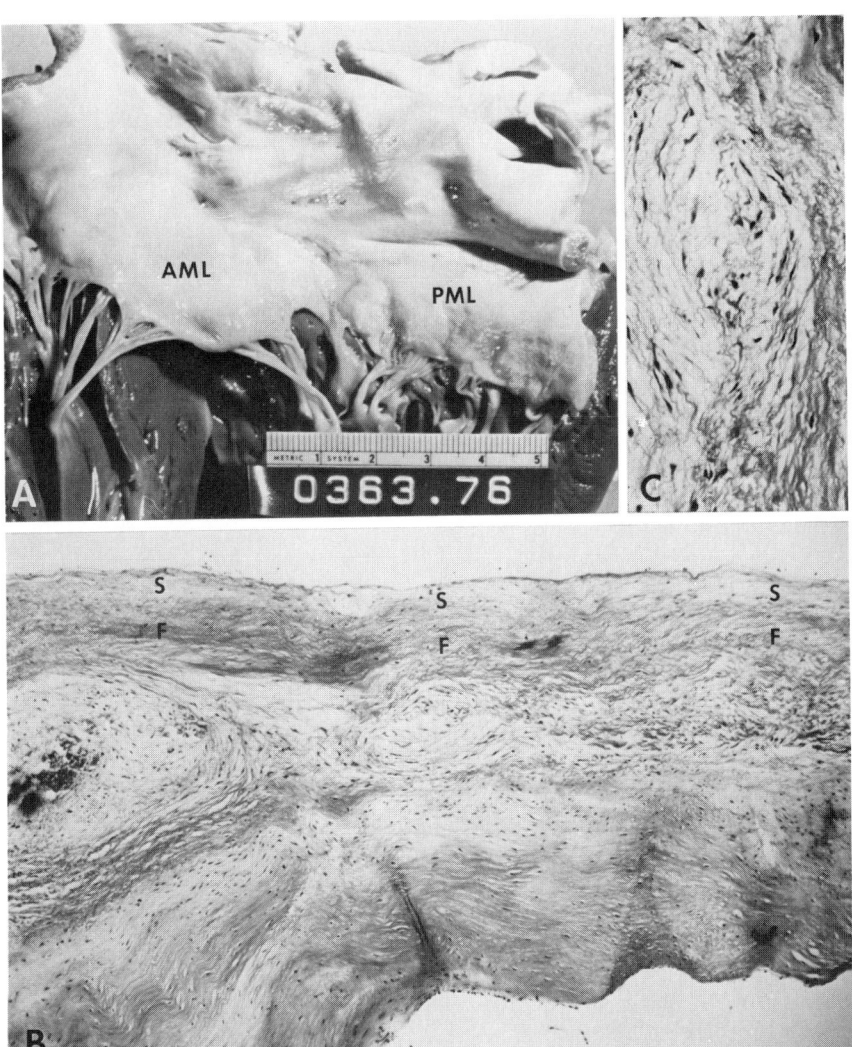

FIGURE 9-2. Sudden death in a 28-year-old white man with myxomatous (mucoid) degeneration of the mitral valve (ME 2402-75). *A.* The mitral valve shows thickening and elongation of the chordae tendineae and leaflets. Note the distinctly abnormal finding of a posterior mitral leaflet (PML) equal in length to the anterior mitral leaflet (AML). *B.* Histologically, the spongiosa (S) of the leaflets is intact, but the fibrosa (F) is markedly thickened due to accumulation of loose mucoid and dense fibrous tissue. *C.* Higher magnification view of the characteristic mucoid tissue. (*B*, hematoxylin and eosin stain ×66; *C*, hematoxylin and eosin stain ×166.)

sections of myocardium, with particular emphasis on the left ventricular wall. Histologic examination is important for evaluating the extent of myocardial fibrosis (particularly interstitial fibrosis which might not be obvious grossly), the pattern of myocardial hypertrophy (Fig. 9-3), the presence of inflammatory infiltrates indicative of myocarditis, and the presence of myocardial necrosis. Documentation of myocardial necrosis, however, becomes increasingly difficult as the interval between onset of irreversible myocardial injury and death shortens. It is generally recognized that histologic diagnosis of myocardial necrosis cannot be made

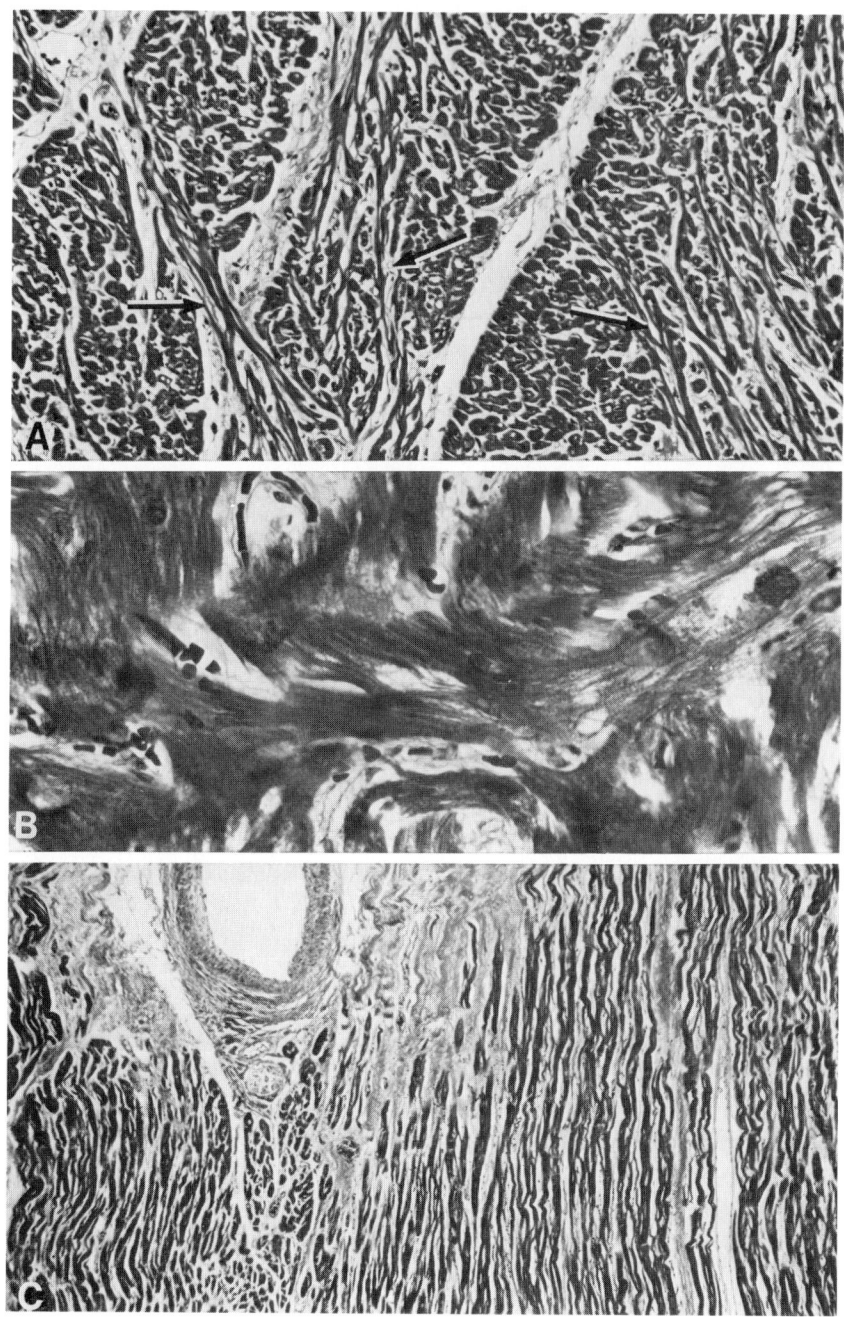

FIGURE 9-3. Sudden death in a 6-year-old black girl with hypertrophic cardiomyopathy (ME 1753-75). The heart weighed 160 gm (expected weight 82-101 gm), but the ventricles were not dilated. There was no evidence of disproportional septal thickening. A. The myocardium throughout the left and right ventricles shows a disorganized arrangement with criss-crossing of muscle bundles (arrows). B. This high magnification view shows the bizarrely shaped, hypertrophied muscle cells charcteristic of hypertrophic cardiomyopathy. C. Section of control ventricular myocardium from another patient shows the normal parallel alignment of muscle cells. (A, hematoxylin and eosin stain ×166; B, hematoxylin and eosin stain ×425; C, Masson trichrome stain ×66.)

with confidence if the interval between onset of myocardial necrosis and death is less than 6 to 8 hours.[33,34] Documentation of myocardial infarcts of somewhat longer duration also can be complicated by the problem of sample selection since gross changes of myocardial infarction usually do not become obvious until approximately 24 hours after the onset of necrosis. Localization of early myocardial infarcts over 6 to 8 hours old can be aided by incubation of gross heart slices in tetrazolium solutions.[34,35]

A variety of staining and histochemical procedures, including hematoxylin–basic fuchsin–picric acid (HBFP) and other methods, have been tried as aids in the diagnosis of early myocardial infarction. In general, however, histochemistry has been found to be unhelpful or unreliable in the definitive diagnosis of early acute myocardial infarction, particularly in the most difficult category of lesions less than 6 hours old.[36-39] The finding of wavy myocardial fibers also appears to be nonspecific.[40,41] Measurement of myocardial electrolyte abnormalities appears promising, but needs further evaluation in the forensic autopsy setting.[42-46]

Some additional comments are warranted to place into proper perspective the problem of pathologic documentation of acute myocardial infarction in forensic pathology. Recent clinicopathologic studies have now made clear, as forensic pathologists have long maintained, that the vast majority of cases of sudden death prior to hospitalization in patients with coronary heart disease are not associated with acute coronary occlusion and do not occur during early stages of classic acute myocardial infarction.[47-50] Rather, sudden death prior to hospitalization in patients with coronary heart disease usually results from ischemia-induced electrical instability of sudden onset, most often ventricular fibrillation.[47-50] Acute coronary thrombosis is more likely to be found in a patient with acute myocardial infarction, particularly transmural infarction, than in the patient with a sudden death–ventricular fibrillation syndrome.[51,52] These recent studies have reinforced the role of acute coronary thrombosis in the pathogenesis of transmural acute myocardial infarction.

Examination of the Cardiac Conduction System

In order to perform a thorough examination of the cardiac conduction system, serial histologic sectioning and examination of the conduction tissue are required.[3,53-55] It is evident that serial sectioning of the conduction system is not a feasible undertaking as a routine procedure in a forensic or general autopsy service. Nevertheless, sudden cardiac death can result from certain relatively rare disorders involving the conduction system, such as Wolf-Parkinson-White syndrome and prolonged Q-T syndromes.[56] The decision to perform histologic examination of the conduction system rests with the discretion of the individual pathologist during the evaluation of a given case of sudden death.

THE SCENE INVESTIGATION AND HISTORICAL DATA

A general conclusion from the above discussion is that autopsy examination of the cardiovascular system can document the presence of relatively chronic cardiovascular disease which may be responsible for sudden death, but such examination alone cannot confirm that the cardiac disease in fact gave rise to pathophysiologic phenomena which caused death.

The major cardiac causes of pain, fear, apprehension, and those sensations that cause dysfunction or inability to respond to a demanding situ-

TABLE 9-3. CARDIOVASCULAR CAUSES OF SUDDEN DEATH

Carotid sinus syncope
Stokes-Adams attack
Paroxysmal dysrhythmias
Aortic stenosis
Pulmonary stenosis
Severe pulmonary hypertension
Left atrial myxoma
Cardiac tamponade
Constrictive pericarditis
Muscular infundibular stenosis (hypertrophic cardiomyopathy)
Barlow's syndrome (floppy mitral valve syndrome)

ation may occur without a definite anatomic counterpart. Table 9-3 lists many of these entities and points out how few can be recognized by autopsy techniques alone. Not discussed in this chapter are those other causes of loss of control (such as epilepsy) which might eventuate in an accident of fatal nature. Designation of cardiovascular disease as the primary cause of death with reasonable certainty requires evidence confirming an association between symptoms and signs of acute cardiac dysfunction and death (Table 9-4). In forensic pathology, this task is often not easily accomplished, and it becomes especially difficult in cases associated with accidents or trauma.

For complete evaluation of a case of sudden death, the autopsy examination should be supplemented by a thorough scene investigation, including documentation of the physical surroundings of the death as well as collection of historical data from any witnesses of the death. This is important for all cases of sudden death, whether or not trauma or accident is associated. The latter point may be emphasized by consideration of the rare but real category of instantaneous physiologic death due to vasovagal reaction or ventricular fibrillation. Requirements for this diagnosis include witnessed sudden death in tense circumstances devoid of immediate physical trauma and autopsy examination excluding any morphologic lesions or toxicologic abnormalities.[57]

In cases of concomitant heart disease and trauma, evidence obtained from witnesses may provide convincing evidence of the primary cause of

TABLE 9-4. OBSERVATIONS PERTINENT TO DIAGNOSIS OF THE PRIMARY CAUSE OF DEATH IN CASES OF CONCOMITANT CARDIOVASCULAR DISEASE AND TRAUMA

Observations favoring cardiovascular disease as the primary cause of death:

1. Witnessed historical observations of symptoms, signs, actions, or inaction consistent with acute cardiac dysfunction preceding accident
2. Physical evidence from scene investigation consistent with acute cardiac dysfunction preceding accident
3. Autopsy documentation of a specific cardiovascular disease
4. Secondary considerations
   a. Autopsy documentation may or may not reveal potentially lethal traumatic lesions
   b. Toxicologic examination may or may not be abnormal

Observations favoring accident or trauma as the primary cause of death:

1. No evidence of acute cardiac dysfunction observed by surviving witnesses (internal witnesses) or bystanders (external witnesses)
2. No evidence of acute cardiac dysfunction obtained from scene investigation
3. Toxicologic evaluation may (or may not) be abnormal
4. Autopsy may reveal potentially lethal traumatic lesions

death. Cardiac disease can reasonably be considered the primary cause of death on the basis of observations by witnesses of symptoms and signs of acute cardiac dysfunction which preceded an accident and appeared to cause the victim to perform inappropriate actions or fail to react. Such evidence would include reports that the victim complained of severe chest pain or headache or clutched the chest prior to apparent loss of consciousness.

The witness has a key role to play in the unraveling of the accident being caused by death, disability, pain, syncope, contusion, or fear due to cardiovascular disease or heart disease. Because witnesses are human, the statements made must not be taken at face value. The account given by the witness may be accurate and true, or it may be a grossly distorted story. Variations from the truth may be deliberate or they may be the result of honest mistake, poor observation, or carelessness. The witness who deliberately slants his story so as to conceal the truth or part of the truth may do so because of fear, desire to gain, or the wish to protect someone. The historical data may be influenced by considerations relating to whether the witness was a participant in the accident (internal witness) or a bystander (external witness). The task of the medical examiner or other investigator into the facts surrounding the accident is difficult. The truth may never be ascertained, even after the most meticulous investigation.

Many cases of sudden death may go unwitnessed, or the witnesses may die in the ensuing accident. In these cases, certain physical evidence may point to cardiac disease as the primary cause of death of the chief victim of an accident (Fig. 9-4). This would include autopsy documentation of significant cardiovascular disease, the absence of potentially lethal traumatic lesions at autopsy, and evidence collected at the scene of inappropriate response in the circumstances of an accident. In the face of such evidence, the primary cause of death of the principal accident victim may be reasonably designated as heart disease of a specific type determined by the autopsy examination.

Investigation into the past medical history of the apparent accident victim with concomitant heart disease is another route to be explored. Clues to heart disease precipitating the accident may be sought by examination of hospital, clinic, and physicians' records maintained on the deceased individual. Heart disease history denied by surviving relatives may be uncovered. Again, as in the case of witnesses, denials by family members may be deliberate with intent to cover up, or made in ignorance of the true physical condition of the dead person. Many an individual has concealed his illness from his spouse and children.

In accident or trauma cases without historical or physical evidence of acute cardiac dysfunction prior to initiation of traumatic events, we believe the reasonable procedure is to assign accident or trauma as the primary cause of death and to consider chronic cardiac disease as a secondary diagnosis.

Four brief case studies are given below. They are in two groups. The first pair illustrates the severe motor vehicle crash precipitated by heart disease but without injury, and the converse. These cases underscore the need for investigation as well as for autopsy. The leading case is also used as an illustration of what we consider a reasonable and sufficient description of the autopsy and subsequent microscopic examination of the heart.

The second pair of cases are presented as examples of a different type of heart disease. Both victims had widespread subacute and chronic my-

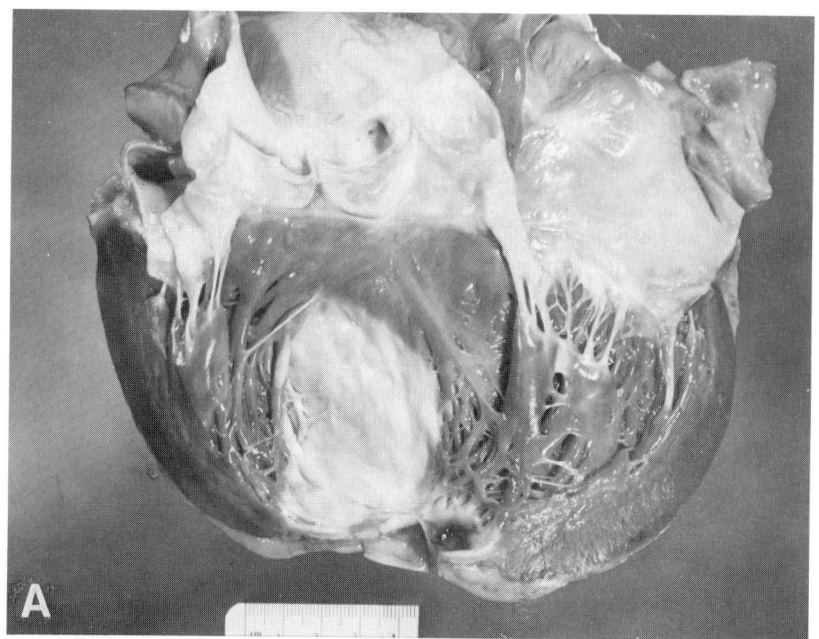

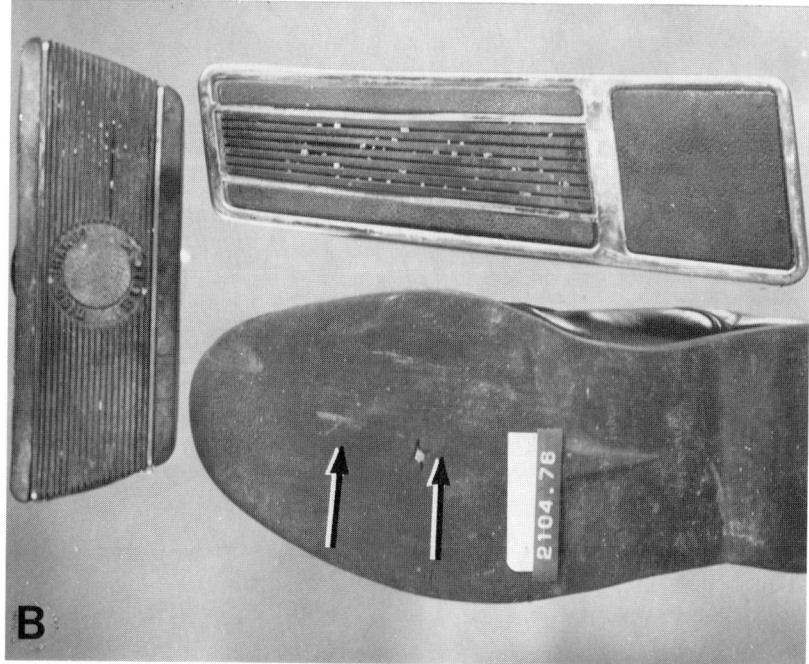

FIGURE 9-4. Concomitant coronary heart disease and automobile fatality in a 60-year-old white male (ME 2104-76). *A.* The heart is enlarged (530 gm) and shows a large, healed, apicoanteroseptal myocardial infarct. *B.* Scene investigation of the fatal automobile accident showed that the subject died with his foot on the accelerator. The photograph shows an imprint of the accelerator on the sole of the victim's shoe (arrows). This was interpreted as evidence of a lack of appropriate response consistent with fatal cardiac dysrhythmia prior to the crash.

ocarditis. In the first case the severe myocarditis was but an incidental finding in a man who crashed his airplane shortly after takeoff and who died of massive injuries. In the second instance, the driver of a motor vehicle suddenly lost consciousness and control of the automobile which eventually sustained moderate damage. Death was due to the myocarditis. These two cases are used to point out the need for questioning of the witnesses of the crash.

Case 1

A 60-year-old white man was driving west on an intracity freeway. It was after dark, but the road was dry and well illuminated, and only moderate traffic was present. The wife of the driver was in the front passenger seat of the heavy, late model sedan. As reconstructed after the crash, by following the tracks of the automobile on the medial strip, it left the inside lane of the westbound traffic, gradually veering across the median into the inside lane of the eastbound traffic. Shortly after its arrival, there was a head-on collision with a large, tractor trailer truck. The truck driver was not injured badly, but both the other driver and his wife were found to be dead, still contained in the automobile. There was no obvious reason for the driver of the sedan to have left his own traffic lane and to have entered the stream of traffic traveling in the opposite direction.

Because of the apparent traumatic origin of the deaths, both bodies were inspected by the medical examiner. The driver's wife was found to be dead of multiple injuries. The driver, however, had only two fractured ribs and minor abrasions of the knees, face, and hand. There were no manifestations of traumatic asphyxia or pneumothorax. It was the opinion of the medical examiner that the driver's death had resulted from severe heart disease.

A description of the heart follows in sufficient detail to permit a reviewing pathologist to read and understand the degree of cardiac abnormality. It is our opinion that this description (gross and microscopic) is adequate. Further documentation by photographs would be considered ideal, but is not absolutely necessary.

The aorta exhibited moderately severe arteriosclerosis. The kidneys showed changes of mild arteriolonephrosclerosis. The heart weighed 530 gm and exhibited moderate hypertrophy and dilatation of the left ventricle (see Fig. 9-4). The coronary arteries showed a balanced distribution with the posterior descending coronary artery originating from the right coronary artery. Examination of the coronary arteries at multiple cross-sectional levels revealed extensive involvement by old arteriosclerotic plaques. The coronary ostia and left main coronary artery were widely patent, but the left anterior descending, left circumflex, and right coronary arteries had approximately 75 percent narrowing of their luminal areas by old plaques. No foci of acute coronary occlusion were present. The heart was opened according to the direction of blood flow. No valvular or congenital lesions were noted. Approximately one-third of the left ventricular myocardium was replaced by an old, healed myocardial infarct which was localized to the apex and anteroseptal region (see Fig. 9-4). The involved myocardium was markedly thinned and contained dense, white, fibrous tissue. The endocardium over the infarct also was thickened, and a small mural thrombus was present at the apex. No foci of acute myocardial necrosis were identified.

Histologic examination of decalcified sections of coronary arteries confirmed the gross findings of severe arteriosclerosis without acute lesions. Sections of myocardium showed a completely healed, transmural region of myocardial replacement fibrosis. Other regions of the left ventricle revealed extensive interstitial and replacement fibrosis as well as nuclear enlargement and hyperchromasia, and marked variation in size of muscle cells, indicative of ischemic atrophy and compensatory hypertrophy. No foci of myocardial necrosis were identified.

Thus the heart of this accident victim showed evidence of severe coronary heart disease similar to that observed in many subjects with sudden natural death (Figs. 9-4 and 9-5). It should be noted, however, that examination of the shoe soles of the driver, and comparison of the ridged pattern on the sole of the right shoe with the pattern on the accelerator, showed that at the time of the head-on collision the driver's right foot was on the accelerator (see Fig. 9-4).

The remaining three cases will be given in less detail. All four illustrative cases are presented in tabular form (Table 9-5).

Case 2

A 61-year-old black woman was driving her sedan down a street with a moderate downhill slope. An adult cousin of the driver was in the front passenger seat. At the foot of the hill, the street ended in a cross street. The surviving passenger related that the driver failed to apply the brakes,

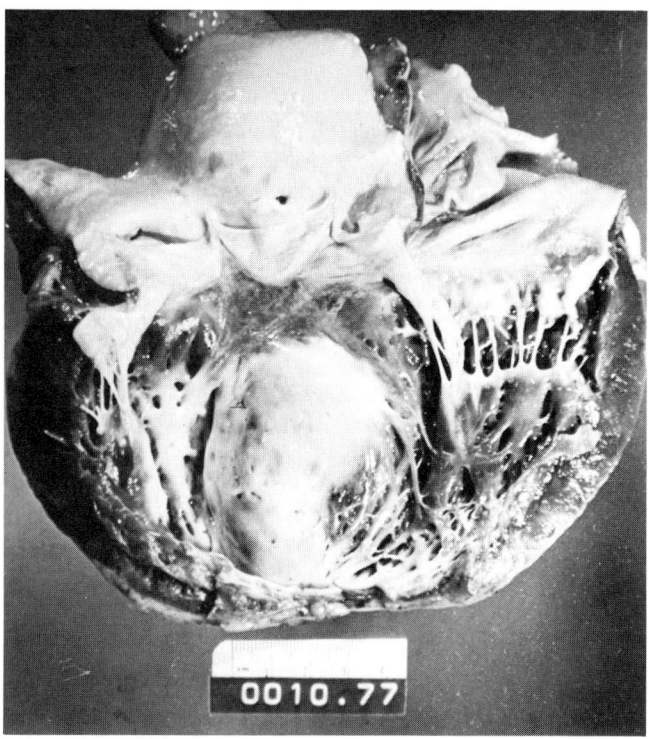

FIGURE 9-5. Sudden natural death due to coronary heart disease with old apicoanteroseptal myocardial infarct (ME 0010-77). The subject was a 64-year-old man with a history of hypertension who collapsed in the bathroom and died shortly thereafter.

TABLE 9-5. FOUR CASE STUDIES

	Case 1	Case 2	Case 3	Case 4
Cause of crash:	Heart disease	Undetermined	Heart disease	Vehicle failure (fuel delivery, light plane)
Cause of death:	Heart disease	Ruptured aorta	Heart disease	Multiple injuries
Injuries, external:	Bilateral knee abrasions Small lacerations and abrasions, face and left hand	Bilateral knee abrasions	Moderate laceration of face	Multiple, severe
Injuries, internal:	Not fatal degree—fractures of right ribs 2 and 3	Fatal degree Multiple fractured ribs: right 1, 2, 3, 4, 5, 6 and left 4, 5, 6 Ruptured aorta—alpha location Left hemothorax—1400 cc blood	None	Multiple rib fractures Rupture of aorta Bilateral hemothorax
Heart disease present:	ASCVD Myocardial hypertrophy (LV) Myocardial infarction Mural thrombus, apex LV Severe coronary artery atherosclerosis Severe arteriosclerosis of aorta Moderate arteriolarnephrosclerosis	HCVD and ASCVD Myocardial hypertrophy (LV) Moderate coronary artery atherosclerosis Mild arteriosclerosis of aorta Marked cerebral arteriosclerosis	Myocarditis, subacute and chronic	Myocarditis, subacute and chronic
Blood alcohol level:	0.00%	0.090%	0.00%	0.00%
Manner of death:	Natural disease	Accident	Natural disease	Natural disease

and although he shouted warnings to the driver, she did not slow down, and the automobile impacted a tree after jumping the curb at the foot of the hill.

No resuscitative measures were applied by the emergency medical technicians who responded to the accident, and the body was taken to the medical examiner's office after being pronounced dead on arrival at a hospital.

The cause of death was determined at autopsy to be a ruptured aorta with an associated massive left hemothorax. The aorta was ruptured for approximately three-quarters of its circumference at a point about 1.5 cm inferior to the site of the obliterated ductus arteriosus. Right ribs 1, 2, 3, 4, 5, and 6, and left ribs 4, 5, and 6 were fractured in the anterior axillary lines.

The heart weighed 330 gm (the body was 64 inches in length and weighed 130 pounds). The left ventricular wall was hypertrophied and measured 2.2 cm in thickness. The heart was a balanced coronary type, and a moderate degree of soft, yellow, subintimal atherosclerotic plaquing involved all of the major coronary arteries and narrowed their luminae to less than 35 percent of normal at many points. Much of the thickening of the coronary artery walls was symmetrical. No scarring of the myocardium was noted, and there were no valvular abnormalities. Only a very mild degree of aortic arteriosclerosis was present, and no arteriolonephrosclerosis was noted. The blood alcohol level was 0.09 percent. No other toxic substances were found in the blood.

The cause of the accident was not determined. The failure of the deceased to apply the brakes was not explained. She must have turned the steering wheel at least partially to the right because the automobile's point of impact (against the tree) was located to the right and somewhat up a slight grade, and the surviving passenger stated that he did not attempt to steer the vehicle. Therefore, the deceased must have been alive and reacting to a degree just before the impact. The cause of death was the rupture of the aorta with massive internal hemorrhage. The manner of death was considered, therefore, to be "accident."

Case 3

A 40-year-old, healthy white man was the pilot of a small, single-engine private airplane that took off from a well-equipped airport with three passengers. The weather was warm, calm, and sunny. The airplane was witnessed to be climbing. When it was about 300 feet off the ground, the engine sputtered. The plane began to turn left, apparently stalled, and crashed with the left wing low.

The pilot was dead when the ambulance arrived at the crash scene a few minutes later. All three passengers were seriously injured. All stated that the engine suddenly stopped after a momentary sputter.

The pilot sustained multiple injuries—multiple rib fractures, fracture of the sternum, partial transection of the aorta with bilateral hemothorax, and multiple contusions and lacerations of the face and legs. His heart weighed 405 gm. There was a moderate degree of soft, yellow, atherosclerotic plaquing of the subintima of the major coronary arteries. The myocardium was a normal reddish brown everywhere except for a 2.5 × 1.5 cm area in the posterior basal portion of the interventricular septum, where it was a mottled tan, but not softer than elsewhere. On microscopic examination, myocarditis was visible in all areas of the myocardium.

At the time of autopsy, it seemed that the heart disease (myocarditis) might well have disabled the pilot and thus precipitated the crash. However, the witnesses were all in accord in regard to the engine's stopping before the pilot's loss of control. Examination of the aircraft revealed a completely clogged fuel filter in the gasoline line leading to the engine from the full tank in use at the time of the crash. It was concluded that a mechanical failure had caused the accident. Therefore, the widespread myocarditis was only an incidental finding, neither the cause of the crash nor the cause of death.

Case 4

A 26-year-old woman was driving in an urban area. The four passengers in the vehicle stated that she suddenly slumped against the window of the driver's door, and that the automobile swerved and sideswiped several signs and another car before coming to rest against a post.

At autopsy, the only sign of trauma was a laceration of the face. Grossly, the heart was unremarkable except for slight dilatation of the left ventricle. It weighed 290 gm. Histologically, every one of the 20 sections examined revealed a widespread myocarditis, with the inflammatory cells composed mainly of lymphocytes and plasma cells. No other disease process was noted. The myocarditis in this case was considered to be the cause of death and the cause of the crash.

Interpretation

By means of case summaries, we wish to emphasize the extreme importance of these cardinal steps of proper interpretation of the victim of trauma who has coexisting heart disease:

1. Investigation
   a. medical history
   b. circumstances of death (crash)
   c. examination of crash vehicle
2. Witness interview (part of the investigation, but isolated to emphasize importance)
3. Autopsy
4. Toxicologic examination
5. Documentation
6. Correlation
7. Interpretation

The goal of all of the above steps is to evaluate the entire heart disease–trauma situation so as to determine properly the cause of accident and death and to resolve the manner of death. Nevertheless, it is necessary to document all of the details and interpretative processes so as to form a firm foundation for all legal and paralegal phases, including litigation if such results. The intermediate goal is to describe in sufficient detail the heart and entire cardiovascular system so that a reviewing pathologist can understand and mentally construct a reasonably accurate image of what was seen. Photographs and diagrams are most useful for this purpose, as are slides prepared for histologic examination.

REFERENCES

1. Reiner, L.: Gross Examination of the Heart, in Gould, S. E. (ed.): *Pathology of the Heart and Blood Vessels.* ed. 3. Charles C Thomas, Springfield, Ill., 1968.
2. Hudson, R. E. B.: Structure and Function of the Heart, in *Cardiovascular Pathology.* Vol. 1. Williams & Wilkins, Baltimore, 1965.
3. Davies, M. J., Pomerance, A., and Lamb, D.: Techniques in Examination and Anatomy of the Heart, in Pomerance, A., and Davies, M. J. (eds.): *The Pathology of the Heart.* Blackwell Scientific Publications, Oxford, 1975.
4. Roberts, W. C., and Buja, L. M.: The Frequency and Significance of Coronary Arterial Thrombi and Other Observations in Fatal Acute Myocardial Infarction. A Study of 107 Necropsy Patients. *Am. J. Med.* 52:425–444, 1972.
5. Schwartz, J. W., Kong, Y., Hackel, D. B., and Bartel, A. G.: Comparison of Angiographic and Postmortem Findings in Patients with Coronary Artery Disease. *Am. J. Cardiol.* 36:174–178, 1975.
6. Lawrie, G. M., Lie, J. T., Morris, G. C., Jr., and Beazley, H. L.: Vein Graft Patency and Intimal Proliferation after Aortocoronary Bypass: Early and Long-term Angiopathologic Correlations. *Am. J. Cardiol.* 38:856–862, 1976.
7. Vlodaver, Z., Neufeld, H. N., and Edwards, J. E.: *Coronary Arterial Variations in the Normal Heart and in Congenital Heart Disease.* Academic Press, New York, 1975.
8. Friedman, M.: The Coronary Thrombus: Its Origin and Fate. *Hum. Pathol.* 2:81–128, 1971.
9. Shipley, R. E., and Gregg, D. E.: The Effect of External Constriction of a Blood Vessel on Blood Flow. *Am. J. Physiol.* 141:289–296, 1944.
10. Wegira, R., Segers, M., Keating, R. P., and Ward, H. P.: Relationship Between the Reduction in Coronary Flow and the Appearance of EKG Changes. *Am. Heart J.* 38:90–96, 1949.
11. Weale, F. E.: The Haemodynamics of Incomplete Arterial Obstruction. *Br. J. Surg.* 51:689–693, 1964.
12. Gould, K. L., Lipscomb, K., and Hamilton, G. W.: Physiologic Basis for Assessing Critical Coronary Stenosis. Instantaneous Flow Response and Regional Distribution During Coronary Hyperemia as Measures of Coronary Flow Reserve. *Am. J. Cardiol.* 33:87–94, 1974.
13. Grande, F., and Taylor, H. L.: Adaptive Changes in the Heart, Vessels, and Patterns of Control under Chronically High Loads, in Hamilton, W. F., and Dow, P. (eds.): *Handbook of Physiology, Section 2: Circulation.* Vol. 3. American Physiological Society, Washington, D.C., 1965, pp. 2615–2677.
14. Linzbach, A. J.: Heart Failure from the Point of View of Quantitative Anatomy. *Am. J. Cardiol.* 5:370–382, 1960.
15. Morganroth, J., Maron, B. J., Henry, W. L., and Epstein, S. E.: Comparative Left Ventricular Dimensions in Trained Athletes. *Ann. Intern. Med.* 82:521–524, 1975.
16. Roeske, W. R., et al.: Noninvasive Evaluation of Ventricular Hypertrophy in Professional Athletes. *Circulation* 53:286–292, 1976.
17. Bulkley, B. H., and Roberts, W. C.: Dilatation of the Mitral Annulus (MA): A Rare Cause of Mitral Regurgitation (MR). *Circulation* 48 (Suppl. 4): IV–150, 1973.
18. Lamb, D.: Cor Pulmonale and Pulmonary Hypertension, in Pomerance, A., and Davies, M. J. (eds.): *The Pathology of the Heart.* Blackwell Scientific Publications, Oxford, 1975.
19. Kannel, W. B., et al.: Role of Blood Pressure in the Development of Congestive Heart Failure. *N. Engl. J. Med.* 287:781–787, 1972.
20. Badeer, H. S.: Pathogenesis of Cardiac Hypertrophy in Coronary Atherosclerosis and Myocardial Infarction. *Am. Heart J.* 84:256–264, 1972.
21. Gould, K. L., Lipscomb, K., Hamilton, G. W., and Kennedy, J. W.: Left Ventricular Hypertrophy in Coronary Artery Disease: A Cardiomyopathy Syndrome Following Myocardial Infarction. *Am. J. Med.* 55:595–601, 1973.
22. Buja, L. M., Ferrans, V. J., and Roberts, W. C.: Drug-induced Cardiomyopathies. *Adv. Cardiol.* 13:330–348, 1974.

23. Roberts, W. C., Ferrans, V. J., and Buja, L. M.: Pathologic Aspects of the Idiopathic Cardiomyopathies. *Adv. Cardiol.* 13:349–367, 1974.
24. Roberts, W. C., and Ferrans, V. J.: Pathologic Anatomy of the Cardiomyopathies: Idiopathic Dilated and Hypertrophic Types, Infiltrative Types, and Endomyocardial Disease. *Hum. Pathol.* 6:287–342, 1975.
25. Roberts, W. C., Dangel, J. C., and Bulkley, B. H.: Nonrheumatic Valvular Cardiac Disease: A Clinicopathologic Survey of 27 Different Conditions Causing Valvular Dysfunction. *Cardiovasc. Clin.* 5:333–446, 1973.
26. Pomerance, A.: Ageing and degenerative changes, in Pomerance, A., and Davies, M. J. (eds.): *The Pathology of the Heart.* Blackwell Scientific Publications, Oxford, 1975.
27. Swartz, M. H., Herman, M. V., and Teichholz, L. E.: Dermatoglyphic Patterns in Patients with Mitral Valve Prolapse: A Clue to Pathogenesis. *Am. J. Cardiol.* 38:588–593, 1976.
28. Chappell, S. E., Marshall, C. E., Brown, R. E., and Bruce, T. A.: Sudden Death and the Familial Occurrence of Mid-systolic Click, Late Systolic Murmur Syndrome. *Circulation* 48:1128–1134, 1973.
29. Goodwin, J. F.: ? IHSS ? HOCM ? ASH: A Plea for Unity. *Am. Heart J.* 89:269–277, 1975.
30. Maron, B. J., et al.: "Malignant" Hypertrophic Cardiomyopathy: Identification of a Subgroup of Families with Unusually Frequent Premature Deaths *Am. J. Cardiol.* 41:1133–1140, 1978.
31. Bulkley, B. H., Weisfeldt, M. L., and Hutchins, G. M.: Isometric Cardiac Contraction. A Possible Cause of the Disorganized Myocardial Pattern of Idiopathic Hypertrophic Subaortic Stenosis. *N. Engl. J. Med.* 295:135–139, 1977.
32. Maron, B. J., et al.: Quantitative Analysis of Cardiac Muscle Cell Disorganization in the Ventricular Septum of Patients with Hypertrophic Cardiomyopathy. *Circulation* 59:689–706, 1979.
33. Mallory, G. K., White, P. D., and Salcedo-Salgar, J.: The Speed of Healing of Myocardial Infarction: A Study of the Pathologic Anatomy in 72 Cases. *Am. Heart J.* 18:647–671, 1939.
34. Lie, J. T., and Titus, J. L.: Pathology of the Myocardium and the Conduction System in Sudden Coronary Death. *Circulation* 52 (Suppl. 3): III–41–III–52, 1975.
35. Anderson, J. A., and Hansen, B. F.: Autolytic Changes in the Human Myocardium, Particularly with a View to Detecting Acute Myocardial Infarction by the Nitro-BT Method. *Acta Pathol. Microbiol. Scand.* (Section A) 82:337–344, 1974.
36. Morales, A. R., and Fine, G.: Early Human Myocardial Infarction: A Histochemical Study. *Arch. Pathol.* 82:9–14, 1966.
37. Lichtig, C., et al.: Basic Fuchsin Picric Acid Method to Detect Acute Myocardial Ischemia: An Experimental Study of Swine. *Arch. Pathol.* 99:158–161, 1975.
38. Van Reempts, J., Borgers, M., and Reneman, R. S.: Early Myocardial Ischaemia: Evaluation of the Histochemical Haematoxylin–Basic Fuchsin–Picric Acid (HBFP) Staining Technique. *Cardiovasc. Res.* 10:262–267, 1976.
39. Rajs, J., and Jakobsson, S.: Experiences with the Hematoxylin Basic Fuchsin Picric Acid Staining Method for Morphologic Diagnosis of Myocardial Infarction: An Experimental Study in Forensic Pathology. *Forensic Sci.* 8:37–48, 1976.
40. Bouchardy, B., and Majno, G.: Histopathology of Early Myocardial Infarcts: A New Approach. *Am. J. Pathol.* 74:301–330, 1974.
41. Hoch-Ligeti, C., and Lan, C. W.: Morphology and Frequency of Early Myocardial Damage in Various Diseases. *Am. J. Clin. Pathol.* 62:455–460, 1974.
42. Zugibe, F. T., Bell, P., Jr., Conley, T., and Standish, M. L.: Determination of Myocardial Alterations at Autopsy in the Absence of Gross and Microscopic Changes. *Arch. Pathol.* 81:409–411, 1966.
43. McVie, J. G.: Postmortem Detection of Inapparent Myocardial Infarction. *J. Clin. Pathol.* 23:203–209, 1970.

44. Lie, J. T., et al.: Time Course and Zonal Variations of Ischemia-induced Myocardial Cationic Electrolyte Derangements. *Circulation* 51:860–866, 1975.
45. Rose, A. G., Opie, L. H., and Bricknell, O. L.: Early Experimental Myocardial Infarction: Evaluation of Histologic Criteria and Comparison with Biochemical and Electrocardiographic Measurements. *Arch. Pathol. Lab. Med.* 100:516–521, 1976.
46. Rammer, L., and Janson, O.: Determination of Electrolytes in the Myocardium as a Tool for the Post-mortal Diagnosis of Recent Infarction. *Forensic Sci.* 8:127–130, 1976.
47. Liberthson, et al.: Pathophysiologic Observations in Prehospital Ventricular Fibrillation and Sudden Cardiac Death. *Circulation* 49:790–797, 1974.
48. Liberthson, R. R., Nagel, E. L., Hirschmann, J. C., and Nussenfeld, S. R.: Prehospital Ventricular Defibrillation: Prognosis and Follow-up Course. *N. Eng. J. Med.* 291:317–321, 1974.
49. Baum, R. S., Alvarez, H. A., and Cobb, L. A.: Survival after Resuscitation from Out-of-Hospital Ventricular Fibrillation. *Circulation* 50:1231–1235, 1974.
50. Weaver, W. D., Lorch, G. S., Alvarez, H. A., and Cobb, L. A.: Angiographic Findings and Prognostic Indicators in Patients Resuscitated from Sudden Cardiac Death. *Circulation* 54:895–900, 1976.
51. Chandler, A. B., et al.: Coronary Thrombosis in Myocardial Infarction. Report of a Workshop on the Role of Coronary Thrombosis in the Pathogenesis of Acute Myocardial Infarction. *Am. J. Cardiol.* 34:823–832, 1974.
52. Davies, M. J., Woolf, N., and Robertson, W. B.: Pathology of Acute Myocardial Infarction with Particular Reference to Occlusive Coronary Thrombi. *Br. Heart J.* 38:659–664, 1976.
53. Hudson, R. E. B.: The Conducting System, in *Cardiovascular Pathology*. Vol. 1. Williams & Wilkins, Baltimore, 1965.
54. Lev, M., and Bharati, S.: Lesions of the Conduction System and Their Functional Significance. *Pathology Annual* 9:157–208, 1974.
55. James, T. N.: Anatomy of the Conduction System of the Heart, in Hurst, J. W., et al. (eds.): *The Heart, Arteries and Veins.* ed. 3. McGraw-Hill, New York, 1974.
56. James, T. N.: Order and Disorder in the Rhythm of the Heart. *Circulation* 47:362–386, 1973.
57. Petty, C. S.: Instantaneous "Physiologic" Death, in Risher, R. S., and Petty, C. S. (eds.): *Forensic Pathology: A Handbook for Pathologists.* National Institute of Law Enforcement and Criminal Justice, Washington, D.C., 1977.

CHAPTER 10

William A. Meissner is the former Chairman of the Department of Pathology at the New England Deaconess Hospital in Boston, and is Professor of Pathology at Harvard Medical School. Dr. Meissner completed both his undergraduate and medical studies at the University of Oregon. He is Past President of the Massachusetts Division of the American Cancer Society, receiving its Award for Outstanding Contributions to Cancer Control in 1965. Dr. Meissner was the 1976 recipient of the Distinguished Service Award for Continuing Education of the American Society of Clinical Pathologists. He is the author of many papers, articles, and chapters treating various aspects of the pathology of cancer.

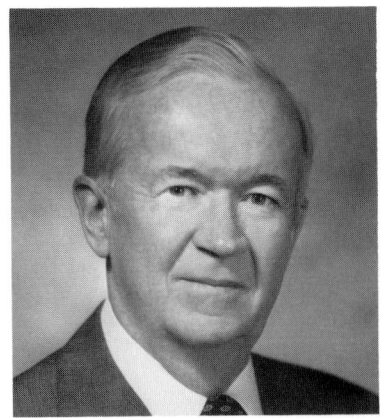

TRAUMA AND DEATH RELATED TO NEOPLASTIC DISEASES

William A. Meissner, M.D.

SIGNIFICANCE OF TRAUMA

The role of trauma in initiating or stimulating the process of neoplasia has been debated for many years. Half a century ago a relationship between the two processes was considered by many to be not only possible, but probable. With succeeding decades, however, more and more competent observers with much experience in the field of cancer have concluded that such a relationship is either rare or nonexistent.

The consideration is complicated by two factors. First, trauma is such a common event in everyday living. Hardly a day passes without some part of the body receiving at least a minor injury. One could speculate that if trauma were a common cause of cancer, the human race might not have survived over the centuries. Second, the exact nature of cancer remains a complex problem, and its causes still are incompletely understood. It is tempting, therefore, to assume a relationship when the two processes of trauma and tumor seem to be temporally related. Compensation claims for the development of tumor thought to be secondary to trauma often have been settled in favor of the injured party merely because of such an apparent temporal relationship, but this does not prove that it was a factual one. Most reports of tumor caused by trauma are of individual cases; exhaustive studies by experienced observers always reach an opposite conclusion.

Even if trauma is never or only infrequently a factor in the causation of tumors, the possibility still must be examined. But before a discussion of such a possibility, it is necessary to define what is meant by trauma and to review the neoplastic process in the light of current concepts as to its nature, pathogenesis, and etiology.

In a broad sense, trauma may mean bodily injury from any cause. A more precise medical definition is as follows: "Trauma is an injury or wound to a living body caused by the application of external force or violence." By implication the injury is of sufficient degree to produce a break in continuity of one or more of the body tissues, with an accompanying release of chemicals and with varying degrees of hemorrhage, edema, and cell destruction. Then follow the processes of repair and regeneration, both of which involve proliferation of cells. Repeated minor trauma is called chronic irritation. Injuries from chemicals, minerals, ionizing radiation, ultraviolet radiation, and from occupational hazards are not properly encompassed in the definition.

RELATIONSHIP OF TRAUMA TO TUMORS

Much of the older accumulated literature concerning the relationship of trauma to tumor development and growth antedates by many years current knowledge and concepts of the nature, etiology, and development of tumor. Tumors (neoplasms) represent masses of body cells that have developed a permanent defect in their metabolism, causing them to proliferate in an abnormal, persistent, and excessive fashion. The neoplastic process is thought to be induced by a variety of etiologic agents, frequently working in combination, that produce a series of alterations of intracellular metabolism, often in a steplike manner, until a permanent defect that is passed on to the cells' progeny results. Possible causes of tumors, many of which have been proved experimentally, include a great diversity of factors and agents such as heredity, sex, age, immunologic status, hormones, dietary habits, chemicals, dusts, solar and ionizing radiation, and viruses. Many cancer scientists now believe that chemical agents are the most important of the various possible etiologic agents and account for a majority of tumors. The induction time of tumors is quite variable and in some instances is many years. For example, the induction of leukemia in Japanese exposed to the ionizing radiation from the atomic bomb was first noted after 3 years and reached a peak after 6 years. The shortest possible induction time is debatable and varies with type of tumor, but probably should never be less than a month.

Tumors arise in and from essentially all body tissues, and the number of varieties is almost limitless. It is customary to name tumors according to the tissue or cells from which they appear to arise and to classify them further according to anticipated behavior. *Benign* tumors grow slowly, remain localized, and seldom have ill effects on the patient. *Malignant* tumors, also called *cancers,* tend to grow rapidly, destroy adjacent tissues, and spread to distant parts of the body where the cells set up independent colonies called *metastases.* The problem of tumors is essentially due to the malignant variety because the relentless growth of cancer, unless adequately treated, will ultimately result in death of the patient.

Neoplasms, especially cancers, have great variations in growth habits so that the course is not consistently predictable, even for tumors of the same general type. Since it is impossible to predict with certainty how an individual tumor will behave, it follows that it is difficult to evaluate consistently the influence of extraneous factors, even clinical treatment, on the course of the disease.

Because many processes such as inflammation may mimic tumor, confirmation is essential. The confirmation is reached by a pathologist after microscopic study of the suspected lesion or a part of it (i.e., biopsy).

The consideration of the possible relationship between trauma and tumor involves three questions: (1) Can trauma to normal tissue cause tumor? (2) Can trauma to abnormal tissue induce tumor? (3) What effect may trauma have on an already existing tumor?

TRAUMA TO NORMAL TISSUE

There are several theoretical explanations for possible induction of tumor in normal tissue by trauma. Since trauma produces a breakdown of normal tissue, a chemical substance might be released from the tissue to induce a permanent change in the metabolism and growth of some local cells. This must remain as a highly hypothetical speculation since no such substance has been demonstrated.

Another possibility, with more appeal, is based on the theory that tumors may arise from somatic cell mutations. If, therefore, trauma acted as a mutagen (an agent producing the cellular mutation), it might induce tumor. While such a possibility cannot be entirely denied, there is little evidence that trauma can act in this fashion. Most experimental work on tumors has shown that trauma to normal tissues has no tumor-producing effect, and, indeed, there are reports that trauma may even inhibit the development of some experimental tumors.

Trauma also results in physiologic cellular proliferations called regeneration and repair. Because tumor is also a cellular proliferation, induction of tumor by way of the reparative process following trauma may be considered. Again, however, such is not found experimentally; only in cases of chronic irritation is there evidence for tumor induction from chronic repair. Formation of excessive scar tissue (keloid) is not tumor.

The most conclusive evidence against a relationship between trauma and tumor formation is the great frequency of trauma and the rarity of a tumor related to it. Trauma is frequent in children, yet the incidence of tumor is low. Neoplasia is not an occupational hazard of professional athletes. There has been no increased incidence of tumor formation following traumatic injuries in either of the two world wars. Tumors do not arise from fractured bones or in surgical excisions.

The evidence would seem to be overwhelming that trauma does not induce neoplasia and that the coexistence of the two processes is purely coincidental; certainly coincidence is not a synonym for causal relationship.

The nature and development of cancer is still a complicated subject, and its causes are not completely defined. It is necessary, therefore, that an occasional case be evaluated for a possible relationship of trauma to tumor. Rarity does not necessarily mean that there is never a relationship. In order to allow selection of cases for more detailed evaluation, minimal criteria have been developed over the years. Most instances will fall far short of the minimal criteria for various reasons. The criteria suggested by Ewing and by Warren (see p. 212) are among the better known.

It is often difficult to establish that the injured part was previously normal. Only rarely has a patient had a carefully documented examination immediately before an injury; the previous integrity of the part is often assumed rightly or wrongly if it had normal function and appearance. It should be stressed that trauma, being such a common event, often merely calls attention to a pre-existing tumor that had not previously been noted.

The authentication and adequacy of trauma are easier to assess, particularly if the patient obtained documented medical treatment for the in-

> **MINIMAL CRITERIA NECESSARY FOR CONSIDERATION OF RELATIONSHIP BETWEEN TRAUMA AND CANCER**
>
> *Ewing*
> 1. The authenticity and adequacy of the trauma must be shown.
> 2. The wounded part must have had previous integrity.
> 3. The tumor must arise from the exact point of injury.
> 4. A reasonable time must exist between injury and appearance of tumor.
> 5. There must be a positive (pathologic) diagnosis of the presence and nature of the tumor.
>
> *Warren*
> 1. Integrity of the tumor site prior to injury must be established.
> 2. The injury must be sufficiently severe to disrupt the continuity of the tissue at the site and so initiate reparative proliferation of cells.
> 3. The tumor must follow the injury by a reasonable length of time.
> 4. The tumor must be of a type which might reasonably develop as a result of the regeneration and repair of those tissues which had received the injury.

jury. The authentication cannot be based on a vague recollection of an injury weeks or months before appearance of the tumor.

The time interval between trauma and the appearance of tumor must be in a range long enough to allow tumor transformation. Probably a month at least should lapse; the maximum time is difficult to state. Certainly the tumor must not be apparent immediately after the injury.

One example of a relationship between trauma and neoplasia often cited concerns the development of meningioma of the brain following traumatic injury. About 40 years ago Cushing and Eisenhardt concluded that trauma to the head was a significant etiologic factor in about a third of their cases of intracranial meningioma. Because of the great reputation of these authors, the relationship was widely quoted. A recent opinion, however, states "this theory has not gained wide acceptance, but is from time to time revived in case reports in which such a relationship, although still inferential, appears to rest on fairly substantive circumstantial evidence." In a follow-up study of 2,858 cases of head injury cited by Parker and Kernohan, there was no instance of brain tumor developing.

One of the most compelling arguments against production of tumor in normal tissue by trauma is the opinion of competent, experienced pathologists who have studied the subject:

> *Ewing* (1935): It is generally agreed that a single trauma never produces a malignant tumor in previously normal tissue.
> *Warren* (1943): So far as a single mechanical injury producing cancer is concerned, the evidence rests chiefly on reasoning from *post hoc ergo propter hoc*—all too often fallacious.
> *Stewart* (1946): The normal wear and tear of life induces a multiplicity of traumas which are rarely noted or quickly forgotten until the time arises to make something out of them.
> *Willis* (1967): Simple injury of healthy tissues is rarely, if ever, a sufficient cause of neoplasia.

Moritz (1975): There is no conclusive evidence that trauma is more than fortuitous in sequential relationship.

EFFECT OF TRAUMA ON ABNORMAL TISSUE

It is a little more plausible to accept the suggestion that trauma to tissue already abnormal might induce neoplasia. With the current theory that tumor induction often occurs in a steplike fashion, one can postulate that trauma could be one of several initiating or promoting factors, a cocarcinogen. There is, indeed, some experimental evidence that trauma under certain circumstances can precipitate the formation of tumor if the cells have been previously conditioned with a chemical carcinogenic agent. That the repair process resulting from trauma might promote cancer induction in a predisposed tissue cannot be denied.

There are several problems with such reasoning. In the first place, while it might be possible experimentally, it is difficult to determine in an individual instance of human tumor whether tissues are truly preconditioned; precancerous lesions and states are not that well defined. Furthermore the trauma would have to occur at an appropriate time in the stage of tumor development. Thus, from the practical point of view, it remains very difficult to prove that trauma plays any role in tumor development in abnormal tissue, even though it remains a theoretical possibility. Minimal criteria similar to those described for normal tissues need to be applied.

Another question might concern traumatic aggravation of a benign tumor so that it becomes malignant. Spontaneous transformation of benign to malignant tumors always has been considered a possibility and sometimes can be well documented and confirmed. The type of malignant tumor produced by transformation should be similar in histologic type to the pre-existing benign one. Current concepts, however, hold that most cancers are malignant from their inception rather than passing through a benign neoplastic phase. Proof that such transformation to malignant tumor was caused by trauma would be most difficult to document in an individual case.

REPEATED MINOR TRAUMA AND CHRONIC IRRITATION

Although repeated minor trauma and chronic irritation do not fall within the scope of the accepted definition of trauma, a brief discussion is warranted since, with repeated minor trauma and disruption of tissue, the cellular proliferations of regeneration and repair become continual; in a few instances cancer develops from the process, usually only after many years. One example is cancer arising in the skin adjacent to a chronic osteomyelitic sinus that has drained for a number of years. While such a draining sinus does not conform to the definition of trauma, it might nevertheless have been originally a contributory cause of its production.

Another type of injury—thermal—is an occasional cause of cancer of the skin. Skin cancers developing in burn scars have been well documented; both squamous and basal cell carcinomas may arise. The cancers develop in from 4 months to as long as 30 plus years after the injury with the average time about 20 years. It is not clear why thermal burns predispose to cancer development; scars from other types of injuries, including surgical incisions, rarely show tumor.

Since trauma disrupts tissue and causes edema, hemorrhage, and repair, it would seem quite possible that it might activate a pre-existing tumor, particularly a cancer, to grow and spread more rapidly. The act of trauma might also force tumor cells into lymphatic or blood vessels so that they could metastasize more readily. All of this reasoning is difficult to apply to an individual case. Tumors, like normal tissues, are exposed to multiple traumas daily; to be significant, the traumatic event would have to be an unusual one and out of the ordinary, such as a rupture of the capsule of the tumor or production of severe hemorrhage. Sudden growth of any tumor, without trauma, is common and is due to the spontaneous occurrence of hemorrhage, edema, and necrosis.

In order to establish that trauma has contributed to an accelerated course of a tumor, one needs to establish what the predicted course would have been without trauma. As noted previously, such predictions of the course of individual tumors are likely to be unreliable. Activation of a pre-existing tumor by trauma, therefore, seems a distinct theoretical possibility, but difficult to prove in an individual case.

A few instances have been reported in which metastases from a cancer have appeared at sites of trauma. Presumably the hemorrhage and tissue disruption provided a favorable situation for deposition of circulating tumor cells and their subsequent growth. Such an event could only happen in the late stages of cancer and could have no bearing on the causation of the primary tumor and little influence on the course of the disease in the patient.

ROLE OF THE MEDICOLEGAL INVESTIGATOR

There are no specific or unusual problems for the medicolegal officer in investigating death due to tumor that is suspected to have been induced by trauma. An autopsy should be performed so that the tumor can be verified and classified and its extent determined both grossly and microscopically. The stated trauma site should be evaluated for its relationship to the primary tumor location and for evidence of residual injury, regeneration, or repair.

CONCLUSION

Based on current concepts concerning the nature, causes, and development of tumor, especially cancer, trauma to normal tissue does not cause neoplasia. The possibilities that trauma might act as a promoting factor in previously abnormal tissues and that trauma might accelerate the growth of an existing tumor are theoretically acceptable, but difficult to prove in an individual instance. An occasional anecdotal case seeming to support a relationship between trauma and tumor is probably merely coincidental, yet the tumor process is so complex and so incompletely understood that such a relationship cannot be denied categorically. For the evaluation of a given case, data should be collected and documented according to established criteria.

Case 1

A 47-year-old moderately obese woman was injured while riding on a streetcar. She was standing when the streetcar stopped abruptly and was thrown off balance against a metal support bar, hitting it with her left shoulder and breast. That evening, she noted a bruise of the skin of the left shoulder and felt a nodule in her breast at about the region of the trauma. After 2 weeks the bruise had disappeared, but the breast nodule remained, and she sought medical advice. A mastectomy was performed. The breast nodule proved to be an adenocarcinoma; there were metastases in two axillary lymph nodes. The patient sought compensation for tumor induced by the trauma.

Comment: Neither the injury nor its degree and extent were documented. More important, a 2 cm adenocarcinoma of the breast which already had metastasized to axillary lymph nodes is not an "early" cancer and could not have reached such development in a few weeks' time. The trauma merely called attention to a pre-existing mass, not recognized before.

Case 2

A 54-year-old man developed a nodule on his left lower leg. The mass was excised and was diagnosed as cancer—a fibrosarcoma. The patient stated that 6 years before he had been injured at work by a metal pipe falling on his leg; he had reported the injury and x-rays had been taken. The documented injury, however, had been to the right leg, not to the left where the tumor developed.

Comment: Injuries are common and are easily recalled when the time is appropriate. Historical data, unless well documented, are often unreliable.

Case 3

A 60-year-old man slipped on greasy stairs, fell, and injured his right thigh. X-rays showed a fracture of the femur. The leg was placed in a cast, but the fracture did not heal. Six weeks later surgery was performed on the fracture site, and a biopsy of edematous tissue was taken. The biopsy showed cancer, but the specimen was not sufficient to allow further classification. The fracture still did not heal, and a month later nodules were found in the lungs by x-ray examination and were interpreted as metastatic cancer. The patient had a progressively downhill course and died with bronchopneumonia 4 months after the initial injury. Autopsy showed a primary tumor of the left kidney which had metastasized to the lungs, to the vertebrae, and to the right femur.

Comment: The autopsy was important for the exact determination of the site and type of the primary tumor. The metastasis to the femur undoubtedly had occurred before the trauma, and fracture might well not have occurred if the metastasis had not been present. Such a fracture is called a "pathologic fracture," meaning that disease existed before the trauma. The tumor clearly was not caused by trauma, nor did it accentuate the tumor growth. It cannot be stated conclusively, however, that the pathologic fracture would have occurred without the trauma.

REFERENCES

1. Bereston, E. S., and Ney, C.: Squamous Cell Carcinoma Arising in a Chronic Osteomyelitic Sinus Tract with Metastasis. *Arch. Surg.* 43:257, 1941.
2. Bizzozero, O. J., Johnson, K. G., and Ciocco, A.: Radiation-related Leukemia, Hiroshima and Nagasaki, 1946–1964. I. Distribution, Incidence and Appearance Time. *N. Engl. J. Med.* 274:1095, 1966.

3. Brown, K. L.: Medical Problems and the Law. Charles C Thomas, Springfield, Ill., 1971.
4. Cowdry, E. V.: *Cancer Cells*. W. B. Saunders, Philadelphia, 1955.
5. Crane, A. R., and Decker, J. P.: Trauma and Neoplasia, in Brahdy, L. (ed.): *Disease and Injury*. J. B. Lippincott, Philadelphia, 1961, pp. 302–341.
6. Cushing, H., and Eisenhardt, L.: *The Meningiomas*. Charles C Thomas, Springfield, Ill., 1938.
7. Dunham, L. J.: Cancer in Man at Site of Prior Benign Lesion of Skin or Mucous Membrane: A Review. *Cancer Res.* 32:1359, 1972.
8. Ewing, James: Bulkley Lecture. Modern Attitude Toward Traumatic Cancer. *Arch. Pathol.* 19:690, 1935.
9. Gaeta, J. F.: Trauma and Inflammation, in Holland, J. F., and Frei, E., III (eds.): *Cancer Medicine*. Lea & Febiger, Philadelphia, 1973, pp. 102–106.
10. Moritz, A. R., and Morris, R. C.: *Handbook of Legal Medicine*. C. V. Mosby, St. Louis, 1975.
11. Parker, H. L., and Kernohan, J. W.: Relation of Injury and Glioma of the Brain. J.A.M.A. 97:535, 1931.
12. Rhoads, J. E., Howard, J. M., and Jannetta, P. J.: *The Chemistry of Trauma*. Charles C Thomas, Springfield, Ill., 1963.
13. Rigdon, R. H.: Trauma and Cancer: A Relationship Based upon Cell Mutation. *South. Med. J.* 55:341, 1962.
14. Rous, P., and Kidd, J. G.: Conditional Neoplasms and Subthreshold Neoplastic States. *J. Exp. Med.* 73:365, 1941.
15. Rubenstein, L. J.: Tumors of the Central Nervous System, in *Atlas of Tumor Pathology* (Second Series, Fascicle 6). Armed Forces Institute of Pathology, Washington, D.C., 1972.
16. Shear, M. J.: Studies in Carcinogens. *Am. J. Cancer* 33:499, 1938.
17. Stewart, F. W.: Occupational and Post-traumatic Cancer. *Bull. N.Y. Acad. Med.* 22:145, 1947.
18. Stoll, H. L., and Crissey, J. T.: Epithelioma from Single Trauma. *N.Y. J. Med.* 62:496, 1962.
19. Treves, N., and Pack, G. T.: The Development of Cancer in Burn Scars. *Surg. Gynecol. Obstet.* 51:749, 1930.
20. Warren, S.: Minimal Criteria to Prove Causation of Traumatic or Occupational Neoplasms. *Ann. Surg.* 117:585, 1943.
21. Willis, R. A.: *Pathology of Tumours*. ed. 4. Appleton-Century-Crofts, New York, 1967.
22. Willis, R. A.: *The Spread of Tumours in the Human Body*. Butterworth, London, 1973.

ADDITIONAL READING

Adelson, L.: Injury and Cancer. *Western Reserve Law Rev.* 5:150–173, 1954.
Courville, C. B.: Trauma and Intracranial Tumors—with Particular Reference to the Gliomas. *J. Forensic Med.* 3:16–26, 1956.
Eidman, K. W.: Defense of Traumatic Cancer Cases. *Defense Law J.* 9:59–94, 1961.
Gottlieb, A.: Can Trauma Produce Malignant Bone Tumors? A Medico-Legal Answer. *Med. Legal J.* 50:1–4, 1933.
Gowing, N. F. C.: Relationship of Trauma and Tumor Formation. *J. Forensic Med.* 8:116–121, 1961.
Ladanyi, D. J.: Impact Trauma as 'Legal Cause of Cancer.' *Cleveland State Law Rev.* 20:409–419, May 1971.
March, J. T.: Traumatic Cancer in Workmen's Compensation Cases. *Cleveland-Marshall Law Rev.* 115:501–511, 1962.
Russell, W. O., and Clark, R. E., Jr.: Medico-Legal Considerations of Trauma and Other External Influences in Relationship to Cancer. *Vanderbilt Law Rev.* 6:868–882, 1953.
Small, B. F.: Gaffing at a Thing Called Cause: Medico-Legal Conflicts in the Concept of Causation. *Texas Law Rev.* 31:630–659, 1953.
Warren, S.: Criteria Required to Prove Causation of Occupational or Traumatic Tumors. *U. Chicago Law Rev.* 10:313–322, 1943.

CHAPTER 11

William Q. Sturner is Chief Medical Examiner of the State of Rhode Island, as well as Professor of Pathology and Laboratory Medicine and Director of Forensic Medicine at Brown University. He is a member of the Executive Committee and Board of Directors of the National Association of Medical Examiners and was President in 1978–1979. Between 1969 and 1974, Dr. Sturner was a medical examiner in Dallas County, Texas, and earlier served as Associate Medical Examiner for the City of New York. In 1967 and 1968, he was Assistant Director of Pathology for the Cook County Coroner's Laboratory in Chicago. After completing his undergraduate studies at the College of St. Thomas, in St. Paul, Minnesota, Dr. Sturner entered St. Louis University, taking his medical degree in 1959. He earned the Diploma in Medical Jurisprudence from the London Society of Apothecaries (Pathology) in 1970. Dr. Sturner has conducted scientific research on sudden infant death syndrome under a co-awarded grant at Brown University.

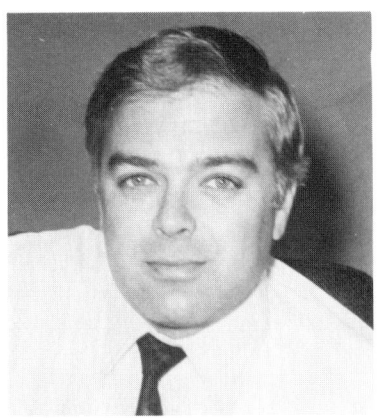

PEDIATRIC DEATHS

William Q. Sturner, M.D.

It is well known that the majority of fatalities, both from organic disease and external trauma, apply to children as well as to the adult population. By the same token, there are sufficient differences in the investigation and examination of infant deaths to warrant a special chapter dealing with problems peculiar to this young age group. We shall be pointing out, for example, the number of hazardous substances and paraphernalia which can be lethal weapons for a young infant, whereas they may be only incidental objects in an adult fatality.

With reference to the medical historical aspects of such investigations, we would recommend securing the records of the family physician as well as the birth and delivery charts of the infant and mother. In some instances, the origins of symptomatology, if not frank disease, are outlined in written form even prior to the body inspection and the performance of the autopsy.

It should be further stressed that an examination of the scene should be conducted in every instance, even if the decedent has been moved to the hospital or elsewhere. This is especially true if the decedent is a young infant and a compromise in the bed or crib space is a possibility as the mechanism of death.

Society's ills appear to be having an adverse impact on the young in increasing numbers with homicide, suicide, vehicular accidents, drug abuse, and sudden natural death all playing a role in the statistics of childhood fatalities. Special emphasis throughout this chapter will be given to the differentiation of modalities and circumstances that are particularly associated with young people.

ABORTION CASES

Since the landmark Supreme Court decisions concerning abortion, a different spectrum of death cases has been reported and seen by medical examiners. In previous decades, maternal fatalities from secondary infection following illegal abortion were as frequent an event as the discovery of a discarded fetus or premature infant. With the advent of legal interruption of pregnancy, maternal mortality has decreased dramatically so that only 44 women died from all forms of abortion in 1975, half that reported just 3 years earlier.[1] Some fatalities have been associated with saline injections with the solution passing into the maternal bloodstream, often resulting in fatal asymmetric brain hemorrhages.[2]

Now that the courts have determined that any fetus of over 20 gestational weeks is presumed alive and capable of independent existence with all the rights of a person, it is becoming necessary to formulate guidelines for medicolegal investigation of therapeutic abortions in this age range. Of course, where the mother's health is a consideration, such a procedure can be authorized in most hospital facilities, provided that appropriate consultation is obtained. However, the medical examiner may have a duty to investigate cases which appear to have been aborted without an apparent maternal health problem.

A concomitant issue, and a very thorny one during the past several years, has been that of fetal research. Following standards developed by the National Institutes of Health,[3] many university medical centers and other health care facilities have revised their codes of procedures and have promulgated rules pertaining to fetal research acceptable under the NIH guidelines. Such considerations involve not only biomedical problems of scientific research, but also legal issues such as "informed consent." Alterations in permission forms for disposal of tissues have been adopted, no doubt enhanced by a recent court decision.[4]

STILLBIRTHS

The issue of stillborn versus live-born infants continues to be a major point of controversy. The famous Edelin case, albeit categorized as an "abortion trial," was nonetheless prosecuted on the charge of manslaughter. Evidence given by the medical examiner indicated that the infant was indeed alive at the time of removal from the mother as interpreted from the microscopic examination of the baby's lungs. The fact that two independent experts, both neonatologists, rendered contrary opinions as to the viability of the child, did not persuade the jury to find for the physician. The Massachusetts Supreme Judicial Court overturned the conviction.[5] It is a well-known fact that the lung tissue from those infants who are stillborn compared to that from live-born infants succumbing shortly after birth cannot be readily distinguished.[6]

Stillbirths continue to occur in utero, especially following automobile trauma.[7] It is difficult to judge the amount of maceration and the length of time in utero following such deaths, but some approximation can be made (Fig. 11-1). Toxicologic analysis can play a corollary role in the interpretation of circumstances in these fatalities. In a recent case, a macerated infant's liver and blood revealed 0.15 percent ethyl alcohol, the amount probably in the mother's system at the time of an automobile accident 2 days prior to the stillborn delivery. Other cases pose even more difficult interpretive problems (Fig. 11-2).

SUDDEN NATURAL DEATHS

A number of natural disease processes during the first few months of life can produce a fatal outcome in infants.[8] Such findings will also occur,

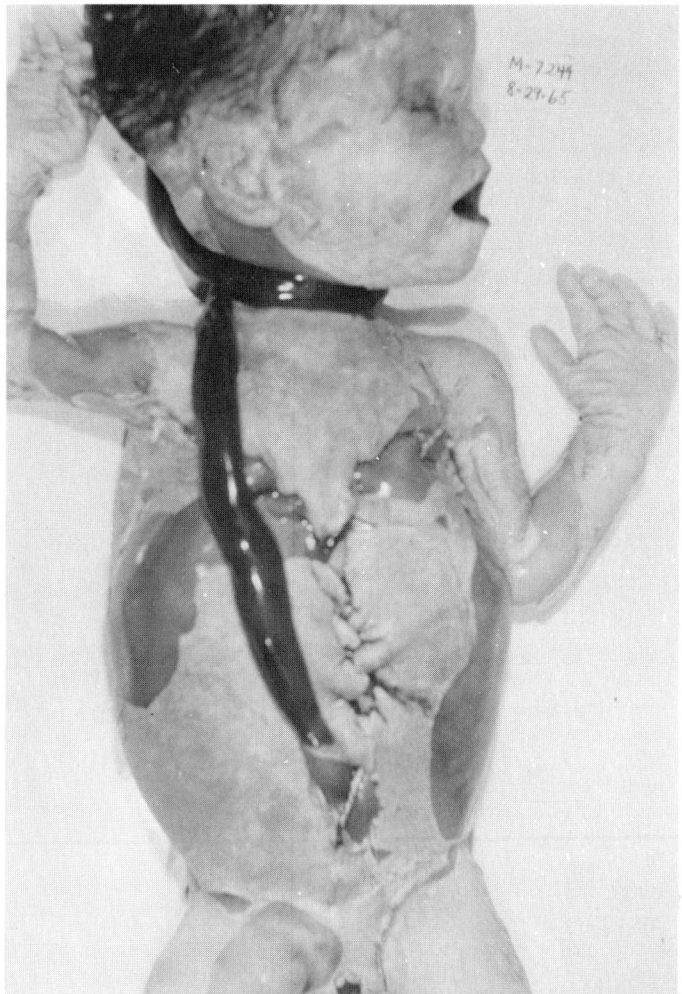

FIGURE 11-1. A near-term fetus that died in utero following maternal vehicular trauma. Note the umbilical cord wrapped around the neck, a not uncommon finding in normal births.

though to a lesser extent, in young children and teenagers. Two of the more common varieties in the younger age group are congenital abnormalities and infections. Sudden unexpected deaths have been known to occur in the newborn nursery, with the majority of deaths due to unsuspected hereditary conditions or complications following a difficult birth process. Some of the latter deaths are related to respiratory distress syndrome and similar conditions. Among the cases in our experience has been that of a newborn infant succumbing shortly after an uncomplicated delivery. The autopsy revealed a congenitally absent hemidiaphragm on the left side, allowing the intestinal tract to protrude into the chest cavity, causing incomplete development without aeration of the left lung and subsequent acute cardiorespiratory failure (Fig. 11-3). Another cardiac condition causing sudden death in the first few months of life is endocardial fibroelastosis. The pathogenesis of this condition has yet to be elucidated. It appears that hypoxia, infection, or a combination of etiologic agents may be responsible.[9]

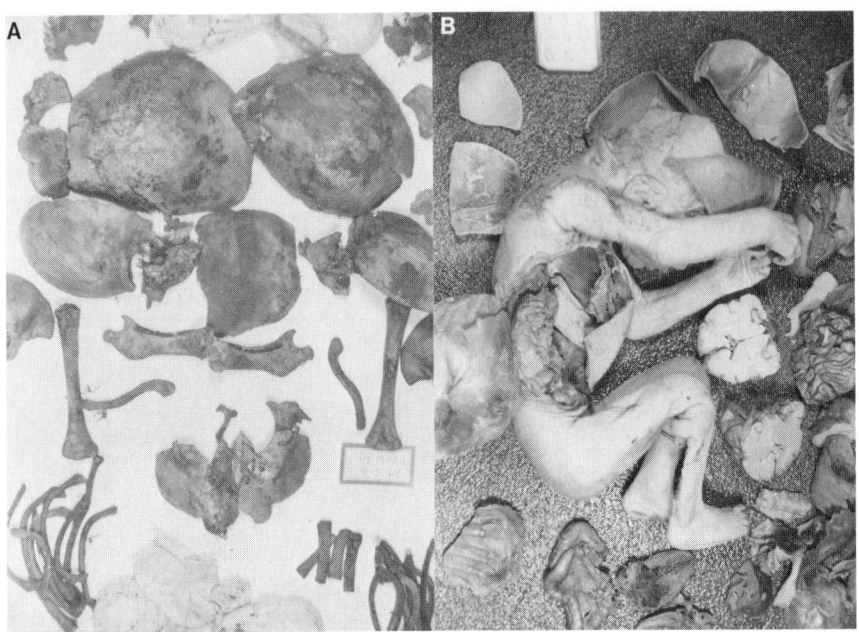

FIGURE 11-2. *A.* The skeletal remains of a 3-month-old infant, the supposed victim of "crib death." The mother led police to a cemetery where she had buried the child. The father, stationed overseas, was not told of the birth. Note the toys buried with the infant. No trauma was noted, and the case was certified as "undetermined." *B.* A near-term infant found as shown in a large vat of preservative (formaldehyde) in the basement of a coed dormitory on a university campus. "Autopsy" was performed, and no injuries were noted. The case was certified as "undetermined."

In the older child, a variety of infectious disease processes are responsible for untimely deaths. Common among these are respiratory infections varying from isolated lesions such as epiglottitis to diffuse pulmonary infections involving large and small air passages (Fig. 11-4). Acute bronchiolitis is not an infrequent condition in infants several months of age who die suddenly and unexpectedly. It is characterized by multifocal neutrophilic infiltration of the terminal alveolar ducts. Isolated tracheobronchitis without pneumonitis can also cause sudden death. We have seen focal isolated lobular pneumonias with the remaining lung parenchyma free of disease. Rarely, a diffuse viral pleuritis can be also demonstrated; occasional chronic and subacute aspiration pneumonias are seldom responsible for demise.

Lesions of the lung with involvement of other tissues can be found in conditions such as cytomegalic inclusion disease. The salivary gland and kidney must be carefully studied along with the lung if such a condition is suspected, with constant screening of the former undertaken in all cases.

Organ systems involved in infectious disease deaths in children include the heart, liver, gastrointestinal tract, central nervous system, and the blood. The latter is evidenced as generalized sepsis, often arising from an isolated focus such as the middle ear. It may produce a high fever and sudden death with little or no histologic expression in the tissues. In such instances, pure cultures of the offending organism, often *H. influenzae*, may be recovered from the ear, blood, lung, and other tissues. In a recent

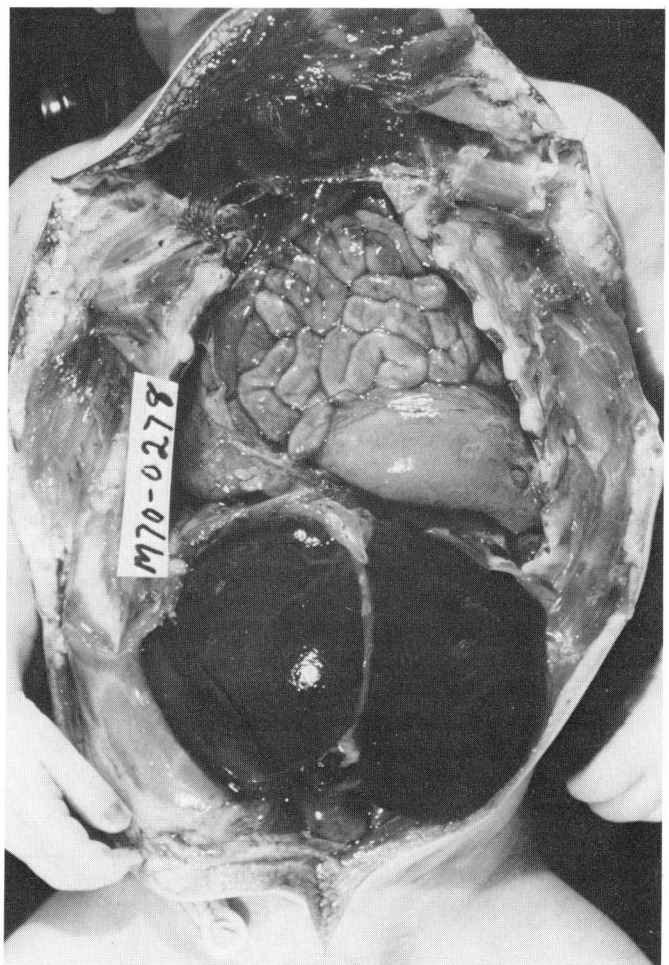

FIGURE 11-3. A newborn infant at autopsy. Primary incision reveals the intestine filling the left thoracic cavity.

series of cases, acute hepatitis has been documented, indicating that the liver should not be overlooked as a primary focus of an infectious disease process.[10] Severe pyogenic infection has long been known to produce hemorrhagic changes in the adrenal glands, referred to as the Waterhouse-Friderichsen syndrome. The latter condition may or may not be accompanied by a purulent meningitis.

Gastrointestinal tract disorders are caused by a variety of organisms, many of which are not easily cultured after antibiotic and other therapy. Rarely will a child succumb abruptly from a gastrointestinal infection, and more often it is the secondary effects of dehydration and electrolyte imbalance that will precipitate the demise. Gross lesions may be apparent in either small or large intestines; Peyer's patches may be accentuated and the mesenteric lymph nodes enlarged. Pseudomembranous enterocolitis is more often seen in hospitalized patients than in sudden deaths referred to the medical examiner.

A variety of other conditions, such as hematologic diseases including sickle cell anemia, still account for sudden death as well as secondary

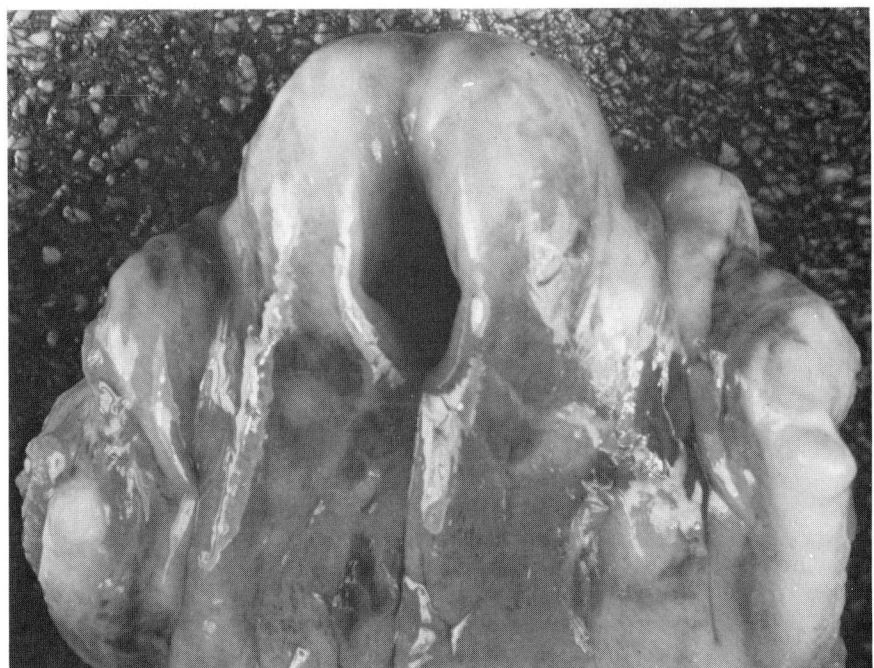

FIGURE 11-4. A young child with marked swelling, inflammation, and induration of the epiglottis.

infectious complications. Endocrine abnormalities are rarely seen but should be suspected, especially when a suggestive family history exists. A recent case, initially suggesting malnutrition and dehydration, was ultimately confirmed, with chemical corroboration and a subsequent sibling workup, as congenital adrenal hyperplasia. In older children, sudden and unexpected death from conditions such as asymmetric hypertrophy of the heart should not be overlooked, and the public health and familial consequences of diagnosing this condition should be kept in mind.[11] In the teenage population, arteriovenous malformations are a common cause of sudden death, especially during or immediately after physical activity. An isolated cerebellar hemorrhage at autopsy, for example, should be viewed as a likely vascular malformation, with a histologic study readily confirming (or excluding) this process. Rupture of the aorta from cystic medial necrosis may initially present as a potential and suspicious traumatic death (Fig. 11-5).

SUDDEN INFANT DEATH SYNDROME

Among the deaths that take place in the first year of life which are sudden and unexpected, the majority fall into what has been variously called crib death syndrome, sudden infant death syndrome (SIDS), or cot death, as it is commonly known in the United Kingdom.[12] Such cases are defined as the unexpected death of a previously healthy infant in which no findings relative to the cause of death are obtained following a thorough postmortem examination. Following a rate of approximately 3 per 1000 live births, the incidence in the United States has fallen dramatically in the mid 1970s to approximately half that figure. The majority of such infants fall into an age range of from 1 month to 9 months with the peak at 3 months. Slightly

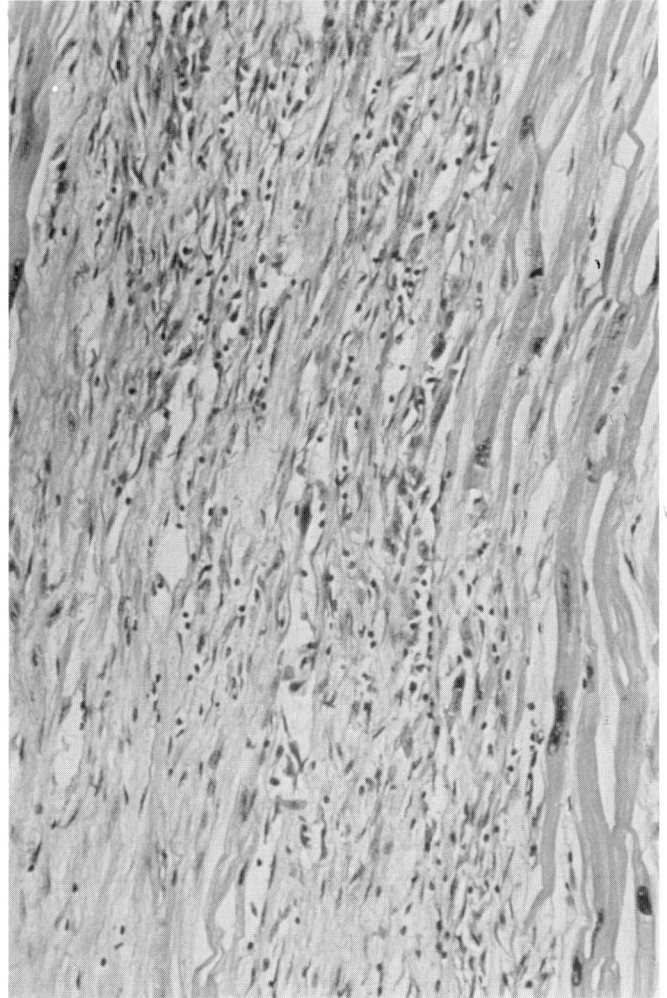

FIGURE 11-5. Histologic section of the aorta of a 13-year-old male initially reported as following an altercation. No external trauma was noted. The youth died from hemorrhagic shock following aortic rupture 1 day after hospitalization. Cystic degeneration of media was observed at autopsy.

more males have been involved, and premature babies have been affected more than full-term infants. There seem to be more fatalities during the winter months, and the time of death is most often the early morning hours as the infants are found dead in their cribs following a supposedly uneventful night's sleep. Many infants show froth in the air passages and facial pallor (Fig. 11-6).

The factors involved in such fatalities still remain obscure, although certain mechanisms have been demonstrated which may be at least partially responsible. These include sleep apnea, first illustrated by Steinschneider,[13] in which a group of infants presented with lengthy apneic episodes, several of whom ultimately died a sudden and unexpected death. More recently, Naeye[14] demonstrated thickening of the pulmonary blood vessels, along with increased heart weights, and suggested that chronic hypoxia is the physiologic mechanism responsible for the telltale histopathologic changes generally found in such cases. Naeye,[15] Valdez-

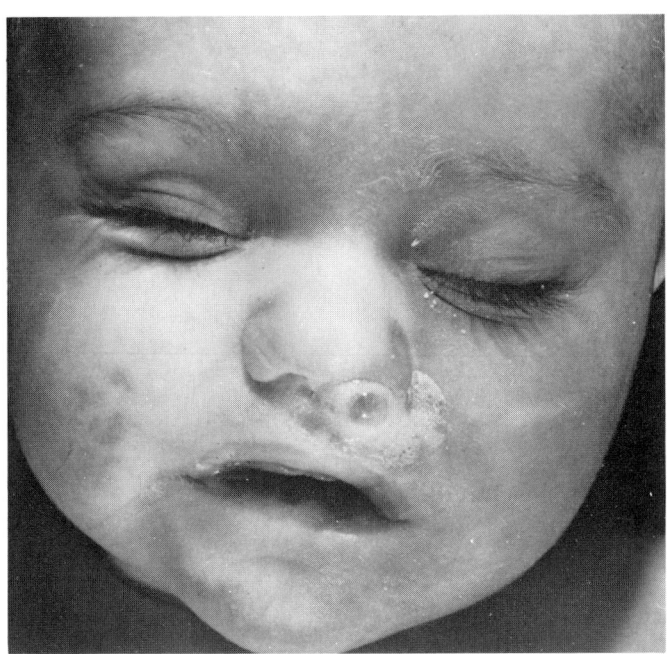

FIGURE 11-6. A young infant found face down in his crib. Note the nasal froth and pallor of the nose and right cheek, characteristic of sudden infant death syndrome.

Dapena,[16] and others have also documented an increase in extramedullary hematopoiesis in the liver and the fetal fat surrounding the adrenal glands, suggesting further evidence of chronic hypoxia.

Other theories with less extensive research to support them continue to be popular. These include hypersensitivity reactions, viral infections, elemental deficiencies, metabolic and endocrine abnormalities, digestive indiscretions, and more recently, postural asphyxia.[17]

The single most important responsibility for the forensic pathologist in sudden infant death cases is proper and thorough examination. This includes investigation and documentation at the scene of occurrence, including a survey of the home, clothes, toys, and bed or other contrivance in which the infant was found.[18] A thorough past medical history, including the hospital records of the mother and child, along with the case notes of the pediatrician or the family practitioner, and a complete autopsy including toxicologic, chemical, hematologic, and microbiologic studies should always be included, leading ultimately to a sympathetic discussion with the family. This conversation should take the form of peer or professional counseling to allay the fear, guilt, and other emotional reaction which follows the unexpected death of the infant. Information concerning sudden infant death is now readily available in pamphlet form and written especially for grieving families.[19]

ASPHYXIA IN CHILDREN

Death from asphyxia in infants and children is one of the most difficult diagnoses to confirm at autopsy. In most instances, the key to the diagnosis lies in the circumstances and, therefore, the scene investigation at or close to the time of occurrence is of paramount importance.[20] Such an investigation will reveal the location and type of bed, crib, or other contrivance in which the infant was found; objects in and about the crib, playpen, or other area which may have caused one of several forms of mechanical obstruction; a bathtub, swimming pool, or other water-containing device capable of causing drowning; and scenes of conflagration where the cause of death is most likely smoke inhalation.

The dangers of "bed-sharing" have been emphasized, and the condition of "overlaying," or compression suffocation, still occurs, albeit infrequently.[21] The majority of these victims are in the younger age group, usually less than 1 month of age, and they may be brought from the crib to the parents' bed in order to soothe and quiet their "fussy nature."[22] The careless and/or intoxicated parent can easily roll onto the child, and the weight of his or her body will inhibit respiration, whether or not the nose and mouth are covered. An unusual lividity pattern and absence of petechial hemorrhages may be the only postmortem findings at autopsy.

Cases of suffocation from extrinsic objects are generally confined to bags and wrappers made out of nonporous plastic. A particularly lethal object is the ever-present dry cleaning bag, which should be tied into knots and disposed of immediately when infants and small children are household members. Children in the second 6 months of life seem to be particularly susceptible. The contents of the bed and crib should be carefully examined with this in mind (Fig. 11-7).

Wedging of a young infant can occur in several circumstances, the most recently publicized being a defective crib.[23,24] The manufacture and design of such cribs are now regulated,[25] but older cribs which are ill-repaired with spaces enabling infants to "wiggle through" remain in use and are perilous. Even the hospital is not immune from such occurrences (Fig. 11-8). Other perilous circumstances occur when inadequate "bumpers" in cribs are fitted with small mattresses which are otherwise normal in design. Adult beds, situated several inches from the wall where infants can become wedged in the crevice, are not immune from suspicion. Fur-

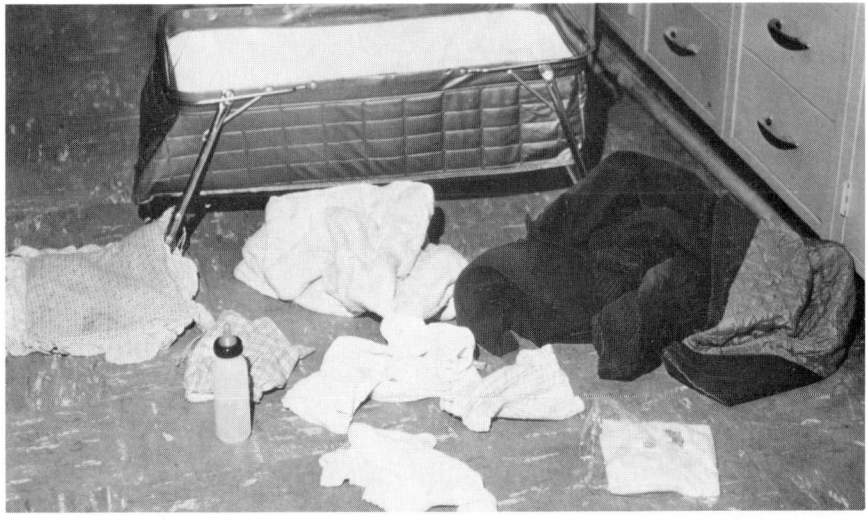

FIGURE 11-7. The bassinet of a young infant with its contents noted in the foreground. Note the plastic bag in the right foreground, a potentially lethal object.

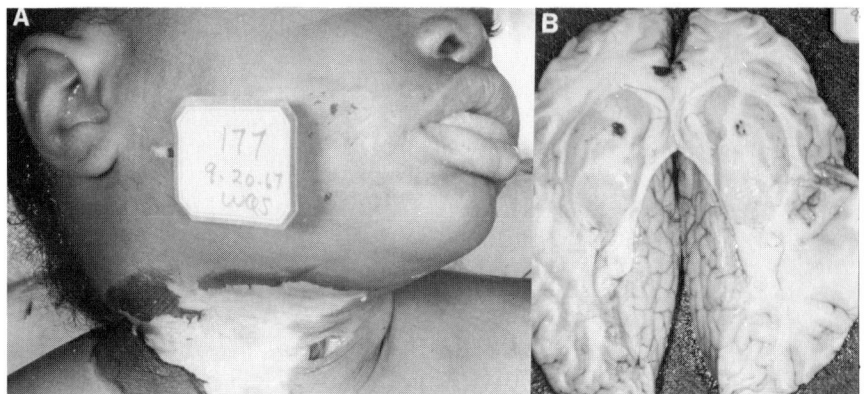

FIGURE 11-8. *A.* Incomplete healing 8 days following suspension in "oversized" crib slats in the emergency room, awaiting repair of a cut foot. *B.* Hemorrhagic necrosis of the globis pallidum and corpus callosum.

niture such as bureau drawers can compress infants to death. Play articles in the home and on playgrounds can result in death. Once again, the scene investigation and the exact location of the child are absolute imperatives. Patterned abrasions, abnormal lividity patterns, alterations in pallor, and congestion of various organs are the key postmortem findings (Fig. 11-9). Petechial hemorrhages may be lacking in many such cases where death ensues rapidly from anoxia.[26]

Accidental hanging can be caused by strings of toys, pacifiers, and other elongated items becoming entangled in the infant's clothing and/or crib.[27] Such cases usually occur in the second half-year of life. Choking on foreign objects such as food, toys, and other objects can occur as early as the first year, but is more common in later life. Balloons, whether recently inflated and ruptured or existing in parts, are particularly dangerous, and children should be discouraged from playing with them altogether. Autoerotic hangings occur in young teenagers during masturbation and other sexual pleasure-seeking.

Deaths from smoke inhalation, carbon monoxide intoxication, and other mechanisms of fires are most frequently caused by older siblings playing with matches. Rare instances of lightning, automobile trauma, and electrical malfunctions can be the cause of such conflagrations. Smoke alarm systems are highly advisable devices for family dwellings, but are no substitute for the habits of safety which should be instilled in young children. Unrecognized pulmonary burns can be extremely hazardous (Fig. 11-10).

BLUNT FORCE TRAUMA

A variety of injuries from different sources can be responsible for blunt force trauma in infants and young children. The more common conditions producing such injuries are falls, either from heights or down stairs while playing, and vehicular-related trauma. Small infants have been known to sustain craniocerebral trauma in falls from adult beds, high chairs, and other objects. Such conditions should be carefully separated from instances of battered child syndrome. Nevertheless, we are impressed with the paucity of head injuries, especially fractures, found in young children who are said to have "struck their heads" in this manner.

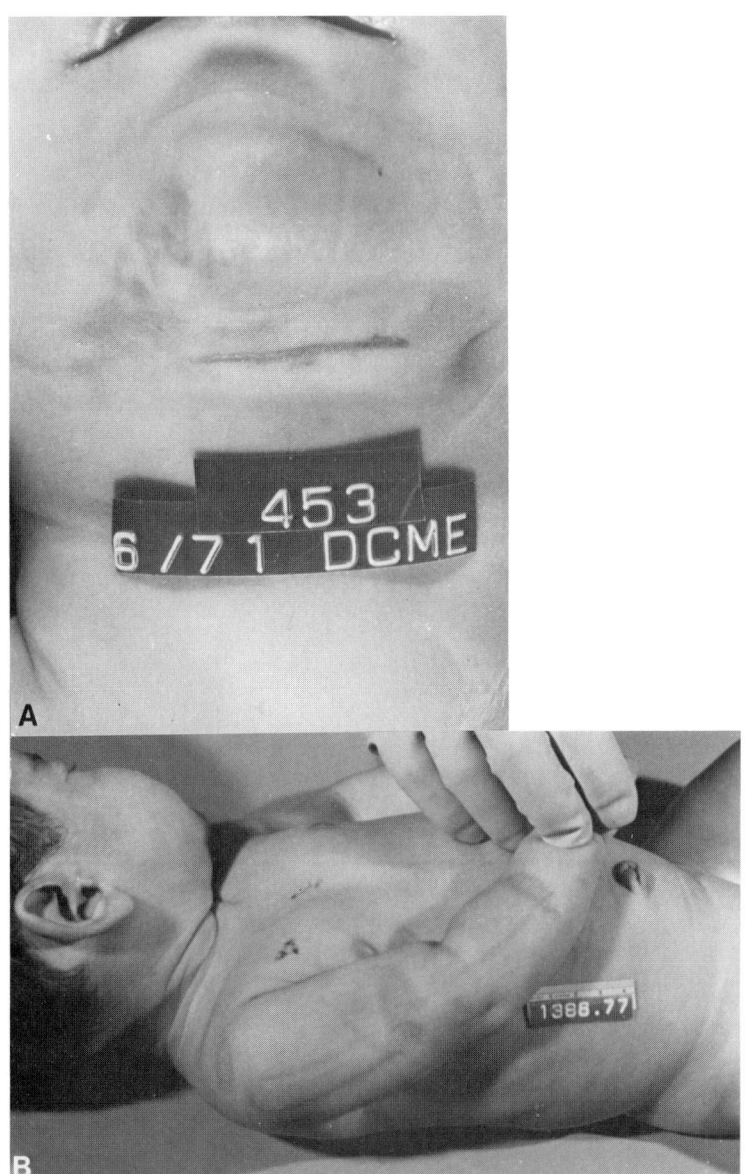

FIGURE 11-9. *A.* Chin abrasions resulting from suspension between a mattress spring and sideboard. *B.* Patterned contusions of arm during compression and suspension of the body in a defective crib.

Once again, the pattern of the injury is of extreme importance in reconstructing the circumstances of the trauma, especially when the pathologic findings do not substantiate the available information. We have seen an instance of two patterned circular abrasions of the midanterior chest, suspiciously resembling cigarette burns, in a 19-month-old infant in apparent good health. The autopsy findings revealed a ruptured septum of the heart with resultant cardiac tamponade (Fig. 11-11). Only when an extension gate across the stairwell was examined at the scene was the conclusion reached that the youngster had climbed over this gate to the top of the steps and then tumbled down into two cylindrical brads pro-

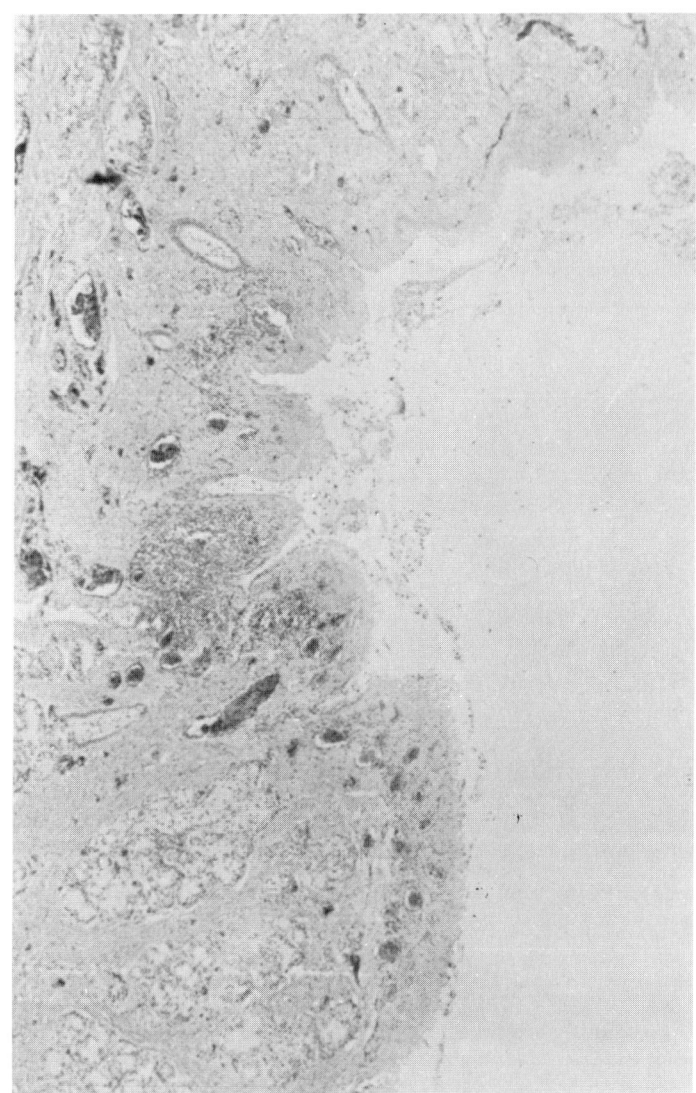

FIGURE 11-10. An unrecognized "pulmonary burn." The trachea of a 2-year-old child following an 8 percent surface area burn of the neck and "face." The child was treated in the emergency room and released, but was dead on arrival 3 days later. Note sloughing of the epithelium of hemorrhagic necrosis and inflammation of the submucosa.

truding from the gate at exactly the width of the circular chest injuries. The gate had provided sufficient resistance upon impact to produce this unusual, but nonetheless typical, deceleration trauma upon impact.

Abdominal trauma is frequently confined to the mesentery and its vasculature, but ruptures of the parenchymal organs, especially the spleen, are seen with certain types of accidents. The author is familiar with cases of snow-sledding accidents in which youngsters have injured themselves, either on the sled at impact, or from falling and striking the ground or other fixed object. Recently, two separate and distinct teenage cases of splenic rupture, sustained while engaging in athletics, demonstrated an

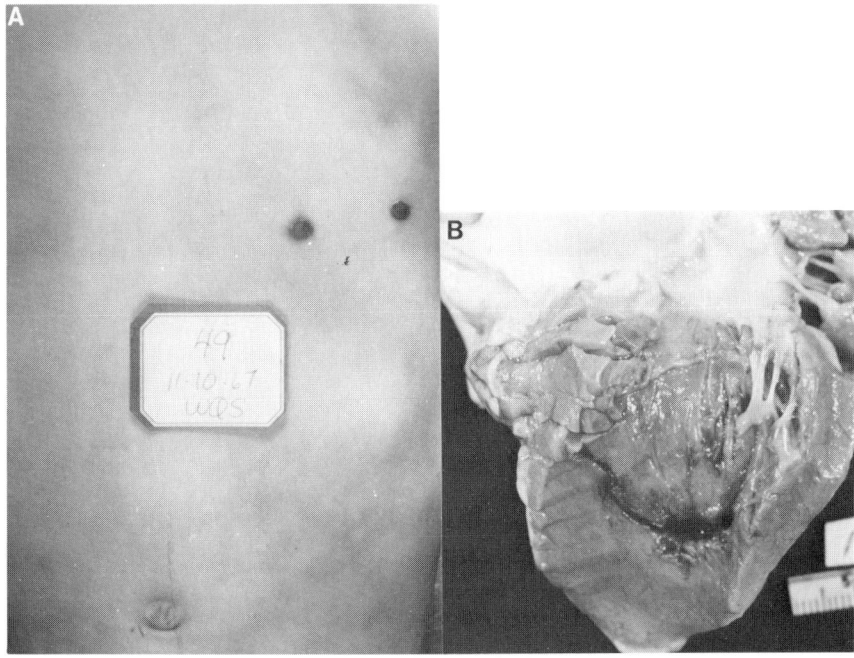

FIGURE 11-11. *A.* Skin of chest showing circular abrasions. *B.* Laceration of the septal wall of the heart.

underlying infectious mononucleosis with accompanying splenomegaly and thus greater "exposure" during abdominal trauma.

A wide variety of head injuries can be seen in infants, children, and teenagers. Young school children have been known to sustain minor head injuries producing an unsuspected epidural hematoma. One such instance occurred when a child swung on a chain from a flagpole at school. Upon returning home, the child felt weak and tired and went to bed early without noticeable craniocerebral symptoms other than a headache. The child was found dead in bed the next morning due to a unilateral epidural hematoma without external markings on the skin. Firearm injuries to the head are rare but do occur in the very young (Fig. 11-12).

Vehicular injuries constitute the largest category of blunt force trauma to infants and children as well as to adults. Such injuries include stillbirths following maternal auto accidents, skate-board fatalities, and motorcycle and bicycle injuries. The author has seen a case of a circular fracture of the skull resulting when a portion of a tricycle was thrown from three stories above the sidewalk where the child victim was found (Figs. 11-13 and 11-14). The diameter and the matching pattern of the handlebar with the skull fracture were essential in documenting the offending agent and apprehending the teenage assailants.

An unusual form of head injury seen on occasion consists of massive swelling without intermeningeal hemorrhage or fracture, most often seen when a flat, broad surface has struck the head. Such a case occurred when a teenage youngster carrying his musical horn case was struck deliberately with its flat, broad surface. He fell to the ground abruptly and was dead in 15 to 20 minutes, as documented by an arriving rescue unit. The brain weighed approximately 1750 gm and showed massive swelling, but no intermeningeal or brainstem hemorrhage. A small subgaleal bleed was

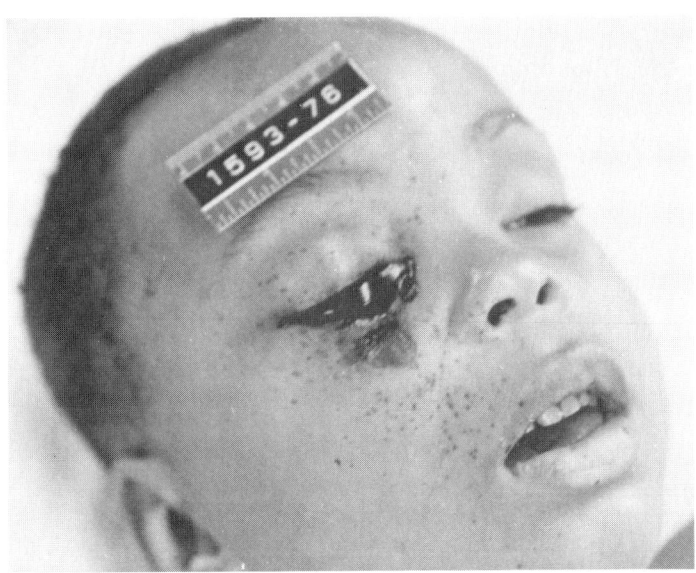

FIGURE 11-12. A 3-year-old child who had obtained his mother's loaded .38 caliber revolver from her purse; the pistol discharged while held in his lap. Note stippling of the cheek and abraded inferior margin beneath entrance in the right eye.

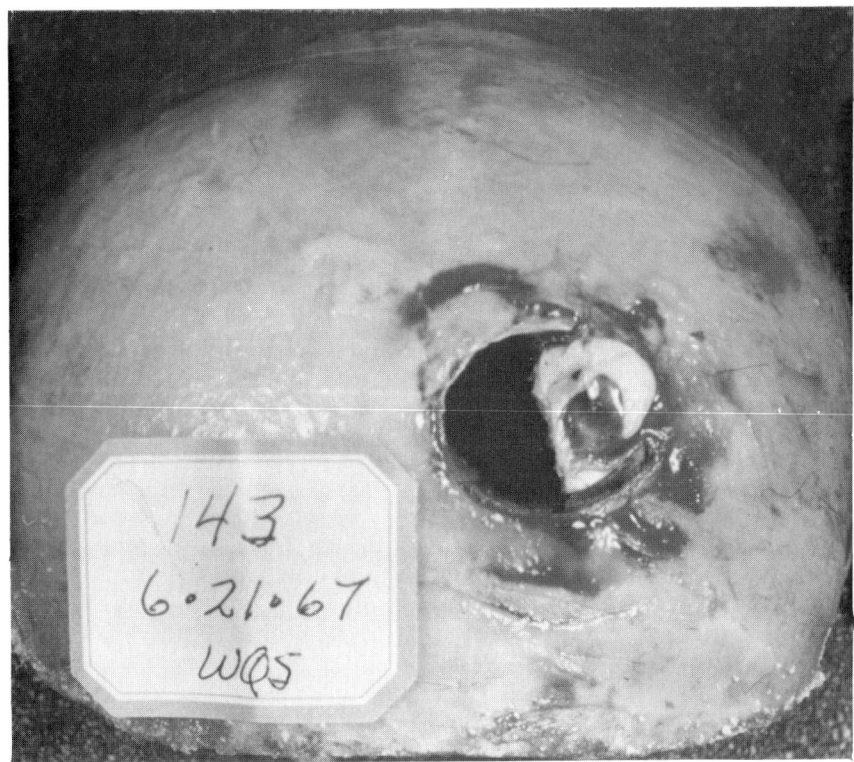

FIGURE 11-13. Blunt force trauma in a young child. Note the circular skull fracture.

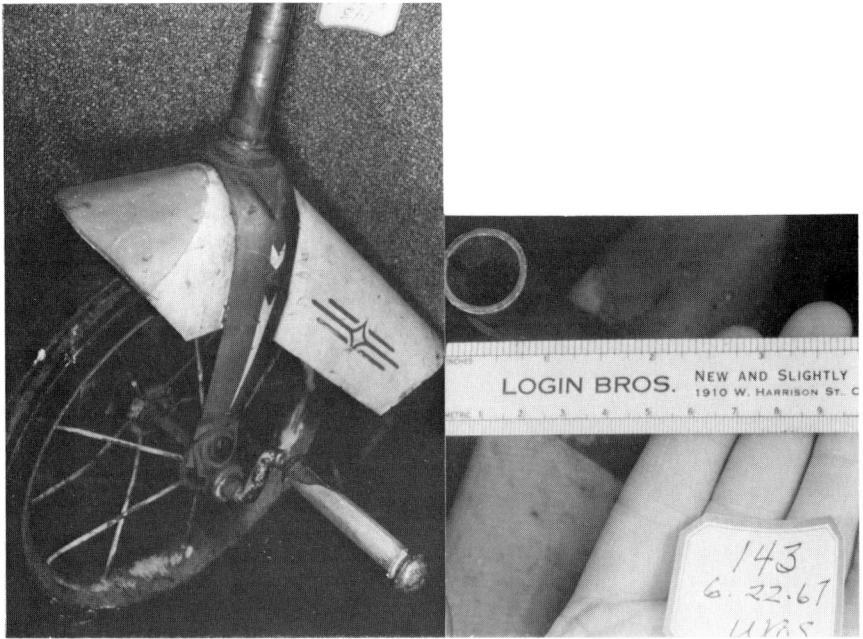

FIGURE 11-14. Tricycle recovered at the scene of the accident cited in Figure 11-13. Note the shape and diameter of the open-bar pedal, which conforms to the injury pattern shown in Figure 11-13.

the only indication that trauma had been inflicted. This dramatic response to injury has also been seen in a fall downstairs by a 2-year-old infant, the head probably striking the flat, broad surface of uncarpeted hardwood.

Other nonfatal injuries must be considered in these cases since some lead to secondary infection and sepsis. A recent article described how children accidentally injure themselves with staplers which do not protect against trauma to the digits of the untrained user.[28]

CHILDHOOD POISONINGS

The number of accidental poisonings in children has decreased dramatically over the last few years, primarily due to safety caps on pill vials. Fatal poisonings that do occur have also been managed with more effectiveness at the clinical level. On the other hand, older children, especially teenagers, have indulged more generously in alcoholic beverages as well as medications, occasionally with self-destructive intent. This latter category of suicide has substantially increased over the last decade, and seems to account for the majority of poisoning fatalities in young people today.

Ethyl alcohol intoxication has been seen in the small infant whose parents, guided by country folklore or other spurious wisdom, have administered brandy and other spirits to alleviate "teething," "colic," and other nondescript complaints. The adolescent who experiments in his father's liquor cabinet learns all too quickly the acute depressive effects of alcohol intoxication. Other volatile poisonings are rare and unusual, although the author has seen a teenager who soaked his clothing and a surrounding blanket in gasoline and inhaled the vapors with a fatal outcome.

The dangers of gaseous substances, with special reference to carbon monoxide, cannot be overemphasized. Defective mufflers in automobiles, inadequate space heaters, and conflagrations of all sizes produce rapid and lethal concentrations of carbon monoxide which are often fatal. Another substance known to produce sudden death is freon, the propellant for many aerosol products presently on the market. The volatile potential of the constituents of airplane glue (particularly toluene) is dangerous, especially with the additional anoxia produced by employing a plastic

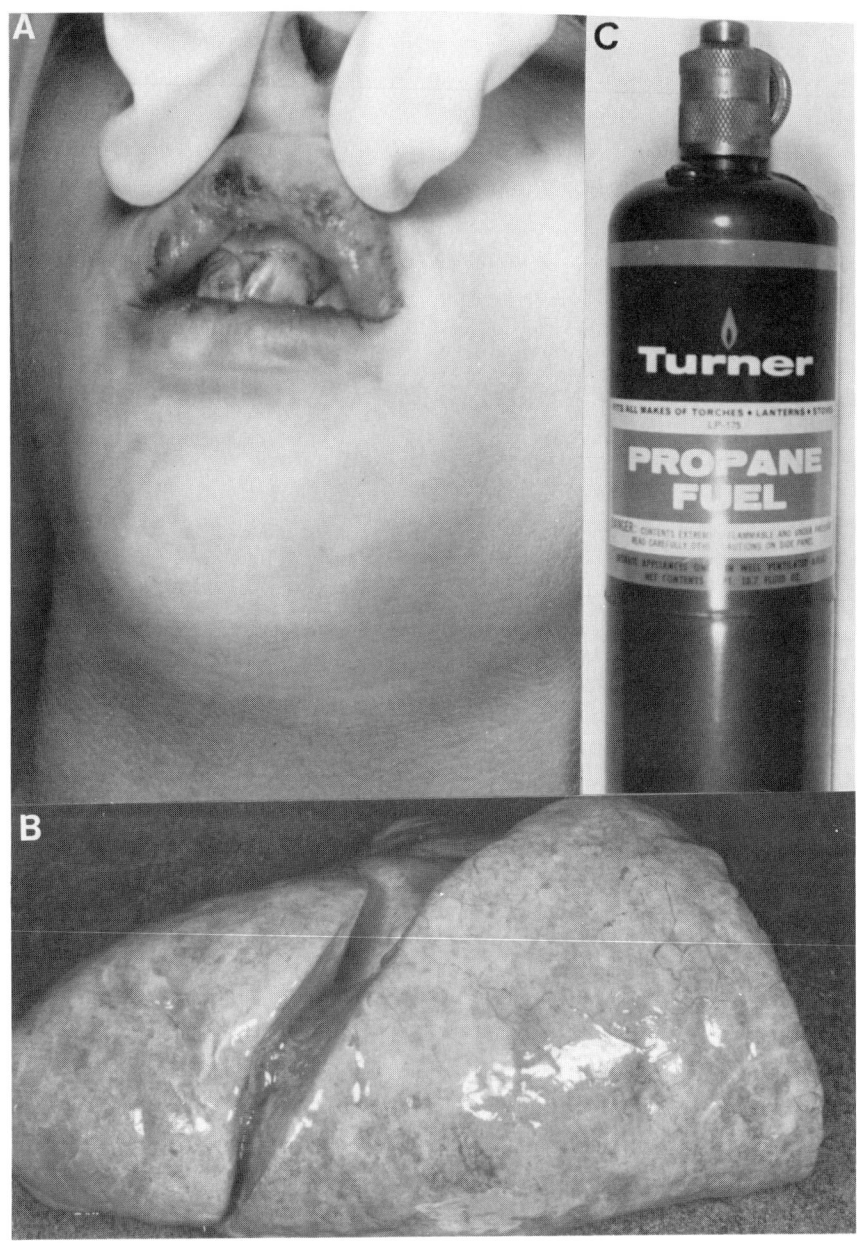

FIGURE 11-15. Fatal inhalation of propane by a 13-year-old youth. A. Lip abrasions noted on external examination. B. Hyperinflation of lung noted at autopsy. C. Propane tank found at the scene.

bag over the head. The author has seen a 13-year-old boy succumb from inhaling propane from a bottled tank, ostensibly acquired as an adjunct for model airplane and ship building (Fig. 11-15).

Narcotic abuse and accidental death have been recorded in the very young following the ingestion of methadone in fruit juice located in the easily accessible refrigerator of addicted parents.[29] The middle and late teenage population continues to experiment with a variety of inhalants and injectable drugs (Fig. 11-16). The so-called street drugs are perhaps more dangerous, not because of their constituents, but owing to the lack of knowledge of the user about their individual identification and strength. A recent activity condoned by peer groups is the mixture of pills and capsules ("fruit salad") with random ingestion producing unexpected responses.[30]

A variety of household products still remain a deadly source of toxic substances for all ages, but especially for the young. Household cleaners and gardening supplies represent the majority of such agents, and the lack of suitable "child-proof" containers on many of these has kept the number of accidental ingestions and fatal outcomes relatively high. Special dangers arise from inordinately high concentrations of acidic and basic substances in such cleaners.[31] The complications following surgical

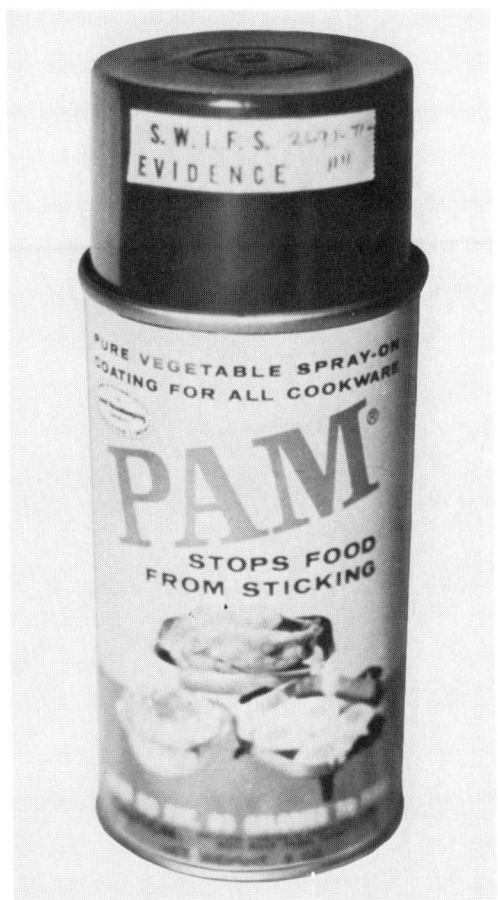

FIGURE 11-16. Spray can used in cooking. Lecithin is the active ingredient. Freon 11 and 12 (propellants) are toxic to the cardiorespiratory system.

repair of esophageal stricture resulting from lye ingestion vary widely; a fatal case of pancake-syrup ingestion in such a child has been documented by the author.[32]

The most common variety of chronic poisoning in children remains lead intoxication. A great number of products and circumstances of ingestion have been documented, from toys and drinking glasses to glazed pottery and, most recently, accidental inhalation of lead-containing gasoline from power lawn mowers and herbal medication.[33] Teenagers are not immune from ingestion of prescription drugs, especially during trying circumstances and with little personal circumspection as to the outcome.[34] Instances of initial suspicion of toxic effects can prove otherwise with careful investigation and thorough autopsy (Fig. 11-17).

CHILD ABUSE

Child abuse, including the "battered baby syndrome," takes the lives of over 4,000 infants and children each year in the United States. Much has been written about the psychological and physical aspects of such trauma, the team treatment methods, and various other facets of the problem.[35] The pathologic features are reasonably well defined and can generally be divided into cases of repetitive trauma, single-episode trauma, and starvation or other severe neglect.[36] Sexual abuse may be a component in any or all of these patterns.

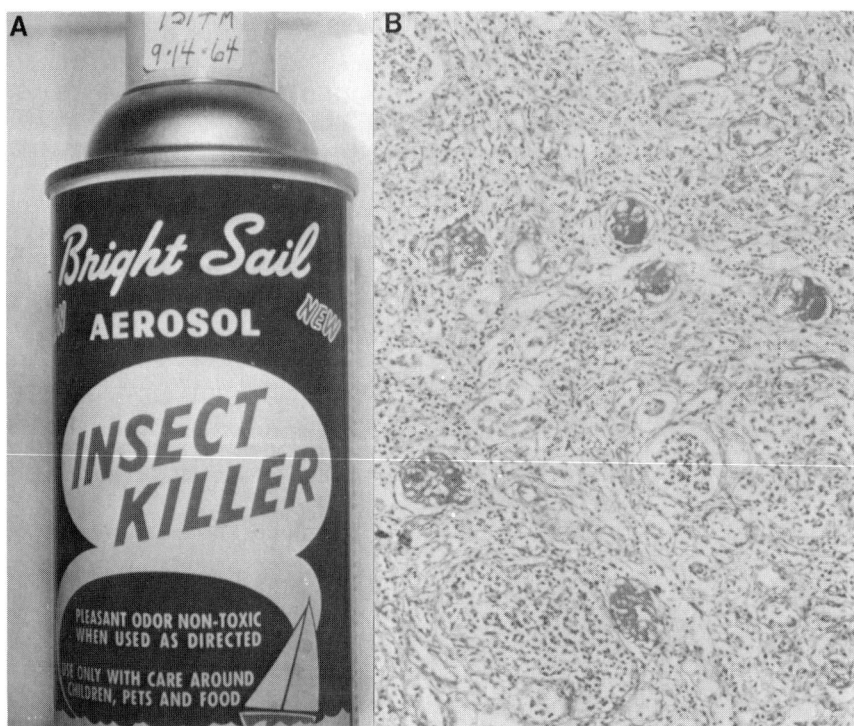

FIGURE 11-17. A. A can of "insecticide" said to have been sprayed indoors several hours prior to the sudden "illness" of a 3 year old. B. PAS stain of kidney. Autopsy 1 week later showed glomerulonephritis, chronic and subacute, but no tubular disease, the latter usually associated with insecticides. Kidney biopsy on the fourth hospital day yielded finding of "toxic nephritis."

Repetitive trauma, the classic pattern of the "battered baby syndrome," consists of both recent and older injuries. The marked callous formation of old fractures and the resolving bruises of the skin and soft tissue may be so diffuse as to cover the majority of the surface area of the body. On the other hand, small lacerations and subtle bruises of the vital organs, including the brain, may be barely perceptible until fine dissection of the tissues is undertaken (Fig. 11-18). Deeper bruises, which are often inapparent on external examination of the skin, can reveal large areas of hemorrhage and fat necrosis, and even "pooled pockets" of blood in areas such as the lower buttocks and thighs. The more common mechanisms of death found at autopsy include hemorrhage from ruptured parenchymal organs as well as mesenteric fat and blood vessels; subdural hemorrhage from head trauma, which may or may not include fractures; multiple soft tissue injuries without parenchymal trauma; and skeletal damage with hemorrhage in subcutaneous and intramuscular locations throughout the trunk and extremities (Fig. 11-19). The latter condition inevitably becomes labeled as the "difficult case." The inexperienced pathologist and the prosector will often feel that they have "insignificant findings" following the standard medicolegal autopsy, not realizing that the shock following trauma and blood loss in a young person is a readily acceptable mechanism of death.

The single episode of trauma tends to occur in families in which the mother, often emotionally and physically exhausted from a new birth, turns out of frustration to strike an older child who has been pestering her for attention. The author has seen two such instances in which a child struck his head on the corner of a fireplace hearth and the edge of a table, respectively, resulting in fatal head trauma. In these cases the children are

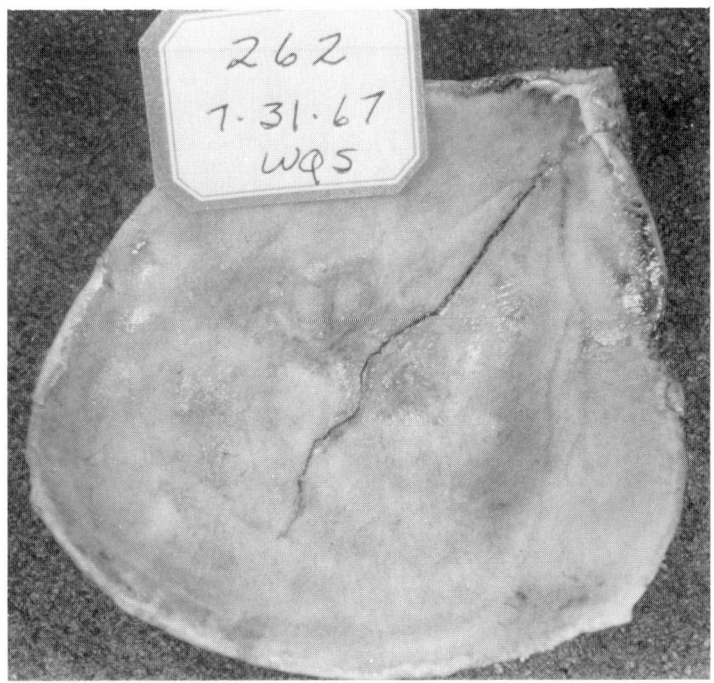

FIGURE 11-18. Healing skull fracture in a 6-month-old child said to have been "dropped" by his mother, who lived above a tavern where she worked as a "dancer."

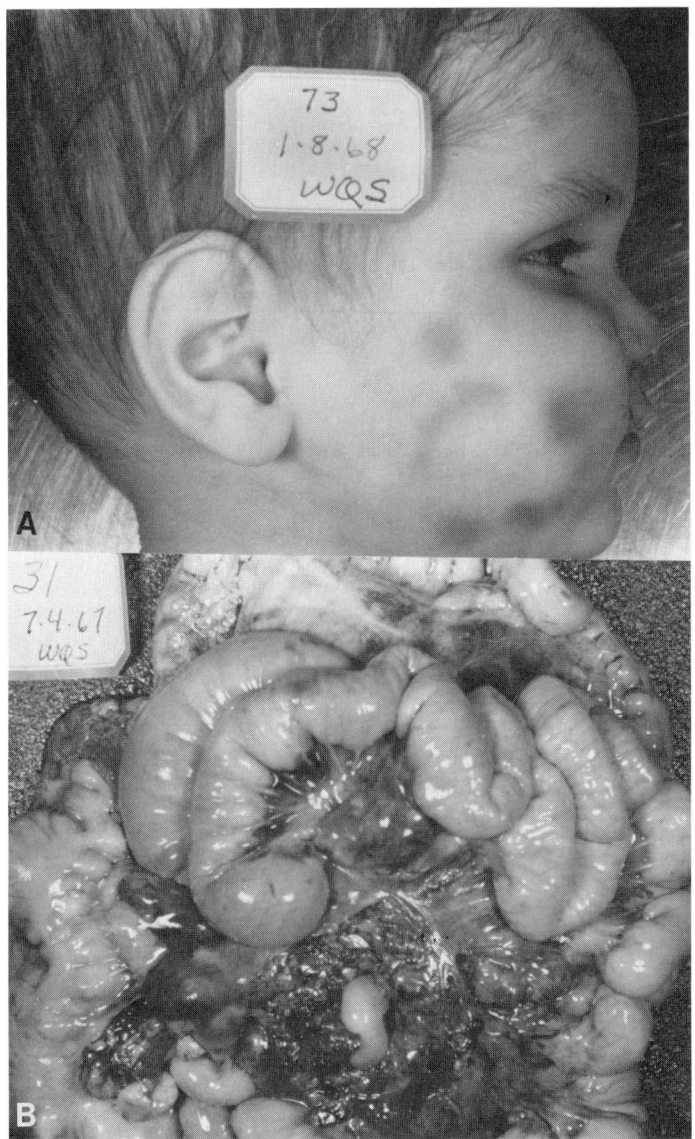

FIGURE 11-19. Child Abuse. *A.* Patterned contusion of the cheek; shoe incriminated but "bite mark" not excluded. *B.* Laceration of mesentery with contusion of intestine. Blunt force trauma to abdomen present.

usually well cared for, show good hygiene and nutrition, and, most importantly, seldom show any marks of previous injury, much less sexual abuse. In one recent study, approximately 25 percent of child abuse deaths fell into this category.[36]

The final category, that of starvation and other severe neglect, approximates one-fourth of child abuse cases (Fig. 11-20). Injuries of a blunt force nature and skeletal fractures are not common on the neglected child, but have been noted to occur. These children are often very young, can be the first or subsequent child in a family, and appear severely wasted to the point of an absence of subcutaneous fat. Pathologic findings include fatty metamorphosis of the liver, iron deposits in the liver and spleen, thymic

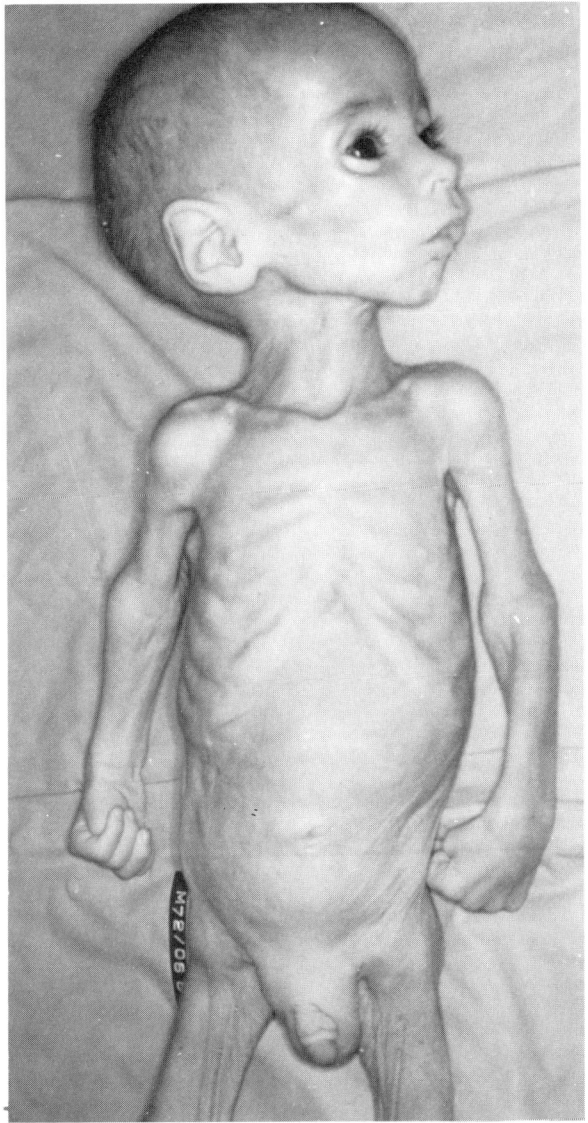

FIGURE 11-20. Starvation and neglect of a 5-month-old child. Note the absence of any overt trauma. Congenital and acquired disease producing a similar picture must be excluded.

atrophy, and empty intestinal tract and secondary pneumonia. Terminal dehydration can often be diagnosed with vitreous electrolyte studies. It must be remembered that religious beliefs may prohibit some parents from seeking care of an injured or sick child, with the resulting death due to inanition and wasting.

In all the above cases, careful search of the genital organs for burns, foreign material, and injuries as a result of insertion of objects should be conducted. Older children are particularly vulnerable, but the author has recently seen a 1-year-old child with the characteristic striatal lacerations of the anorectal junction producing subsequent hemorrhage and death. Swabs for spermatozoa and acid phosphatase should be taken from the body orifices, but unusual sites such as the axillae and legs should not be overlooked for potential foreign stains. Atypical findings and circumstances of child abuse may occur and should be kept in mind.[37]

Gastric contents should always be saved in cases of child abuse. The timing of the injury may be of critical importance in court, and the last meal ingested by the child may be of paramount importance in ascertaining the sequence of the fatal trauma.

The projection of transparent photographic slides in the courtroom has become more frequently utilized as a method of demonstrating the pattern of injuries to the jury. The author has participated in a trial where such exhibits were offered and accepted notwithstanding the previous introduction of the physical evidence (objects used to strike the child) and photographic prints, both of which were already distributed to the jury (Fig. 11-21).

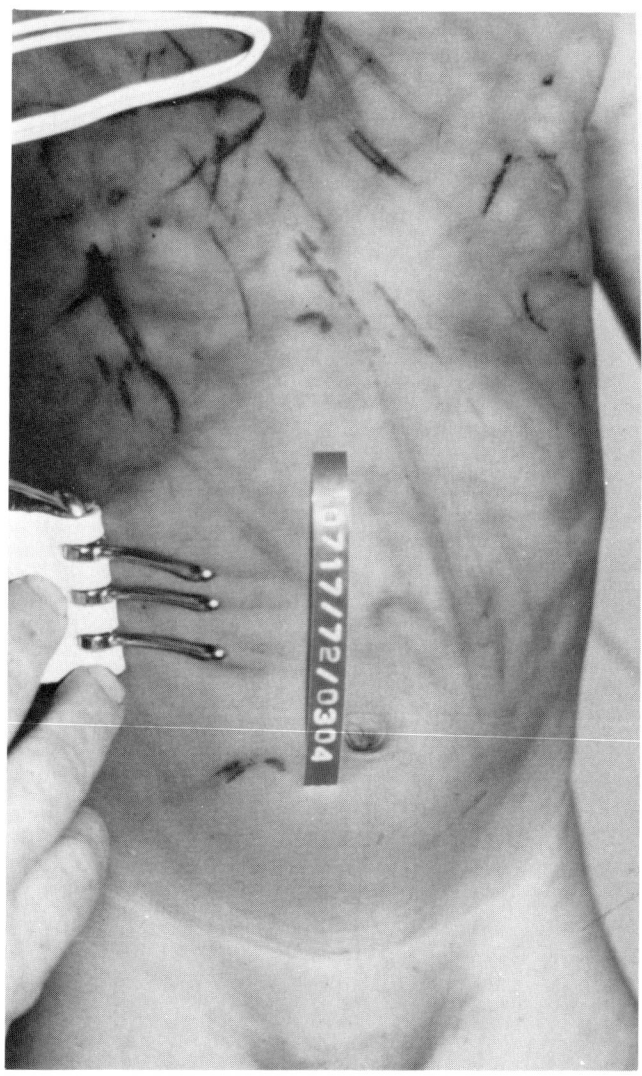

FIGURE 11-21. Patterned abusive injuries to the skin of a child with nearby offending agents. Note the shape and similarities of the contusions.

CHILDHOOD DROWNING

Each year there are approximately 8,000 drownings in the United States with over 6,000 of these involving swimming, wading, playing, or falling into the water. Drowning is the third leading cause of accidental death, and in the age range of 1 to 44 ranks second only to motor vehicle accidents.

Accidental drowning is infrequent under the age of 1, but it rises rapidly in early childhood to peak at ages 15 to 19 in males and 10 to 14 in females. The incidence of drowning among males is over ten times that of females during the teenage years. The peak incidence of females is registered at preschool ages 1 to 4. Four out of five swimming fatalities take place at unorganized facilities (i.e., places not officially designated as swimming areas). This reinforces the belief that only a small proportion of those who swim are skilled enough to take care of themselves in situations they are likely to encounter. There are less than 100 drownings a year among scuba divers and skin divers, although this estimate is misleading since deaths in this group are also from other causes.

In the 100 or so drownings annually among persons taking a bath, over 60 are of children. Preschool children also account for more than two-thirds of the drownings of people playing adjacent to water.

We have noted the dangers to very young children from diaper pails and wash buckets, especially those of the 3- to 5-gallon size, into which a head-first topple is easily accomplished.[20] Blackbourne's study of infant drownings in bathtubs over a 10-year period calls attention to little-realized dangers such as scalding (three cases showing this type of burn pattern) and instances where older siblings were left alone with the young infant, inadvertently causing submersion and drowning.[38]

A complete autopsy is mandatory in all cases of infant drowning, with the time-honored sign of fluid-filled lungs usually present. A more important consideration at autopsy is the documentation of pre-existing natural disease which may have played a role in the submersion. The author has recently noted an advanced case of diffuse myocarditis, apparently asymptomatic, in a 3-year-old child found in a tub half filled with lukewarm water.

Instances of drowning, with or without scalding, must always be examined as potential child abuse cases (Fig. 11-22). In one instance, the author examined the case of a diabetic mother who claimed to have had an "insulin reaction," and for a period of time was asleep in her bedroom. Her 20-month-old child was in the bathtub and apparently adjusted the hot water to scalding temperatures and was severely burned. An examination of the heat capabilities of the hot water system at the house with appropriate temperature recordings of the water, the depths in the tub, and the length of time taken for such occurrences made it clear that it was impossible for the mother to have adjusted the hot water herself, and her story was accepted as factual. Such instances emphasize the importance not only of the scene investigation, but also of the attempt to recreate the conditions, if possible, that led to the terminal event.

Other circumstances which lead to accidental submersion are falls through thin ice, inadvertent stumbling into outdoor swimming pool areas in unfenced and unprotected areas, the occasional accidental submersions in supervised swimming pools, and the drowning due to slipping out of flotation toys and other such devices. It seems redundant to stress the importance of swimming lessons and water safety procedures for children from the earliest ages.

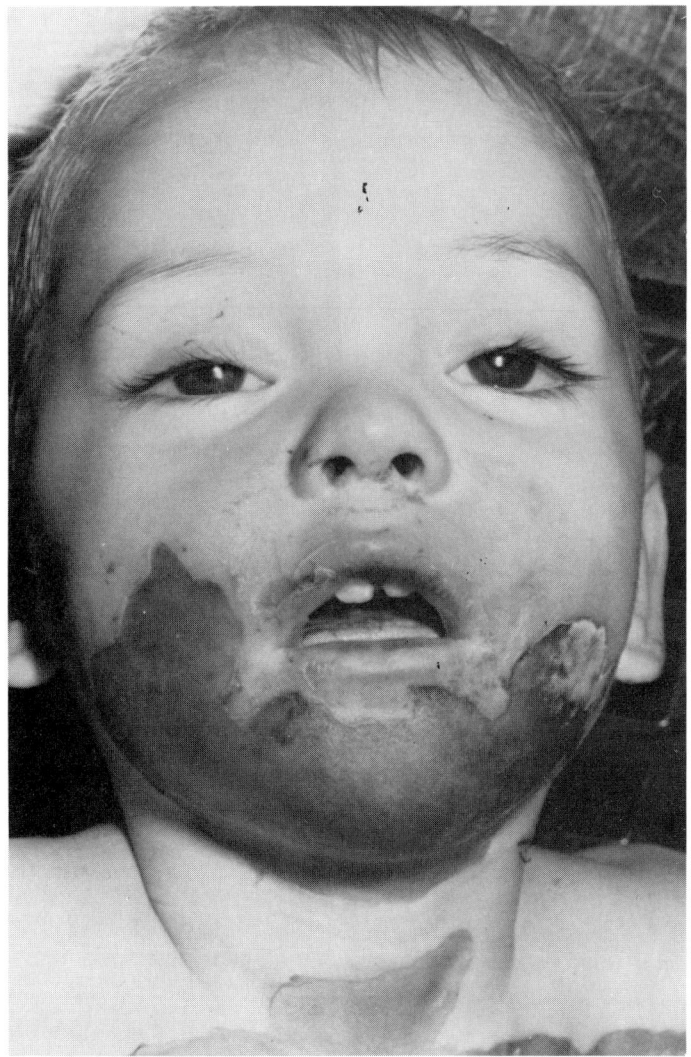

FIGURE 11-22. Scald burns on the face of a child following submersion in hot bath water. This case was probably accidental, and no sibling was involved.

CHILDHOOD SUICIDES AND HOMICIDES

The number of suicides of young children and teenagers has dramatically increased over the last decade. A wide variety of modalities have been employed with all of the methods utilized by the adult population also seen in young people. These include firearms, jumps from heights, inhalation of auto fumes, drug overdoses, and hangings. Less frequent instances are those from incised wounds and submersion. Children and teenagers can also be under the influence of alcohol and occasionally drugs at the time of their self-destructive act.

The reasons for such suicides are many and varied, but standard responses to inquiries bring answers such as disappointment in the home, including parental breakup; failure at school in either academic or athletic endeavors; inability to be accepted by peer groups; disappointment or rejection in a love affair, often for the first time; and more recently, preoccupation with death, especially involving other young members of a fatalistic group.[39]

Many young suicides leave notes, often addressed to their friends and family, some very voluminous and a few rather incoherent. A greater tendency to tape-record messages has also been demonstrated in recent years.

It would seem that very few of these children have received psychiatric help, counseling, or any other assistance at this critical time in their lives. Some tend to end their lives seemingly "on the spur of the moment" without being recognized as troubled, and do not leave any messages indicating their final intentions.

The homicidal deaths of infants, young children, and teenagers, other

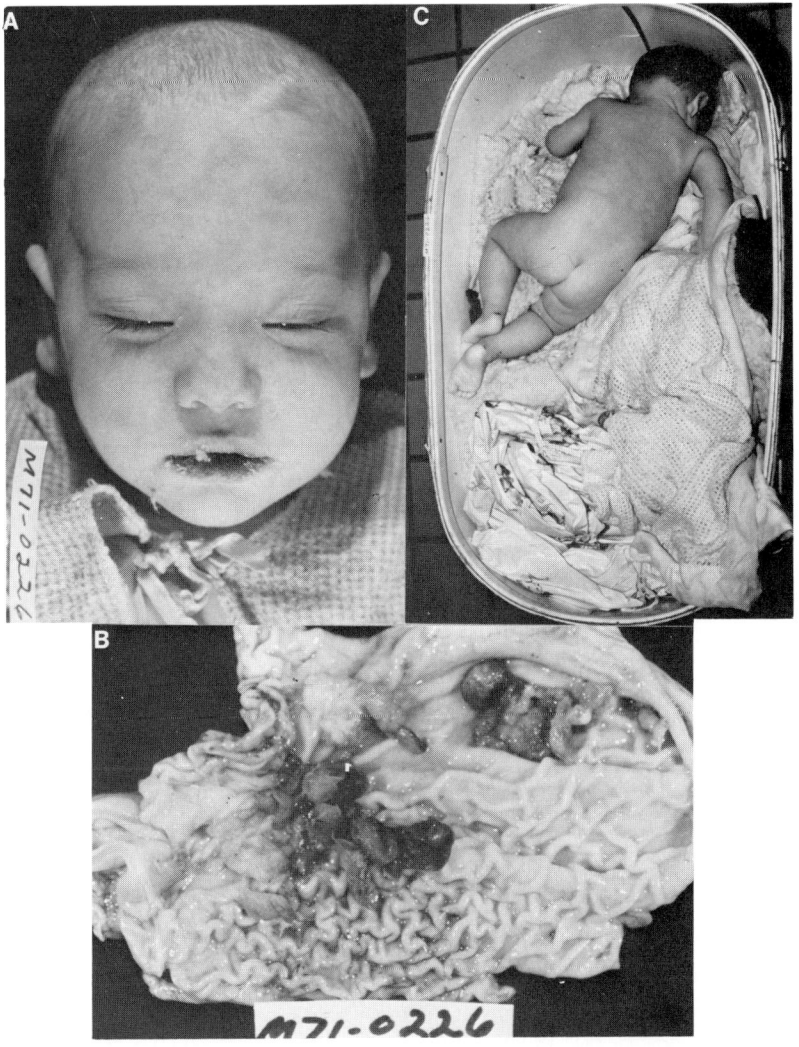

FIGURE 11-23. Deliberate suffocation of a 5-month-old child. A. Cotton fibers over face and about mouth. B. Cotton fibers mixed with gastric contents. C. Simulation of the child's position in the bassinet with open cotton padding prominent.

than those categorized as child abuse, are relatively infrequent but remain constant. The majority of cases occur outside of the family circle with a stranger or an acquaintance.[40]

A few of the cases of homicide are those of infants found in their beds and are reported initially as crib deaths. The author has investigated a case in which cotton fibers were found in the air passages as well as the stomach of a 5-month-old child lying face down in a bassinet (Fig. 11-23). The plastic covering on the bedding had been partially torn away, exposing the fibers. The male baby sitter in question, an acquaintance who was placed in charge of the household while both parents worked, had stolen

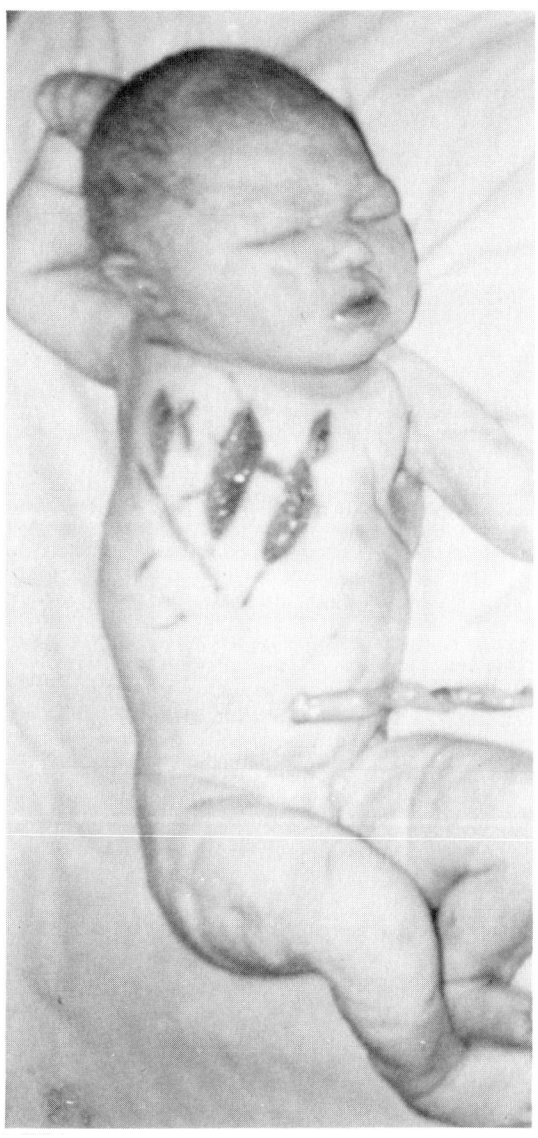

FIGURE 11-24. A stillborn term infant recovered from a toilet. Note the slash marks on the chest, shown to be superficial at autopsy. The lungs were unaerated, and there were no other signs of independent existence. The distraught mother admitted to having wounded the lifeless child immediately after home delivery.

the father's car and, after returning it 48 hours later, told the story that he was unable to stop the baby from crying and so "held its head down firmly against the bedding" until the crying had ceased. A murder indictment was filed against this man and he was tried and convicted. Several murders masked as "crib deaths" and committed by the parents of the children have been documented.[41]

In inadequately supervised centers such as hospitals, orphanages, and children's homes, instances involving negligence occasionally occur. A case is recalled in which a 5-year-old child on a hospital ward without professional attendance suffocated a newborn infant because the older youngster was "unable to sleep amidst the crying." Stillborn infants who are unattended at home may be "assaulted" and disposition attempted, thus masquerading as "infanticide" (Fig. 11-24).

The other large group of homicides perpetrated against the young involves teenagers. Many cases arise out of homosexual relationships, often inadvertent for the younger child. Other deaths are caused by "friends" while playing with firearms or other weapons. Fatalities occurring during juvenile "gang wars" are different examples of this type of behavior.

There are numerous documented cases of hitchhikers who are seen in one locality but, after accepting a ride with a stranger, are never seen alive again. Only later the body is discovered in a wooded area. Pathologic findings are often those of blunt force injuries and/or strangulation with sexual assault usually occurring just prior to death. Emasculation and other more bizarre sexual activities before, during, and even after death are known to occur in homicides perpetrated by small juvenile "gangs." Such exhibitionism, especially to female gang members, or sometimes to a female captive, is a frequent accompaniment of these crimes.

REFERENCES

1. *Abortion Surveillance, 1975.* Center for Disease Control, Atlanta, p. 7.
2. Cameron, J. M., and Doyan, A. D.: Association of Brain Damage with Therapeutic Abortion Induced by Amniotic Fluid Replacement: Report of Two Cases. *Br. Med. J.* 1:1010–1013, 1966.
3. Additional Protections Pertaining to Research, Development and Related Activities Involving Fetuses, Pregnant Women and Human in vitro Fertilization. *Code of Federal Regulations,* Sections 46(201–46), 211, October 1, 1976.
4. *Johnson v. Woman's Hospital,* 527 S.W. 2d 133 (Tenn. App. 1975).
5. *Commonwealth v. Edelin,* 359 N.E. 2d 4 (Mass. 1977).
6. Adelson, L.: *The Pathology of Homicide.* Charles C Thomas, Springfield, Ill., 1974, pp. 628–632.
7. Crosby, W., and Costiloe, J. P.: Safety of Lock Belt Restraints for Pregnant Victims of Auto Collisions. *N. Engl. J. Med.* 284(12):632–636, 1971.
8. Naeye, R. L.: Causes of Perinatal Mortality in the U.S. Collaborative Perinatal Project. *J.A.M.A.* 23(3):228–229, 1977.
9. Blackbourne, B. D., and Failing, R. M.: Sudden Death Due to Endocardial Fibroelastosis. *J. Forensic Sci.* 11(3):384–389, 1966.
10. Sturner, W. Q.: Some Perspectives in Cot Deaths. *J. Forensic Med.* 18(3):96–107, 1971.
11. Sturner, W. Q., and Spruill, F. G.: Asymmetric Hypertrophy of the Heart in Two Cases of Sudden Death in Adolescents. *J. Forensic Sci.* 19(3):565–572, 1974.
12. Beckwith, J. B.: The Sudden Infant Death Syndrome. *Curr. Prob. Pediatrics* 3(8):1–36, 1973.
13. Steinschneider, A.: Prolonged Apnea and the Sudden Infant Death Syndrome: Clinical and Laboratory Observations. *Pediatrics* 50:646-654, 1972.

14. Naeye, R. L.: Pulmonary Arterial Abnormalities in the Sudden Infant Death Syndrome. *N. Engl. J. Med.* 289:1167–2270, 1973.
15. Naeye, R. L., Whalen, P., Ryser, M., and Fisher, R.: Cardiac and Other Abnormalities in the Sudden Infant Death Syndrome. *Am. J. Pathol.* 82(1):1–7, 1976.
16. Valdez-Dapena, M. A., Gillane, M. M., and Catherman, R.: Brown Fat Retention in Sudden Infant Death Syndrome. *Arch. Pathol. Lab. Med.* 100:547–549, 1976.
17. Simson, L. R., Jr., and Brantley, R. E.: Postural Asphyxia as a Cause of Death in Sudden Infant Death Syndrome. *J. Forensic Sci.* 22(1):178–187, 1977.
18. Sturner, W. Q.: Sudden, Unexpected Infant Death, in Tedeschi, C. G., et al. (eds.): *Forensic Medicine: Trauma and Environmental Hazards.* W. B. Saunders, Philadelphia, 1977, pp. 1015–1032.
19. *Facts About Sudden Infant Death Syndrome.* DHEW Publication (NIH) 76–225, Washington, D.C.
20. Sturner, W. Q., et al.: Accidental Asphyxial Deaths Involving Infants and Young Children. *J. Forensic Sci.* 21(3):483–487, 1976.
21. Francisco, J.: Smothering in Infancy: Its Relationship to the Crib Death Syndrome. *South. Med. J.* 63:1110–1114, 1970.
22. Luke, J. L., Blackbourne, B. D., and Donovan, J. W.: Bed-Sharing Deaths Among Victims of the Sudden Death Syndrome: A Riddle within a Conundrum. *Forensic Sci. Gaz.* 5(2):3–4, 1975.
23. Blackbourne, B. D.: Accidental Injuries in Children. *Clin. Proc. Child. Hosp. Nat. Med. Center* 30(4):83–91, 1974.
24. Bass, M.: Asphyxial Crib Death. *N. Engl. J. Med.* 296:555–556, 1977.
25. Requirements for Full Size (and Non-Full Size) Baby Cribs. *Code of Federal Regulations,* Sections 1508, 1509, 1977.
26. Sturner, W. Q., and Dempsey, J.: Sudden and Unexpected Infant Death: Postmortem Chemistry Studies of the Vitreous Humor. *J. Forensic Sci.* 18(1):12–19, 1973.
27. DiMaio, V. J. M.: Accidental Hanging Due to Pacifiers. *J.A.M.A.* 226(7):790, 1973.
28. Laughlin, R. A., and Habal, M. B.: The Stapled Finger Syndrome: Another Health Hazard. *N. Engl. J. Med.* 296(17):1005, 1977.
29. DiMaio, D. J., and DiMaio, T.: Fatal Methadone Poisoning in Children: A Report of Four Cases. *J. Forensic Sci.* 18(2):130–134, 1973.
30. Baden, M.: Investigation of Deaths from Drug Abuse, in Spitz, W., and Fisher, R. (eds.): *Medicolegal Investigation of Death.* Charles C Thomas, Springfield, Ill., 1973, p. 509.
31. Leape, L. L., Ashcraft, K. W., Scarpelli, D. G., and Holder, T. M.: Hazard to Health—Liquid Lye. *N. Engl. J. Med.* 284(11):578–581, 1971.
32. Sturner, W. Q., and DiMaio, V. J. M.: Fatal Hyperglycemia and Acidosis due to Pancake Syrup Ingestion in a Child with Colonic Interposition for Esophageal Stricture from Lye Ingestion. *Aaction* 1(1):3–5, 1973.
33. Lightfoote, J., Blair, N. J., and Cohen, J. R.: Lead Intoxication in the Adult Caused by Chinese Herbal Medication. *J.A.M.A.* 238(14):1539, 1977.
34. Sturner, W. Q., and Garriott, J. C.: Deaths Involving Propoxyphene (Darvon): A Review of Forty-One Cases over a Two-Year Period. *J.A.M.A.* 233(10):1125–1130, 1973.
35. Weston, J.: The Pathology of Child Abuse, in Helfer, R. E., and Kempe, C. H. (eds.): *The Battered Child.* University of Chicago Press, Chicago, 1972, pp. 77–100.
36. Weston, J.: The Childhood Maltreatment Syndrome, in Spitz, W., and Fisher, R. (eds.): *Medicolegal Investigation of Death.* Charles C Thomas, Springfield, Ill., 1973, pp. 385–419.
37. Palmer, C. H., and Weston, J. T.: Several Unusual Cases of Child Abuse. *J. Forensic Sci.* 12(4):851–855, 1976.

38. Blackbourne, B.: Danger—Baby's Bath. *Forensic Sci. Gaz.* 3(2):1–3, 1972.
39. Sturner, W. Q., and Sisti, J., Jr.: Suicide Perspectives in Rhode Island in 1974. *R.I. Med. J.* 59(8):364, 1976.
40. Luke, J. L., Lyons, M. M., and Devlin, J. F.: Pediatric Forensic Pathology in Death by Homicide. *J. Forensic Sci.* 12(4):421–430, 1967.
41. DiMaio, V. J. M., and Bernstein, J. D.: A Case of Infanticide. *J. Forensic Sci.* 19(4):744–758, 1974.

CHAPTER 12

Joseph H. Davis is Chief Medical Examiner of Metropolitan Dade County, Florida, and Professor of Legal Medicine at the University of Miami. He is also Chairman of the Medical Examiner's Commission of the State of Florida. Dr. Davis pursued undergraduate studies at Lehigh University, Virginia Polytechnic Institute, and Princeton University, and received his medical degree in 1949 from the Long Island College of Medicine. He is a Past President of the National Association of Medical Examiners and of the Dade County Medical Association, and has for many years been a consultant for the Federal Aviation Association. Dr. Davis is the author of numerous papers, articles, and chapters on various aspects of forensic pathology and traumatic death.

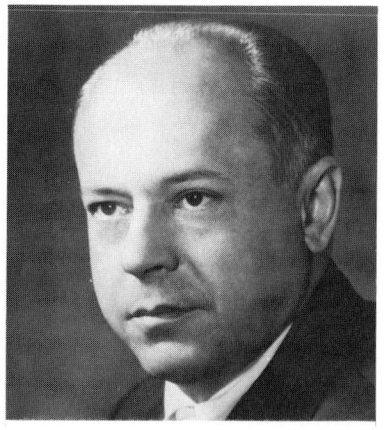

ASPHYXIAL DEATHS

Joseph H. Davis, M.D.

The term asphyxia has acquired a rather broad definition quite different from its etymological derivation of "pulselessness." Adelson has defined asphyxia as "the physiologic and chemical state in a living organism in which acute lack of oxygen available for cell metabolism is associated with inability to eliminate excess carbon dioxide."[1] Critical consideration of this definition indicates that it is common to almost all modes of death. It may also be considered from a mechanistic standpoint as anoxic anoxia, or prevention of oxygen from reaching the lungs; anemic anoxia, or inability of hemoglobin to transport sufficient oxygen; stagnant anoxia, or lack of oxygenated blood transport to the affected tissues; and histotoxic anoxia, or interference with the oxidative process at the intracellular level. A mechanical categorization can be described as that based upon physical interference with the breathing process. Certain poisons can interfere with oxygen transport or utilization, such as carbon monoxide, aniline, or hydrogen cyanide; other poisons depress the respiratory center; and some atmospheres become deficient in oxygen. All of the above can be considered variants of asphyxia. Nevertheless, one should refrain from the use of the term asphyxia except where one is obliged to speak in broad generalities. It is better to use the specific asphyxial variant such as choking, strangulation, barbiturate intoxication, or drowning.

Mechanical asphyxias may be considered according to the location of the respiratory blockage. When the mouth or nose is occluded, the terms suffocation, smothering, and gagging fall into this category (Figs. 12-1 and 12-2). Occasionally, a violent beating results in sufficient facial injuries to accomplish the same result. When the inner portion of the airway is occluded, the term choking applies, whether caused by a foreign body or by inflammatory swelling of the tissues (Figs. 12-3 and 12-4). Pressure on the exterior of the neck is seen with hanging, manual strangulation,

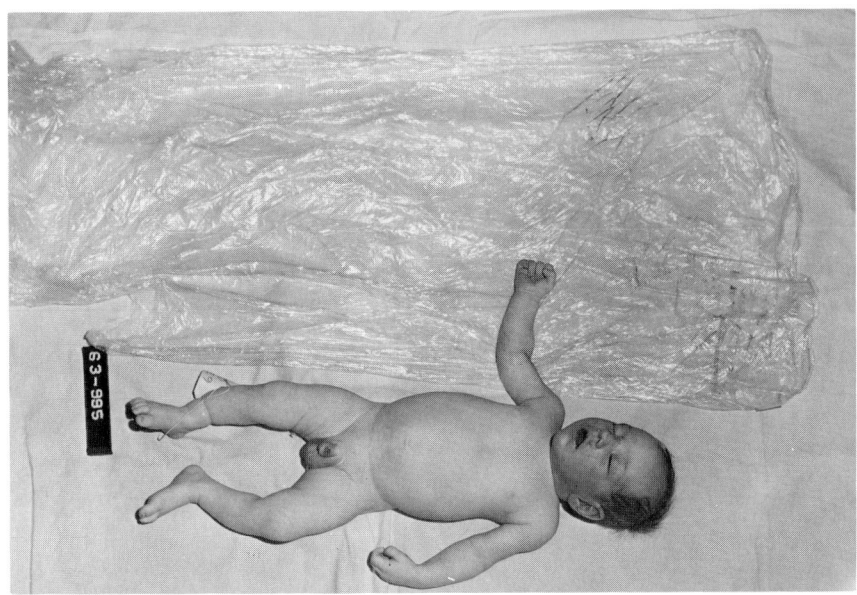

FIGURE 12-1. Suffocation. This 2-month-old infant was placed upon a mattress covered by a thin plastic wrap on which a sheet had been spread. The sheet was loose and the child's mouth and nose became occluded. The infant was able to tear a small piece of plastic free; this was found clenched in the left hand. The small blood stain on the plastic is the result of hemorrhagic pulmonary edema.

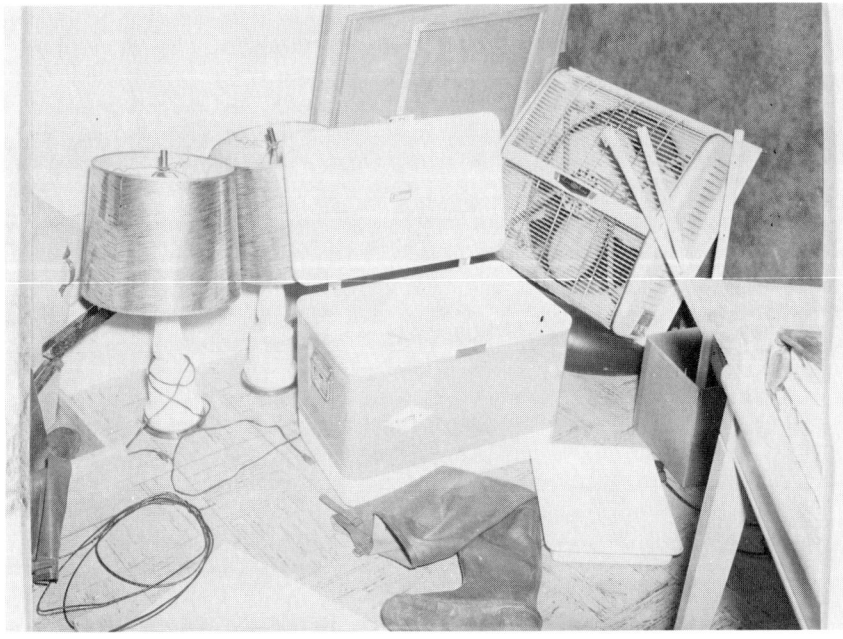

FIGURE 12-2. Suffocation. A 3-year-old child had placed herself inside this insulated chest and closed the lid.

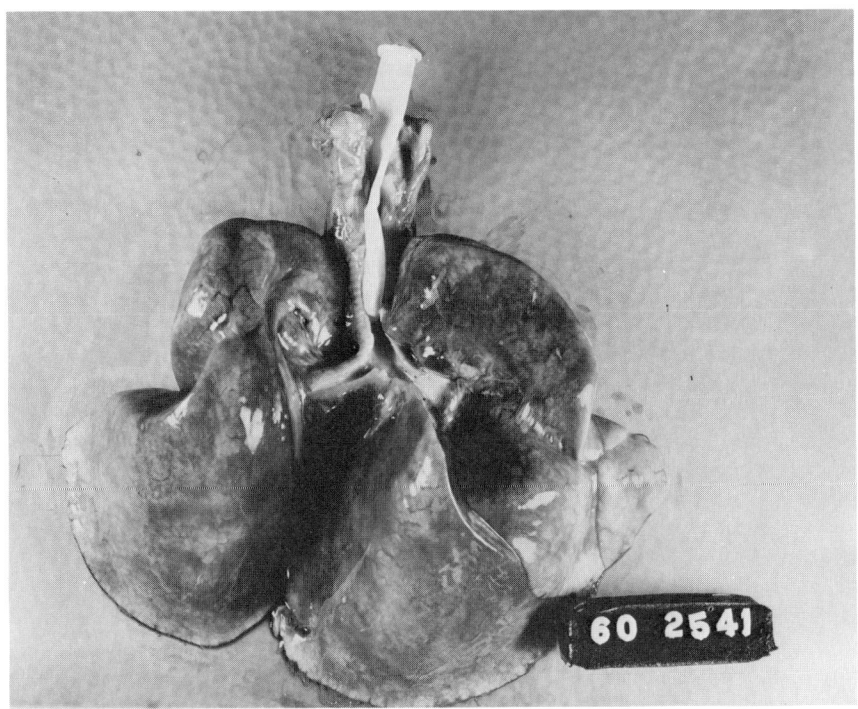

FIGURE 12-3. Choking. The lungs of an 8-month-old infant who had been playing with a deflated toy balloon.

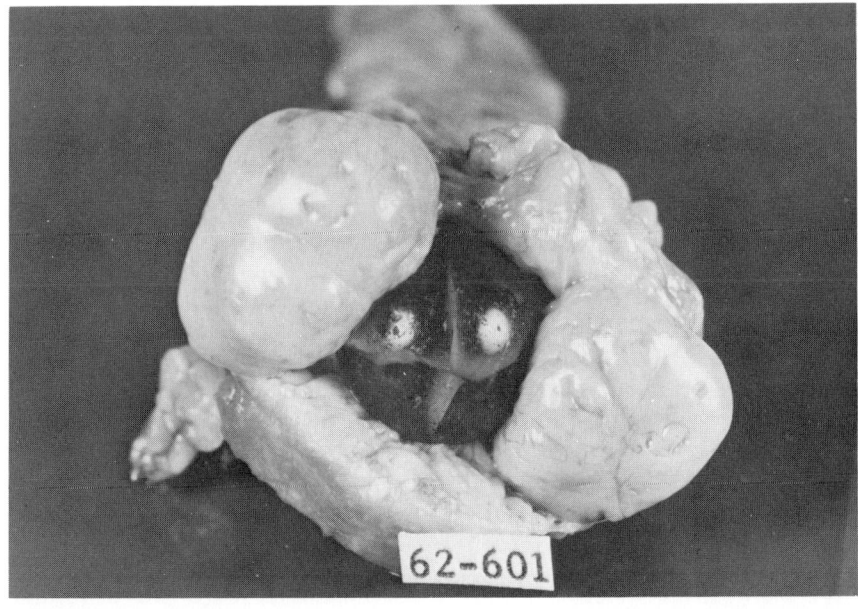

FIGURE 12-4. Choking. The palatine tonsils of a 4-year-old child who had been playing with a marble when it became firmly lodged between the hypertrophied masses.

and ligature strangulation. For some peculiar reason, the term traumatic asphyxia has been applied where there is a mechanical fixation of the chest sufficient to cause death. A complex form of mechanical asphyxia is that due to submersion (i.e., drowning).

SUDDEN DEATH MECHANISMS

There are three basic variations of sudden death mechanisms in an otherwise well-functioning individual. Exsanguination is usually self-evident as to presence and cause. Another mechanism is when the heart suddenly ceases to pump. A third mechanism is when respirations suddenly cease. When either of these latter two mechanisms occur, there ensues a systematic shutdown sequence of the whole organism. Certain subtle and not so subtle circumstantial and autopsy findings indicate the mechanism involved in the death which, in turn, sheds light on the underlying cause. Differential diagnosis is not always simple for there may be other forces which modify or obscure the findings. Most frequently seen are post-collapse efforts at resuscitation which can sometimes re-establish circulation even though the brain has undergone irreversible damage. Resuscitation may also result in visceral injuries with hemorrhage which may be mistaken for an effective intervening cause of death, which it certainly is not.[2]

Sudden onset of heart stoppage, ventricular fibrillation from electrocution, and coronary artery disease ischemia generally result in sudden collapse after a short lag period of 10 to 13 seconds of consciousness. A few short, ineffectual respiratory gasps and scant seizure activity may be observed. When breathing suddenly stops due to interference with the respiratory center, the heart, capable of a fair amount of anaerobic function, continues to beat and pump blood through the circulatory system. Lacking the circulatory assistance of respiratory excursion of the chest, blood tends to pool within the lungs. This leads to the congested, hemorrhagic, and edematous lungs of an acute asphyxial death. The continued function of the heart in the absence of respirations has been well documented. Consider the following circumstances:

> Henry Cobler Moselmann was executed by judicial hanging in the Jail Yard of Lancaster County, Pennsylvania, in 1839. He had murdered Lazarus Zellerbach and was afforded proper justice. Doctor Washington L. Atlee approached Sheriff Anthony E. Roberts a month prior to execution and received permission for study upon the soon to be dead body of Moselmann. A committee of several physicians and medical students was divided into subcommittees to carry out observations. Studies of pulse, heartbeat, expired air, temperature, etc., were followed by galvanic experiments upon the body and the interior of the body after dissection. A complete phrenological study (of lumps and contours of the head) indicated, incidentally, a large "love of life." Judicial hanging causes death by sudden destruction of the junction of the medulla with the cervical spinal cord. This results in sudden loss of respiratory activity. On Friday, December 20, at 17 minutes past 2 p.m., the drop fell: "Two or three successive emprosthotonoid efforts of the body were the only motions observed. These spasms were confined to the muscles on the anterior part of the body, from the pelvis up, and they gave a gently swinging motion to the body. Three minutes after execution there was a slight spasmodic action, which was the last perceived."

A careful external examination of the thorax of the hanged man indicated no respiratory activity. Four minutes after the execution, the sound of the heart was obscure but the rhythm was perfect. Four and one-half minutes after execution the heart was "less confused." Five minutes after execution the pulsations of the heart were so frequent that they could not be counted. At five and one-half minutes the sounds of the heart were scarcely audible and the pulsations were very frequent. At seven minutes the pulsations of the heart were 120 per minute. At seven and one-half minutes they were 132 per minute and at ten minutes they were 60 per minute. At twelve minutes the pulsations of the heart were 54 per minute and at thirteen minutes the sound was entirely gone. In the meantime the peripheral pulse could be detected and counted through seven minutes.[3]

The weight and appearance of the lungs may assist in differentiation of the mechanism of death when there has been no distorting, pre-existing natural disease process, putrefaction, or extensive resuscitative attempts. The light lungs (about 300 gm) are more compatible with sudden rhythm disturbance and cessation of pumping action of the heart. Heavier lungs (450 to 500 gm or more) may be indicative of cessation of respiration with continuance of the heartbeat for several minutes (e.g., slow heart stoppage). Some of the heaviest lungs are to be found in those individuals dying from an acute intravenous injection of heroin and its diluents. The opiates, being primary respiratory depressants, can be expected to operate within this framework of respiratory cessation with continued heartbeat. Complicating factors are those of demonstrable and nondemonstrable damage to the lungs by the previous and terminal intravenous injection of chemicals which, in bolus form, pass through the lungs on their way to the opiate receptors in the brain.

AUTOPSY FINDINGS

General Observations

The nonspecific autopsy findings of an asphyxial death have been categorized as pulmonary congestion and edema, discussed above; petechial hemorrhages of serosal surfaces; and fluidity of blood. Petechial hemorrhages may be an expression of sepsis, hemorrhagic diathesis, or postmortem lividity. In an uncomplicated mechanical asphyxia such serosal hemorrhages are hypothesized as a reflection of the effects of hypoxia upon pre- and postcapillary sphincters with postrespiratory arrest circulation aggravating the capillary congestion.

Fluidity of the blood is nothing more than an expression of sudden death in an otherwise healthy individual with no pre-existing malignant disease or necrotic tissue. The processes which maintain fluidity in life continue after death with any clots that have formed becoming lysed for the most part. Such fluidity may be seen in sudden death from cardiac stoppage such as ventricular fibrillation in an individual with myocardial fibrosis or in mechanical obstruction of the airway. If the victim has active infection or a focus of necrotic tissue, such as an acute myocardial infarct, pneumonia, or some other process invoking a hypercoagulable state, postmortem clots may be expected to be rich in fibrin and have the classic chicken fat appearance. Inasmuch as most victims of strangulation or choking are in good health, one would expect fluid blood, and conversely, if ill, clots.

Mechanical Asphyxia

The autopsy findings in death from mechanical asphyxia are modified by the circumstances under which the victim died. It should be appreciated that textbook descriptions of autopsy findings of mechanical asphyxia include those which result from forces above and beyond what is necessary to kill. Concomitant natural disease changes do not assure that natural disease was the cause of death. The ultimate determination of cause results from a very careful investigation of the circumstances of death. A carefully investigated, well-documented set of circumstances is far more valuable in evidentiary weight than an unsupported series of autopsy observations. The autopsy surgeon may be faced with a circumstance in which the plastic bag was removed from the face and no mention of this was made prior to the autopsy. The findings of physical trauma would be absent. In some mechanical smotherings with hands, or even manual strangulations, traumatic hemorrhages of the lips or neck viscera are totally absent. Usually the forces applied, whether accidental, suicidal, or homicidal in nature, are above and beyond what is needed to result in death. Excessive force results in soft tissue hemorrhages, fractures of the thyroid cartilage and hyoid bone, and petechiae above the line of the airway, even when the agent of death has been removed.

Smothering and Gagging

In smothering or gagging deaths, the object frequently remains or was applied with sufficient force to produce distortion of tissues. Special attention should be paid to the mouth and lips to search for evidence of chafing of the mucosa or even more serious injury from the teeth. The tongue may exhibit evidence of injury. Gags, usually homicidal, are most commonly tied with extreme cruelty or tension, resulting in pronounced distortion of the mouth and cheeks, particularly in edentulous victims. If the gag has been removed, some foreign matter such as lint may still be present.

Foreign Body Inhalation

Death by inhalation of foreign bodies often is caused by food, the "cafe coronary," a popular term coined by Dr. Roger Haugen, former Medical Examiner of Broward County, Florida.[4] The victim may be observed to slump over at the dining table or get up and walk across the room only to collapse on the way to, or after arrival at, the restroom facility. Noteworthy is the absence of coughing, gagging, or other obvious signs of distress. This is the result of the accompanying drunkenness on the part of the victim as well as the occlusion of the airway by the large mass of food. In general, there are three findings of note: the impaction, the presence of dentures or no teeth at all, and a fairly high level of alcohol, usually in excess of 0.20 gm percent concentration in the blood. Due to popularization of the term "cafe coronary," resuscitative attempts frequently result in removal and loss of the critical evidence, even when the victim has succumbed. Beefsteak is the most common agent, but bread with peanut butter, vegetables, and even flavored crushed ice have been observed in our experience. Again, the pathologist must be alert to the fact that death while eating may be such a case and must assure himself that the offending agent has been accounted for. A frequent point of confusion is the presence of vomitus within the airway. Regurgitation and aspiration of vomitus are common to many modes of dying or resuscitation attempts. As such it is not a primary cause of death from mechanical asphyxia. It should be looked upon in the same light as an involuntary micturition or defecation during the dying process and should be considered a result, not a cause.

Hanging and Strangulation

External pressure upon the neck may be applied by hanging or strangulation. Hangings may involve any form of suspending device—ropes, string, belts, wearing apparel, chains, and so forth. Commonly, it is a rope or insulated electrical wire, as these are most readily accessible. A matching imprint of the surface of the cord may be visible on the skin. Usually there is a parchment-like compression groove about the neck. The degree of pressure placed upon the veins does not affect the underlying carotid and vertebral arterial system, which is quite well protected. Hemorrhages and congestion may be seen above the point of compression within the neck viscera. Fractures of the thyroid cartilage or hyoid bone may be present, although usually not in the younger individual. Suicidal hanging (Fig. 12-5) may be effected with the victim lying prone or supine

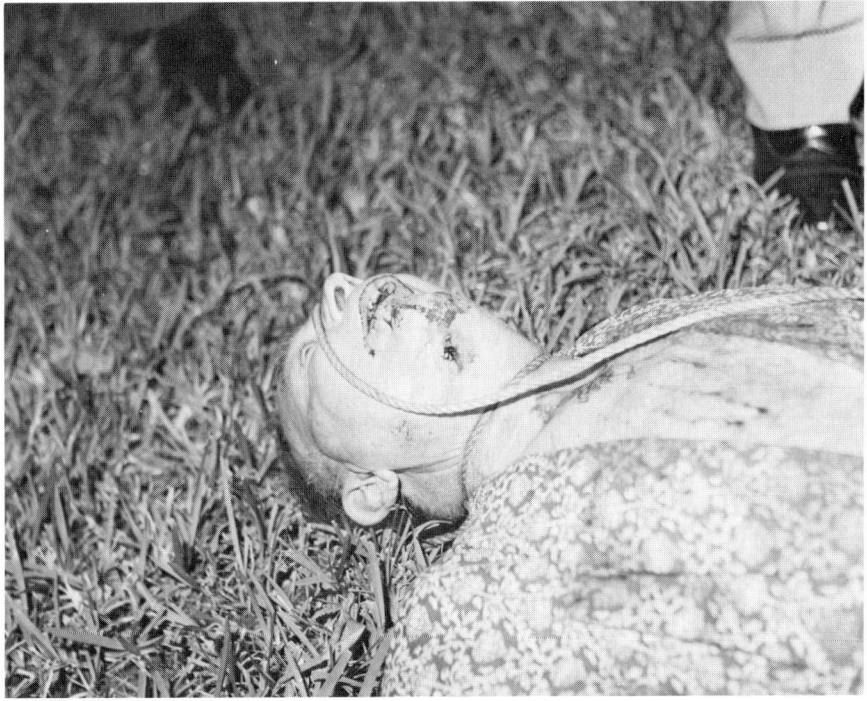

FIGURE 12-5. This 72-year-old man had shot himself under the chin with a .22 caliber rifle. He then slashed both wrists repeatedly with a double-edged razor blade. Following this he walked 100 feet to a tree and hanged himself. The rope slipped from the branch, but the neck knot remained snug. He was found on the ground beneath the tree with the ligature tight as shown.

upon the floor with the head barely raised. In one instance, a hospitalized patient stretched his bathrobe sash between the arms of a chair, leaned from his bed, and rested the front of his neck upon the sash. He died.

Homicidal hanging, including judicial hanging, is quite rare. The latter is more nearly akin to decapitation in that there is severe musculoskeletal and soft tissue damage with fracture dislocation of the upper cervical spine and transection of the spinal cord or medulla. It is possible for an individual to be hanged after death from any cause with marks on the neck being indistinguishable from some suicidal hangings. Obviously every case of apparent death from hanging should be carefully investigated with particular attention given to the circumstances and the physical evidence left by the rope upon the upper point of suspension where it was tied to the pole, board, rafter, or whatever. At the lower point of suspension the hanging body produces a mark which extends upward at that point of the neck where suspension takes place. With ligature strangulation, either suicidal or homicidal, the constricting device is placed around the neck and tends to leave a circular mark without an upward extension (Figs. 12-6 and 12-7).

Homicidal asphyxias usually involve manual strangulation or blows to the neck with loss of integrity of the supporting structures. From the evidentiary standpoint it is fortunate that most assailants apply much greater force and most victims struggle with sufficient strength to result in mechanical disruption of the cartilaginous bony and soft tissues within the neck. It must be emphasized that gentle manual strangulation can result in death with absolutely no sign of local tissue damage on the surface or within the neck and no petechiae above the line of constriction. Some might postulate that the mechanism of death is bradycardia associated with an unusually sensitive carotid sinus reflex mechanism. Such strangulation deaths with almost no objective signs within the neck are unusual and more likely associated with a gentle pressure application rather than a carotid sinus bradycardia. The best evidence is oftentimes available from the assailant who may be quite willing to describe in detail exactly how the crime was committed.

Occasionally the question arises as to whether an individual can manually strangle himself. Another question concerns the rapidity with which a person dies. As for the former, it is impossible to strangle oneself manually unless the position of the victim allows the weight of the body to press the neck against a ligature which in turn is supported with the hands.[5] The best response to this allegation is that there is no evidence to support such a speculation.

The rapidity of unconsciousness may be inferred from human and animal experimentation. Modell has described the sequential blood gas changes in anesthetized dogs.[6] Craig has studied breath-holding and loss of consciousness in humans.[7] With humans it is difficult to acquire other than scantily supported anecdotal information pertaining to respiratory occlusion resulting in death. The assailant can sometimes offer clues. In one circumstance where three victims had been abducted, killed, and buried by the assailant, the medical examiner, the police, and the assailant spent several days together traveling from one grave site to another. The description and demonstration of the killings are summarized as follows:

The assailant developed a technique of killing quickly with minimal evidence of trauma in the event that the body were to be found. His

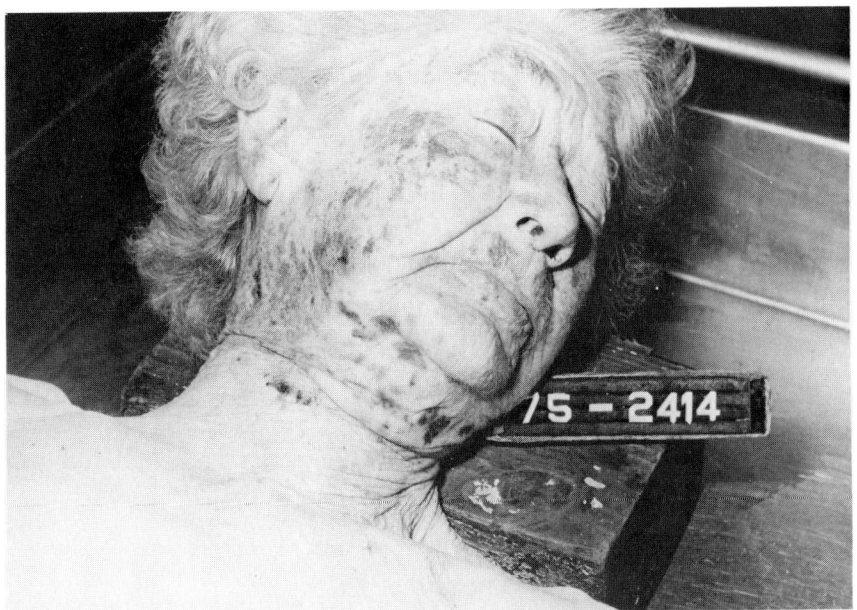

FIGURE 12-6. An 84-year-old woman, the victim of manual strangulation. Note the fingernail abrasions under her chin. An insulated electric wire was also used as a ligature. After its removal, only a faint horizontal indentation remained.

technique was to tie the victim's hands behind his back and make him kneel on the front seat of the car, facing the rear. While holding the back of the victim's neck with the left hand, he would grasp the trachea and lower larynx between his thumb and fingers and then compress and rotate them clockwise. In three cases of children aged 11 through

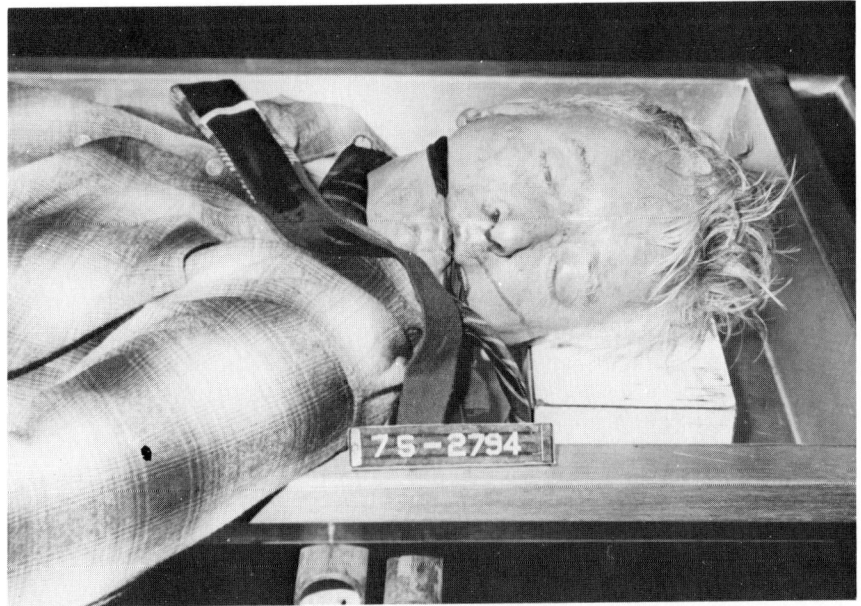

FIGURE 12-7. A 59-year-old man strangled with two neckties, one across his mouth.

16, he described loss of consciousness in 3 to 4 minutes, preceded by significant struggle which he controlled by his weight from behind. He then would turn the victim around and reposition him on the seat of the car, now rotating the larynx and trachea to the right. This was required because in each case respirations resumed after turning the victim. He reported loss of carotid pulse and heart sounds after an additional 5 to 10 minutes of compression. In the one body where decomposition was minimized such that neck hemorrhage, if present, would have been expected to be observed, no evidence of hemorrhage was present. The killer demonstrated his technique upon the medical examiner, Dr. Ronald K. Wright, who noted essentially no pain associated with complete inability to inhale or exhale.

Traumatic Asphyxia

Traumatic asphyxia, fixation of the chest by mechanical compression, produces variable findings. Where the victim is caught by machinery or by building collapse, the compressive pressures may result in a most striking hemorrhagic purple suffusion above the point of compression. Where the pressure is scant or evenly distributed, external findings may be negligible. For example, two boys, aged 13 and 15, were tunneling into a sandpile which collapsed. Other than soiling by sand there were no external pressure signs. Internally there was, in addition to fluid blood and some serosal hemorrhages, a demonstrable degree of partial atelectasis coupled with pulmonary edema. In another example, a laborer for a house-moving business was under a house when the load shifted slightly and held him immobile. When extricated he was dead with no internal or external visible effects of trauma. Usually such events involve more severe forces, and the purple suffusion of the skin above the point of compression is in sharp contrast to the compressed area.

Further Clinical Findings

Clinical observations of survivors of hanging, ligature or manual strangulation indicate that there is considerably more small vessel trauma than is usually visible at autopsy when the victim has died during the attack. Severe hoarseness may develop as well as stridor secondary to traumatic edema of the larynx and supraglottic tissues. Even more striking is the development of bilateral ecchymoses caused by coalescence of petechial hemorrhages which continue to bleed in the survivor following relief of the neck constriction. This observation may be generalized for most physical injuries where an element of survival provides time for reactive hemorrhage to occur. It is reactive hemorrhage which calls attention to most blunt trauma damage sites. The full extent of tissue damage cannot be appreciated when effective circulation to the injured area has ceased at the time of injury or immediately thereafter.

INVESTIGATION AND REPORTING OF ASPHYXIAL DEATHS

Scene Investigation

The investigation of an asphyxial death demands autopsy and circumstance correlations with anticipation of future allegations. It is preferred that the autopsy pathologist participate in the scene investigation and that the police investigators and crime laboratory technicians participate in the autopsy study. By now it should be apparent that the autopsy findings are subtle and pattern variabilities are great. Every consideration should be given to the circumstances of injury, the position of the victim in the dying and postmortem state, manipulations of the body, and laboratory findings which may be significant. Consider this case:

> A wealthy businesswoman was found dead in bed, face down on her pillow. The history indicated an injection of meperidine shortly before retiring the evening before. Autopsy revealed pulmonary congestion and edema as well as evidence of injectable drug abuse with extreme fibrosis and chronic and subacute inflammation of the buttocks. Toxicologic results on the blood revealed 0.06 mg percent meperidine (Demerol), 0.25 mg percent promethazine (Phenergan), and 0.82 mg percent ethchlorvynol (Placidyl). Alcohol was negative. The presence of food in the stomach along with fixed lividity and rigor indicated that she probably died closer to the time of retiring than to the time of discovery. After meticulous investigation of circumstances, past history, and correlation of all factors, it was concluded that postural asphyxia while sedated with multiple drugs had resulted in death. The autopsy and toxicologic tests, by themselves, are meaningless unless correlated with all circumstantial information.

Interpretation of Autopsy Reports

How should a medicolegal consultant, pathologist, police officer, or attorney interpret the reports prepared by a pathologist or police investigator in an asphyxial death? The problem may be compounded by the subtleness of physical damage to be found in the victim and an unfortunate lack of appreciation of the need for total case investigation. Some gunshot autopsy reports are self-evident, but homicidal suffocation with a plastic bag does not result in clear-cut autopsy findings. Initial review of the autopsy report should indicate whether or not the pathologist was expanding his dissection and documentation of clues crucial to the cause and mechanism of death. All too frequently the autopsy report is a stereotype with meaningless phraseology that is repetitious from one report to another. One may wonder who or what performed the autopsy. As for the "what," bear in mind that automated programed typing machines can grind out beautifully spaced and printed documents wherein most of the wording is identical in form regardless of the nature of the case. These "counterfeit" autopsy reports are to be deplored. Another serious problem is the preprinted autopsy form where space for adequate description is restricted and the entries lack the qualitative and quantitative variation necessary to suit the needs of the individual case. Police and other investigative reports likewise may lack information which could help differentiate between an unnatural or a natural death or which is essential to interpret autopsy findings. The recent expansion of rescue squad and emergency room life support activities creates data of great assistance in interpretation of the dying mechanism while simultaneously creating problems on injury interpretation. Intravenous and intra-arterial insertion of needles into the neck may lead to hemorrhage in addition to hemorrhages resulting from previously inflicted trauma. Resuscitation may add materially to the weight of the lungs and may produce interstitial emphysema and additional rib fractures. Valuable witness information, whether lay, paramedical, or medical, must be actively sought in order to document observed physiologic events of assistance in diagnosis.

Gathering Evidence

It should be realized that the autopsy report is only part of the total constellation of positive and negative evidence of mechanical asphyxia. Therefore every available scrap of preliminary information pertaining to the victim, the circumstances of death, and his environment should be made available to the pathologist prior to and during the autopsy. Preferably, a scene visit or at least review of available photographs, in conjunction with a police investigator, is advisable. The techniques of autopsy data documentation include photography, specialized dissections, and toxicologic or other laboratory tests. External and internal color photographs complement and sometimes supplement the written observations. Orientation of the photographs and their composition should serve to tell the story rather than to confuse. Wet sponges lead to hemolysis and pronounced hemoglobin staining of tissues. Careful blotting with dry absorbent paper can better prepare the object for photographic documentation. The high quality and relatively low cost of photographic equipment should result in no untoward delay in taking photographs.

Key Aspects of Clinical Findings

In many autopsies upon victims presumed dead of natural disease, the target organ is examined first. On the other hand, should strangulation be a serious consideration, the neck organs should be examined after removal of the intrathoracic and intracranial viscera. This permits blood to drain from the neck vessels. The subtleties of strangulation hemorrhage within the neck mandate that individual strap muscles be designated in the description with the precise location, size, and appearance of the hemorrhage being documented. Manual strangulation in young individuals, even with struggle, may result in no appreciable damage to the highly resilient supportive structures of the neck. In older individuals calcification of the thyroid cartilage and fixation of the normal joints of the hyoid bone complex set the stage for fractures of these objects. The most common fracture site is a superior horn of the thyroid cartilage. Careless dissection may lead to a fracture or transection of the superior horn by the scalpel. Absence of hemorrhage at the damage site tends to support the opinion that the damage was autopsy artefact. The junction between the body and the greater horn of the hyoid bone frequently is composed of dense fibrous strands. Mobility in this area is normal in such hyoids. Careful shaving of the tissue from the anterior portion of this joint may disclose hemorrhage associated with traumatic distortion of the joint as evidence of applied force. With fist or karate blows to the neck there may be severe destruction of the superior horns of the thyroid cartilage with vertical fracturing of the main portion of cartilage. This indicates a violent lateral displacement or compression of the supporting tissues.

Laboratory Tests

There should be careful consideration of needed toxicologic and other laboratory tests prior to the commencement of the autopsy. Transfer evidence upon the body may be present and should be documented. The strangulation may be incidental to sexual assault or other motives, and the evidence for same should be considered.

Autopsy Report

The autopsy report should be the objective documentation of the positive and negative findings. There is no room in the field of medicolegal death investigation for the autopsy report to incorporate masses of hearsay, speculation, and the inept "clinical pathological correlation" so frequently included by pathologists. Every effort should be made to consider correlative aspects during the investigative phase, but the report should describe only objective findings suitable for subsequent correlation when all the circumstances are known.

DEATH CERTIFICATION

Careful Terminology

Death certification in a mechanical asphyxial case should be simplified. Complex mechanisms and speculation about physiologic derangements secondary to the underlying proximate cause should not be included in the death certificate. If the patient died as the result of a homicidal manual strangulation, the cause of death should indicate "manual strangulation" or simply "strangulation." If the patient hanged himself, the connotation of "hanging" is sufficient. Suffocation by a plastic bag need only read "suffocation." Elsewhere on the certificate is room for a very simple designation of the circumstance, such as "patient placed plastic bag over head." Sometimes the information is not sufficient to pinpoint a specific simple term, and the cause of death must be expressed within a broad framework. Under some circumstances the phrase "consistent with" is necessary, such as "decomposed remains consistent with asphyxia," where circumstances and evidence aside from the body, coupled with absence of alternative injury patterns, lead logically to this conclusion. There is no basis for the ridiculous terminology of "No anatomical cause of death." When one considers that disease-state structural aberrations most often demonstrated at autopsy are identical to structural aberrations found in living individuals, it readily becomes apparent that the circumstances surrounding the death are essential determinants of interpretation. For example, the majority of people who die from coronary artery disease complications have rhythm disturbances rather than spontaneous rupture of an infarct. The anatomic findings in the individual dead of a lethal rhythm are frequently less alarming and severe than findings in live patients with similar disease processes. Autopsy findings are clues, not causes. The cause is within the sum total of all available information.

Findings and Conclusions

Occasionally the pathologist must play a role more legal than medical. This arises when the autopsy findings, *by themselves,* are equally consistent with homicide, accident, suicide, or natural causes. Most frequently such events occur where the body is decomposed or skeletonized, or the mechanism of death is drowning with no autopsy evidence to differentiate between intentional and unintentional drowning. However, the circumstances under which the victim disappeared and the environment in which the victim is found will indicate whether there is sufficient evidence to furnish presumption of death from criminal causation. A forensic pathologist *experienced in scene investigations* may be qualified to offer an opinion that the death was of probably criminal causation. Obviously this should depend upon careful examination of the evidence at the scene of death compared with that found upon and within the body. Such an opinion may be crucial when other facets of investigation have resulted in an otherwise valid confession of guilt. Before a confession may be introduced into court, the corpus delicti, the body of the crime, must be demonstrated. It is necessary to show that the death circumstances indicate criminal causation and are inconsistent with accidental, suicidal, or natural means. An opinion that the death is of criminal causation need be expressed only to the level of a preponderance of evidence. For that matter, this is the legal test for most opinions of causation rendered by physicians, including medical examiners.

DROWNING

Drowning is not a simple entity but is a complex condition with wide variations of occurrence and resulting clinical and structural findings within the victim. Each drowning episode results from an adverse reaction of man and his environment. Each of these in turn is highly variable. Accordingly, the best definition of drowning is the simplest: death due to submersion.

The Victim and the Environment

The approach to a drowning case is twofold—a consideration of the victim and of the environment. All too frequently the victim is considered but the environment is not. It is this incomplete approach which leads to unanswered questions as to whether or not the victim died of drowning and, if so, why. Victims have wide variations in age and in physical and functional findings. The watery environment may be extremely variable, hazardous for many or only for a select few. The circumstantial findings, the autopsy findings, and the determination of why the individual got into and could not get out of difficulty are variable from one case to another. The complexity of these variable patterns is proportional to the lack of a complete investigation of the drowning incident.

Environmental situations may be hazardous for a few but not for all. Home swimming pools are common, yet few adults drown accidentally in these pools. Small children, aged 1 to 3 years, do. A benign environment for a reasonably sober adult with swimming ability becomes deadly for the toddler. Sometimes the water environment may change so as to be extremely hazardous at one point in time but not another. In Miami Beach the occurrence of an "apparent drowning" of an adult during a prevailing southeast mild breeze indicates a probably serious human factor deficiency—heart disease or acute alcoholism. When the wind shifts to the northeast, treacherous offshore currents may carry an unwary victim out to sea, indicating the potential for a major environmental causative factor. It is a grave mistake in investigation to consider only the victim to the exclusion of the environment. The best approach is to study the circumstances and arrive at a probable hypothesis as to which factors interacted to lead to the adverse result. The autopsy is then performed in order to test the hypothesis, bearing in mind the variations in autopsy findings based upon age, pre-existing disease processes, chemical impairment of the victim, resuscitation effects, and variabilities of the amount of water inhaled and the chemical composition of the water.

Pathophysiology of Drowning

Drowning pathophysiology has been inferred from autopsy and experimental evidence. Relatively few physicians have studied, on a personal basis, animal experiments, treatment of the near drowning or postimmersion syndrome, and the death-investigative aspects of each of these. One such experienced physician is Modell, upon whose studies much of these pathophysiologic comments are based.[6] Three broad variables influence human physiologic and anatomic reactions to the drowning process: the pre-existing physical condition of the victim, the salinity or other chemical components of the water, and the amount of solution inhaled. All vary widely from one incident to another.

The small child with normal lungs and intact protective cough and laryngeal reflexes cannot be equated with the alcohol-anesthetized victim with tobacco-abused lungs or the unconscious epileptic. In the former, the amount of water inhaled may be slight, and in the latter there may be far greater amounts of water aspirated. The chemical nature of the water may be a factor. Swann's older experimental evidence[8] and Modell's more recent findings[6] indicate that there are differences, assuming that the same amount of water has been aspirated. Modell's publications are recommended as a reference in this regard, inasmuch as the frequently cited experiments of Swann are based upon limited studies of only a few animals.

Fresh water destroys surfactant with resulting alveolar shunting. Thus hypoxia and the effects of water upon the alveolar cell membranes produce pulmonary edema. When very large amounts of fluid are aspirated, hemodilution may accentuate the pulmonary edema.

Hypertonic sea water aspiration has less effect upon surfactant. However, the hypertonicity causes osmotic transfer of water from the blood stream into the alveoli and results in a relatively more profuse pulmonary edema. In addition there may be sufficient aspiration to induce some hemoconcentration which, at autopsy, may be manifest by the dusky hue of the cerebral and cerebellar cortices seen more frequently in salt water drowning than in fresh.

Inasmuch as the amount of water actually inhaled is variable, the degree of reaction to the aspirated water, regardless of salinity, is also variable. The major problems do not involve electrolyte and hemodilution or hemoconcentration changes but are concerned with persistent arterial hypoxemia, a process which required minimal aspiration.[9] It is within this group that the laryngeal spasm of older drowning literature is to be found. Even as little as one milliliter of aspirated water per pound of body weight in dogs results in prolonged arterial hypoxia.[10,11]

Autopsy Findings

There are certain autopsy findings which should be looked for in drowning, although they may be extremely variable in occurrence:

1. Pulmonary edema
2. Inhalation of foreign material into the airway
3. Swallowed water
4. Water in the sphenoid sinus
5. Hemorrhagic edema of the middle ears and petrous sinuses

Hemorrhagic edema of the middle ears is a reflection of the pressure changes during the drowning struggle and may be seen as a result of energetic resuscitation in the nondrowned victim of a heart attack. Foreign matter in the airway may occur as a result of postmortem migration of sand or silt long after death as the body is buffeted by wave action. Usually it results from active aspiration.

Laboratory tests to prove drowning have been searched for but never found because these are dependent upon a theory of drowning with a standard amount of water inhaled by a standard victim whose body is recovered in a standard time and whose body has not been subjected to resuscitation attempts or decomposition.[12] Aspiration of diatoms may be helpful, but these may also be inhaled by the breathing of sea air without the victim being in the water.[13]

Each case must be carefully approached with correlation of all circumstances and consideration of hypotheses as to the causative factors before the performance of the autopsy and laboratory tests and their interpretation. The following case delineates these complexities:

> A decomposed body of an adult male was found in a salt water bay ineffectually weighted with a 10-pound anchor. The autopsy revealed approximately 120 ml of blood-tinged fluid in the right pleural space and 100 ml in the left. The collapsed lungs had a combined weight of 600 gm. A fine linear fracture was noted, extending from the right maxillary bone upward into the ethmoid region. The facial bone structure was quite thin. The discolored decomposing flesh could be easily stripped from the bone, and no differentiation between traumatized soft tissue and decomposed tissue could be made. The semisolid brain was not stained with blood. The medical examiner's preliminary investigative report was only "evidence of a head injury." Subsequent investigation disclosed the victim to be a burglar who was punched in the face during an altercation with a friend. He was then silenced with a strip of adhesive over the mouth. Subsequently the reactive soft tissue swelling closed off his nasal airway, resulting in death. His alarmed antagonist removed the tape, attempted mouth-to-mouth resuscitation to no avail, and then furnished an equally ineffectual "burial at sea." Obviously, only careful follow-up investigation could determine such a series of events, for the evidence of the blow and the occluded airway had been altered by the assailant and subsequent decomposition.

The temperature of the water likewise plays a role in the drowning process. Cold water may result in a rapid loss of body temperature and loss of control, even with adequate flotation support.[14] Helium-oxygen mixtures in scuba diving may likewise result in rapid hypothermia due to the more efficient thermoconductivity of helium as compared to nitrogen or compressed air.

SCUBA DEATHS

The investigation of a scuba death cannot be piecemeal, but must be interpreted with the same person, or team, investigating the environment, the victim, the equipment, and the circumstances simultaneously. In our experience, some of the following factorial situations have been noted:

1. Environmental hazards most commonly seen involve those associated

with cave diving in northern Florida. These underground fresh water channels extend hundreds of feet into the earth in complete darkness, a most hazardous situation even for the expert diver.
2. Human factors generally involve lack of experience which may result in panic and drowning. More frequently seen is entrapment of air within the lungs on rising from the depths, producing fatal or nonfatal *extra-alveolar air syndrome*. Air escapes from the alveoli and may result in interstitial emphysema, pneumothorax, or air embolism. This is caused by disproportionate expansion of air-containing alveoli as compared to the adjacent fluid-filled vascular channels during too rapid an ascent. The pathophysiology has been well discussed in the classic monograph of Macklin and Macklin.[15] Autopsy findings are not as clear-cut as would be expected because of resuscitation efforts in the immediately recovered victim or decomposition changes in the victim with delayed recovery. In addition, recovery of a dead victim from a great depth (i.e., 60 to 200 feet) will result in a dramatic expansion of dissolved gases, leading to copious froth from the mouth and vascular bubbles, even to the point of complete distention of blood vessels by gas under pressure. Only a careful and critical appraisal of all circumstances, including interrogation of witnesses and consideration of the experience of the victim, may lead to an estimation of what triggered the event, whether it be nitrogen narcosis or whatever.
3. Equipment failure, other than poor weight-belt release mechanisms and lack of flotation, is unusual as a causative factor, although we have encountered a loss of oxygen in a rusted tank.[16] In this instance the victim breathed an air mixture of 1.5 percent oxygen.

Postimmersion Syndrome

Near drowning, or postimmersion syndrome, results when resuscitation has resulted in survival or a period of survival. The organ systems most seriously affected are the lungs and, to a lesser degree, the brain.[17] The damage to the latter is usually manifest at the time of the drowning episode. The pulmonary autopsy findings in a postimmersion case will depend to a great extent upon the amount of initial insult to pulmonary parenchyma by aspirated water or vomitus and the duration of survival with its concomitant oxygen therapy. In short survival of less than 24 hours, the lungs may be identical in appearance, both grossly and microscopically, to those of a drowning victim without survival. Usually the delayed death cases have survived several days, and the lungs are solidified with extensive fibrinous exudate within the alveoli. Steroid therapy, secondary infection, and gastric content serve to modify the appearances. The brain changes in those with prolonged neurologic deficit run the gamut of cerebral anoxic effects.[18]

In summary, the investigation of a drowning episode is not an exercise in autopsy technique as that is only a small, albeit essential, ingredient of such an investigation. The pathologist who cannot think clinically should not attempt to deduce why a person drowned if he has not concerned himself with the total circumstances surrounding the unfortunate event. After consideration of all environmental and human factors, as revealed by the circumstantial and autopsy investigations, the death certificate may reflect such alternative choices as drowning, or drowning with a contribution by heart disease, or heart disease with an agonal contribution by aspiration of water. In the final analysis we should strive to answer the basic question: Why did the victim get into difficulty in the water?

REFERENCES

1. Adelson, L.: *The Pathology of Homicide.* Charles C Thomas, Springfield, Ill., 1974, p. 521.
2. Stephenson, H. E.: *Cardiac Arrest and Resuscitation.* Part Eight: Pitfalls, Precautions and Complications in Cardiac Resuscitation. C. V. Mosby, St. Louis, 1974.
3. Atlee, W. L.: Report of a Series of Experiments Made by the Medical Faculty of Lancaster, upon the Body of Henry Cobler Moselmann, Executed in the Jail Yard of Lancaster County, Pennsylvania, on the 20th of December, 1839. *Am. J. Med. Sci.,* No. 51, May 1840, pp. 2–34.
4. Haugen, R.: "The Cafe Coronary"—Sudden Death in Restaurants. *J.A.M.A.* 186(2):142–143, 1963.
5. Rupp, J. D.: Suicidal Garrotting and Manual Self-Strangulation. *J. Forensic Sci.* 15(1):71–77, 1970.
6. Modell, J. H. (ed.): *The Pathophysiology and Treatment of Drowning and Near-Drowning.* Charles C Thomas, Springfield, Ill., 1971.
7. Craig, A. B.: Causes of Loss of Consciousness During Underwater Swimming. *J. Appl. Physiol.* 16(4):583–586, 1961.
8. Swann, H. G., and Spafford, N. R.: Body Salt and Water Changes During Fresh and Sea Water Drowning. *Texas Rep. Bio. Med.* 9(2):356–382, 1951.
9. Modell, J. H., et al.: Blood Gas and Electrolyte Changes in Human Near-Drowning Victims. *J.A.M.A.* 203(5):337–343, 1968.
10. Modell, J. H., and Moya, F.: Effects of Volume of Aspirated Fluid During Chlorinated Fresh Water Drowning."*Anesthesiology* 27:662–672, 1966.
11. Modell, J. H., et al.: Effects of Fluid Volume in Seawater Drowning. *Ann. Intern. Med.* 67(1):68–80, 1967.
12. Davis, J. H.: Tests for Drowning, in Modell, J. H.: *The Pathophysiology and Treatment of Drowning and Near-Drowning.* Charles C Thomas, Springfield, Ill., 1971.
13. Spitz, W. U., and Schneider, V.: The Significance of Diatoms in Diagnosis of Death by Drowning. *J. Forensic Sci.* 9:11–18, 1964.
14. Spitz, W. U.: Drowning, in Spitz, W. U., and Fisher, R. S.: *Medicolegal Investigation of Death—Guidelines for the Application of Pathology to Crime Investigation.* Charles C Thomas, Springfield, Ill., 1973.
15. Macklin, M. T., and Macklin, C. C.: Malignant Interstitial Emphysema of the Lungs and Mediastinum As an Important Occult Complication in Many Respiratory Diseases and Other Conditions: An Interpretation of the Clinical Literature in the Light of Laboratory Experiment. *Medicine* 23:281–358, 1944.
16. Temple, J. D., Bosshardt, R. T., and Davis, J. H.: Scuba Tank Corrosion As a Cause of Death. *J. Forensic Sci.* 20(3):571–575, 1975.
17. Fandel, I., and Bancalari, E.: Near-Drowning in Children: Clinical Aspects. *Pediatrics* 58(4):573–579, 1976.
18. Courville, C. B.: *Contributions to the Study of Cerebral Anoxia.* San Lucas Press, Los Angeles, 1953.

CHAPTER 13

James A. Benz is Associate Professor of
Pathology at Indiana University and is
Chief of Pathology Services at Wishard
Memorial Hospital in Indianapolis. A 1952
graduate of Indiana University, Dr. Benz
entered the University's School of
Medicine in Indianapolis, receiving his
medical degree in 1955. He was the
Director of the Laboratory for the
Commission on Forensic Sciences of the
State of Indiana and is a state consultant in
forensic pathology. Dr. Benz also teaches
an Introduction to Forensic Sciences in the
Department of Forensic Studies of Indiana
University. Dr. Benz was the chairman of
the Council of Forensic Pathology of the
American Society of Clinical Pathologists
from 1972 to 1978, and presently serves as
Commissioner of the Commission on
Continuing Education of that society.

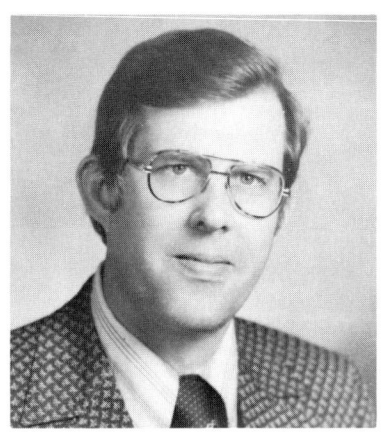

THERMAL DEATHS

James A. Benz, M.D.

SCOPE OF INVESTIGATION

Thermal deaths are those which result from the effects of systematic and/or localized exposure to excessive heat or cold. The vast majority of these deaths result from fires or contact with hot liquids, steam, or hot objects. Deaths due to heat exhaustion, heat stroke, and cold exposure are generally less common, being more prevalent in those areas where climatic conditions exist to promote such deaths.

The scope of investigation of thermal death requires careful review in order to resolve the medicolegal questions which result from this tragic event. It is important that the death investigator be aware of the medicolegal issues involved and direct the investigation to insure *factual* answers wherever possible. Too often a charred body is removed from a conflagration and the grotesque remains promptly buried with little investigative effort expended in the "obvious accidental death." In such a case only a few days may pass before the insurance company, contemplating payment of a large accidental death benefit, asks the embarrassing question, "How did you establish identity of the deceased?"

The death investigation of a person exposed to excessive heat or cold should be directed toward providing factual answers to these questions:

1. How was identification of the deceased established?
2. Was the victim dead or alive at the time of the exposure?
3. What were the circumstances of the event which caused the exposure?
4. What injuries or disease does the victim exhibit and how do they relate to:
   a. Exposure to the excessive heat or cold (direct effect)—extent and severity.

    b. The circumstances of the exposure—injuries produced by the surroundings, such as collapse of structures upon the incapacited victim.
    c. Injuries and disease present before the exposure and their relationship to the death.
    d. Injuries due to medical treatment or recovery of the body—resuscitation, surgical procedures, postmortem injuries, etc.
5. What caused the victim's death and is the cause of death related to the exposure?
6. Why didn't the victim escape?

Adequate death investigation is a team effort which involves many people. The team includes the scene investigator, photographer, evidence technician, law enforcement officers, pathologist, morgue attendant, and clerical help. Occasionally, ancillary help from specialists such as anthropologists, laboratory technicians, toxicologists, criminologists, and dentists will be required. No one person alone can conduct a proper death investigation. The overall success of the investigation is dependent upon the weakest member of the team.

The investigation of thermal deaths exemplifies the necessity of a well-organized, functioning team to answer the critical medicolegal questions. In deaths due to systemic hyperthermia (heat exhaustion and heat stroke) and systemic hypothermia (cold exposure), the anatomic findings observed on or within the dead body may be meager and certainly not pathognomonic in implicating the cause of death. The nonspecific autopsy findings correlated with laboratory findings and extensive investigation concerning the circumstances of death will be needed to provide a logical conclusion. Similarly, in a conflagration, the extensive destruction of the body, as well as the scene, dictates exhaustive studies by all members of the team in order to reach a satisfactory conclusion. In the absence of such investigative efforts, the medicolegal issues are open to extensive challenge and debate in the courtroom, and a verdict must be rendered on conjecture rather than facts. Case 1, at the end of this chapter, illustrates such a situation.

There are four basic steps involved in any death investigation. These are:

1. Gathering detailed information concerning the circumstances of the death;
2. Processing the body;
3. Ancillary laboratory and/or x-ray studies;
4. Correlation of the above for a satisfactory conclusion.

All members of the investigative team contribute to these basic procedures. In the performance of each step, certain team members play a key role in providing factual information leading to a successful end result. The total investigation is only as good as the weakest link in the fact-finding procedural scheme. Each step of the investigation is subject to close legal scrutiny in the courtroom and to criticism by counsel for the plaintiff or defense. Serious errors can be avoided only if the investigative team is well organized, cooperative, and coordinated. The strengths and weaknesses of the local death investigative system may be sought out by the attorney and used to his advantage. He should examine the investigative efforts of each case, concentrating on these basic procedural steps to assess the completeness of the death inquiry. The basic goals of identifying the deceased, estimating the time of death, and deciding the cause and manner of death must be factually documented.

Utilizing the systematic inquiry outlined above, the investigation of thermal deaths will be discussed, emphasizing the role of the various forensic team members.

DEATHS DUE TO FIRES

Deaths due to fires are a common occurrence. Exposure to the heat and flame of the fire usually produces burns, but some victims in fires within closed structures (house fires, burning buildings, etc.) may die from secondary effects of the fire (carbon monoxide intoxication and smoke inhalation) without any evidence of thermal injury. In other instances, postmortem burns may occur before the fire is extinguished or the victim is removed from the burning dwelling. In such circumstances, the severe cutaneous burns observed in the postconflagration subject may have nothing to do with the cause of death. Thus the mechanism of death of the fire victim is variable and dependent on a number of factors, including proximity to the fire, duration of exposure, protection of the body surface (clothing, blankets, contact with the floor, etc.), toxic substances produced by the fire, structural damage caused by the fire, availability of rescue services and medical care. Any of these factors which influence the mechanism of death in a fire victim may be the cause of court action to settle a medicolegal issue. Is the cause of the fire a liability or negligence issue? Did the smoke and toxic gases gain entry into the ventilating system, spread through the building, and cause the death of a sleeping victim located several floors away because of malfunction of the system or smoke detector equipment? Were fire detection and escape systems functional? Was there a prolonged delay in the arrival of fire-rescue equipment? Was medical treatment adequate? These are examples of issues which may be raised for litigation purposes. Furthermore, deaths due to fires may occur quite rapidly in cases of overwhelming exposure, or be delayed weeks or months, resulting from complications of the thermal injury or even medical mismanagement. All of these factors must be carefully assessed and documented by proper death investigation before the medicolegal issues can be rationally evaluated. Referring back to the basic investigational scheme previously described, the fire death inquiry will now be discussed.

Gathering Information Concerning Circumstances of Death

The importance of the on-the-scene investigators cannot be overemphasized. They are responsible for determining the cause of the fire and establishing whether the fire resulted from arson, accident, or negligence. The legal ramifications of this determination are obvious. Furthermore, the results of their inquiry will seriously influence the procedural steps of the death investigation which will follow. For instance, if the scene investigators are suspicious of an arson fire, then any deaths resulting from the fire are possible homicide victims. Thus an extensive homicide inquiry will ensue, requiring meticulous detail to fulfill the court requirements necessary for prosecution. This type of investigation will be very time-consuming and expensive. On the other hand, if the scene investigator reports a purely accidental origin of the fire, due entirely to the negligence of the deceased, the succeeding steps of the investigation will be relatively simple to accomplish.

In addition to establishing the cause and details of the fire (method of spread, extent of damage, evidence of negligence or crime), the on-the-scene investigator also provides other vital correlative information to the other members of the death investigation team. Facts concerning presumptive identification of the deceased; evidence of his movement about the premises before his death; location of the victim in relationship to structural damage of the building; postmortem injuries incurred during attempted resuscitation or while fighting the fire (high-pressure hose water directed on charred remains), or during removal of the body are necessary in arriving at a satisfactory conclusion of the death investigation. The scene investigation may reveal why the victim did not escape from the fire. The field investigator should always be alert to those instances where a fire has been started to conceal a homicide or suicide, or to perpetrate fraud. He must carefully exclude these possibilities during his inquiry.

The competency of the scene investigation is subject to close scrutiny during litigation of the legal issues. The training and experience of the scene investigator and fire laboratory analyst will be questioned. As knowledge and techniques concerning fire investigation have broadened, the demands placed on these individuals have increased proportionately. Proper documentation of their findings to insure the admissibility of the evidence into the courtroom is essential.

Processing the Body

Detailed examination of the body is primarily the responsibility of the pathologist. However, information concerning the location and position of the body at the scene and the possibility of postmortem injuries caused by the firemen, fire-rescue members, or during transportation to the morgue must be provided to the pathologist prior to his examination. Known information concerning the circumstances of the fire must be available to him since this may seriously influence the details of his inquiry. Hopefully, adequate documentation of facts concerning the body at the scene has been accomplished by good photography and scene diagrams. These items may become extremely important in the overall evaluation and conclusion concerning the victims' injuries and their relationship to the cause and manner of death. Under no circumstances should the body be stripped, transported to a funeral home, and embalmed prior to the pathologist's examination. Such action should be strenuously opposed since factual resolution of many medicolegal issues may be rendered impossible.

Observations of the pathologist should be documented by photography, body diagrams, and description in the autopsy protocol. The documentation should include detailed information concerning any injuries, presence or absence of natural disease, comparative data to help establish identification, smoke and burn distribution, and severity of burns. If no burns are present, this should be so stated.

Specific medicolegal issues requiring factual evidence documented by the pathologist processing the body are discussed below.

IS THIS AN ATTEMPT TO CONCEAL A HOMICIDE?

This possibility must always be considered in examining the fire victim. Attempting to conceal a homicide by conflagration of the victim is a well-recognized, time-honored criminal act. If only a cursory examination of a charred body is made, the homicidal character of the death may be overlooked. Detailed autopsy examination should exclude the most common homicidal causes of death (i.e., gunshot wounds, stabbing, blunt trauma). Asphyxia due to suffocation and certain types of strangulation may be extremely difficult to ascertain in the burned body. Anatomic evidence that the victim was dead at the time of the fire may provide the only clue to the possibility that death was due to asphyxia, provided no other cause of death is found. In such cases, scene investigation and information concerning the circumstances of death may furnish the proper solution. Case 2, at the end of this chapter, is an example of an attempt to conceal multiple homicides by setting a house on fire.

WHO IS THE BURNED VICTIM?

The subject of establishing identification is lengthy and will not be discussed in detail. Positive identification requires fingerprint, footprint, or dental comparison studies. These studies are best accomplished by other specialists of the death investigation team (fingerprint and dental experts). If these studies are not possible (e.g., in the case of an edentulous body with severely burned extremities), then identification must be considered presumptive. Absence of positive identification may cause serious medicolegal problems. In badly charred victims, dental identification may be the best hope, since the teeth are relatively resistant to fire. It is the duty of the pathologist, however, to furnish other comparative data (e.g., physical characteristics, evidence of old trauma or operative procedures). He should also obtain postmortem x-rays, blood, and hair samples for additional studies.

WAS THE VICTIM ALIVE OR DEAD AT THE TIME OF THE FIRE?

This question must be answered by the pathologist. In cases where dead bodies have been found in a conflagration, only the pathologist can render this decision. Factual information provided by postmortem studies should furnish the answer to this question. These facts are derived from examination of the respiratory tract and/or laboratory studies. Indications that the victim was alive at the time of the fire include the following:

1. *Presence of smoke particles in the distal respiratory tract.*
   This proves that the subject inhaled smoke and was breathing during the fire. The soot must be located distal to the nose or mouth (Fig. 13-1).
2. *Evidence of thermal injury of the respiratory tract.*
   Inhaled hot gases or heat usually cause thermal damage of the mucosa and acute laryngeal edema. If the edema develops quite rapidly, asphyxiation may quickly result.
3. *Elevated blood carbon monoxide saturation.*
   This blood level must be greater than 10 percent saturation since it has been shown that heavy smokers can attain a level of 7 to 10 percent. The majority of fire victims who were alive at the time of the fire exhibit significantly elevated carbon monoxide levels. However, the absence of an elevated carbon monoxide level does *not* mean that the subject was dead at the time of the fire. Instances are recorded of victims who were suddenly enveloped in extremely hot

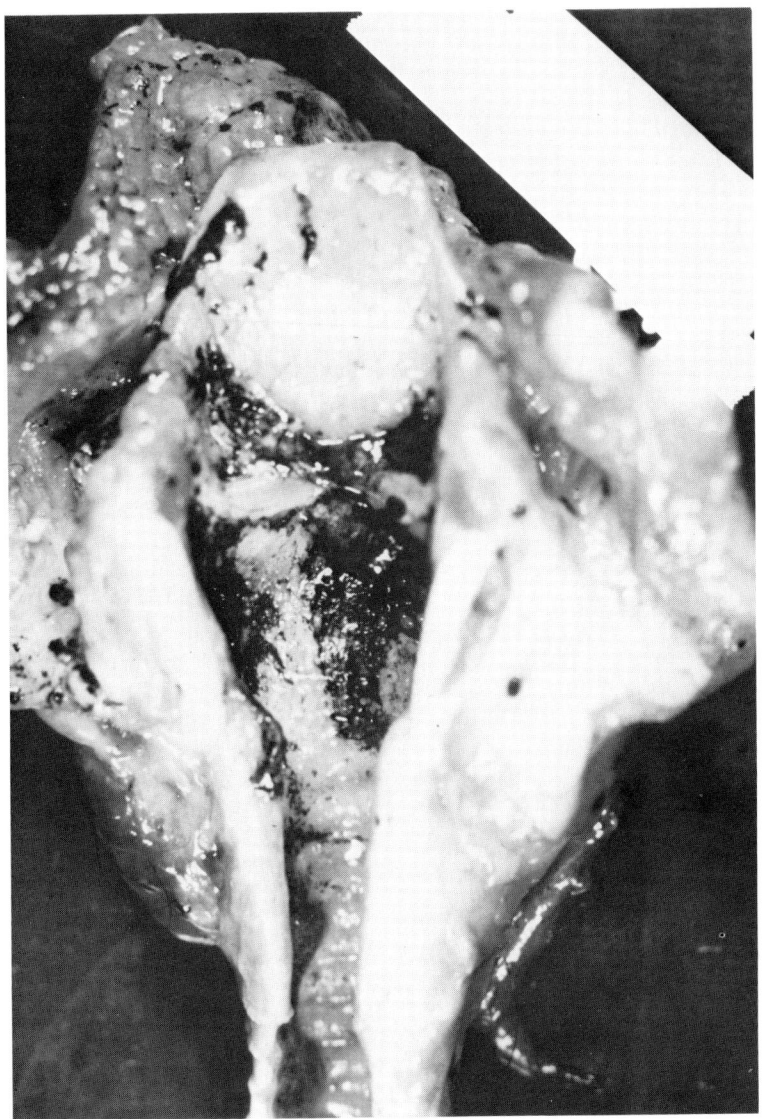

FIGURE 13-1. Soot deposits in the larynx and trachea of a fire death victim, indicating that the subject was alive during the fire. Blood carbon monoxide saturation was 72 percent.

flames which caused thermal injury to the upper respiratory tract (Fig. 13-2) and rapid development of laryngeal edema and asphyxiation, with no significant elevation of carbon monoxide levels. This is particularly true in explosive-type fires. Moreover, the presence of elevated carbon monoxide saturation of the blood *alone* does not prove that the victim was alive at the time of the fire. Death may have resulted from carbon monoxide intoxication from some other source (e.g., auto exhaust fumes) before the fire started. Findings of smoke inhalation and an elevated carbon monoxide saturation together are absolute proof that the subject was alive at the time of the fire.

One must be aware that the level of carbon monoxide saturation

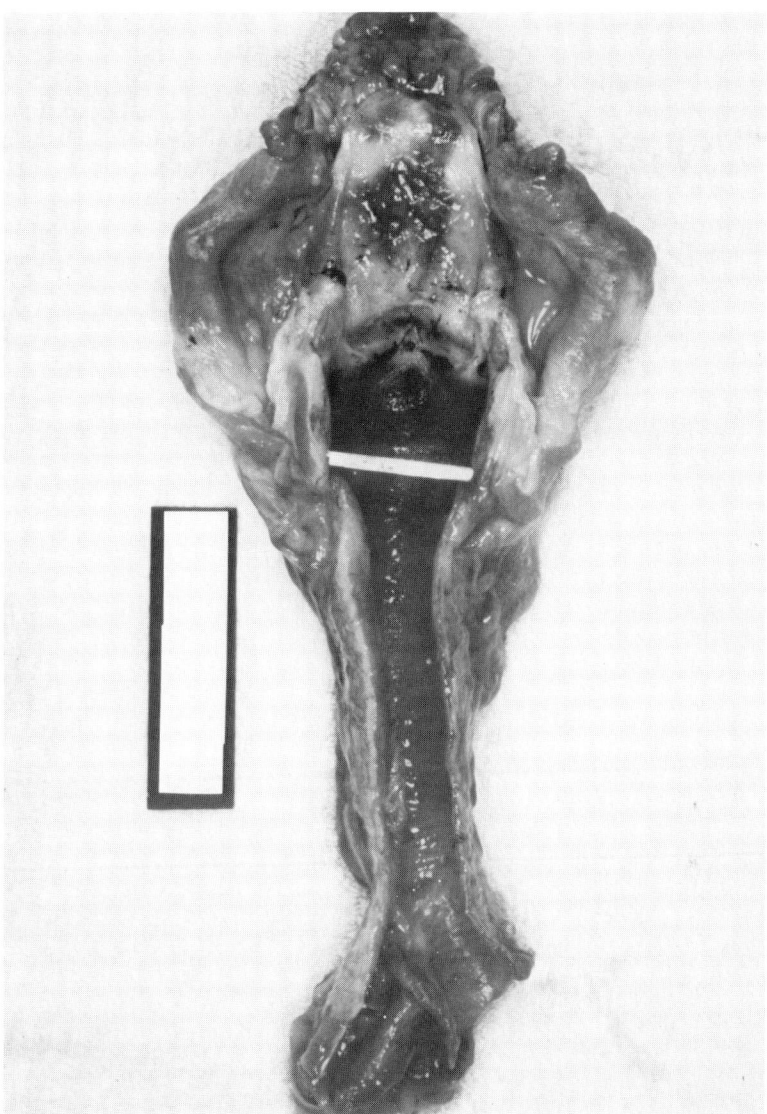

FIGURE 13-2. Thermal injury of the respiratory tract of a fire death victim. Note erythema and scorching of the epiglottis and larynx. A very small soot deposit is present. Blood carbon monoxide saturation was 7 percent. (See Figure 13-20 for a detailed view.)

of the blood is dependent on a number of factors including the concentration of carbon monoxide in the inhaled air, the duration of exposure, the rate and depth of respiration, and the hemoglobin content of the blood. Conditions effecting any of these factors will therefore increase or decrease the rate of carbon monoxide absorption. For example, in a smoldering-type fire in a closed room, the accumulation of carbon monoxide in the air may be rapidly increased to a high concentration. Therefore, one would expect the absorption of carbon monoxide in the victim to be increased correspondingly. By contrast, in a flame-type fire in an open field, the accumulation of carbon monoxide would be expected to be less, and, therefore, the absorption within the body would be correspondingly less rapid. Activity of the individual within an atmosphere containing carbon monoxide also increases the rate of absorption. Anemic individuals or those with heart disease may reach a fatal saturation more rapidly than a normal person. Thus the interpretation of the results of a carbon monoxide blood analysis in the fire victim must be correlated with the scene investigation, the anatomic findings, and all other known facts in order to reach a logical conclusion.

4. *Cutaneous reaction to heat and flame.*

Some authors state that formation of fluid-filled vesicles (blisters) and reddening of the skin associated with burns occur only in the live person subjected to thermal injury. Other authors dispute this observation and state that vesicles having erythematous margins can be produced post mortem. These findings, therefore, are argumentative as far as resolving the dead or alive question. If histologic examination reveals an inflammatory response associated with the wound, the evidence for antemortem origin becomes more positive for that particular burn. It does not necessarily follow that this victim's death resulted from the fire. For example, the victim may have sustained several localized burns a day or so preceding his final fatal experience.

WHAT INJURIES OR DISEASE DOES THE VICTIM EXHIBIT AND WHAT IS THEIR SIGNIFICANCE?

The postmortem examination should document all injuries present on or within the body. The pathologist must differentiate those injuries which are a result of direct exposure to the elements of the fire (e.g., flame, heat, toxic gases) from those which occurred prior to the fire, during the exposure, or post mortem. Injuries due to antemortem trauma such as gunshot wounds, stabbing, and blunt trauma will be the same as those described elsewhere in this book. The characteristic features of these wounds may have been altered due to burning of the tissues, rendering recognition and detailed evaluation difficult or impossible. This is particularly true if incineration of the tissues has occurred. In such cases, post mortem x-ray studies may be helpful. Early detection of foreign bodies within the deceased (e.g., bullets, broken knife tips) or unsuspected fractures may be accomplished by these x-ray studies. This type of examination is particularly recommended if the remains are badly charred.

If the fire victim is burned, the extent and severity of the cutaneous burns should be carefully documented. Photographs and description in the autopsy protocol serve this purpose; however, the use of body diagrams is strongly suggested as a supplementary method. (Fig. 13-3). Such diagrams are usually available at hospital burn units. The burned areas can be easily mapped on the diagrams and an assessment of the percentage of total body surface area involved in the burns can be made. In making this determination, the commonly used values assigned to the various body parts is as follows: head and neck—9 percent; each upper extremity—9 percent; anterior trunk—18 percent; posterior trunk—18 percent; each lower extremity—18 percent; and the perineum comprises 1 percent of the total body surface area. The determination of the extent of cutaneous burns is of particular importance in cases of delayed death,

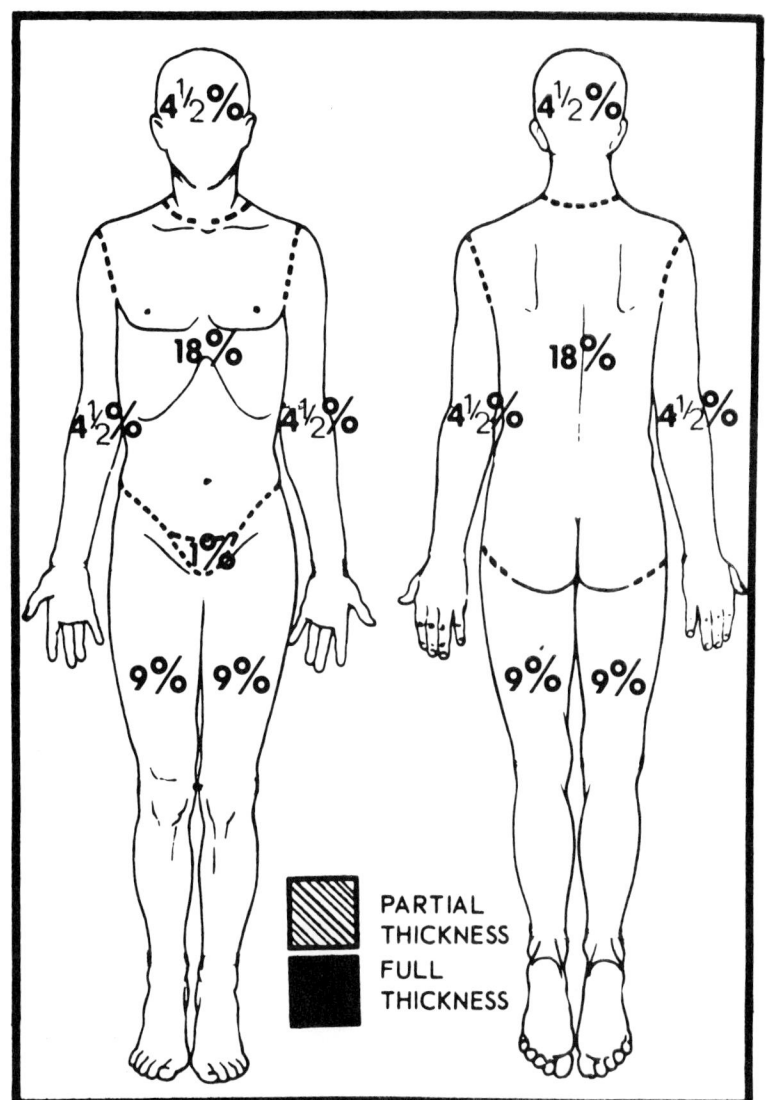

FIGURE 13-3. Body diagrams illustrating estimated percentages of total body surface areas.

since this factor is most influential in the prognosis and medical treatment. Severity of a cutaneous burn usually refers to the depth of the thermal injury. Some authors classify the depth of the burn as first, second, or third degree. The *first-degree* burn is characterized by reddening of the skin. The superficial layers of the skin (epidermis) remain intact. The skin is reddened due to vasodilatation of the vessels in the deeper layers (dermis). The subepithelial tissues may become swollen and edematous. If the victim survives for a period of time following the injury, microscopic examination of the skin will show an inflammatory response. The *second-degree* burn is characterized grossly by blister (vesicle) formation. The epidermis has been destroyed without significant irreversible damage to the dermis. Fluid exudes into the epidermal-dermal junction, elevating the epidermis to form a blister. If the victim survives for a period of time, microscopic examination of the tissues will reveal an inflammatory response. The *third-degree* burn is characterized by irreversible damage to the full thickness of the skin and may extend into the underlying soft tissues. If the exposure is prolonged, the skin and subcutaneous tissues may be incinerated and charred. Extensive exposure of the body after death to heat and flames may produce charring of the entire body surface with cooking of the musculature and internal visera, and finally partial incineration of these structures, particularly the extremities, genitalia, and ears. The variability of the extent and degree of burning is dependent entirely upon the area exposed to the heat and flames as well as the temperature and duration of the exposure.

Other authors characterize the depth of burns into only two categories: full-thickness, in which there is irreversible damage to all skin elements, and partial-thickness, in which some dermal elements having regenerative capabilities have survived the thermal injury.

Burns resulting from a flame usually cause burning or singeing of the hair. Burns caused by hot liquids or hot gases usually do not cause this damage. Similarly, chemical and radiation burns usually do not cause thermal alterations of the hair and are rarely of full-thickness severity. Flame burns frequently have a patchy distribution and vary in size and shape, or "geographic pattern" (Fig. 13-4). "Flash burns" refer to thermal injury due to sudden, brief exposure to flame (Fig. 13-5). This type of exposure is common in explosions or upon ignition of highly flammable liquids. Fairly severe burns limited to one side or part of the body with prominent singeing of the hair is suggestive of this type of circumstance, particularly if the burn is sharply limited to the exposed areas with scorching of the adjacent clothing.

Blunt trauma injuries and incised wounds of recent origin must be

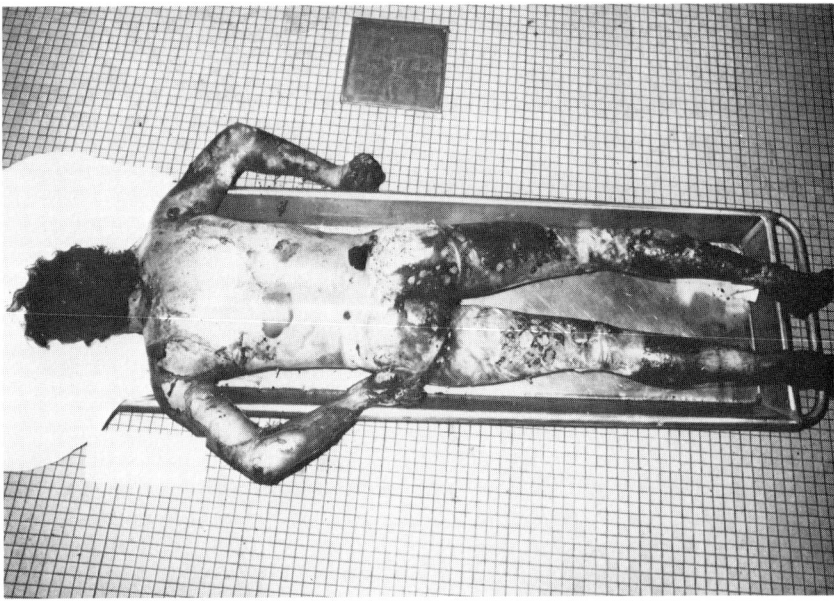

FIGURE 13-4. A "fire death victim" exposed to flames, showing a "geographic" burn pattern. The intensity of the fire was greater in the area of the lower extremities. The victim's head was covered and thus protected from the flames, and the hair was not burned. Blood carbon monoxide saturation was negative, indicating that the victim was dead at the time of the fire.

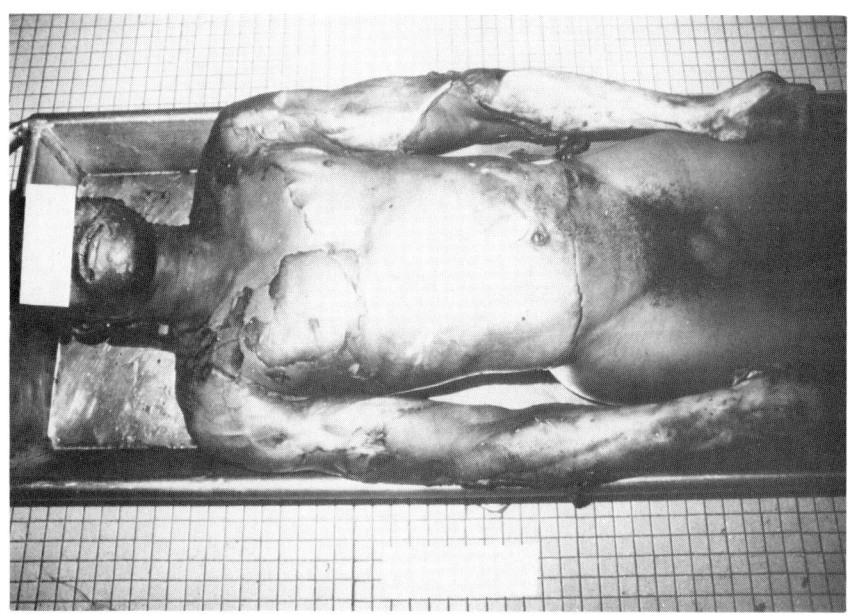

FIGURE 13-5. "Flash burns" in a victim of an explosive gasoline fire. The burns were limited to the front of the body. The subject was wearing trousers which protected the lower body from brief exposure to intense heat. His head hair, moustache, and beard were singed. His blood carbon monoxide level was 18 percent. Extensive thermal injury of the larynx caused obstructive edema. A small soot deposit was present.

evaluated in context with the known circumstances of the death. Location of the body in relationship to structures which may have collapsed and fallen onto the deceased must be known. Evidence at the scene may indicate that the subject attempted to break out windows with his unprotected extremities, providing an explanation for incised wounds in these locations. Lethal blunt trauma without such explanation of antemortem origin should arouse a definite suspicion of homicide. Gunshot wounds and sharp instrument wounds having suicidal characteristics also require meticulous inquiry into the circumstances of the death before homicide can be excluded, and in some circumstances the manner of death in these cases is best classified as "undetermined." Suicide by self-immolation must also be considered.

Significant antemortem incapacitating injuries or natural disease must also be documented. Their importance lies in a possible explanation for reasons that the victim was unable to escape the fire. Immobility of these persons due to their injury or natural disease makes them much more susceptible to succumb in the fire.

During his processing of the body, the pathologist must differentiate certain postmortem artifacts which may occur in a dead body exposed to heat and flame from antemortem injuries. The novice death investigator sometimes misinterprets the "pugilistic" attitude of the burned body to indicate that the deceased was engaged in combat at the time of death (Fig. 13-6). It is the cooking of the muscles which produces this frequent postmortem position of the burned victim. Contraction of the burned tissues often causes splitting of the skin in the charred body. The resulting artifacts greatly resemble incised wounds and may be so misinter-

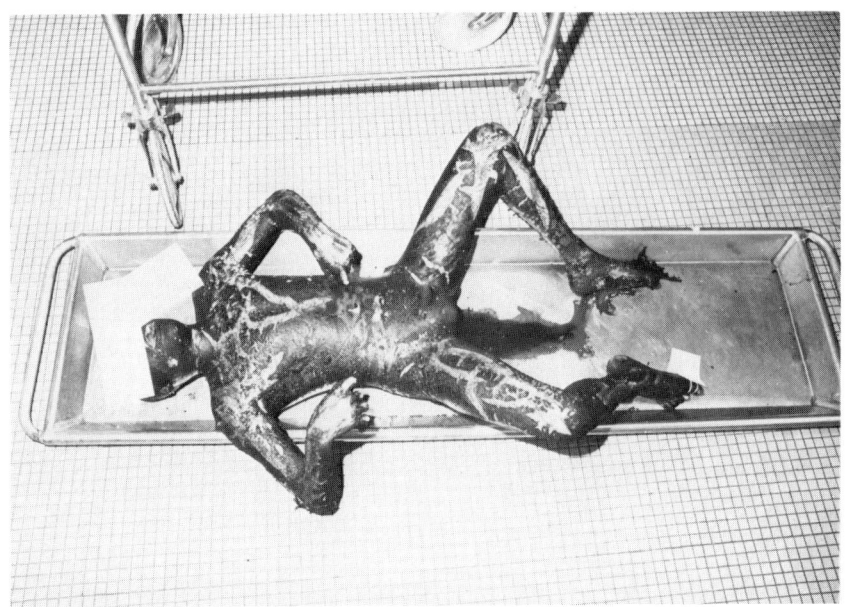

FIGURE 13-6. Examples of fire artifacts. Note the "pugilistic" attitude resulting from heat contracture of the cooked musculature, and the skin splits due to contraction of the skin.

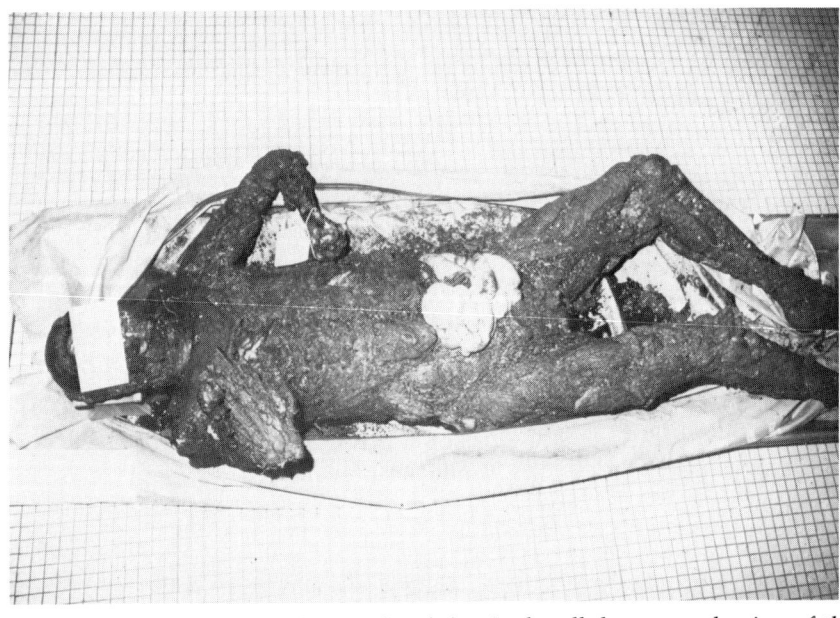

FIGURE 13-7. Artifactual defect in the abdominal wall due to weakening of the wall, caused by burning, and heat expansion of the intestinal gas. The intestine has ruptured through the partially incinerated abdominal wall. Note also the "pugilistic" attitude.

preted. Absence of hemorrhage and location only in areas damaged by the fire help differentiate these defects from antemortem incised wounds. Partial incineration of the abdominal wall associated with gas expansion within the intestine may produce an artifactual rupture of the abdominal wall in the charred burn victim (Fig. 13-7). Frequently, the intestines protrude through this defect. Again, lack of hemorrhage, either externally or internally, in a body with a charred abdominal wall differentiates this artifact from antemortem injury. The badly burned and charred head may exhibit artifactual skull fractures or separation of nonunited cranial sutures (Fig. 13-8). The artifactual fractures occur most commonly in areas where the scalp has been incinerated and the underlying skull severely

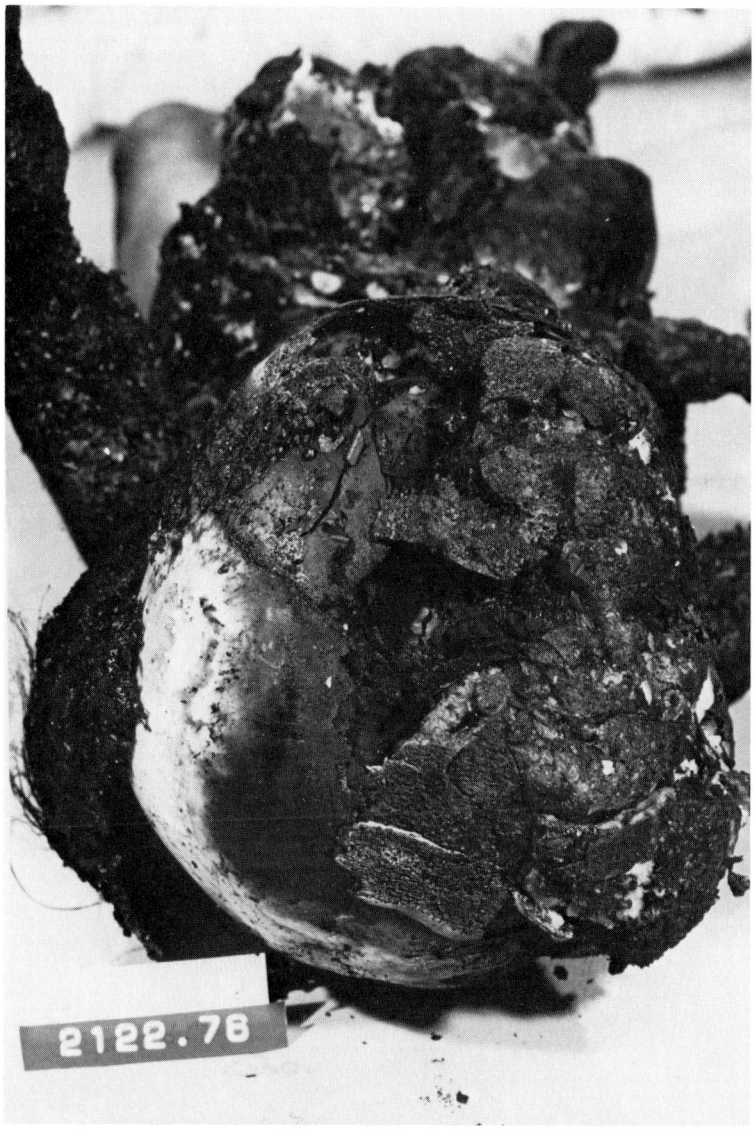

FIGURE 13-8. Artifactual skull fractures of a fire death victim. Note outward deviation of the bone fragments, caused by increased pressure within the skull during the fire.

burned. All skull fractures in a charred body must be evaluated cautiously. Artifactual fractures of the bones of the extremities are also frequent findings in a badly charred, partially incinerated body where there has been prolonged exposure to flame and heat (Figs. 13-9 and 13-10). The charring of the bones of the skull and extremities also renders these structures more susceptible to postmortem trauma which may occur in body transportation to the morgue or during attempts to extinguish the fire by use of a water stream from a high-pressure hose. Another common postmortem artifact is the apparent epidural hematoma which sometimes occurs with prolonged postmortem exposure of the head to heat and fire, resulting in the extrusion of blood between the dura and the inner table of the skull (Figs. 13-11 and 13-12). The artifactual hematoma is more common in heads which are charred. Differential features are listed in Table 13-1.

Wounds caused by surgical procedures, medical management, or resuscitative attempts must be documented by the pathologist, and their relationship to proper medical treatment should be established by critical review of the medical records. Any discovery of possible malpractice should be further investigated.

WHAT CAUSED THE VICTIM'S DEATH AND IS THE CAUSE OF DEATH RELATED TO THE FIRE?

Although most dead bodies removed from a conflagration died as a result of the fire, the pathologist processing the body should be cognizant that this indeed may not be the case. Serious medicolegal questions can arise if his investigation is incomplete. Precise determination of the cause and manner of death depends on correlation of autopsy and laboratory findings and details of the circumstances of the death. Most victims who die rapidly within the conflagration do so as a result of smoke inhalation, carbon monoxide intoxication, and/or thermal burns. Death usually is

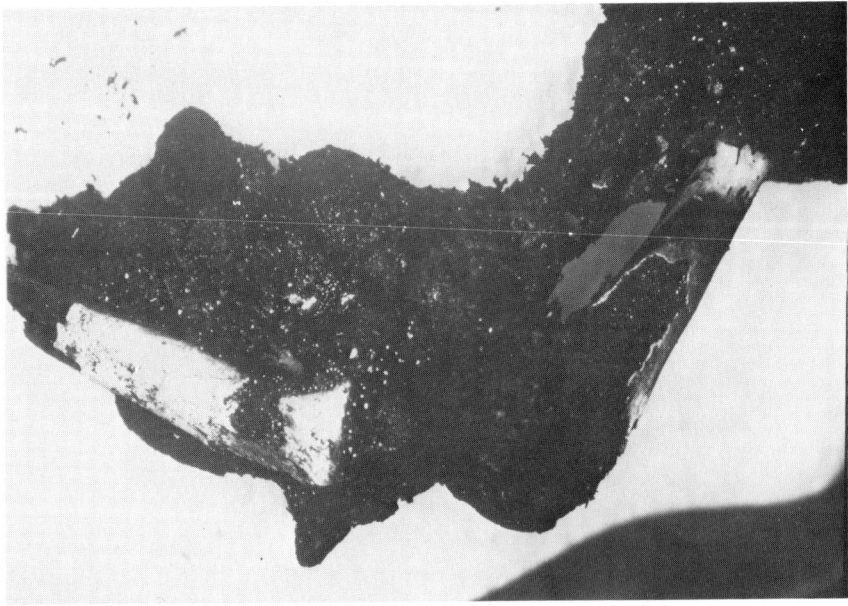

FIGURE 13-9. Fire fractures of the bones in the arm of a fire victim.

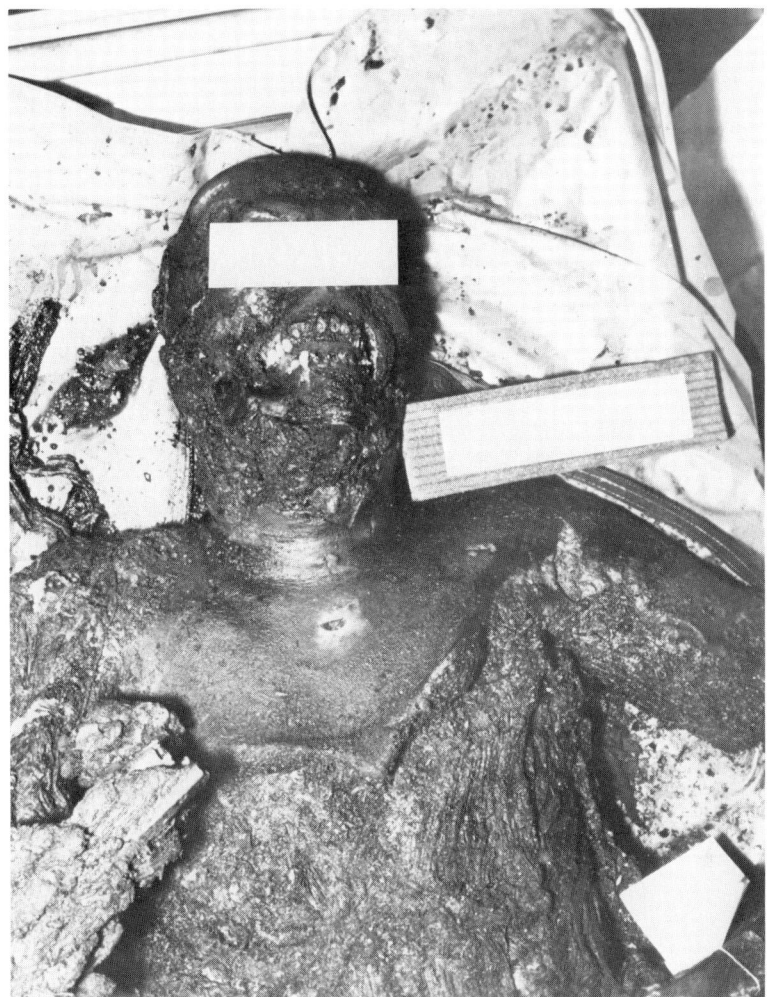

FIGURE 13-10. Fire fractures of the bones of the right forearm. Note the stab wound in the chest which perforated the heart and resulted in death. No soot was present in the respiratory tract, and the negative blood carbon monoxide indicated that death occurred before the fire. This case was determined to be an attempt to conceal murder by means of arson.

associated with a combination of these factors. Carbon monoxide intoxication and smoke inhalation are most frequently responsible in smoldering-type fires. However, the extent and severity of thermal injury and the saturation of the blood with carbon monoxide must be carefully appraised to establish their relationship to the cause of death. Some causes of death unrelated to the fire have been previously discussed. A man may have a heart attack or stroke and die, dropping his smoking materials and causing a fire which may produce extensive postmortem burns. A woman may take an overdose of sedatives and drop her smoking materials as she lapses into coma, producing the same sequence of events. Adequate postmortem examination, however, should resolve these cases. Reference Cases 1 and 5 illustrate these points.

Fire victims who survive for a period of time may pose complex medicolegal problems since they may die for a variety of reasons which may or

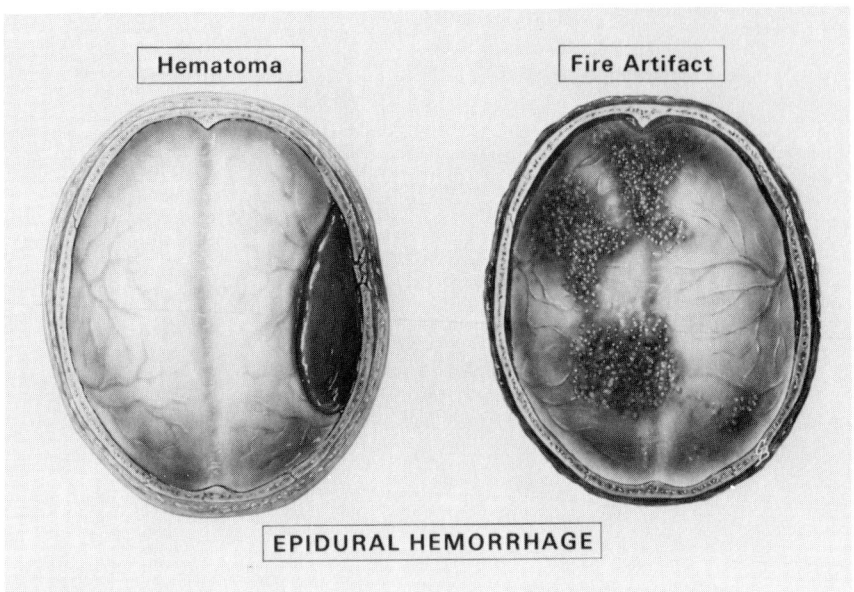

FIGURE 13-11. Coronal view of the skull, illustrating the differential features of traumatic epidural and fire artifact hematoma. (Drawings by George Buckley, Department of Clinical Pathology, Indiana University School of Medicine.)

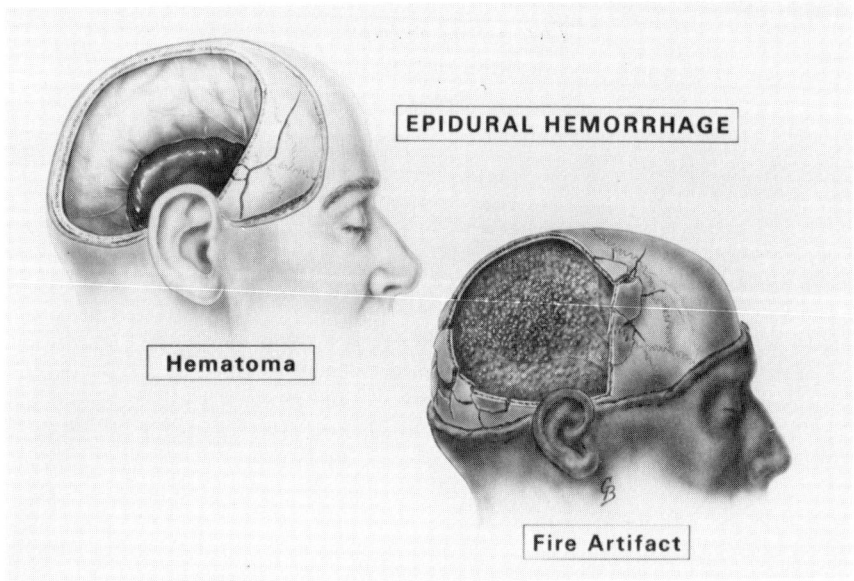

FIGURE 13-12. Temporal view illustrating the differential features of traumatic epidural and fire artifact hematoma. Note the presence of fire artifact skull fractures. (Drawings by George Buckley, Department of Clinical Pathology, Indiana University School of Medicine.)

TABLE 13-1.

Artifactual Epidural Hematoma	Antemortem Epidural Hematoma
1. Usually bilateral	1. Usually unilateral
2. Diffuse	2. Well-circumscribed
3. Usually thin, granular, friable, evenly distributed or sickle-shaped, chocolate brown	3. Discoid shape, localized more rubbery consistency, reddish-purple
4. Skull may be fractured	4. Associated skull fracture in temporal area
5. Located anywhere	5. Usually located adjacent to sylvian fissure
6. No injury to CNS	6. Frequently has injury to CNS

may not be related to the fire—at least conclusions may be argumentative. Delayed death of the majority of fire victims is caused by complications of the cutaneous burns or thermal injury to the respiratory tract. Infection of the thermally damaged areas is the major complication causing death. Pneumonia, septicemia, renal failure, ulceration of the gastrointestinal tract with hemorrhage or perforation, embolism, therapeutic mismanagement, and serum hepatitis are other common complications which may result in death. Unless it can be demonstrated within reasonable medical certainty that the lethal complication was caused by the initial fire injury, death cannot be attributed to the fire. Death caused by mechanical trauma and events related to collapse of the structure surrounding the victim, caused by fire damage, is certainly related to the fire. Inhalation of smoke and toxic gases, producing irreversible pulmonary edema, must also be considered. The asphyxial aspects of carbon monoxide have been discussed, but the anoxic effects due to prolonged nonlethal exposure are also noteworthy and may contribute significantly to the patient's demise. Other noxious gases and fumes may be produced in a fire, depending on the material burned, particularly if these materials contain one or more plastic substances such as polystyrene, polyvinyl chloride, polyurethane, polyethylene, or polypropylene. These gases may include hydrogen cyanide, ammonia, sulfur dioxide, hydrogen sulfide, nitrogen oxide, and carbon dioxide. All of these substances are toxic and potentially lethal. Thus, knowledge of the possibility of inhalation of toxic gases and fumes is essential for proper medical care, not only of burn victims, but also of firemen who are "overcome" while engaged in fire-fighting activities.

WHY DIDN'T THE VICTIM ESCAPE?

The presence of significant immobilizing antemortem injury or disease as a cause for the victim's inability to escape the fire has been previously discussed. In addition, complete toxicologic analyses are necessary to rule out the possibility of a toxic substance as a cause for inability to escape. The relationship between alcohol abuse and fires is well known. Drug abuse may be equally important and should be evaluated by toxicologic studies. Carbon monoxide intoxication is another frequent reason for irrational behavior in a fire.

Ancillary Laboratory and X-Ray Studies

From the foregoing discussion, it is apparent that ancillary laboratory and/or x-ray studies are mandatory to elucidate the medicolegal issues.

These studies may include analyses of the body fluids and tissues of the fire victim for toxic substances, analyses of materials removed from the scene for inflammable substances, evaluation of materials removed from the scene by the fire laboratory for evidence of mechanical or electrical failure, analyses of blood and hair removed from the fire victim to aid in identification, and examination of materials removed from the body by criminologists. Postmortem x-ray examination may be necessary for identification purposes and discovery of unsuspected injury or foreign objects within the body.

Correlation of Data

After all members of the death investigation team have collected and evaluated their data, the pooled information can be analyzed to determine if all medicolegal issues and problems of the case have been answered. The cooperation between the various members of the death investigation team is essential to provide sufficient answers. The pathologist, for example, may have discovered findings necessitating further on-the-scene investigation as well as toxicologic studies. Similarly, the field investigator may be helpful in directing certain studies of the pathologist or the fire laboratory analyst. Scientific objective investigation by each team member and coordinated effort by the team as a whole are necessary to reach definitive conclusions.

DEATHS DUE TO THE THERMAL INJURY CAUSED BY HOT LIQUIDS, STEAM, OR HOT OBJECTS

Deaths caused by hot liquids, steam, or hot objects are less common than fire deaths. Scalding injuries are more common in young children than in adults. Accidental spillage of hot water or grease is a frequent cause of scalding injury. Burns caused by contact with hot objects are more frequent in children and in industrial accidents. Deaths caused by contact with hot objects are infrequent, owing to the limited area of the burn usually produced in this manner. Debilitated persons, of course, are more susceptible to death as a result of burns, no matter how the injury occurred. Deaths due to steam burns are usually of industrial origin. In order to produce cutaneous burns, the hot material is usually in excess of 55°C (130°F).

The scalding burns produced by hot liquids and steam are similar. The burn injury is limited to the area of contact and is more severe at the point of the initial contact. The hair is not singed. The burn severity may be first, second, or third degree, depending on the temperature of the inflicting agent, the duration of exposure, and the part of the body involved. The skin of the face and abdomen, for example, is more easily burned than the calloused areas of the hands or the soles of the feet. Age of the victim is also important; the skin of the child seems to be more susceptible than that of the adult. Charring of the skin or overlying clothing does not occur. Since clothing dissipates heat, it affords protection against scalding, and, therefore, the exposed areas of the body are more frequently involved. However, scalding can occur through clothing. Inhalation of steam may cause thermal injury of the respiratory tract, producing asphyxial death secondary to airway obstruction by the edematous mucous membranes. Ingestion of hot liquids rarely produces death unless the liquid is aspirated into the respiratory tract while drinking, thus producing thermal injury of the airway.

Burns caused by hot objects are limited to the area of contact and may leave a burn imprint identical to the shape of the object. Severity of the burn, again, is determined by the temperature of the hot object, the duration of exposure, and the body part involved. Singeing of the hair is generally not present unless the temperature of the hot object is sufficient to produce this change. Although inhalation of hot vapors may cause a rapid demise, death due to contact with hot liquids, steam, or hot objects is usually delayed and results from complications of the burn injuries.

Gathering Information

Death due to these thermal injuries is usually delayed. Therefore, historical information concerning the circumstances of the injury is usually available to the investigators, unless the victim is comatose, an infant or a child, or an attempt has been made to conceal the facts. Examination of medical records may be necessary to obtain this information. Most of these deaths are accidental. Occasionally, however, homicidal or suicidal scalding occurs. The investigator should be aware of these possibilities. Immersion of infants or children in boiling water or throwing of boiling liquids onto a victim as a means of revenge are examples of such a homicidal intent. Purposeful scalding as a means of suicide has been reported. The author has been involved in the investigation of a case in which a mentally deranged woman ingested boiling coffee in sight of her family as a means of suicide. Death resulted from aspiration of the hot liquid.

The field investigator must ascertain details concerning how the injuries occurred. The determination of the manner of death will be based primarily on this evidence. Problems involving negligence or liability are also largely dependent upon this information for solution. Product liability cases resulting from malfunction of a heating pad or an electrical appliance are examples of common medicolegal issues. The relationship between time of injury causation and time of seeking medical treatment is also of primary importance since infection of the wounds is the beginning of the usual lethal sequence. Details of medical therapy and past medical history are also of much significance.

Processing the Body

Details of thermal injury should be documented by photography, body diagrams, and autopsy protocol description. Distribution and severity of the burns should be adequately recorded to be certain that they coincide with the history of the injury. This is particularly true in cases of apparently abused children where all sorts of stories are contrived to explain burns caused by immersion in hot water or lighted cigarettes. In such cases, the establishment of burns of varying ages may be critical in supporting a charge of child abuse.

If hot material has been thrown onto the subject, the direction from which it was thrown or splashed may be indicated by detailed examination of the burn. At the point of initial contact, the burn will be more severe and will then become less so as the material cools in spreading across the surface. Correlation of this information with related facts concerning the circumstances of the "accident" may support or disprove the story.

The possibility that the burns are not of postmortem origin must also be evaluated by the pathologist. Elderly individuals, for example, may have sustained a terminal heart attack or stroke and collapsed into a tub of hot water, sustaining minimal or moderate burns only as a result of prolonged exposure in the postmortem state (Figs. 13-13 to 13-15).

Additional responsibilities of the pathologist include collection of data concerning establishment of identification, establishment of the relationship between cause of death and the thermal injury, collection of postmortem materials for ancillary laboratory studies, and determination of natural disease present within the deceased. The relationship of natural disease to the cause of death must also be evaluated. Details of these responsibilities have been previously described.

Ancillary Laboratory and/or X-Ray Studies

These studies are essentially those described earlier in this chapter concerning deaths due to fires. The extent of these studies will be markedly influenced by the nature of the information gathered.

Correlation to Establish a Logical Conclusion

This step is essentially the same as previously described. In contrast to fire deaths, neither the scene nor the body has been drastically altered by the excessive exposure. Since historical information from the burned victim is usually available, the solutions to the medicolegal problems are hopefully conclusive.

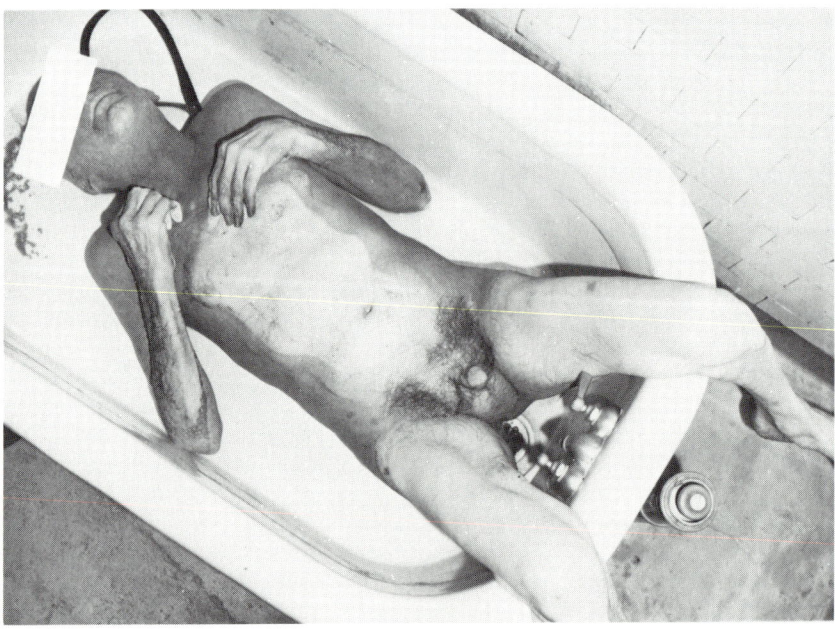

FIGURE 13-13. Scene picture of an elderly male who had a fatal heart attack, collapsed, and fell into a bathtub containing scalding hot water in which he had been preparing to bathe.

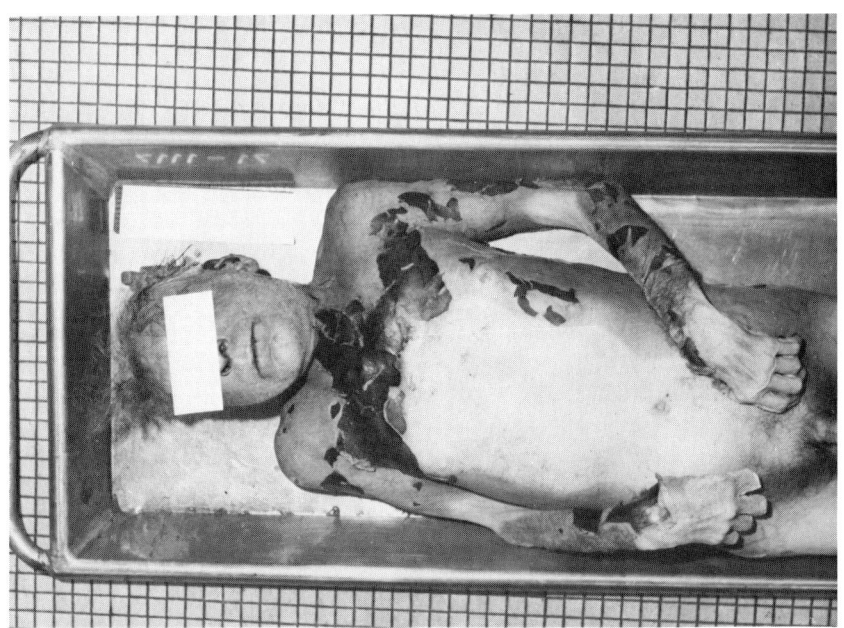

FIGURE 13-14. The same victim as shown in Figure 13-13. Note the sharp demarcation of thermal damage to the skin, limited to areas contacted by the scalding water. The subject's hair was not burned.

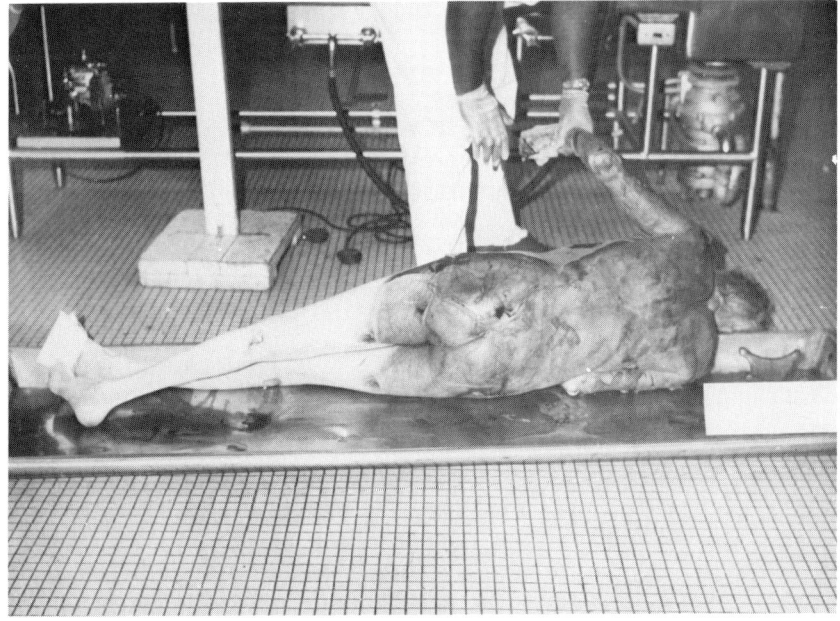

FIGURE 13-15. The scald-burn victim shown in Figure 13-14. This posterior view illustrates extensive thermal injury to the submerged portion of the body.

DEATHS DUE TO HEAT EXHAUSTION AND HEAT STROKE

Deaths due to systemic hyperthermia result from a malfunction of the physiologic mechanisms which maintain the normal body temperature. The heat regulatory mechanisms of the human body which maintain thermal homeostasis with the environment are principally alterations in peripheral blood flow, sweating, and metabolism. When the body is subjected to an elevated environmental temperature, heat production within the body is reduced by a lowered metabolism, and heat loss is promoted by peripheral vasodilatation and increased sweating. Evaporation of the sweat cools the body. The vapor pressure of the skin and air and the motion of the air greatly influence the rate of evaporation. Thus the external temperature, humidity, and air motion are important factors in causing heat exhaustion and heat stroke. This is particularly true in the person who is not acclimatized to these conditions. Strenuous physical exercise is also important since this increases the production of body heat.

When certain environmental conditions of elevated temperature and/or humidity exist, the heat regulatory mechanisms of the body may fail resulting in systemic hyperpyrexia. Obviously, prolonged exposure, exercise, and relatively still air will help promote the breakdown. If untreated, the condition can be fatal. Muscular cramping, nausea, vomiting, weakness, and lethargy are common prodromal symptoms warning of the impending, more serious disorder of heat exhaustion or heat stroke.

In the clinical condition of heat exhaustion, continued exposure produces additional symptomatology and fainting due to vasomotor instability. The body temperature may be slightly elevated, but the skin is moist, due to the profuse sweating.

Heat stroke represents complete deterioration of the heat regulatory system. Sweating ceases and the skin becomes dry. Body temperature becomes markedly elevated to levels of 106 to 108° F. Progressive central nervous manifestations of irrationality, lethargy, coma, and convulsions become more apparent. The subject may die suddenly if vigorous medical treatment is not instituted.

The environmental conditions and pathophysiology involved in the development of these heat disorders are such that certain population groups are more susceptible. These include elderly persons with degenerative cardiovascular disease, poorly conditioned individuals engaged in prolonged strenuous exercise (particularly if wearing heavy clothing), and those taking atropine-like or diuretic hypotensive drugs. Alcohol abuse also predisposes to these clinical conditions.

Gathering Information

Since the autopsy findings are nonspecific, detailed documentation of the circumstances of the death are essential in establishing the correct diagnosis. Since death is usually delayed, it is important that the investigator trace the sequence of events back to the prolonged exposure to the excessively hot environment. Precise details of this exposure must be documented, including the exact temperature and humidity of the environment and duration of exposure. Facts concerning ventilation (air motion) and physical activity are also necessary. Information concerning the amount of physical effort actually exerted and what was required may also be needed to evaluate the possibility of compensation and/or liability in industrial cases. The question as to whether the victim was forewarned of the possible dangers of overexposure to these conditions may have to be factually answered. The availability of supervision, rescue equipment, and medical treatment may also be questioned. Information concerning proper physical conditioning and supervision may be needed in evaluating athletic deaths due to these heat disorders. The medical records of the deceased must be closely scrutinized by a knowledgeable investigator concerning present and past medical history and the details of the medical treatment.

Processing the Body

There are no pathognomonic autopsy findings enabling one to precisely diagnose a heat disorder. A detailed, complete autopsy is of importance, however, in excluding other causes of death or documenting conditions which may have predisposed this individual to a heat disorder. Other diseases known to produce hyperpyrexia must be carefully eliminated from consideration. Terminally, these patients may present a clinical status similar to a stroke, and thorough examination of the central nervous system is necessary to exclude this possibility. The pathologist must collect body fluids and tissues at the time of autopsy for toxicologic analyses. Of equal importance is the collection of vitreous humor from the eyeball for postmortem chemical analyses to indicate evidence of electrolyte abnormalities.

Ancillary Studies

Toxicologic and chemical studies on materials collected post mortem are necessary as indicated above. The possibility of death due to toxic substances must be excluded.

Correlation of Data to Reach a Logical Conclusion

The absence of specific autopsy findings or toxicologic findings to explain death often necessitates further detailed inquiry concerning the circumstances of death in order to reach a satisfactory conclusion in these types of cases. Studies during the clinical phase of the illness or post mortem chemical studies indicating a serious electrolyte abnormality may provide the only clue in some circumstances. See reference Case 3 for an example.

DEATH DUE TO COLD EXPOSURE

When heat loss of the body is greater than heat production, the body becomes hypothermic. Prolonged somatic hypothermia eventually causes circulatory failure, ventricular fibrillation of the heart, and death. Most deaths associated with prolonged exposure to cold are accidental and occur in regions where adverse climatic conditions exist. Occasional deaths occurring in commercial freezers or similar industrial settings have been reported. Homicidal and suicidal deaths solely due to cold exposure are unusual, and a death associated with hypothermic medical procedures is extremely rare. Hypothermia of significant degree is usually associated with some underlying disease, injury, or toxic agent. Prolonged exposure to a cold environment causing death is frequently caused by an immobilizing injury, a natural disease condition which lowers the resistance of the exposed person, or depressant toxic agents (e.g., alcohol, drugs). As a generality, infants and the elderly are more susceptible than young adults. The damage produced by cold exposure is markedly influenced by wetness. The body can tolerate dry cold much better than wet cold (immersion). Wetness increases heat loss dramatically.

Gathering Information

Since the pathologic abnormalities observed at autopsy are not specific, the evidence concerning the circumstances of the death must substantiate the diagnosis. Detailed information concerning the environmental temperature and humidity, wetness of the body, duration of exposure, windchill factors, clothing, medical history, and evidence of alcohol or drug abuse must be carefully evaluated. This information is needed not only to establish the correct diagnosis, but also is a factor affecting the length of survival in cold exposure. Facts concerning the victim's physical conditioning, degree of exhaustion, and history of antecedent disease or injury must also be considered. If there was a period of hospitalization prior to the subject's demise, the medical records must be extensively reviewed by a knowledgeable individual. Adequacy of rescue work or medical management may become a medicolegal issue. It is of particular importance to note whether the severity of the hypothermia of the hospitalized patient was adequately documented since most standard clinical thermometers will not record a reading below 95° F (35° C). During cold exposure, peripheral vasoconstriction and shivering are the two major means of regulating body heat. The shivering reaction usually ceases at a body temperature of about 86 to 90° F (30 to 32° C), and it is also at about this level that the patient usually becomes somewhat insensitive to cold. Thus accurate documentation of the body temperature upon admission is essential in establishing a diagnosis of hypothermia, particularly when one is confronted by a confused elderly individual who has been exposed to a low environmental temperature.

The symptoms and signs of hypothermia may be related within the medical record, and if an electrocardiogram was taken during the hypothermic episode, it may show changes which some authors regard as pathognomonic of this condition. These changes include lengthening of the PR and QRS intervals and a distinctive "J" deflection in the left ventricular leads.

Processing the Body

It is the opinion of this author that there are no specific pathologic findings diagnostic of death due to cold exposure. The diagnosis can be established with some degree of certainty only when correlated with circumstances of death related to prolonged exposure to cold. Some authors list a variety of anatomic abnormalities which have been observed with increased frequency in deaths related to cold exposure. Most of these series of cases are small and include both subjects found dead and those who survived for awhile, various age groups, and/or those who had other injuries, disease, or toxic substances which contributed to the death. The reported findings include pulmonary congestion and edema, extensive visceral congestion, right heart dilatation, pancreatitis, parotitis, focal hemorrhages or small ulcerations of the gastrointestinal mucosa, acute tubular necrosis of the kidney, brain edema, and petechial brain hemor-

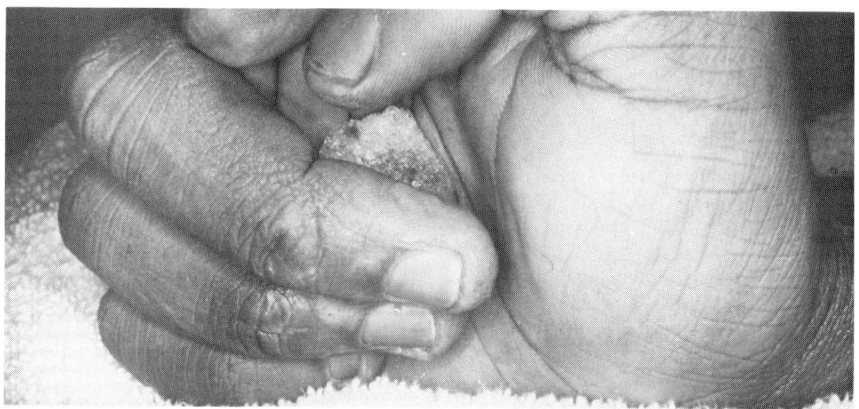

FIGURE 13-16. The hand of a cold exposure victim. Note the "frostbite" injury to the fingers, indicating that the subject survived for a period of time while exposed to frigid temperature. The presence of snow tightly clutched in the hand (cadaveric spasm) also indicates that the subject was alive while lying in the snow.

rhages. None of these abnormalities is pathognomonic of cold exposure. Many of these findings are related to terminal cardiovascular failure and can be seen in numerous conditions unrelated to cold exposure.

Although the autopsy findings may not be specific that *death* was caused by hypothermia, there may be factual findings of localized injury ("frostbite" or "immersion foot") indicative of excessive exposure to cold while the victim was alive (Fig. 13-16). These findings may be of importance in suggesting a sequence of events or estimating time of death in bodies found in a frozen condition. The pinkish color of the lividity and internal tissues may also be suggestive of antemortem exposure, but carbon monoxide and cyanide intoxication must be excluded.

The localized hypothermic injury may vary in severity, including blotchy reddish-purple discolored areas of the skin usually located on the extremities, swelling of the ears and face, or the lesions of "frostbite." Manifestations of "frostbite" differ from simple redness and swelling of the damaged tissue to variable depths of necrosis with blister formation and gangrene (Figs. 13-17 and 13-18). The exposed areas of the body usually

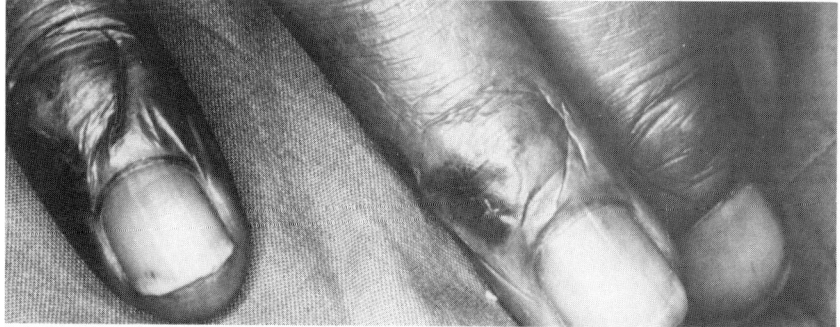

FIGURE 13-17. Localized cold injury ("frostbite") of the fingers. Note the formation of blisters and the presence of swelling and superficial necrosis.

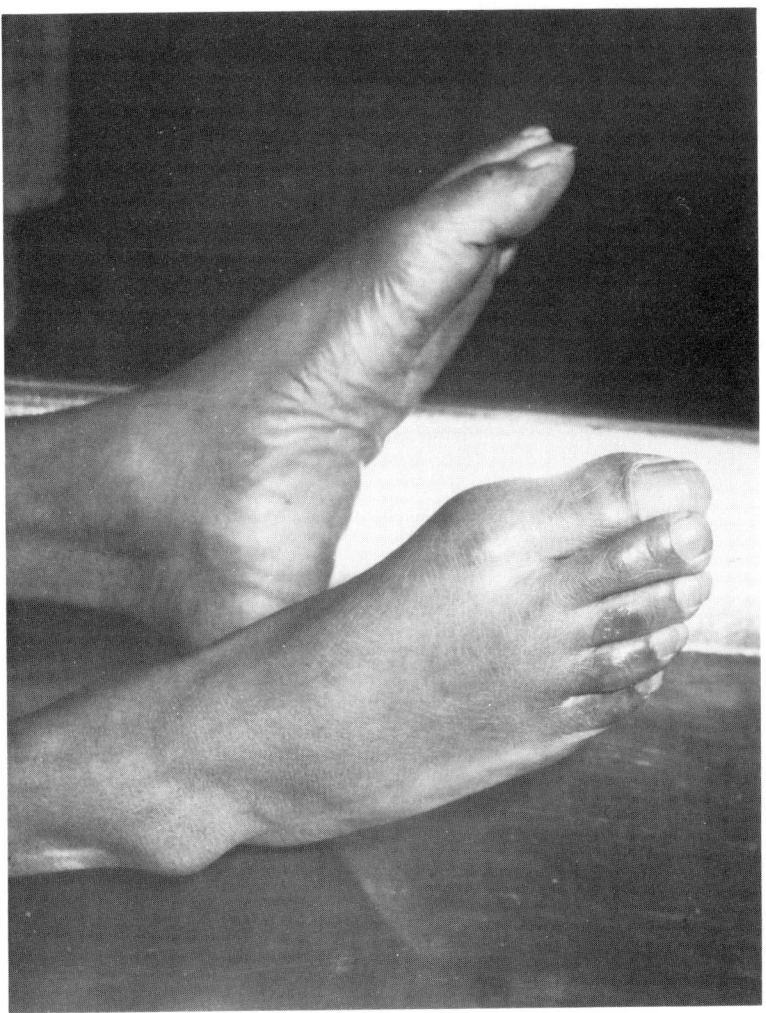

FIGURE 13-18. Localized cold injury of the toes.

exhibit the most severe damage. The pathologist must document the presence or absence of these localized hypothermic injuries.

The major importance of the autopsy in the cold exposure death is to exclude other causes for the subject's demise, including natural disease, trauma, or toxic agents. Other items included in processing of the body, such as data collection for identification, documentation of the presence of other injuries or disease, and collection of specimens for toxicologic studies have been discussed previously.

Ancillary Studies

Toxicologic studies are necessary to determine if toxic substances may have produced a clinical state predisposing to prolonged exposure. The frequent relationship to alcohol abuse mandates analysis for this substance. Specimens for analysis include those collected post mortem and, if the subject was hospitalized prior to death, any antemortem specimens that may still be available. Of the latter, those specimens collected at the time of admission would be the most important. Other special studies would be dictated by the particulars of the case (e.g., unidentified person, evidence of possible homicide or suicide, etc.).

Correlation of Data

Documentation of the circumstances of the exposure is essential in establishing the correct diagnosis and providing factual data to resolve the medicolegal issues. Since the autopsy findings are nonspecific, the history of cold exposure is indispensable. Detailed information concerning the circumstances of the death must be carefully evaluated and correlated with the clinical, autopsy, and laboratory findings. If there is good correlation, then the probability of a logical, correct conclusion is excellent.

The series of cases which form the concluding section of this chapter illustrate various problems encountered in the investigation of thermal death. The case may introduce one or more medicolegal problems which were difficult to solve. The cases demonstrate the necessity for detailed input from the various members of the death investigation team in order to arrive at a satisfactory conclusion. The axiom that "death investigation is a team effort" is adequately shown. No one person solves a case; the contribution of each individual member is of equal importance.

CASE 1

Death in a house fire; incomplete investigation resulting in questionable cause of death.

An elderly physician in a small town returned home at approximately 2 a.m. after completing a house call to find his house filled with smoke. The origin of the fire was in his wife's bedroom which he found ablaze when he opened the door. The local volunteer fire department extinguished the fire approximately 1 hour later.

The body was removed from the premises by the local coroner and was embalmed and buried the following day. The distraught physician stated that his wife slept in a separate bedroom so that she would not be awakened by phone calls from his patients. She was known to be a smoker, and it was presumed that the fire resulted from her smoking in bed. The physician stated that she frequently smoked while reading in bed after retiring, and on several occasions had fallen asleep while smoking, causing minor fires.

Several weeks later a double indemnity claim for $100,000 was filed by the husband for the accidental death of his wife. Investigation by the insurance company revealed that there had been marital problems between the husband and wife and that on several occasions the wife had attempted suicide by drug overdose. Relatives also suggested the possibility of homicide. Furthermore, it was learned that this elderly lady had a history of "heart disease." The insurance company therefore refused to pay the double indemnity claim on the basis that (1) it was not proven that death resulted from the fire, and (2) there was a suicide exclusion clause in the insurance policy. The insurance company insisted that the body be exhumed for autopsy before any double indemnity payment be instituted.

Reluctantly, the husband consented to exhumation and autopsy of his wife. Although the body was severely burned, carbonaceous material was demonstrated to be present within the respiratory tract. A small amount of blood was recovered within the dural sinuses, and analysis of the blood revealed a carbon monoxide saturation of 70 percent. No significant coronary artery disease was found. Toxicologic analyses for other substances was seriously hampered by the embalming procedure. However, secobarbital was found to be present within the blood in therapeutic quantities only. No other toxic substances were found to be present.

Arson investigators were also seriously impaired in their investigation since the majority of the burned furniture and interior of the room had been removed from the premises, as the possibility of homicide was not entertained until several days after the fire. Although charred remnants of the mattress, bedclothing, and rug were available for analysis for flammable substances, these materials had been laid in an open dump, allowing evaporation to take place. They had also been exposed to several heavy rainfalls during that period of time.

Although the circumstances of this death suggested that the wife had taken a sedative after retiring and had been smoking in bed and fallen asleep, and that the fire had been started by her smoking materials, this conclusion could be derived only after extensive, needless cost for an exhumation. The allegations of "drug overdose" or suspicion of homicide by conflagration could not be conclusively excluded. The autopsy findings, however, did provide factual evidence that the victim (a) was alive at the time of the fire; (b) died as a result of carbon monoxide intoxication, smoke inhalation, and thermal burns; (c) had no significant heart disease; and (d) had no other evidence of demonstrable trauma.

The insurance company paid the double indemnity settlement.

CASE 2

Attempt to conceal homicidal deaths by arson house fire.

The fire department was summoned to a residential home about 2:30 a.m. when neighbors reported smoke coming from the dwelling. Firemen entered the house through the locked (non-deadbolt type) front door. Dense smoke filled the home. The fire was confined to a family room adjoining the living room. The fire was rapidly extinguished using water hoses.

A 28-year-old man and his 26-year-old wife were found dead, lying face down on the floor of the family room. The man was dressed in trousers and undershorts; the woman was nude. The couch in this room was partially incinerated, and partially incinerated clothing lay on top of both victims. Other furniture in the room was only slightly burned, but covered with soot. The clothes closet in this room was empty, and no drapes were on the windows. Wire clothes hangers and drapery hooks were included in the burned rubble, and several of these items lay on top of the victims. Both individuals had burns over the exposed body surfaces.

In a small bedroom in the back of the house a dead 6-month-old male dressed in pajamas was found lying on his back in his crib. Soot covered the exposed skin surfaces and bed clothing, but no thermal injury was observed.

An empty overturned 5-gallon gasoline can was found in the family room, and the spout from this can, stuffed with a paper towel, was found in the adjoining living room. Because of these findings, an arson fire was strongly suspected.

Autopsy findings of both adults were similar. Partial-thickness, flame-type cutaneous burns involved predominantly the posterior aspects of the bodies with patchy burned areas on the face. Burning of the lower extremities was more severe with charring of the posterior aspects of the legs and feet. Soot covered the exposed areas of the body and was present in the nares. A few petechial hemorrhages were found in the conjunctivae of both persons. No soot or thermal injury was found in the respiratory tracts, and analysis for carbon monoxide and other toxic substances was negative. Evidence of focal blunt trauma was observed on the head and chin area of the male and also focal abrasions on the forehead and nose. The female had evidence of focal blunt trauma on the head, chin, and left side of neck. Pulmonary congestion and edema, visceral congestion, and a few petechial hemorrhages in the pleural and epicardial surfaces were the only significant internal findings in either victim. No internal trauma was present.

Postmortem examination of the infant revealed no thermal injury of the skin or respiratory tract. An abundance of soot covered his exposed surfaces and was present in the nose, mouth, and entire respiratory tract. No evidence of internal trauma was found. Pulmonary congestion and edema, visceral congestion, and pinkish discoloration of all tissues were the only significant internal observations. Toxicologic analysis of the blood revealed a carbon monoxide saturation of 67 percent as the only positive finding.

Further inquiry revealed that the couple had attended a social engagement on the night of their death, returning home about 1 a.m., after picking up the infant from a baby sitter. The man was to appear as a key witness in a theft trial against a known criminal the following week.

Laboratory analyses of partially incinerated materials from the scene revealed the presence of inflammable substances consistent with gasoline. The gasoline can was traced to the criminal involved in the theft trial.

Conclusions derived from the investigation were that the victims had returned home, put the sleeping infant in his crib, and prepared to go to bed. They were confronted by the suspect (a known burglar), who apparently entered through the front door by successfully opening the non-deadbolt lock with a plastic card. Both adults were then taken to the family room, apparently rendered unconscious by blows to the head, and asphyxiated. Several neckties which were knotted and cut were found near the bodies, suggesting that their hands may have been tied. The positions of the bodies suggested that they were lying face down with their hands tied behind their backs. The mild blunt neck trauma of the female suggested that she may have been strangled. The relative absence of any signs of struggle in the male suggested that he may have been suffocated by holding his face into a pillow while he was in an unconscious state. A burned pillow was found near his head. The knotted neckties which bound their hands were then cut loose. Clothing from the closet in the family room and the window draperies were piled on top of the dead victims, gasoline was poured over the clothing and the couch, and the room was set on fire. The assailant left through the front door with the spring-loaded lock automatically securing as the door was closed.

During the murder trial it was admitted that the precise mechanism of the asphyxial deaths could not be ascertained by autopsy findings, but the ancillary evidence strongly suggested the above stated method.

The anatomic evidence did prove conclusively that these two healthy young adults were both dead at the time of the fire, and that natural and toxicologic causes of death were definitely excluded. The infant died as a result of cabon monoxide intoxication and smoke inhalation during the arson fire and thus was clearly a homicidal death.

Evidence was also presented to show that the suspect was in the neighborhood, inquiring about the location of the victims' house several days before, and had purchased 5 gallons of gasoline at a nearby gas station on the night of the fire. The gasoline was dispensed into the container found at the scene. The gas station attendant who sold him the capless gasoline can clearly recollected stuffing a paper towel into the spout of the can to prevent spillage. The jury convicted the assailant of first-degree murder on three counts.

CASE 3

Apparent fire death with identification problem; arson fire for purpose of fraud.

A volunteer fire department was called to the scene of a garage fire. The garage was located about 40 yards from the house and was burning extensively upon their arrival. Before the fire could be extinguished, the garage was almost completely destroyed. An automobile parked in the garage was also badly damaged. The firemen discovered an extensively charred body lying face up on the floor of the garage adjacent to the car. The remains of a 16-gauge single-barrel shotgun lay across the body.

Presumably, the body was that of a 52-year-old white male who lived at this residence. A ring belonging to this man was found adjacent to the body in the smoldering rubble. The man had incurred severe financial debts in the past few years and had become somewhat introverted. It was presumed that this individual had set the garage on fire and then shot himself, reasoning that his insurance claims would solve the family's financial problems.

The local coroner removed the body to a funeral home. Since the anterior aspects of the body were partially incinerated, exposing the majority of the thoracic and abdominal viscera, the coroner explored the body in an attempt to recover shotgun pellets. He found none. He obtained a blood specimen from the heart. The remains were then covered with embalming compound (powder) and placed in a plastic bag for burial.

The insurance death claims on this individual totaled almost one million dollars. Several of the insurance companies immediately inquired how identification of the deceased was established. They requested further investigation as to the circumstances of the death and autopsy examination of the deceased.

The charred remains were delivered to the morgue in a zippered plastic bag. Embalming powder covered the external aspects of the body and was deposited within the body cavities. The remains consisted of an extensively charred, partially incinerated torso and head. Much of the skull in the superior aspect of the head, portions of the anterior thoracic and the entire abdominal wall, and the majority of the extremities were incinerated and absent. The external genitalia and ears were incinerated. The cranial cavity was exposed, and the majority of the brain was absent from the skull and submitted separately. The right lung exhibited thermal injury to the surface. The heart and left lung had been previously excised, were submitted separately, and also exhibited surface thermal injury. The larynx, esophagus, and aorta were intact. The majority of the abdominal viscera were present in the body with burned, exposed surfaces. The cecum, ascending colon, and right kidney could not be found as this area of the body was incinerated. Several apparent incineration defects, 1 to 2 inches in diameter, were located in the left lateral abdominal wall.

Postmortem x-rays revealed no bullets or shotgun pellets within the body. Autopsy failed to reveal any evidence of internal traumatic injury. Specifically, there was no evidence of shotgun pellet or missile wounds. No natural disease was found to explain the death. The internal tissues and organs had a pinkish color. A 15- to 20-ml blood specimen was collected by aspiration from the aorta, inferior vena cava, deep pelvic veins, and dural sinuses. Analysis of the blood specimen revealed a carbon monoxide saturation of 80 percent, and a blood ethanol content of 137 mg percent. No other toxic substances were found.

Although the larynx and upper respiratory tract were cooked, no soot deposits were found within these structures, nor was there evidence of antemortem thermal injury.

Based on the autopsy and toxicologic studies, it was concluded that this individual died as a result of carbon monoxide intoxication. However, absence of soot deposit or antemortem thermal injury of the respiratory tract strongly suggested that this man was dead at the time of the fire.

The identity of the deceased had not been established. Detailed comparative physical data needed to be obtained by the field investigators. Further studies by the pathologist was also necessary to accomplish this goal. The blood specimen was available for blood typing procedures by the serologist. A small amount of hair was collected posteriorly at the base of the neck as well as axillary hair. These were submitted to the criminologist for hair comparison studies. Extensive postmortem x-ray examination was performed to obtain films for comparison studies and to determine bone age by the radiologist. This included fluoroscopic examination for evidence of old skeletal injuries and unerupted or impacted teeth. The pathologist found only one tooth lying free within the plastic bag, mingled with fragments of charred tissue. A forensic dentist was solicited to perform further dental examination. An anthropologist was engaged to evaluate the skeletal remains. The field investigators carefully searched the scene for evidence of other personal effects or teeth. None was found.

After several weeks of further inquiry, the data were assimilated and reviewed. The details are summarized as follows:

1. Blood obtained from the burned victim was major blood grouping AB. The presumed victim had a blood group of B.
2. Various dental experts (forensic odontologists) identified the only tooth found to be tooth 31 (right lower second molar). The tooth had been extracted from the presumed subject several years earlier. This fact was confirmed by dental reports and dental x-rays maintained by his dentist. Also, the presumed subject had additional teeth, none of which was ever found. The jaws of the burned body were consistent with an individual who had the majority of his teeth extracted.
3. The presumed subject was a 52-year-old white male, 5 feet 8 inches tall and weighing approximately 160 pounds. Anthropologic and x-ray studies determined the burned victim to be a Caucasian male approximately 50 to 55 years old. Due to the extensive burning, stature could not be estimated.
4. Two radiologists independently examined the numerous postmor-

tem x-rays and compared them with x-rays of the presumed subject which were obtained from a local hospital and from his insurance carrier. Both radiologists rendered an independent opinion that on the basis of nine separate skeletal differences, the remains were not those of the presumed subject.
5. Examination of the hairs by the crime laboratory revealed the hair from the burned body to be of Caucasian origin, medium brown in color, and probably from a person having straight hair. Hair comparison studies indicated that the hair from the burned victim was not consistent with hair from the presumed subject who had dark black, curly hair.
6. Examination of the ring found at the scene near the burned body revealed the name of the presumed deceased inscribed on the inner surface. It was known that the presumed subject also wore a gold wedding band. Despite careful search, the wedding band was never located. It was suggested that the wedding band may have melted in the fire. Therefore the melting point of the ring found at the scene was ascertained. The type of metal present in the gold wedding band was determined by records of the jeweler who sold the band to the presumed victim. It was determined that the melting point of the wedding band would be almost identical to that of the ring found at the scene. Thus it was determined that the presumption that the wedding band melted in the fire was incorrect. The question as to why both rings were not present remained unanswered, but correlated with the above information, it suggested that the ring with the inscribed name had been left on or near the body to cause misidentification.
7. The blood specimen which had been removed by the coroner was subjected to studies which revealed toxicologic and blood type findings identical with those previously reported.

To date, this case remains unsolved. The identity of the burned body has never been established. The presumed subject has never been located. The insurance companies have refused to make death benefit payments.

CASE 4

Death due to heat stroke in a nursing home.

An 86-year-old female died in a nursing home during a mid-afternoon in July in a midwestern city. She had been hospitalized at this institution for several years with a diagnosis of senility. She was bedfast in a four-bed room. Her clinical condition had deteriorated rapidly in the 2 days prior to her death. Although she was not examined by a physician, several nurses had telephoned her doctor, reporting that she was "doing poorly," had a low-grade fever, and had lung findings suggestive of an early developing pneumonia. Therefore, the physician had prescribed antibiotic therapy via telephone conversation. Terminally, the patient spiked a temperature of 105° F.

At her demise, the physician refused to sign the death certificate and asked for further investigation of the case, since this was the third elderly woman to die under similar circumstances in the past 2 days.

Autopsy revealed no evidence of pneumonia, nor any disease to explain her elevated temperature. Arteriosclerotic cardiovascular disease of moderate to advanced severity involved the coronary arteries and vasculature of the brain. The kidneys revealed only mild to moderate disease secondary to arteriosclerosis. The pathologist also was of the opinion that this woman was dehydrated. No other significant anatomic findings were found.

Toxicologic studies were negative. Chemical studies of the vitreous humor removed from the eyeballs at the time of autopsy revealed findings indicative of a severe electrolyte imbalance and dehydration.

Further investigation then revealed that the air conditioning system of the nursing home had broken down 3 days prior to the patient's demise and remained inoperable for 4 days while repairs were being accomplished. During this period of time the temperature of the room averaged 96 to 98° F. Relative humidity was extremely high, and efforts to increase ventilation within the room were quite minimal. No medical treatment had been instituted in an attempt to reduce the patient's body temperature.

Death was attributed to heat stroke. Negligence and liability suits were instituted against the nursing home and the physician.

CASE 5

Fire death with low carbon monoxide blood level.

Early one Sunday afternoon, a fire was reported to be present within an apartment. The apartment house was located only two blocks from the fire station. Upon entry into the apartment, the firemen quickly extinguished the fire which was confined to the bedroom. A dead man was found lying on his back on the floor adjacent to the bed which had been ablaze. The majority of the subject's red silk pajamas had been burned from the body, and there were extensive, cutaneous burns (Fig. 13-19).

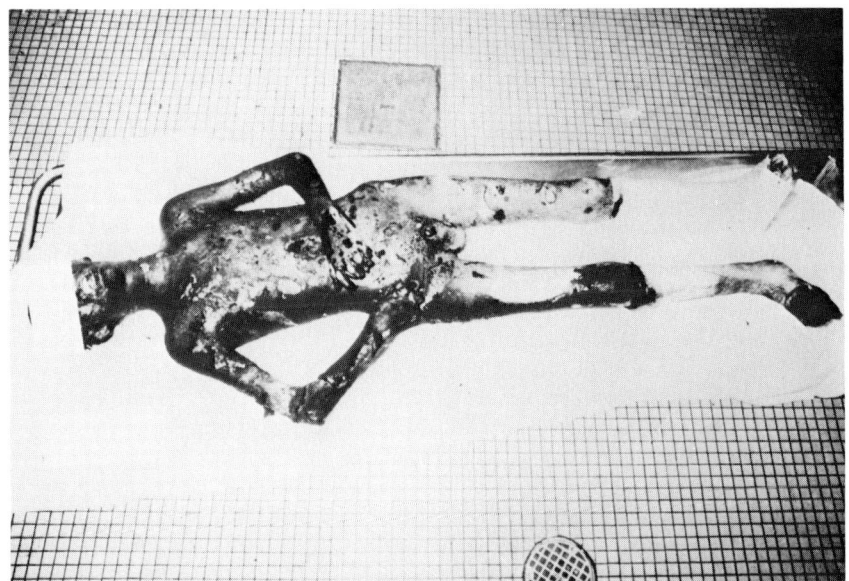

FIGURE 13-19. Flame burns of a fire death victim (see Case 5). The right side of the body was closer to the source of the fire. The victim's pajamas were burned off his body.

Plaster casts were present on both legs, extending from below the knee to the distal aspects of the foot.

In the past, the subject had attempted suicide on three occasions. Two of the unsuccessful attempts involved ingestion of an overdose of barbiturates. The last attempt occurred several months before when he jumped from a fourth story window in a hotel, sustaining fractures of the ankle and heel bones of both legs and a back injury. The back trauma caused partial paralysis of both lower extremities. He was released from the hospital only 1 day prior to his death.

Examination of the body revealed second- and third-degree burns involving approximately 95 percent of the total body surface area. There was extensive thermal injury to the upper thorax and face.

A blood specimen was obtained immediately upon arrival at the morgue. Analysis of the blood revealed a carbon monoxide saturation of only 7 percent. This finding confused investigators because the subject was reported to be alive when the fire was initially discovered.

Postmortem x-rays confirmed the presence of healing fractures of the ankle and foot bones and a compression fracture of lumbar vertebrae L-2 and 3. No foreign objects (bullets, etc.) were found.

Autopsy findings consisted of the cutaneous thermal burns previously mentioned, extensive pulmonary congestion and edema, sutured surgical wounds of the feet and ankles, congestion of the internal viscera, healing fractures of the ankle and heal bones, a compression fracture of lumbar vertebrae L-2 and 3, and hematomyelia of the lumbar spinal cord.

Examination of the upper respiratory tract revealed information explaining the low carbon monoxide level. Extensive reddening and edema (swelling) of the uvula and adjacent pharyngeal structures, and thermal injury to the epiglottis, vocal cords, laryngeal mucosa, and proximal trachea were present. A small quantity of soot was deposited on the mucosal surface of the vocal cords, upper larynx, left pyriform sinus, and surface of the tongue (Fig. 13-20). The thermal injury to the upper respiratory tract indicated that this man was alive at the time of the fire and had inhaled a small amount of smoke and extensive heat (possibly flame), causing the thermal injury to the respiratory tract and asphyxia. This sequence of events had apparently occurred quite rapidly, producing death before a significant rise in carbon monoxide saturation of the blood.

Further details of the circumstances of the fire were necessary before this conclusion could be accepted. Subsequent inquiry revealed the following story. The neighbor who lived across the hallway was leaving his apartment when he heard the subject cry for help. He attempted to enter the subject's apartment, but found the door locked. The subject related that he had fallen asleep while smoking in bed, and that his bed clothing was on fire. The neighbor immediately called the fire department located nearby. The neighbor, aware of the subject's incapacitating physical condition, forced open the apartment door. The neighbor stated that there was a very small quantity of smoke near the ceiling. He found the subject lying on the floor on his back, right side against the bed. The subject was alive and moaning. The bed was smoldering. By this time, the fire department was arriving outside the building. Unfortunately, the neighbor thought it was desirable to get some fresh air into the apartment, and he opened a large window in the bedroom. When this was done there was a sudden flash fire and the entire bed was immediately engulfed in flames, also igniting the subject's pajamas. The subject screamed in pain as the neighbor ran from the room. At that time, the firemen entered the apart-

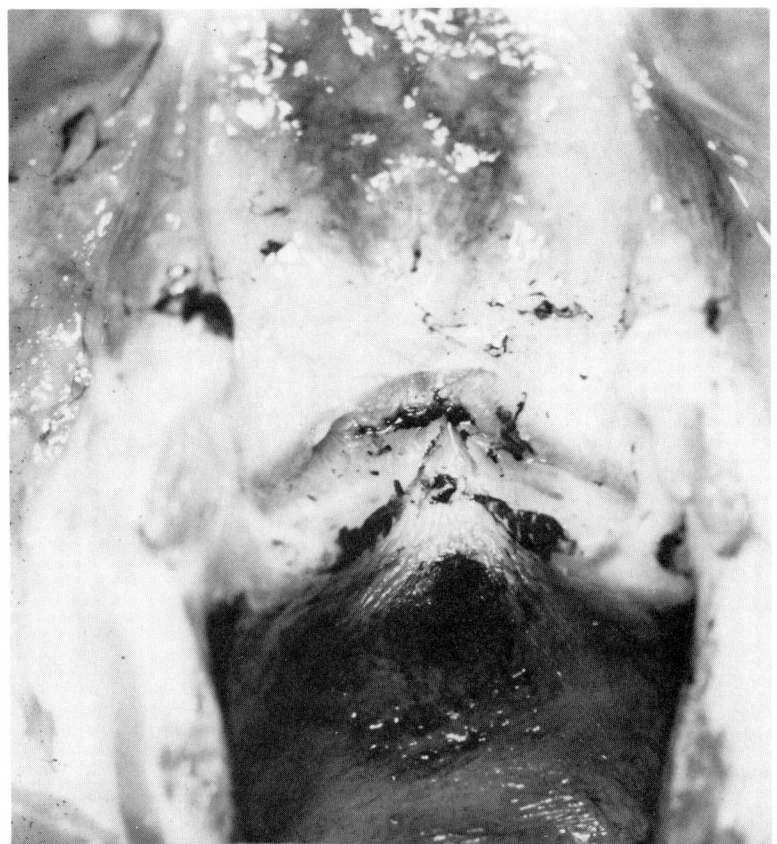

FIGURE 13-20. Close-up view of the larynx of the fire victim shown in Figures 13-2 and 13-19. Note the small amount of soot deposits and the extensive thermal injury to the mucosa with edema. The blood carbon monoxide level was found to be 7 percent. Death was attributed to asphyxiation and thermal burns.

ment and quickly extinguished the fire. Following his scream, the subject had inhaled the flame and a small amount of smoke, causing the rapidly fatal thermal injury to the upper respiratory tract.

Analysis failed to reveal other toxic substances within the blood or body tissues.

ADDITIONAL READING

Adelson, L.: *The Pathology of Homicide.* Charles C Thomas, Springfield, Ill., 1974.
  Superb coverage of all aspects of fire deaths. Excellent coverage of fire artifacts.
Benz, J.A.: *Investigation of Deaths Due to Fires.* Workshop in Forensic Pathology. American Society of Clinical Pathologists, Chicago, 1976.
Camps, F.E. (ed.): *Gradwohl's Legal Medicine.* ed. 3. Wright & Sons, Bristol, 1976.
Dominquez, A.M.: Problems of Carbon Monoxide in Fires. *J. Forensic Sci.* 7:379–393, 1962. Excellent review of factors affecting CO levels of fire victims.
Early Bronchoscopy, Blood Gas Levels Show Airway Smoke Injury (Medical News). *J.A.M.A.* 238:293–294, 1977. Describes use of early fiberoptic bronchoscopy and blood gas analysis in evaluating patients with smoke inhalation problems.
Ek, N., Maehly, A., and Rudh, E.: Arson Investigation, in Tedeschi, C. G., et al.

(eds.): *Forensic Medicine.* Vol. 1. W.B. Saunders, Philadelphia, 1977. Excellent review of arson investigation.

Fink, P.A.: Exposure to Carbon Monoxide, in Tedeschi, C.G., et al. (eds.): *Forensic Medicine.* Vol. 2. W.B. Saunders, Philadelphia, 1977. Excellent complete review of entire subject of carbon monoxide intoxication. Extensive reference list.

Gonzales, T.A., Vance, M., Helpern, M., and Umberger, C.J.: *Legal Medicine, Pathology, and Toxicology.* ed. 2. Appleton-Century-Crofts, New York, 1954.

Harvey, A.M., Johns, R.J., Owens, A.H., and Ross, R.S. (eds.): *The Principles and Practice of Medicine.* ed. 12. Appleton-Century-Crofts, New York, 1972.

Hirsch, C.S., and Adelson, L.: Absence of Carboxyhemoglobin in Flash Fire Victims. *J.A.M.A.* 210:2279–2280, 1969. Excellent article reporting a series of cases of death due to fires in which there was no significant elevation of carboxyhemoglobin.

Hirvonen, J.: Systemic and Local Effects of Hypothermia, in Tedeschi, C.G., et al. (eds.): *Forensic Medicine.* Vol. 1. W.B. Saunders, Philadelphia, 1977. Excellent complete review of hypothermic injuries. Very extensive reference list.

Hughes, D.J.: *Homicide Investigation Techniques.* Charles C Thomas, Springfield, Ill., 1974. Written primarily for the police officer.

Parikh, C.K.: *A Simplified Text Book of Medical Jurisprudence and Toxicology.* Medical Publications, Bombay, 1970.

"Plastic Fires" Create New Hazards for Both Fireman and Public (Medical News). *J.A.M.A.* 234:1211–1213, 1975. Describes dangers of toxic gases produced by burning of plastic-containing materials.

Polson, C.J.: *The Essentials of Forensic Medicine.* ed. 2. Charles C Thomas, Springfield, Ill., 1965.

Spitz, W.U., and Fisher, R.S.: *Medicolegal Investigation of Death.* Charles C Thomas, Springfield, Ill., 1973.

Tedeschi, C.G.: Systemic and Localized Hyperthermic Injury, in Tedeschi, C.G., et al. (eds.): *Forensic Medicine.* Vol. 1. W.B. Saunders, Philadelphia, 1977. Excellent complete review of hyperthermic injury. Very extensive reference list.

Wetherell, H.R.: Occurrence of Cyanide in the Blood of Fire Victims. *J. Forensic Sci.* 11:167–173, 1966.

Winters, P.M., and Miller, J.N.: Carbon Monoxide Poisoning. *J.A.M.A.* 236:1502–1509, 1976. Reviews pathophysiology, clinical signs and symptoms, laboratory findings, and treatment of CO intoxication.

CHAPTER 14

Joseph H. Davis is Chief Medical Examiner of Metropolitan Dade County, Florida, and Professor of Legal Medicine at the University of Miami. He is also Chairman of the Medical Examiner's Commission of the State of Florida. Dr. Davis pursued undergraduate studies at Lehigh University, Virginia Polytechnic Institute, and Princeton University, and received his medical degree in 1949 from the Long Island College of Medicine. He is a Past President of the National Association of Medical Examiners and of the Dade County Medical Association, and has for many years been a consultant for the Federal Aviation Association. Dr. Davis is the author of numerous papers, articles, and chapters on various aspects of forensic pathology and traumatic death.

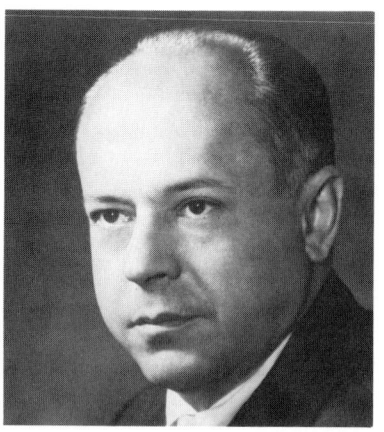

AUTOMOBILE DEATH INVESTIGATION AND PREVENTION PROGRAMS*

Joseph H. Davis, M.D.

HISTORY

Motor vehicle surface transportation commenced with Cugnot's steam tricycle in 1769. Benz and Daimler of Germany and Selden of the United States, in 1885 and 1886, brought forth the earliest automobile concept. However, it was not until Duryea sold his American-made automobile in 1896 that the industry was born in the United States. In 1899, the first traffic fatality occurred in the United States. By 1915, there were 3 million motor vehicles in use in the United States; the national population of 100 million suffered 7,000 motor vehicle deaths that year.

Because the initial incidents were public disturbances and police were the initial responders, traffic accident investigation became the lot of the police officer. Detroit police formed a special unit, the Accident Investigation Bureau, in 1920. In 1929, the National Safety Council created its Traffic Safety Division. The following year there were 26 million motor vehicles on the road and a total of 31,000 related deaths. Although some studies had been conducted to determine cause and prevention, public interest did not really become aroused until 1935, when *Reader's Digest* published "And Sudden Death" by J. C. Furnas. Following World War II, crash survival, in addition to concern over driver control, became a sub-

---

*The author wishes to thank Dr. William Fogarty, School of Engineering, University of Miami, for suggestions pertaining to crash investigative techniques; Dr. William Haddon, Jr., Insurance Institute for Highway Safety, Washington, D.C., for making available prepublication data of significant value; and Fred Folger, Department of Pathology, University of Miami School of Medicine and Donald W. Calhoun, Southwestern Institute of Forensic Sciences, Dallas, for their assistance in preparation of the illustrations used in this chapter.

ject of study with the Cornell Aeronautical Laboratories Automotive Crash Injury Research Project.[1]

Public interest lagged behind until Ralph Nader's book *Unsafe at Any Speed* was widely publicized in 1965. Since then, with the creation of the National Highway Safety Bureau, increasing emphasis has been placed upon studies of cause and prevention of automobile accidents. A major thrust has been to utilize the influence of Federal monies and regulatory power in major highway design improvement. This effort was sorely needed in view of the callous disregard of the rudiments of safety in highway construction. The early freeways and interstate highways were designed with obvious flaws in engineering, totally incompatible with the increasing speeds of automobiles and traffic density. In Dade County, Florida, the first major expressway constructed for high-volume traffic at 70-mph speeds had numerous busy intersections controlled only by stop signs. The result was carnage. Eventually, Federal laws and regulations have begun to be applied to highway and vehicular design standards.

PROBLEMS

Transport accidents are the major cause of accidental death each year in the United States. Motor vehicles consitute approximately 40 percent, and the next most frequent cause (about 17 percent) is attributed to falls.[2] The major burden rests with young persons up to age 37. Each year this represents in excess of 1 million years of lost future life expectancy! Two million traffic deaths occurred in the United States from 1899 to the mid-1970s. The traveling population is at risk of death or injury. In 1976, transportation fatalities included 44,807 highway deaths (90 percent), compared with all other transport deaths (general aviation, railroad grade crossings, railroad, marine, air carriers, and pipelines), which totaled 4,778 (10 percent). These figures do not reveal the full story of risk. Estimates based upon deaths per 100 million passenger miles reveal that general (private) aviation and motorcycles rank highest (13), followed by automobile (1.4), bus (0.2), and passenger train and scheduled passenger plane (0.1 each).[3] Expressed in economic terms, the annual cost of motor vehicle injuries is estimated at $10 billion, more than 1 percent of the Gross National Product.[4]

Motor vehicle crashes account for a major source of multiple trauma treated in surgical practice. In one study, 87 percent of 168 consecutive surgical clinic multiple trauma cases were automobile associated.[5] A 16-year study of hospitalized chest injury patients in Denver, Colorado, revealed that 73 percent were due to automobile crashes.[6] The death-injury ratio of 1:60 attests to the extensive losses associated with motorized transport.[7]

Editorializing has no effect on this problem. Stricter laws have little direct influence. No programs will impact favorably until individual incidents are properly documented, the results utilized properly in court, and the resultant data utilized for constructive criticism of the participants involved in the motor vehicle scene, including government, industry, roadway engineering, licensing agencies, drivers, and pedestrians. What may we expect of an investigative system which condones the absence of simple photographic documentation of major crashes, the deliberate refusal to utilize chemical tests on offending drivers, and the inane court histrionics which seem to vacillate between "cash register" justice and the deliberate freeing of overtly recidivistic criminal drivers? Of what use is a system of coroners and medical examiners whose major effort is to "sign out" fatalities or—if autopsy is performed—to furnish only a list of injuries with little or no attempt to ascertain the pre-crash interaction of driver, vehicle, and environmental causative factors?

Despite this dismal outlook, much has been accomplished. Many police jurisdictions, formerly incompetent in crash investigation, have improved themselves by the utilization of trained investigators. Many traffic court systems have instituted innovative programs for the delineation of chronic offenders and have established specialized training programs for such offenders. Currently, Dade County has a program of driver education, conducted by the Dade County Citizens Safety Council, which is mandatory for drivers whose licenses have been suspended. The lobbying activities of local safety councils have improved governmental responsibilities. Improved performance of medical examiners has resulted in better case investigation. Specialized engineering research programs have served to raise the standards of investigation, vehicular design, and highway engineering. The tools and knowledge needed for case investigations and program implementations are already known. The basic problem is to raise the standards of performance in those areas in need without detriment to those programs of excellence which may already exist.

The initial step toward traffic injury problem-solving is a dedication by all participants to a spirit of cooperation. Each participant must be well trained in his own discipline, but must also assist those in other disciplines who are involved. Some individuals may be found within the system who exert themselves to activate the system. A proper combination is a motivated individual with investigative and record collation capability.

Regardless of fiscal support or caseload experience, each person involved in the crash investigation must endeavor to answer three key questions:

1. Why did this automobile crash occur?
2. What remedies are suggested to prevent a recourse?
3. What pragmatic political means may be employed to implement a program of prevention of recurrence?

THE CAUSE OF THE CRASH

For purposes of discussion we shall consider an automobile which crashes out of control into another vehicle or into a fixed object. The investigative principles described herein apply in all crash situations, whether they involve automobiles, trucks, trains, bicycles, or pedestrians. The familiar nine-cell analytic matrix is an excellent investigative tool. This is based upon standard epidemiologic methodology concerned with considerations of host, agent, and environment.[8] It consists of three main components—the pre-crash, the crash, and the post-crash phases, each having three components—the human, the vehicular, and the environmental factors. Included is the concept that damage and injuries result from abnormal exchanges of energy between persons, vehicles, and environments. Note that these factors are plural and may be considered in terms of major and minor. With consideration of these points, the factors of causation (the pre-crash phase), the factors of injury and damage causation during the crash, and the factors of post-crash complications are less apt to be overlooked. Of additional importance is the logical organization of data which lends itself to the development of programs for improvement in the administrative, legislative, and engineering aspects of automobile accident prevention.

PRE-CRASH FACTORS

Before assessing the role of the participants in the crash causation, it is necessary to identify the driver and the passengers. It is axiomatic that a surviving driver, given the opportunity, will claim that the dead passenger was the driver. This is especially true if the surviving driver has a record of previous criminal or serious traffic charges. Correlative to this is the willingness of some investigators to accept the statement of the prevaricating driver even when the at-fault vehicle is known to be owned by the surviving "passenger." All too frequently, the scene investigator is eager to accept such prevarication without question. Accordingly, there are certain investigative presumptions which need confirmation or denial by impartial witness or physical evidence. It should be presumed that the occupant-owner was the driver, especially if the owner survives and has a past record of driver's license revocation. Physical evidence should serve to clarify the issue of vehicular operation. Transfer evidence, blood and hair, from the occupant to points within the vehicle will indicate occupant position prior to the crash when correlated with the crash kinematics. Transfer patterns from vehicular components to occupants may likewise indicate relative position. Frequently overlooked are shoe sole imprints which may indicate brake pedal application by the driver (Fig. 14-1). In suicides, the accelerator pedal imprint adds additional evidence of the deliberate nature of the crash.

Certain injury patterns help to differentiate the right front passenger from the driver. Steering wheel impact injuries with knee injuries from the undersurface of the dashboard are characteristic (Figs. 14-2 to 14-4). Older model vehicles with rigid steering posts can produce severe chest injuries to the point of near impalement. Dental injury and tooth imprints on the upper margin of the steering wheel may occur. Deep abdominal injury, liver rupture, and trauma to the intestinal mesentery and pancreas may result from the lower margin of the steering wheel. Windshield head impacts, over-the-windshield head contact points, and "A pillar" (the post between the windshield and front door) injuries are also found. Careful correlation of vehicle interior with occupant-injury patterns serve to indicate occupant positions prior to the crash.

Human factor loss of control must be correlated with the environment. The greater the driver's skill, the more hazardous the roadway environment must be before the driver loses control. The more impaired the driver, the less hazardous need be the driving conditions before the driver is unable to cope. In general, it is the impaired driver who demonstrates the environmental hazards. For example, the easily confused elderly tourist with marginal eyesight is more apt to enter a poorly marked expressway exit against the flow of traffic than is the less impaired driver. The same applies to alcoholic impairment. As blood alcohol concentration rises, the driver becomes less able to cope, speeding beyond capabilities and failing to appreciate changes in traffic flow, curves, or signal devices. It is for these reasons that minimal standards of driver capability (or conversely, maximal allowable standards of driver impairment) are derived. From these considerations, the relative degree of weight assigned

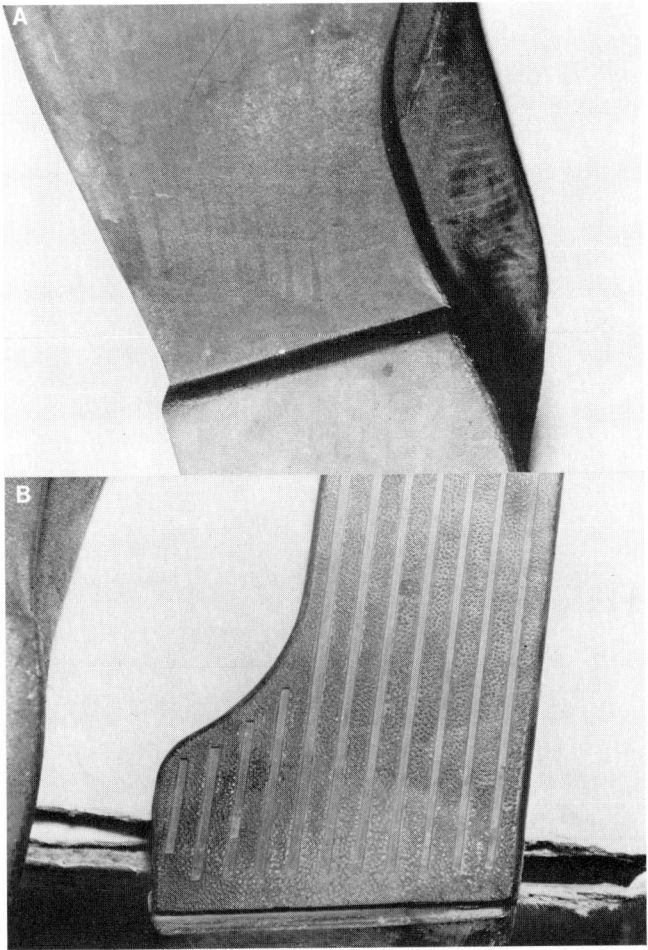

FIGURE 14-1. Shoe imprint. *A.* The shoe sole imprint coincides with the accelerator pattern. An additional pattern on the inner side of the shoe corresponds with the floor mat design. *B.* The accelerator which matched the shoe sole pattern.

to the role of driver causation may be considered. For example, a running-off-the-roadway crash on a clear, dry day with moderate traffic flow indicates either human or vehicular factors as most likely. On the other hand, in the darkness of night, a posted speed close to the environmental limits of tolerance, accompanied by confusing signs or poor lighting, may serve as an engineering trap for even mildly inattentive drivers. Two examples personally investigated by the author serve to illustrate these points.

1. A sole occupant was killed when his automobile crashed over a guardrail alongside an expressway. The weather was sunny. Traffic conditions were light. The vehicle had adequate brakes, tires, and steering mechanism. Accordingly, the main area of consideration was human factor impairment. The alcohol, carbon monoxide, and common drug screens were negative. Medical inquiry revealed the victim to be epileptic. This, coupled with the absence of antiepileptic medication in the blood, provided the most reasonable hypothesis to explain loss of driver control. When witnesses were subse-

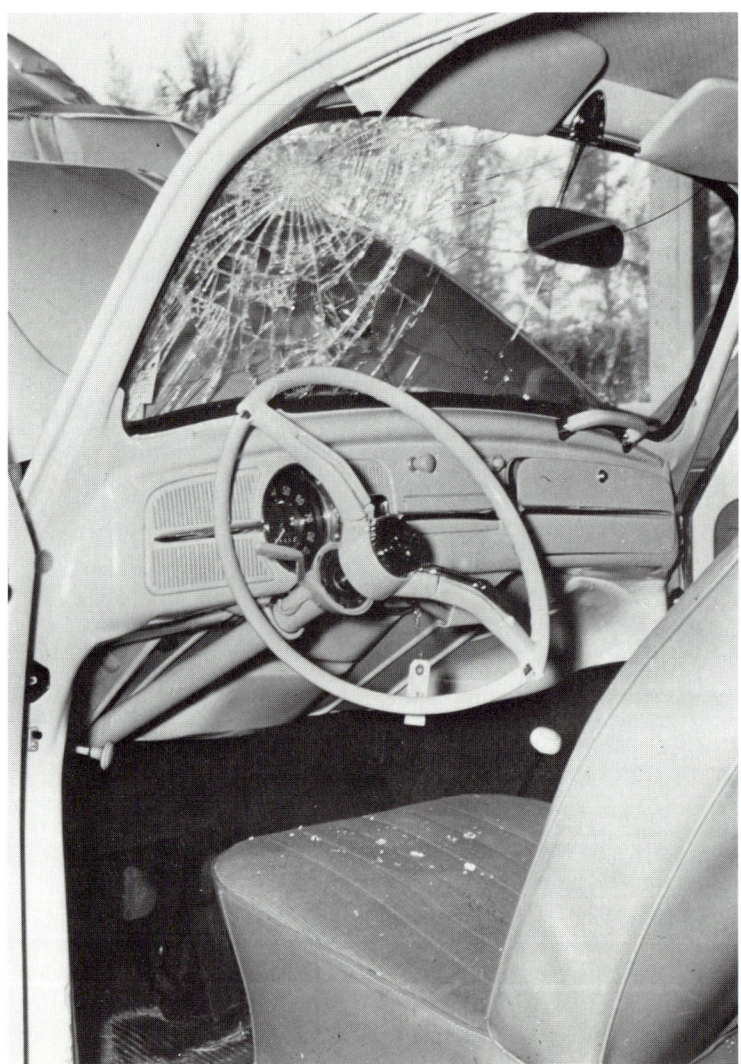

FIGURE 14-2. Steering wheel deformation. Deformation of the steering wheel rim from impact with the driver torso is present along with windshield damage from the head. The driver failed to utilize his seat belts.

quently queried as to the precise activity of the driver within his vehicle, it was determined that he, impatient and aggressive, had been restrained from violating the speed limit by a driver who blocked the passing lane. After much horn-blowing, the median lane driver slowed, creating an opening. At this moment the victim passed the driver on his left and accelerated into the median lane in order to pass the vehicle in the outside lane. While executing this maneuver, he turned rearward toward the driver he was passing

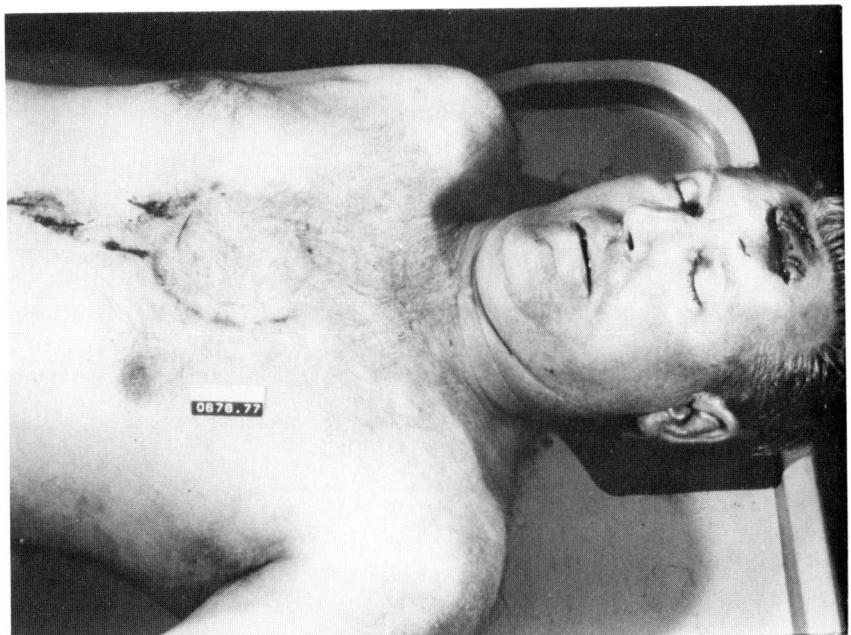

FIGURE 14-3. Driver injury pattern. The steering wheel imprint on the thorax identifies the victim as having been in the driver position at the time of frontal impact. The forehead laceration coincides with the upper edge of the windshield. Not shown are the knee injuries from the dashboard. The triad of chest, head, and knee injuries proves this to be the driver.

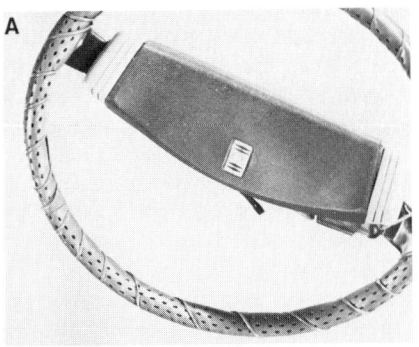
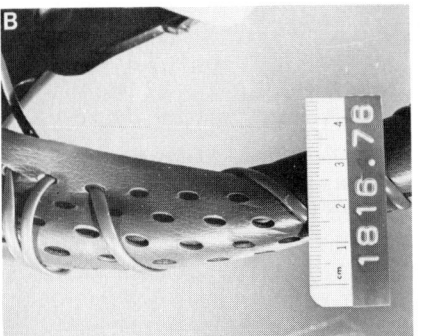
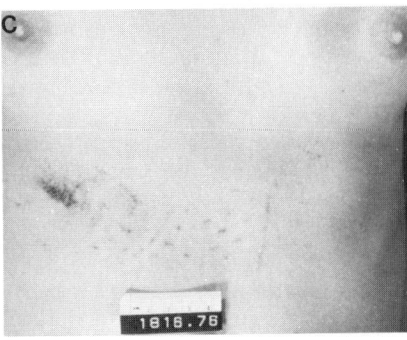

FIGURE 14-4. Steering wheel pattern. The fine skin pattern is quite specific when compared with the pattern of the wrapped steering wheel (A). A closer view (B) reveals the source of both the circular and the linear patterns (C).

AUTOMOBILE DEATH INVESTIGATION

and made a gesture with his extended middle finger. Immediately, he was out of control, struck the curb, and went over the guardrail. The major cause of his crash was indeed a human factor, but it was a product not of epilepsy, but of his aggressive personality expressed by an obscene gesture.

2. A small car entered into a turn at expressway speed in order to transfer the vehicle from one expressway to another. Immediately beyond a brightly lit overhead sign was an unlighted roadway division into curves leading to other expressways. The driver, attempting to choose the righthand alternative, turned sharply, tipped over, and slid sidewise up a gradual curb and over an embankment. The push-button door latch, being disengaged, allowing him to be thrown out as the vehicle rolled in midair. He was killed when his head struck a concrete culvert. Human factor analysis indicated inexperience, the exuberance of youth (the victim was 17 years old), and alcohol (0.07 percent). The vehicular component factors were a relatively high center of gravity, allowing for roll-over, and a push-button door handle. The most significant factor, however, was roadway design. As the investigation progressed, other vehicles approached the area with tires screeching from attempts to negotiate the confusing curves. This area of highway was posted at maximum expressway speed. Immediately beyond the well-lit overhead sign, the roadway division was in pitch blackness. There were no guardrails. The gully contained numerous gouges and fragments of debris from previous wrecks. Despite all this evidence, there had been no attempts to improve this blatant example of thoughtless roadway design.

These two cases serve to indicate how human factors correlated with engineering and vehicular factors to determine crash causation.

The most common and readily identifiable human factor in fatal crashes is alcohol impairment. Prior to the epic report to Congress in 1968[9], there had been little evidence of national concern with this problem. Two main reasons can be cited for such apathy: the lack of Federal involvement in the safety aspects of highways constructed with Federal funds, and the lack of any state or national system of adequate traffic accident data collection and analysis. Prior to 1968, the only national data were those derived from the states as reported on the uniform motor vehicle traffic accident report form. Unfortunately, this report was only the work product of the initial officer upon the scene and served to indicate that an incident had occurred. Contributing circumstances, the closest approximation to causative factor estimation, included such inane choices as failure to keep the vehicle under control. It is little wonder that the true involvement of alcohol, especially in fatal crashes, came as a revelation to many when a limited number of police, coroner and medical examiner agencies produced in-depth data. Although anonymous, the 1968 report should be credited to William Haddon, Jr., M.D., a practicing public health officer, who realized that traumatic death and injury studies follow the same epidemiologic principles as studies of contagious disease. Fortunately, he had been chosen as the first director of the newly created National Highway Safety Bureau within the Department of Transportation.

In Dade County, Florida, alcohol involvement in fatal crashes has been studied since the Office of the Medical Examiner was created in 1956. Table 14-1 indicates the presence of alcohol in all fatally injured drivers.

Excluded from the test were those drivers who died after prolonged hospitalization or whose remains were found after extensive decomposition. The table includes drivers killed by other drivers who may or may not have been drinking.

TABLE 14-1. AGE INCIDENCE AND ALCOHOL: ALL DRIVERS (1956–1977)

Age Group	Number Killed	Number Tested	Number Positive	Percent Positive
0–17*	233	99	17	17
18–24	427	331	162	49
25–34	401	317	197	62
35–44	329	255	153	60
45–54	299	234	119	51
55–64	225	154	59	38
65–74	171	112	33	29
75–84	69	38	4	11
85–94	8	3	1	33
Total	2,162	1,543	745	48

*This age group includes all children on bicycles killed by automobiles.

The fact that 48 percent of all fatally injured drivers had been drinking becomes highly significant when we realize that the percentage of drinking drivers with a blood alcohol of 0.10 percent or greater, who were uninvolved but passing by crash sites, averages approximately 1 to 4 percent.[10] If we consider only fatal single-vehicle crashes, with only one driver at fault, we note the greater percentage of alcohol involvement (Table 14-2).

TABLE 14-2. AGE INCIDENCE AND ALCOHOL: SINGLE DRIVERS

Age Group	Number Killed	Number Tested	Number Positive	Percent Positive
0–17*	46	37	12	32
18–24	184	146	93	64
25–34	184	154	116	75
35–44	117	101	74	73
45–54	116	101	69	68
55–64	72	52	33	63
65–74	42	33	11	33
75–84	8	5	1	20
85–94	2	2	–	–
Total	771	631	409	65

*This age group includes all children on bicycles killed by automobiles.

Sixty-five percent of these drivers had measurable blood alcohol. Of these, almost half had in excess of 0.10 percent. Approximately half of those in excess of 0.10 percent exceeded 0.20 percent blood alcohol concentration.

In a personal study involving six average males weighing approximately 180 pounds (82 kg), each test subject was given one-half pint (8 fluid ounces, 250 ml) of 100-proof whiskey to drink as fast as possible during the course of a driver ability demonstration. Among this group, the maximum observed blood alcohol concentration ranged from 0.09 to 0.13 percent. A 0.10 percent blood alcohol, for practical purposes, means that the individual has consumed a large amount of alcohol. Most drinking adults carry out their activities over a period of time, often with some food which delays absorption. Accordingly, a 0.10 percent finding indicates much more alcohol consumption than that which would be determined from Widmark's formula:

$$\text{Fluid ounces of alcohol} = \frac{\text{Ounces of body weight} \times 0.68 \times \text{Blood alcohol concentration}}{0.8}$$

This formula would indicate that a 180-pound male would need only 5 fluid ounces of 100-proof whiskey to achieve a blood alcohol of 0.10 percent.[11] In real life it takes more than what the Widmark formula would indicate. The formula is a handy tool to estimate the absolute minimum number of "drinks" consumed by the offender in order to achieve the observed concentration. A quick and easy consolidation of the formula involves the following equation: 13.6 × weight in pounds × concentration of blood alcohol = minimum fluid ounces of pure alcohol (200-proof) to achieve the blood concentration. Double this and one has the fluid ounce equivalence of 100-proof whiskey.

Obviously, 0.10 percent is too high a permissible concentration for drivers on a public highway. In 1924, Norway established 0.05 percent as the maximum permissible concentration. This must be the goal of legislative and judicial reform in the matter of chemical test law. It should be noted, however, that simple enactment of legislation does not cure a problem. From legislation must spring programs of identification and control of the chronic offender. Even in the Scandinavian countries, a significant proportion of fatal and serious crashes continues to involve drinking drivers.[12]

Although alcohol excess ranks highest as the chemical impediment to driving, other drugs can be quite dangerous. Garriott and coworkers[13] found that the blood of 127 fatally injured drivers contained alcohol in 52 percent, other drugs plus alcohol in 9 percent, and drugs alone in 9 percent. They conclude that psychoactive drugs are a significant contributory factor in motor vehicle crashes. The most common chemically encountered psychotropic drug was diazepam. We now encounter cases where the crash circumstances are those of obvious driver impairment of the alcohol type, such as a youthful driver returning from an evening party and crashing into an automobile halted at a stop light. The blood alcohol concentration is only 0.05 or 0.07 percent. These circumstances indicate the probability of an additional impairment factor, namely, illicit drug abuse such as that involving methaqualone or marijuana. Methaqualone blood concentrations of 0.7 percent indicate serious impairment of driver capability. More common in our experience is marijuana impairment superimposed upon the effects of alcohol. Marijuana does impair driver capability.[14] At the point of hallucination, the impaired driver may not manifest overt signs of intoxication to the arresting officer.[15] Current interest in this problem has lagged behind its importance. Radioimmunoassay methodology needs to be perfected and standardized in regard to specificity and reproducibility of test results. In the absence of acceptable blood testing methods, the investigator must rely upon scene and circumstance in order to implicate the role of the drug. Additional evidence may be obtained by swabbing the lips and fingers for the presence of marijuana resin. The defeatism which arises from courtroom antics intended to cast doubt on scientific methods should not deter investigators from following an investigative protocol which can indicate the probability of drug involvement in crash causation.

Carbon monoxide must always be considered as a potential causative factor in crashes where the engine is known to have been operational. Natural death may be accentuated by carbon monoxide. Cases in which the alcohol-intoxicated driver is found dead from carbon monoxide in a parked automobile with the engine idling are not at all unusual. Often it is the last few inches of rusty tailpipe which allow the exhaust to be directed upward through rust defects of the vehicle body (Fig. 14-5). Less frequently the driver of a moving vehicle is made overtly ill or crashes as a result of a similar mechanism. A well-operating air conditioning system should not result in such contamination because the intravehicular pressure is higher than that beneath the vehicle, and air intakes are located in front of the windshield.

Carbon monoxide in the blood need not indicate a defective exhaust system. It may result from a post-crash fire. Most frequently carbon monoxide is the result of cigarette smoking. The average blood concentration is 4.58 percent hemoglobin saturation for smokers and 0.85 percent for nonsmokers.[16] Smokers with habits of 25 cigarettes per day average 8.55 percent saturation, which can rise to 17.0 percent with rapid continuous smoking.[17] The chronic alcoholic who chain-smokes cigarettes may exceed 20 percent carbon monoxide hemoglobin saturation, especially if highly intoxicated by alcohol. Subtle defects of neurologic function may be encountered with such carbon monoxide concentrations. However, a carbon monoxide saturation of 18 to 22 percent must not be falsely used to excuse culpability arising from blood alcohol excess.

It is important when interpreting the role of drugs or physical impairment in crash causation to correlate test results with true circumstance;

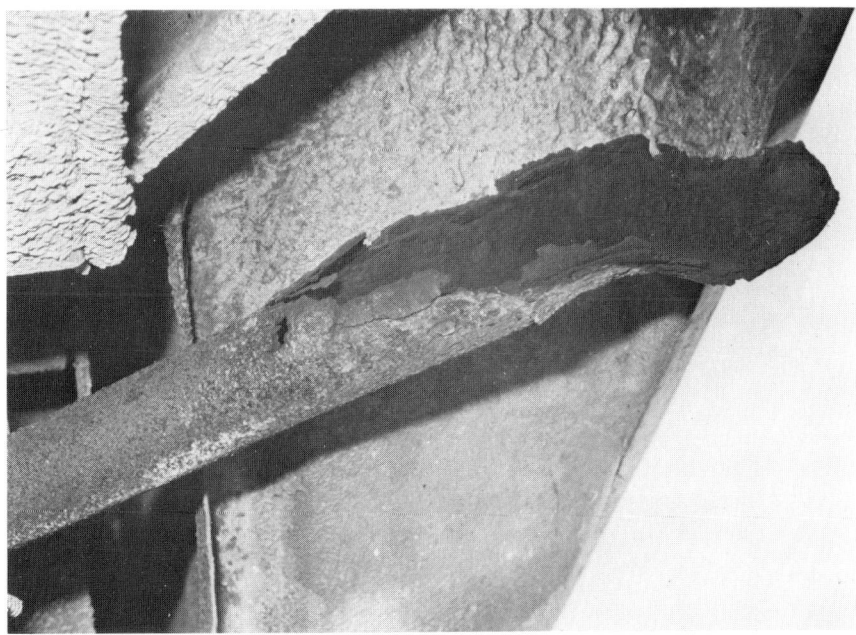

FIGURE 14-5. Lethal rusting of the exhaust pipe. Deterioration of the last 6 inches of the tail pipe directed corrosive exhaust fumes against the vehicle body with resultant entry into the occupant compartment.

otherwise serious errors of opinion will ensue. For example, the driver or pedestrian with a very high concentration of alcohol may have been in a proper traffic configuration and totally innocent. On the other hand, one must never forget that the intoxicated, not-at-fault driver or pedestrian, by traffic enforcement standards, might well have been capable of evasive action if alert and not impaired. It is not at all unusual to find that all crash participants were under the influence of one or more drugs, including alcohol.

Certain pre-crash and crash patterns suggest the expected degree of driver impairment by alcohol. For example, the driver with a concentration between 0.05 and 0.15 percent is apt to drift off the pavement and overcompensate by pulling back onto the roadway into the opposing lane of traffic. In the range of 0.15 to 0.30 percent, the tendency is to find a much slower response to drifting off the roadway. With a concentration greater than 0.30 percent, there may be little evidence of prompt or delayed evasive action. Under no circumstances should driver impairment be excused as "falling asleep at the wheel" when in fact the driver is anesthetized by alcohol, a chemical with a molecular configuration similar to ethyl ether, formerly the most commonly used surgical anesthetic.

Crash investigation requires close, cooperative discussion between police and medical investigators in order to accurately reconstruct the circumstances. The following case exemplifies the value of such procedures:

> A motorcyclist returning from a party was killed in a single-vehicle crash on a clear, dry night. Cocaine was found in the blood, but the crash kinematics indicated a sudden deviation as if the front wheel had suddenly failed. It obviously had not, for the vehicle had only minor scratches and dents. The crash circumstance was inconsistent with careless loss of control by the driver. The vehicle had acted as if it had struck something in the roadway which was found afterward to be clear and unobstructed. The most logical hypothesis was that the cyclist struck an animal which had left the scene prior to arrival of the police. Subsequent examination of the front wheel revealed opossum hair between the rim and tire.

Appreciation of the role of natural disease as a significant causative factor is dependent upon the totality of investigation. Demonstration of cardiac disease by history or autopsy, or a history of epilepsy, does not necessarily implicate a disease process as a causative factor. However, it certainly raises the issue. As noted in the prior examples, exact reconstruction of the crash sequence is needed in order to assess the role of disease or other human factors in crash causation. One should answer the question: Did the vehicle act as if it had no driver at the controls? If affirmative, natural disease, very severe intoxication, or another cause of total driver incapacitation must be sought.

The frequency of sudden death causing fatal crashes has been of concern. Peterson and Petty[18] reviewed sudden death from natural disease in operators of motor vehicles in the Baltimore area over a 4-year period. Of the 81 cases, 36 were involved with some degree of minor collision damage. Subsequently, Baker and Spitz[19] reviewed cases of 275 fatally injured drivers over a 4-year period and found the number of accidental deaths attributable to natural causes to be too small to be measured as a proportion of all accidents. Hossack[20] studied 102 consecutive drivers who died at the wheel during 1 year in the Melbourne metropolitan area. In 11 cases (9.2 percent), the driver died of natural disease, five with no injury or property damage, and six with only minor property damage and minimal injury to the driver. No other person was injured.

The largest postmortem series was that of Dalton, Davis, and Blackbourne.[21] We reviewed 1,171 Dade County driver fatalities investigated over a 12-year period. Included were all cases where the driver of a motor vehicle died with or without fatal injuries. The group was subdivided by segregating those who were not at fault, having been struck by another offending driver who may or may not have been killed. The not-at-fault drivers numbered 237 and were not further considered as they were obviously alive prior to the crash. The 934 drivers of vehicles which went out of control and crashed or went off the side of the roadway were divided into two categories. There were 305 whose injuries were not of fatal type and who had obviously suffered a fatal heart attack while driving. Evaluation of this group revealed that 193 cases resulted in no property damage, the dying driver managing to control the vehicle to a stop. There were 112 drivers who lost sufficient control for the vehicle to sustain or cause moderate damage, usually coming to rest against a sign post or power pole. Serious property damage or injury to others occurred in 11 cases. One innocent driver was killed when an out-of-control vehicle occupied by a dead driver crossed the center line and crashed into oncoming traffic. The remaining 629 drivers were those who lost control and sustained fatal injuries. Their total records and autopsies were carefully examined as to sudden incapacitation by disease. The majority of the 629 "at-fault" drivers had alcohol as the major human factor of control loss. However, careful evaluation revealed 37 crashes where the driver had lost control through sudden incapacitation by disease, 29 cases due to coronary atherosclerosis, one case due to a witnessed pre-crash rupture of a vascular malformation of the brain, and seven cases associated with epileptic seizures. Accordingly, it may be stated that 5.9 percent of "at-fault" drivers suffering fatal injury patterns in single- or multi-vehicle crashes lost control because of a sudden unconsciousness from disease. Two-thirds of these are cardiovascular and one-third are epileptic in nature. One of the seizure cases, a man witnessed to stiffen up suddenly with head back and subsequent acceleration into a truck ahead, was found to be suffering from Lissauer's lobar sclerosis of the brain. Although Hossack found that 9.2 percent of his 102 drivers was dead of natural disease, our total deaths certified as natural were 305 out of 1,171 or 26 percent. If we add the 37 cases of fatal crash instigated by natural disease, the figure rises to 29 percent of all drivers dying at the wheel. Obviously, comparison must include age corrections, data which were impossible to obtain from the licensing agencies at that time.

At this point it is well to note that motor vehicle administrators responsible for issuance of licenses may incur liability if a third party is injured as a result of their knowingly issuing a license to a driver at high risk of sudden incapacitation from physical disease. Well-intentioned, disease-oriented volunteer health organizations may press for the elimination of license restriction on epileptics, but the evidence is unequivocal—automobile crashes from sudden loss of control due to natural disease and epileptic seizures do occur. Stringent, fair, physical requirements for licensure are a necessity. Equally necessary are impartial medical boards to evaluate the fitness of a driver in question. It is fallacious to depend upon the private physician of the licensee to assume the responsibility for such a determination.

CRASH PHASE INVESTIGATION

Crash kinematics are determined from witness testimony, physical evidence at the scene, and victim injury patterns. Each modality is limited and correlation becomes essential. Witnesses vary widely in their ability to perceive because the sudden total sensory input is overwhelming. All ordinary witness testimony should be subject to critical question. What a witness honestly recalls may, in fact, be far from the truth.[22] Furthermore, a crash sequence of 0.1 second is too fast for the average person to observe everything. A rear-seat passenger may be thrown forward, strike the rearview mirror, revert to the rear seat, and have no recollection of having left the seat. In view of anticipated civil and criminal litigation, deliberate prevarication by one or more of the participants or their experts is not uncommon. Fraud, involving an illegal alliance between physicians, hospitals, and attorneys, has been well documented in our experience in Florida, and there is no reason to believe it has not existed elsewhere.

Physical evidence, based upon physical laws of motion, material deformation, heat, and electricity constitute valuable information. Interpretative opinions must be expressed within the limits of such laws.

Impact decelerative forces may be calculated from the formula

$$G = \frac{Kv^2}{d}$$

where G is expressed as gravitational force, v is the initial impact speed, d is the stopping distance, and K is a constant (0.034) with speed in miles per hour and distance in feet.[23] With kilometers per hour and meters, K is 0.0039. An approximately 30-mph impact with a 3-foot stopping distance will apply a force of approximately 9.75 times gravity (i.e., the body weight would be increased 9.75 times). Such forward decelerative G forces may be tolerated by healthy individuals. However, the stopping distance of the outside of the vehicle is not the critical distance. It is the secondary impact of the occupant—continuing at the same initial speed to impact against the vehicle interior—which is critical. The interior residual stopping distance of the occupant may be only 2 inches, not 3 feet. The resulting force would be about 20 times that of the 3-foot stopping distance, well beyond body tolerance to injury.

Estimates of initial speed may be calculated from physical evidence after the crash, including skid marks and vehicular deformation. A rule of thumb for contemporary average-sized American automobiles in frontal impact is 1 inch of crush per mile per hour. With smaller vehicles the increased rigidity results in less crush per unit of speed with resulting increased decelerative forces transmitted to the vehicular interior.

The skid mark formula for vehicular speed estimation is:

$$v = 5.5 \sqrt{fd}$$

where v is velocity in miles per hour, d is the skid mark in feet, and f is a drag factor erroneously considered the coefficient of fiction. Coefficient of friction in this instance pertains to dynamic coefficient which changes according to speed as compared with static coefficient of friction. For example, steel on steel coefficient of friction is 0.2, but railroad drag factor values turn out to be 0.04 to 0.07. Standard American automobiles with good tires on good, dry pavement have drag factors in the range of 0.6 to

0.9, but with wet pavement this shifts to 0.5 to 0.7. With change of speed the drag factor may change 0.003 per mile per hour. This may imply scientific accuracy, but roadway conditions of wear and petroleum contamination vary widely. Intersection pavement has a lower drag factor because of petroleum contamination. The outside lane of a well-traveled expressway has more wear and oil deposition than the median lane. A motorcyclist traveling between automobile tire pathways is riding on a different roadbed, less worn but more oil-soaked. Tire wear complicates the formula. A smooth tire or racing slick has more drag factor on dry pavement than tread tires have. On wet pavement the converse is true as surface water is diverted into the space between treads, allowing for tread rubber to grip dryer surface. At higher speeds, hydroplaning is expected with rapid decrease of the drag factor.

Measurement of skid marks is fraught with error for the marks may be the result of yaw or acceleration. On wet pavements the skid marks may be "inverted" or "reverted," lighter in color than the pavement instead of darker. The friction heats the water, effectively "steam-cleaning" the pavement. In every case the marks should be photographed to allow for subsequent evaluation as to their true nature. It is apparent that retrospective speed evaluation requires skill and is not a matter of simple arithmetic. The ideal situation would be to perform experiments using the same vehicle under identical conditions of place and climate. The impracticality is apparent.

In sudden vehicular deceleration or change of angle, the momentum of the occupants requires that they continue in their original direction until sufficient force is applied to alter their momentum and/or angle of travel. The secondary impacts within the vehicle result in injury. Given adequate and properly worn seat and shoulder harness restraints, or airbags, the forces applied to the victim are distributed over a sufficiently wide area and during a sufficiently prolonged duration of time to assure minimal injury even though the vehicle may be demolished. Conversely, a minimal impact with forces locally applied may result in a fatality:

> A 22-year-old pregnant woman at term who was a right-front passenger in a small European car was thrown forward during a 15-mph intersection impact. Her head struck and cracked the windshield. The left breast area struck and broke the protruding radio control knob on the dashboard (Fig. 14-6). A slight bruise and two cracked ribs resulted. Because of pregnancy, she was admitted to a hospital for observation. Two weeks later she suddenly complained of faintness, collapsed, and had cessation of effective heartbeat. Although the pericardial sac was intact, the impact force had contused the myocardium, which ruptured, resulting in cardiac tamponade. Incidental cesarian section was successful. The child has developed normally for several years.

Vehicles are constructed of diverse materials including metals, plastic, glass, cloth, and paints. Their energy-absorbing and deformation character varies considerably. Moreover, the initial shape of the material affects its reaction to stress. The interaction of such materials with occupants and pedestrians is variable. However, general rules apply under similar circumstances of impact.

Examination of the interior of the vehicle, along with consideration of the crash circumstances, should suffice for ready correlation. Accordingly, hair, blood, brain, teeth, or bone samples will indicate impact points of

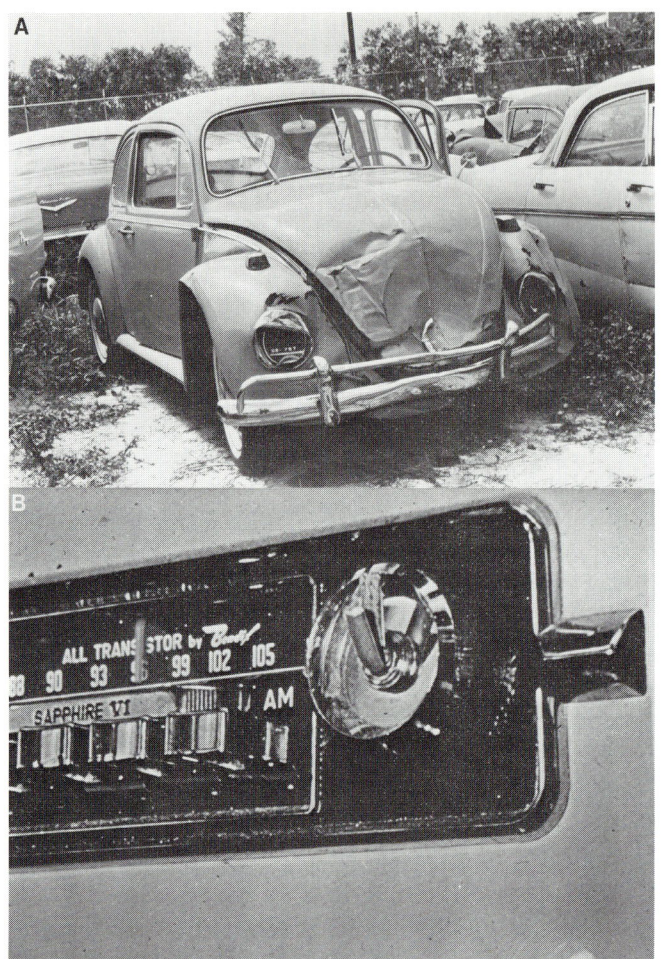

FIGURE 14-6. Fatal injury from protruding object. A low-speed impact of 15 mph, evidenced by mild frontal damage, resulted in the unrestrained passenger being thrown forward *(A)*. The protruding radio knob *(B)* was broken off by impact with the chest wall, causing delayed rupture of the heart.

occupants within the vehicle. Deformation of vehicular components can be associated with injury patterns upon the victims. Paint, glass, and metal knobs can be expected to leave such patterns. There is a considerable difference in patterns of skin injury from impact against laminated safety glass, tempered glass, or, if the victim is ejected, roadway gravel (Fig. 14-7). Forward impacts obviously result in anterior patterns. Lateral impacts result in corresponding injuries to that side of the body.

With impact injuries there must be consideration of tissue strength as well as the shape and strength of various materials. Human tissues vary widely in elasticity and strength, according to the effects of disease and age. These factors and the internal configuration of viscera influence the ability to withstand or suffer from the effects of auto-crash impacts.

The spectrum of automobile occupant injuries is immense. In a collective review of 94 references, Sims and coworkers covered the spectrum of secondary impact injuries.[24] These have been listed for windshield, steering wheel, dashboard, seat belt, whiplash, and miscellaneous interior

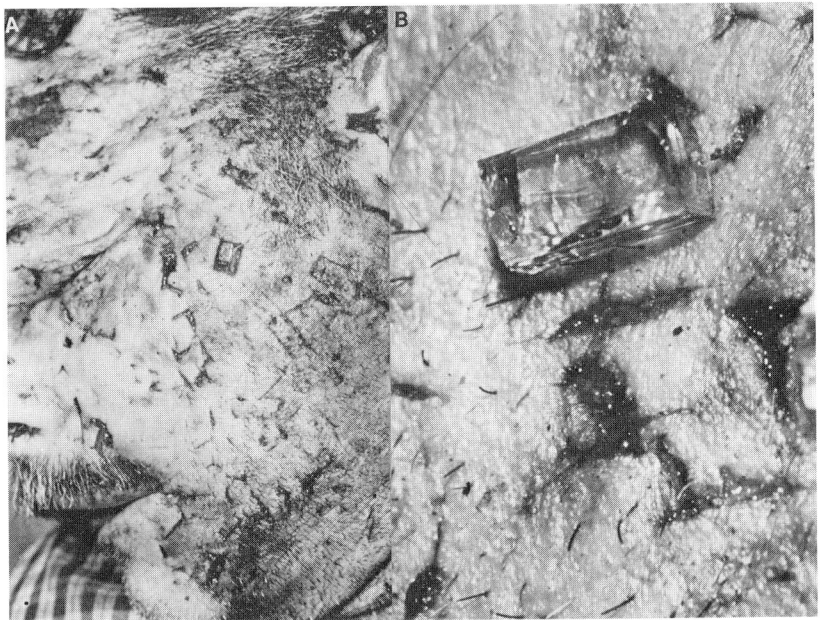

FIGURE 14-7. Tempered glass pattern. Tempered glass "dicing" pattern *(A)* indicates lateral impact into the side window. The close view *(B)* reveals the typical rectangular margins of the fragments.

categories (Figs. 14-8 and 14-9). Fifty-four separate, severe injury patterns from the head to the urinary bladder are enumerated and referenced for the steering wheel alone. Fifty-one categories are associated with dashboard impacts. These exemplify the magnitude of injury production.

In any study of injuries it is essential to correlate the location and lethality in uniform fashion in order to gain the most value from autopsy or medical records. The Abbreviated Injury Scale, developed by the Committee on Medical Aspects of Automotive Safety of the American Medical Association, is a valuable tool for study.[25] However, it is of little value if tissue damage is not documented. Proper documentation demands some expectations of what is apt to be found, based upon prior knowledge of the crash circumstance. The common practice of investigative separatism by police and forensic pathologists is deplorable.

MOTORCYCLE DEATHS

The injuries to motorcyclists are in accord with the laws of physics. However, the cyclist lacks the energy-attenuating surroundings of an automobile and is usually injured by primary impact with the opposing vehicle, an object, or the ground. Craniocerebral injury, crushing chest injuries, and major extremity fractures are common. There is no doubt whatsoever that enactment of motorcycle helmet laws has favorably altered the craniocerebral injury statistics. Unfortunately, political pressure by misguided motorcyclists has caused a rescinding of these beneficial statutes in many jurisdictions. The results have been regrettable. Few persons comprehend the high risk of motorcycle transport and the significant speeds at which these vehicles carry their unprotected riders. Most persons would not venture forth upon a tenth-story window ledge for fear of falling. Assuming 10 feet per story, this is a height of 100 feet. The impact of such a fall

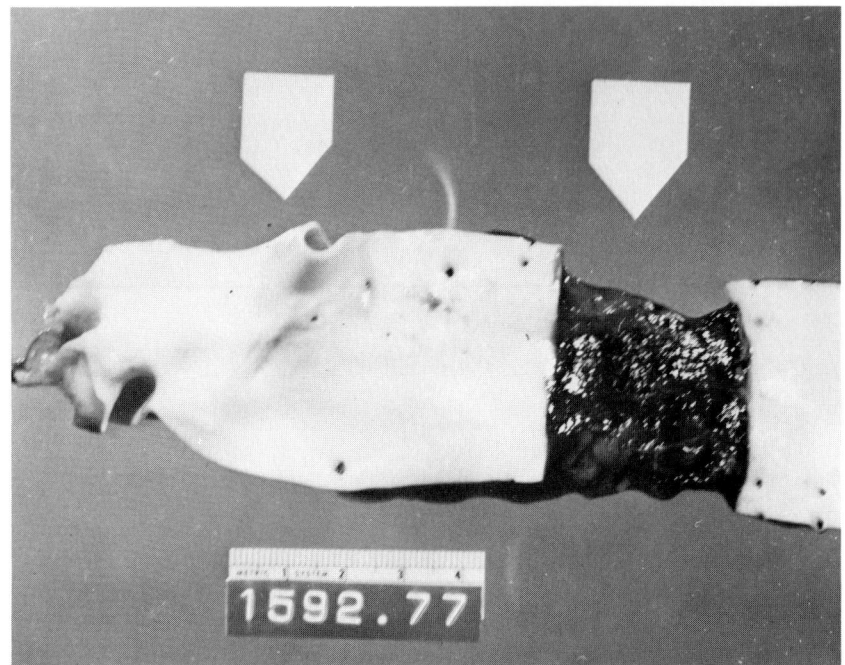

FIGURE 14-8. Traumatic rupture of aorta. Severe frontal chest impacts against the steering wheel may result in aortic rupture close to the ligamentum arteriosum.

is about 54 mph, a common motorcycle speed. Although helmets do decrease fatalities, their greatest value is protection at lower speed or tangential impacts.[26] Frank[27] describes a case of a college merit scholar who fell from a motor scooter when it stopped suddenly in heavy traffic. He sustained a mild blow to the head with resulting progressive deterioration of intellect to the point of being unable to perform grade school arithmetic. A helmet would have prevented this tragedy. If helmet requirements are to be voided, so also should public and insurance industry liability for the custodial care of those whose injuries are aggravated by such lack of self-concern. Legislators who espouse the repeal of helmet requirements should first consider this statement by the Federal District Court in Massachusetts in a case subsequently affirmed by the United States Supreme Court:

> While we agree with plaintiff that the act's only realistic purpose is the prevention of head injuries incurred in motorcycle mishaps, we cannot agree that the consequences of such injuries are limited to the individual who sustains the injury. . . . The public has an interest in minimizing the resources directly involved. From the moment of the injury, society picks the person up off the highway; delivers him to a municipal hospital and municipal doctors; provides him with unemployment compensation if, after recovery, he cannot replace his lost job, and, if the injury causes permanent disability, may assume the responsibility for his and his family's subsistence. We do not understand a state of mind that permits plaintiff to think that only he himself is concerned.[28]

Worse yet is a plethora of product liability suits against motorcycle helmet manufacturers. The allegation is that neck injuries occur as a result

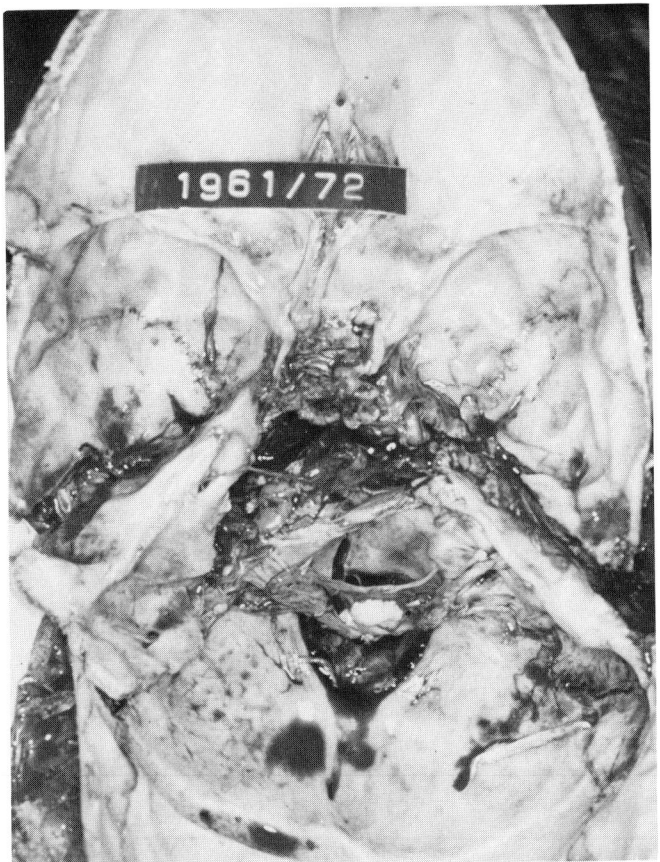

FIGURE 14-9. Basal skull fracture. Transverse basal skull fractures may occur with frontal impacts of the head against the interior of the vehicle.

of helmet design even though the victim was propelled at high speed against a firm and unyielding object. It is usually alleged that the posterior rim of the helmet impinged the neck and caused the injury. Radiographic motion picture studies indicate that this is not so. It is pointless to assess helmet design fault responsibility when the human body has been propelled through the air at 40 to 60 mph into a motor vehicle, a tree, or the roadway.

PEDESTRIAN FATALITIES

In our experience pedestrian deaths constitute 29 percent of motor vehicle fatalities. These ratios may vary from one jurisdiction to another depending upon availability of public transportation and the relative mix of motor vehicles and pedestrians. Children and elderly are at highest risk for obvious reasons. Pedestrians have their own peculiar injury patterns which assist in determining whether or not a victim found by the roadside was indeed struck by an automobile. The most common finding is the bumper fracture of the legs, occurring when a pedestrian is struck by the front of an average motor vehicle. Headlight rim patterns or other front end patterns are of similar significance. Because the center of gravity of the average adult is pelvic,[29] and modern automobiles are low to the

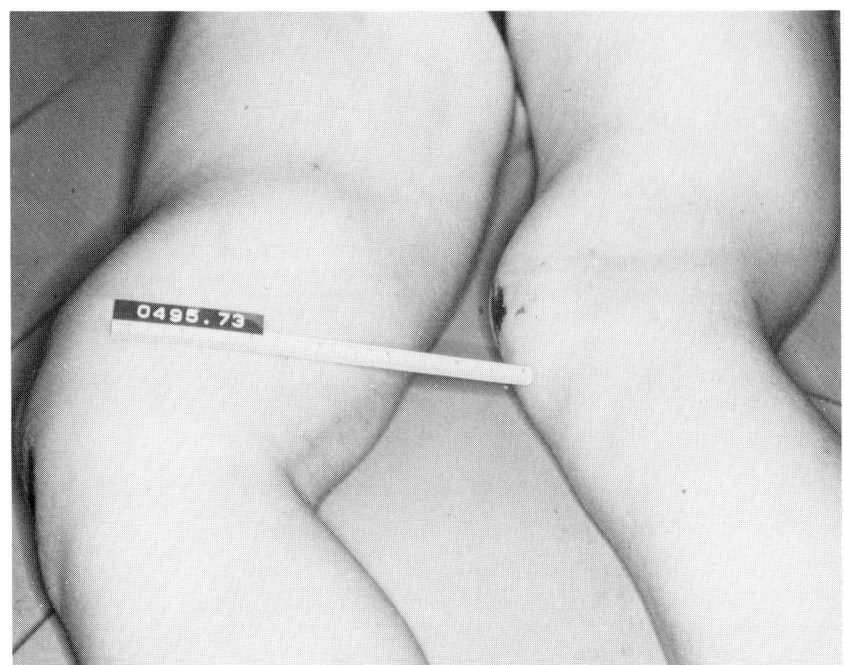

FIGURE 14-10. High bumper fractures. Bumper fractures above the knees indicate that the brakes of the automobile were probably not applied prior to impact.

ground, the usual sequence of a frontal impact is leg injury from the bumper (Fig. 14-10), thigh patterns from the front of the vehicle (Fig. 14-11), and head injury from the victim's having been thrown back against the hood or windscreen (Fig. 14-12). There may be stretch marks on the groin from hyperextension of the legs when struck from the rear (Fig. 14-13). With higher-speed impacts the victim's body may be propelled completely over the top of the vehicle. The elasticity of skin and tissues tends to keep the body in one piece, albeit broken. At very high speeds (80 mph, 130 km per hour), impacts may be expected to exceed the skin elastic limits and result in hemisection of the victim. In unwitnessed hit-and-run cases this observation may offer evidence of the impact speed.

The short stature of children facilitates a knock-down, run-over pattern

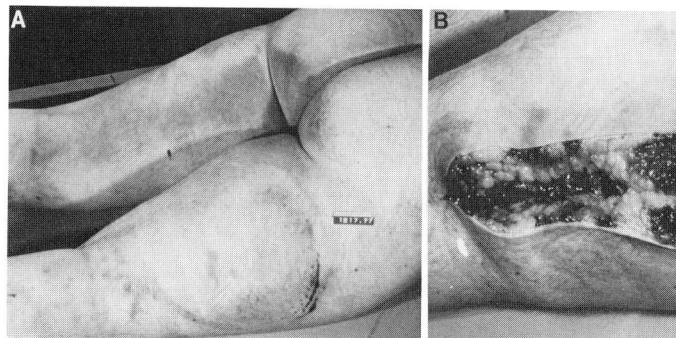

FIGURE 14-11. Headlight pattern injury. The pattern of injury (A) coincides with portions of the suspect vehicle, a headlight in this case. The deeper contusion injury (B) is much greater than the surface pattern might indicate.

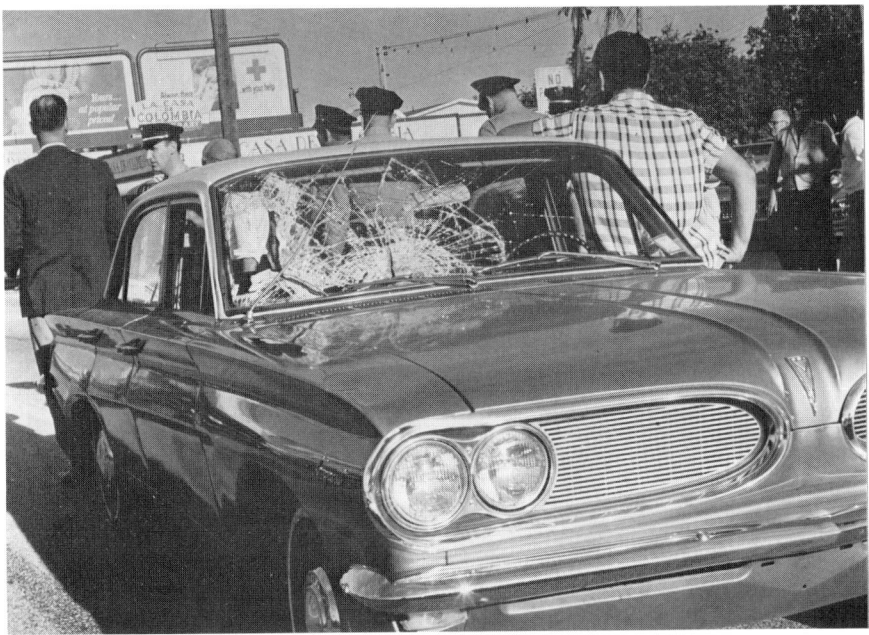

FIGURE 14-12. Vehicle which struck pedestrian. Low-speed impact resulted in minimal headlight trim damage, but the victim's head and elbow struck the windshield. Brain tissue was found inside the passenger compartment.

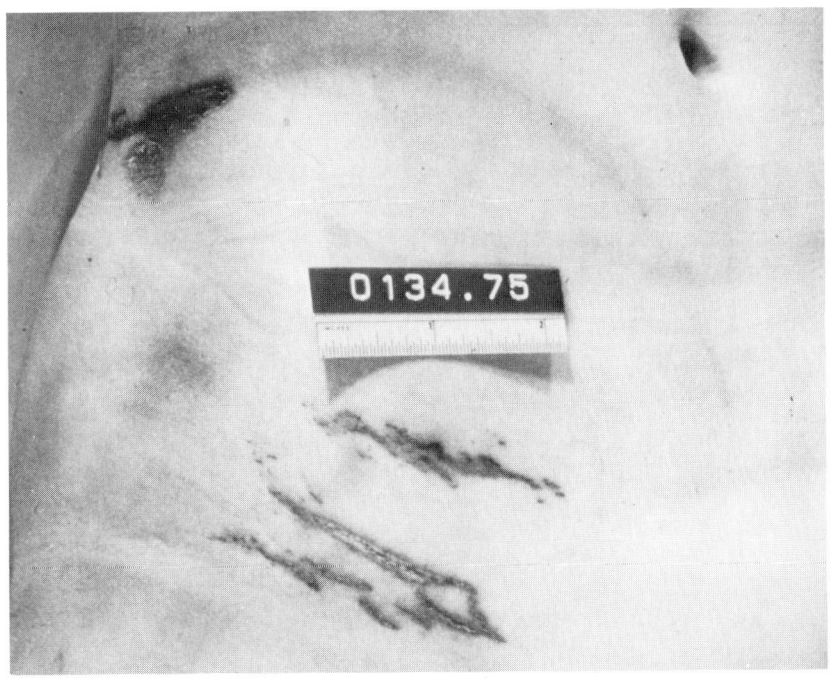

FIGURE 14-13. Stretch marks of skin. A pedestrian struck from the rear may have skin stretch marks in the groin due to the bending backward of the torso upon the hood of the automobile.

rather than a scooping up into the air as seen in adults. The body's rolling under the vehicle results in extensive abrasions, grease soiling, and burns from the exhaust system. These findings likewise are noted in drunken adults run over while lying in the road. Children are apt to run into the side of slow-moving vehicles and fall beneath a rear wheel with resulting wheel patterns. Tire imprints upon the skin are indicative of this event (Fig. 14-14).

The body of a pedestrian and the suspect vehicle should be meticulously examined for transfer evidence or significant pattern injuries or defects. In hit-and-run or potential manslaughter cases, physical evidence documentation and chain of evidence preservation are essential (Fig. 14-15). Blood and hair for comparison must be retained. Prior to the examination of the victim there must be some appreciation of the relative direction of travel of the victim and the vehicle. From this information an estimate of the areas of anticipated major injury is made. After this the body is examined to see if the patterns do correlate. A pedestrian known to be crossing from west to east and struck by a south-bound automobile would be expected to evidence more severe injuries on the left side of the body than the right. A simple listing of injuries revealed by the autopsy is unprofessional and useless. The pathologist should be mindful of correlative aspects. It is essential to describe the injuries in detail and in meaningful groups so that the report clearly indicates the direction of force application to the body. The investigative process is a continuous mix of correlation with observation as new findings are noted.

"THE FLORIDA ACCIDENT"

Vehicles recovered from water constitute a special problem. It must be ascertained whether the vehicle was inadvertently driven into the water or was disposed of with or without an occupant. In South Florida the high

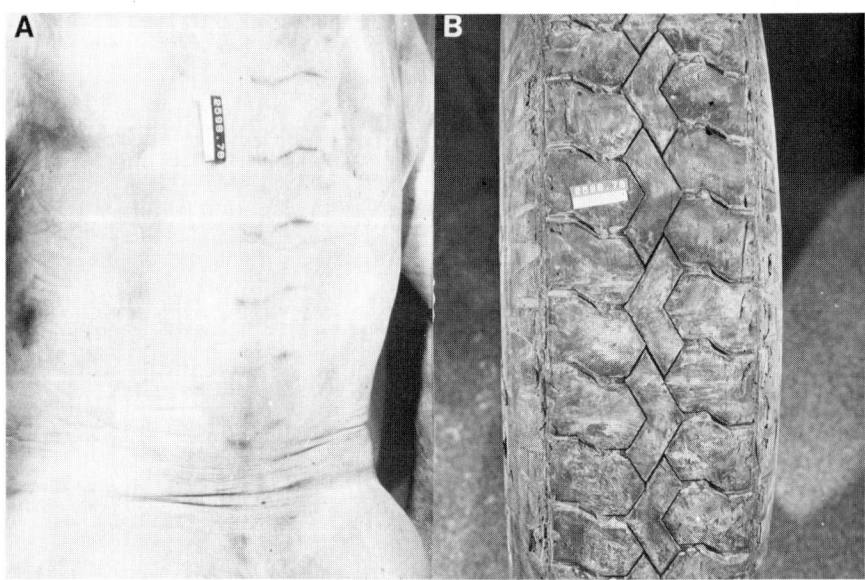

FIGURE 14-14. Tire tread pattern of skin. Tire tread patterns (A) are easily recognizable by their repetitive nature. Photographic overlays revealed this tread (B) to coincide with the skin pattern.

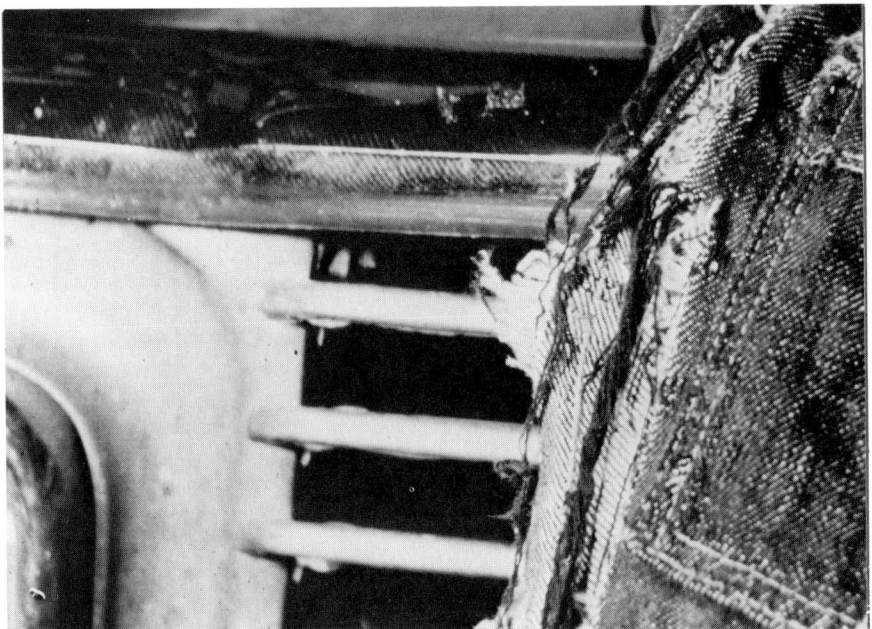

FIGURE 14-15. Clothing pattern transfer. The dust on the chrome trim imprinted the cloth pattern. The introduction of this photograph resulted in the defendant's plea of guilty to leaving the scene of a fatal accident.

water table necessitates excavation of fill from alongside roadways. This results in canals parallel to the roads. Some of these canals have depths of 20 feet to 40 feet. Not until the last decade were guardrails utilized along heavily traveled highways. The resulting fatalities were legion and colloquially known as "the Florida accident," a term coined by the late Dr. Jack Mickley, former medical examiner for Broward County, Florida. Such crash incidents have a unique characteristic, the relative sparing of the vehicle and the occupants from severe decelerative deformation and injuries. Sometimes the vehicle is recovered long afterward. Decomposition complicates the assessment of human causative factors and determination if the victim were alive or dead prior to water entry. A careful total assessment of scene circumstance and vehicle is crucial in order to rule out an intentional death.

Such accidents are not, of course, limited to South Florida, or to such particular road conditions. They can occur wherever a vehicle passes off a road or a narrow bridge without guard rails into a body of water alongside the road.

POST-CRASH FIRE HAZARD

Post-crash fire is another complication of motor vehicle crashes, 1.5 percent of our 3,518 occupant deaths during years 1956 through 1977. Specific questions arise as to whether the victim was alive or dead prior to the crash, the identity of the victim, and the presence or absence of sufficient autopsy or witness and circumstantial evidence to indicate whether or not pain and suffering occurred during the fire. One must examine the airway with great care for evidence of smoke inhalation. It must be realized that a flash fire from gasoline may result in death with surprisingly low carbon monoxide concentrations. Hirsch and coworkers[30] report in detail the deaths of eight victims of a single multivehicular crash in which six were proven to have died exclusively from the gasoline-fueled flash fire. Carboxyhemoglobins were not significantly elevated, nor was soot noted in the airway. Accordingly, a very careful assessment of total autopsy findings with the crash circumstances is essential before expressing interpretive opinions. It must be assumed that a body found burned beyond recognition in an automobile might well be a homicide where the vehicle owner has killed a victim; placed false identification on the body, including jewelry; and set fire to the vehicle. Such cases occur with regularity. Sometimes putrefaction indicates the body to have been dead prior to the fire. What is amazing is the frequency with which such events escape detection at the hands of the initial investigators who seem, in such cases, determined to support the deception despite variance with published reports on the characteristics of fire spread within automobiles.[31]

INTENTIONAL AUTOMOBILE CRASHES

An intentional motor vehicle crash can involve a suicide by a supposed "victim" struck by the automobile, a suicide by the driver who intentionally crashes his vehicle in order to cause his own death, and various types of homicidal actions by drivers, resulting in death to others.

Among a total of 2,650 suicides in a 15-year period in the Miami area, we determined 12 deaths of pedestrians run over by motor vehicles to have been suicides. Two other deaths during this same period were determined to be intentional actions by drivers to cause their own deaths.

Suicide Death by Drivers

The characteristic of a driver-suicide death is a head-on collision with a roadside object, pole, or bridge support at a high rate of speed without evidence of an effort to apply the brakes or to evade striking the object. Suspicion of suicide should exist in any single-vehicle, single-occupant crash. The investigation is not complete until suicide has been ruled out. The human factor analysis is essential. The presence of an incisional wrist scar or medicinal tranquilizers, along with a prior abnormal psychological history, should result in an intensive investigation of suicide as the major causative factor. The same applies to accelerator pedal imprints upon a shoe sole. Petty and coworkers[33] reviewed the various interpretations of shoe sole imprints, including determination of the actions of the driver at the moment of impact, the actions of drivers in two-vehicle crashes, and the determination of the actual driver when all occupants are killed and ejected (see Fig. 14-1). Sometimes two-vehicle crashes may be suicidal, as we have observed. There need be no haste in certifying a single-vehicle crash as an accident. The death certificate and the police conclusions may remain pending until all motives for suicide have been explored.

Homicide by Motor Vehicle

Vehicular-associated homicide may be considered in four major categories:

1. Wanton and culpable negligence of the driver, resulting in death of another person (manslaughter in most statutes).

2. Utilization of a false motor vehicle crash to conceal a prior homicide.
3. Deliberate utilization of the vehicle as the weapon.
4. Deliberate shooting of an operator of a moving vehicle.

Vehicular manslaughter usually involves excessive speed or drunk driving behavior where operator performance is offensive in the extreme, yet there is not deliberate intent to cause the fatal crash. The victim, therefore, must be carefully examined to rule out any defense objection that the death was the result of an intervening cause. Likewise careful attention should be paid to events including trace evidence transfer. A charge of homicide is dependent upon the establishment of the corpus delicti, the body of the crime, in order to establish a successful prosecution. This involves the identification of the victim, the ruling out of natural disease as a cause, and the demonstration that the death is the result of the criminal act of another. In those jurisdictions where the norm is a casual approach to investigation, such cases may not be successfully prosecuted.

1. The driver escaped when his automobile drove through a parking lot, across a wharf, and into the Miami River. His female passenger drowned. He claimed to have made a wrong turn in the darkness. It developed that he had just acquired a large accidental death insurance policy on his friend, although there was no legal interest on her life. His vehicle was equipped with outside locks sufficient to keep his passenger within. He was the son of a leader of a murder-for-insurance ring formerly operating in the northern part of the state. He was tried and convicted of murder.
2. The police report indicated that the driver struck a dog and then "swerved to right in a belated evasive action." The automobile struck a power pole head-on. A steering column impact pattern was prominent on the right anterior chest. Blood alcohol concentration was 0.24 percent. Autopsy revealed, in addition to a fractured larynx and rib fractures, a transverse left to right ragged laceration of the vertex of the scalp with penetration of the calvarium by a bullet. Subsequently it was learned that the driver verbally insulted an occupant of an automobile to his left, who retaliated with a gunshot. Even the newspaper had reported the crash as an "accident" (Fig. 14-16). The assailant was convicted of murder.

POST-CRASH MEDICAL CARE

As a general rule, the post-crash medical treatment of crash victims affects morbidity rather than mortality. In this author's opinion, most dead victims of crashes have sustained such serious injuries, including ruptured hearts or crushed heads, that survivorship is nil. However, not all are initially doomed. Frey and coworkers, in a retrospective study, judged that 17.6 percent of occupants dead of automobile injuries were probably salvageable.[33] Sevitt correlated injury to death times according to organ system involvement.[34] Delayed deaths usually involve central nervous system injury complications. On the other hand, each autopsy should be assessed carefully for evidence of the need for improved emergency and definitive medical care. Some crash victims, dead upon arrival of rescue personnel or after arrival at the hospital emergency room, may exhibit surprisingly little evidence of overt fatal trauma. In such circumstances the solution to this enigma is to be found in the events which transpired

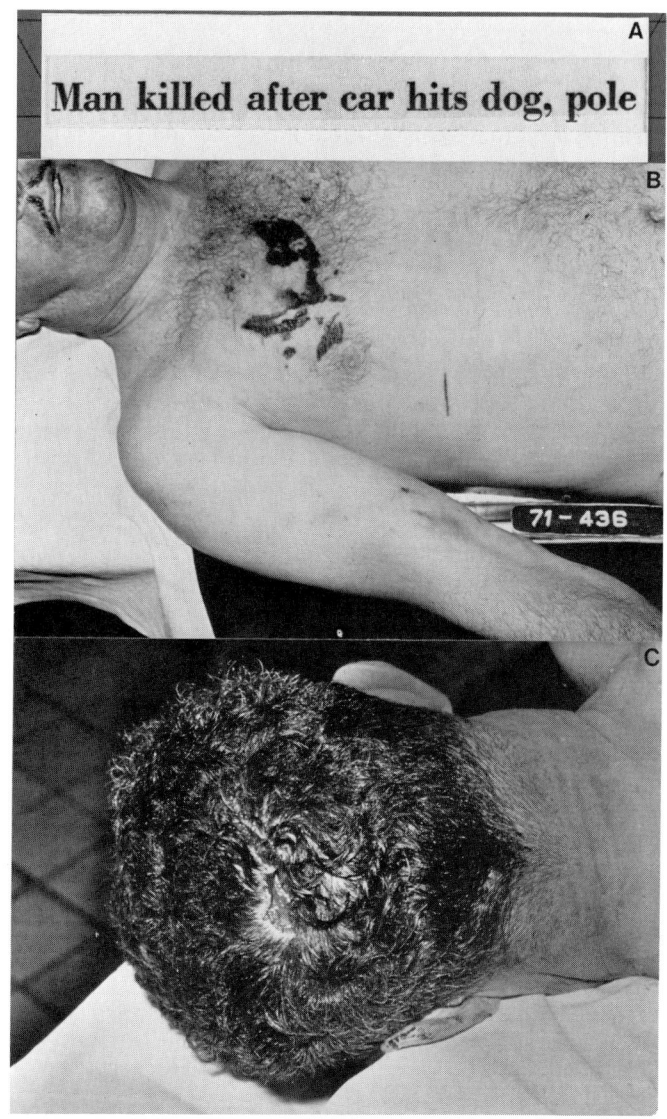

FIGURE 14-16. Murder thought to be accident. Newspaper headline *(A)* is based upon the initial "accident" investigation. The steering wheel impact *(B)* correlates with the frontal impact into a power pole. The easily overlooked or misinterpreted wound of the scalp *(C)* is from a bullet. Without careful autopsy scrutiny, such murders must be overlooked.

prior to arrival at the hospital. The victim was either fixed in an awkward position with resulting respiratory compromise before the rescue units arrived, or airway interference occurred as a result of poor rescue techniques. Wright and Harris[35] describe a right front-seat passenger rendered unconscious when his head struck the windshield. He was breathing quite well on rescue. After application of a Thomas splint, he was placed into the rear seat of an automobile for transport, rather than awaiting the arrival of an ambulance. The victim, 6 feet 2 inches in height, died from the neck flexion resulting from his compromised position in the "rescue" vehicle, an excellent example of postural asphyxia.

Post-crash hazards may exist for rescuers or nearby residents if the vehicular cargo is flammable, explosive, or poisonous. Liquified petroleum gas is especially dangerous as it spreads invisibly away from the crash site. Aircraft cargos are also potentially very dangerous. In Dade County, cargo aircraft ferry dynamite to South America in 40,000-pound lots. In another aircraft example, an agricultural-spray plane crashed and its 2,500 pounds of ammonium nitrate fertilizer detonated as police approached the smouldering wreckage. One officer was permanently disabled.

TORT LIABILITY

Today, it is axiomatic that remote liability is to be alleged in every automobile crash with injuries or death. By remote is meant liability against a party not involved in the original crash. This is especially so when the insurance coverage of the offending driver is absent or marginal. The courts often hold liable the employer of an offender when his on-the-job status is extremely tenuous. A recent example was the employee of a large corporation, who was attending a convention. He rented an automobile and was driving to a friend's home when he failed to halt at a stop sign. He struck a panel truck whose unbelted youthful driver sustained permanent central nervous system injury following ejection from the vehicle. The employer was judged liable to the extent of two million dollars, despite the fact that the at-fault driver was not strictly engaged in company business. His employer had the money, colloquially known in the courthouse as the "deep pocket." Product liability against the automobile manufacturer is an expected occurrence where the at-fault driver insurance coverage is poor.

Roadway engineering design is likewise becoming grounds for high judgments, regardless of the culpability of the injured driver. In one such case, resulting in a multimillion dollar verdict against a municipality, the drinking driver returning home from a cocktail party had already been stopped by the police and allowed to proceed. He crashed into a rock-decorated medial strip and became quadriplegic. The crash investigation officer, totally untrained, neglected to press for a blood alcohol study upon the injured driver. This officer was employed by the same municipality which was held liable for construction of a road-beautification rock garden in the medial strip.

Even where the victim is manifestly at fault, the doctrine of comparative negligence permits some juries to set astronomical verdicts and only to reduce these by a minor percentage for the contributing negligence of the driver with results still measured in millions of dollars. As publicity continues and legal precedent expands, more such product liability cases may be expected. The recent post-crash gasoline fire litigation has added fuel to these events. It is essential that each fatal auto crash be investigated to the utmost so that correct and adequate evidence is collected. No governmental agency may justify any investigation less than complete if court decisions are to be just and equitable.

The medical examiner and forensic pathologist must be concerned with the totality of crash reconstruction which involves human factors as they interface with other causative factors, kinematic factors, and preventive factors. Positive as well as negative evidence must be documented. Every effort must be made to ascertain the psychological, physical, and chemical factors which played a role in poor driver performance. Adequate toxicologic and autopsy evidence is essential. Wound correlation with the kinematics of the crash will clarify the role, if any, of design deficiencies which may be alleged in a forthcoming product liability action. Finally, and most important to social welfare, is the value of detailed investigation to the prevention of death and injury. A constant search for improvement in vehicle and highway design and in medical care to the injured is essential. It should be apparent that simplistic solutions do not exist. Roadway engineering and vehicular design improvements have clearly resulted in decreased morbidity and mortality. Driver attitude modification utilizing all resources, including advertising techniques for modification of public beliefs, is very much needed. Least desirable is a laissez faire attitude on the part of government employees who rationalize their own failures and deficiencies as "public apathy."

PREVENTION OF TRAFFIC FATALITIES

A highway crash occurs when the mix of human, vehicular, and environmental factors reaches a critical hazard point at a precise moment. An omission of a single minor factor may result in a "near miss." The principles of epidemiologic investigation apply to the concepts of prevention with consideration of person, place, and time.

Although pertinent factors may be identified in most crashes, prevention is not simple. Human factors, including inebriation and aggressive personality, result in speeding and gross carelessness. Even if aberrant behavior patterns or personality defects could be readily identified, behavior modification is one of the most difficult and least cost-effective solutions. This is not to say that law enforcement, trial, and post-conviction programs are useless. On the contrary, such programs aimed at behavior modification do help. Moreover, the enforcers gain deeper insight into the problems they face by being involved in such programs.

Without a doubt, the most cost-effective approach is achieved by roadway and vehicular engineering improvement. Ideally, pedestrians, bicyclists, and motor vehicles should be kept apart in every feasible circumstance. The use of traffic death and injury statistical data, coupled with study of highway traffic patterns, is an ideal way to pinpoint problem locations. However, each study area should be qualitatively evaluated in order that the crash data are properly interpreted. For example, a study by this author resulted in the construction of pedestrian channeling and control devices on one stretch of a major highway. In actual fact the pedestrian deaths elsewhere on the highway were more frequent than the one which triggered the study. However, it could be demonstrated that the cost benefit was greatest close to the university, where numbers of students had to cross the highway in order to reach a shopping pavilion. Ultimately, the agility of youth could no longer cope with the traffic density pattern. The population at risk had reached the critical point. In a rural area to the south, the pedestrian deaths, although more frequent, were the result of drunk pedestrians "passing out" on the roadway at night when traffic was relatively sparse.

Crashworthiness of motor vehicles was discussed earlier. However, crashworthiness of highways is an equally valid concept. Modification of guardrail construction and location has resulted in a definite decrease in severity of crashes (Fig. 14-17). Most dramatic has been the effect of energy attenuators, such as collapsible barrels, at the apex of expressway divisions and next to fixed objects. In some circumstances, formerly fatal,

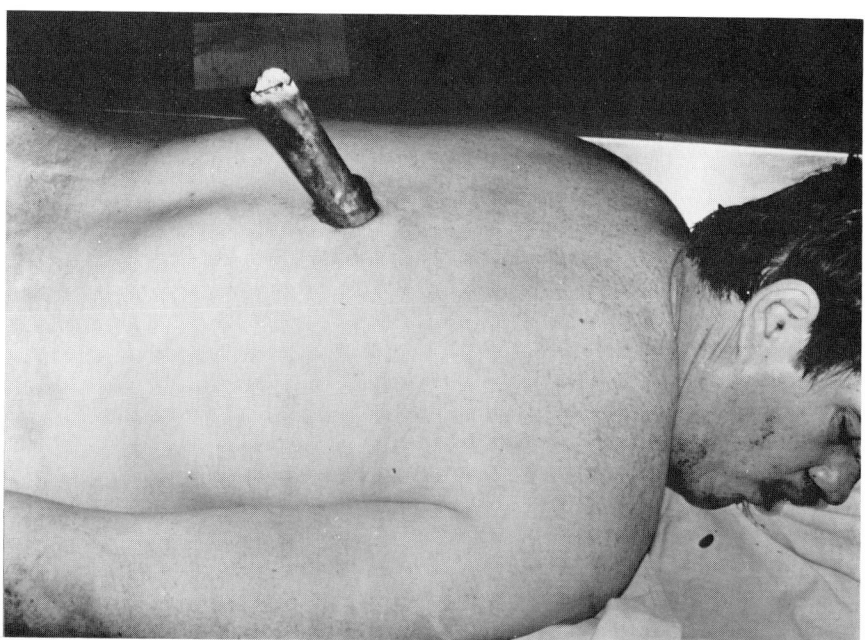

FIGURE 14-17. Improper guardrail design. The top rail of a roadside chain-link fence impaled this errant motorist. A properly installed guardrail prevents such needless deaths.

the motorist has driven away from the scene, leaving behind only the damaged energy attenuators, a little glass, and some chrome strips as mute evidence of an earlier drama. The cost-benefit of improved crashworthiness in highway design has been proven beyond any question.

National design standards assume that attention to such detail will prevail in new construction. The problem remains with highways constructed before improved standards were instituted. These deteriorate and traffic flow patterns increase, owing to highway changes elsewhere or new housing nearby. A constant monitoring of crash and traffic problems is essential in order to delineate the needed sites of improvement. Monies will be in short supply and must be allocated properly. Accordingly, it behooves medical examiners, coroners, and others in the death case investigation and enforcement chain to associate themselves with politically active safety councils and other groups who can exert influence upon those who allocate highway funding. Only when data derived from adequate case investigations are used effectively may one consider that the worth of investigative agencies has been established.

REFERENCES

1. Eames, W. G., Lee, S. N., and Fell, J. C.: State of the Art, Motor Vehicle Accident Studies, 1970. *International Automobile Society Conference Compendium*, Society of Automotive Engineers, New York.
2. McFarland, R. A.: Injury—A Major Environmental Problem. *Arch. Environ. Health* 19:244–256, 1969.
3. Haddon, W., Jr., and Baker, S. P.: *Injury Control.* Insurance Institute for Highway Safety, Washington, D.C., 1978 (Subsequently published in Clark, D. W., and MacMahon, B. (eds.): *Preventive Medicine.* ed. 2. Little, Brown, Boston, 1978).

4. *To Prevent Harm.* Insurance Institute for Highway Safety, Washington, D.C., 1978, p. 59.
5. Stoppa, R., Ossart, J. L., Henry, X., and Samarq, B.: Thoracic and Abdominal Injuries in Multiple Trauma. *Internat. Surg.* 62(1):8–14, 1970.
6. Ashbaugh, D. G., et al.: Chest Trauma, Analysis of 685 Patients. *Arch. Surg.* 95:546–555, 1967.
7. Kihlberg, J. K.: Multiplicity of Injury in Automobile Accidents, in Guardjian, E. S., et al. (eds.): *Impact Injury and Crash Protection.* Charles C Thomas, Springfield, Ill., 1970.
8. Gordon, J. E., The Epidemiology of Accidents. *Am. J. Public Health* 39:504–515, 1949.
9. *1968 Alcohol and Highway Safety Report.* Committee of Public Works, 90th Congress, 2nd Session, U.S. Government Printing Office, Washington, D.C., 1968.
10. Ibid., p. 12.
11. Muehlberger, C. W.: Medicolegal Aspects of Alcohol Intoxication, in Gradwohl, R. B. H (ed.): *Legal Medicine.* C. V. Mosby, St. Louis, 1954.
12. Ross, H. L.: The Scandinavian Myth: The Effectiveness of Drinking-and-Driving Legislation in Sweden and Norway. *J. Legal Studies* 4:285–310, 1975.
13. Garriott, J. C., DiMaio, V. J. M., Zumwalt, R. E., and Petty, C. S.: Incidence of Drugs and Alcohol in Fatally Injured Motor Vehicle Drivers. *J. Forensic Sci.* 22:383–389, 1977.
14. Moskowitz, H.: Marijuana and Driving. *Accident Analysis and Prevention* 8:21–26, 1976.
15. Klein, A., Davis, J. H., and Blackbourne, B. D.: Marijuana and Automobile Crashes. *J. Drug Issues* 1:86–89, 1971.
16. Davis, G. L., and Gantner, G. E.: Carboxyhemoglobin in Volunteer Blood Donors. *J.A.M.A.* 230:996–997, 1974.
17. Miller, L. C., Schilling, A. F., Logan, D. L., and Johnson, R. L.: Potential Hazards of Rapid Smoking as a Technique for the Modification of Smoking Behavior. *N. Engl. J. Med.* 297:590–592, 1977.
18. Peterson, B. J., and Petty, C. S.: Sudden Natural Death Among Automobile Drivers. *J. Forensic Sci.* 7:274–285, 1962.
19. Baker, S. P., and Spitz, W. H.: An Evaluation of the Hazard Created by Natural Death at the Wheel. *N. Engl. J. Med.* 283:405–409, 1970.
20. Hossack, D. W.: Death at the Wheel, A Consideration of Cardiovascular Disease as a Contributory Factor in Road Accidents. *Med. J. Australia* 1:164–166, 1974.
21. Dalton, T. V., Davis, J. H., and Blackbourne, B. D.: *Natural Disease as a Cause of Fatal Vehicular Accidents.* Thesis sponsored by Universities Associated for Research and Education in Pathology, Rockville, Md., 1968.
22. Buckhout, R.: Eyewitness Testimony. *Sci. Am.* 231:23–31, 1974.
23. Cullen, S. A.: The Prevention of Injury in Vehicular Accidents, in Mason, J. K., (ed.): *The Pathology of Violent Injury.* Year Book Medical Publishers, Chicago, 1978.
24. Sims, J. K., Ebisu, R. J., Wong, R. K. M., and Wong, L. M. F.: Automobile Accident Occupant Injuries. *JACEP* 5:796–808, 1976.
25. *The Abbreviated Injury Scale (AIS).* American Association of Automotive Medicine, Morton Grove, Ill.
26. *Highway Loss Reduction Status Report* 13(16):6, Nov. 17, 1978. Insurance Institute for Highway Safety, Washington, D.C.
27. Frank, E. D.: The Motor Scooter. *N. Engl. J. Med.* 271:834–835, 1964.
28. *Simon v. Sargent,* 346 F. Supp. 277, 279 (D. Mass, 1972), affirmed, 409 U.S. 1020 (1972).
29. Duggar, B. C.: The Center of Gravity of the Human Body. *Human Factors* 4:131–148, 1962.
30. Hirsch, C. S., et al.: Carboxyhemoglobin Concentrations in Flash Fire Victims. *Am. J. Clin. Pathol.* 68:317–320, 1977.
31. Hyrnchuk, R. J.: A Study of Automobile Fires. *J. Can. Soc. Forensic Sci.* 11:15–19, 1978.

32. Petty, C. S., Smith, R. A., and Hutson, T. A.: The Value of Shoe Sole Imprints in Automobile Crash Investigations. *J. Police Sci. Administration* 1:1–10, 1973.
33. Frey, C. F., Huelke, D. F., and Gikas, P. W.: Resuscitation and Survival in Motor Vehicle Accidents. *J. Trauma* 9:292–310, 1969.
34. Sevitt, S.: Fatal Road Accidents in Birmingham: Times to Death and Their Causes. *Br. J. Accident Surg.* 4:281–293, 1973.
35. Wright, R. K., and Harris, L. S.: Auto Fatalities by Postural Asphyxia. *Proceedings of the 18th Conference of the American Association of Automotive Medicine,* 1974, pp. 104–107.

CHAPTER 15

Laurence R. Simson, Jr., is Associate Pathologist at the Edward W. Sparrow Hospital in Lansing, Michigan. He is also Adjunct Professor in the School of Criminal Justice and Associate Clinical Professor of Pathology at Michigan State University. Dr. Simson received his undergraduate education at Denison University and studied medicine at the University of Cincinnati, graduating in 1962. Since 1968 he has been Lecturer in Aviation Pathology at the U.S. Air Force School of Aerospace Medicine, and is presently Civilian National Consultant (Aviation and Forensic Pathology) to the Surgeon General of the Air Force.

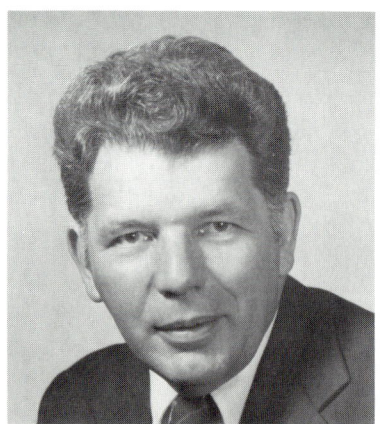

AIRCRAFT DEATH INVESTIGATION: A COMPREHENSIVE REVIEW

Laurence R. Simson, Jr., M.D.

Aircraft accidents are not random events. Rather, they present recurring themes and epidemiologic patterns. Specific types of aircraft tend to have specific kinds of accidents. Airframe and power-plant malfunctions are statistically predictable. Similarly, aircraft operators "malfunction" in characteristic ways conditioned by human physiology and behavior in the flight environment. When a crashed aircraft finally comes to rest, the occupants exhibit patterned injuries from dynamic interaction with aircraft structures. The role of the medical investigator and pathologist includes documentation and interpretation of the dynamic interaction between man and machine.

Few pathologists deal routinely with traumatic injuries of the severity commonly encountered in aviation accidents. Injury patterns, which reflect crash dynamics, are generally unfamiliar. The overlap of official investigative authority is often confusing; yet the pathologist's interpretations of his autopsy findings may have far-reaching effects in accident prevention, flight operations, equipment design, and in crash-related civil litigation.

The following remarks are intended to provide an orientation to aircraft accident investigation and a conceptual framework within which to conduct the medical/pathologic component of such investigations.

AIRCRAFT CRASH INVESTIGATION: DEVELOPING PRINCIPLES

Aircraft accident investigation is strongly oriented toward engineering and flight operations. The underlying assumption is that the cause of a given accident is, in principle at least, discoverable. Motivation is the hope of preventing similar accidents. This "hardware" approach to accidents was entirely appropriate during the early years of aviation. In the days of "wooden airplanes and iron men," aircraft crashes were not unexpected. Engines were unreliable. Airframes were of unproven design and uncertain fabrication. Pilots who "flew by the seat of their pants" were often poorly trained. During World War I, medical rejects from the horse cavalry readily qualified for pilot training. About 90 percent of all air casualties were caused by accidents, not enemy action. "Pilot error" was, and to a large extent remains, the catchall category for unexplained accidents, especially if the pilot is among the fatalities.

As engineers developed aircraft which could fly higher and faster, physicians and physiologists had to devise ways to keep aviators and their passengers alive and well in an increasingly hostile environment. Hypoxia, extreme cold, fatigue, vestibular and visual illusions, accelerative forces, and fear had to be overcome. The medically unfit, the unintelligent, the unreliable, and the reckless had to be excluded from the cockpit. Physicians began to play an integral role in aircrew selection, equipment design, and flight operations. These efforts to increase the safety of flight, however, were almost exclusively directed toward accident prevention. Injury or death was accepted as the inevitable outcome of a crash.

By the end of World War II, the notion of "pilot error" was being reexamined. A pathology laboratory had been established in the United States Army School of Aviation Medicine. In 1944, G. M. Hass, the laboratory's director, wrote: "The attitude was taken that the phrase 'pilot error,' which is the assigned cause of most aviation accidents, should be replaced for analytical purposes by the phrase 'why did a particular pilot make a particular error under a particular set of circumstances?'"[1] Thus, at the close of aviation's fourth decade, crash investigators were finally beginning to explore the limitations and failures of the human operators of the hardware.

Crash injury and survival aspects of accidents had earlier antecedents which, significantly, were largely ignored. DeHaven, an engineer and former military aviator, who had himself suffered severe injuries in an aircraft crash, wrote about the Royal Air Force experience during World War I: "Observations made at the time, during investigation of air crashes, gave strong indication that the range of the traumatic results of aircraft and automobile accidents could be avoided. Structures and objects, by placement and design, created an inevitable expectancy of injury in even minor accidents."[2]

During the late 1930s, an institute devoted to aviation pathology was founded in Germany. Scientific crash injury analysis was conducted, and medical/pathologic data were applied to aircraft and equipment design.[3] Similarly, American military physicians studied the relationship between major injuries and aircraft structures, and recommended design modifications to improve safety.[4]

Systematic analysis of crash injuries and crash injury prevention began in the United States during the early 1940s. The pioneering work of John Stapp on human tolerance to short-term deceleration demonstrated that a properly restrained aircraft occupant can withstand forces equal to or greater than that which can be resisted by a modern aircraft fuselage.[5] It became apparent that "safe transportation of people in any type of vehicle must of necessity apply the practical principles which are used by every packaging engineer to protect goods in transit."[6] Given the premise that crashes will occur, proper design of the aircraft, its structural characteristics, accessory equipment, seats, and restraint systems will significantly decrease the likelihood of injury or death. Recommendations were made to improve the crash-protection capability, or "crashworthiness," of light aircraft without objectionable weight, cost, or performance penalties.[7] Some of these design features have been incorporated into general aviation aircraft, especially aerial-applicator aircraft, the so-called crop dusters.

Although the general aviation accident rate has declined remarkably during the past several decades, the survivability of crashes remains low. Unlike automobile crashes, wherein serious injuries are about 10 times more common than fatalities, in general aviation crashes a fatal outcome is twice as likely as a serious injury.[8]

The majority of air travelers have no choice but to stay with the aircraft in the case of impending disaster. Military aviators generally have provision for in-flight escape. Studies of mishaps involving the high-performance, propeller-driven aircraft of the 1940s revealed that few aviators were able to escape by parachute from aircraft moving at more than about 250 mph. Nor was escape likely from an aircraft at low altitude, diving, spinning, or otherwise out of control. Crewmen were unable to extract themselves from the aircraft, or failed to clear the aircraft, so that they were struck and killed by aircraft structures. Bail-out at low altitude allowed insufficient time for parachute opening.[9] Therefore, it was necessary to develop devices to assist in escape from aircraft in flight. These devices, at first ballistic charge–propelled "ejection seats," have evolved into the various types of rocket-powered ejection seats and escape modules of modern military aircraft.

As the civil air transport system has developed in the decades since World War II, first incorporating aeronautical advances stimulated by wartime research and, more recently, technology of the "space age," there has been increasing awareness of the problems of passenger escape from crashed aircraft. Clearly, an accident involving the disintegration of an airliner at high altitude, or its impact into the ground at high speed, is not survivable. But such crashes are uncommon. The majority of crashes occur during the takeoff and landing phases of flight, at relatively low speed, and with shallow angles of ground impact, so that decelerative forces are attenuated. Fire and toxic combustion products are the danger. Properly "packaged" passengers, who survive the decelerative forces of a crash, must extricate themselves through a maze of physical and human barriers from the rapidly lethal thermotoxic environment of aircraft wreckage.[10]

Beginning in the late 1950s, flight safety increased remarkably. A number of major technologic advances received widespread application almost contemporaneously. Turbine engines, more reliable than the reciprocating engines then available, powered the new generation of military and civil transport aircraft. Quantum advances in aeronautical engineering and metallurgy were incorporated into aircraft structures. Electronic navigation aides, especially radar, greatly improved weather forecasting capability, and improved air traffic control procedures became generally available.

The "Human Factors" Concept

Sustained interest in the application of the techniques of pathology to the understanding of fatal aviation accidents began in 1955. Two British Comet aircraft, part of the first jetliner fleet in civil air transport service, had crashed under obscure circumstances. Analysis of the injury patterns of the crash victims contributed to recognition of the aircraft design deficiencies and metal fatigue-induced structural failure that were the underlying causes of the crashes.[11] Investigations of these accidents also revealed the serious lack of basic knowledge about aircraft accident pathology. As a direct consequence, the Joint Committee on Aviation Pathology (JCAP), headquartered at the Armed Forces Institute of Pathology (AFIP) in Washington, D.C., was established to serve as a clearinghouse for aviation accident pathology.[12] Each of the military services subsequently included "life science" groups in their flying safety centers. The Aeronautical Center of the Federal Aviation Administration, in Oklahoma City, Oklahoma, became the repository for life science data in civil aviation. Some of the fundamental concepts of aviation accident pathology were developed by investigators associated with these agencies. However, many other organizations and individuals have also made major contributions to the present understanding of human function and malfunction in the flight environment, crash biodynamics, and crash injury analysis.

Thus has evolved the "human factors" concept in aviation accident investigation. This concept holds that the proximate, or contributory, cause of an accident may have been a human failure, and that such failure can be explicitly defined. Moreover, these human factors include all interactions between man and machine during the crash sequence and in the immediate post-crash environment. The various life science disciplines, including pathology, aviation medicine, physiology, toxicology, psychology, physical anthropology, and radiology, may be called into play. The pathologist's documentation of mechanical and thermotoxic injuries, together with manifestations of natural disease processes, provides the basic raw material for the human factors analysis. Human factors can now be interpreted within the context of the overall aircraft accident investigation.

MAGNITUDE OF THE PROBLEM

Aircraft accidents can be broadly grouped as air carrier, general aviation, or military. The National Transportation Safety Board (NTSB) statistics for 1976 list 45 air carrier fatalities and 1,273 deaths in general aviation.[13] Although no figures are available for military accidents during this period, another 500 to 600 fatalities seems to be a reasonable estimate.

The American air-transport fleet, including certificated air carriers, supplemental carriers, and commerical operators of large aircraft, had 28 accidents during 1976. Four of these accidents resulted in fatal injuries to passengers and/or crew members.[14] In 1970 there were no fatal accidents involving American flag air carriers. The collision of two fully loaded "jumbo" jetliners on the runway at Tenerife, Canary Islands, in 1977, caused the death of nearly 600 people. On the basis of recent trends, however, about 45 accidents, resulting in the death of 150 to 200 people, should be expected each year.

General aviation, in this discussion, refers to "light aircraft" operations involving personal, executive, air taxi, commuter, and aerial applicator aircraft. Over the past 5 years the number of accidents has been in the range of 4,250 to 4,650 per year, with 14 to 16 percent resulting in fatal injuries. Parenthetically, the number of people killed each year in general aviation accidents is about the same as die at railroad grade crossings (1,124 in 1976).[13]

A wide variety of aircraft are used by the military services. Many of these are passenger and/or cargo aircraft and light aircraft similar to those used in civil aviation. In addition, the military operates large numbers of high-performance fighter-type aircraft, large bombers, and many kinds of rotary wing aircraft (helicopters).

This potential caseload of about 2,000 aviation accident fatalities each year is distributed throughout the United States. By no means are all these crash victims examined at autopsy. Crew members of air carrier and military aircraft are routinely autopsied. Passengers of air carrier and military aircraft are often autopsied; however, these autopsies are frequently limited to the problems of victim identification and determination of a "cause of death." Only about one-third of fatally injured pilots of general aviation aircraft are autopsied, and few passengers.[15]

Autopsies of aviation accident victims are generally performed by local pathologists. Even in military accidents about one-half of all autopsies are conducted by civilian pathologists from nearby communities. Few pathologists, military or civilian, are experienced in the pathology of trauma. Fewer still are familiar with the injury patterns associated with specific types of aircraft and flight operations. The inexperience of the pathologists is, in large part, a function of relatively few fatal accidents distributed over a large geographic area. The low autopsy rate is a function of the organization and philosophy of the official investigating agencies.

INVESTIGATIVE AUTHORITY

The National Transportation Safety Board (NTSB), an independent agency of the United States government, has responsibility under federal law for investigating all civil aircraft accidents which occur within the territorial limits of the United States, and for determining the "probable cause" of each accident.[16,17] Safety Board personnel also act as accredited representatives to assist other governments in the investigation of accidents involving American flag or American-built aircraft. The NTSB Bureau of Accident Investigation investigates all civil airline and air-taxi accidents, all midair collisions, and most fatal general aviation accidents. Authority for investigating nonfatal general aviation accidents, involving aircraft having a gross weight of 12,500 pounds or less, is usually delegated by the NTSB to the Federal Aviation Administration (FAA).[18] However, the NTSB reviews all FAA-investigated accidents and determines the "probable cause."

In cases of accidents involving both military and civilian aircraft, military authorities participate in the NTSB investigations.[16] If an accident involves only military aircraft, but there is a possible association between the accident and an FAA employee, facility, or procedure, the FAA must be given an opportunity to participate in the military investigation.[19]

Although the formal "cause" determining process may vary from one country to another, the organizational format for on-the-scene investigations of major civil aviation accidents has been largely standardized by the International Civil Aviation Organization. This organization, with more than 100 contracting members, headquartered at Montreal, Canada, has worked to achieve uniformity of accident notification, investigation, and reporting procedures.[20]

In recognition of the importance of the autopsy as an integral part of the investigation of aircraft accidents resulting in fatalities, and to circumvent the problems encountered by federal investigators in obtaining prompt authorization for autopsies in the multitude of local jurisdictions, an amendment to the Federal Aviation Act of 1958 was enacted in 1962 that provided:

> In the case of any fatal accident, the Board is authorized to examine the remains of any deceased person aboard the aircraft at the time of the accident, who dies as a result of the accident, and to conduct autopsies or such other tests thereof as may be necessary to the investigation of the accident; provided that to the extent consistent with the needs of the investigation, provisions of local law protecting religious beliefs with respect to autopsies shall be observed.[21]

Investigations of accidents involving military aircraft are the responsibility of the branch of service owning the aircraft. Service regulations, directives, and instructions define the composition, authority, and function of the aircraft accident investigation boards.[22-25] Although the regulations differ in detail, each of the uniformed services is empowered to obtain autopsies of military personnel killed in aviation accidents when these accidents have occurred in areas of exclusive federal jurisdiction.[26] When a fatal accident occurs on property not exclusively federal, the military investigators must interact with state and local medicolegal investigative systems.

State and local medical examiners and coroners clearly have an interest in fatal aviation accidents. That death resulted from a mishap with an aircraft makes it no less sudden, unexpected, and violent than had some other type of vehicle been involved. Most states have medical examiner or coroner statutes broad enough to give local authorities jurisdiction over the remains of aircraft crash victims and to order the performance of autopsies without requiring authorization of a spouse or next of kin.[27] It is the local medicolegal authorities who must ultimately certify the deaths of crash victims.

NTSB authority to order the performance of autopsies is permissive and does not require that autopsies be performed on the victims of civil aircraft accidents. The military services do not share this independent autopsy authority; consequently, military accident investigators must be especially cognizant of local laws and establish cooperative relationships with local medicolegal authorities.

Investigations of military aircraft accidents which occur outside the territorial limits of the United States are subject to the local laws and status-of-forces agreements with the host nation.

ORGANIZATION OF CRASH SITE INVESTIGATIONS

Civil Aircraft Accidents

The nature and seriousness of an accident determine the character and magnitude of the investigative response of the NTSB. Most fatal general aviation accidents (650 to 750 per year) are investigated by a single air safety investigator from a regional NTSB field office. A catastrophic accident, such as an airliner crash, results in an investigative team of 10 or more specialists being dispatched from the Safety Board's Washington office. This investigative team is composed of specialists in aircraft structures, systems, power plants, maintenance, flight operations, air-traffic control, weather, and human factors. Obviously, only a few such full-scale investigations are conducted each year. It is also apparent that few pathologists will have occasion to be involved in the investigation of a major aviation accident.

As a practical matter, the air safety investigator seldom takes part in the initial activities at the scene of a fatal general aviation accident. By the time he reaches the crash site, many hours may have elapsed. Local fire and law enforcement authorities, together with the medical examiner or coroner, may have, of necessity, assumed jurisdiction. Wreckage may have been disturbed. Survivors may have been rescued and transported for medical treatment. The deceased may have been removed, possibly already embalmed or, less frequently, subjected to conventional "hospital-type" autopsy. Such autopsies are directed toward discovery of natural disease processes with little or no attempt to correlate injury patterns with crash dynamics.

The work product of the air safety investigator is a report designed to document the hardware and operations aspects of the accident, including the history of the flight, physical damage to the aircraft, type of equipment aboard, flight plan, weather conditions, airport specifications, and the adequacy of communications systems and navigation aids. The human factors portion of the report lists the pilot's training and experience, together with the raw statistics of survival, injury, and death. Comments are made about the relationships between gross injuries sustained, seating positions of pilot and passengers, and the failure of structures such as seat belts or seat-belt restraints. Reports of autopsies, if performed, and toxicologic analyses are included.[28]

Medical assistance is to be provided for the air safety investigator by the FAA regional flight surgeon or the local FAA aviation medical examiner (AME). Sometimes these consultants assist in the analysis of injuries. Seldom are they able to visit the crash site or provide guidance for the local pathologist.

These comments are not intended as criticism of the professionalism or competence of the air safety investigators or the local authorities who suddenly have to deal with fatally injured people in an unfamiliar physical and dynamic setting. In some jurisdictions, medical examiners, coroners, AMEs, and pathologists are extremely proficient in the assessment of the human factors aspects of aviation accidents. In general, however, the human factors analysis of fatal general aviation accidents is less than optimum.

A full-scale investigation of a catastrophic accident is directed by an NTSB investigator-in-charge, with Bureau of Technology specialists serving as the head of each of the working groups. These working groups are supplemented by "designated parties" including "those persons, Government agencies, and associations whose employees, functions, activities, or products were involved in the accident and who can provide suitable qualified personnel who will actively assist in the field investigations."[29] Investigators are provided by the airline concerned; the aircraft, powerplant, and equipment manufacturers; the professional associations of pilots, flight engineers, and cabin attendants; and several governmental agencies.

The "human factors group" consists of a number of knowledgeable and experienced investigators from a variety of organizations and specialties, including representatives of the airline, the professional associations, and the FAA regional flight surgeon. Additional personnel are sometimes provided by the FAA Civil Aeromedical Institute and the AFIP. Local fire department and civil defense representatives, the medical examiner or coroner, and local pathologists are also assigned to this working group.

Although initial fact-finding activities are directed toward specifically defined areas, these investigations are conceptually based on the principles of systems analysis and are oriented toward understanding the human, machine, and environmental factors which interacted before and during the crash sequence. The human factors group is concerned with:

1. The role of medical, human engineering, or behavioral factors in the causal sequence of events leading to the crash.
2. The relationships between crash dynamics and other factors in causing injury or death.[30]

NTSB investigations of major accidents can be conducted with extreme thoroughness because of the enormous investigative resources which may be brought to bear.

The factual sections of all NTSB aircraft accident reports (Group Chairman Reports; Reports of Investigations) are intended as public documents and are available from the NTSB. The Safety Board also issues formal reports on catastrophic accidents (Accident Reports; Briefs of Accidents).

Military Aircraft Accidents

Most fatal military aircraft accidents are investigated by Aircraft Accident Investigation Boards. Generally these boards are ad hoc committees of active duty military personnel assigned to the installation which operated the aircraft. Board members will include experienced aviators; specialists in flying safety, operations, and maintenance; and a physician. Representatives of aircraft, power-plant, and equipment manufacturers may participate in the field investigation. The Board, through its President, may enlist the assistance of various other federal agencies.

The medical member of the Board is usually a flight surgeon. A flight surgeon is a physician who has graduated from a specified course in aerospace medicine conducted by one of the military services, and who is assigned to flying-related duties. His specialized training is directed toward aviation physiology and the special medical problems associated with the flight environment. He will have had minimal training in aviation pathology. Usually he will have the assistance of an aviation physiologist who is expert in the specialized life support equipment used in high-performance military aircraft.

Although the AFIP, the military schools of aerospace medicine, and the military flying safety centers provide consultative services, they seldom offer direct assistance during the field investigation. Thus the flight surgeon, aviation physiologist, medical examiner, coroner, and local pathologist often comprise the entire human factors group.

AVIATION ACCIDENT PATHOLOGY

Patterns of Injury

Aircraft and, consequently, aircraft accidents come in many sizes and degrees of complexity. A medical investigator or pathologist familiar with the various types of aircraft and their flight operations (missions) can, in large measure, anticipate the general patterns of injury which will be exhibited by crash victims. Although this simplified classification of aircraft does not correspond to that used by the FAA for issuing type or airworthiness certificates, it is useful in discussing crash injury patterns and interpretative problems likely to be encountered.

LIGHT AIRCRAFT

These airplanes comprise the vast majority of the general aviation fleet and, properly, are what come to mind when one thinks of "private flying." They are also used for a variety of other purposes including nonscheduled passenger and cargo services, flight instruction, aerobatics, and special industrial and agricultural operations (the special problems of "crop dusters" will be discussed separately). Most business and executive aircraft are in this category. The military services also operate a large number of these aircraft.

Light airplanes have "fixed wings," meaning that the wings, which may be mounted above or below the fuselage, are attached in such a way that wings and fuselage move through the air at the same speed. The force (lift) which keeps the aircraft airborne is a function of the speed at which it moves through the air. Thus these aircraft are properly called "airplanes." Most light airplanes weigh between 2,000 and 4,000 pounds, although they may weigh as much as 12,500 pounds. Typically they are powered by one or more reciprocating engines. Most accommodate two to six people. Usually they are equipped with two sets of flight controls. Takeoff and landing speeds are generally on the order of 60 to 100 knots (kts.) Most cruise between 100 and 200 kts.

Since the majority of accidents take place during the landing and takeoff phases of flight, at relatively low speed, fatal injuries are often qualitatively similar to those seen in high-speed automobile accidents. Angles of ground impact are commonly rather shallow, so that the aircraft bounces or slides along the ground, reducing peak-decelerative loads, but subjecting occupants to forces in both vertical and horizontal planes.

During the crash sequence the victims are seated and wearing restraining devices, either lap belts or lap belt–shoulder harness combinations. Injuries of head, neck, and upper torso are related to the degree of upper torso flailing and structural deformation of the passenger compartment.[8]

Flailing injuries of extremities are commonplace. Legs may be injured by upward collapse of the passenger compartment floor. Vertical and lateral decelerative forces complicate the injury patterns.

In some instances, such as a crash in a flat spin, decelerative forces may be almost entirely in the vertical axis. Such forces commonly cause compressive injuries to the axial skeleton, together with traction and compression injuries of the internal organs.

Circumstances of the crash may result in relatively low peak-decelerative loads. A light airplane becoming entrapped in electric power lines may be gradually slowed and rather gently lowered to the ground. On the other hand, crash forces generated by a light airplane at cruising speed colliding with a fixed object, such as a mountain, may produce injury patterns similar to those seen in crashes of high-performance aircraft. Occasionally a light airplane experiences a major structural failure in flight,[31] or a midair collision. Crash forces in such accidents may approximate those which occur on ground impact from free-fall (about 115 to 120 ft/sec).

Fire is a major hazard in the crash of any powered aircraft. People who survive the decelerative forces of the crash are still threatened by the possibility of post-crash conflagration. Many factors determine whether or not a fire will occur. For this discussion it is sufficient to say that aviation fuel is readily volatilized during a crash, that there are many possible ignition sources, and that post-crash fires are common. Thermal damage complicates victim identification and assessment of mechanical injuries. The medical investigator or pathologist must differentiate premortem from postmortem burns and determine the relative importance of thermal (thermotoxic) and mechanical injuries. The possibility of in-flight fire, with thermotoxic injury and incapacitation having occurred prior to ground impact, must also be considered.

AERIAL APPLICATOR AIRCRAFT ("CROP DUSTERS")

Aerial applicator aircraft are specifically designed to carry and dispense chemical agents such as fertilizers, herbicides, defoliants, and insecticides. Occasionally they are used for seeding crops. Most are low-wing monoplanes. However, some designs have the wings mounted above the fuselage. Others are biplanes. (Helicopters are also occasionally used as aerial applicators.) Most "crop dusters" are powered by one reciprocating engine and have a single seat. Since these aircraft are routinely operated heavily loaded and close to the ground, in the vicinity of electric power lines, utility poles, trees, and other obstructions, there is ample opportunity for mishap.

The general concepts of crashworthiness[7] have been most extensively incorporated in the design and construction of aerial applicator aircraft built since the early 1960s.[32] These crash safety design features include:

1. A cockpit or cabin located as far back on the fuselage as possible to provide a maximum of energy-absorbing structure forward of the occupant(s).
2. Design of the cockpit or cabin as the strongest part of the airplane to prevent its collapse on impact or during roll-over.
3. Providing for rearward displacement of the engine during a crash without compromise of cockpit or cabin integrity.
4. Locating heavy structural components below and forward of the cockpit or cabin to prevent crushing of the occupant areas by inertial loads acting on these components during a crash.
5. Placement of a strong, smooth keel beneath the aircraft to prevent the aircraft from digging into or "plowing" the ground, and permitting deceleration time to be prolonged.
6. Locating fuel tanks away from the cockpit or cabin and engine to reduce the possibility of spilled fuel ignition and to increase escape time when a fire does occur.
7. Providing occupants with seat belt and upper torso restraints of sufficient strength to resist failure up to the point of complete collapse of the cockpit or cabin area.

Most injuries and deaths of aerial applicator pilots are not attributable to crash-induced failures of cockpit structures. Both lethal and nonlethal injuries more commonly result from failures of restraint equipment, seats, and roll-over structures.[33]

The toxicity of some of the materials carried and dispensed by these aircraft poses a major hazard. Among the insecticides are a variety of chlorinated hydrocarbons, arsenic compounds, nicotine salts, dinitrophenols, carbamates, and organophosphates. Paraquat is a commonly used contact herbicide. During the handling of bulk quantities of these materials, as in loading an aircraft's spray tanks, there is opportunity for toxic exposure of the pilot (and his ground crew). Thus the possibility of pilot poisoning, especially with an organophosphate, must be considered as a possible cause factor in any "crop duster" crash.

Toxic materials dispersed from ruptured cargo hoppers or spray tanks during a crash may contaminate the pilot, causing serious injury or death. Persons in the vicinity of the crash site, including rescue and investigative personnel, may be exposed. Consequently, the medical investigator or pathologist should promptly determine the nature of the aircraft's cargo, and if a toxic hazard exists, take appropriate measures to minimize exposure and ensure prompt treatment of poisonings. In nonfatal accidents it is essential that the physicians attending crash victims be informed of possible toxic exposure, since prompt and specific treatment may be lifesaving. For example, poisoning with a cholinesterase inhibitor, such as methyl parathion, may require treatment with large doses of atropine and pralidoxime (Protopam).

It should be noted that while considerable attention has been given to improving crash survival and occupant escape in military fighter-type aircraft and helicopters, and, recently, to improving crash safety standards for automobiles and other ground vehicles, rather little work has been directed toward providing similar protection for air transport passengers and crews.[35]

Fire may envelop a crashed airliner in a matter of a few seconds, or it may take several minutes. The cylindrical fuselage may act as a flue or chimney, drawing fire through the passenger compartment with gale-force winds. In addition to large quantities of smoke and carbon monoxide, a wide variety of other combustion products are liberated from burning fuel, lubricants, hydraulic fluid, and the plastic materials used in aircraft interiors. Among these combustion products are HCN, NO_x, HF, and HCl. The toxicology of these various combustion products, and their effects in combination with the inevitably present carbon monoxide, are the subject of research presently being conducted by the FAA Civil Aeromedical Institute,[36] the National Aeronautics and Space Administration (NASA), and others.

FIGHTER-TYPE AIRCRAFT

These high-performance airplanes are operated primarily by the military services. Most are advanced training or combat aircraft which carry either one or two aviators. Two-place aircraft may have side-by-side or tandem seating and two sets of flight controls. Takeoff and landing speeds of 150 to 170 kts are common. Cruising speeds are generally in the range of 500 to 600 kts. Many of these aircraft types are capable of sustained supersonic flight. Operating altitudes in excess of 40,000 feet are not unusual. However, some fighter-type aircraft are also routinely flown at high speed and low altitude, as on gunnery range or terrain-following missions.

As with other types of aircraft, mishaps terminating in crashes most often occur during the takeoff and landing phases of flight. However, specific kinds of missions of specific types of aircraft are also associated with an increased incidence of accidents. Fighter-type aircraft are frequently operated near the limits of human physiologic and psychomotor capability. Similarly, the aircraft are sometimes operated near the limits of their aerodynamic and structural capability. The Aircraft Accident Investigation Board has access to the accident history of the aircraft type involved in each crash. This well-documented "epidemiology" of military aircraft accidents is extremely useful to the crash investigators because it alerts them to the common "failure modes" of both the machine and its human operators.

Since unassisted bail-out is unlikely to be successful, fighter-type aircraft are equipped with "ejection systems." Occupants who fail to achieve in-flight escape will almost certainly be killed in a crash. Although some operational aircraft are fitted with modular escape systems, "ejection seats" are the standard escape device.

Ejection seats are designed to propel the seat and its occupant clear of the aircraft, release the restraining harnesses, separate the occupant from the seat, and initiate parachute opening. Typical vertical velocity during ejection is 50 to 70 ft/sec, with peak velocity being achieved in about 4 feet. The aviator is subjected to an 18 to 20 G acceleration. Elapsed time from initiation of ejection to parachute opening is about 1 second. During bail-out at high altitude, parachute opening is automatically delayed, and the aviator free-falls to lower altitude (about 15,000 feet) before an aneroid device deploys the parachute.

Modern ejection systems have an excellent record of reliability when used within the so-called ejection envelope; that is, within the limits of altitude, airspeed, aircraft attitude, and sink-rate for which the system was designed. Most fatalities occur either because the ejection system is activated so late in the accident sequence that effective parachute opening cannot be achieved prior to the victim's striking the ground, or because the circumstances of the accident preclude the opportunity to attempt bail-out. Occasionally, ejection is successfully accomplished and parachute opening achieved, but the aviator, nevertheless, is seriously injured or killed. The parachutist may, for example, land in trees or electric power lines, be dragged across the ground by high winds, land in a body of water and drown, or descend into the flaming wreckage of his own aircraft.

Paraquat is toxic on contact with skin and mucous membranes, and is extremely poisonous if ingested. Acute renal and liver failure may occur. Proliferative alveolitis sometimes develops. Since there is no effective antidote available, avoidance of exposure is of paramount importance.

The FAA aviation medical examiner and local poison control center may provide assistance in determining the degree of toxic hazard and in the management of poisonings.

ROTARY WING AIRCRAFT (HELICOPTERS)

Fixed-wing aircraft must maintain considerable forward speed to move the wings (airfoils) through the air rapidly enough to produce sustaining lift. Helicopters have wings, called "rotor blades," which are rotated at high speed in the horizontal plane above the fuselage. This rotating wing provides force for both sustentation and translational motion. There is no relationship between rotor blade speed and fuselage speed. Helicopters can rise and descend vertically, hover (remain stationary in flight over a spot on the ground), and fly forward, backward, or sidewise.

Most helicopters have a single rotor with two or more blades. Some of the larger or special purpose helicopters have two separate rotors. Power is provided by one or two engines which may be of either reciprocating or turbine type. Forward cruising speeds are generally between 80 and 150 kts.

Safety design considerations are complicated by the necessity of positioning the large and rapidly revolving rotor blades over the fuselage, and the need for locating heavy engines, gear boxes, fuel tanks, and occupants near the center of gravity beneath the gyroscope-like rotor. Weight limitations restrict the degree of structural stiffening of occupant areas. The need for unobstructed forward and downward vision places the pilot(s) in the nose of the aircraft where little aircraft structure is available to attenuate crash forces.

There are no injuries sufficiently distinctive to be called characteristic of a helicopter accident as opposed to a fixed-wing aircraft mishap.[34] Multiple fatal injuries are commonly caused by horizontal and vertical crash forces, collapse of cockpit or cabin structures, and crushing beneath engines and gear boxes. Head injuries are especially common among the pilots, associated with their exposed forward location. Protective helmets, which considerably reduce the likelihood of head injury, are routinely used by military aviators, but seldom by civilians.

Fire is of special concern in helicopter crashes. The fuel cells cannot be located any great distance from the occupants, and are usually directly beneath or behind the cockpit/cabin. Many victims survive the crash forces only to die in the subsequent conflagration. Consequently, considerable attention has been given to the development of crashworthy fuel systems which will withstand crash forces without fuel spillage.

AIR TRANSPORT AIRCRAFT

A wide range of aircraft types are used in transport operations. Small "airliners" are similar to the larger general aviation aircraft. At the other extreme are the enormous wide-bodied "airbuses" and the aircraft used in intercontinental service. The "typical" modern airliner is powered by two, three, or four turbine engines. It carries from a few people (as on training flights) to several hundred. Takeoff and landing speeds are on the order of 150 kts. Commonly these aircraft cruise at 400 to 600 kts, at altitudes between 20,000 and 40,000 feet. Occupant areas are pressurized to provide breathable air at high altitude.

Accidents terminating in ground impact at high speed result in disintegration of the aircraft and its occupants. Intermingled aircraft and human remains may be scattered over thousands of square yards. Fortunately, such crashes are uncommon. Much more frequently accidents occur during takeoff or landing, with shallow angles of ground impact. Deceleration time is prolonged, and peak G-loading is reduced. Energy is dissipated as the aircraft slides along the ground and its structural components are deformed by crash forces. The fuselage may remain relatively intact.

About one-half of the fatalities which occur in air transport accidents are not the result of impact injuries. Rather, they result from thermotoxic injuries during the post-crash fire.[10] To escape from the wreckage, passengers and crew must successfully reach, open, and pass through doors, emergency exits, or rents in the fuselage. As many as three-quarters of the exits are not used because of jamming, blockage, fire, smoke, or other factors.[35] Having escaped the confines of the aircraft, the survivors must move, or be moved, to a safe distance.

Injuries sustained during the decelerative phase of a crash, such as legs broken by flailing against seats, head injuries from impact against seats and tray tables, or perineal and buttocks injuries associated with downward failure of seats, may have incapacitated the victims. Correlation of injury patterns with crash dynamics and structures in the vicinity of each victim is essential to understanding the mechanisms of injury. Understanding of how injuries occur is the starting point in the development of more crashworthy equipment.

When a modern fighter-type aircraft crashes, even at relatively low speed and with a shallow angle of impact, it is likely to disintegrate. Fire commonly envelops the crash site. High speeds and/or high angles of ground impact produce crash scenes aptly described as "smoking holes." Thus, if in-flight escape was attempted but unsuccessful, the victim's body tends to be relatively intact. Injury patterns, then, reflect lethal events which occurred during or subsequent to bail-out. If the victim remains in the aircraft at ground impact, the body is likely to be fragmented.

Aviators who operate high-performance military aircraft wear life-support equipment including protective helmets, oxygen masks, parachutes, and G-suits. For extreme high-altitude flight, they are also fitted with partial-pressure or full-pressure suits similar to those used by astronauts. Malfunction of any of this equipment may be a "cause factor" in an accident, or may preclude successful in-flight escape from an impending crash. Thus it is essential that the medical investigator or pathologist have the expert assistance of a military flight surgeon and/or aviation physiologist when examining and removing the life-support equipment from a fatally injured aviator. Even in high-speed crashes, when the victim and his equipment are fragmented and widely distributed over the crash site, the experienced flight surgeon or aviation physiologist is often able to recover and assess the functional state of key life-support components.

A note of caution is warranted. Military aircraft sometimes crash with live ordnance, such as bombs and rockets, aboard. Unfired ejection seats contain ballistic and rocket charges which may remain capable of causing serious injury or death should they be inadvertently activated. The military services provide ordnance specialists who will disarm these devices. Personnel not essential to rescue and fire-fighting operations should not approach aircraft wreckage until it has been declared "safe" by the fire marshal and/or the ordnance specialists.

General Considerations

As in the investigations of other modes of violent death, autopsies of aviation accident victims are usually performed while only incomplete and sometimes inaccurate information is available from the death scene. Consequently, free exchange of information between pathologist and crash-site investigators is essential. Premature conclusions based solely on autopsy findings must be avoided.

The hardware and operations investigation at a crash site may extend over days or weeks. Components of wrecked aircraft, such as engines, flight instruments, and specific structural or functional components (plus flight data and cockpit voice recorders of air transport aircraft), are commonly removed from the crash site and forwarded for laboratory analysis by technical experts. The pathologist, because his subject matter is perishable, has only a single opportunity and a rather short time to make and document his observations.

Having received autopsy authorization from the local medicolegal authority or the NTSB, the pathologist should familiarize himself with the general features of the aircraft involved, the nature of the accident, and the specific interpretative problems likely to be encountered. A tour of the crash site, in company with the air safety investigator or flight surgeon, is especially helpful. An appreciation of the physical setting and some concept of crash dynamics greatly assist in the interpretation of injury patterns. Discussion with the primary investigators may alert the pathologist to medical, pathophysiologic, crash injury, or toxicologic problems of special concern. If possible, the investigating flight surgeon or aviation medical examiner should attend the autopsy.

The pathologist seldom is able to make an initial examination of aircraft crash victims while they are still in the wreckage. Usually the bodies will have been removed by rescue or firefighting personnel, often at the direction of the medical examiner or coroner. All too frequently the locations of victims within the aircraft will not have been recorded. Since interpretation of the postmortem examination depends on detailed knowledge of each victim's immediate surroundings and possible role in aircraft operation, this type of scene disturbance, innocently motivated, can jeopardize the entire human factors investigation. Therefore, the pathologist's first task is to establish the seating position or location of each victim within the cabin or cockpit. Sometimes photographs will have been taken of the victims in the wreckage. Often it will be necessary to identify and interview the people who moved the bodies. Although this matter may seem trivial, it is the author's experience that failure to firmly establish the seating positions of victims is a common deficiency which largely destroys the value of the most meticulous autopsies.

In no other type of death investigation is the pathologist more dependent on highly specialized technical assistance to interpret his observations. Injury patterns not understood at the time of autopsy may have critical significance when related to specific aircraft structures and crash dynamics. Natural disease processes which are "cause factors" in one accident sequence may be of little consequence in another. Similarly, the hardware and operations investigators and the flight surgeon must base many of their conclusions on autopsy and toxicologic findings. Clearly, documentation of observations made during postmortem examination, through photographs, roentgenograms, diagrams or drawings, and written narratives, is of extreme importance.

Comments on Documentation

Autopsy findings are eventually reduced to a written narrative, with accompanying anatomic drawings or diagrams, which constitutes the work product of the pathologist. These materials become part of the accident report prepared by the air safety investigator or the military Aircraft Accident Investigation Board. Photographs and roentgenograms of crash victims are not ordinarily forwarded as part of the official record, but rather are retained in the files of the medical investigator. Photography and roentgenography not only provide additional means of documentation, but when properly used are powerful investigative tools.

PHOTOGRAPHS

Photographic documentation begins at the crash site. The primary investigators take numerous photographs of the aircraft wreckage and surrounding terrain. Some of these photographs, which depict damage to aircraft structures but not the injuries to aircraft occupants, are included in the accident report. Additional photographs are usually taken for law enforcement, fire department, and medical examiner or coroner records. The medical investigator is well advised to take his own photographs of the crash scene with emphasis on the cockpit or cabin area of the aircraft and the locations at which bodies were recovered. Ideally, this photographic record begins before the bodies of the victims are removed. Crash sites, especially those of general aviation accidents, are seldom secure. Wreckage soon is disturbed and the value of scene information rapidly degraded.

Photographs of crash victims, clothed and then unclothed, with special attention directed toward external manifestations of injuries, even those injuries which appear inconsequential, should be taken under the good lighting conditions of the morgue. During the course of the postmortem examination, internal injuries and significant natural disease processes should be photographed. Thorough photographic documentation of broken hardware and human injuries greatly facilitates retrospective analysis of crash injury patterns.

ROENTGENOGRAMS

Roentgenographic examination of crash victims can provide significant information which is difficult or impossible to obtain by other means. Roentgenograms can be used to establish positive identification of crash victims when fingerprint or dental comparisons are not feasible. Anatomic sites, such as maxillary and frontal sinuses which are important in aviation physiology but seldom examined at autopsy, are readily visualized.[37] Radio-opaque foreign objects imbedded in bodies, such as bits of flight instruments or bomb fragments, are readily demonstrated. In the investigation of high-speed crashes, the author has used roentgenograms of debris collected at the crash site to locate fragments of human skeletal remains amid the rubble.

Certain roentgenographically demonstrable injuries are of special importance. For example, posterior dislocation of the thumb is characteristically found in the hand(s) gripping the control yoke or stick of an aircraft at the instant of impact. Upwardly displaced comminuted fractures of the metatarsals, with preservation of the integrity of the os calcis and phalanges (so-called aviator's fracture) occurs when the foot is being pressed with force against a rudder bar at impact. Such skeletal injury patterns, easily documented roentgenographically, may establish who was physically in control of the aircraft at the instant of impact.[38]

Roentgenography permits a more comprehensive examination of the axial skeleton than is possible during autopsy. Vertebral compression fractures, associated with high vertical loads, are readily demonstrated. Flexion and/or extension fractures can be categorized. Combinations of flexion and vertebral shearing fractures allow rough quantification of maximum crash forces.[38]

The frangible skeletal system records magnitude, direction, and rate of onset of mechanical force more vividly and more permanently than soft tissues. In a sense, roentgenography provides a means of observing and recording human "structural failure" caused by mechanical loads in excess of the "design limits." Unfortunately, the roentgenographic literature does not include a comprehensive catalogue of skeletal injuries incurred in aircraft accidents. Interpretation must, in large part, be based on extrapolation from roentgenographic experience with motor vehicular trauma, falls from height, and from the rather few published observations.

Toxicology in Aviation Accidents

Toxicologic analysis of body fluids and tissues of persons fatally injured in aviation accidents is an essential part of the human factors investigation. Collection of appropriate specimens is part of the autopsy. Chemical agents of primary concern are ethanol, carbon monoxide, prescription and over-the-counter medications, and illicit drugs. In special circumstances other toxic substances may be of importance, such as cyanide levels in certain air transport accidents. Blood cholinesterase, as an indirect indicator of exposure to certain insecticides, may be useful in aerial applicator accidents.

ETHANOL

Even mild degrees of ethanol intoxication significantly impair a pilot's ability to perform the intellectual and psychomotor tasks necessary to operate an aircraft safely. The NTSB considers blood ethanol levels of 0.050 percent or more as "possibly contributing factors" in aircraft accidents.

When the cadaver is in good condition, and clean blood, urine, and tissue samples are properly collected, preserved, transported, and analyzed by appropriate laboratory methods, problems of interpretation are minimized. When bodies are putrified, fragmented, immersed in water for prolonged periods, or contaminated with soil, vegetation, or aviation fuel, there are many opportunities for error and artifact.[39] Considerable research has been devoted to the problems of specimen contamination, especially by bacteria, and false ethanol determinations.[40]

CARBON MONOXIDE

Carbon monoxide is an emission product of aircraft engines and a combustion product of in-flight and post-crash fires. Faulty reciprocating engine exhaust systems or defective cockpit or cabin heaters may leak carbon monoxide into the occupant area. The toxicity of carbon monoxide increases as the partial pressure of oxygen decreases at higher altitudes.[41] Thus postmortem blood levels of carbon monoxide which might be of little significance at sea level produce significant pilot incapacitation at altitude. An elevated blood carbon monoxide level and soot in the airway may result from an in-flight fire or inhalation of combustion products in a post-crash fire. Thus interpretation of postmortem carbon monoxide levels requires detailed knowledge of the crash sequence and the other autopsy findings.

DRUGS

Toxicologic examination of pilots (and other aircrew members) should include a "drug screen" and quantification of any drug(s) detected. A pharmacologic agent may be present in sufficient concentration to be incapacitating and, therefore, a "cause factor" in an accident. The presence of therapeutic levels of certain drugs may provide clues to symptomatic natural disease. For example, an antihistamine would suggest the possibility of an upper respiratory tract infection which might predispose to acute barotitis media or barosinusitis, the attendant pain of either being capable of causing distraction or partial incapacitation during a critical phase of flight. Detection of quinidine would suggest a history of heart disease not documented in the victim's FAA or military medical records. Similarly, finding one or more of the various tranquilizers would prompt further inquiry into the aviator's psychological and psychiatric history.

The victim's personal effects should be searched for medication containers, and in instances where prescription drugs are discovered, the prescribing physician should be contacted in an effort to develop further medical history.

Not infrequently aircraft are used to convey bulk quantities of illegal drugs, such as cocaine, heroin, and marijuana. Occasionally the aircraft crash. The possible in-flight use of these pharmacologic agents must be considered.

SAMPLE COLLECTION AND PROCESSING

The importance of proper collection and preservation of fluid and tissue samples for toxicologic analysis cannot be overemphasized. Common errors include failure to collect any specimens, to collect scant specimens, to put multiple specimens in the same container, and to identify inadequately the specimens collected. In some medicolegal jurisdictions, bodies are routinely embalmed prior to autopsy, with blood samples, if taken at all, being pumped out of the cadaver by the pressure of injected embalming fluid. Clearly, the pathologist or medical investigator must attempt to protect the bodies of crash victims from both embalming and decomposition prior to autopsy. When adequate refrigeration is not available, the postmortem examination and specimen collection must be performed promptly.

Specimens which can be used for toxicologic analysis will vary, depending upon the circumstances of the accident. In high-speed crashes, for example, only fragments of skeletal muscle and marrow-containing bone may be available. In the majority of aviation accidents, however, rather complete sampling can be achieved. When possible the investigating AME, the FAA regional flight surgeon, or the military flight surgeon should be consulted concerning specimens to be collected and their subsequent disposition. Consultation with the toxicologist who will perform the analyses can be extremely helpful when "routine" samples are not available.

The following specimens, obtained from each fatally injured victim, will suffice in most cases:

Blood: 20 ml, or more, from heart, peripheral blood vessels, or body cavities (if uncontaminated by gastric contents or urine).
Urine: 100 ml, if available.
Visceral organs: 50 to 100 gm of each—liver, kidney, spleen, lung, skeletal muscle, and brain. (Each specimen should be packaged separately.)
Gastric contents: as available up to 100 ml. (Be sure to record total volume.)

All specimens, except blood, should be immediately frozen. The blood should be collected in sodium fluoride (NaF), 0.1 gm/10 ml of blood. Blood for cholinesterase determination must be collected in heparinized tubes.[42] Additional blood, collected in a "clot tube," may be used for blood typing. Blood samples should be refrigerated.

The FAA regional flight surgeon, AME, or military flight surgeon can arrange for toxicologic analysis of the collected materials. Specimens from fatally injured military personnel will be forwarded to the Armed Forces Institute of Pathology, in Washington, D.C. In civil accidents, local toxicologic services may be used, or the specimens may be shipped to the Aviation Toxicology Laboratory of the FAA's Civil Aeromedical Institute, in Oklahoma City, Oklahoma.

VITREOUS HUMOR

While collecting specimens for toxicologic analysis, the pathologist is well advised to obtain samples of vitreous humor from the eyes of each fatally injured victim. Several milliliters of vitreous, easily obtained with a syringe and small needle, can be analyzed for a variety of substances. In the author's laboratory, vitreous is routinely analyzed for glucose, acetone, urea, sodium, potassium, chloride, and ethanol. These chemical determinations are especially useful in "ruling out" metabolic states such as diabetic ketoacidosis and acute ethanol intoxication.[43]

Natural Disease in Aviation Accidents

Pilots (and other aircrew members) are required to have periodic physical examinations. Physical standards are prescribed and the examining physicians designated by the FAA or the military services. Persons found to have natural diseases which might compromise their ability to operate an aircraft, or which might result in their sudden incapacitation, are disqualified from being in primary control of an aircraft in flight. Occasionally, aviators conceal manifestations of serious chronic illness, such as angina pectoris, diabetes mellitus, idiopathic epilepsy, or malignancy from their AME or flight surgeon. Others choose to fly while suffering from acute conditions, such as respiratory tract infections, gastroenteritis, or migraine headache.

Minor degrees of physiologic or psychologic upset may reduce a pilot's level of judgment or physical coordination. Pain, such as odontalgia, may produce significant distraction. Physiologic aberrations, such as the nausea of airsickness, spatial disorientation, and the respiratory alkalosis of anxiety-induced hyperventilation, may seriously compromise an aviator's ability to perform the complex intellectual and physical tasks required for safe aircraft operation.[44] Sudden collapse and/or death may result from such afflictions as acute coronary arterial insufficiency, ischemic or hemorrhagic cerebral infarcts, ruptured intracranial aneurysms, or spontaneous pneumothorax. Incapacities ranging from mild physiologic disturbances[37,45] to sudden death[46] have been clearly established as the causes of specific accidents.

At autopsy, pilots manifest the same range of natural diseases as their passengers or any other group of reasonably healthy adults who die violent deaths. To avoid serious error, autopsy findings must not be interpreted out of context. For example, severe coronary arterial atherosclerosis and a healing myocardial infarct in a pilot might mean that a crash occurred because of in-flight incapacitation and/or death of the aircraft operator. The interpretation is quite different, however, if the engineering analysis of the aircraft wreckage, corroborated by the flight data recorder, indicates that the aircraft, while in straight and level flight, sustained a major structural failure due to a design deficiency and metal fatigue. A brain tumor might have initiated a grand mal seizure, causing complete incapacitation of the pilot, loss of control, and crash. The tumor might be an incidental finding if that pilot could not have been in control of the aircraft at any time in the crash sequence.

The pathologist's primary responsibility is to observe and to document. Final interpretation should be a collaborative effort between the pathologist and the other human factors investigators, within the framework of the entire accident investigation.

Objectives of the Autopsy

The objectives of the autopsy examination of aircraft crash victims can now be summarized in a series of questions:

1. Who died?
2. What was the "cause of death"?
3. What was the manner of death?
4. What specific interactions between victim and aircraft structures or components resulted in fatal injuries?
5. If the aircraft had provisions for in-flight escape, why did the victim(s) fail to escape?
6. If the victim(s) survived the decelerative forces of the crash, why did they fail to escape from the lethal post-crash environment?
7. What role, if any, did the victim(s) play in causing the crash?
    a. Who was flying the aircraft?
    b. Was the pilot incapacitated?
    c. Were physiologic aberrations initiating or contributory cause factors in the accident?

The first three questions are addressed during the course of every medicolegal autopsy since the answers are required for issuance of a death certificate. The remaining questions define the basic subject area of aviation pathology.

Comments on Death Certification

Identification of persons fatally injured in aircraft crashes is of great importance to the living. Insurance policies, estates, wills, remarriages, business partnerships, and fraudulent attempts to simulate death all depend on positive identification. The usual means of identifying victims include:

1. Visual recognition by relatives or friends;
2. Fingerprint comparisons;
3. Dental comparisons;
4. Roentgenographic comparisons;
5. Clothing, documents, and jewelry on or near the body;
6. Exclusion.

In most general aviation accidents, victim identification presents few difficulties. Crashes of high-performance and air transport aircraft present formidable identification problems.[47] The pathologist should not hesitate to ask for assistance. Law enforcement agencies, including the Federal Bureau of Investigation, provide the most direct and immediate help. The NTSB or the military service can arrange for whatever additional assistance is required. However, the pathologist should retain responsibility for coordinating victim identification.

"Cause of death" can usually be expressed in a phrase such as "multiple injuries" or "craniocerebral injuries," which summarizes the detailed documentation of these injuries in the pathologist's records. On rare occasions, death from natural disease will have preceded the crash.

The phrases "aircraft crash" and "aircraft accident" are commonly used interchangeably, as in the present discussion. However, all aircraft crashes are not accidents, nor is the "manner of death" necessarily the same for all victims found in the wreckage. A pilot may suffer a "natural death" while at the controls of an aircraft. The passengers in that same aircraft will die "accidentally" in the ensuing crash. On occasion, aircraft are used as instruments of suicide[48] and/or homicide. Thus determination of the "manner of death" cannot be based solely on autopsy findings, but rather requires knowledge of the overall circumstances of the crash.

Summary

Autopsy of aircraft accident victims has several interrelated objectives. The legal and moral requirement is positively to identify the decedents and to establish the cause and manner of their deaths. Beyond this, the pathologist and medical investigator are concerned with understanding those interactions between the aircraft and its occupants which may have been factors in causing the accident and which contributed to injury and/or death during the crash sequence. Participation in the human factors investigations of these accidents offers the pathologist opportunity to make significant contributions to aviation safety.

REFERENCES

1. Hass, G. M.: Types of Internal Injuries of Personnel Involved in Aircraft Accidents. *J. Aviation Med.* 15:77–84, 92, 1944.
2. DeHaven, H.: Mechanical Analysis of Survival in Falls from Heights of Fifty to One Hundred and Fifty Feet. *War Med.* 2:586–596, 1942.
3. Strughold, H.: Development of Aviation Medicine in Germany, in *German Aviation Medicine, WW II.* Vol. 1. U.S. Government Printing Office, Washington, D.C., 1950.
4. Hass, G. M.: Relations Between Force, Major Injuries and Aircraft Structures with Suggestions for Safety in Design of Aircraft. *J. Aviation Med.* 15:395–400, 1944.
5. Stapp, J. P.: Human Exposures to Linear Decelerations. Part II—The Forward-facing Position and Development of a Crash Harness. Air Force Technical Report No. 5915. Wright Air Development Center, December 1951.
6. DeHaven, H.: Accident Survival—Airplane and Passenger Automobile. Crash Injury Research, Cornell University Medical College, New York, January 1952.
7. DeHaven, H.: Development of Crash Survival Design in Personal, Executive and Agricultural Aircraft. Crash Injury Research, Cornell University Medical College, New York, May 1953.
8. Swearingen, J. J.: General Aviation Structures Directly Responsible for Trauma in Crash Decelerations. Special Report AM-71-3, Federal Aviation Administration, Washington, D.C., January 1971.

9. Mason, J. K.: Escape from Aircraft in Flight, in *Aviation Accident Pathology*. Butterworth, London, 1962, pp. 22–44.
10. Snow, C. P., Carroll, J. J., and Allgood, M. A.: Survival in Emergency Escape from Passenger Aircraft. Special Report AM-70-16, Federal Aviation Administration, Washington, D.C., October 1970.
11. Armstrong, J. A., Fryer, D. I., Stewart, W. A., and Wittingham, H. E.: Interpretation of Injuries in the Comet Aircraft Disasters—An Experimental Approach. *Lancet* I:1135–1144, 1955.
12. Reals, W. J.: Concepts and Development of Aviation Pathology, in Mason, J. K., and Reals, W. J. (eds.): *Aerospace Pathology*. College of American Pathologists Foundation, Chicago, 1973.
13. National Transportation Safety Board: Special Report SB 77–26, Washington, D.C., May 14, 1977.
14. National Transportation Safety Board: Special Report SB 77–2, Washington, D.C., January 13, 1977.
15. Personal communication.
16. The Federal Aviation Act of 1958, August 23, 1958, as amended (72 Stat. 731, 49 U.S.C. 1301).
17. The Transportation Safety Act of 1974, Title III: Independent Safety Board Act of 1974 (88 Stat. 2156, 49 U.S.C. 1901).
18. *Code of Federal Regulations.* Vol. 14, Section 400.45.
19. Title 19, U.S.C. Section 1442.
20. *International Standards and Recommended Practices for Aircraft Accident Inquiry.* Annex 13 to the Convention on International Civil Aviation. International Civil Aviation Organization, Montreal, Canada. ed. 2. March 1966.
21. Title 49, U.S.C., Section 1441(c).
22. AFR-127-4: *Investigating and Reporting USAF Mishaps.*
23. AFM-127-1: *Aircraft Accident Prevention and Investigation.*
24. AR 95-5: *Aircraft Accident Prevention, Investigation, and Reporting.*
25. OPNAV 3750-6: *Naval Aircraft Accident, Incident, and Ground Accident Reporting Procedures.*
26. Lilienstein, O. C.; Jurisdictional Problems in the Autopsy of Aircraft Accident Victims. *Aerospace Med.* 43:675–678, 1972.
27. Wecht, C. H.: *The Medico-Legal Autopsy Laws of the Fifty States, the District of Columbia, American Samoa, the Canal Zone, Guam, Puerto Rico, and the Virgin Islands.* rev. ed. American Registry of Pathology, Armed Forces Institute of Pathology, Washington, D.C., 1971.
28. FAA AC 70-3541: *Basic Aircraft Accident Investigation Procedures and Techniques.* Training Manual, Course N-IPT-1, National Aircraft Accident Investigation School, Federal Aviation Administration Aeronautical Center, Oklahoma City, Oklahoma, May 1970.
29. National Transportation Safety Board: Procedural Regulation 14 CFR (5), Part 431: *Rules of Practice in Aircraft Accident Inquiries.*
30. Bruggink, G. M., and Danaher, J. W.: International and Domestic Aspects of Aircraft Accident Investigations, in Mason, J. K., and Reals, W. J. (eds.): *Aerospace Pathology*. College of American Pathologists Foundation, Chicago, 1973.
31. Snyder, R. G.: Inflight Structural Failures Involving General Aviation Aircraft. *Aerospace Med.* 43:1132–1140, 1972.
32. Walhout, G. J.: Crashworthiness Observations in General Aviation Aircraft Investigations—A Statistical Overview, in Saczalski, K., Singley, G. T., Pilkey, W. D., and Houston, R. L. (eds.): *Aircraft Crashworthiness.* University Press of Virginia, Charlottesville, 1975.
33. Swearingen, J. J., Wallace, T. F., Blethrow, J. G., and Rowlan, D. E.: Crash Survival Analysis of 16 Agricultural Aircraft Accidents. Special Report AM-72-15, Federal Aviation Administration, Washington, D.C., 1972.
34. Miller, D. F., and Sand, L. D.: Helicopter Deaths, in Mason, J. K., and Reals, W. J. (eds.): *Aerospace Pathology*. College of American Pathologists Foundation, Chicago, 1973.

35. Synder, R. G.: Advanced Techniques in Crash Impact Protection and Emergency Egress from Air Transport Aircraft. Report AGARD-AG-221, North Atlantic Treaty Organization, Advisory Group for Aerospace Research and Development, 1976.
36. Personal communication.
37. Simson, L. R.: Investigation of Fatal Aircraft Accidents: Physiological Incidents. *Aerospace Med.* 42:1002–1006, 1971.
38. Simson, L. R.: Roentgenography in the Human Factors Investigation of Fatal Aviation Accidents. *Aerospace Med.* 43:81–85, 1972.
39. Wootton, D. G.: Error and Artifact in Postmortem Toxicological Analysis. *Aviat. Space Environ. Med.* 46:1280–1283, 1975.
40. Smith, P. W., Lacefield, D. J., and Crane, C. R.: Toxicological Findings in Aircraft Accident Investigation. *Aerospace Med.* 41:260–262, 1970.
41. Heim, J. W.: The Toxicity of Carbon Monoxide at High Altitudes. *J. Aviation Med.* 10:211–215, 1939.
42. Handbook 8025.1: *Aviation Medicine Participation in Aircraft Accident Investigations.* Federal Aviation Administration, Washington, D.C., March 30, 1970.
43. Coe, J. I.: Postmortem Chemistries on Human Vitreous Humor. *Am. J. Clin. Pathol.* 51:741–750, 1968.
44. Simson, L. R.: Physiological and Psychological Investigations of Fatal Aircraft Accidents, in Mason, J. K., and Reals, W. J., (eds.): *Aerospace Pathology.* College of American Pathologists Foundation, Chicago, 1973.
45. Rayman, R. B.: Sudden Incapacitation in Flight. *Aerospace Med.* 44:953–955, 1973.
46. Leighton-White, R. C.: Airline Pilot Incapacitation in Flight. *Aerospace Med.* 43:661–664, 1972.
47. Jerman, A. C., and Tarsitano, J. J.: The Identification Dilemma. *Aerospace Med.* 39:751–754, 1968.
48. Jones, D. R.: Suicide by Aircraft: A Case Report. *Aviat. Space Environ. Med.* 48:454–459, 1977.

CHAPTER 16

Charles S. Petty is Director of the Southwestern Institute of Forensic Sciences at Dallas, Chief Medical Examiner of Dallas County, Director of the Dallas County Criminal Investigation Laboratory, and Professor of Pathology and Forensic Sciences at the University of Texas Southwestern Medical School at Dallas. Dr. Petty holds degrees in pharmacy and physiology from the University of Washington and received his medical education at Harvard Medical School. He is a diplomate of the American Board of Pathology in pathologic anatomy, clinical pathology, and forensic pathology. Dr. Petty is former President of the American Academy of Forensic Sciences and is a Fellow of the American Association for the Advancement of Science, the American College of Physicians, the American Society of Clinical Pathologists, and the British Academy of Forensic Sciences.

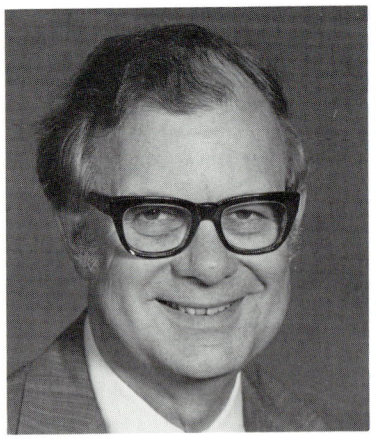

DEATH BY TRAUMA: BLUNT AND SHARP INSTRUMENTS AND FIREARMS*

Charles S. Petty, M.D.

This chapter is concerned with trauma-related deaths generally and with certain types of trauma in particular. Included in the latter group is trauma resulting from blunt or sharp instruments and firearms. Several other chapters in this text examine other types of trauma-related death due to various causes of significance in medicolegal investigation.

Trauma, or injury, in the usual forensic sense, implies the application of a trauma-producing agent in such a manner that the victim's state of healthy equilibrium is suddenly altered from the norm. Thus the healthy and normally functioning individual suffers immediately from the effects of the trauma-producing agent. The result is a wound, with attendant bleeding and/or shock, or an alteration or cessation of function. It is unusual, although not unknown, for a succession of small traumas to aggregate their effects over a prolonged period of time, so as to eventually alter the victim's function and thus his health.

Trauma-producing agents of forensic importance have been classified in many ways. They have been grouped under headings such as mechanical force, thermal actions, chemical agents, electromagnetic force, asphyxia, and embolic trauma. As seen in medicolegal practice, combinations of trauma frequently occur, caused by a single agency. Thus the trauma resulting from a motor vehicle crash can be of several types: mechanical and thermal, and occasionally chemical, electromagnetic, and/or asphyxial. The classification of trauma becomes, of necessity, a mixture depending upon the producing agency and also the producing force or event.

---

*The author is indebted to Donald W. Calhoun, forensic photographer at the Southwestern Institute of Forensic Sciences in Dallas, for providing most of the photographs which illustrate this chapter.

BLUNT-FORCE TRAUMA

Two major varieties of blunt force trauma are frequently encountered: the moving blunt instrument which impacts the relatively unmoving victim, and the moving victim who directly encounters the unmoving object. In some instances the results are similar; in others they are quite different. In some cases it may be possible for the examining pathologist to determine whether the wounding object or the body was in motion at the time of the application of force. In other situations such a determination will not be possible.

Regardless of the object or the instrument causing the injury, there are but few ways in which the tissues or organs of the body can exhibit damage. An injury caused by mechanical force results in one or more of the following:

1. Abrasion,
2. Laceration,
3. Contusion or rupture,
4. Fracture,
5. Compression,
6. Bleeding.

These six hallmarks associated with, but not necessarily exclusive to, blunt force injury are in themselves overlapping and in a real sense not pure denominators of such trauma.

Abrasion

Abrasion implies a rubbing away of the skin. It may be superficial, when only the external skin (epidermis) is rubbed away, or the injury may be deeper and extend into the underlayer of skin (dermis) or still deeper into the soft tissue beneath the skin (subcutaneous layer). If the abrasion extends further than simply the epidermis, blood vessels may be entered and bleeding will ensue. The direction in which the force was applied may be determined by an examination of the abraded area. Two clues may be observed. First is the direction in which the epidermis is rolled up. Figure 16-1 shows an abrasion in which the direction of force is from the lower right to the upper left. The second clue is the presence of parallel deeper portions of the abrasion, indicating the irregularities of the abrading object. Thus, as is shown in Figure 16-2, the direction of force is in the horizontal dimension of the figure, rather than the vertical. This, combined with the topography of the body area involved (the "shadows" of no abrasion in the low and somewhat protected areas), would indicate that the force was from right to left in the figure, rather than from left to right.

Note that in each illustrated instance either the body itself or the abrading instrument could have moved. All that is required to produce the effect of abrasion is that there be relative motion between the two.

The pattern of the abrasion may indicate the shape or something of the nature of the abrading object. Thus the edge of a piece of five-layer plywood may cause an abrasion that has five separate ridges (Fig. 16-3). The age of the abrasion cannot be determined with certainty by an examination of the wound with the naked eye. When the epidermis alone has been rubbed away, a slight color change and roughening may be the only

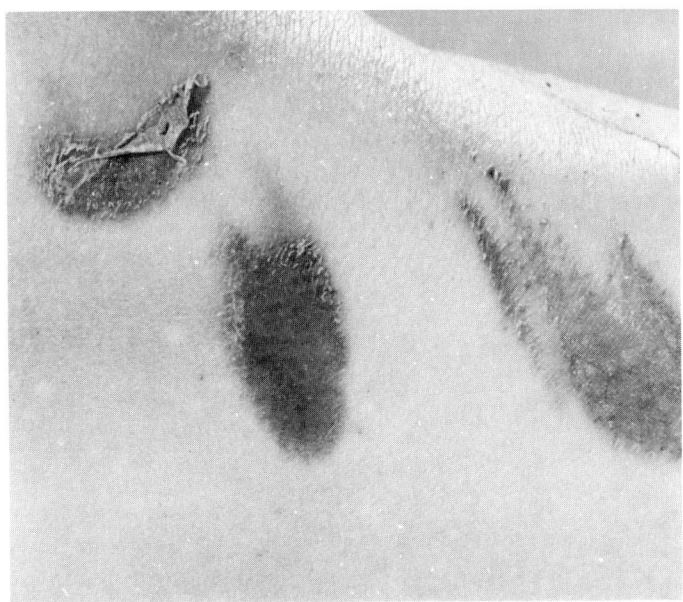

FIGURE 16-1. Superficial abrasion. The direction in which the force was applied is from the lower right to the upper left of the figure as evidenced by the rolling-up of the epidermis.

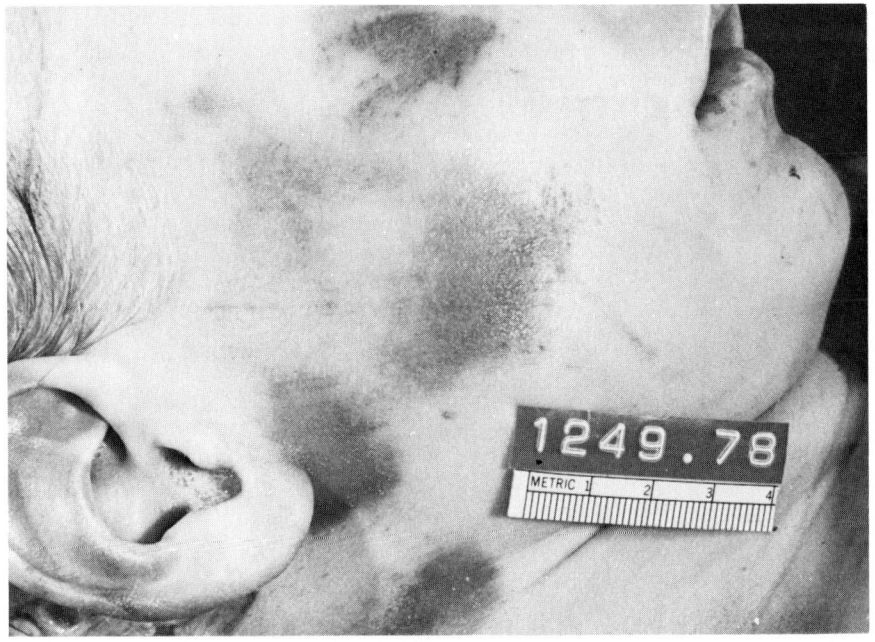

FIGURE 16-2. Abrasion of face and neck. The parallel deeper portions indicate the direction of application of force from right to left. Had the direction of force been from left to right, the shadowing effect would have been different.

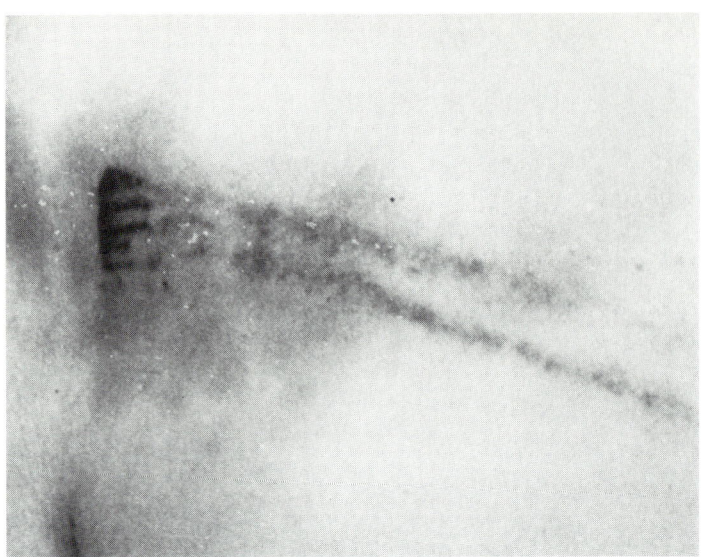

FIGURE 16-3. Abrasion of the chest and shoulder. The victim was struck by a piece of five-layer plywood. The layers of the plywood have produced a pattern of abrasion on the skin. The faint discoloration of the skin adjacent to the left (patterned) end of the abrasion is due to contusion.

difference to be noted between the abnormal area and the surrounding normal skin. Rapid return to the natural state is expected with epithelial cells replacing themselves in a normal manner. When the dermis has been entered, tissue fluids admixed with red blood cells and those cells of repair called forth by the injury (white blood cells) rapidly form an eschar (also termed crust or scab) which covers and protects the injured area while regrowth of the epithelium takes place from the periphery and those remaining isolated epithelial islands more centrally located. In the instance of an abrasion which extends into the subcutaneous tissue, the bleeding may be more noticeable, and tissue fluid loss is more marked. Here epithelialization is from the periphery unless islands of epidermis remain centrally; eschar formation is conspicuous.

A rough estimate of the age of an abrasion may occasionally be made upon a painstaking microscopic examination of the area of the abrasion. The age, however, cannot be determined with precision. For practical description, it may, at best, be categorized as of very recent origin (within a few hours), recent (a few hours to a day), a few days old, or older than several days. More precision is not possible because of the variation in the nature (depth, area, location, extent of infection) of differing wounds and the variability of the reaction of the individual to wounds.[1]

Remote effects of abrasions are relatively rare. Bleeding is not severe because only tiny blood vessels are involved. Loss of tissue fluids is usually also minimal. Hemorrhage and tissue fluid loss are not productive of remote effects unless the abraded area is extremely large. Infection can take place and may cause generalized (remote) effects. Because of the surface nature of the wound, bacteria whose growth is depressed by oxygen are not expected to establish a foothold. However, foreign material rubbed from the abrading object may be contaminating and may not only bring bacteria to the area, but also cause nidi of tissue (foreign body) reaction and continuing bacterial growth. The festering wound may then

TABLE 16-1. ABRASIONS—MEDICOLEGAL SIGNIFICANCE

Affect skin surfaces or rarely mucous membranes

Force:
  An indication that force has been applied to the surface.
  May indicate the direction in which force was applied:
    from parallel deeper portions of the abrasion;
    from rolled-up superficial skin (epidermis).
Pattern:
  May indicate something of the nature of the abrading object (weapon, tire, etc.).
Alteration with age:
  Depends to large extent upon depth of abrasion.
    Very superficial (epidermis) heals by simple growth of cells.
    Deeper (involving dermis) heals by gradual filling in from islands of remaining epidermis, and the peripheral epidermis.
    An eschar (scab or crust) may form over the weeping surface.
    Deep abrasions, with total destruction of central epidermis, will heal from the periphery with the pink rejuvenating epidermis growing toward the center under the eschar or scab.
    Microscopic examination may enable a very rough approximation of age to be made.
Pathophysiology:
  Bleeding not severe because large blood vessels not involved.
  If integrity of epidermis is lost, a portal of entry for bacteria will result.
  Large, more than just epidermal-deep abrasions may allow much leakage of protein and electrolyte-containing tissue fluids. Only in extreme instances does this cause metabolic upset.

continue to serve as a source for bacteria to be distributed throughout the body (Table 16-1).

Superficial (Subcutaneous) Contusions

The lay term for superficial contusion is "bruise." The force responsible for the contusion causes very rapid tissue compression over a very short time period. This results in tearing and rupturing of small blood vessels in the tissue (subcutaneous, muscle, etc.) or organ (lung, heart, liver, kidney, etc.) involved. It is the subsequent bleeding that is noted as a bruise when the subcutaneous tissue is involved. The hemorrhage is noted through the overlying intact skin as a blue-black-purple discoloration and, in some instances, swelling of the involved area.

Unlike some abrasions, examination of a superficial contusion cannot reveal the direction in which the contusing force was applied, nor can the examination of the contusion alone indicate whether the moving body struck the object or vice versa. However, the location of contusions involving the subcutaneous tissue can indicate certain things of forensic importance. Bruises on the backs of the fingers, hand, and forearms may indicate a defensive action or posture on the part of the victim (Fig. 16-4). Multiple small contusions on the arms just below the level of the shoulders, sometimes in the expected pattern of fingerpads, indicate forceful grasping of the arms during a struggle or during the act of rape (Fig. 16-5).

Bleeding beneath the skin, the "bruise" of the layman, is readily visible because of the discoloration due to the red blood. In persons with heavily pigmented skin, the subcutaneous accumulation of blood may not be readily visible; indeed, contusions may be better felt (because of swelling of the tissue) than seen. As the bruise becomes older and the accumulation of blood ceases, body mechanisms come into action which cause

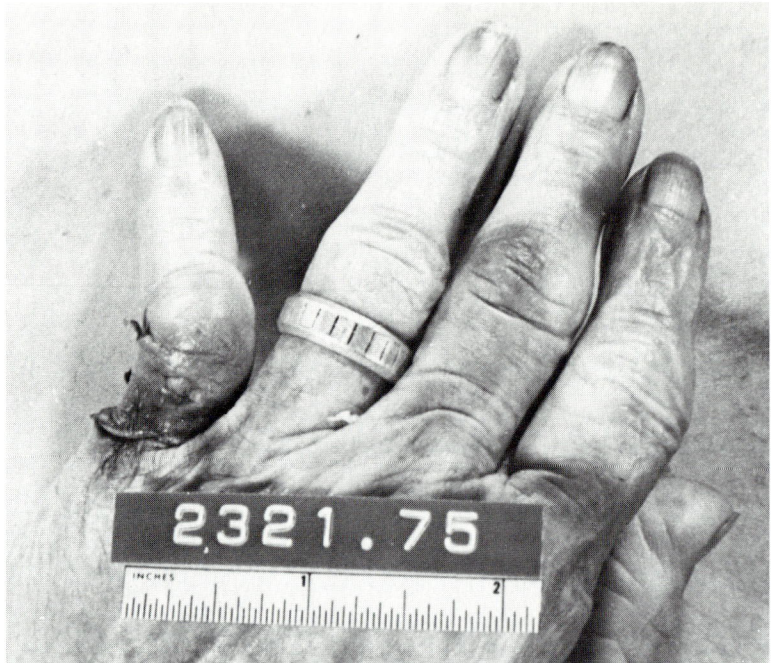

FIGURE 16-4. Contusions on fingers and hand. The fingers are discolored and somewhat swollen by the contusions sustained when the victim attempted to ward off the blows of her assailant. There is a fracture of a bone of the fifth finger.

breakdown of the hemoglobin (the red pigment of the blood) to other colored pigments, which are then eventually removed. Thus it is that the original blue-purple-black contusion (bruise) changes in color and then eventually fades. The color change is most easily seen at the periphery of the wound, where the change is first to green, then yellow, with gradual

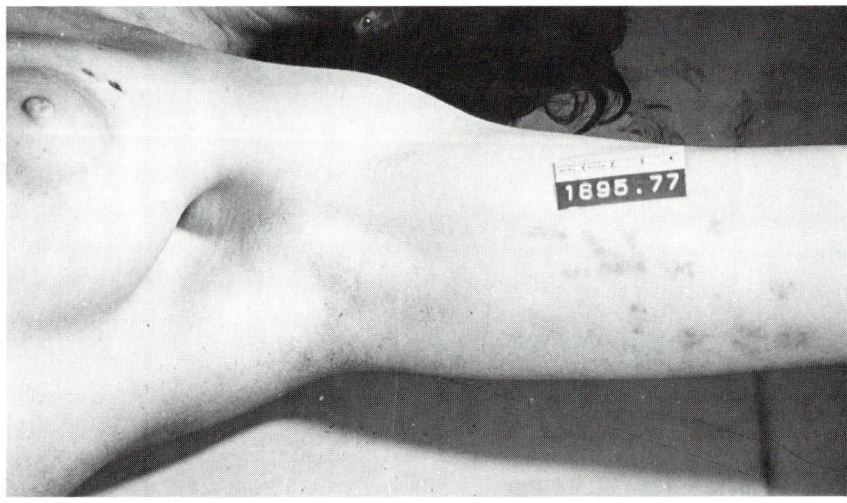

FIGURE 16-5. Contusions of arm. The small, discrete contusions of the inner aspect of the arm resulted when the subject was grabbed and held by the arm while being attacked.

alteration of the color of the entire contusion, then fading, and eventual disappearance.

Both the color change and fading of the wound are time-related. Obviously a yellow-green contusion is older than a blue-purple one. But how much older? Unfortunately the time sequence of the color change varies greatly from one wound to another, and from one person to another. No precise rate of color change can be accurately predicted. By external examination alone, no more precision can attend the determination of the age of the subcutaneous contusion than is possible for the aging of abrasions.[2] One important source of misinformation about contusions affecting the subcutaneous tissue is photography. Contusions appear much more pronounced in black and white photographs than by direct observation of the wounds themselves. It follows, then, that color photographs (with proper color balance) more truly reproduce contusions than do black and white photographs. This is true notwithstanding the fact that some courts reject color photographs in favor of black and white photographs, perhaps because of a desire to eliminate the color of blood, without realizing that blood, even beneath the skin, will appear black on the colorless (black and white) photograph.

A factor to be kept in mind in relation to the appearance of subcutaneous contusions (bruises) is the time after death of the viewing of the wounds. Every pathologist who has had the opportunity to observe a contused body newly dead and then to re-examine the body several hours later has noted the sometimes marked increase in the darkness and therefore the visibility of contusions. In some such instances contusions may be observed that were not noted at the time of the first examination. Thus the interval between death and observation of the body has some bearing upon the appearance of the contusion. The necessity to wait for the arrival of the photographer, increasing the time between death and photography, coupled with black and white photographs of the wounds, may yield rather different-looking contusions than those described originally by the pathologist.

Microscopic examination of contusions is a technique that is used to gain some idea of the time that elapsed from the infliction of the wound to death. However, as is the case with abrasions, only a very general approximation of the interval may be gained by such examination. Minute and hour delineation cannot be made.[3,4] During the first few hours, the so-called very recent injury presents little or no observable alteration from one just inflicted. After 3, 4, or more hours, beginning changes in the cellular reaction to the injury are observable upon microscopic examination. As more time elapses, more pronounced changes are seen. The cellular reaction present may be totally due to the body's reacting to the injury alone, or to a mixture of reaction to injury and to an incidental infection which may be present. Earliest scar tissue formation may not be observable until 2, 3, or even 4 days have elapsed. It cannot be overemphasized that the determination of the duration of the interval between contusion and death is without precision even when carried out by highly skilled and experienced pathologists. Indeed, the degree of reluctance of the examiner to pinpoint the time interval may be a measure of his competence.

The remote, or pathophysiologic, effects of contusions are several. Since a contusion is the result of the tearing of blood vessels with escape of blood into the soft subcutaneous tissue, the volume of the remaining circulating blood is depleted by each contusion. Multiple and massive contusions can so severely decrease the amount of circulating blood that shock, with mental confusion, fainting, and even death may result. Such cases are rare, but are seen by medicolegal investigators, as the following examples point out:

Example 1. A young woman (Fig. 16-6), being severely beaten with fists, withstood the pummeling well for many minutes. She then gasped, "Honey, you have hurt me," became confused, and soon lost consciousness. The assailant then drove her to a hospital. Shortly after arrival, she died. Autopsy revealed only massive, widespread contusions of the head, trunk and extremities. There were no internal injuries. Death was due to the loss of circulating blood into the subcutaneous tissue. The manner of death was homicide.

Example 2. A middle-aged man, working as an elevator maintenance man, tumbled through an open elevator shaft door and fell two stories. He was found dead at the bottom of the shaft. Extensive, huge contusions involved the subcutaneous tissue of the back, buttocks, thighs, and arms. Distortion due to the bleeding into these bruises was extreme. No internal injuries and no fractured bones were found. Death was ascribed to the extensive loss of blood into the subcutaneous tissues noted above. The manner of death was certified as accidental.

A second remote or pathophysiologic effect of subcutaneous contusions is aggregation of blood beneath the skin, resulting in an interruption of the return of venous blood from that part of an extremity (arm or leg) further from the trunk than the contusion itself. Since circulation is thus denied to the part, gangrene and death of tissue can result.

A third remote effect of a contusion is the formation of a place for bacterial growth in the medium of pooled or sequestered blood. Many bacteria grow well in blood, and a focus of serious infection can result. Associated with the extravascular blood is the tissue destruction and dead tissue due to the crushing of the tissue incident to the production of the contusion itself. The dead tissue, together with slowed or absent circula-

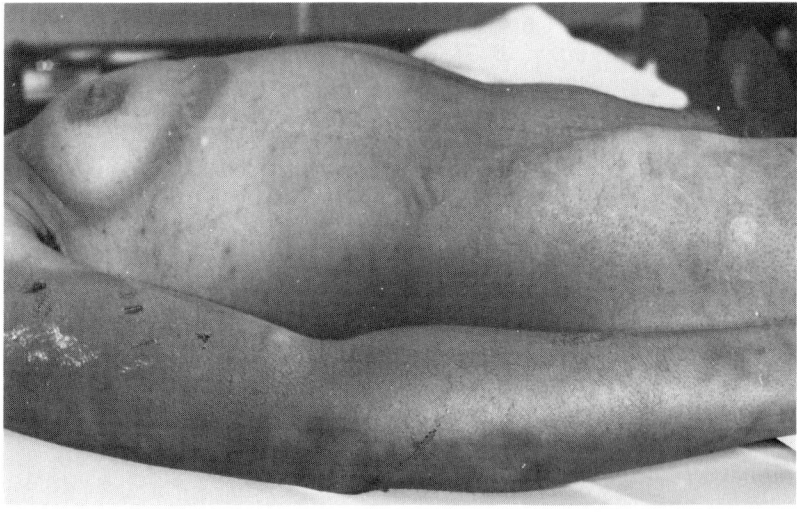

FIGURE 16-6. Massive contusions of upper extremity. Both the arm and forearm are discolored and swollen because of bleeding into the subcutaneous tissue.

tion, furnishes an appropriate growth area, low in oxygen, for anaerobic bacteria. Of especial note are members of the clostridial group which can produce gas gangrene. Such an infection may result in the subject's death due to the toxic substances formed by the bacteria. Of course, bacteria are not ordinarily present in the subcutaneous tissue. To gain access, there must be some portal of entry. It should be understood, however, that contusions frequently do not occur as a single type of wound, but in combination with others which might then allow for bacterial penetration.

Another remote or pathophysiologic effect of contusion applies only in the instance of a severe sudden compression of the subcutaneous tissue. Such can occur as a result of an individual's being struck by a motor vehicle. The striking part of the moving motor vehicle injures the subcutaneous tissue so severely that the fat is expressed from the fat cells (Fig. 16-7). The liquid fat then enters the injured and torn blood vessels to be borne to the lungs by the returning venous blood, resulting in pulmonary fat embolism.[5] In some instances the fat may pass through the pulmonary filter to enter the systemic circulation to various organs, the brain being the most important, and death can be the result (Fig. 16-7).

The shape of the contusion may mirror the striking object. Figure 16-8 illustrates some patterned contusions of a particular shape on the back of a child who has been beaten repeatedly with a coat hanger. The shape of the bent end of the coat hanger can easily be compared with the contusions it has made (Fig. 16-9). The nature of the weapon can thus be determined.

Some contusions may be situated so deeply in the subcutaneous tissue that they may not be seen by observation of the overlying intact skin. This is especially true of contusions in those who have highly pigmented

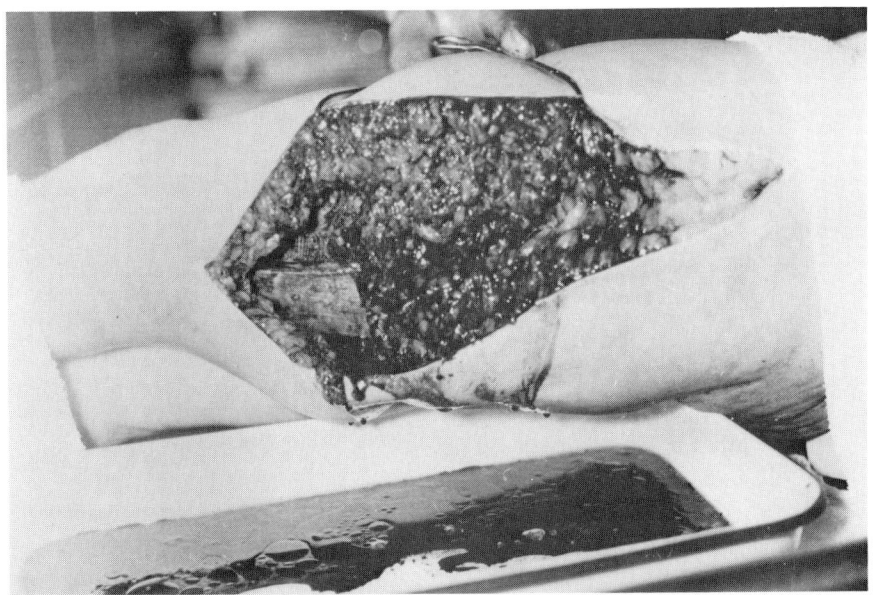

FIGURE 16-7. Liquid fat from thigh. The primary impact point (thigh) has been incised; a large quantity of liquid fat has escaped and can be seen floating on the surface of the blood collected in the pan. The victim was a pedestrian struck by a motor vehicle.

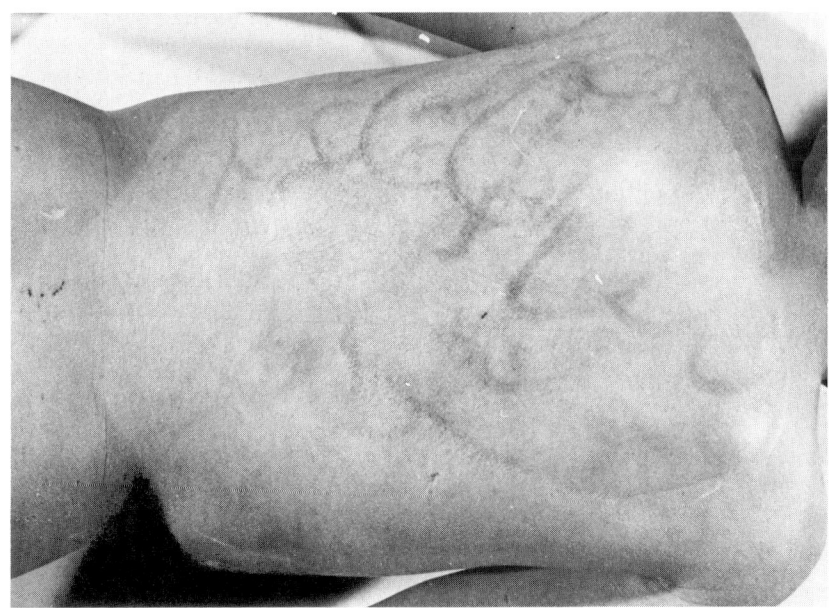

FIGURE 16-8. Contusions in shape of wounding object. The back of the beaten child has been marked by narrow, patterned contusions. The nature of the wounding object is not apparent in this view.

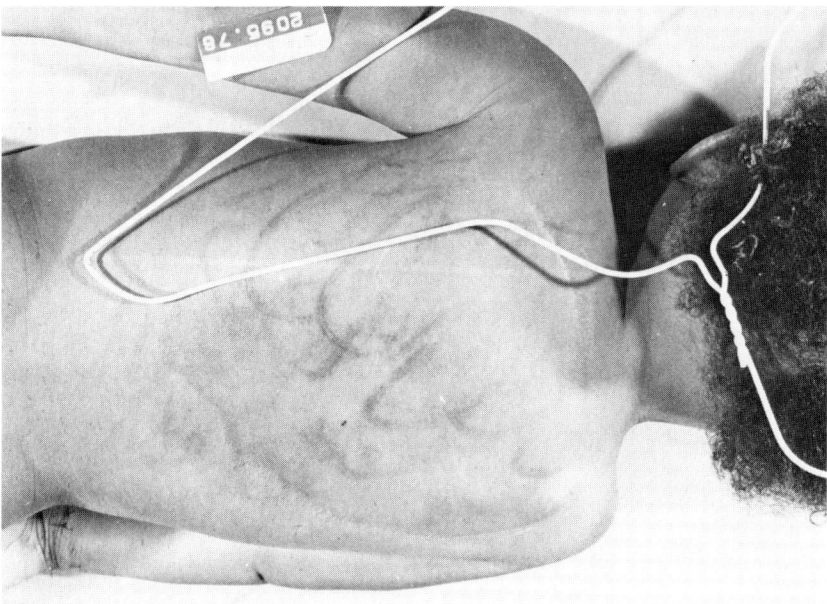

FIGURE 16-9. The same child shown with a coat hanger similar to the one used to inflict the wounds. The similarity in shape of the object and the contusions is marked.

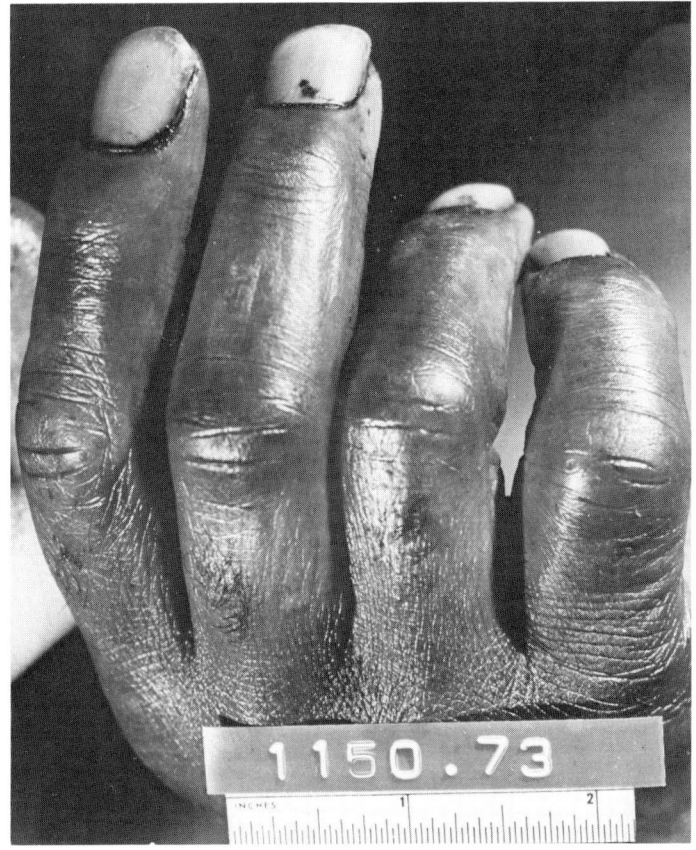

FIGURE 16-10. Contusions of hand. The contusions of the finger joint areas are barely visible due to the highly pigmented skin of the black victim of a beating. This is an example of defense wounding.

skins (swarthy skinned persons, or those with deep tans) (Fig. 16-10). Incision with a knife through the skin into the subcutaneous tissue is an honored technique for search and demonstration of such deep, invisible contusions. This technique is also useful to employ to examine primary impact points in pedestrians struck and killed by moving motor vehicles.

Deep Tissue and Organ Contusions

All organs can be contused. Contusions of different organs assume different degrees of importance. Obviously a vital organ such as the heart or the brain (and especially the brain stem), when contused, may suffer marked derangement of function and even death may result.

A contusion of the brain, with bleeding into the substance of the brain, may initiate enough swelling with gradual accumulation of acid byproducts of metabolism that further swelling and impairment of function results.[6] A vicious circle is then established which, in the absence of relief, causes confusion, then coma, then death (Fig. 16-11). It is sometimes surprising to note, at the time of the autopsy, the relatively small size of the contusions of the brain which alone cause death. This is particularly true of contusions which are situated in certain vital centers, such as

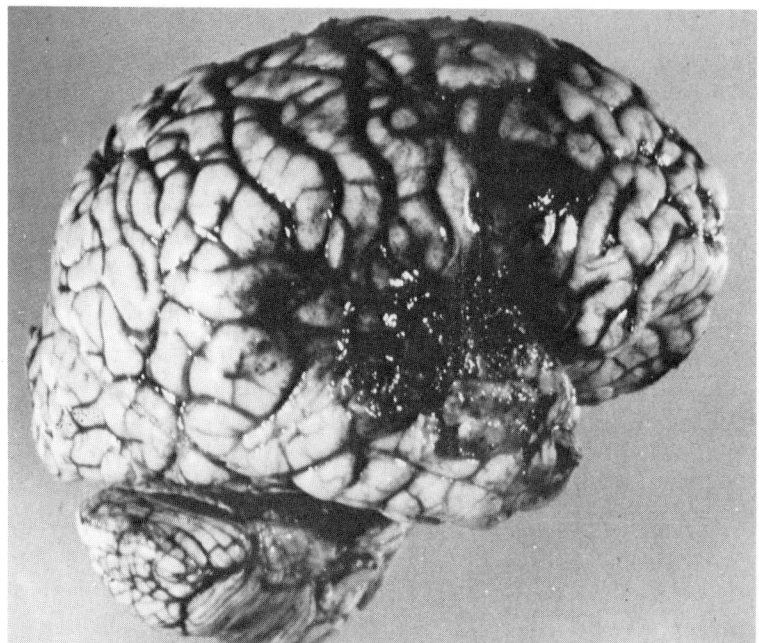

FIGURE 16-11. Contusion of the brain. A large contusion of the right side of the brain (temporal lobe) has caused discoloration. The brain was fixed in formalin prior to photography.

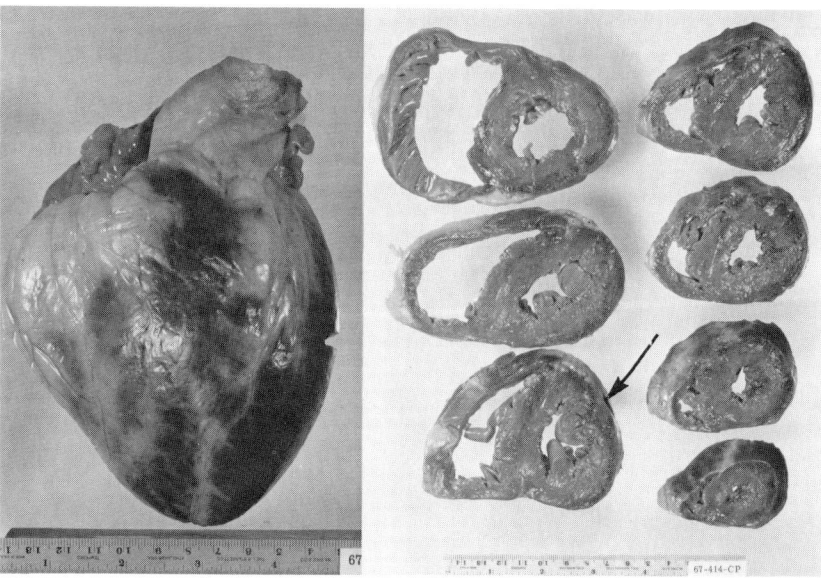

FIGURE 16-12. Massive contusion of the heart. The anterior surface of the heart is discolored centrally; this is due to a contusion. The multiple slices through the ventricles show also the deep contusion. This is indicated by an arrow adjacent to one slice. The victim was the driver of a motor vehicle which left the roadway and struck a fixed object.

those which control respiration and blood pressure. Here a tiny contusion, perhaps smaller than a match head, can be fatal.

The heart is also highly vulnerable. A small contusion, placed so as to affect those areas of the heart responsible for the initiation and transmission of the impulse to cause it to beat, can cause serious disruption of normal rhythm or cessation of cardiac action altogether. Large contusions, by virtue of swelling and interference with muscle action, often prevent adequate cardiac emptying and lead to heart failure (Fig. 16-12). In some instances, the muscle fiber injury itself, as a result of the contusing force, may contribute to inadequate cardiac muscle action and heart failure. Another hazard of contusion of the heart is that, as the contusion ages, the damaged area becomes weaker; rupture of the heart and loss of blood into the pericardium (the containing sac investing the heart) results in death due to cardiac tamponade.[7]

Contusions of other organs may eventually cause rupture of that organ's cellular covering with resulting bleeding, either slow or brisk, into the body cavity containing that organ. Disability due to the hemorrhage may be severe and death may ensue. Frequently such contusions are associated with tears or lacerations of the organ (see below). Contusions of the liver, kidney, and spleen, and sometimes other organs may be seen (Table 16-2).

Laceration

When the crushing force necessary to produce a contusion of the subcutaneous tissue is applied over a relatively small area, such as by an edge of a piece of lumber or the end of a length of household waterpipe, the striking surface is narrow enough to cause a tearing of the skin, the production of a laceration. Thus the tear or laceration is produced by a narrow but not truly sharp object crushing the skin and underlying tissue with force and actually disrupting to a greater or lesser extent the continuity of skin and subcutaneous tissue. Because of the forcing and tearing nature of the birth of the laceration, the edges of the laceration are irregular and rough (Fig. 16-13), and frequently the immediately adjacent skin surface is abraded, caused by the flatter portions of the striking object rubbing against the skin as it is indented by the forceful blow (Fig. 16-14). Since bleeding is an invariable effect of a laceration, a contusion or pseudocontusion accompanies the tear or laceration of both a skin area and a mucous membrane.

In some instances the tearing of the skin or mucous membranes and the underlying tissue is incomplete, and bridges of tissue (usually skin) cross the valley of the laceration (Fig. 16-15). This bridging, together with the irregular, rough edges of the laceration, and the adjacent abrasion sometimes seen, owing to the flat nature of the striking object, usually distinguish a laceration from an incised wound caused by a very sharp object such as a knife.

The edges of the laceration may give an indication of the direction in which the force or blow was applied to effect the laceration. The more undermined edge of the laceration is the side toward which the force of the striking object was directed; the sloped side of the laceration is that side from which the blow was directed (Fig. 16-16). Similarly, the side of the laceration with the adjacent contusion is often the side from which the force of the blow was directed.

The shape of the laceration may indicate something of the nature of the

TABLE 16-2. CONTUSIONS—MEDICOLEGAL SIGNIFICANCE

Subcutaneous (beneath skin—termed bruises)
- Visible:
  - Discolored and swollen.
  - Except in highly pigmented blacks.
  - Not all such discolored, swollen areas represent true contusions:
    - periorbital (fracture of frontal bone);
    - Battle's sign (fracture of base of skull).
- Alteration with age:
  - Naked eye detects color change.
  - Microscopic examination reveals tissue damage repair.
  - Neither color change nor damage repair proceeds at a standard, reproducible rate (see text).
- Pathophysiologic effects:
  - Can drain the circulatory system of blood to produce shock to cause weakness, confusion and even (rarely) death (see text).
  - Can cut off circulation to distal parts of extremities.
  - The pooled sequestered blood can serve as a good site for bacterial growth.
  - The fat expressed from subcutaneous tissue fat cells can cause fat embolism.
- Shape:
  - May mirror striking object. The so-called patterned contusion. Useful in weapon, tire identification, etc.
- Location:
  - May indicate action of the victim.
  - Backs of hands and forearms may show defensive posture (so-called defense wounds).
  - May indicate action of assailant:
    - finger pad pattern;
      - about neck in holding or strangulation;
      - about arms near shoulder in holding, shaking, raping;
      - on buttocks of infants and children when spanked.

Deep contusions—involving tissues and organs other than the subcutaneous tissues
- Not visible:
  - Presence may not be suspected by medical personnel.
- Location:
  - May be located in any organ or tissue:
    - brain, lung, heart, liver, muscle, etc.
- Pathophysiological effects depend upon:
  - Location:
    - Vital organs—brain (particularly brain stem) and heart markedly altered in function, with confusion, unconsciousness and death possible results.
  - Size:
    - Large areas of involvement may alter the function of the organ.
    - Rupture of containing membrane or tissue.
    - This may lead to uncontrolled bleeding into a body cavity with shock and eventual death.

object that caused it (Fig. 16-17). However, because of the resiliency of the target tissues, much stretching may result before the tearing of tissues results. So it is that hammer blows do not necessarily cause hammer face-shaped or even semicircular lacerations. Tearing at the ends of lacerations, at angles diverging from the main laceration itself, so-called swallow tails, are frequently noted (Fig. 16-18). Experience shows that many different objects can produce similar patterns in a given laceration.

The altered appearance of a laceration due to age follows, to a degree, the changes noted in abrasions and contusions. The first change, however, is a blood clot, which tends to overfill the valley of the laceration and to spread out into the surrounding skin or mucous membrane. This clot, together with aggregated tissue fluids and body cells of response to injury, and sometimes damaged tissue combine to form an eschar, or scab.

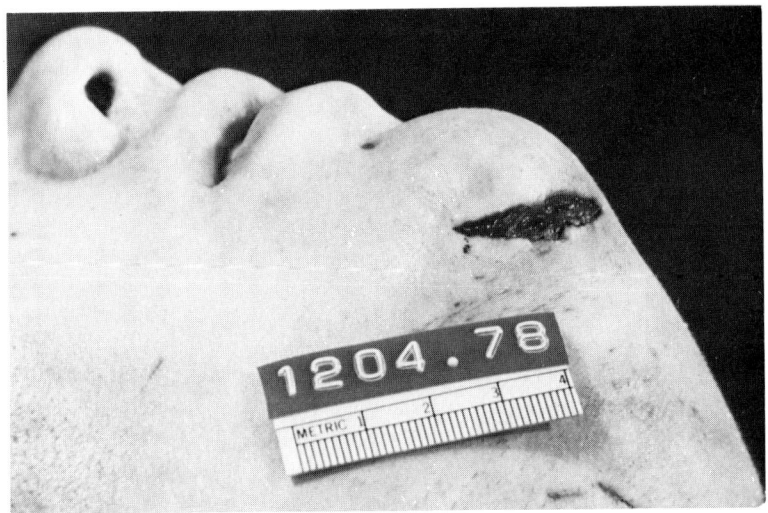

FIGURE 16-13. Laceration of the chin. The edges of this laceration are irregular, a typical feature of lacerations. Near the top of the label some "stretch laceration" or tears of the skin indicate something of the force of the blow which caused the injury. The victim was involved in a motor vehicle crash, striking his chin against an unyielding object.

Scar tissue growth begins in the depths of the laceration, gradually filling the valley as silt would be carried in by a brook. Finally, the external skin (epithelium) begins to grow down onto the new scar tissue and repair then is complete. The scar never contains the so-called skin appendages, including sweat glands, hair, and other such structures.

Estimation of the time from infliction to examination of lacerations is no more precise than that possible with abrasions or contusions. The best that can be hoped for in most instances is an educated estimate of very recent, recent, a few days, and older than several days. Lacerations occur-

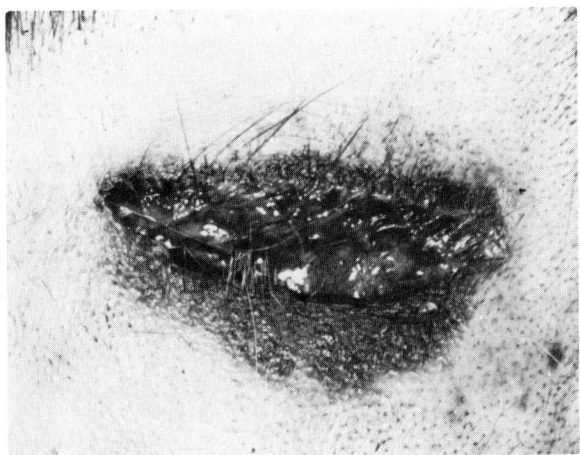

FIGURE 16-14. Laceration with adjacent abrasion. This typical laceration is nearly surrounded by an abraded area, more visible adjacent to the lower margin than the upper. The object used to inflict the wound compressed and abraded the skin as the skin was torn.

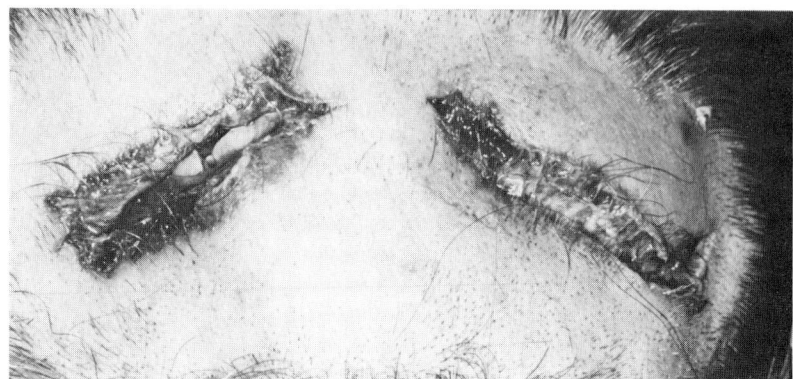

FIGURE 16-15. Laceration with bridging. Two lacerations are shown. Some tissue bridging is present in the wound on the right.

ring after death can be distinguished by the absence of bleeding (Fig. 16-19).

Remote, or pathophysiologic, effects of lacerations can be far reaching. The laceration may be the source of severe, perhaps even fatal bleeding. A single laceration, even in the absence of the tearing of a large artery or vein, may result in slow bleeding which, if continued over a prolonged period, can be fatal. Multiple lacerations, involving only the skin and subcutaneous tissue, each causing some hemorrhage, may combine to cause shock due to blood loss, and eventual death. The disruption of the skin or mucous membrane allows bacteria on the wounding object to be swept into the deeper layers of tissue, and also allows for the introduction of bacteria derived from the skin or mucous membrane surfaces themselves. A portal of entry thus established may persist until sufficient healing has taken place to seal the opening to further bacterial penetration. The presence of the laceration, particularly if located over or near a joint, may cause considerable pain, especially when the joint is activated,

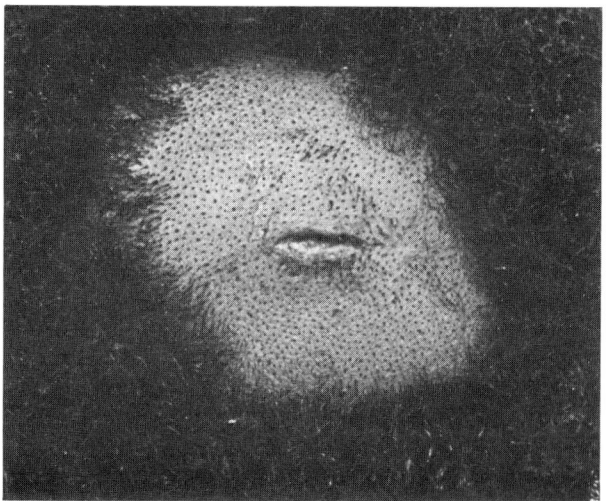

FIGURE 16-16. Undermining of laceration. The upper edge is undermined; the lower edge has a slope. The object that caused the laceration was directed from below upward.

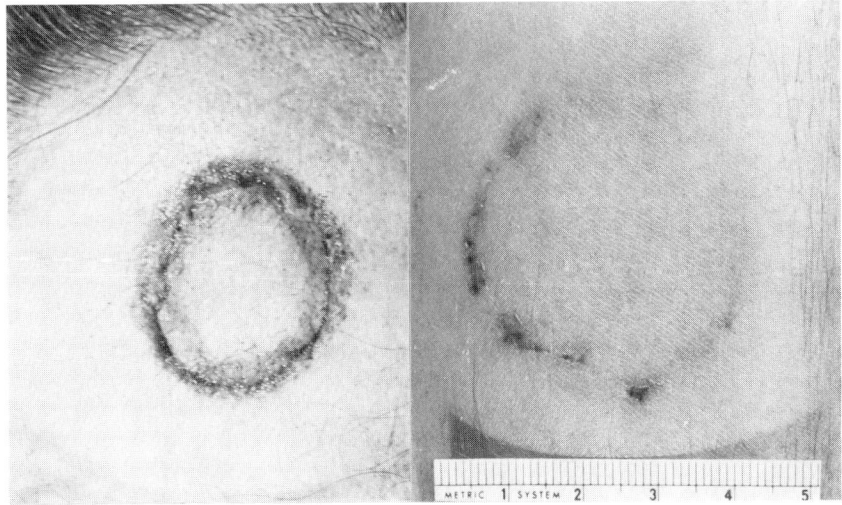

FIGURE 16-17. Shape of wounding object. The figure on the right shows the small, individual superficial lacerations (with some abrasion and contusion) caused by biting. This injury is sometimes specific enough to permit precise comparison with the assailant's teeth. The laceration caused by a lug wrench is shown on the left. The external circular shape and the internal hexagonal outline of the wrench may be seen.

stressing and pulling the torn sides of the laceration. The pain may, therefore, cause dysfunction, another pathophysiologic effect of the wound. Additionally, crushing of the fat-containing subcutaneous tissue may result in the entrance of liquid fat into the circulation and pulmonary or systemic fat embolism as described earlier.

Lacerations involving deep tissues and organs can and do occur. Some tissues and some organs tear or rupture simply as a result of the pressure inflicted. Other organs tend to behave much as do fluid-filled bags and burst as the pressure wave reaches them. This is particularly true of the heart (in diastole, when filled with blood), the aorta, the liver (Fig. 16-20), and the spleen. The determination of the presence of rupture or laceration of any deep organ or tissue is often difficult, especially when multiple other effects of trauma are observable, affecting several areas of the body.

One often unanticipated effect of a laceration-causing trauma is tissue

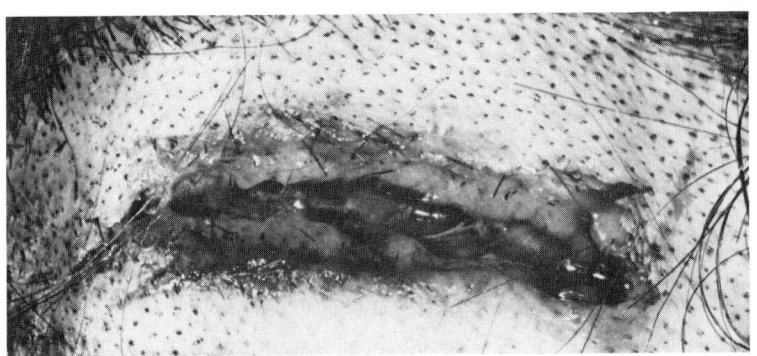

FIGURE 16-18. Laceration with swallow tails. The tearing of the ends of the laceration, producing "swallow tails," is frequently noted, especially when there is a layer of bone situated beneath the overlying skin and subcutaneous tissue.

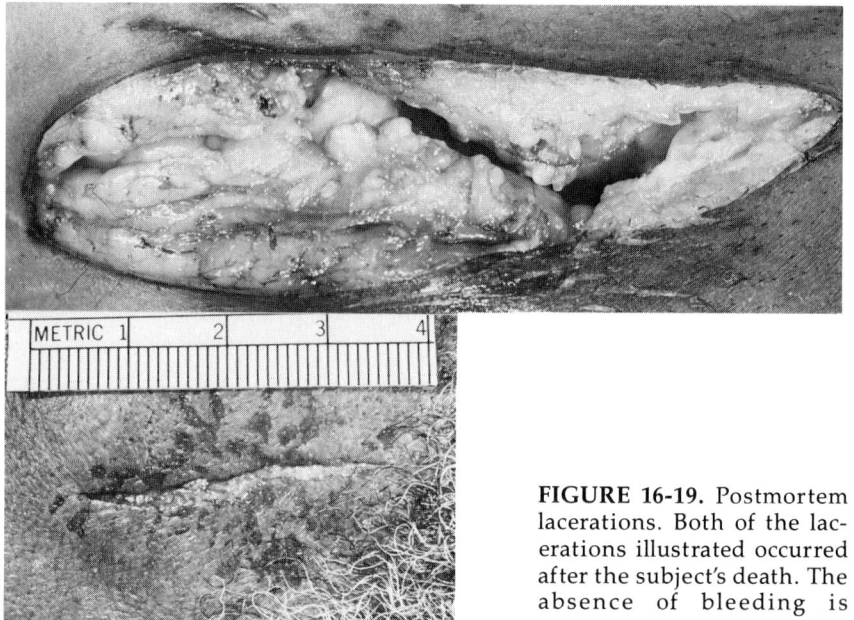

FIGURE 16-19. Postmortem lacerations. Both of the lacerations illustrated occurred after the subject's death. The absence of bleeding is apparent.

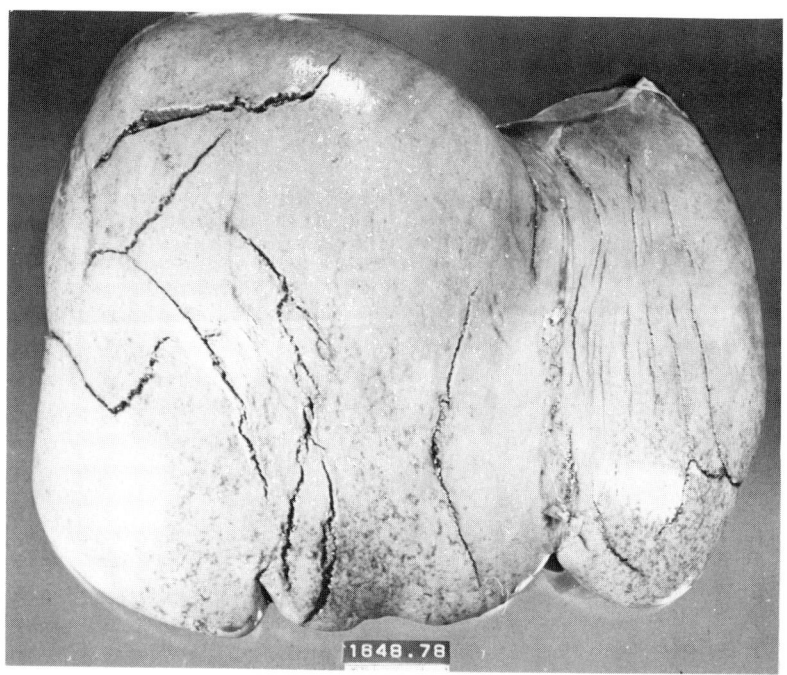

FIGURE 16-20. Rupture of liver. This liver is obviously ruptured. The term "fracture" is also applied to this type of injury. In the example shown, the liver is enlarged and fatty; the normal liver may also rupture due to the application of blunt force.

damage with complete tearing or serious laceration occurring long after the blow was struck. Lacerations of the heart, aorta, liver, and spleen are most apt to behave in this manner. The laceration is incomplete but the tissue is weakened, and after hours or days the affected tissue may suddenly give way to allow for unanticipated bleeding which can be fatal (Table 16-3).

Combinations of Abrasions, Contusions and Lacerations

As has already been implied, abrasions, contusions, and lacerations frequently are seen together or as integral components of one another. The same object may cause a contusion with one blow, a laceration with the next, and an abrasion with a third (Fig. 16-21). Alternatively, all three types of injury may result from a single blow. The body may be in motion with the wounding object stationary, or vice versa, for any of the three types of injuries to occur. In some instances, an impression or imprint may result from the impaction of the offending object, and it may be difficult to determine whether the imprint is primarily an abrasion or a contusion.

Fracture

More than one forensic meaning is assigned to the term fracture. As usually used, it implies a break or disruption of bone. Surgical classification of the types of fractures of bone have little forensic import. The surgical terms "simple fracture" and "compound or open fracture" are in general use. The former term refers to a fracture of the bone but with intact skin overlying it, and the latter term indicates that the fracture site

TABLE 16-3. LACERATIONS—MEDICOLEGAL SIGNIFICANCE

Skin and mucous membranes

    Character:
        May indicate direction in which the blow was struck, with undermining of the skin margin on the side toward which the blow was directed.
        Associated, contiguous abrasions may also help indicate direction in which blow was struck.
    Shape:
        May (sometimes) clearly indicate the nature of the striking object (e.g., hammer, pipe).
    Alteration with age:
        Blood clot, eventually eschar (scab) fills wound.
        Scarring (replacement of void with connective tissue commences at depth of wound. Scar eventually bridges the gap between sides of laceration with epithelium overgrowing from sides. No hair or other skin appendages in scarred area. Age estimation potential not precise, as with fractures.
    Pathophysiologic effects:
        May be the source of severe, even fatal bleeding.
        Opens a portal to bacteria with possible resulting local or generalized infection.
        If located where skin stretches or is wrinkled (over joint areas, particularly), repeated and continuing oozing of tissue fluids and blood may cause irritation, pain, and dysfunction.
        Crushing of subcutaneous tissue may result in liquid fat entering the circulatory system (fat embolism).

Organs

    Hemorrhage with severe dysfunction and perhaps death. Ultimate total rupture may be delayed, sometimes for days. The interval may be so long that no association between trauma and death is apparent.

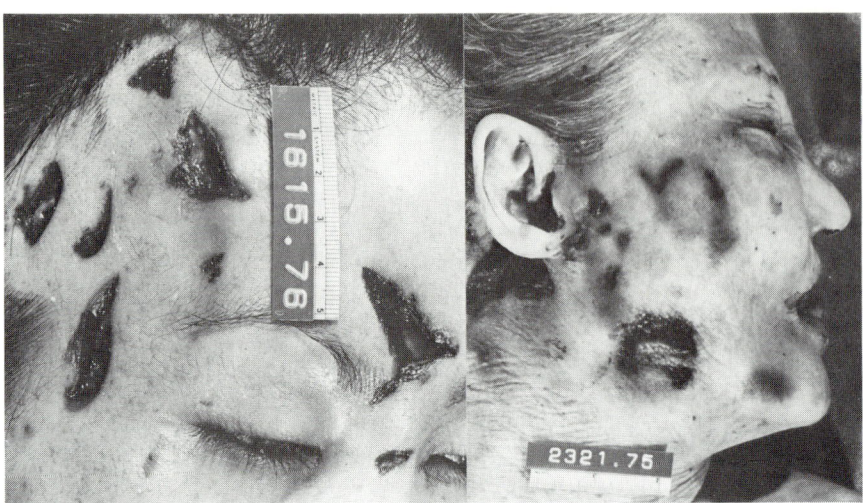

FIGURE 16-21. Different injuries from one weapon. Two examples are shown. In the panel on the right are abrasions, contusions, and lacerations. In the left-hand panel, abrasions and different-shaped lacerations are evident.

has an open pathway to the air (as in an ice pick wound) or that the fractured and usually jagged ends of the bone have penetrated the overlying skin. The pathophysiologic importance of the latter type of fracture is that bacteria easily gain entrance to the deep tissues, including the bone itself. The term may also be used to describe the rupture of an organ; in this sense, the spleen or liver could be "fractured."

The propensity of a bone to fracture is based upon many factors. In the very young individual, bone (particularly the skull) may be quite resilient and may suffer great momentary deformity, due to the application of force, without fracturing. With reference to the rib cage, in younger adults and children, the costal cartilages are not calcified and therefore not firm and unyielding. Thus more force may be absorbed by the rib cage, with more temporary deformity, during the application of force, than that found in an older individual with calcification (bone formation) of the cartilages. In older individuals, usually in women but not limited to females, decalcification and thinning of bone may occur (osteoporosis), and fractures may result from the application of force that might not cause fracturing of bones of persons without osteoporosis. Thus, in the production of a fracture, not only the force, but also the nature of the bone itself must be considered.

In the absence of obvious deformity, one useful way to demonstrate the presence of fractures is to examine the bones by x-ray techniques. Many variations of the basic x-ray examination can be utilized. The object of the scrutiny can be viewed either directly by means of fluoroscopy or image intensification, or indirectly by an examination of a photographic film exposed during the x-ray examination. Xeroradiography is another technique which can be used to demonstrate fractures of bone. With this technique, considerable fine detail of bone and fractures can be developed. It should be emphasized that no x-ray technique always demonstrates an existing fracture of bone. Perhaps as many as 20 percent of linear fractures of bones of the skull are not found, despite careful and painstaking search by various x-ray techniques. Incident to the examination of a dead person, the bone may be exposed at the time of autopsy if

TABLE 16-4. FRACTURES—MEDICOLEGAL SIGNIFICANCE

Character

    The shape of the fracture may indicate:
        Nature of striking object. This is particularly true of fractures of the skull, where hammers and hatchet-like objects leave telltales of their presence, and also indicate the direction of force.
    The fragmentation of bone may indicate the direction in which the force was applied.

Changes with age

    As healing of the fracture site takes place, a fibrous "splint" (callus) is formed about the fracture site and extending along the bone for a distance on either side. This later becomes calcified. Can be detected by direct or by x-ray examination. Within some limits, fairly accurate age estimation can be made.

Pathophysiological effects

    Hemorrhage, internal in simple fractures, internal and external in compound fractures.
    Pain and dysfunction.
    Damage to surrounding structures by tearing of tissues and organs by jagged bone ends.
    Marked shock, not necessarily related to the extent of fracture.
    Portal of entry for bacteria (compound fracture).
    Fat and bone marrow embolism, usually pulmonary but may be systemic.
    Depressed fractures of the skull, with a fragment of bone pressing on the underlying brain may cause severe dysfunction, confusion, convulsions, coma, death.

---

visualization of a fracture or suspected fracture site is considered to be of enough importance. It is, of course, impractical to skeletonize the body and search every bone for possible fracture. Such searches are much more easily conducted by whole-body x-ray search with great saving in time and the preservation of the body in satisfactory condition for later viewing at the funeral. The failure of x-ray techniques to demonstrate all fractures, especially small ones with no displacement of the fractured bone edges, must be kept in mind.

Fractures are of considerable forensic importance (Table 16-4). The shape of a fracture (especially fractures of the skull) may indicate the nature of the striking object. Thus the fracture-defect made by a hammer may resemble half or more of the face of the striking portion of the hammer (Fig. 16-22). The shape of fractures of the skull may also indicate, to some degree, the direction the force exerted and the direction from which the blow was struck. This is particularly true when a chopping instrument is used. The undermined edge of the fracture defect is the direction in which the lateral force vector is exerted, and the slanted edge is the side from which the force was directed. In the instance of long bones, the direction in which a severe blow was struck (such as by an automobile striking a pedestrian) can be determined by x-ray or direct examination of the fragments, with the fragments being loosened on the side opposite that from which the force came. In regard to fractures of the pelvis, the direction of the force vector can be determined in some instances. This occurs when there are fractures of the bony pelvis beneath the primary impact site (as might be determined by the presence of abrasions, contusions, or lacerations, or a combination of these) and also fractures of the opposite side of the pelvis. A line drawn across the pelvis to connect both fracture sites will indicate the direction of force, and perhaps also determine in which direction the victim was facing at the time of being struck.

Fractures of bones heal well under usual circumstances. The rate of healing varies somewhat from one individual to another, but can be predicted within broad limits. Visual examination of the fracture may reveal

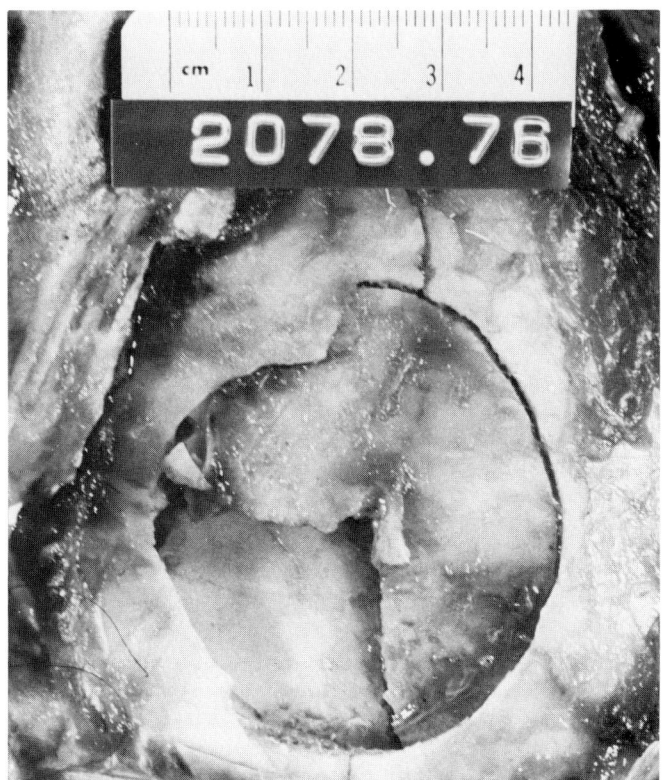

FIGURE 16-22. Hammer fracture of the skull. The general outline of the hammer face is apparent.

it to be fresh, healing, partially healed, or healed. Radiographic examination can yield information as to state of healing (and, therefore, an estimate of the span of time between injury and examination), based upon the gradual accumulation of calcium (ossification) of the callus. Microscopic examination of the fracture site and the healing area may be of use in estimating the age of the fracture. The greatest accuracy results from the integration of all methods of examination.[8] It should be noted that no healed fracture site ever quite resembles the original bone configuration, and knowledge of old, healed fractures may be used to help in the identification of badly burned or decomposing bodies and of skeletal remains.

The pathophysiologic effects of fractures are legion. Hemorrhage is an inevitable result of fracture of bone. If the overlying cover of the bone (periosteum) remains intact over the fracture site, the subperiosteal hemorrhage may be extremely painful and may contribute to great dysfunction. If much blood escapes from beneath the periosteum, or if the broken bone ends tear blood vessels of other than very small size, blood may flood the soft tissues surrounding the fracture area with swelling of the tissues and possible decrease in the venous return of blood from the portion of the extremity farthest away from the site of injury. Interruption of the circulation to the part may result. If a very large artery is torn by the fractured bone, circulation will suffer, loss of blood will be marked, and if the fracture is open or compounded, exsanguination and death may result. Shock due to the bone injury may be severe, may not bear any relationship to the degree of fracturing, and may cause marked dysfunction of the individual.

The hollow central portions of long bones contain an admixture of fat cells and bone marrow, both of which can enter the blood stream and be carried by the blood to the lung or to other organs. Thus marrow or fat embolism takes place. Cerebral fat embolism, with symptoms beginning 2 to 4 days after fractures occur, can result in death (Fig. 16-23). Pulmonary fat embolism, with symptoms of respiratory distress beginning 14 to 16 hours after the fracturing, is not usually of a fatal nature, but may be so.[5] Pulmonary fat and marrow embolism is so frequently an accompaniment of bone fracture that a search for such emboli may be one possible way to determine if a fracture was made prior to or after death. Bone marrow embolism and/or fat embolism (in the absence of significant soft fatty tissue injury) would indicate the antemortem nature of the fracture.

With reference to fractures of the skull, if the fracture is linear, with no depression of the edges of the bone, the fracture is not necessarily of great significance insofar as body function is concerned (Fig. 16-24). In some locations a linear fracture causes tearing of arteries on the inner aspect of the skull, with bleeding in the extradural space (Fig. 16-25). Such hemorrhage is of great importance (see below). Depressed fractures of the skull are also very serious clinically. When the bone edge or fragment presses inwardly upon the brain, the fragile and sensitive brain is often damaged (Fig. 16-26). Localized and even generalized brain swelling usually results

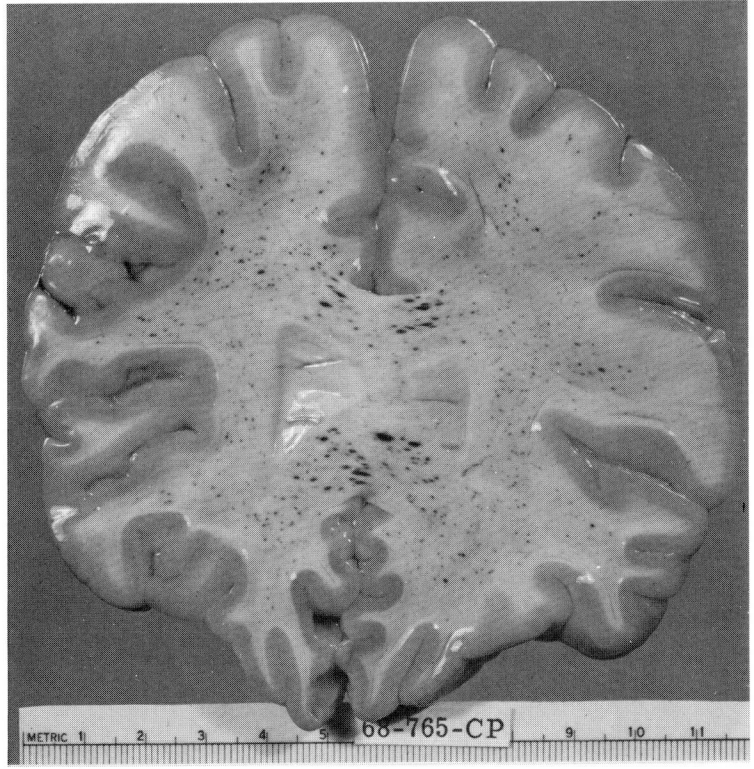

FIGURE 16-23. Cerebral fat embolism. A cross section of the frontal portion of the brain is shown. The small, nearly punctate, hemorrhagic areas in the white matter are characteristic but not pathognomonic of fat embolism.

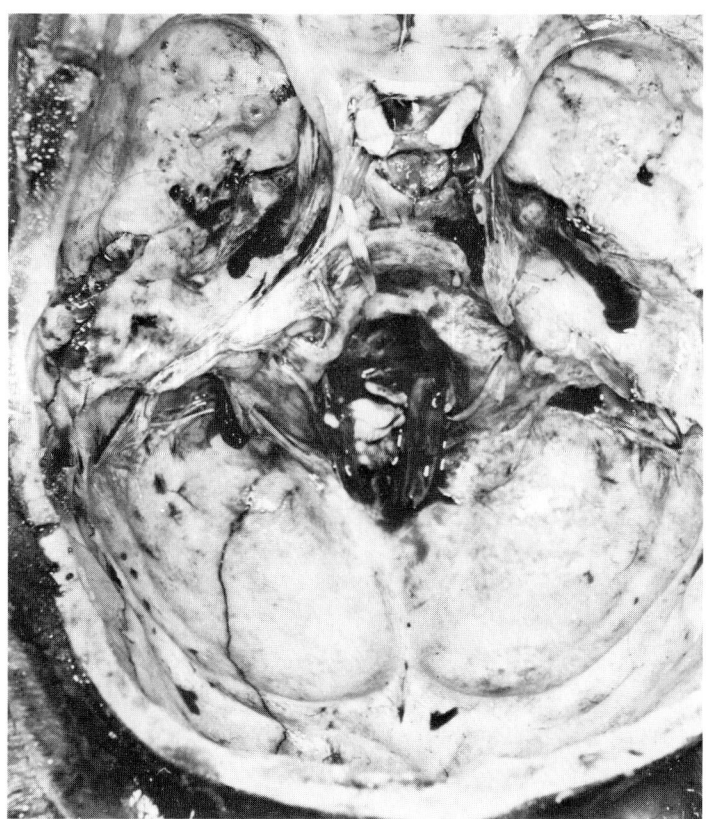

FIGURE 16-24. Linear fractures of the skull. A linear fracture of the skull, involving the left posterior cranial fossa, is easily recognizable.

with corresponding dysfunction of the brain. Confusion, convulsions, coma, and death can be the result. It is also possible that the sharp, depressed bone edge will tear or lacerate the brain with marked and irreversible damage. The depressed skull fracture may result in swelling of the brain, contusion of the brain, or actual laceration of the brain.

Compression

Continuing compression, the prolonged application of force, can cause both local and remote effects. The classic result of compression is the not infrequently encountered traumatic asphyxia. Here a heavy weight presses against the chest, preventing the victim's muscles of respiration from exerting their usual bellowslike action on the chest (Fig. 16-27). Death is due to asphyxia, no respiratory air exchange being possible.

Continuing and prolonged compression of local areas of the body may contribute to a closing off of the circulation to an area or to an entire limb with resulting tissue death, gangrene, and eventual loss of the part. Compression by means of hemorrhage into the soft tissues has already been noted. Table 16-5 can be reviewed for other effects of compression upon other body parts.

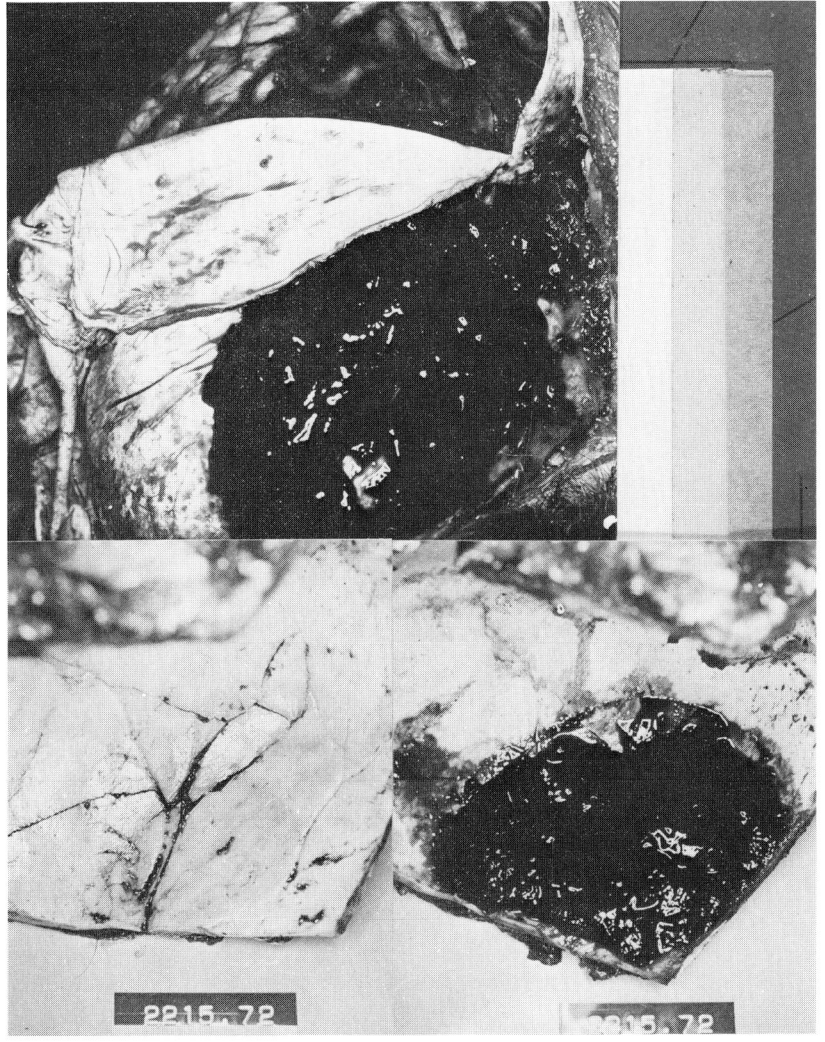

FIGURE 16-25. Epidural hemorrhage. In the upper panel, the epidural (extradural) hemorrhage is to be seen external to the dura and obviously pressing upon the dura and underlying brain. The lower two panels show the portion of the epidural hemorrhage adherent to the inner surface of the skull and the fracture of the skull after removing the bloodcake.

Hemorrhage

Some of the effects of hemorrhage have been discussed under the headings of contusion, laceration, fracture, and compression. Other forensic implications of hemorrhage, however, need examination.

The amount of blood contained in the circulatory system is related to the size of the person. There are tables available to allow for the prediction of the blood volume based upon body weight. Average-sized adult males have a blood volume of 5 to 6 quarts of blood. The loss of one-tenth of this, such as might result from the donation of blood at a blood bank, does not cause any significant difficulty. Millions of individuals donate blood each

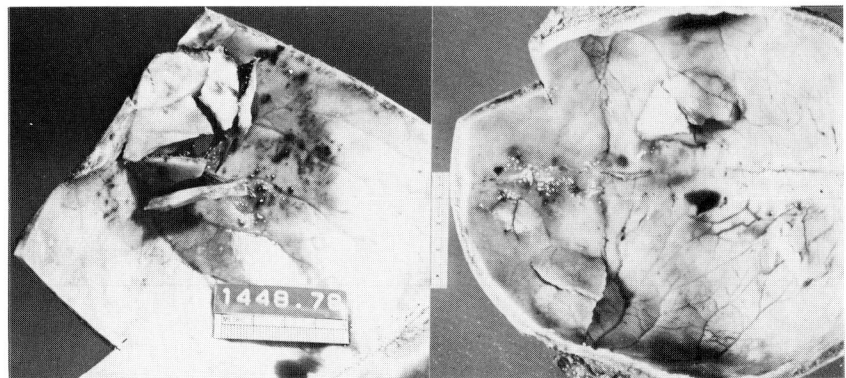

FIGURE 16-26. Depressed fracture of skull. In the right-hand panel, the skull cap is viewed from the inside. Four depressed fractures can be seen. These resulted from four separate blows struck with the butt of a heavy revolver. The left-hand panel shows a large depressed fracture made by a blow with a heavy branch from a tree.

year and suffer nothing other than slight transient lethargy or weakness. The loss of 1 quart of blood, twice the amount usually donated, frequently causes fainting, even when the subject is lying down. The loss of even more blood will inevitably result in fainting. Shock, then death, will result if blood loss is greater. The latter occurs when approximately one-half of the blood volume is suddenly lost. Weakness, confusion, and then fainting consequent to the loss of 1 or 2 quarts of blood place the victim in a position where he cannot defend himself or take action to prevent further

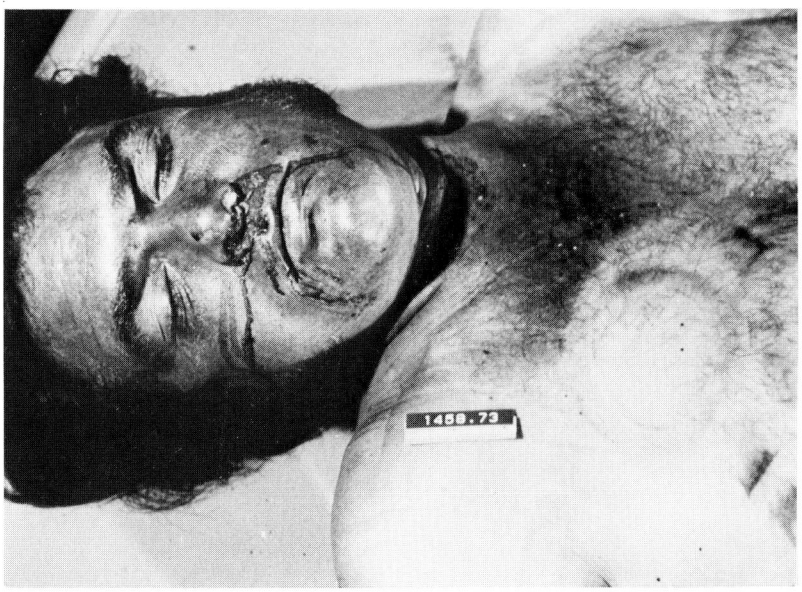

FIGURE 16-27. Traumatic asphyxia. The appearance of the face and chest of the victim is indicative of traumatic asphyxia; note the dark-colored face and the impression on the chest. The driver was pinned against the steering wheel when the load in the truck suddenly shifted and a very heavy steel beam compressed him so severely that he could not breathe.

TABLE 16-5. INJURIES DUE TO CONTINUING COMPRESSION

Entire body compression	
Immobility	Traumatic asphyxia
Chest compression	
Air exchange impossible	Traumatic asphyxia
Head compression	
Brain dysfunction	Confusion, convulsions, coma, death
Compression of arteries conducting blood to head, or veins conducting blood away from head	Asphyxia
Compression of airway (larynx, trachea)	Asphyxia
Compression of spinal cord	Paralysis of body below spinal level
Compression of extremity	Cutoff of circulation to or from extremity with tissue death, gangrene. Compression of nerve with dysfunction resulting
Compression of any soft tissue	Soft tissue destruction, bleeding, fat embolism

blood loss. Thus the victim may, despite apparently nonfatal wounds, go on to bleed further, with fatal consequences.

The rapidity with which bleeding occurs is a function of the size and nature of the blood vessels that have been cut, as well as the type of defect made by the object inflicting the wounds. When a large artery is cut across, or transected, the open end will discharge blood with little possible natural or bodily method of control. If the wound to a large artery is slitlike, such as would be made on the side of the artery by a knife, the bleeding will be slow and perhaps intermittent. A gunshot wound of a large artery will cause a stellate-shaped wound with less self-closing of the artery wall than with a knife wound.

As is commonly understood, bleeding from an artery, with the blood under considerable pressure, will be much more brisk than bleeding from a vein of similar size where the blood is under little pressure.

Not truly part of the discussion of trauma, but needing some detailing is the appearance of the scene of wounding of the victim. Discontinuous spots of blood on the walls of the room may not only indicate splashing of blood from the victim, the assailant, or the weapon, but in some instances may indicate spurting of blood from a divided artery, the blood spurting out each time the heart beats. Ordinarily, the amount of blood present cannot be measured and, because of the highly colored nature of blood, the amount present is apt to be overestimated. It is likewise impossible to measure the amount of blood remaining in the body at the time of autopsy. Thus neither from the scene nor from the body can the amount of blood lost be accurately determined. This is also true of estimates of the rapidity of bleeding. The terms rapid or slow may be the only ways to describe the rate at which blood loss apparently occurred.

Hypertension may cause excessive and rapid bleeding from a given arterial wound. Inadequate blood clotting mechanisms can also cause prolonged bleeding. Such a condition is encountered among persons who have hemophilia and other clotting disorders, or among those being treated with anticoagulants. Individuals with chronic alcoholism frequently fail to form blood clots in the normal manner. The investigation of death due to hemorrhage of whatever means must, therefore, include a total body examination with search for those diseases or conditions which might contribute to the bleeding situation (Table 16-6).

TABLE 16-6. SOME CONDITIONS PREDISPOSING TO PROLONGATION OF BLEEDING CAUSED BY TRAUMA*

Clotting System Malfunction

    Cellular failure
        Decreased platelet production
            e.g., leukemia
        Abnormal platelet function
            e.g., aspirin
    Clotting factor failure
        Decreased clotting factor production
            e.g., cirrhosis, hemophilia
            e.g., drugs such as Warfarin
        Increased consumption of clotting factors
            e.g., infection, cancer

Vascular Integrity Malfunction

    Vitamin deficiencies
      (especially Vitamin C)
    Infection
        e.g., meningococcemia
    Drugs
        e.g., steroids
    Endocrine disease
        e.g., Cushing's disease

*This table outlines the most frequently encountered conditions that may cause prolongation of hemorrhage once it is begun. Very few examples are given; many others could have been cited.

HEAD INJURY

Of special importance among all of the injuries caused by blunt force are injuries to the head. Reference to Table 16-7 will indicate the complex nature of the head (excluding the face) and the great potential for different types of injuries caused by blunt force. Injuries of the scalp, including abrasions, contusions, and lacerations, have been covered in the preceding discussion. Fractures of the skull have also been examined. It is to those injuries associated with the coverings of the brain and contusions of the brain that this further discussion is directed.

Head Injuries Associated with Coverings of the Brain

The brain is invested in three separate layers of tissue. The most external, or outer, layer is named the dura mater. Frequently the term is shortened simply to "dura." This membrane is thick and tough and is not closely applied to the surface of the brain or spinal cord. The dura mater is applied much more closely to the inner aspect of the skull than to the brain itself. Between the skull and the dura is a potential space, the so-called epidural or extradural space. This space is of considerable forensic importance as will be shown below.

The layer most closely investing the brain is called the pia mater. This fragile membrane is adherent to the brain and extends into the clefs (sulci) on the surface of the brain. This layer has little forensic importance attached to it, and further mention of it will not be made.

Immediately external to the pia mater is a wispy, weblike thin layer termed the arachnoid. The name derives from the Latin term for spider, because of the spider web appearance of the tissue. This layer fairly

TABLE 16-7. CHARACTERISTICS OF CENTRAL NERVOUS SYSTEM HEMORRHAGE

Type	Location	Type of Bleeding	Usually Associated with Fracture	Aggregation of Blood	Blood in CSF	Demonstrated by CT Scan
Traumatic						
Epidural (extradural)	Epidural space (extradural space)	Arterial	Yes (skull)	Rapid	No	Yes
Subdural	Subdural space	Venous	No	Slow	No	Not unless massive
Subarachnoid (of two types; see text)	Subarachnoid space	Arterial and venous	No	Rapid	Yes	Not unless massive
Subarachnoid rupture (vertebral artery)	Subarachnoid	Arterial	Yes (vertebra)	Very rapid	Yes	Probably not
Intracerebral contusion	Brain substance	Arterial or venous	No	Rapid	Often	Yes
Nontraumatic						
Subarachnoid rupture (berry aneurysm)	Subarachnoid space	Arterial	No	Very rapid	Yes	Only if massive
Intracerebral A/V malformation-rupture	Brain substance or ventricle or subarachnoid space	Arterial and/or venous	No	Rapid	Sometimes	Yes, if large enough
Intracerebral hemorrhage (hypertensive or apoplectic type)	Brain substance	Arterial and/or venous	No	Variable	Variable, usually not	Yes

closely follows the contour of the brain, but does not dip as deeply into the sulci and smaller surface irregularities as does the pia mater. Separating the arachnoid layer from the dura mater is a space termed the subdural space. This is variable in depth, in some areas very thin, in others many millimeters in depth. It should also be noted that the clear, thin fluid which surrounds the brain is contained in the subarachnoid space and not in the subdural space.

It is possible for bleeding to occur in any of the three spaces noted—epidural, subdural, or subarachnoid space—as well as into the brain substance itself. See Table 16-7 for an outline of characteristics of these areas; all are of particular forensic importance.

Epidural (Extradural) Hemorrhage (Hematoma)

Epidural hemorrhages are associated with skull fracture. If the fracture line crosses the course of one of the small arteries closely applied to the inner aspect of the skull, usually the middle meningeal artery or a branch thereof, the artery may be torn and brisk bleeding ensues (see Fig. 16-25). The accumulating blood gradually forces the dura away from the skull, and the space occupied by the blood enlarges. Although the bleeding is brisk, the artery is small and some force of the accumulating blood is necessary to force the dura mater away from the skull. The dura is pushed inward and the brain is compressed. As the bleeding is very localized, the hematoma (aggregate mass of blood) is relatively thick, and pressure upon the underlying brain is severe; headache, then confusion, stupor, and finally coma are expected and seen. Death will ensue if no therapy is applied. An interval of many minutes to many hours may exist, spanning the time between the injury which caused the fracture and initiated the bleeding and the onset of detectable symptoms. This period is sometimes called the "lucid interval," and if prolonged, the victim may neither recall the initial injury nor relate it to his symptoms.

Subdural Hemorrhage (Hematoma)

Subdural hematoma implies hemorrhage into the subdural space. Such usually occurs when a "bridging vein," one passing from the dura through the subdural space to the brain, is torn and blood aggregates in the subdural space. Because of the midsagittal falx cerebrae, a single subdural hemorrhage is confined to one side or the other (Fig. 16-28), although bilateral subdural hemorrhages can and do occur, each side originating separately. As the blood aggregates, increasing pressure is exerted upon the underlying brain. Since the blood accommodates to the shape of the brain, the pressure phenomenon is best seen by the examination of the contralateral cerebral hemisphere which will present a flattened gyral surface because this hemisphere is pressed directly against the dura by the ever-expanding hematoma on the opposite side of the cranial cavity. Because the accumulation of blood is slow (since the blood is of venous origin), the "lucid interval" is long, usually many hours to days in duration. The amount of blood found in fatal subdural hemorrhages is very rarely more than 120 cc, and sometimes considerably less (Fig. 16-29). Neurosurgeons who estimate the size of subdural hemorrhages at the time of surgical evacuation usually estimate the amount as considerably larger. This may be because of the continued bleeding subsequent to the relief of intracranial pressure incident to the operative procedure, or due

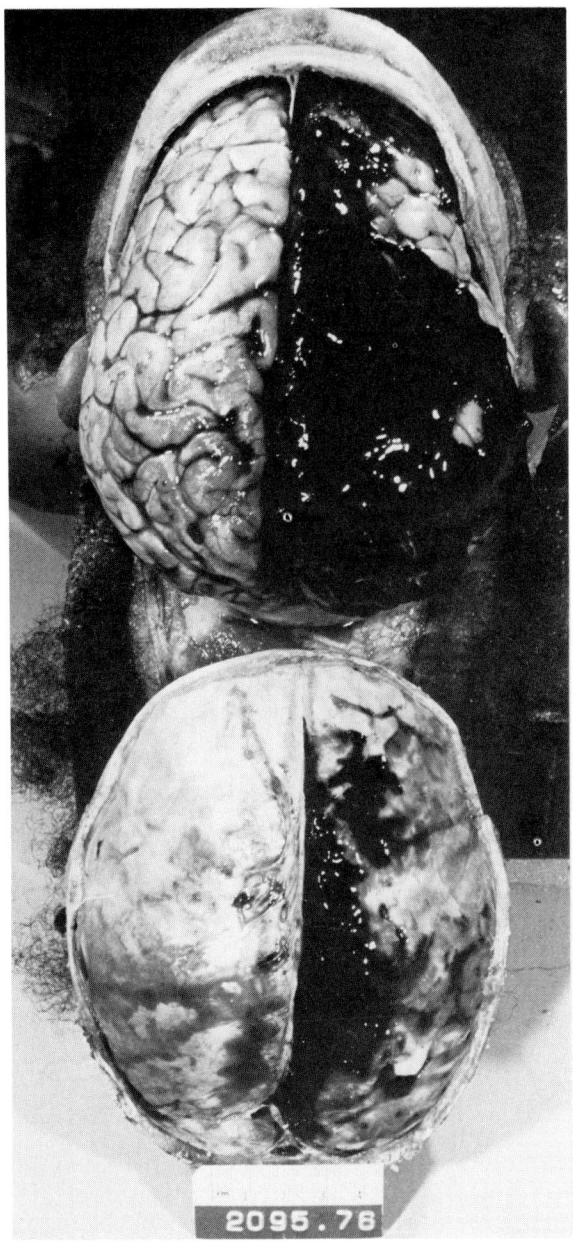

FIGURE 16-28. Subdural hemorrhage. The hemorrhage is confined to the right-hand side of the cranial vault by the midline falx cerebri. Flattening of the opposite cerebral hemisphere is obvious.

to the irrigating fluid used to wash out the subdural space. No attendant fracture of the skull is expected or necessary as in the case of the epidural hematoma.

Not all epidural or subdural hemorrhages are lethal. Some never grow to a sufficient size to compress the brain to produce more than mild symptoms. Some are evacuated surgically and the brain compression is relieved before the hematoma grows to a lethal size.

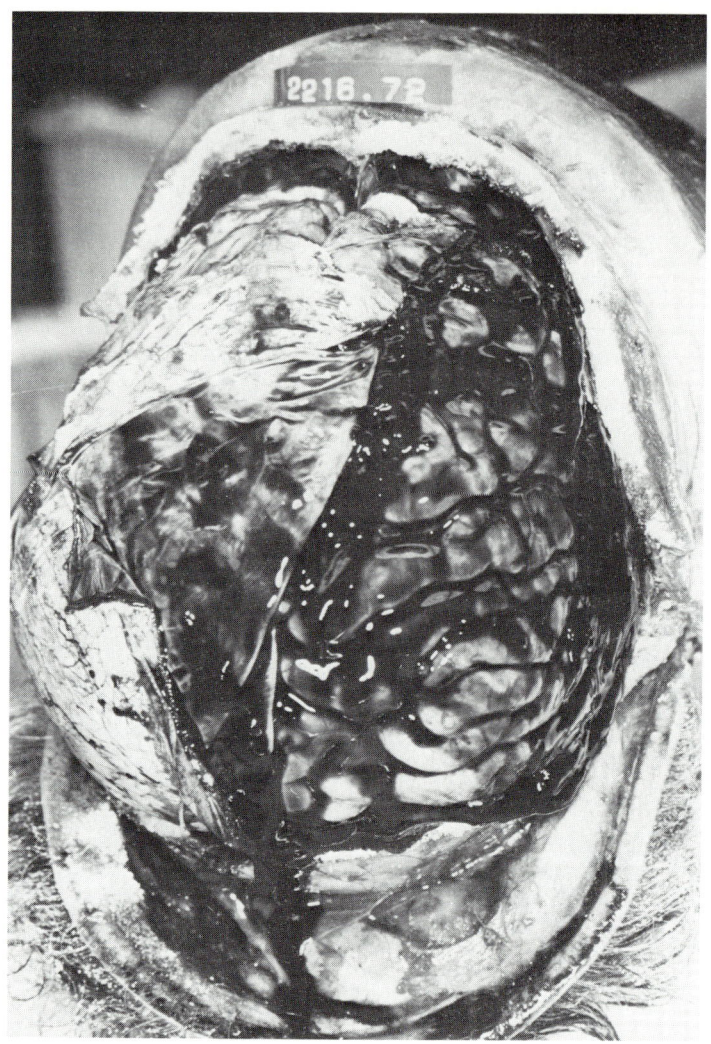

FIGURE 16-29. Acute subdural hemorrhage. The semiliquid blood of a very recent (acute) subdural hemorrhage is revealed by reflecting the dura mater.

Healing of subdural hematomas has been well studied, and the healing process passes through several well-recognized stages.[9,10] The blood, at first fluid, undergoes clotting. Organization (scar formation) begins on the dural side of the clot and gradually extends to encompass all surfaces of the clot, while at the same time the contained blood begins to break down. The final result is a thin mass of soft scar tissue adherent to the dura, but so thin that it does not significantly press against the underlying brain (Fig. 16-30). Frequently, large vascular channels remain in the scar, making it vulnerable to further injury with resulting bleeding. Although the time sequence of the reparative phases of a subdural hemorrhage would appear to be precise, just as in other body reparative activities, there is considerable variation from one individual to the next. Perhaps the most accuracy that can be expected in the dating of the age of a subdural hemorrhage is the same order of precision that has been indicated earlier in this chapter regarding contusions and lacerations.

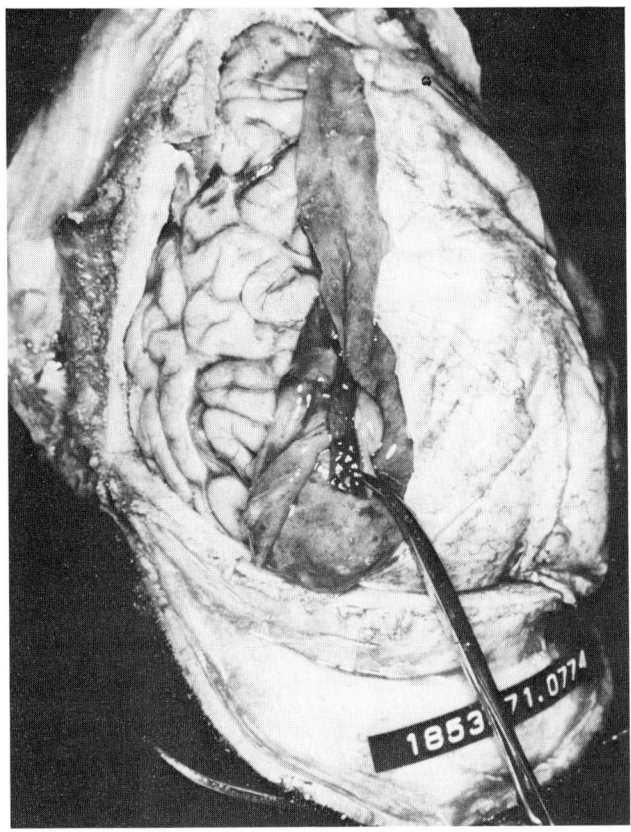

FIGURE 16-30. Old subdural hematoma. This left-sided old (chronic) subdural hemorrhage has been partially reflected with the clamp to show its nature. This hematoma is many months of age.

Epidural hemorrhage, with the associated fracture of the skull and bleeding from the tearing of an artery, is invariably of traumatic origin. Subdural hemorrhage is usually of traumatic origin. Occasionally the trauma which caused either type is not recalled. Despite this, external (scalp) injury may be noted by the examiner, and the origin by trauma of the hematoma may then be suggested.

Rarely, subdural hemorrhages may not be related at all to trauma. Bleeding beneath the dura mater may be seen in individuals with disorders of the blood clotting mechanism, or in chronic alcoholics. In the latter instance the amount of blood may be small and not contributory to death. In the former instances, the hemorrhage may have followed an incident of trauma so trivial as to be unimportant to the normal person, but fatal to one who cannot properly initiate blood clotting so as to stop hemorrhage.

Occasionally a subdural extension of hemorrhage occurs when an intracerebral hemorrhage (the cause of apoplexy or stroke) breaks through the brain substance through the pia mater, and then into and through the arachnoid layer to reach the subdural space.

Subarachnoid Hemorrhage

There are five common causes for subarachnoid hemorrhage, two nontraumatic and three associated with trauma. They may be listed as follows:

1. Nontraumatic subarachnoid hemorrhage:
   a. rupture of an aneurysm of an artery supplying the brain with blood;
   b. rupture of an intracerebral hemorrhage of nontraumatic origin (apoplectic hemorrhage or stroke) into the subarachnoid space.
2. Traumatic subarachnoid hemorrhage:
   a. direct trauma to the brain with focal areas of subarachnoid hemorrhage;
   b. trauma to the side of the face and neck with fracture of a cervical vertebra with tearing of the enclosed portion of a vertebral artery;
   c. tearing of one of the thin-walled arteries at the base of the brain due to sudden hyperextension of the head upon the neck.

Since the rupture of the aneurysm of an artery (vertebral, basilar, internal carotid or a branch thereof) is "nontraumatic" in origin, little discussion would seem warranted here. However, an artery with a weak and bulging spot in its wall is much more fragile than a normal artery. Hence, relatively slight traumatic force can cause the rupture of the aneurysm with the flooding of the subarachnoid space with blood, leading to serious dysfunction and even death (Fig. 16-31). A classic forensic puzzle is sometimes seen in this regard: Did the trauma of a fist fight cause the rupture of the already existent aneurysm, or did the individual suffer headache and become bellicose because the aneurysm had already begun to bleed? In another example, did a fall from a considerable height cause the rupture, or did the rupture and subarachnoid hemorrhage cause the person to lose control of himself and fall? In some instances correlation of investigatory and autopsy findings may solve the puzzle. In other cases no resolution seems possible.

Traumatic subarachnoid hemorrhage is usually of the type first listed above. Focal areas of mild subarachnoid hemorrhage result from force applied to the head, usually accompanied by shaking of the brain and its coverings within the skull (Fig. 16-32). Small blood vessels are torn in the subarachnoid layer and small, usually nonconsequential hemorrhages ensue. In the absence of other possible cause, such as poor clotting ability, the hemorrhages will be telltales of force applied somehow to the head.

Rarely, a blow to the side of the head and neck in the area under the lobe of the ear may result in a fracture of one of the lateral processes of one of the superior cervical vertebrae (Fig. 16-33). Since the vertebral arteries pass upward in small circular defects in the lateral processes of the upper vertebrae of the neck, a fracture in that area may result in tearing or laceration of the artery with massive hemorrhage which usually dissects upward into the subarachnoid layer of the upper cervical portion of the spinal cord and the adjacent brain stem and results in flooding of the subarachnoid space with blood.[11] The upward flow of blood may be extensive and may extend over the base of the brain and onto the lateral sides of the cerebral hemispheres. Some such cases are confused with nontraumatic hemorrhage of ruptured aneurysmal origin. Usually, al-

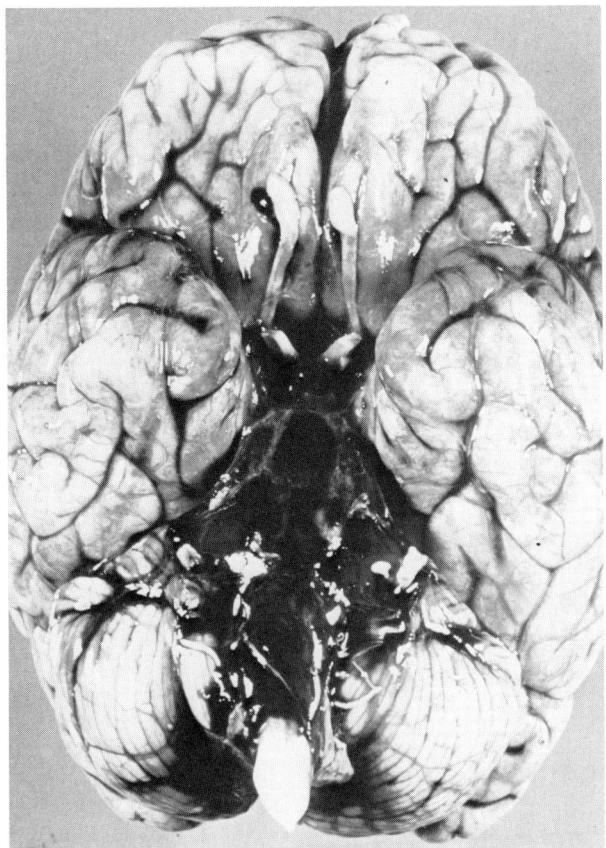

FIGURE 16-31. Massive subarachnoid hemorrhage. This basilar subarachnoid hemorrhage resulted from the rupture of a malformed artery at the base of the brain. Such hemorrhage may be even more extensive in some instances. No trauma was implicated in the illustrated case.

though not always, there is an overlying contusion or contusion-abrasion of the area below and near the ear lobe, pointing to the need for consideration and examination of the upper cervical and vertebral artery area.

The other type of traumatic subarachnoid hemorrhage listed earlier is actually very rare and of a nature that may easily confuse the pathologist. This type is massive subarachnoid hemorrhage, involving the base of the brain and extending onto the lateral sides of the brain, just as does hemorrhage associated with a ruptured aneurysm of one of the large arteries at the base of the brain. However, careful examination fails to reveal any aneurysm, and the vertebral arteries are intact. The cause of the hemorrhage appears to be a rupture of a thin-walled, nonaneurysmal artery at the base of the brain.[12,13] Sometimes the site of rupture can be demonstrated by injecting fluid under some pressure into the arteries at the base of the brain. In such instances, a point of leakage may be detected. This is not an ideal method, however, because the process of removal of the brain and its attendant arteries from the skull can cause small, apparent sites of rupture. Two other bits of evidence, not always present, support the view that an actual rupture has taken place. The first is that there is a history of sudden hyperextension of the head on the neck just prior to collapse

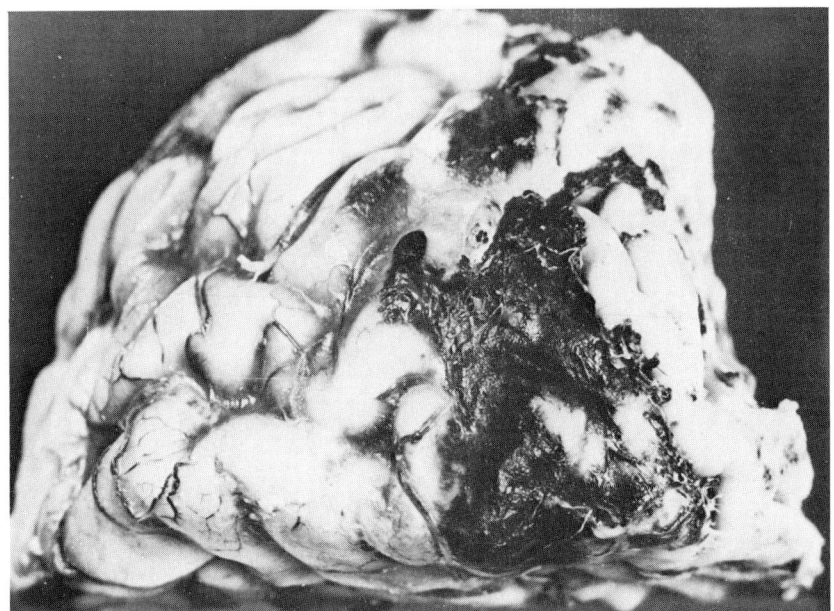

FIGURE 16-32. Focal subarachnoid hemorrhage. A small focal area of subarachnoid hemorrhage is visible, partially overlying a small contusion of the brain.

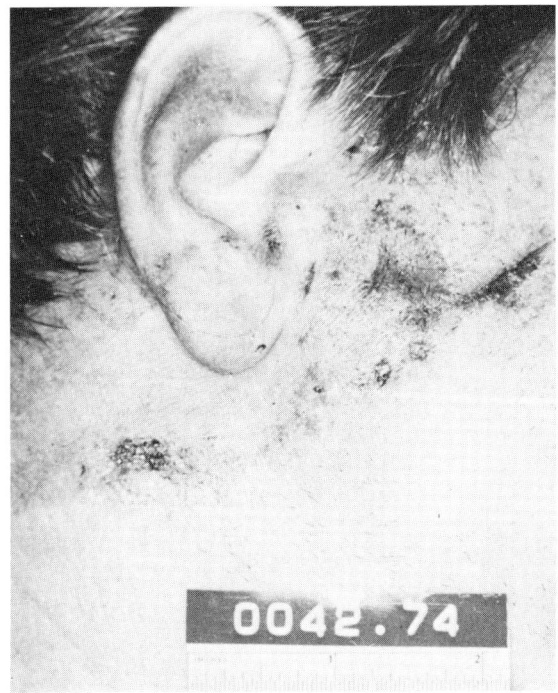

FIGURE 16-33. Contusion and abrasion of face and neck. The contusion and abrasion of the face and neck were caused by a blow administered by a heavy, blunt instrument. This caused a fracture of the lateral process of one of the upper cervical vertebrae, with tearing of the vertebral artery and massive, sudden subarachnoid hemorrhage.

and death. This sort of sudden hyperextension can be suffered by an individual being struck a hard blow on the point of the chin, causing extreme upward and backward movement of the head on the neck. The second condition is that the arteries at the base of the brain in such persons are often extremely thin-walled. The history of the type of blow and the discovery of thin-walled blood vessels with an apparent point of leakage occur often enough in instances of subarachnoid hemorrhage to suggest that causal links can be established, though very rarely, in traumatic deaths.

One difference of considerable clinical importance that separates epidural and subdural hemorrhages from subarachnoid hemorrhage is that only in the latter type of hemorrhage is frank blood found in the cerebrospinal fluid when a spinal tap is performed. Because of the local nature of bleeding in epidural and subdural hemorrhages, with compression of the brain, such conditions are subject to diagnosis, demonstration, and delineation by a C.T. scan. Subarachnoid hemorrhage of the severe basilar type is less precisely demonstrated by this technique, but the presence of bloody cerebrospinal fluid can be expected. Examination of the cerebrospinal fluid coupled with a C.T. scan should prove diagnostically useful.

Brain Contusion

Most contusions of the brain are superficial, occupying only the gray matter (Fig. 16-34). Some are deeper, involving the white matter of the brain (Fig. 16-35). Superficial or gray matter contusions are of great forensic importance.[14] The tearing of blood vessels with subsequent loss of blood into the brain tissue causes swelling and, as noted earlier, a vicious circle may ensue so that if the contusions are extensive enough, brain

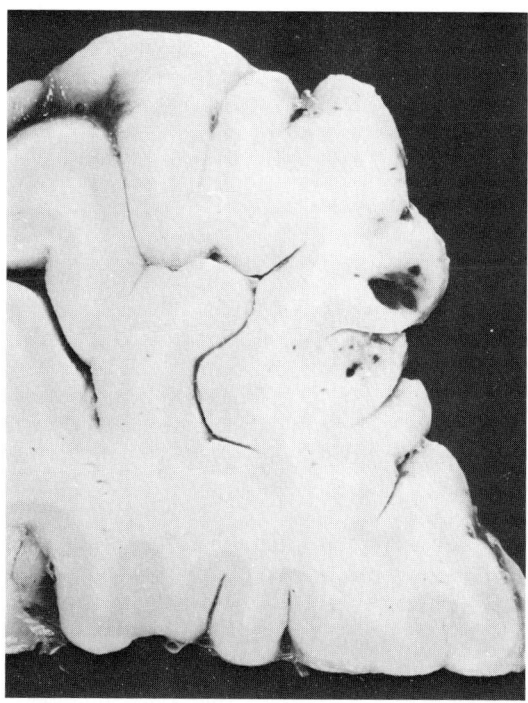

FIGURE 16-34. Contusions of brain. Small, streaklike contusions of the brain, confined to the gray matter. The subject was an automobile crash victim.

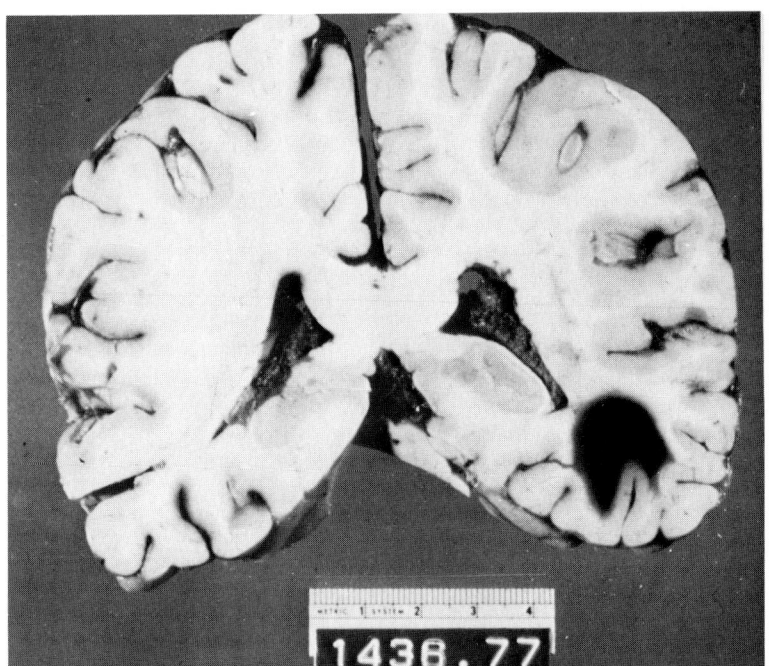

FIGURE 16-35. Deep contusion of brain. Although most contusions of the brain are superficial and are situated in the gray matter, some are more deeply located such as this one in the white matter. The subject was beaten about the head with a heavy, blunt instrument.

swelling may cut off circulation to the brain, resulting in brain death, coma, and eventually the total death of the subject. A second point of considerable medicolegal importance is that the healing of the contusion may result in scarring which later serves as a focus for epileptic seizures.

Another important consideration is the location of the superficial type of contusion in relation to the direction of application of the force that caused it. This point is significant only when the pattern of injury is discovered upon examination of the head and those components which are the sites of trauma: the scalp, skull, and brain.

When a stationary head is struck by a firm, heavy object such as a hammer or a beer bottle, the point of impact will be, to a greater or lesser extent, marked by abrasion, contusion, or laceration of the scalp. The skull underlying the impact point may or may not be fractured. If the underlying brain is contused, the maximum point of superficial contusion will be immediately underlying the point of impact. This type of contusion has long borne the French term "coup" (Fig. 16-36). It is the demonstration of the pattern of injury that enables the examiner to state with certainty that a blow was struck to the head while the head was relatively motionless.[15]

We should also consider the alternate situation where a moving head impacts a firm, fixed object. In this instance, damage to the scalp and possibly to the skull can be similar or even identical to that present in the moving object-fixed head situation. However, the underlying contusion, instead of being immediately under the impact point, will be on the opposite side of the brain. This is the so-called contracoup contusion (Fig. 16-37).

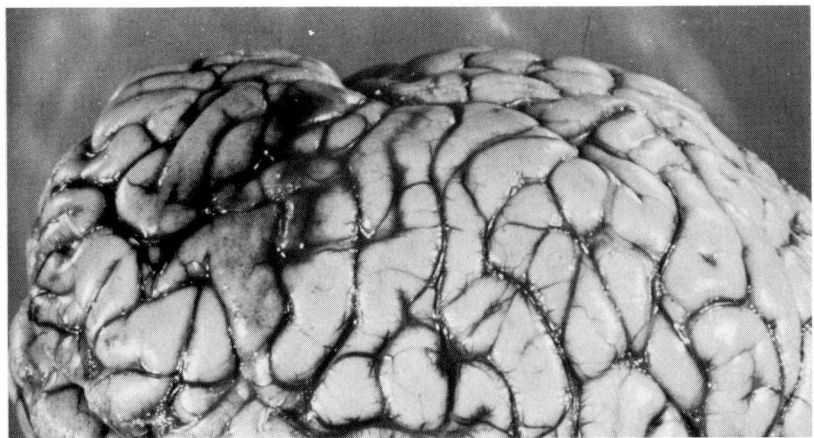

FIGURE 16-36. Contusion of brain (coup type). The contusion was situated directly under the impact point in the head. The victim was struck a blow with a heavy, blunt instrument. There is subarachnoid hemorrhage overlying part of the contusion. The recognition of the contusion as of "coup" type is only through knowledge of the relationship to the overlying scalp (skull) injury.

As with most matters medical, a pure situation is rarely encountered. A small amount of contracoup contusion is frequently encountered in the fixed head-moving object instance, and a small amount of coup contusion is frequently encountered in the moving head-fixed object situation (Fig. 16-38). Nevertheless, the relatively large coup contusion is a telltale of the fixed head-moving object, whereas the large contracoup contusion indicates the other head-object relationship. Note that an examination of the

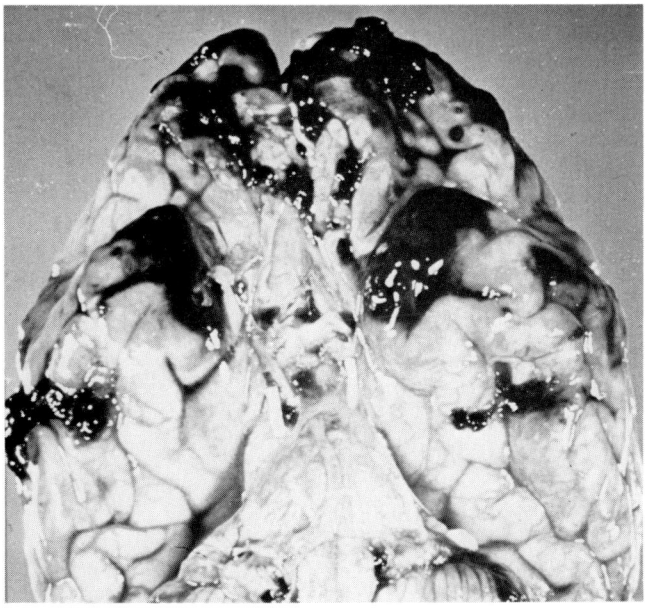

FIGURE 16-37. Contusion of brain (contrecoup type). The contusions shown here involve the inferior surfaces of the frontal and temporal lobes. These are contrecoup contusions resulting from the moving head striking the concrete sidewalk during a fall.

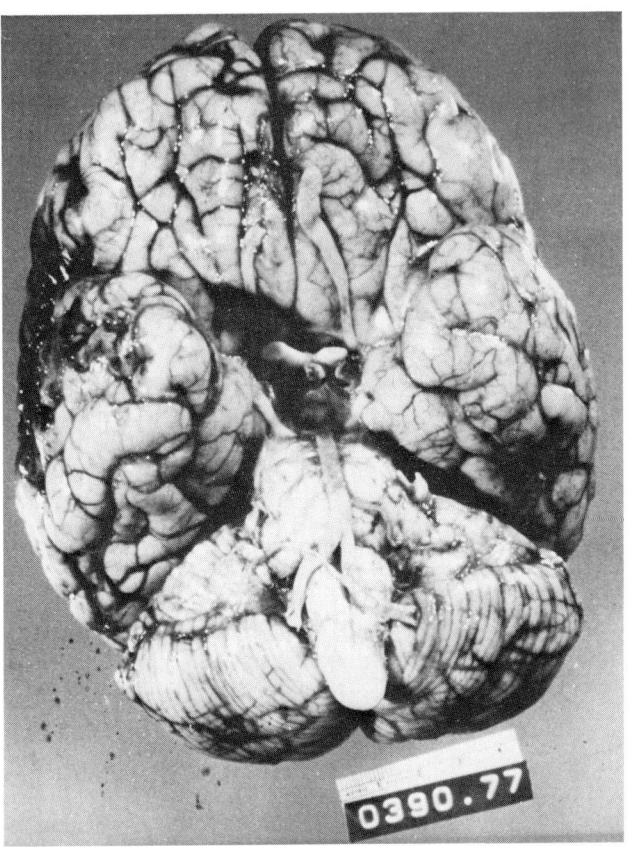

FIGURE 16-38. Contusion of brain (coup and contrecoup). The coup contusion is on the right side of the figure; the larger contrecoup contusion is on the left side. The victim was a motorcyclist who slid against a curbing when the vehicle skidded.

head, including the scalp and skull, is necessary to establish the entire pattern of injury. Because photographs of all of the components of the head injury of whatever type are not ideally suited for the demonstration of the trauma pattern, diagrams may be better employed to illustrate the relationships.

The purity of the injury situation may be confusing, not only because of a minor component of contracoup in the still head-moving object situation and vice versa, but also because the blow to the fixed head may cause a fall onto a hard object. Thus the pattern may be mixed, confused, and not necessarily open to clear interpretation.

Another type of contusion is encountered in medicolegal investigations. This type is relatively deep in penetration, usually involving the deep gray matter or the white matter, covered with an overlying layer of apparently normal brain substance, and large or small hemorrhages (Fig. 16-39). The small hemorrhages are frequently termed "ball hemorrhages" due to their spherical shape. They may be confused with focal hemorrhages that sometimes are seen in individuals with marked hypertension. The larger and deeper hemorrhages are often more irregular in shape and may be confused with apoplectic hemorrhage or stroke.[16] An adequate

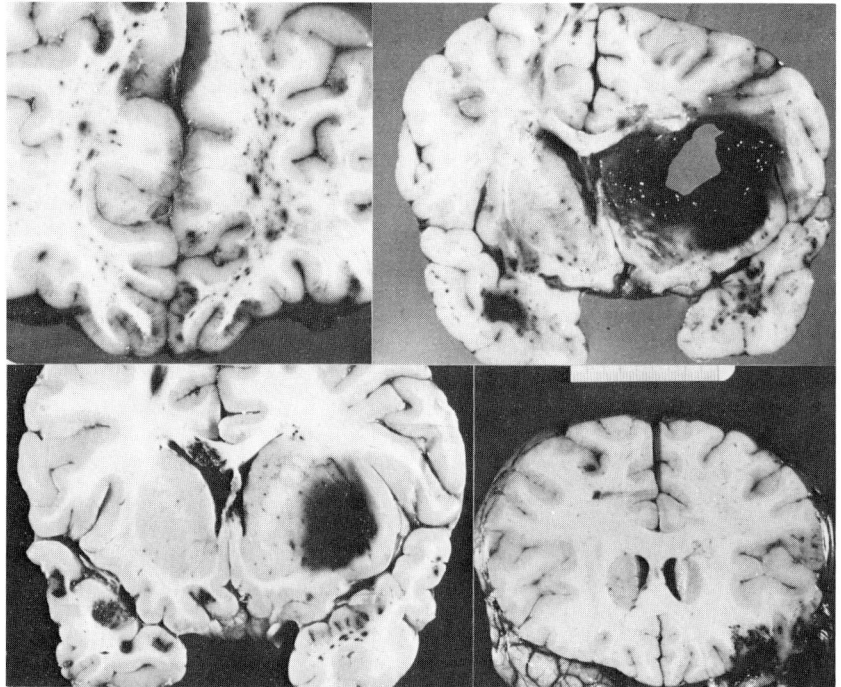

FIGURE 16-39. Multiple contusions of brain. Cross-sectional views of four different brains are shown. Different patterns of deep and superficial contusion can be seen. In the upper left panel, the direction of force is from the top to bottom of the photograph, and extending from the back of the brain to the front. The contusions seem to follow the force vector. The upper right and lower left panels illustrate large, deep contusions in the basal ganglia. This site is that expected in a nontraumatic cerebral hemorrhage; the presence of other contusions and, in the lower left panel, a tear of the corpus callosum are indicative of traumatic origin of the contusions. In the lower right panel, the force vector is from the lower right to the upper left side.

history of the circumstances surrounding death, the presence or absence of other signs of head trauma, and an assessment of diseases affecting the deceased may help to differentiate between trauma and other causes of the deep hemorrhage.

Intracerebral hemorrhage of the apoplectic type not associated with trauma usually involves areas not ordinarily involved with the deep hemorrhages of trauma. The usual sites of predilection are deep in the basal ganglia, the pons, and the cerebellum, with the first-listed location the most frequently involved. Those hemorrhages associated with arteriovenous malformation may occur anywhere within the brain. Unlike the apoplectic hemorrhage, the victim is usually young rather than middle aged and does not have a history of hypertension.

Pulmonary edema of the so-called neurogenic type often accompanies head injury. The external manifestation commonly found is the "foam cone," a mass of frothy white or pink foam exuding from the nostrils and mouth (Fig. 16-40). Such a foam cone is also found in deaths due to drowning, overdoses of drugs, and in heart disease deaths accompanied by gradual decompensation of the heart. The presence of froth does not, therefore, prove that a closed head injury exists.

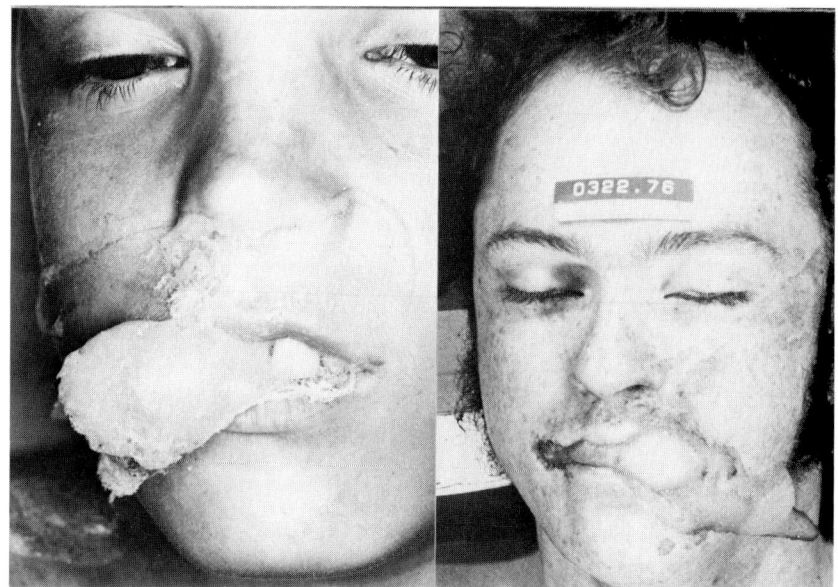

FIGURE 16-40. Pulmonary edema in head injury. The "foam cone" of pulmonary edema is shown arising from the mouth and nostrils of the two subjects. Note that the injury of the head is not apparent in the views shown; neither individual had any injury visible upon external examination alone.

Patterns of Injury

There are many patterns of blunt force injury that can be recognized, leading to the solution of questions of medicolegal importance.[17] A few examples follow:

1. A dicing pattern can be found on the skin, caused by the victim's striking a side window of a motor vehicle at the time of a crash. The side windows of motor vehicles in the United States must be made of tempered glass. When impacted, this glass breaks up into small, cube-shaped fragments. The injury sustained by an individual striking such a glass window with force enough to cause it to shatter will manifest in the form of small abrasions, contusions, and lacerations which have square shapes or angles (Fig. 16-41) (see also Chapter 14).
2. Pedestrians while standing and struck by motor vehicles will frequently sustain fractures of the long bones of the legs (Fig. 16-42). These are sometimes termed "bumper fractures." The presence of such fractures, coupled with other injuries, on a body found by the roadside, indicates that the subject was a pedestrian, that he was struck by a motor vehicle, and may indicate the height of the bumper from the ground. Since all motor vehicles "nose dive" when the brakes are applied firmly, measurement of the bumper height above ground, and the height of the fractures above the level of the shoe heel, can indicate whether or not the driver was attempting to stop his motor vehicle at the moment it impacted the victim's legs.
3. A sizable percentage of individuals who suffer a sudden, fatal heart attack fall to the surface on which they are standing with such force that they injure themselves. The pattern of the injuries are in and

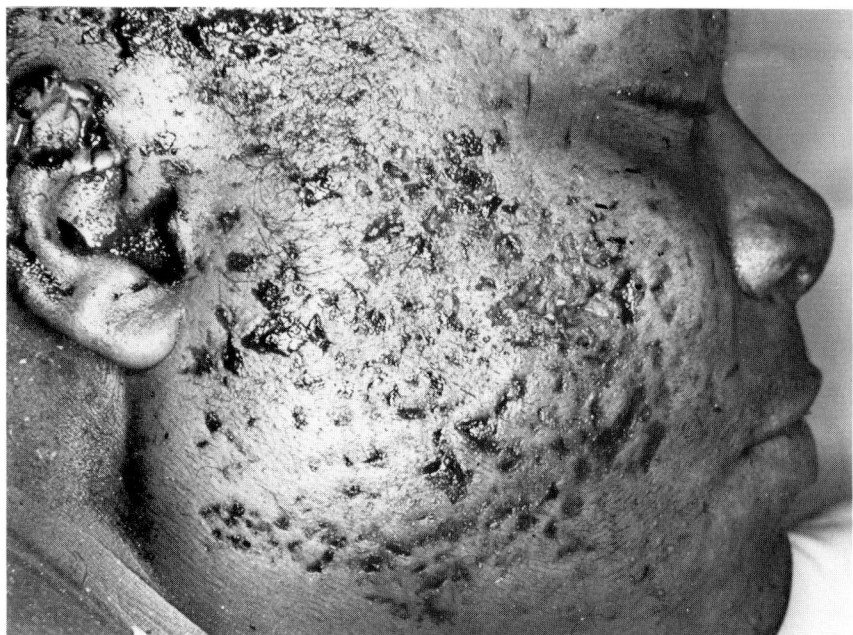

FIGURE 16-41. Dicing pattern of cheek. The "diced" appearance is due to the victim's striking the side window of a motor vehicle at the time of a crash. The tempered glass shattered into small fragments (cubes) which caused the multiple lacerations, abrasions, and contusions.

below the "hat band" area, and usually limited to one side of the face (Fig. 16-43). The presence of such patterned injuries indicates a probable fall as the cause, rather than a blow struck to the face by an assailant.

4. A blow to the mouth area may be much more visible internally than externally. When the blow is struck by a fist, the wounding blunt object may inflict only minor visible damage at the point of contact, but the soft lingular tissues are forced against the teeth (or in the absence of teeth, the dental ridge), and injury to the inner aspects of the lips will result (Fig. 16-44). The frenum of the upper lip is sometimes torn, particularly when the subject is an infant that has been subjected to numerous blows to the head.

Patterns of injury are found in great variety and they tell many tales to the medicolegal examiner. Frequently they are not recognized, not because the victim was not examined, but because the examiner tended to examine in detail, area by area, and failed to recognize the pattern. Photography of the victim, including front and back overview photographs, are often useful in recognizing patterns of injury. The preparation of body diagrams to display graphically the location and nature of injuries is an exercise well calculated to reveal the injury pattern.

SHARP INSTRUMENT INJURY

Sharp instruments such as knives, ice picks, hatchets, axes, meat cleavers, and bayonets cause many of the wounds seen by medicolegal investiga-

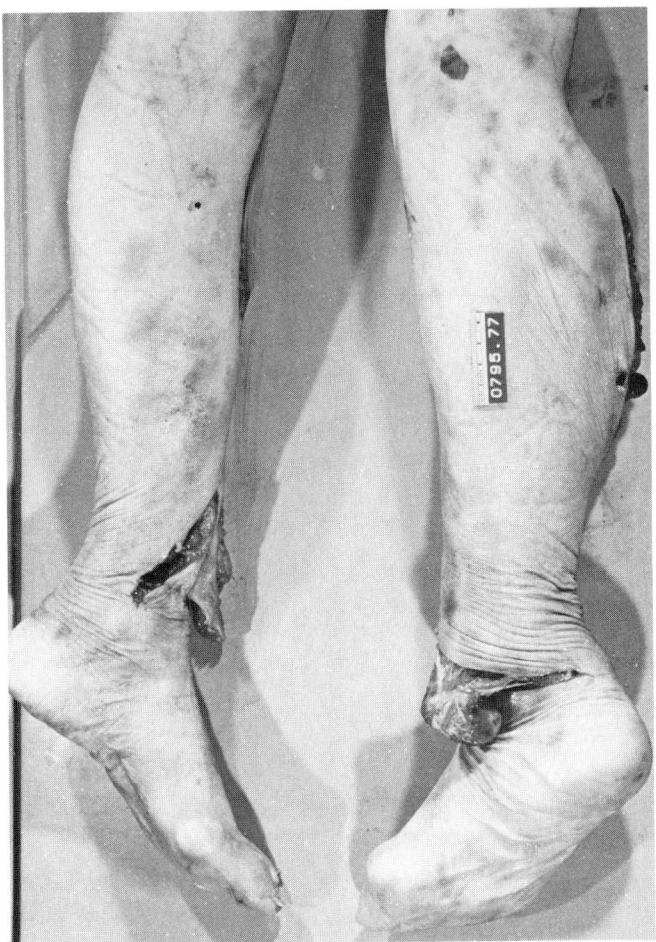

FIGURE 16-42. Bumper fractures of long bones. This pedestrian, struck by the bumper of the motor vehicle, sustained bilateral fractures of the tibia and fibula, and disarticulation at the ankle joints.

tors. The most frequently encountered types of wounds produced by such instruments are discussed in the sections to follow.

Incised Wounds

Incised wounds are those made with a slashing or cutting motion with a sharp instrument such as a knife or a straight-edge razor. Because of the motion of the wounding instrument, the wound is generally longer than it is deep (Fig. 16-45). The length and depth of the wound depend upon the motion of the weapon, the force applied, the sharpness (or dullness) of the wounding instrument, and the nature of the target tissue. The characteristic of incised wounds that sets them apart from lacerations is the smooth edge of the wound. Undermining may be present which indicates the direction from which the slashing stroke was made, but the character of the weapon, other than the fact that it was sharp, cannot be ascertained by an examination of the wound.

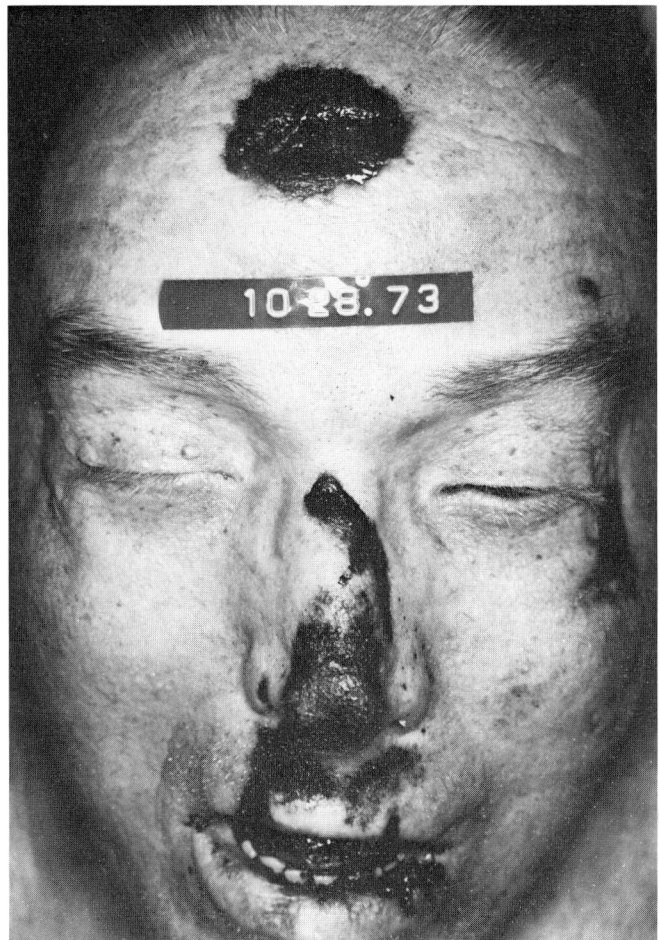

FIGURE 16-43. Pattern of fall. At the time of the fatal heart attack, the victim fell to the concrete walk from a short stepladder, causing the one-sided facial injuries.

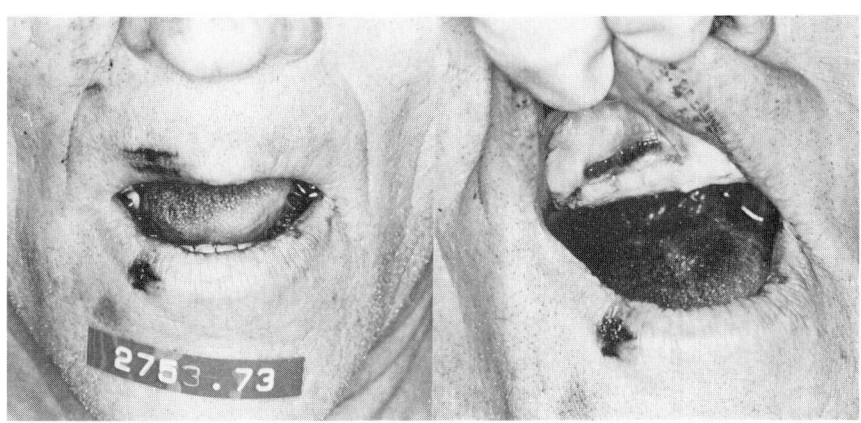

FIGURE 16-44. Blow to mouth. The external and internal injuries to the mouth area are clearly shown. Even in the absence of upper teeth, the injury to the inner aspects of the lip has been caused by the dental ridge.

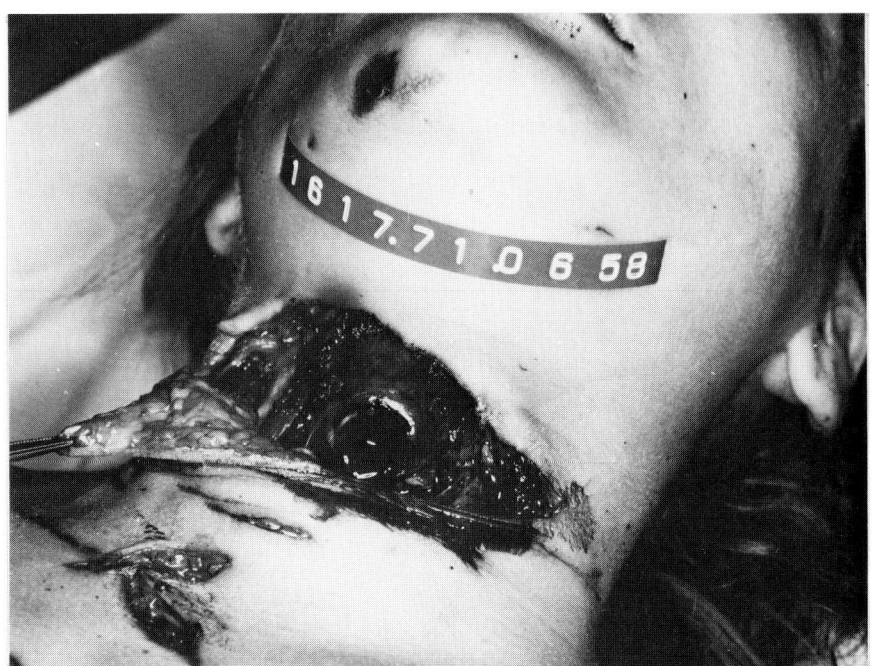

FIGURE 16-45. Homicidal slash wound of neck. This is an example of an incised wound made by a slashing motion with a knife. The adjacent, smaller stab-type wounds are not representative of hesitation marks, but are part of a very extensive mutilation of the victim by the assailant.

Stab Wounds

Stab wounds may be inflicted by any pointed and sharp instrument, including knives, daggers, bayonets, and other manufactured or improvised weapons. The wound caused by such an instrument is made by a thrusting or stabbing motion, or, in the event of impalement, by the victim's falling onto a sharp object. The nature of the wounding instrument may sometimes be ascertained by an examination of the wound. A simple stab wound is produced by a thrusting motion directly into the body and the subsequent outward movement or retraction. Thus the external appearance of the wound may very well resemble the cross section of the weapon. If the knife has one cutting edge, one angle of the wound will be sharp, the other obtuse, blunt, or torn (Fig. 16-46). If the weapon has two cutting edges, as on a stiletto, the angles will both be sharp (Fig. 16-47).

The external appearance of stab wounds does not depend solely upon the cross-sectional configuration of the weapon. The elastic tissue of the dermis, the deeper portion of the skin, has a considerable effect upon the shape of the wound. It should be realized that elastic tissue fibers are arranged in flowing lines in all areas of the body. These lines conform to a pattern described many years ago and generally known as Langer's lines. A stab wound with the long axis at right angles to the elastic tissue of Langer's lines will gape open with the edges pulled apart by the elastic tissue. Thus the wound will appear wide and short. If the wound is parallel to the elastic tissue lines, it will appear narrow and long, and

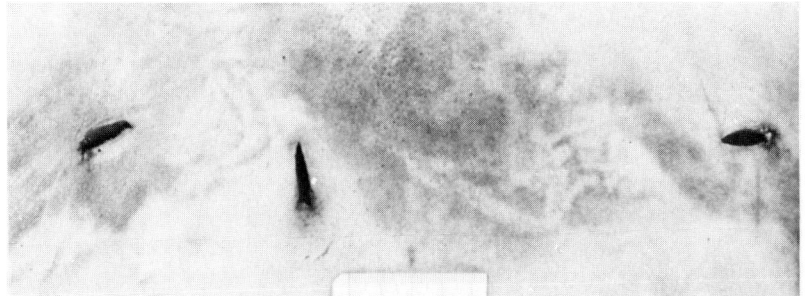

FIGURE 16-46. Single-edge knife wound. Multiple stab wounds have been made with a single-edge knife. The cutting edge has made an acute, sharp angle at one extremity, and the dull edge has made an obtuse angle at the other.

gaping of the wound edges will not be prominent. This phenomenon must be kept in mind at the time of the examination of the wound; the distortion of the wound may be considerable, and single-edged knife wounds may appear to have been inflicted by a double-edged weapon because of this distortion. The effect of Langer's lines on the appearance of awl and ice pick wounds is usually the tearing of the two areas of the margin at right angles to the general plane of flow of the lines. The circular wound caused by the circular cross-section weapon then takes on an elliptical or slitlike appearance. There are, however, other factors that have effect upon the appearance of stab wounds. One of these is the action of the victim. If the victim twists or turns the target portion of the body either during the in-stroke, or during the out-stroke, the external wound may have somewhat serrated edges or be otherwise distorted (Fig. 16-48). Moreover, the weapon itself may be manipulated by other than a simple in and out stroke. Several kinds of wound patterns are likely to be found:

1. The instrument is thrust in, partially out, and in again along a different track. In such situations external wound will be of a com-

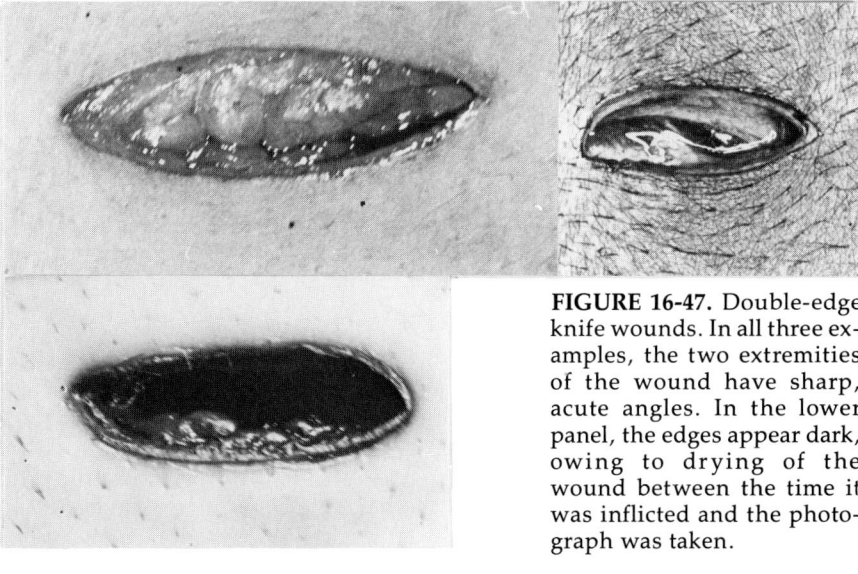

FIGURE 16-47. Double-edge knife wounds. In all three examples, the two extremities of the wound have sharp, acute angles. In the lower panel, the edges appear dark, owing to drying of the wound between the time it was inflicted and the photograph was taken.

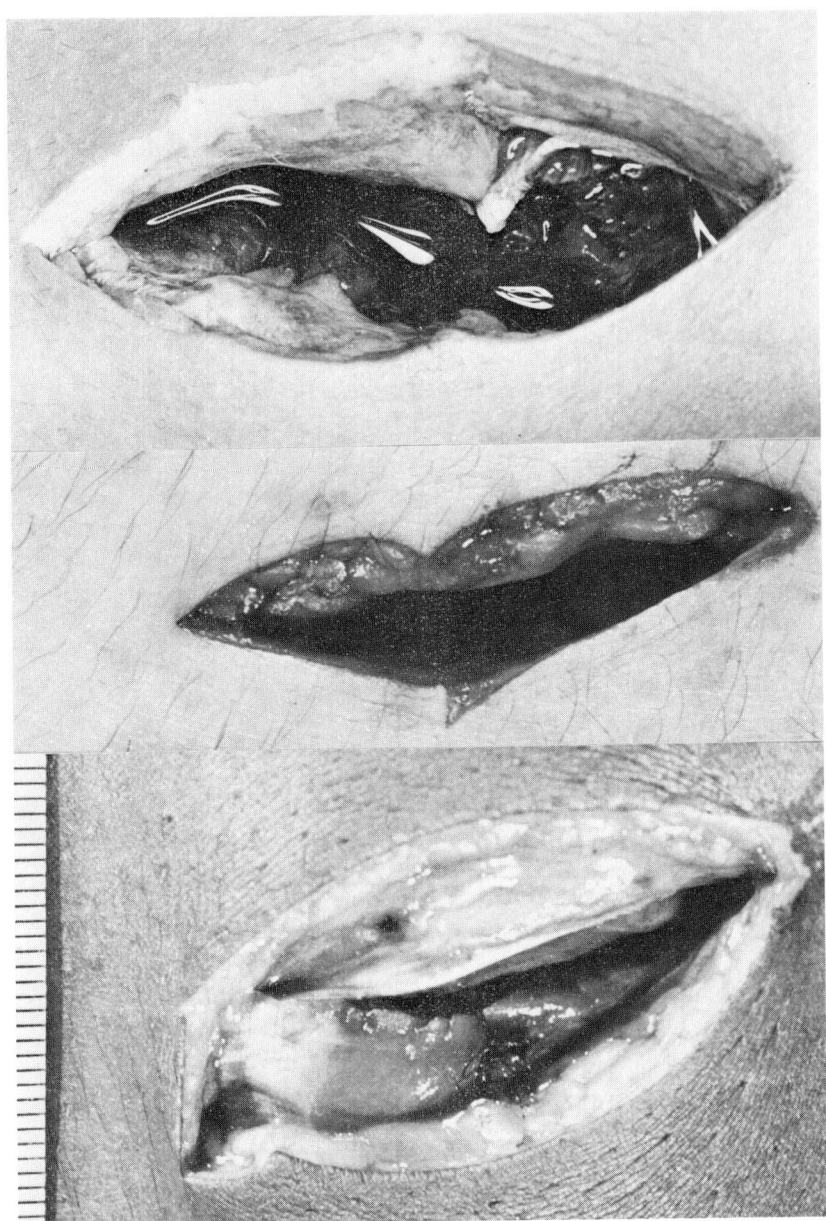

FIGURE 16-48. Compound stab wounds. The wounds shown in these panels are not simple, one-stroke stab wounds. More than one stroke, turning of the sharp instrument, movement of the victim, or other variables have caused alteration in the size and shape of the wound from that expected.

pound nature, and more than one track will be seen in deeper tissues and organs.

2. The instrument is thrust in and then is completely withdrawn with the cutting edge dragging against one extremity or an angle of the wound so as to extend the wound superficially, giving the injury to the skin surface a tail somewhat resembling a teardrop in shape.
3. The instrument is thrust in and then, while still in, it is pulled in

the direction of a cutting edge so that the track and the skin wound are elongated. The external wound will be much larger than the appearance of the weapon would suggest.
4. The instrument is thrust in and then pulled toward a cutting edge, using the point of the knife as a fulcrum, so that the track is narrowest at its deepest point and widest at the most superficial point. Again, the external wound will be larger than the edged weapon itself.
5. The instrument is twisted as it enters or as it is withdrawn, or both. The edges of the external wound will be irregular and large.

In addition to the foregoing, if the weapon has a hilt with a quillon (a bar separating the blade from the hilt), and if the weapon has been used with considerable force, a small contusion may be seen adjacent to the stab wound itself (Fig. 16-49). This contused area will indicate something of the force with which the blow was struck as well. A small abrasion-contusion joining double circular or near circular small punctate defects will indicate that an instrument such as a two-prong barbecue fork has been used (Fig. 16-50).

It would appear that the length of the track made by the stabbing instrument would indicate the minimum length of the weapon necessary to make the track. Some complications, however, attend this estimate. It must be kept in mind that the body of the victim at the time of the stabbing may have been in a position quite different than on the autopsy table. Bending and twisting, leaning foreward, and lifting of the arms may have made the victim vulnerable to stabbing with a weapon considerably shorter than it would appear at the time of autopsy. Manipulation of the body so as to duplicate the body's position at the time of wounding is not always easy or even possible at the time of autopsy because of weight and rigor mortis. Therefore, repositioning of the body so as to permit measurement of the wound track may not be possible. A second point to be considered is the compression of certain parts of the body at the time of stabbing. This compression is readily accomplished by the force of the stabbing blow with the quillon or the hand which holds and manipulates the weapon, compressing the target area so that much deeper penetration is afforded the weapon than would seem possible.

The experienced medicolegal examiner will hesitate to characterize the

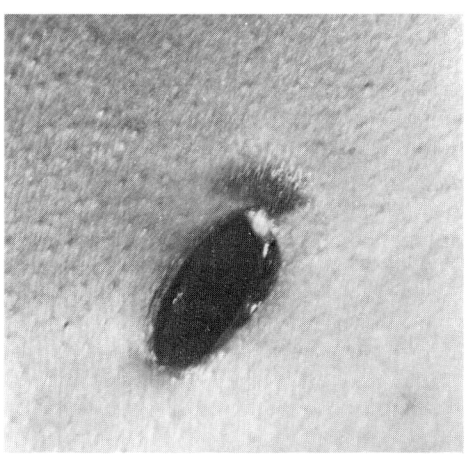

FIGURE 16-49. Quillon or guard mark. Adjacent to the stab wound itself is a small abrasion which was made when the quillon or guard which separated the blade from the handle of the knife impacted the skin. This abrasion is indicative of the force with which the blow was struck.

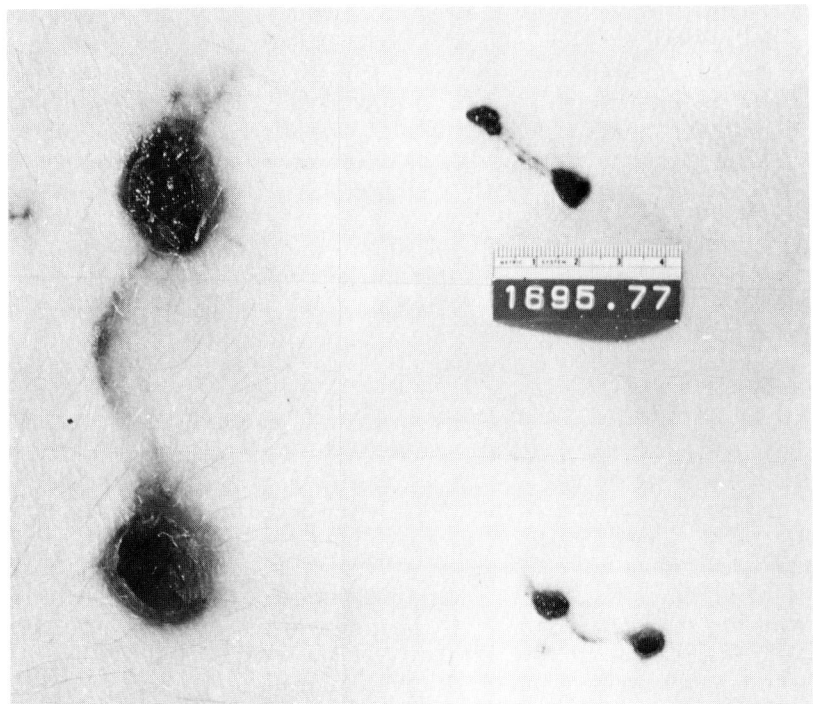

FIGURE 16-50. Barbeque fork wound. Stab wounds made with a barbeque fork may be quite characteristic. The defects made by the tines are more or less joined by faint abrasions made by the part of the fork where the tines are joined.

weapon used in these cases with any great assurance. It is best to say no more than that the wound is consistent with that expected from the weapon at hand.

Stout-bladed knives thrust into the chest wall with some vigor will penetrate costal cartilages, ribs, and even the sternum with relative ease.[18] The cross-sectional characteristics of the weapon are best preserved in bone injury. Occasionally a weak-bladed weapon may break and the broken tip of the weapon will become lodged in bone. It can then be recovered, and the fractured side compared with the broken end of the weapon that was employed.

Chopping Wounds

Chopping wounds result from hacking or chopping motions made with a fairly sharp and relatively heavy instrument such as an axe, hatchet, cleaver, or machete. Sometimes bayonets and very heavy knives are employed in this manner. The nature of the wound caused by such a weapon varies with its sharpness and its weight. The sharper the instrument, the sharper the edges of the wound (Fig. 16-51). As with slash wounds made with smaller sharp instruments, undermining occurs in the direction toward which the chop is made. Adjacent abrasion may accompany such wounds on the side opposite the undermining due to the slap of the flat of the blade. Should the heavy chopping instrument be directed at the head, the angle at which the blade strikes can sometimes be determined by the shape of the skull defect. The flat of the blade may leave a slope to

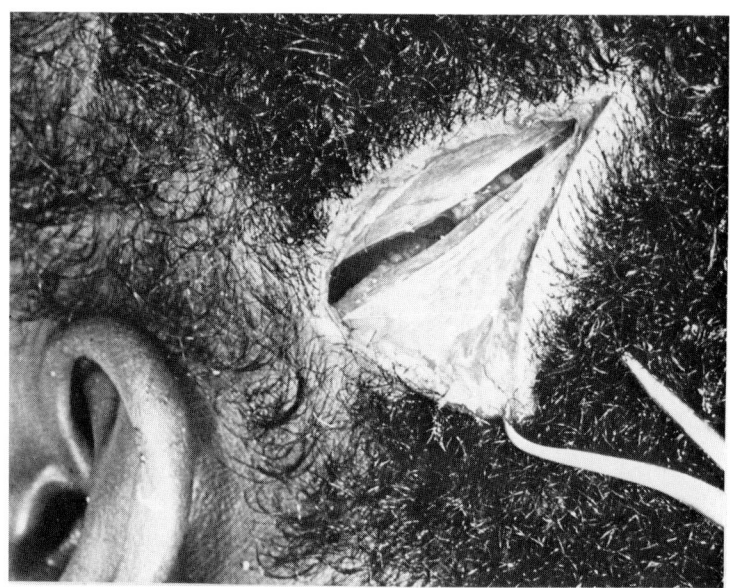

FIGURE 16-51. Chopping wound of scalp. The sharp edges of the wound in the scalp indicate the sharpness of the blade. The underlying skull injury has resulted from the weight of the chopping instrument. The wound was made with a hatchet.

the one side of the defect, while the other side may be sharp or even undermined (Fig. 16-52). The weight of the weapon contributes to its ability to cut through bone underlying the wound itself. The entire thickness of the skull may be penetrated by the heavier chopping or hacking instruments. Instances are recorded where entire teeth have been sectioned by machetes. Severe bone damage is not seen with ordinary knives. Also to be noted is the possibility of a twisting force being employed after the chopping instrument has been embedded in bone and as it is being removed. Such a movement, if conducted with force, can cause splintering of the bone, particularly near the extremities of the chop wound.

The major effect of stab, slash, and chop wounds is hemorrhage. Dysfunction due to severing of nerves of extremities may also be noted. Deep stab wounds may involve any tissue or organ. Very small objects used to inflict stab-type wounds make such small wounds that normal tissue elasticity will close the wound as the weapon is withdrawn, and no bleeding will be noted externally. Ice picks, awls, and hatpins are well known to make this type of wound. As has been noted in the discussion of trauma due to firearms, the slitlike nature of stab wounds of the large arteries and the heart is responsible for slower bleeding than those defects caused by firearms.[19]

Occasionally, unusual weapons are employed to stab, slash, or chop. Razor-sharp hunting arrows have been used as the missiles that they are and also as weapons to hand-stab the victim. Sharp shards of glass, broken bottles, and other sharp glass objects are occasionally employed as slashing or stabbing weapons. Surgical knives, knitting needles, and even large spikes have been employed to cause lethal wounds.

Some mention should be made of the defects caused in clothing by sharp instruments used as stab weapons. When a double-edged knife or

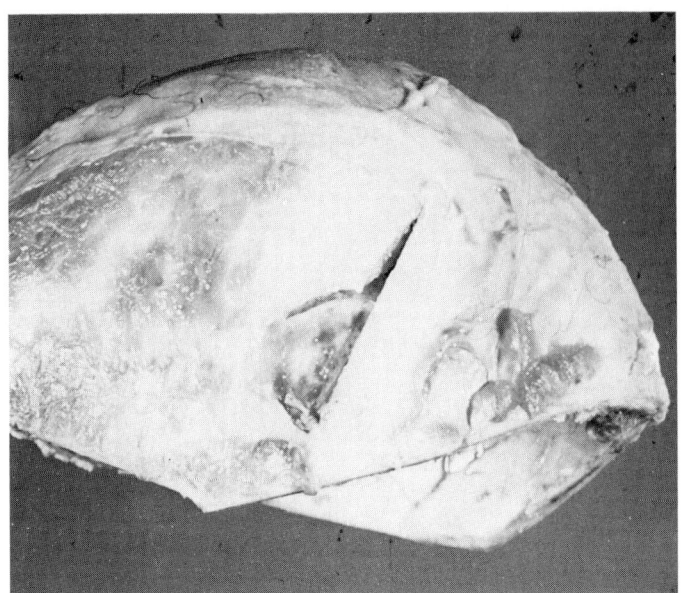

FIGURE 16-52. Chopping wound of skull. This hatchet wound of the skull was inflicted with the blow struck from the left side of the figure. Thus the flat surface of the blade has depressed the left-hand edge of the skull defect, and there is undermining of the right.

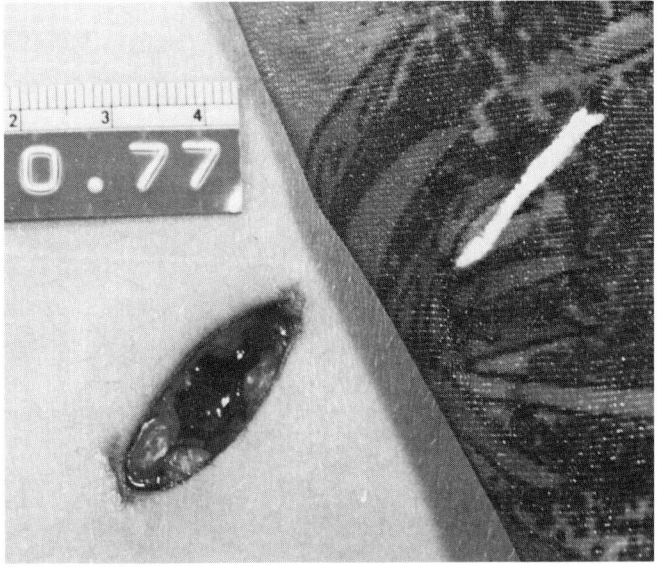

FIGURE 16-53. Clothing defect in stab wound. The shape of the clothing defect can indicate the nature of the weapon. The sharp angle of the clothing defect is similar to the sharp angle of the skin defect. A swallow tail is indicative of the dull edge of the blade. Note the quillon mark adjacent to the sharp angle made by the cutting edge.

similar weapon is used, the sharp, cutting edges cause sharp-angled or acute-angled extremities of the slitlike defect. A single-edged weapon frequently causes one sharp-angled extremity and one swallow-tailed extremity (Fig. 16-53). Thus examination of the clothing of the victim of stabbing may well indicate something of the characteristics of the weapon employed. Such an examination is of particular importance when the stab wound may have been enlarged by the treating surgeon prior to any examination of the victim for medicolegal purposes. Clothing examination may also be useful in determining whether or not the weapon actually penetrated the overlying layers of clothing. Individuals who employ sharp instruments to commit suicide may adjust clothing so that it will not be penetrated by the weapon. The absence of defects in the clothing worn by the victim, yet with wounds in an area that ordinarily would have been covered by that same clothing, may point to death by self-inflicted wounds.

Two types of sharp instrument wounds are well known and both characterize actions taken by the victim. "Hesitation marks" are shallow incised, stab, or chop wounds made before the fatal wound by an individual who is in the act of committing suicide. These hesitation wounds frequently parallel and are close to the deep incised wound of the wrist or neck (Fig. 16-54). They may also take the form of shallow stab wounds near the deep and fatal final stab wound (Fig. 16-55). Although very rarely encountered, superficial chopping wounds of the head may be inflicted before the heavy blow causes unconsciousness and/or death.

Another type of sharp instrument wound is that termed a "defense wound." It is found on the fingers, hands, and forearms (and rarely elsewhere) of victims as they attempt to protect themselves by warding off blows, as by attempting to grab the blade of the sharp instrument (Fig. 16-56).

It should be clear that "hesitation marks" characterize suicide and that "defense marks" indicate homicide. However, it is well to bear in mind that several slashing wounds can be inflicted, usually in or about the neck, by the assailant in homicide cases. Multiple slash wounds of the forearms may also, though rarely, appear to be defense marks, but may actually represent hesitation wounds—multiple attempts by the individual to locate a larger blood vessel, the better to cause rapid and severe bleeding. The interpretation of apparent hesitation or defense marks should be undertaken only after very careful and complete consideration of all of the circumstances surrounding the trauma and death.

FIREARMS INJURY

It must always be kept in mind that when a firearm is discharged, three different substances can be discharged from the muzzle. These are the bullet or other missile, the unburned powder grains of the charge, and gas. It is the burning of the powder that produces the gas that forces the bullet or shot out of the bore of the firearm. The combustion of the powder produces soot, part of it perhaps due to the graphite commonly used to coat the powder grains. Not all of the powder grains actually burn; a fair percentage remain unburned and many, if not most, of these are blown out of the bore as individual grains, each with the same initial velocity as the bullet or other missiles. The mass of the material which blasts out of the muzzle at the time of firing determines the distance it

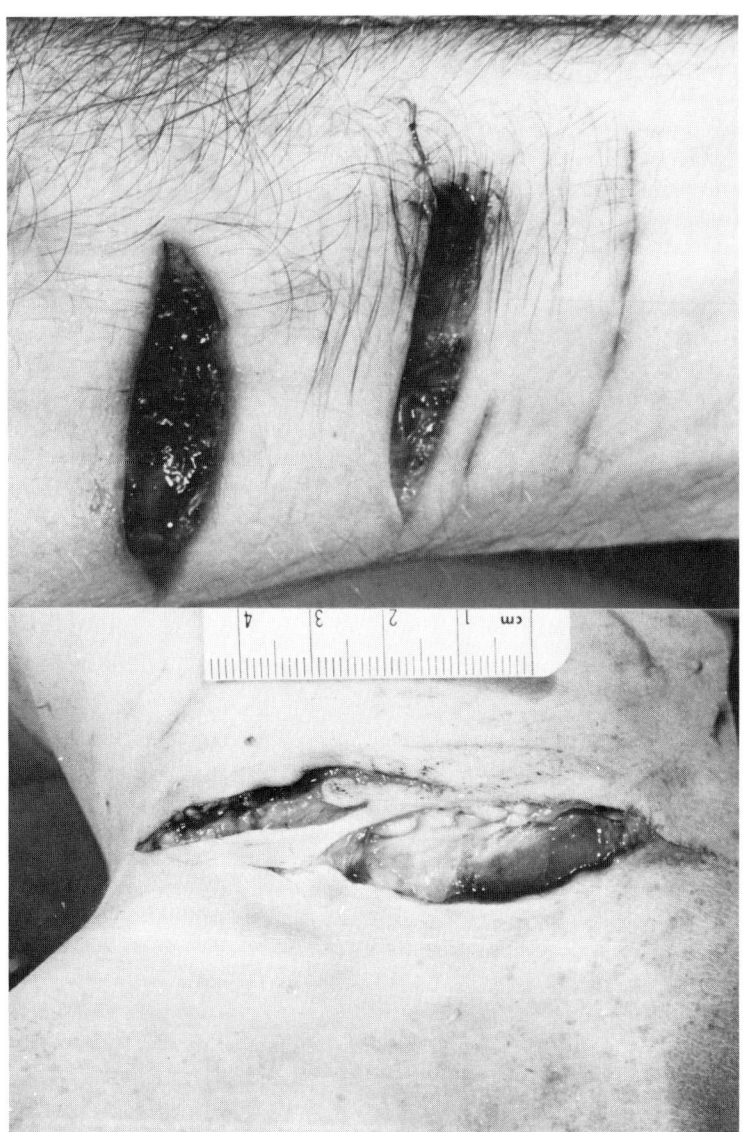

FIGURE 16-54. Hesitation marks. Two examples of hesitation marks are shown, indicating the victim's intent to commit suicide.

will travel. The gas, with its contained soot, is very light and travels a very short distance measured in inches. The unburned powder grains, with greater mass, travel further. Depending upon the type of powder, the distance the powder grains will travel will vary from 2 to 6 feet. The heavy bullet, of course, travels much further on its course to its intended or unintended target.

Range of Fire Determination

The effects on the target of gas, powder grains, and missiles can be used in a forensic scientific manner to estimate the distance from the target at

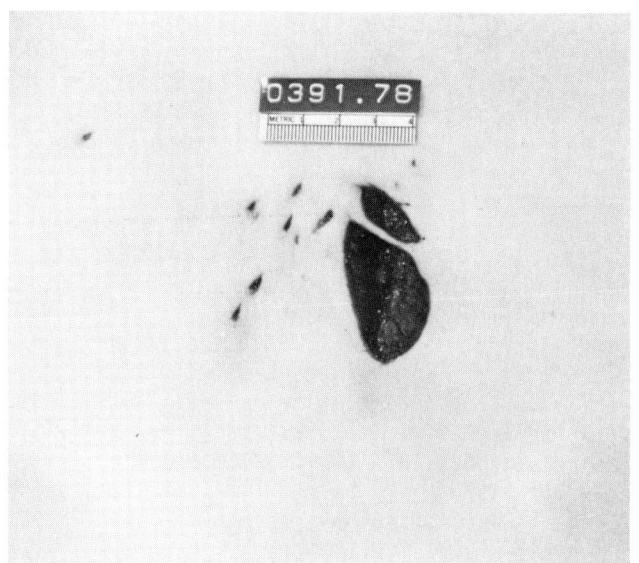

FIGURE 16-55. Hesitation marks. A series of tentative, searching, shallow stab wounds were made prior to the final, fatal wound.

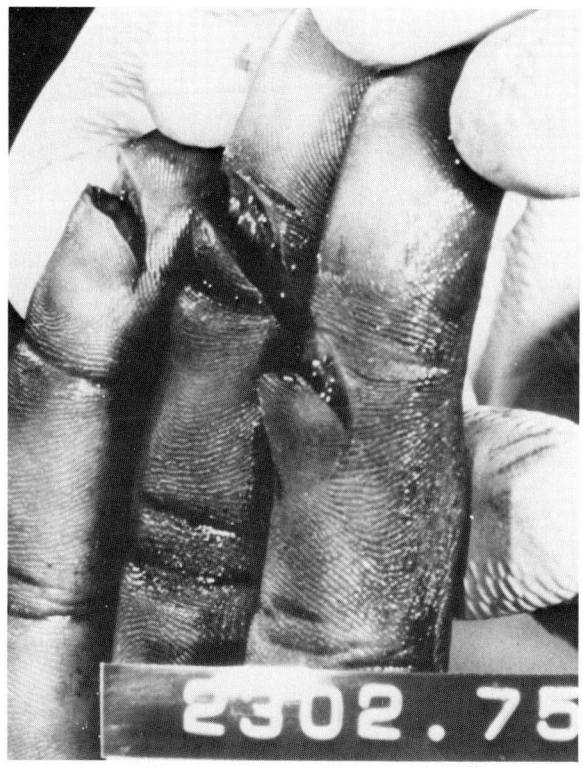

FIGURE 16-56. Defense wound. The victim grabbed the sharp instrument wielded by the assailant, sustaining deep, incised wounds of the fingers.

which the firearm was discharged. Such a determination is of utmost importance: to prove or disprove the statements of the accused; to rule in or out the possibility of suicide; and to help establish the accidental nature of the wound. Although range of fire cannot be determined with absolute precision, the gunshot or shotgun wound can be defined with some accuracy as resulting from a discharge at contact range or at short, medium, or long range. Reference to Table 16-8 will help to classify some of the observable signs that can be used to help determine the range of fire by visual examination of the wound and the skin surrounding the wound. It will be noted that the table deals with both rifled firearms and shotguns. Included among the former are handguns (revolvers and autoloading pistols) and rifles. The common denominator of these weapons consists in the grooves cut in the bore so as to impart a spin to the bullet as it passes down the bore. Shotguns, on the other hand, are without such rifling (smooth bore) and generally are used to fire multiple missiles (spherical shot) at one time. Those interested in a detailed discussion of the different types of firearms are referred to an excellent text by Hatcher, Jury, and Weller.[20] The different types of wounds will be discussed in terms of their medicolegal significance.

Contact-Range Wounds

Many people do not understand that the burning of powder at the time of the discharge of the firearm produces a very large amount of gas. It is the gas that pushes the bullet out of the barrel, and, continuing to expand rapidly, produces the report or noise associated with the discharge. The gas is very hot and another visible result of its presence is the muzzle flash, particularly well seen at night or in a darkened room.

TABLE 16-8. VISIBLE HALLMARKS OF RANGE OF FIRE

	Rifled Firearms	*Shotgun*
I. Contact		
A. Firm, over shallowly situated bone	"Explosive" appearance Soot on edges of defect and deep, in tissue, on bone Muzzle imprint	"Explosive" appearance Soot on edges of defect and deep, in tissues, on bone Muzzle imprint
B. Firm, not over shallowly situated bone	Circular defect Soot in deeper tissues	Circular defect Soot in deeper tissues
C. Loose	Corona (plus same as "B" above)	Same as "B" above
II. Short Range	Soot deposit (powder gas) Free powder grains	Soot deposit (powder gas) Searing (powder gas) Free powder grains Wad prong marks
III. Medium Range	Tattooing (powder grains)	Tattooing (powder grains) Irregular margin to defect Stippling (plastic filler in buckshot loads)
IV. Long Range	Defect alone	Irregular defect with satellite defects Longer range: satellites predominate, wad marks seen

When the muzzle of the weapon is held firmly against the skin, so as to produce a gas seal, the bullet, the unburned powder, and the gas all enter the body at once, the heavy bullet driving deep into the tissues, the unburned powder grains losing velocity rapidly and being deposited along the bullet track and being carried into the tissues and tissue planes surrounding the track by the ever-expanding gas. Soot is deposited, also, along the edge of the wound, along the track made by the bullet, and in the tissues and tissue planes carried there by the gas. As the gas is still very hot upon leaving the muzzle of the firearm, some searing of the edge of the defect is made by the sum of the materials that are blown out of the muzzle.

Three factors operate to vary the nature of the wound produced by the combination of gas and bullet: (1) the amount of gas produced by the burning of the powder; (2) the effectiveness of the seal between the muzzle and the skin; and (3) the presence or absence of bone a short distance below the skin surface. The first of these factors, the amount of gas produced by the burning of powder, bears some relationship to the muzzle velocity of the firearm involved. Obviously, one way in which to increase muzzle velocity is to increase the push imparted to the bullet. Increasing the amount of gas produced by the burning of the powder is the principal way to increase the thrust given to the missile. The second factor involved is the effectiveness of the seal between the muzzle and the skin. The more efficient the seal, the more the gas will fail to blow out around the muzzle and the more gas will be available to expand in the body tissues. The final factor concerns the presence of a layer of bone a short distance beneath the skin, which can prove to be a barrier to the expected massive penetration and expansion of gas in the deeper tissues.

Table 16-8 deals with three types of contact-range situations as follows:

1. Firm or press contact with the skin over shallowly situated bone. The prime example of this type is a contact wound of the head or skull. In such a contact wound, the shallowly located bone serves as a barrier to the rapid, deep expansion of gas. If the gas produced is sufficient in amount, the bone of the skull tends to turn back the ever-expanding cone of gas, which then tends to blast out around the muzzle of the firearm, everting the tissue, and giving it an explosive or eruptive appearance. Under the usual circumstances, firearms, other than .22 caliber (with short, long, or long-rifle cartridges) will cause this type of wound (Fig. 16-57). The amount of gas produced by the three commonly used .22 caliber cartridges is relatively small; a contact wound made with a firearm using such ammunition will not appear disruptive or explosive. Very minor degrees of contiguous skin splitting may occur. It should be recalled, however, that there are other .22 caliber cartridges such as the .22 magnum, designed for use in a firearm specifically chambered for it. Such a cartridge produces much more gas than those mentioned above, and the gas effect on the target at contact range can be considerable.
2. Firm or press contact with the skin, but not over shallowly situated bone. Here there is no layer of bone to divert the expanding cone of gas. As a result, the gas continues to penetrate deeper, ever expanding, to be dissipated in the soft tissues of the body. The wound is not eruptive or explosive in appearance. In fact, the external appearance is similar to a wound made with the firearm held a long dis-

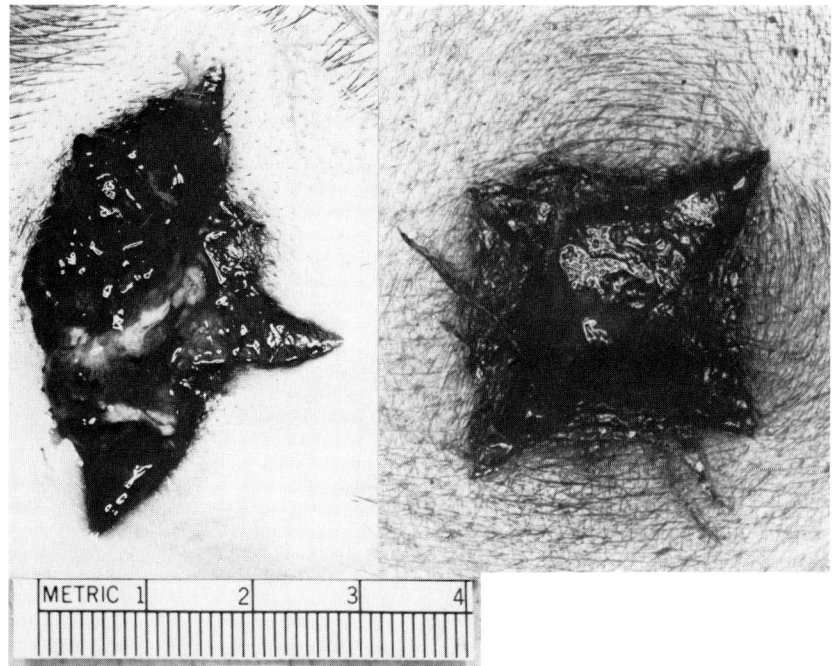

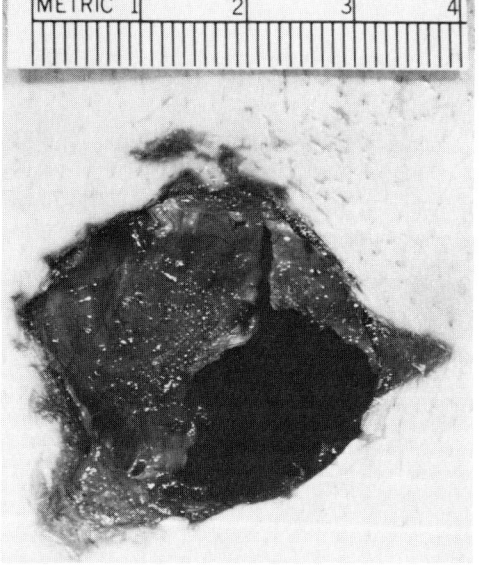

FIGURE 16-57. Explosive contact wounds. The panel in the lower left is representative of an explosive contact wound over shallowly situated bone, in this case the skull. In the upper right is a second example. In the upper left is an explosive contact wound over shallowly situated bone, in this instance the sternum.

tance from the body (Fig. 16-58). Probably this similarity of appearance has been responsible for many misinterpretations of firearms injuries. Careful examination of the tissues should yield evidence of soot or demonstration of intact powder grains in the deeper tissues (see upcoming discussion of firearms residues).

3. Loose or near contact with the skin. The hallmark of this type of wound is the corona, an unusual arrangement of soot on the skin. The corona consists of a circular zone of soot deposit surrounding the missile defect, but separated from it by a band of skin without a deposit of soot. This phenomenon undoubtedly relates to the gas expanding about the muzzle, first at a velocity too high to allow for the settling out of soot, with a subsequent loss in velocity at a short distance from the muzzle, allowing the soot to finally deposit on the

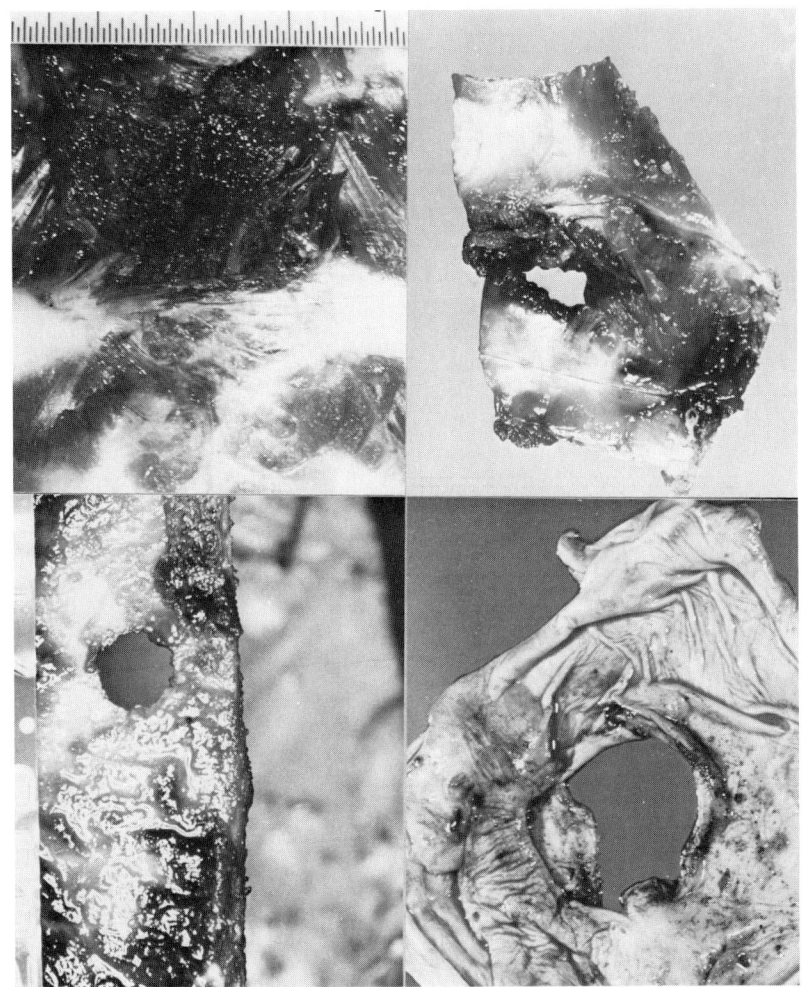

FIGURE 16-58. Visible gunshot residues deep to skin. Four different areas of involvement are pictured: in the upper left panel is shown the deposit of soot and powder grains on the sternum; the upper right panel illustrates the same deposits on the costal cartilages; the lower left, the skull; the lower right, the dura.

skin (Fig. 16-59). The figure also shows an example of a radially arranged streaking to the deposit of soot, sometimes seen when there is a layer of clothing interposed between the muzzle and the skin.

Also noted in Table 16-8 is the phenomenon known as "muzzle imprint." This is found when the muzzle seal is tight, most frequently when the shot is in an area overlying shallowly placed bone, but sometimes seen even when there is no bone directly beneath the inshoot area. The imprint is a more or less complete mirror image of the projecting portions of the muzzle of the firearm. Such an imprint results when the skin is slapped against the muzzle due to the rapid and extensive expansion of the gas within the tissues deep to the skin. Different imprints are illustrated in Figure 16-60.

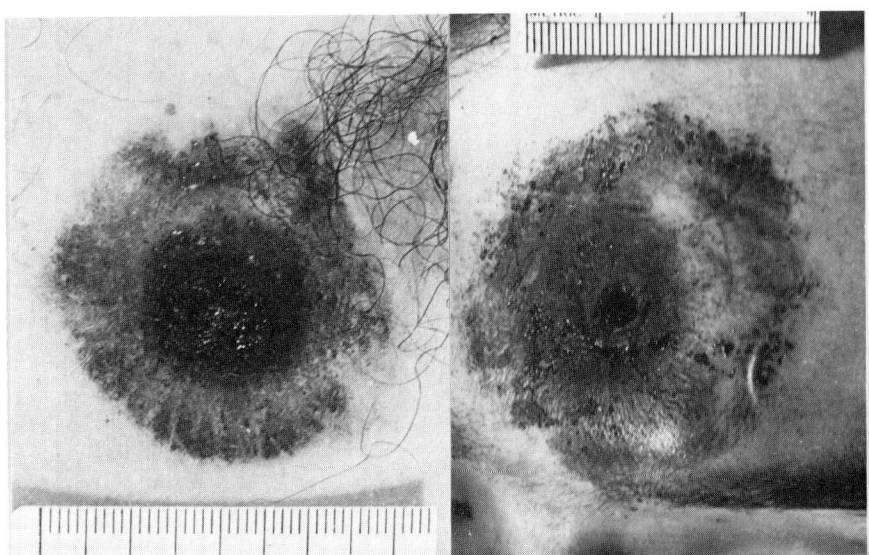

FIGURE 16-59. Loose contact wounds. Loose contact wounds of the forehead (right) and the chest (left) are shown. The corona is clearly visible in each illustration. A layer of clothing overlaid the chest wound. Obviously, no clothing was interposed between the muzzle of the firearm and the forehead.

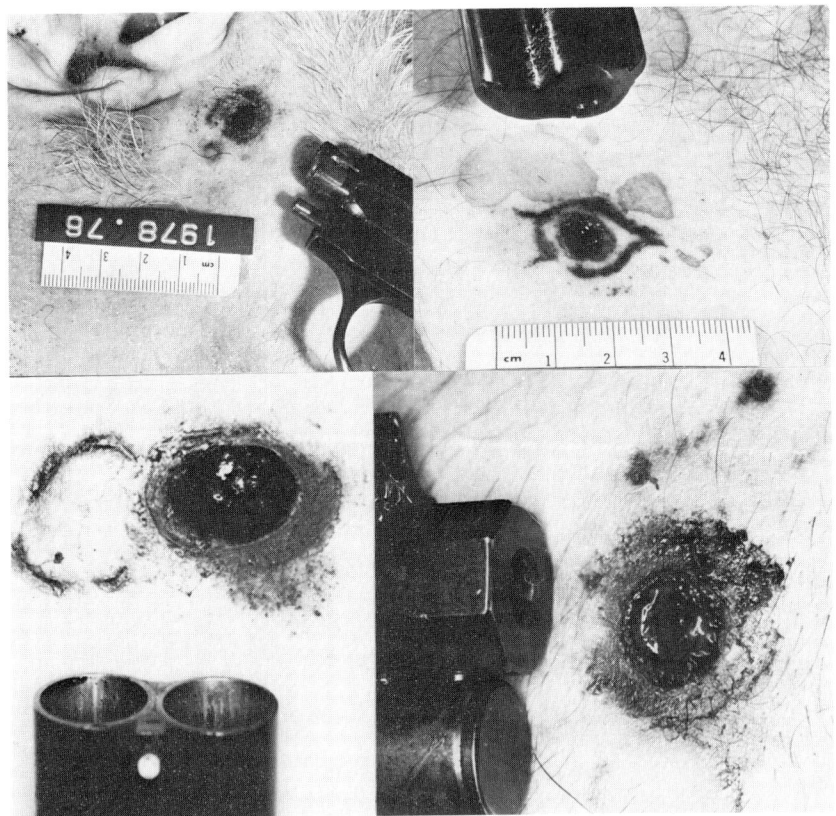

FIGURE 16-60. Muzzle imprints. Imprints of the muzzle are common in contact wounds. Above left is the imprint of an autoloading pistol; above right, that of a revolver; lower left, a shotgun; lower right, a rifle.

Short-Range Wounds

The hallmark of a gunshot wound caused by the discharge of a firearm at a range from loose contact with the skin to a few inches from the skin is the zone of soot deposited about the missile entry point. The gas, being very light, does not carry more than several inches so as to deposit soot upon the skin surface. Unlike the loose contact situation, the soot deposit is a solid zone of blackening more or less concentrically placed about the entrance defect (Fig. 16-61). This zone has sometimes been termed "fouling." The extend of the deposition of soot depends upon the amount of gas produced, the extent of combustion of the powder, and perhaps the amount of graphite used to coat the grains of powder. In such short-range situations, occasional free powder grains may be seen in and on the edges of the defect and deep along the track of the bullet, but "powder tattooing," the characteristic and expected phenomenon of the medium-range wound, is not noted to any significant extent, possibly because of the screening effect of the black deposit of soot (Fig. 16-62).

In short-range wounds resulting from a shotgun, the hot gases in large volume may actually sear the skin itself. The surrounding burns may be visible. Singeing of hair in the region of the soot deposit may occur, but is rarely observed, probably because the singed hair is so fragile that it breaks and is blown away by the muzzle blast and is no longer available for examination after the victim has been treated or the victim's body has been moved. Hair singeing may occur with all manner of firearms.

Medium-Range Wounds

The hallmark for both rifled firearms and shotguns of a medium range wound is "powder tattooing." The individual tattoos are caused by the

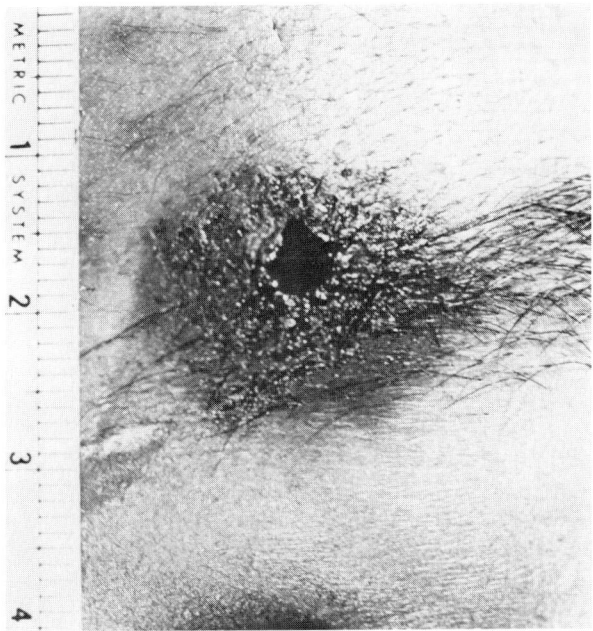

FIGURE 16-61. Short-range wound. A very short-range, almost contact wound characterized by a more or less concentrically placed circular zone of soot deposit.

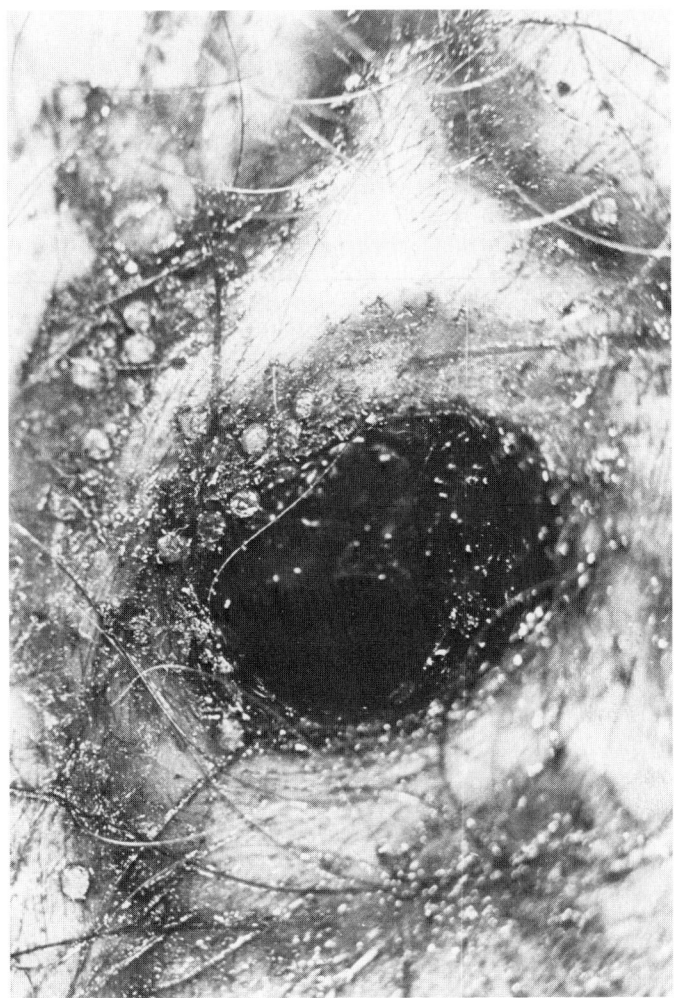

FIGURE 16-62. Powder grains on skin. Free powder grains may be present on the skin, particularly in contact gunshot wounds. The imprint of the muzzle indicates the contact nature of the wound and the disc-shaped powder grains are clearly visible.

individual unburned powder grains being blown into the skin of the victim. Surrounding each tattoo point is a small magenta-colored zone, an actual microcontusion caused by the trauma of the high-speed impaction of the powder grain with rupture of small blood vessels and resulting tiny hemorrhage.

The shape of the individual tattoos gives a clue to the type of powder grain that inflicted the tattooing. Flake powder (grains in the form of discs) causes individual tattoos of varying shape, dependent upon how each grain struck the skin—with the flat side or on edge (Fig. 16-63). Ball powder, either in the form of spheres or flattened spheres, causes more uniform punctate or dot-shaped tattoos (Fig. 16-64). Since the individual grains of ball powder are generally smaller than the grains of flake or disc powder, it follows that the area of tattooing is denser with ball than with flake powder.

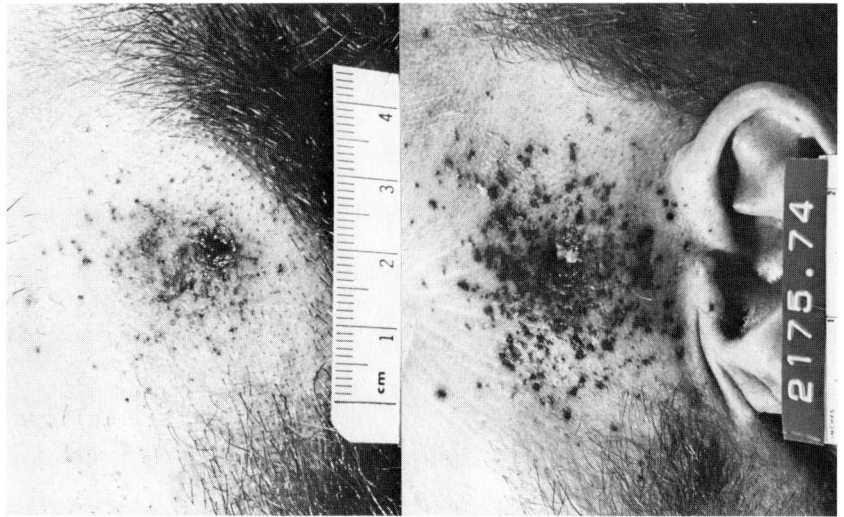

FIGURE 16-63. Flake powder tattooing. Flake powder tattooing is characterized by irregularity of shape of individual tattoos, and it much less dense than that caused by ball powder. Two examples are shown.

The area covered by the tattoo is related to the range of fire. As range increases, the area enlarges and the tattooing becomes less dense. The usual method of determining the size of the tattoo pattern is to measure it in two coordinates, the longitudinal and transverse planes of the body. The comparison of test patterns, fired with the same weapon, the same kind of ammunition and under the same general conditions, with the size of the actual pattern seen on the victim, can result in the determination of the range of fire.

The distance from which different types of powder grains, such as ball, flake, and cylindrical (some rifle ammunition), will cause tattooing varies. Isolated powder grains may carry approximately 8 to 12 feet. However, patterns of tattooing are not seen at a range of over 4 to 5 feet.

Long-Range Wounds

No powder grains and no gas carry to the target at long range. Only bullets or missiles will carry beyond a range of several feet. Therefore, the missile wound consists of the defect made by the bullet (with rifled firearms) itself. There are certain characteristics of the wound that are expected. It usually is circular, or nearly circular, in shape (Fig. 16-65). Just as in the instance of stab wounds, the shape of a bullet wound is altered by the pull of the elastic tissue of the true skin. The margin of the defect is abraded; that is, the epithelium of the skin surface is rubbed away as the bullet strikes the skin against its leading point as it penetrates more deeply. If the bullet is traveling in a fashion that is nonperpendicular to the skin, the abraded margin will be wider on one side than on another (Fig. 16-66). There may actually be undermining of the skin in the direction of the horizontal vector of the bullet flight. Observation of this condition is useful to help determine the general direction taken by the bullet.

At long range, the bullet wound of entrance may appear singularly

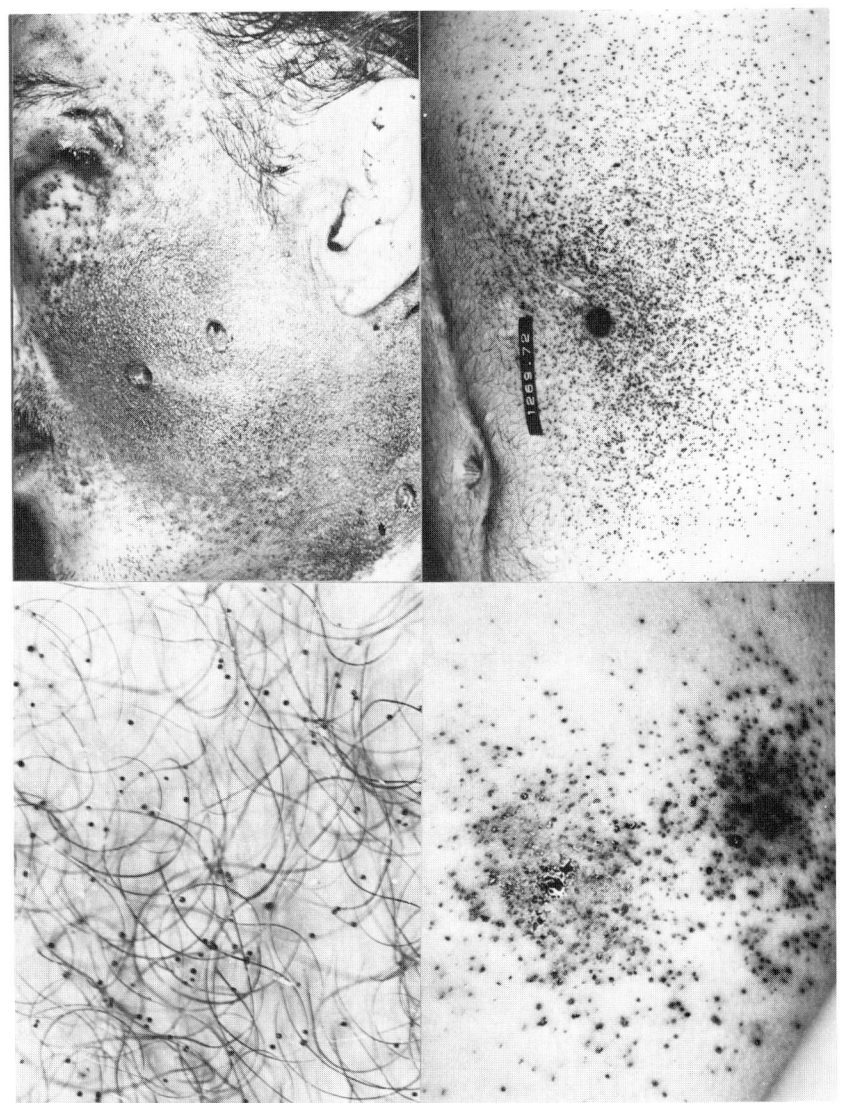

FIGURE 16-64. Ball powder tattooing. Ball powder tattooing is generally more dense than flake powder tattooing. In addition, the individual spots are more uniform in size than those made by flake powder. Three examples are shown. Also shown (lower right) are ball powder grains on the surface of the skin where they came to rest after penetrating clothing.

devoid of characteristics helpful to the interpretation of the case at hand. However, if the wound was inflicted at long range, the possibility of self-infliction, either accidentally or with suicidal intent, can be eliminated, with but four exceptions: (1) a device set up to hold the firearm and to enable it to be discharged at a long range by the victim (Fig. 16-67); (2) a mistake by the examiner of a contact-entry wound with what appears to be a long-range wound (such confusion is most apt to occur when a .22 caliber firearm is employed); (3) confusion caused when clothing is interposed between the victim and the firearm and any soot deposit or powder grains are prevented by the clothing from reaching the skin surface; and

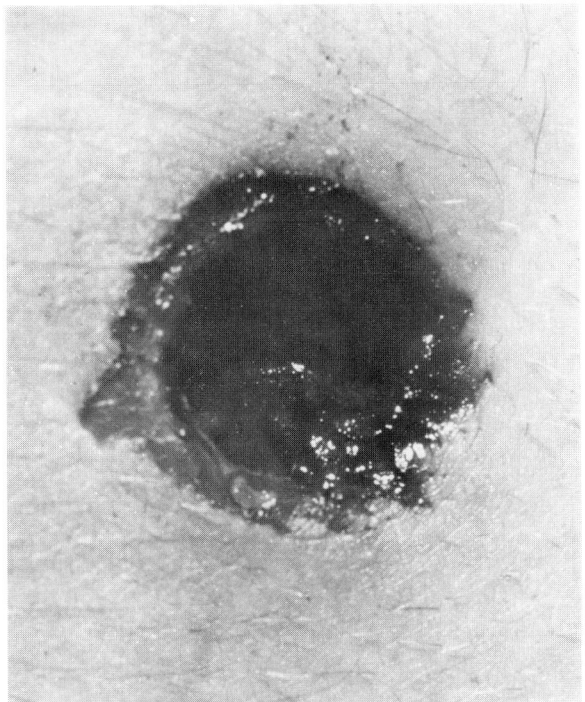

FIGURE 16-65. Inshoot wound (long-range). The abrasion ring is almost perfectly concentric, indicating that the bullet was entering in a nearly perpendicular manner. The small skin splits or tears are not unusual.

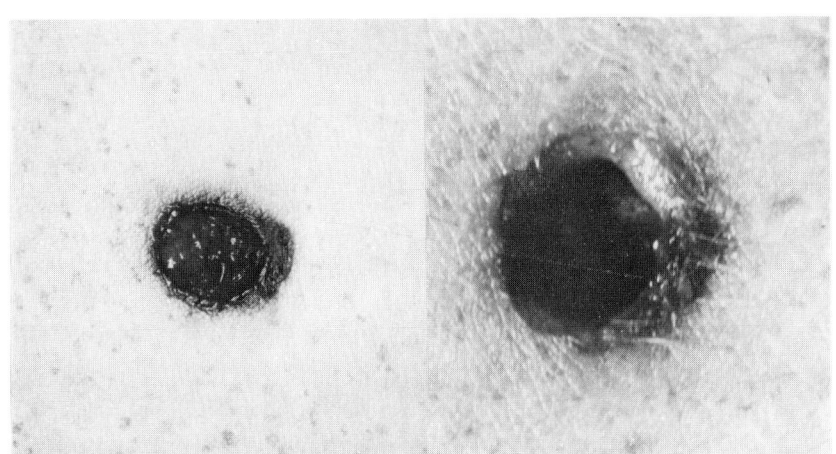

FIGURE 16-66. Inshoot wound (long-range). In the two examples shown, the abrasion ring does not form a concentric pattern about the defect. This indicates that the bullets were traveling at an angle to the skin. The direction of travel is toward the side of undermining.

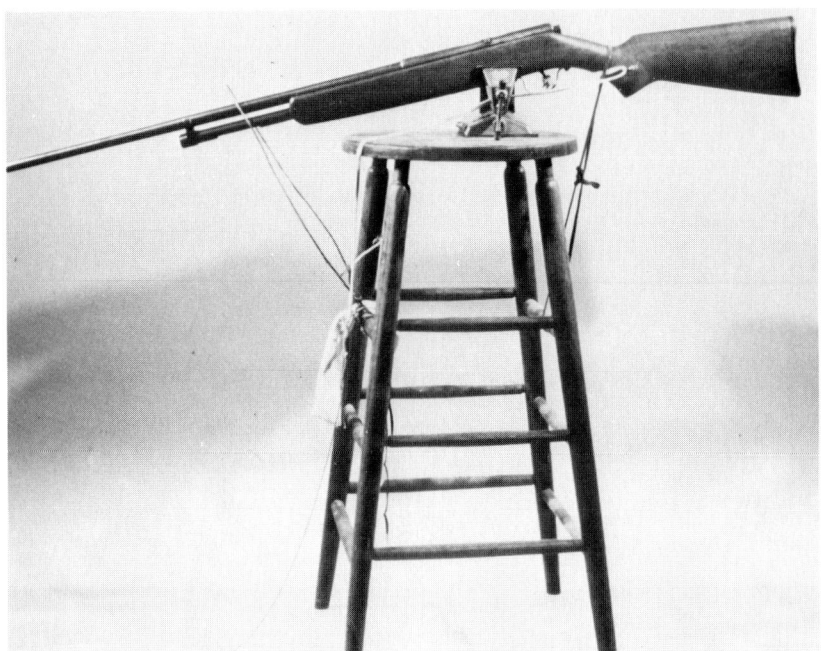

FIGURE 16-67. Suicide device. The firearm has been attached to the stool with a vise and ties. The trigger of the .410 bore shotgun was actuated by a cord.

(4) confusion caused by washing away soot deposit and free powder grains. The latter sometimes occurs without the knowledge of the medical examiner or coroner's pathologist and can be a serious detriment to good medicolegal investigation.

Outshoot or Exit Wounds

Those bullets which pass through the body cause exit wounds, sometimes known as outshoot wounds. Ordinarily, these are of quite a different character than the corresponding wound of entrance. Instead of being circular in shape, or nearly so, outshoot wounds are of varying shapes and can be described as slitlike, stellate, irregular, or gaping. The shape of the exit or outshoot wound cannot be predicted (Fig. 16-68). The reasons for marked variation in the shape of exit wounds are many:

1. The bullet tumbles in the body and fails to exit nose end first.
2. The bullet is deformed during its passage through the body and presents an irregular shape upon exiting.
3. The bullet breaks up in the tissues and exits, not as one mass but rather as several pieces. If jacketed, the jacket may separate completely or in part.
4. The bullet may contact bone and/or cartilage, and fragments of these firm tissues may be blown out of the body with the bullet.
5. When the bullet passes through the skin in exiting the body, the skin will not be supported by anatomic structures. When the elasticity of the skin is overcome by the bullet stretching the skin, it tends to shatter and tear. The resulting defect may bear little relationship in shape to the missile that caused that defect.

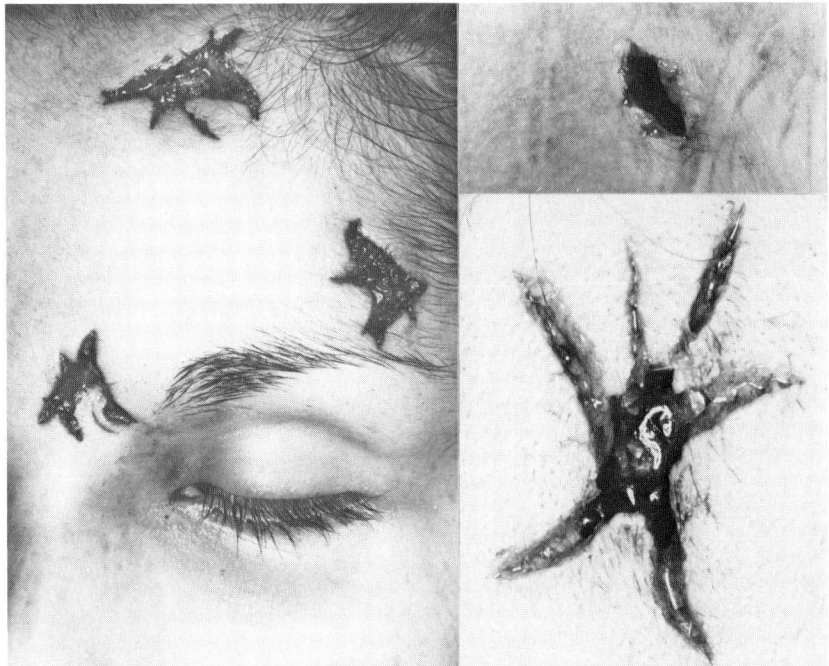

FIGURE 16-68. Outshoot wounds. Three outshoot wounds are present on the forehead of a gunshot wound victim shown in the left-hand panel. The other two panels each show a single outshoot wound. One is stellate-shaped; the other is irregular in shape and rather nondescript.

There is one further consideration regarding exit wounds that is of substantial forensic scientific importance. This involves the characteristics and method of production of the shored or supported gunshot wound of exit. As noted above, one major reason for the irregular shape of exit wounds is the lack of external support of the skin so that the bullet tends to tear or shatter the skin as it exits. However, under some circumstances, the skin is supported and the character of the exit wound is drastically altered. Instead of being irregular in shape, it tends to mirror the shape of the penetrating bullet, usually appearing as a circular or nearly circular defect surrounded by a margin of abrasion resembling a wound of entrance (Fig. 16-69). Indeed, a classic forensic science puzzle is the differentiation of the wound of entrance from the wound of exit, when the latter is of the shored or supported type and the former has been caused by a bullet fired at long range or through clothing that has obscured evidence of firearm residue, or when the firearm is of small caliber (usually .22 caliber) and discharged in contact with the skin at a point where bone is not immediately below the skin surface. Possibly more errors have been made in the interpretation of gunshot wounds because of the presence of shored exit wounds than in any other facet of firearms injuries.

The support of the skin necessary to cause an exiting bullet to make a shored outshoot wound is easily afforded by certain items of clothing, certain anatomic portions of the body, and by the position of the body in relation to items in the surroundings. Many shored exit wounds are caused by tight-fitting clothing: the waist band of trousers, shorts, or

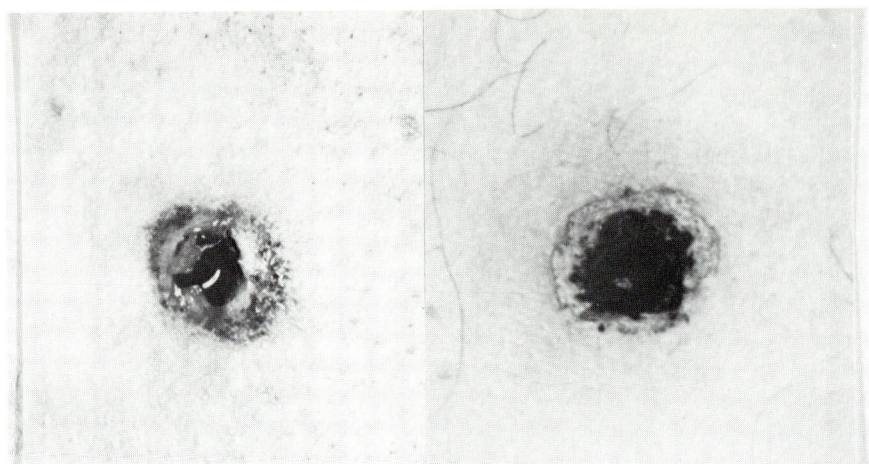

FIGURE 16-69. Shored outshoot wound. On the right is a shored outshoot wound. On the left is the inshoot wound made by the same bullet. The outshoot wound of shored type is larger than the inshoot wound. A slight bullet wipe surrounds the abraded margin of the inshoot wound.

panties; the side panels of a brassiere; support pantyhose; or a man's collar and tie. Similar shored exit wounds can result when the bullet exits from the side of the chest at a point where the inner surface of the arm is being held closely against the chest wall. Other points of anatomic juxtaposition are possible. The same situation of support will result when the victim is lying down, sitting, or leaning against a firm object. The variations are legion.

Not all bullets exit the body. Many strike bone, the tissue which is densest and most resistant to the passage of a missile. Not infrequently the further penetration of the bullet is stopped by bone. Some thin bones do not appear significantly to resist the passage of a bullet (e.g., the thin portions of the wings of the scapula and ilium, and the very thin portions of the skull). In a particular case, of course, the bullet may simply have expended its kinetic energy during its passage through the soft tissues of the body and come to a stop. Many bullets penetrate the body and expend whatever kinetic energy remains in the skin and subcutaneous tissue on the opposite side of the body. The skin is the second most resistant tissue of the body to penetration by a missile. There is much elastic tissue present in the skin, and it behaves much like the catcher who, with his padded baseball glove, stops the hard-thrown ball by allowing his covered hand to move backward somewhat as it absorbs the shock of the ball and eliminates the kinetic energy. Often the bullet can be located in the victim by simply examining the opposite side of the trunk, looking and feeling for the missile just beneath the skin (Fig. 16-70).

Bullets that strike in unusual locations may cause injury and death, but the wound of entry may be extremely difficult to locate. Among areas not anticipated as inshoot points are the ear, nostril, mouth, axilla, vagina, and rectum. Not only may these areas be unanticipated as the points of entry, but, because of blood on the surface of the body, the actual inshoot wound may be obscured (Fig. 16-71).

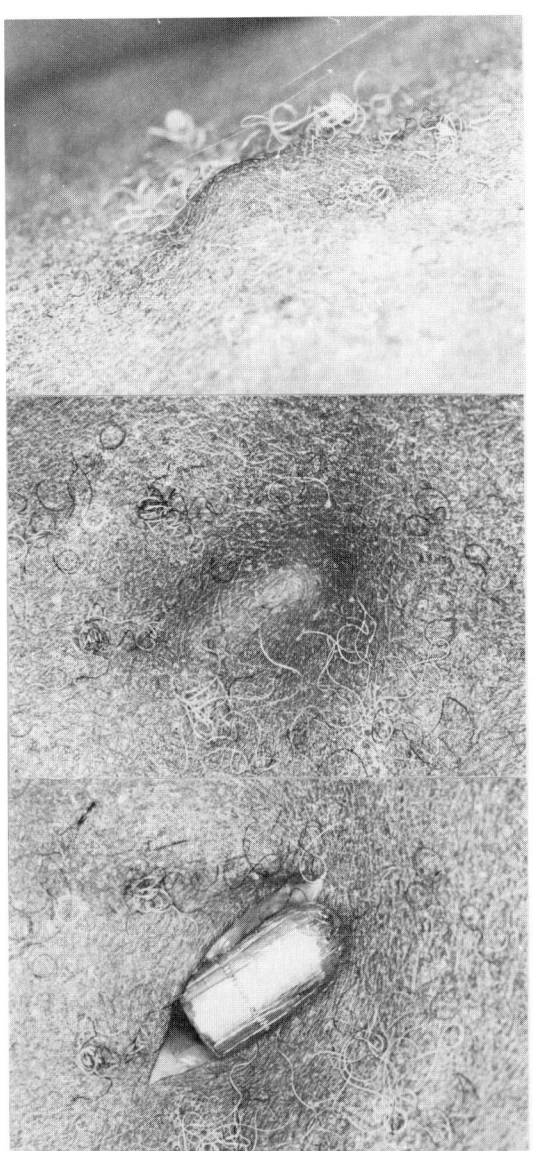

FIGURE 16-70. Bullet beneath the skin. Three views of a bullet located in the tissue just beneath the skin show the general outline of the bullet, the profile of the skin "bulge," and the bullet itself as it came forth through the skin incision made to expose it.

Velocity of Missiles

The range of fire must be taken into consideration in attempting to determine the striking velocity of the missile as it contacts the target. It should be recognized, however, that most homicidal gunshot wounds are inflicted at relatively short range, the great majority within 25 feet. At or under such range, the drop-off in velocity from that achieved at the muzzle is not great. The approximate velocity can be determined by examining the cartridge manufacturer's range tables, or more precisely by determining the velocity with the chronograph, using the weapon and the same type of ammunition employed in the shooting under investigation.

The muzzle velocity of handguns commonly encountered ranges between 350 and 1500 feet per second. Higher velocities can be achieved,

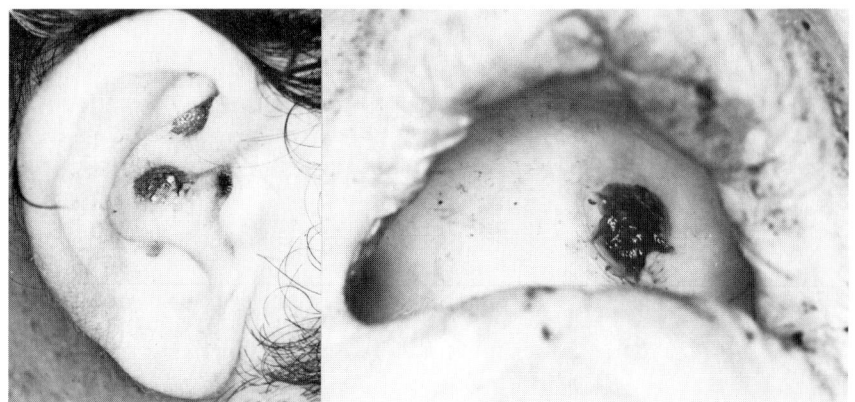

FIGURE 16-71. Sites of bullet entry. The inshoot point in the roof of the mouth (hard palate), and the ear are areas sometimes not considered when searching for the wound of entrance in a gunshot wound victim.

but the recoil and muzzle blast become most marked and physical discomfort is encountered which tends to lead to flinching on the part of the shooter. Pistols, revolvers, and rifles of .22 caliber, employing .22 short, long, or long rifle ammunition fit the same low-velocity category. High-powered or high-velocity rifles such as military rifles and those used for hunting fit the high-velocity category. With such rifles the muzzle velocity may range between 2400 and 4000 feet per second, and occasionally even higher. Between these two extremes is a medium velocity category, best exemplified by the United States Army M-1 carbine with a muzzle velocity of approximately 3000 feet per second.

As the velocity of the bullet increases, so does the degree of tissue and organ damage. Much of the experimental work employing animals (most usually Angora goats) has been carried out by the Wound Ballistics Section of the United States Army Aberdeen Proving Ground. Much of the work is classified and not available to the public; some has been published.[21] Within the low-velocity range the tissue and organ damage can easily be observed by examination of the wound track. Most, though not all, of the damage is present in or very close to the track made by the missile. The so-called shock wave made by a bullet does not really appear until the speed of sound is reached. In dry air this is 1087 feet per second. The dissipation of kinetic energy in the radial direction (at right angles to the path of the bullet) does not begin to be of great significance until the bullet reaches medium velocity, probably above 1500 feet per second. Significant temporary cavity formation then begins to be a factor in the production of tissue damage far in excess of the permanent track caused by the passage of the missile itself. At much higher velocities (2000 feet per second and upward), disintegration of the missile itself may contribute to widespread wounding, each small fragment causing its own track, with huge overall cavity formation.

Wounding is much more dependent upon velocity than upon the weight of the missile, as may be indicated by the kinetic energy formula:

$$KE = \frac{mv^2}{2g}$$

It is the square of the velocity (that is, velocity × velocity) that is the component of greatest influence upon the kinetic energy. In the formula given, m = mass of missile (weight), v = velocity, and g = gravity. Note that the entire formula uses the English system. The kinetic energy is in foot-pounds, the mass is in pounds, and the velocity is in feet per second. To calculate the kinetic energy possessed by a missile weighing 100 grains and traveling 500 feet per second, it is necessary to know that 1 pound = 7000 grains. Substituting in the formula:

$$KE = \frac{mv^2}{2g}$$

$$KE = \frac{\frac{100}{7000} \times 500^2}{2 \times 32.2}$$

$$KE = 55 \text{ foot-pounds.}$$

It would appear that an impact velocity of less than approximately 200 feet per second in a clothed individual will cause only a trivial wound.[21]

The so-called casualty criterion has been determined to be approximately 58 foot pounds of kinetic energy. Thus, in the example given above, the 100 grain missile at a velocity of 500 feet per second is just at the borderline of being a missile capable of converting a normal individual into a wounded, military casualty, unable to react and fight effectively.[21]

Ammunition Types

There is no need here to give more than an overview of the many different types of ammunition available for use in rifled firearms. Many references are available to provide an in-depth coverage of what has become a complex subject.[22]

Disregarding the round ball still used by some muzzle-loading buffs, the traditional bullet is made of soft metal and has a rounded nose. The metal is lead with varying amounts of antimony added to provide hardness. The missile is usually known as the round-nosed, soft bullet. It is the bullet most frequently used in rifles and revolvers. There are some important variations of this bullet. The first is a rather square-nosed, soft metal bullet known as a "wad-cutter" and used primarily for target shooting. The second is a hollow-point variety which has a depression in the nose of the soft metal. This bullet is designed to expand or "mushroom" upon impact (Fig. 16-72). All of these soft metal bullets cause leading of the bore of the firearm used. This wiping of lead onto the bore causes a decrease in accuracy of the firearm, and to overcome this the bullet may be lubricated. The lubricant, made of wax, graphite, or various organic materials, may coat the entire bullet (except the base) or may be applied to the bullet in small grooves or cannelures cut circumferentially into the bullet near the base (Fig. 16-73).

Jacketed bullets are of two types. The first is the full metal jacket bullet in which a tough, heavy jacket covers all but the base where the soft metal interior is exposed (see Fig. 16-72). Such bullets were designed for military reasons. The tough jacket (which may be made of various metals including steel, copper, nickel, and zinc) was intended to withstand the automatic loading process in machine guns and auto-loading pistols. Moreover, the full metal jacketed bullets are not easily deformed when carried by soldiers and exposed to rough handling in combat. The First

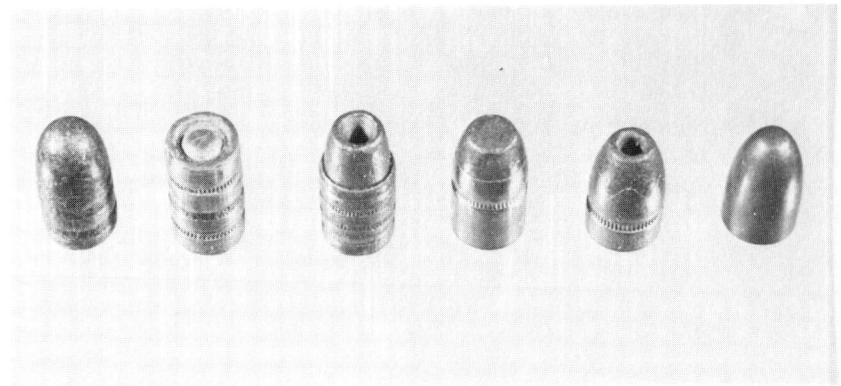

FIGURE 16-72. Commonly used types of bullets. Six different types of bullets are shown. From left to right they are: round-nose, soft-metal; wad-cutter; hollow-point, soft-metal; semijacketed; semijacketed hollow-point; full metal jacket.

Hague Convention of 1899, dealing with "humane" warfare, provided for such bullets in an effort to prevent escalation in the wounding capacity of military rifles and handguns. (It is interesting that the United States was never a signatory to the declaration.) The second type of bullet in this group is only semijacketed. The bullet is provided with a relatively thin but tough jacket which covers the base and the cylindrical portion of the bullet, leaving the nose partly or fully exposed (see Fig. 16-72). This type of bullet was designed to expand or "mushroom" like the soft-metal, hollow-point type described earlier. Indeed, the expected combination of the two is also available, the semijacketed hollow-point bullet combining the potential for expansion of two different designs.

With the exception of ordinary .22 caliber firearms, the general rule is that soft-metal, round-nose bullets are fired from revolvers, full-jacket bullets from rifles and auto-loading firearms, and semijacketed bullets from revolvers and rifles. There are, however, many points of crossover.

Wounding with hollow-point or semijacketed ammunition has been considered by some to be much greater in severity than with nonexpanding bullets. Expanding bullets are designed to accomplish exactly that—

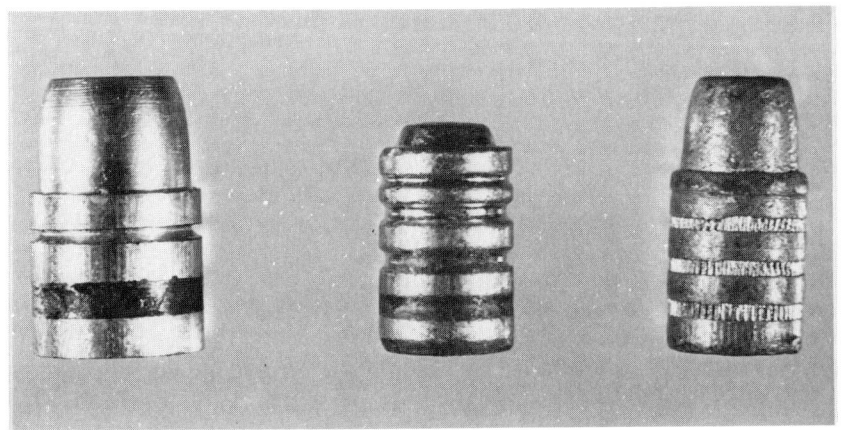

FIGURE 16-73. Lubricant in cannelures. A waxy type of lubricant can be seen in the cannelures of the three bullets shown.

expansion, with increase in diameter and with more rapid slowing within the body and, therefore, a more rapid transfer of kinetic energy to the body. The result is greater "shocking power" or "knockdown power." These terms are not precise. A second result is that the semijacketed and hollow-point missiles tend not to pass entirely through the body to exit and strike a second target. This characteristic alone makes such bullets useful for police use, where perforation of the subject with subsequent wounding of an innocent bystander is an occurrence to be avoided.

It should be noted that mushrooming of semijacketed bullets is often accompanied by a peeling back of the jacket. Both the jacket and the soft metal interior may fragment. In some instances the jacket may peel away and remain nearly intact (Fig. 16-74). Occasionally the soft metal interior may exit, leaving the jacket with the markings so necessary for comparison still in the body. This is one important reason for the examination by x-ray of the body of a firearms wound victim prior to autopsy. To accomplish mushrooming, the velocity of the bullet must meet or exceed approximately 1100 feet per second.[23]

Bullets of .22 caliber may be of the hollow-point variety. Such bullets are rarely known to mushroom. Whether this is due to the marginal velocity achieved, or whether it is a function of size (cross-sectional area) in relationship to the resistance of the body tissues is unknown.

Shotgun Wounds

Some differences in the appearance of wounds caused by shotguns and those associated with rifled firearms have already been noted. The principal difference is caused by the fact that multiple missiles are usually

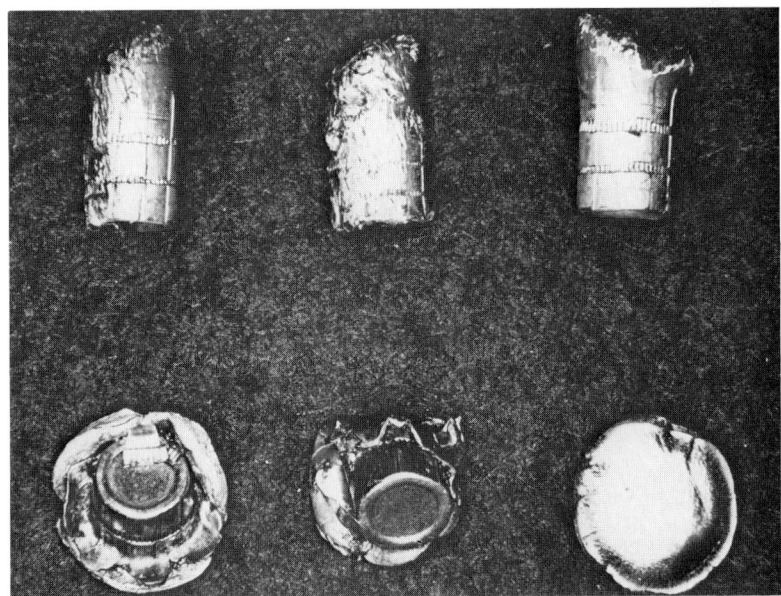

FIGURE 16-74. Mushrooming of bullets. All six of these bullets were fired from one .38 caliber handgun and struck one victim. Only one of the three round-nose, soft-metal bullets (upper right) struck bone, causing it to slightly mushroom. The lower three bullets are all semijacketed; none of them struck bone, but all mushroomed.

discharged each time the shotgun is fired. These may vary in size from approximately the diameter of a .22 caliber bullet to very small, almost sandlike shot. The shape and character of the wound are very dependent upon the range. At short range, the shot and wading enter almost as one massive cylinder-shaped missile, clinging together upon entry to separate only as different resistances of tissue are encountered (Fig. 16-75). The short range type of wound is, then, circular or nearly circular (Fig. 16-76). As the range increases, the shot begin to separate. At medium range, the edges of the wound are irregular, having something of a "moth-eaten" appearance (Fig. 16-77). As the range is increased, the separation of shot becomes greater, and individual (satellite) shot defects are seen, first very close to the main defect, and then gradually spreading (Fig. 16-78). At long range, no large defect is seen, the individual shot each making a single small punctate wound and the entire shot pattern covering a large area (Fig. 16-79).

Soot deposit and powder tattooing occur with shotgun wounds at short and medium range, respectively, just as with rifled firearms injury (see Figs. 16-76 and 16-86).

Three general classes of shot are used in shotgun shells. Birdshot, buckshot, and individual projectiles (usually termed rifled slugs) are employed, with the frequency of use in the order given. Birdshot is generally used for hunting fowl and very small animals. The shot are small, ranging in diameter from 0.050 to 0.150 inch. Because of the small size, many shot are loaded into each shotgun shell, with 200 to 400 shot, depending upon their size, found in 12-gauge shotgun shells. Buckshot is larger than

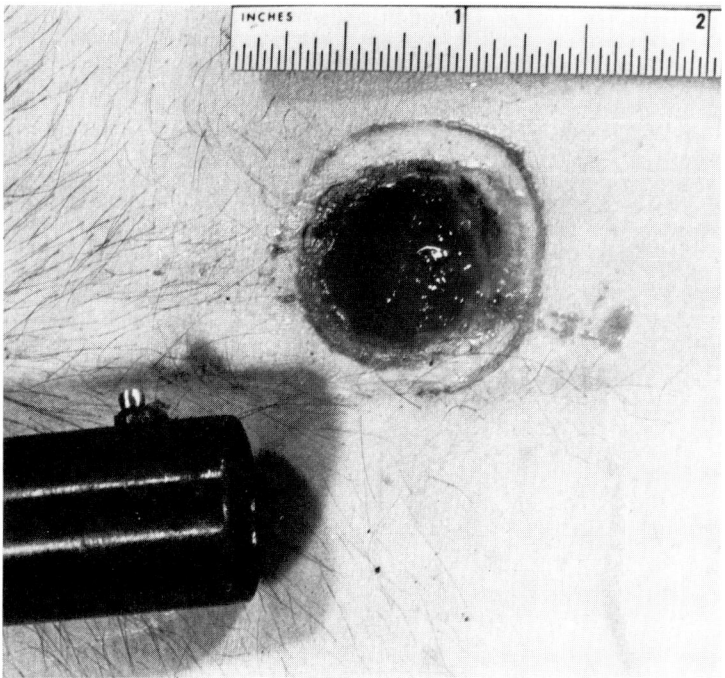

FIGURE 16-75. Muzzle imprint (shotgun). A contact shotgun wound, with the muzzle and sight imprint, is shown. The shot and wads all entered together as a more or less solid cylinder.

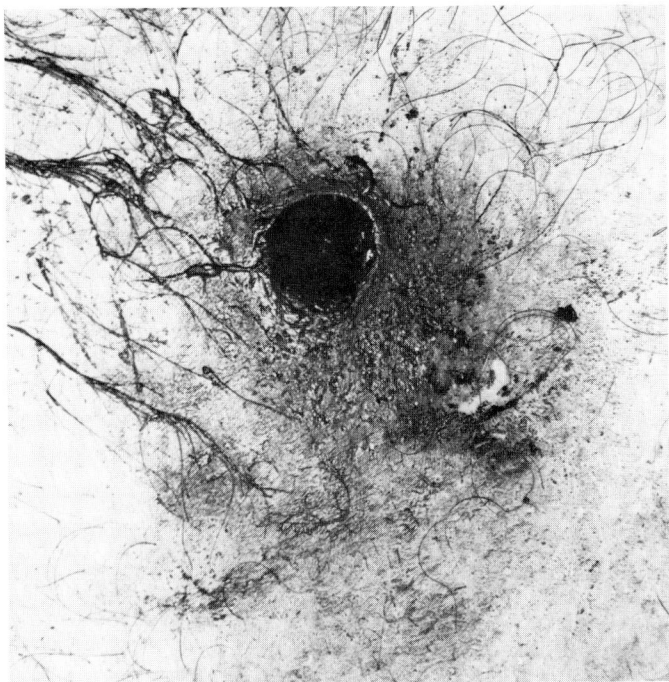

FIGURE 16-76. Short-range shotgun wound. The soot deposit and the circular shape of the defect are both well shown.

birdshot, being from 0.24 to 0.33 inch in diameter. Obviously, many fewer shot are found in buckshot-loaded shells, and when 00 buckshot is employed, a standard 12-gauge shotgun shell will contain only nine shot (Fig. 16-80).

The single projectiles designed to be used in shotguns are termed rifled slugs. Several types are available in the United States.[24,25] Most depend for accuracy upon a heavy leading end and a light trailing end of the

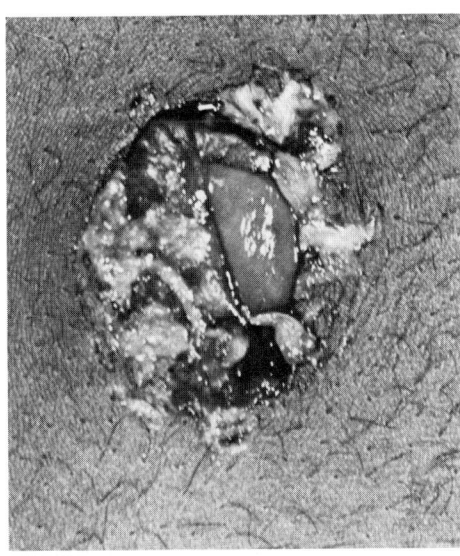

FIGURE 16-77. Medium-range shotgun wound. The edge of the defect is not quite smooth, and two satellite (shot) wounds are present.

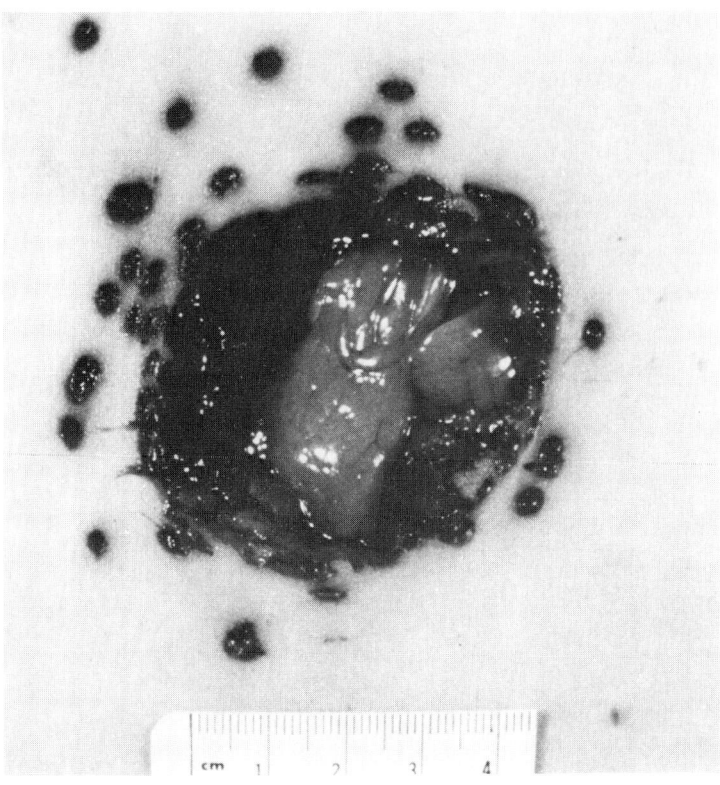

FIGURE 16-78. Medium-range shotgun wound. This wound is characterized by many satellite wounds with the central defect large and with a "moth-eaten" appearance.

missile, such that the rifled slug tends not to tumble but to travel with the heavy front end directed toward the target. The Foster type rifled slug is the one usually used in the United States (Fig. 16-81). Obviously, the wound caused by a rifled slug will consist of a solitary defect, regardless of the range of fire (Fig. 16-82).

A characteristic of shotgun wounds is that exit wounds are not seen except with rifled slugs, larger buckshot, or with birdshot in contact or near contact wounds (Fig. 16-83). The small mass of birdshot permits rapid deceleration of the shot in the body, with insufficient mass and remaining velocity to cause skin penetration in the potential exit area (Fig. 16-84). Therefore, the presence of an exit wound in the instance of a shotgun shooting may nearly define the type of shotgun ammunition employed.

Another wound characteristic of certain shotgun injuries is the "wad mark." This is a separate abrasion or abrasion-contusion, rarely a faint laceration, made by a wad when it impacts against the skin (Fig. 16-85). Wads of various types are used in shotgun shells, primarily to separate the shot from the powder, in some instances to contain the shot within the shell, and for other ballistic reasons. Wads are, or have been, made of cardboard, felt, cork, and plastic; some are disc-shaped and others cup-shaped, and still others have bizarre shapes. Although in cross section wads are of a circular shape, the shape of the abrasion or abrasion-contusion made by the wad depends upon how the wad impacts the skin. At

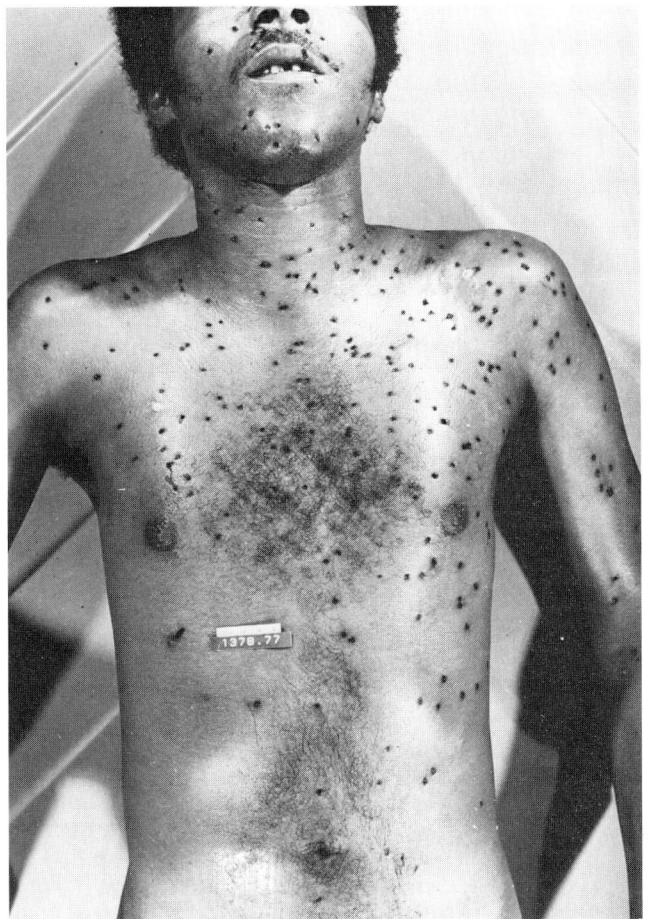

FIGURE 16-79. Long-range shotgun wound. A multitude of individual shot wounds are present from the forehead to just below the level of the umbilicus.

very short range the plastic cup type may be in the process of "opening-up" at the time of impacting the target skin. The prongs then cause some small but distinct radially arranged petal-like marks surrounding the defect made by the column of shot (Fig. 16-86).

Wad marks may be noted in shotgun wounds (with the single exception of prong marks as described above) at any range of fire between two extremes: the shorter range determined by the point at which the wad or wads separate from the column of shot and travel separately, and the longest range being that where the wad fails to impact with sufficient force to mark the target skin, or where the wad has fallen away from the trajectory of the shot and fails to strike the target. It must also be emphasized that at ranges below that at which the wads begin to impact apart from the shot, the wads will penetrate the skin with the shot and may then be recovered from within the body. Obviously the weight and flight characteristics of the wad will have a great effect on the distance it will carry.

Some wads, especially those made of cork or corklike particles, may break up and, at short ranges, the small wad fragments will strike the

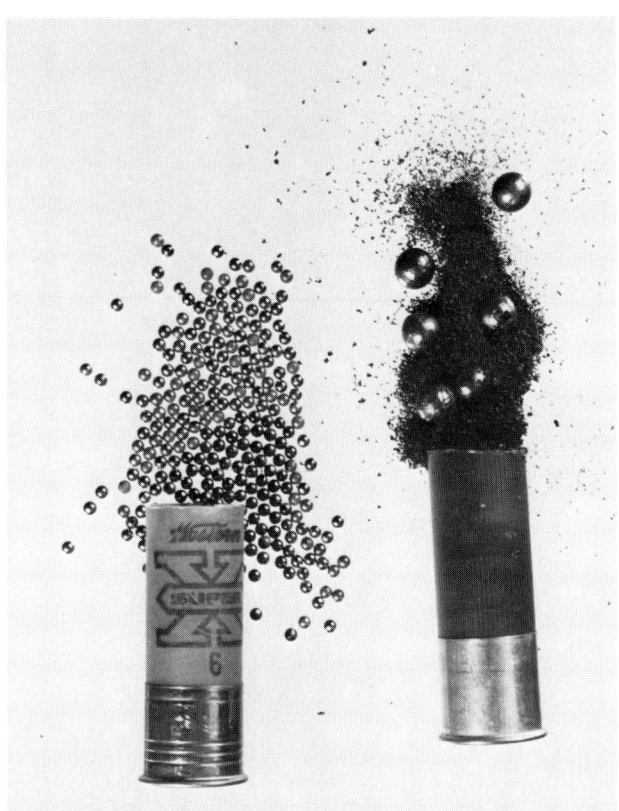

FIGURE 16-80. Birdshot and buckshot. A shotgun shell, cut open to allow the contained birdshot to be displayed, is shown on the left. A shell loaded with buckshot is shown on the right. The fine granular material is the plastic filler sometimes used in shells containing buckshot, but very rarely in shells loaded with birdshot.

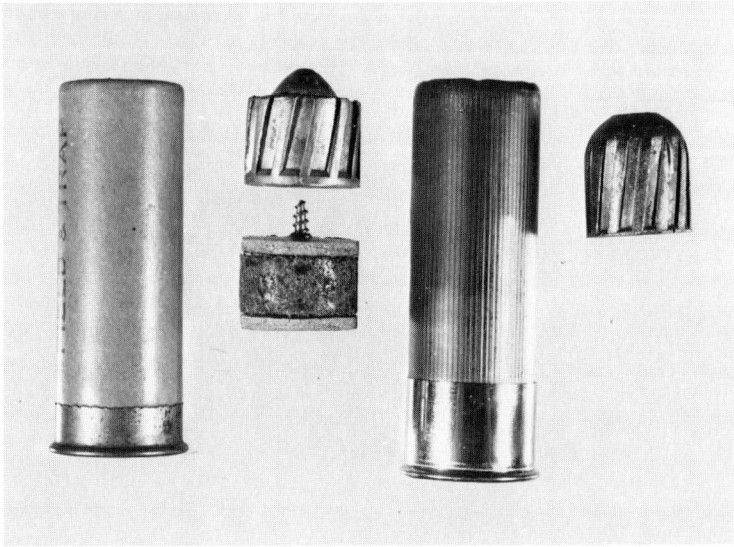

FIGURE 16-81. Rifled slugs. On the left is pictured the Brenneke slug which has wads attached by means of a screw. The Foster type slug is shown on the right.

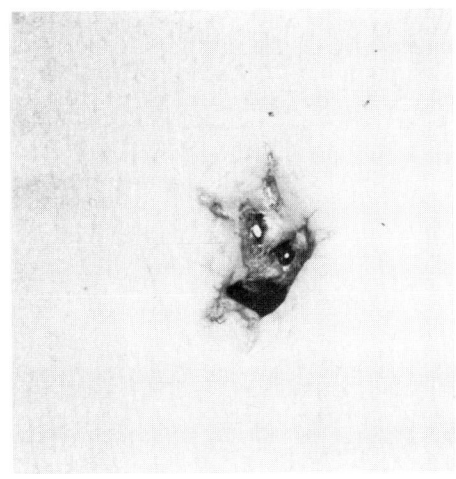

FIGURE 16-82. Rifled slug outshoot wound. An outshoot wound of a 12-gauge rifled slug in the high midposterior thorax is shown. It is of irregular shape and not unlike any single projectile outshoot wound.

skin separately and cause small, irregularly shaped abrasions. Certain fairly heavy plastic over-the-shot wads will perform in the same manner.

After many years of more or less standard production practices, shotgun ammunition manufacturers are making extensive changes in shotgun shells (Fig. 16-87). The choices of ammunition now offered the shotgunner

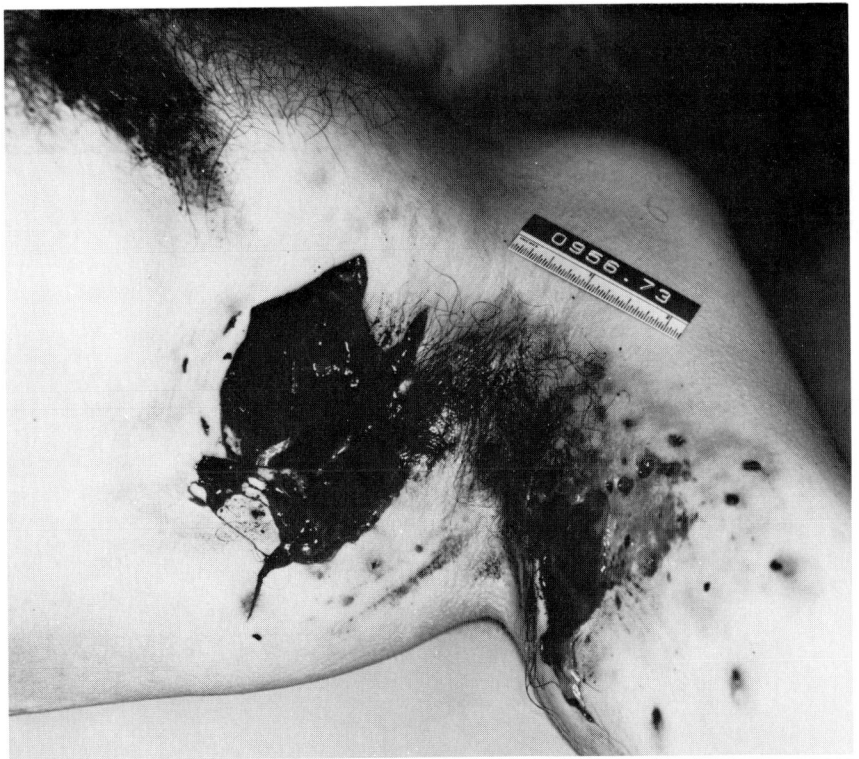

FIGURE 16-83. Near-contact shotgun outshoot wound. The massive outshoot wound on the superior and left lateral chest wall is shown. In the upper left-hand corner of the figure is the near-contact wound. Only the soot deposit is visible. The blast effect has caused re-entry of some shot and a jagged defect on the inner aspect of the left arm where it was in apposition to the side of the chest.

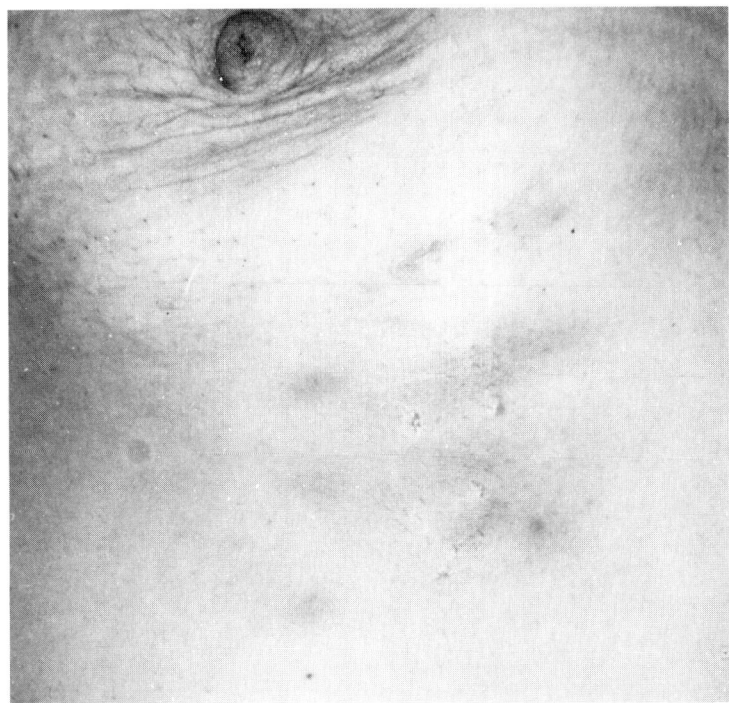

FIGURE 16-84. Shotgun shot beneath the skin. These shot failed to exit, but a telltale of their presence is the series of small, discrete contusions. Most shotgun shot fail to exit because of their small mass.

are many, perhaps so numerous as to confuse the purchaser. A partial list of ammunition variations will be found in Table 16-9.

The diameter of the barrel of a shotgun can be expressed by one of three systems. In the United States the most commonly employed system is that of gauge. The origin of this system is archaic. It refers to the number of

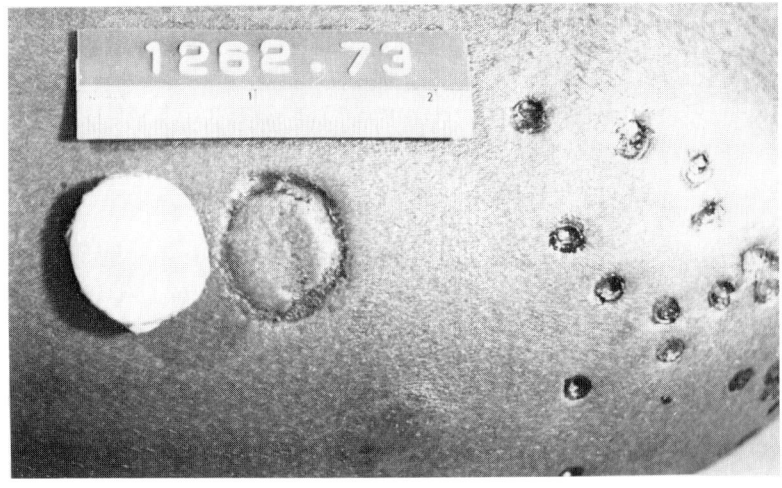

FIGURE 16-85. Wad mark. The felt-type wad struck the skin with sufficient force to cause an abrasion-laceration. An unfired wad of the same kind is shown next to the wadmark.

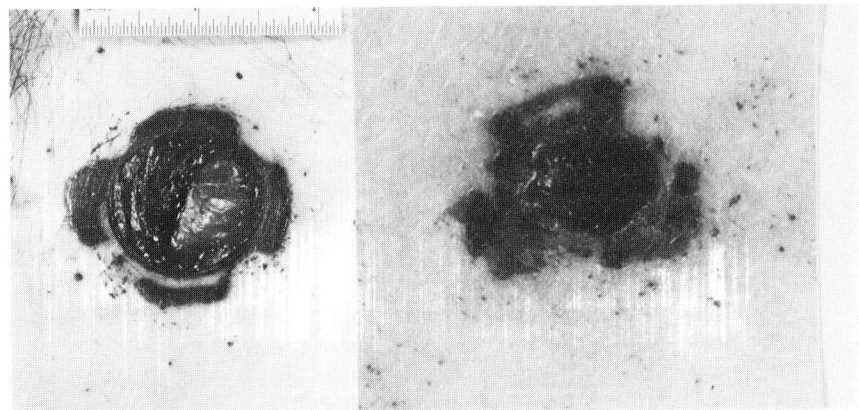

FIGURE 16-86. Wad prong marks. The prongs of the shot cup, a "power-piston" type of plastic wad, make a chracteristic series of marks when they strike the skin and began to open up. Some powder tattooing is present in each of the panels. The right-hand panel illustrates the pattern made by a wad with three prongs; that on the left, four prongs.

lead balls, each fitting the bore, that total 1 pound in weight. Thus a 12-gauge shotgun has a bore diameter such that 12 balls of lead, each just fitting the bore, can be made from a pound of lead. The smaller the gauge designation, the larger the bore. The second system is the expression of bore diameter in inches. The .410 bore shotgun is the only shotgun to be so designated. The metric system with the bore diameter expressed in millimeters is also used. A 10 mm shotgun has a bore diameter of 10 mm.

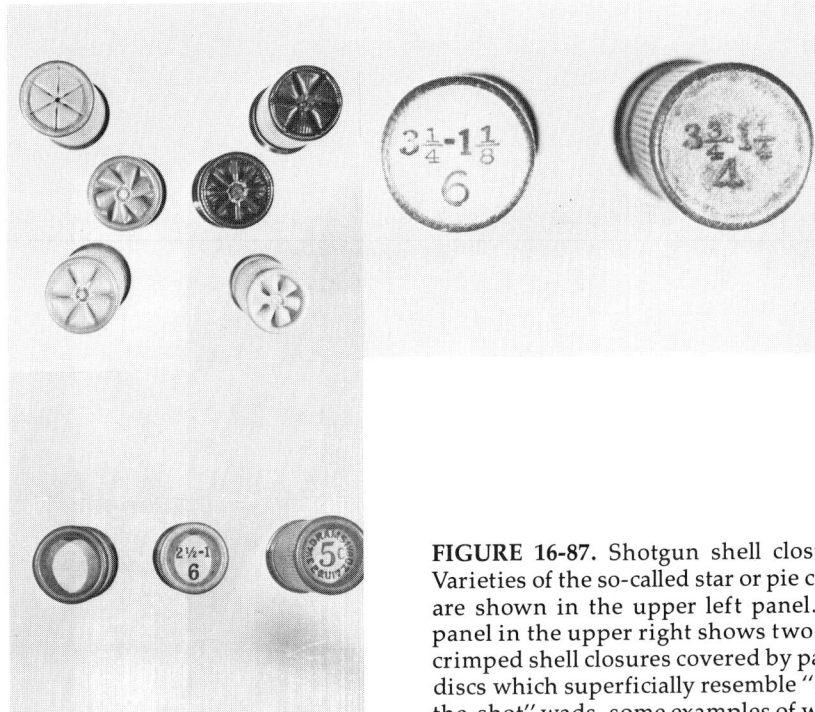

FIGURE 16-87. Shotgun shell closures. Varieties of the so-called star or pie crimp are shown in the upper left panel. The panel in the upper right shows two star-crimped shell closures covered by pasted discs which superficially resemble "over-the-shot" wads, some examples of which are shown in the lower left panel.

TABLE 16-9. AMMUNITION CHANGES: SHOTGUN SHELLS*

Closure		
	Old Standard	Cardboard over-the-shot wads
	New	Star (Pie) crimp
		Plastic over-the-shot wads
Shell case		
	Old Standard	Cardboard, with waterproof coating
	New	Plastic with brass base
		Plastic, entire, without brass base
Shot		
	Old Standard	Chilled shot (lead with antimony)
	New	Plated or coated chilled shot
		Steel shot
Slugs		
	Old Standard	Foster type
		Brennecke type
	New	A variety of slugs including Ball Balle saboted
Wads		
	Old Standard	Felt or cardboard
	New	Plastic, "Power Piston" or variation corklike substance
Packing between shot		
	Old Standard	None
	New	Plastic granules, usually in buckshot loads; in some birdshot loads
Shell liner		
	Old Standard	None
	New	Sheet of plastic between shot and shell wall

*List includes some of the frequently encountered shotgun ammunition modifications of the 20 years prior to 1975.

X-Ray Examination of Gunshot Wound Victims

The usefulness of x-ray examination of the gunshot wound victim is undeniable. The examination of a firearms wound victim cannot be considered complete without x-ray examination. Of course, if no x-ray equipment is available, such examination cannot be undertaken at that site. However, this is an argument for moving the body to a place where the examination by x-ray can be undertaken, not an excuse for waiving its use. There are many reasons for x-ray examination, including the following:

1. To locate the bullet. However, even large bullets are often difficult to find even after they are detected by x-ray (Fig. 16-88).
2. To locate bullet fragments or jackets. Although there may be an exit wound, significant portions of the bullet or bullet jacket may have broken off and may have remained in the body (Fig. 16-89).
3. To delineate the track of the bullet. Internal ricochet, especially frequent within the skull, may be demonstrated. This may be of great importance in the determination of the direction of fire.
4. To determine the breakup pattern of the bullet. This technique may also indicate the type of ammunition used (Fig. 16-90).
5. To determine defects in bone, in areas not easily accessible to direct examination.

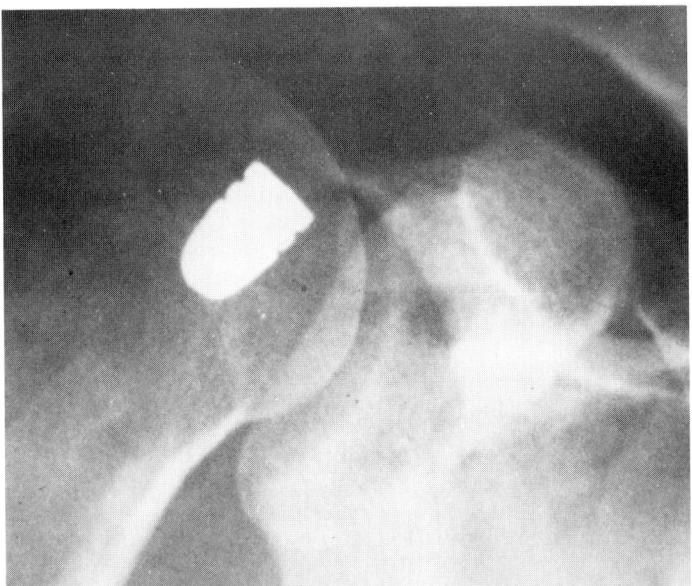

FIGURE 16-88. X-ray of bullet. This large-caliber bullet is in the shoulder joint. The x-ray film reveals that it has two deep cannelures. Presumably, then, it is a cast soft-metal bullet fired from a revolver, not an autoloading pistol.

6. To delineate air embolism accompanying large vessel damage by the missile.
7. To provide documentation that the body was examined, the wound was present, and certain injuries were made by the missile.
8. To rule out the presence of a missile in instances where there is a question as to whether the external wound might have been caused by a firearm.
9. To scan the body for the location of the bullet in instances of bullet embolism or when the missile has been propelled along the gastrointestinal tract by peristaltic action.

Radiography can also be used in living patients to determine some characteristics of a still present bullet in the body. This may be of great use to law enforcement officers, and may resolve problems regarding the weapon used when more than one was available (see Fig. 16-88).

Two somewhat unexpected problems can arise when using radiography in a routine manner in the investigation of firearms injuries. First, the x-ray may reveal the presence of a bullet not related to the shooting under investigation. These surprise missiles may cause some anxiety in the pathologist, who then becomes concerned lest he has overlooked another wound of entrance. Also, since there is no track with hemorrhage near it leading to the surprise bullet, it is difficult to find. The author once examined a dead victim of a single gunshot wound and found two such surprise missiles (Fig. 16-91). Second, the caliber of the bullet cannot be determined with any accuracy by examination of the x-ray film. The actual difference in the diameter of a .22 caliber bullet from that of a .45 caliber bullet is only two times. The distortion by x-ray is great and depends upon the distance of the bullet from the x-ray film and to a lesser extent upon the distance of the x-ray source from the film. It is quite hazardous for the examiner to guess as to the exact caliber of the bullet

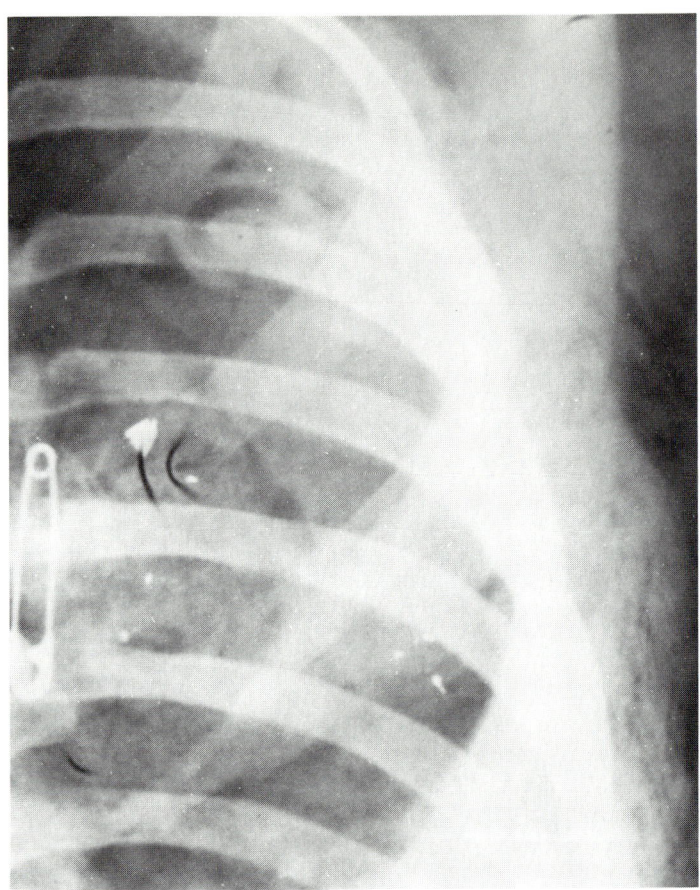

FIGURE 16-89. Fragments of bullet jacket. Several small bullet fragments can be seen in the x-ray film photograph. The bullet entered the thorax in its anterior surface and exited on the posterior surface. Without the x-ray examination, the presence of the fragments would not have been suspected. The largest fragment is of the jacket and it had enough markings characteristic of the weapon to enable matching (comparison) which resulted in the conviction of the murderer.

based upon the appearance of the missile on the x-ray film (Fig. 16-92).

Another type of radiography is sometimes of use in the examination of firearms wounds. This involves soft x-rays, sometimes termed grenz rays. Special apparatus is required; ordinary x-ray equipment will not provide rays of the necessary wavelength, situated toward the ultraviolet end of the electromagnetic spectrum. Because of the low penetration power of these rays, they may be used to demonstrate only mildly radiopaque materials. Powder grains may be detected; the weave of a fabric can easily be delineated (Fig. 16-93). Examination by soft x-ray of the excised, apparent gunshot wound from a decomposing body may demonstrate powder fragments and resolve the problem as to which of several areas of the body represented the inshoot wound (Fig. 16-94).

Examination of Clothing of Gunshot Victims

The examination of the victim of firearms injury is incomplete without a detailed search of the clothing for defects made by missiles and for fire-

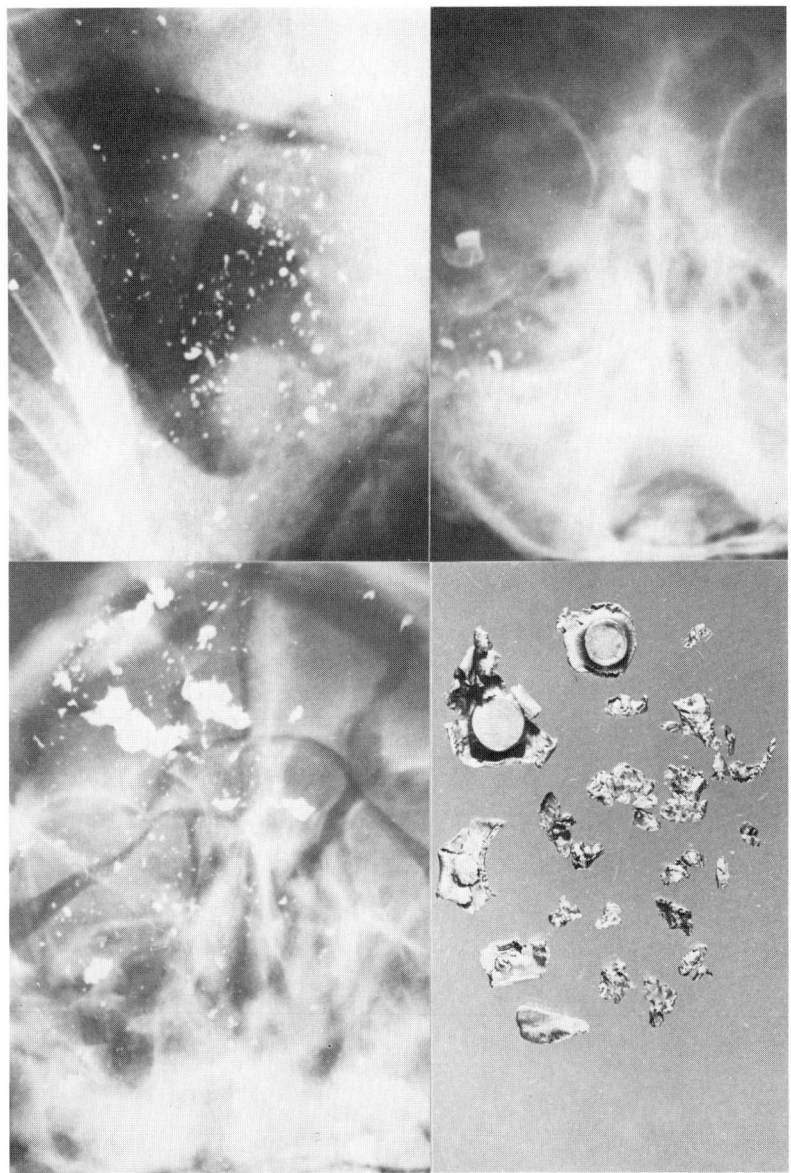

FIGURE 16-90. Fragmentation of bullets. Four different panels are shown to illustrate the breakup of bullets. In the upper left is the "snow storm" effect of the breakup of a high-velocity rifle bullet as seen by x-ray examination. The upper right panel is of an x-ray film of the breakup of a semijacketed revolver bullet; the partially peeled-back appearance of the jacket is easy to recognize. The left lower panel shows the appearance upon x-ray examination of the head of a victim of shooting with a high-velocity rifle. The bullet fragments recovered from the head are shown in the remaining panel. Comparison of some of the fragments with their x-ray film appearance shows great similarity.

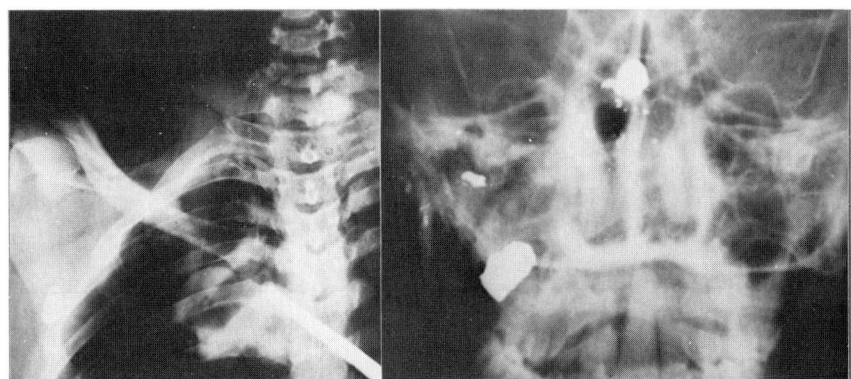

FIGURE 16-91. Unsuspected bullets demonstrated by x-ray examination. The subject had been shot in the face. *Right:* x-ray examination of the head revealed *two* bullets despite only one entrance wound. *Left:* another examination by x-ray undertaken to delineate the depth of the bullets in the head revealed a third bullet near the right shoulder. The fatal bullet was of .22 caliber. The other two bullets were .32 caliber and had remained in the subject following wounding many years before.

arms residues. Indeed, the task of carrying out an autopsy is lightened by an adequate examination of the clothing before the autopsy is commenced. It follows, therefore, that the clothing of the gunshot wound victim must be submitted with the body. In actual practice this is subject to many variations of which some may be exasperating but must be tolerated:

1. Ideally, the clothing should be left on the body, undisturbed; however, this ideal is rarely achieved.
2. The clothing is often left on the body but is subject to search for materials in the pockets that may identify the victim.

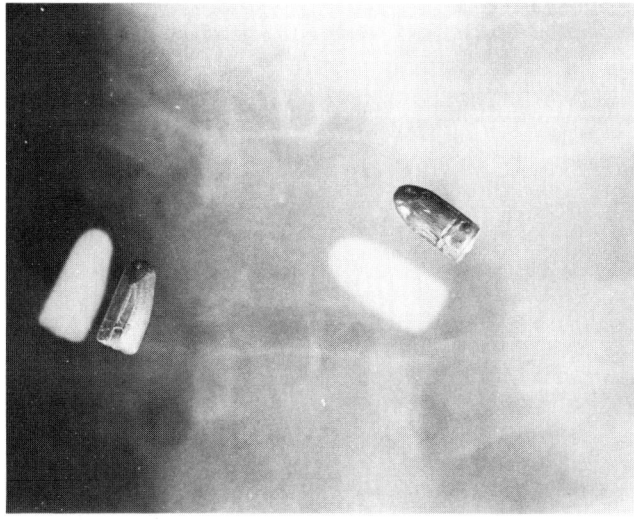

FIGURE 16-92. Distortion of bullet by x-ray. The size of the bullet as shown by x-ray film is compared with actual bullet size. The difference is marked.

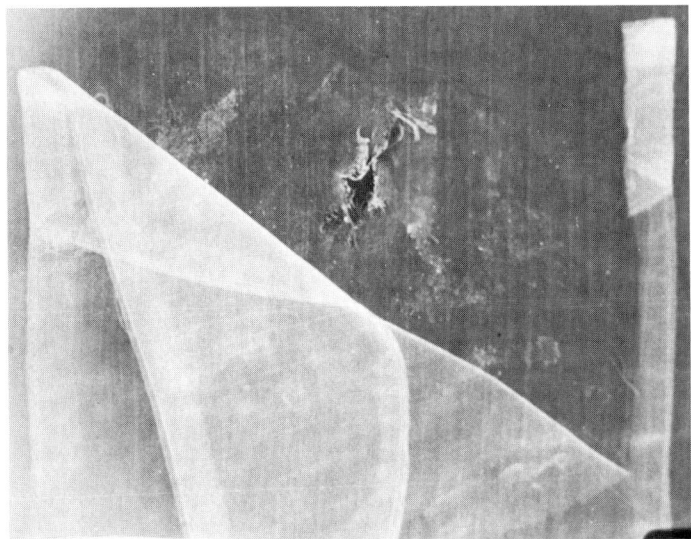

FIGURE 16-93. Soft x-ray of clothing. A pajama top is shown. The gunshot defect behind the pocket is easy to identify (the pocket has been cut on the right and partially folded down). The firearm residues surrounding the defect are clearly shown.

3. The clothing is left on the body but is disturbed or garments are manipulated so that the wound or multiple wounds can be inspected. The latter procedure may or may not be a reasonable action.
4. The dead, dying, or potentially resuscitatable individual is very often subjected to intensive cardiopulmonary resuscitation and

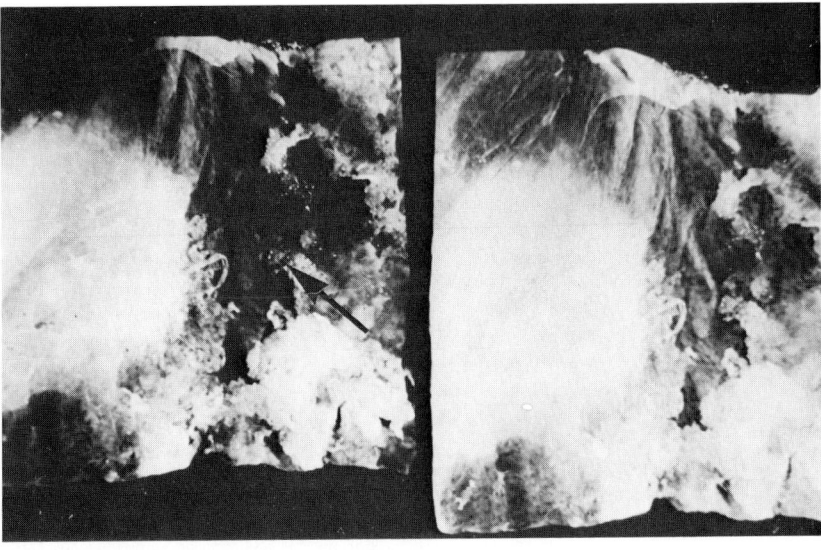

FIGURE 16-94. Soft x-ray of body tissue. The soft x-ray examination of an embalmed and decomposing body, exhumed after nearly 2 years of burial, revealed a gunshot wound with some surrounding powder grains. These are to be seen in the film as very fine granules (see arrow). Two different-intensity soft x-ray exposures of the removed skin and subcutaneous tissue are shown to emphasize that the technique used is delicate and the results are easily varied.

treatment is instituted by the emergency medical personnel. To accomplish this, the clothing is cut and torn away. The removed clothing may not in whole or in part accompany the individual to the hospital emergency room.

5. At the hospital further cutting and tearing away of the clothing will usually occur during emergency procedures. The clothing may be folded down onto either side of the patient, there to become soaked with blood from the wounds made by the firearm and the surgeons. The clothing may be tossed aside, perhaps onto the floor, where it may be walked upon or thrown into a trash container and then sent to an incinerator. At the very best it will be placed in a bag and sent on with the body to the medicolegal officer, usually without any attempt to maintain a chain of evidence. Sometimes it is placed in the hospital property room or turned over to the next of kin. It may be given to a law enforcement officer and eventually turn up in the police property room.

In brief, all manner of things can happen to the clothing outside the control of the medicolegal officer or law enforcement personnel. The defects made by the firearm may be in the line of the cuts made to open the garments (Fig. 16-95). Fragile residues may be flipped off the clothing. The area of the defects may be soaked with blood, body fluids, intravenous fluids, and the like.

If the clothing *is* available for examination by the pathologist or medical examiner, there are several objectives for such scrutiny. The most important of these are as follows:

1. *To help establish the range at which the firearm was discharged.* Soot deposit or powder tattooing on the garments would indicate short and medium range respectively. Tearing of the fabric, fusion of certain artificial (man-made) fibers, or the finding of a corona pattern would indicate discharge of the firearm with the muzzle in contact with the fabric. Since the garments may totally protect the skin from firearms residue, correlation of the clothing and the body examina-

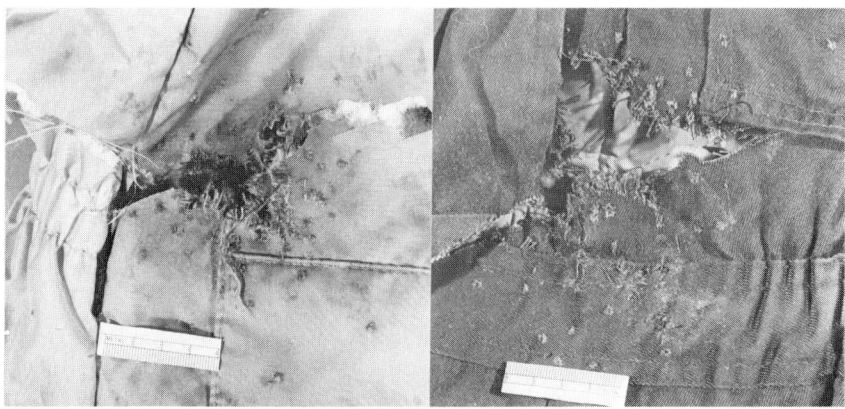

FIGURE 16-95. Clothing cut away through shotgun defects. The two jumpsuits worn by the victim were cut off by emergency medical personnel. The cuts in the longitudinal and transverse planes of both garments passed through the very area that should have been preserved.

tion is essential for an understanding of the range at which the firearm was discharged.
2. *To help establish which defects on the body are of the inshoot type and which are of outshoot origin.* The two can be distinguished because the inshoot defect is surrounded by a more or less concentrically placed bullet wipe. Rarely, the direction of the bullet travel is suggested by inversion of the fabric surrounding the inshoot defect and eversion about the outshoot defect. This, however, is a detail which is not positive and can be altered by manipulation of the clothing.
3. *To help locate the bullet.* If no exit defect exists in the clothing in opposition to the outshoot wound on the body, either the clothing did not cover the area of the exit, or the bullet exited the body with insufficient velocity to pass through the clothing. The bullet may still be in the clothing, or perhaps it fell away from the clothing during the removal of the body, during transport, or during emergency treatment.

Examination of the clothing has many purposes as noted above. The examination itself may be conducted by several different techniques:

1. With the unaided eye;
2. With the help of a magnifying glass;
3. With a binocular microscope;
4. With infrared photography;
5. With ordinary x-ray;
6. With soft x-ray;
7. With energy dispersive x-ray apparatus.

Infrared photography can be used to help delineate soot deposit on dark-colored or black fabrics. Ordinary x-ray can be applied to search for larger metallic fragments of bullets and other missiles. Soft x-ray is useful for these purposes and may also help to identify powder grains. Energy dispersive x-ray techniques can be used to analyze metallic fragments for elemental content. There are other ways in which to examine clothing, but all of those listed above are nondestructive; the clothing remains for subsequent examination or perhaps for use in the courtroom as evidence.

Nonwounding Area Telltales in Gunshot Cases

Four situations will be described in this section. They are somewhat similar in that the missile is related to the visible effect, but the entry point of the missile is apart from the observed abnormality of the body. These situations are as follows:

1. Blood (and sometimes tissue) splatters on the hands. This condition is most often found in suicide victims (Fig. 16-96). Blood (and tissue) splatters on the hand that held the firearm in contact with the head or on the hand that was used to steady the barrel. Brain tissue is the most frequently encountered substance in addition to blood. The hand of an assailant in a homicide can also be found to be covered with blood and tissue, but since contact homicidal wounds are rare, few assailants find it necessary to rid their hands of such reminders after committing a murder.
2. Blood may drip down onto the feet or other parts of a victim's body,

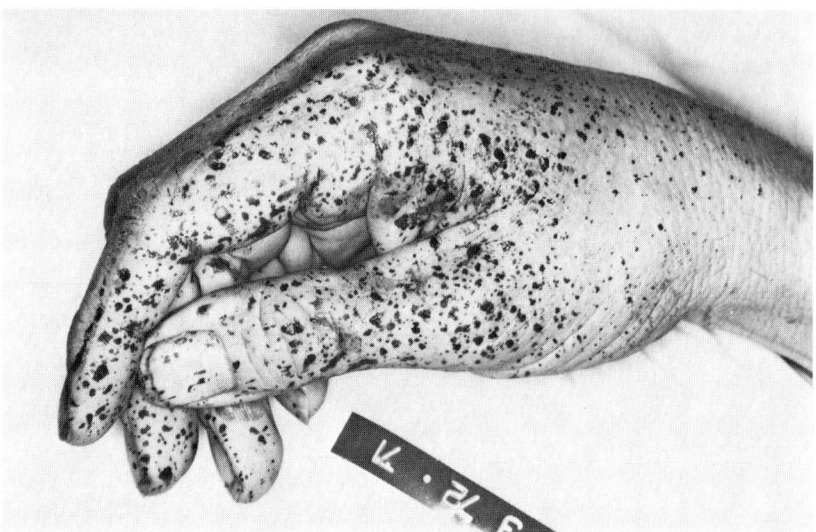

FIGURE 16-96. Blood splatters on hand. The hand of a suicide victim. Obviously, the hand steadied the barrel of the handgun and was close to the near-contact wound of the head.

indicating the more or less upright position of the victim at and after the wounding (Fig. 16-97). Observation and documentation of this phenomenon can be of help in understanding the circumstances of the shooting.
3. Firearm residue on the body in areas other than the actual wound site can indicate the position of the body at the time of shooting. The "flare," or powder gas that escapes from the cylinder gap of a revolver, can indicate the relative position of the body and the weapon (Fig. 16-98); the same is true of powder tattooing or lead-fragment stippling which arises from the leakage of powder grains from the cylinder gap (Fig. 16-99), and from fragments of lead sheared off the bullet as it jumps the cylinder gap and strikes the rear of the barrel to enter the bore (Fig. 16-100).
4. The impingement of powder gas and soot deposit that is found upon the palm of the hand when the same hand has been wrapped about the cylinder of the revolver when the shot is fired (Fig. 16-101) is a hallmark of a firearms suicide victim.

Alteration of Gunshot Wounds

There are many ways in which a gunshot wound can be altered from its appearance immediately after wounding. Alterations can be caused by the following variety of conditions and actions:

1. Drying of margins of the wound opening;
2. Decomposition of the body;
3. Healing of the wound itself;
4. Intervention by emergency care personnel;
5. Surgical intervention;
6. Intervention by nonprofessional personnel at scene of death;
7. Washing or cleansing of the wound after death.

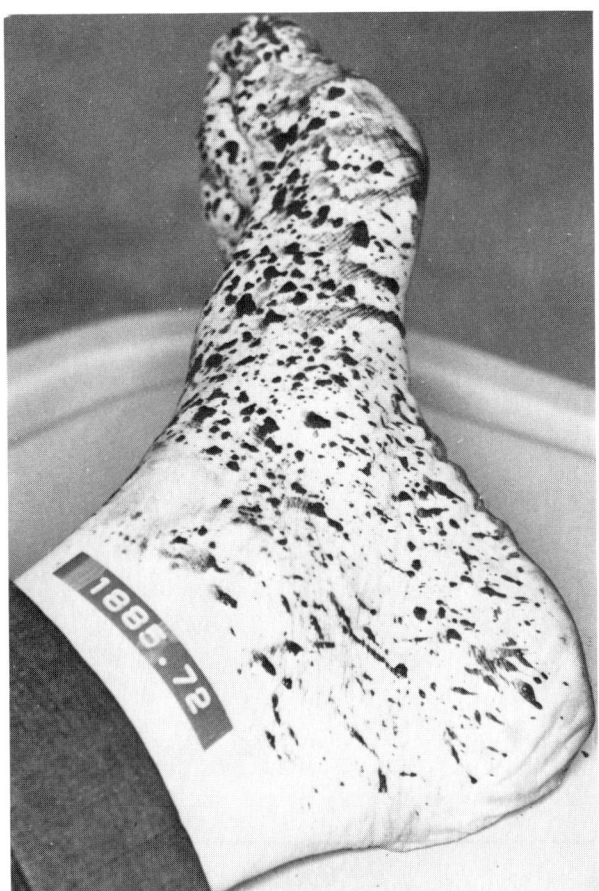

FIGURE 16-97. Blood droplets on foot. The foot of a man who dispatched his wife with one bullet and then shot himself in the head. Blood droplets appear to be originating from two different directions: directly above the foot and from in front of and above the foot. The back-splash from the homicidally inflicted near-contact wound of the head caused one pattern; dripping of blood from the head of the man caused the other.

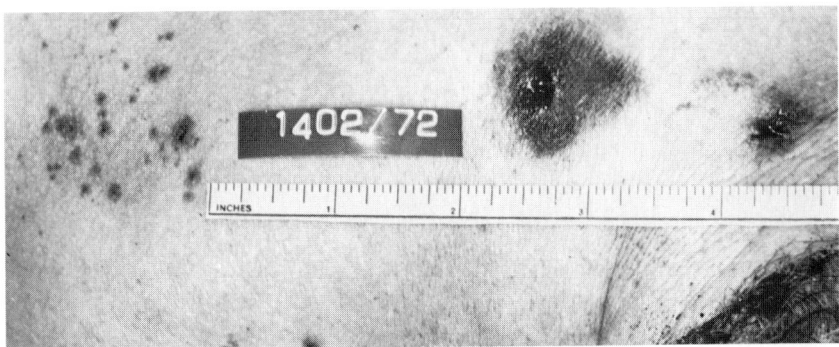

FIGURE 16-98. Revolver flare indicating barrel length. The very short-range wound in the center of the upper back was inflicted with the revolver held nearly parallel to the skin. The exit wound is near the upper right hand corner of the figure. The flare caused by leakage of lead powder particles and gas is situated approximately 3 inches from the inshoot wound, thus indicating the barrel length.

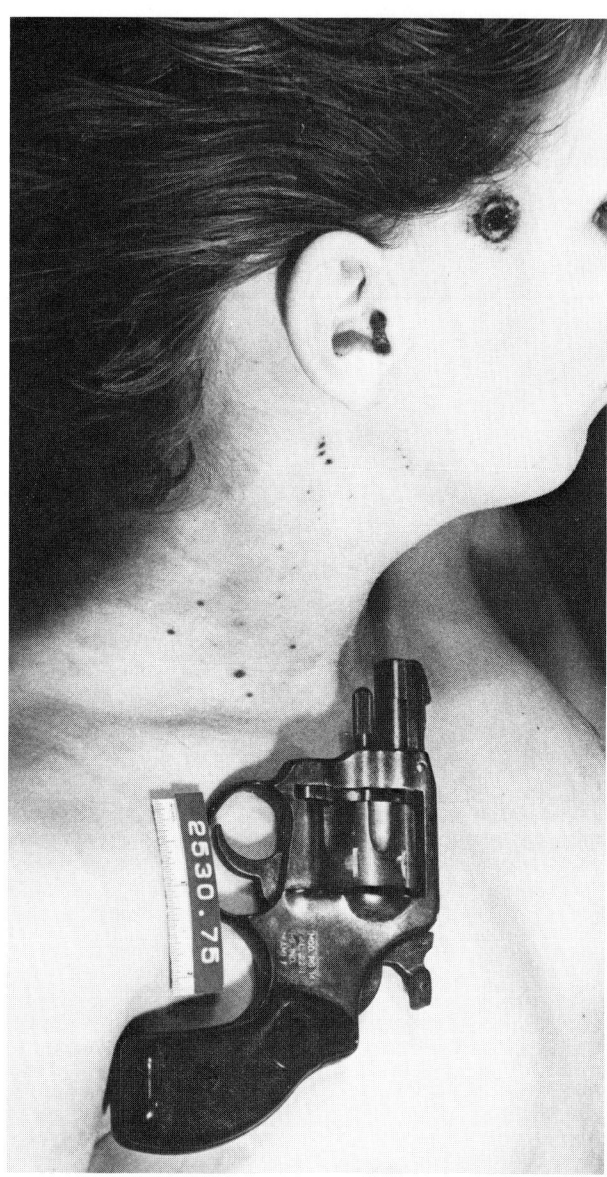

FIGURE 16-99. Revolver flare indicating position of head. This suicide victim must have had her head tipped down to the right at the moment of discharging the firearm as indicated by the flare on the right side of the neck.

Some changes in the appearance of wounds are illustrated in Figures 16-102 through 16-108 (see also Table 16-11).

Firearms Residues

The term residue simply means "something left over." In firearms residue the term has several meanings which will be discussed in this section. Different investigators also tend to be interested in different residues or different locations for firearms residues. Law enforcement officers, for

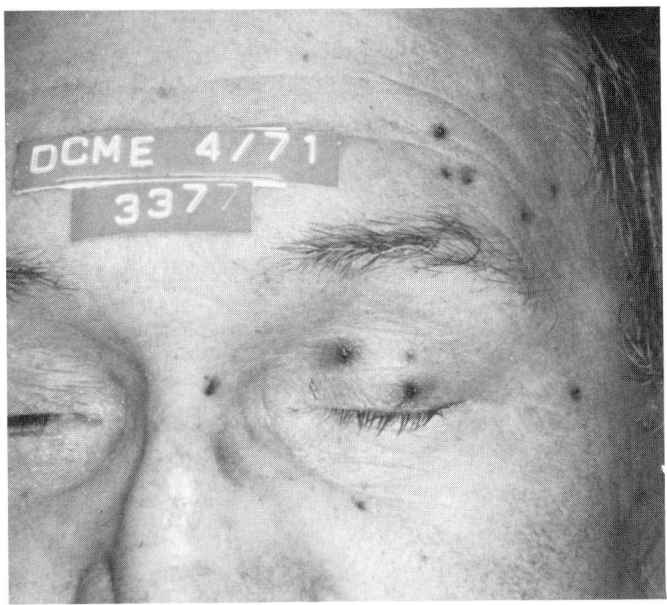

FIGURE 16-100. Stippling from metal fragments. The man pictured was shot many times with a .22 caliber revolver. Fragments of the soft metal bullets were shaved off when the bullet passed from the cylinder to the barrel, impacting the face and causing the stippling pattern. No bullet impacted the body in the facial area.

example, tend to associate the term with residue left on the hands of suspect-assailants in firearm assaults. Firearms examiners, on the other hand, are interested in residues on the firearms themselves. Forensic pathologists tend to deal with residue on the victim's body in association with a discovered gunshot wound.

The subject of firearms residues is quite complex, and the understanding of residue identification, collection, preservation, documentation, analysis, and interpretation is, at best, rather poor. The residues of the discharge of a firearm have traditionally been defined as powder particles and soot caused by the burning of the powder. There are actually many

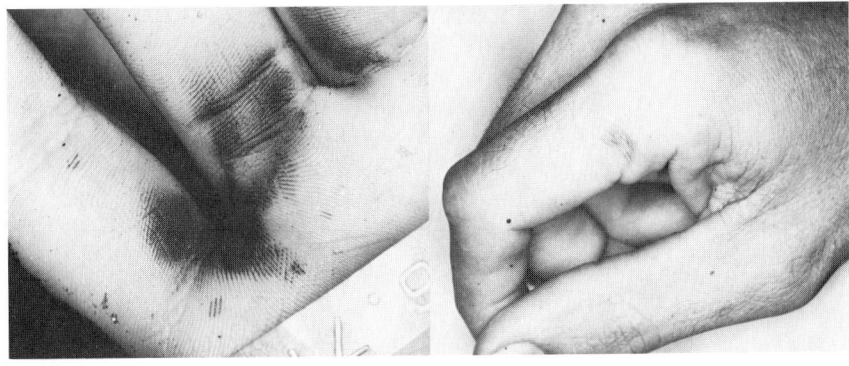

FIGURE 16-101. Soot deposit on hand. Two examples are shown. In that on the left, the hand was wrapped about the cylinder gap at the moment of firing. In that on the right, the forefinger was close to the cylinder gap of the revolver. Both subjects committed suicide.

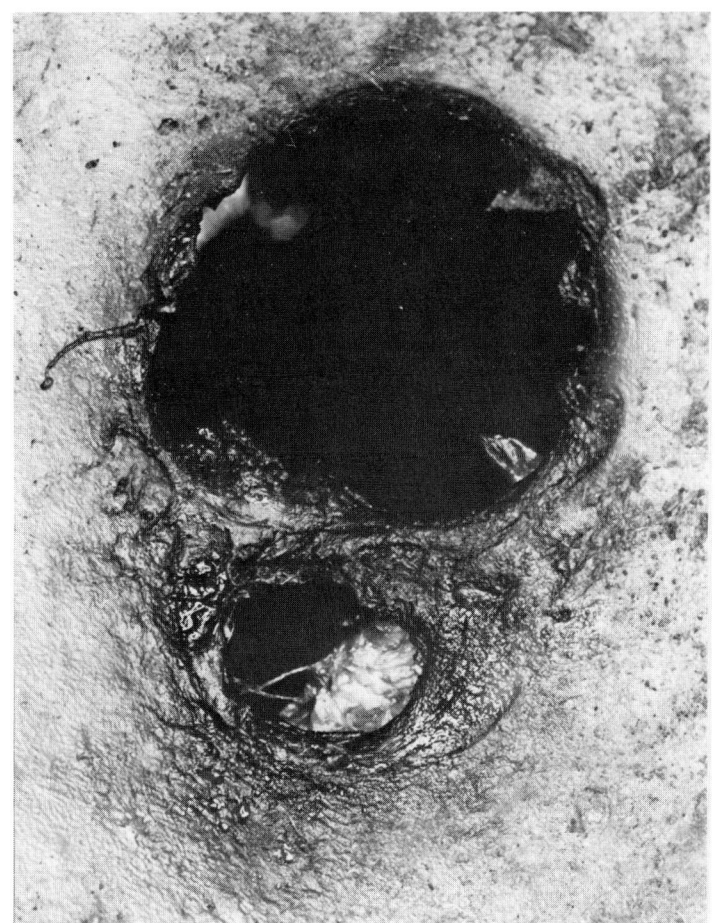

FIGURE 16-102. Gunshot wound in decomposing body. The marked alteration of the ordinary gunshot wound has occurred as a result of extensive body decomposition.

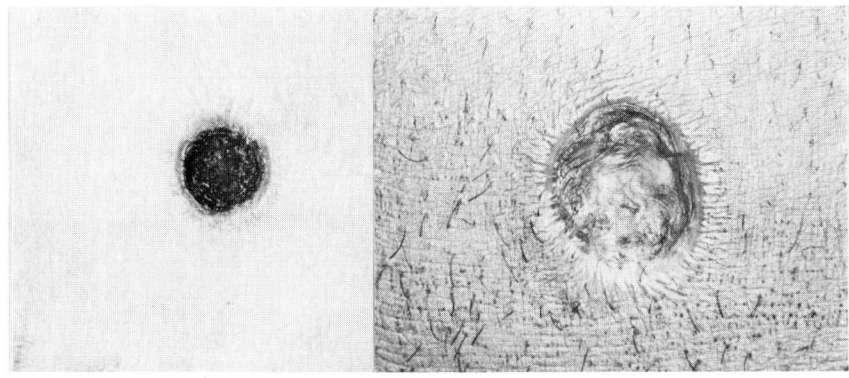

FIGURE 16-103. Healing of gunshot wound. Two examples are shown. Survival was 11 days in the instance of victim shown on the left, 21 days in that on the right.

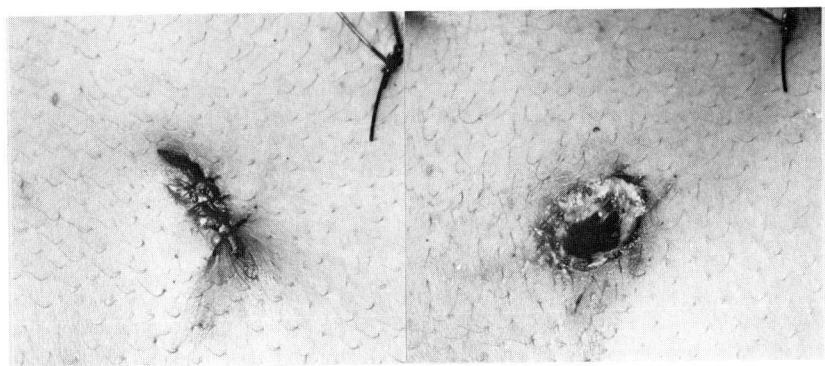

FIGURE 16-104. Suturing of gunshot wound. The surgeon sutured the wound of entrance. The sutured wound scarcely resembling a gunshot wound is shown in the left panel. On the right, the wound is shown following the removal of the sutures.

more residues left after the discharge of a firearm. Table 16-10 lists many of these which are found in medicolegal investigations.

The residues found on the bullet, in and on the cartridge case, and on the firearm itself are expected and rarely are of forensic scientific importance. As will be pointed out later, the examination of the empty cartridge case may be productive of clues concerning the type of powder with which it was filled and may also indicate the nature of compounds used in the primer. This information may be of importance when examining the target for firearms residues since the medicolegal examiner will then have some idea as to what to search for.

Some of the firearms residue on the target is visible and should be described with the wound as soot deposit and tattooing. This is an expected part of a firearms wound picture. There is another invisible and

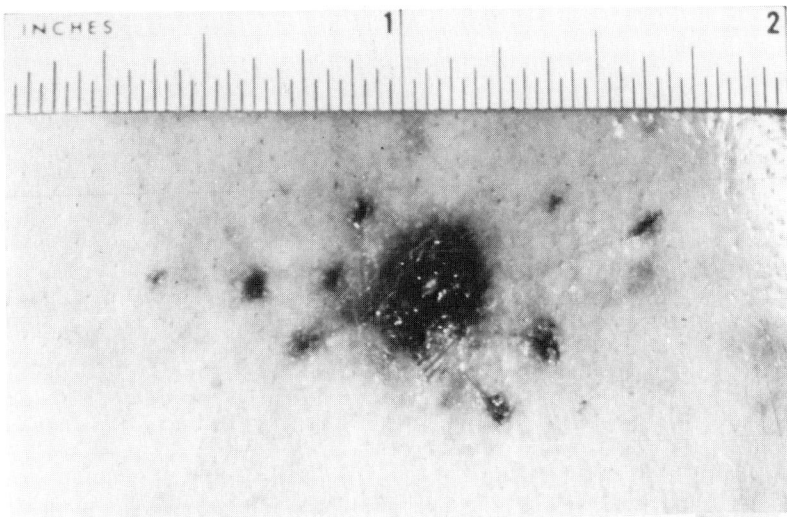

FIGURE 16-105. Sutured gunshot wound. The wound of the forehead was sutured by the surgeon who treated the victim. Removal of the sutures leaves a pattern suggestive of powder tattooing. This is a source of confusion to the examining pathologist and is one reason why communication between the treating physician and the examining pathologist is all-important.

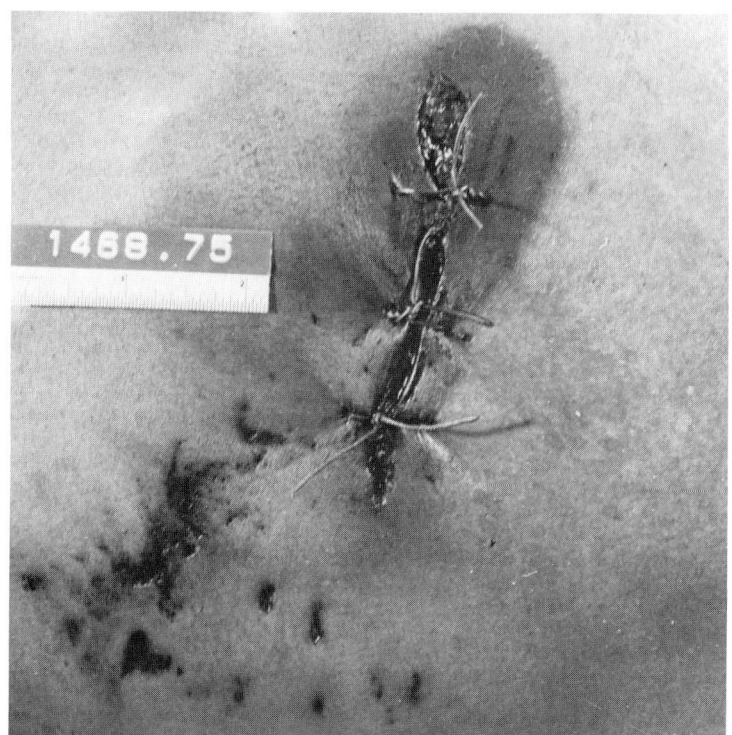

FIGURE 16-106. Incision through shotgun wound. The surgeon has cut through the shotgun wound of entrance and then sutured both the wound and his incision.

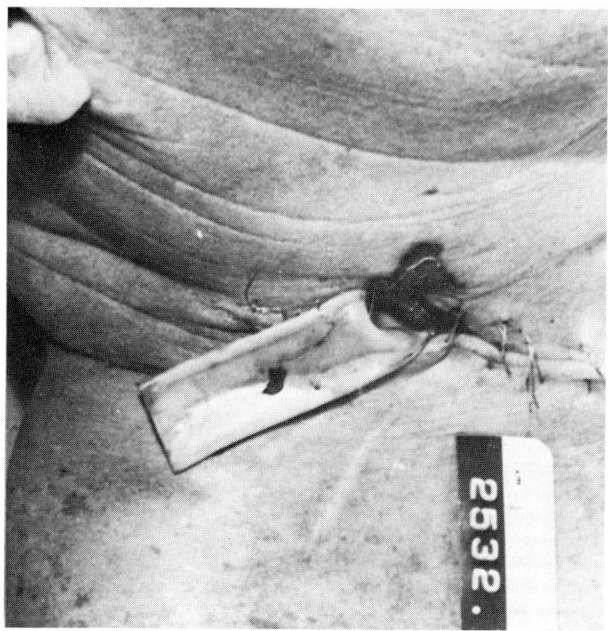

FIGURE 16-107. Drain in gunshot wound. The surgeon has placed a drain in the gunshot wound as well as having made the incision through it.

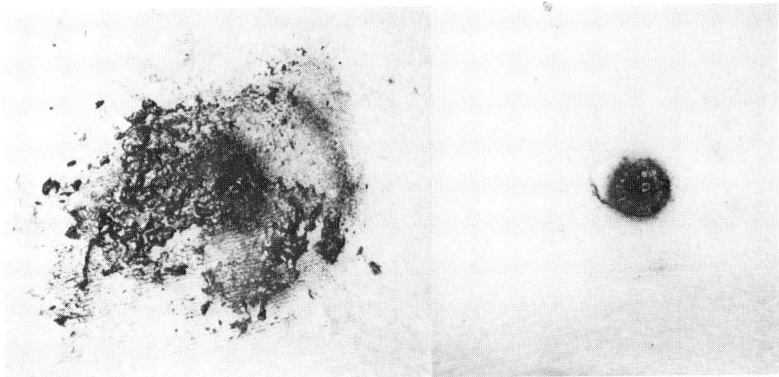

FIGURE 16-108. Alteration of wound by cleansing. The corona, a hallmark of a loose contact wound, is easily obliterated by washing the wound with cold water. On the left is the wound as it originally appeared. The same wound is shown on the right after washing.

less expected component of firearms residue left on the target at varying ranges. This consists of the elemental components of the cartridge case, primer, and bullet. These substances are often deposited on the target in such small quantities as to be invisible. In addition, powder grains and bullet fragments may be visible on the skin surface or may be driven beneath the skin and be unnoticed. A potpourri of residues may be expected at shorter ranges. The study of this aspect of firearms residue is in its early stages, but there is no question that an analysis in detail of whatever residues are present is most useful in estimating the range of fire and in distinguishing inshoot from outshoot wounds in decomposing bodies and in intact bodies where difficulty in examination is encountered.

FIREARMS RESIDUE ON THE HANDS OF THE SUSPECT

Law enforcement officers are usually anxious to check the hands of the individual suspected of discharging the firearm in a murder or assault investigation. The forensic pathologist usually checks the hands of the apparent suicide victim to obtain additional evidence that he did discharge the firearm to cause his own death. The forensic pathologist may also demonstrate by evidence of firearms residue on the hands that the victim threw up his hands in a defensive gesture, or wrestled for control of the firearm.

TABLE 16-10. FIREARMS RESIDUES (RIFLED FIREARMS)*

Residue	Origin	Visible by Naked Eye
Powder particles (grains)	Powder	Yes
Soot	Powder	Yes
Graphite	Powder	Yes, as soot
Carbon monoxide	Powder	Yes, as carboxyhemoglobin / Yes, as carboxymyoglobin
Fragments	Bullet	Yes
Lubricant	Bullet	Yes, as bullet wipe
Lead, antimony, silver, etc.	Bullet	No
Lead, barium, antimony, etc.	Primer	No
Copper, zinc	Cartridge case	No

*Firearms residues that arise from different cartridge components.

Residues on the hands may be visible, in which case their presence is subject to observation and description, and may be photographed for documentation. The term soot deposit or fouling has been applied to such visible residue. The position on the hands may indicate how the individual held the firearm or was exposed to the muzzle gas and other residual material (see Fig. 16-101).

More frequently, the residue is not visible to the unaided eye. Specialized techniques must be employed to demonstrate invisible residues. The first technique to become popular was the so-called paraffin test, introduced in the 1930s.[26] This procedure, which was designed to demonstrate nitrates, employed paraffin as a device for collecting the particles of the sought-for substances. Since nitrates account for the largest share of substances remaining after oxidation of powder, the procedure is not without theoretical merit. The presence of the particles pulled away from the hands after the liquid paraffin had hardened was demonstrated by a color reaction. The chemicals were applied directly to the paraffin casts—a simple, easy, effective technique. Or was it? The high percentage of false-positive determinations caused the Federal Bureau of Investigation Laboratory to undertake a prolonged series of experiments. These were carried out within a few years of the introduction of the procedure in the United States.[27,28] The technique was shown to be unreliable. A second and somewhat similar technique was then developed for the detection of primer components.[29] A dilute acid was used to wash the hands of the subjects. As with the detection of nitrates, the technique was excellent in theory. However, the small quantities of the primer metallic residues found on the hands strained the capability of the procedure. The procedure was not sensitive enough in the situations where it was usually employed. Also, it was cumbersome to carry out.

For reasons not clearly understood, many law enforcement officers and attorneys remain convinced that the "paraffin test" is useful, and crime laboratories are repeatedly asked to undertake the procedure. It is, no doubt, still being performed in the United States.

In the 1960s, a much more useful and accurate test was developed using neutron activation.[30,31] A sample is obtained from the hands by the use of paraffin or by washing the hands with dilute acid. It is then exposed to radiation from a nuclear reactor emitting neutrons. Secondary radioactivity is induced in the materials removed from the hands and, by making appropriate counts at different energy levels, the elemental composition of the residues can be determined with precision and accuracy. The technique is extremely sensitive; very small quantities of primer residues can be detected. However, only a few laboratories in the United States can carry out this procedure and it is expensive. Another drawback is that travel from the laboratory to the court of jurisdiction may be required for the analyst.

Flameless atomic absorption is another useful method for detecting firearms primer residues.[32] This analytical system utilizes high temperatures to vaporize the metallic elements of the primer residues and to detect and quantitate them by absorption spectrophotometry. The technique is quick, sensitive, and employs equipment within the economic means of moderate-sized crime laboratories. Still another method is that brought to perfection by members of the Aerospace Corporation team who utilized scanning electron microscopy as the central analytical tool.[33]

All of the procedures discussed above depend upon one simple and often overlooked step: the protection of the hands of the deceased or the suspect so that the residue will not be lost or contaminated. This step must be initiated and undertaken immediately at the scene of the discovery of the body or the detention or arrest of the suspect. It is easily accomplished in the deceased by placing a paper, not plastic, bag over each hand before manipulation and moving of the body. In the instance of a living person suspected of having discharged a firearm during a robbery or assault, the individual must not be allowed to wash or wipe off his hands, or to place them in his pockets, or to touch anything.

FIREARMS RESIDUE ON THE VICTIM ASSOCIATED WITH THE WOUND OF ENTRANCE

The visible residue, as noted above, consists of soot deposit, bullet lubricant, powder tattooing, powder grains, and occasionally lead stippling and soot from the flare or cylinder gap leakage associated with revolvers. The invisible residue consists of primer materials and vaporized metal from the bullet, its jacket, if any, and the cartridge case.

Ordinarily, the visible residue is noted immediately adjacent to the wound of entry. The actual edge of the defect may be coated or covered with such residues if the firearm was discharged at short range. In contact gunshot wounds, the residues may not be visible externally, except on the edge of the defect which may appear blackened; the residues are deposited along the track of the missile and may even be diffused radially among the tissues. Detection of such residues is best accomplished by removing the skin surrounding the defect, including a core of subcutaneous tissue and perhaps deeper soft structures surrounding the track and searching for powder grains. This is best done by employing the dissecting microscope, an indispensable autopsy room instrument. It is in this way that the wounds of inshoot and outshoot can be distinguished when the body is decomposing or markedly altered by fire, or when there is a question as to whether the wound is of contact type or of long-range type, a problem when dealing with .22 caliber wounds.

Visible residue can sometimes be demonstrated by the use of histologic techniques. Histologic sections made through the wound and wound track at cross section to the track or by making radially oriented sections can be useful in the search for powder particles. A stain for nitrates and/or nitrites is available and may be employed. In the author's experience, however, this method is far less helpful than that utilizing the dissecting microscope to examine the fresh tissue.

When searching for invisible residue in and surrounding the gunshot wound, the removal of tissue and the examination of it by energy dispersive x-ray apparatus is a rewarding activity. By means of this technique, primer components and tiny amounts of metals deposited in vaporized form from bullet, jacket, and cartridge case can be detected and semiquantitated. An estimate of the range of fire may also be derived from such determinations. This approach to the examination of a certain gunshot wounds is most useful, and although a new development, is of great promise.[34]

Mention should also be made of carbon monoxide as a firearms residue. It is found in the gas produced by the burning of powder. When the firearm is in contact with skin, and the gas is deposited beneath the skin and diffuses out into the tissues, the carbon monoxide present will combine with the hemoglobin of the blood and the myoglobin of the muscle to form carboxyhemoglobin and carboxymyoglobin, respectively. It is these substances that cause the bright red color of the tissues, particularly muscle, surrounding the wound track. Since a large amount of gas is formed by rifles other than .22 caliber, by shotguns when they are fired, and by certain handguns such as the .44 magnum, carboxyhemoglobin and carboxymyoglobin may be found in noncontact-type wounds made with these firearms at ranges up to perhaps 1 foot. Therefore, the presence of redness of the tissues or the chemical demonstration of these substances does not necessarily mean that the wound was inflicted at contact range. There is one other seeming anachronism relating to carbon monoxide: occasionally with contact wounds the greatest concentration of carboxyhemoglobin or carboxymyoglobin will be found about the outshoot wound. This is most apt to occur when a high-velocity rifle has been used. Apparently, the cylinder of gas is driven in with such velocity that radial expansion and diffusion do not take place as much in the inshoot area as about the outshoot portion of the bullet track. This is confusing and must be anticipated and not allowed to form the basis of misinterpretation of wounding.

FIREARMS RESIDUE ON THE VICTIM NOT ASSOCIATED WITH THE WOUND OF ENTRANCE

Of course, there must be *some* association of the wound of entry and the residue. What is implied here is that the residue, usually visible, is not circumferentially arranged about the wound. In most such situations the residue is deposited as a result of the leakage of gas, powder particles, and metal shavings from between the cylinder and the barrel of a revolver. This phenomenon may be termed flare or cylinder gap leakage. The visual recognition of such a flare, including metal fragment stippling, is useful to help determine range of fire, the relative position of the revolver and the victim, and in some instances to estimate the length of the barrel of the firearm (see Figs. 16-98, 16-99, and 16-100).

Residues on the firearm, bullet, and cartridge case will not be discussed here. The primary purpose of the foregoing discussion is to indicate that the examination of the victim of firearms wounding is a complex task and may well involve the police investigator, who must protect the victim and his clothing from manipulation and contamination; the forensic pathologist; and many other forensic scientists working in the medicolegal office and the crime laboratory. Without excellent cooperation, incomplete data may easily lead to incorrect conclusions and opinions.

Description of Firearms Wounds

The adequacy of the medicolegal description of firearms wounds will of necessity depend to a large extent upon whether or not the victim is dead. If the victim is alive, the description is apt to be brief and lacking in detail. The treating physician has a primary responsibility to apply emergency therapy. Cleaning of the wound, entering and exploring it, debriding and closing it, and dressing it are all necessary parts of the proper actions of the treating physician. His notes detailing the wound will be made later, and perhaps only after the interposition of other emergency care problems. The description of the wound as made by the treating physician is apt to be brief and lacking in detail. Since little time is devoted in medical school to medicolegal subjects, the physician may well feel no obligation to describe the wound in any detail. A minimum description of the wound in the living victim should include:

1. The location;
2. The size and shape of the defect;
3. The abrasion ring;
4. Contiguous and discontiguous skin splits;
5. Soot deposit, if any;
6. Tattooing, if any;
7. Structures penetrated;
8. The bullet or other surgically removed foreign substance recovered and its disposition;
9. Treatment of the wound, including debridement, suturing, shaving of hair, packing, draining, and surgical extension of the wound.

An example of a brief but adequate description of a gunshot wound in a living victim is given below:

There is an entrance gunshot wound of the midpoint of the anterior surface of the right forearm. The defect is circular with a concentrically placed narrow zone of abrasion. There is no soot deposit or tattooing. A soft metal bullet is recovered in the subcutaneous tissue of the proximal aspect of the dorsal surface of the forearm. It is turned over to Officer J. R. Reilly of the Jefferson Police Department. The bullet track penetrates only the soft tissues, the bone is intact as shown by x-ray. A drain is placed in the wound and the arm bandaged.

In the instance of the dead victim there are no pressures upon the pathologist for emergency care and treatment. However, the body as received may have been subjected to much alteration by the emergency medical care personnel and by others. In addition, the body may be altered by those assigned to prepare the dead body for delivery to the person or agency responsible for receiving it. Further, the body may be washed, cleansed, and even embalmed by the funeral director. He may also suture or otherwise close wounds and cover them with wax or other camouflaging materials. One specific objective of the pathologist must be to determine who has done what, the better to understand the wound picture.

Insofar as the description of the firearms injuries on the body is concerned, the following major points should be included:

1. Location
   a. Distance from the top of the head or the sole of the foot and to right or left of midline
   b. General location in reference to a fixed landmark of the body
2. External wound description
   a. Size and shape
   b. Abrasion ring, thickness and concentricity
   c. Searing
   d. Skin splits, contiguous and noncontiguous
   e. Muzzle imprint
3. Visible firearms residues
   a. Powder grains
   b. Soot deposit, including the corona

c. Tattooing
   d. Metal stippling
4. Alteration
   a. By medical care personnel
   b. By funeral director
5. Track
   a. Organs penetrated
   b. Direction taken
      (1) Front to back (back to front)
      (2) Right to left (left to right)
      (3) Upward (downward)
   c. Secondary damage
      (1) Bleeding
      (2) Wounding near, but not in track
   d. Individual organ damage
6. Bullet recovered
   a. Point of recovery
   b. Type of missile
   c. Identification marks
   d. Disposition
7. Exit wound
   a. Location
   b. Characteristics
8. Bullet fragments recovered
9. Tissues collected for residue examination

The medicolegal description of a gunshot wound must be more detailed than that expected of the treating physician. Moreover, the apparent alterations of the wound by others and by healing should be included as part of the descriptive action. Two examples of a reasonable description are given below:

1. There is a gunshot wound of entrance in the left anterior thoracic wall. This is just above and immediately medial to the left nipple and is situated 40 cm (16 inches) below the top of the head and 10 cm (4 inches) to the left of the midline. The wound is circular in shape, approximately 0.8 cm in diameter, and is made up of a 0.2 cm radial dimensional abrasion ring concentrically placed about a 0.4 cm diameter defect. There is no soot deposit or powder tattooing. A small amount of blood issues forth from the defect upon manipulation of the body.

   A track is established from the gunshot wound of entrance on the left anterior thoracic wall which passes through the third interspace, through the lingua of the left lung, through the aorta, and into the anterior aspect of the body of the seventh thoracic vertebra. Here, embedded in the bone, is recovered a full metal jacketed bullet of approximately .25 caliber. This is marked 'CP-96' and is retained.

   The direction of fire is from front to back, left to right, and downward.

   A left hemothorax of 1500 cc of free and clotted blood is present.

In the above example, the detail of the track made by the bullet in individual organs may be further described.

2. A gunshot wound of entrance is present in the right temple. This is situated approximately 1 cm superior to the midpoint of a line joining the lateral aspect of the right eyebrow and the anterior and superiormost point at which the right ear joins the side of the head. This consists of a 0.7 cm diameter, nearly circular defect with a surrounding symmetrical rim of abrasion measuring 0.1 cm in radial dimension, and further surrounded by a concentrically placed 4.5 cm diameter zone of dense, black, soot deposit. Several grains of powder are seen in the edge of the defect. These are apparently of flake type. Some of these are recovered by the use of cellophane tape, placed on a glass side, and retained.

   There is a track extending from the wound of entry through the scalp, skull, dura, both cerebral hemispheres, the dura, skull, and scalp, and an outshoot wound is present in the left temple situated in a similar location to the inshoot wound.

   The wound of exit is irregular, nearly stellate in shape, and measures 4.0 cm in greatest dimension. A small amount of brain tissue has oozed forth from the wound.

   The inshoot defect in the skull measures 1.0 cm in diameter on the outer table of the skull and is circular. The defect is 1.8 cm in diameter on the inner table of the skull. The beveling is toward the inner aspect of the skull. The outshoot defect in the skull measures 1.5 × 1.0 cm in greatest dimensions on the inner table of the skull, 2.0 × 1.5 cm in greatest dimensions on the outer table of the skull; the beveling is to the outer aspect of the skull.

   Surrounding the inshoot defect on the outer table of the skull there is a radial band of soot deposit measuring 0.5 cm.

In the above example, further detail of the track in the brain and other tissues may be given, but the essentials have been provided.

Autopsy Facilities for Gunshot Wound Victims

Although this section is not intended as a treatise on gunshot wounds, some mention of the facilities necessary for the proper and adequate examination of a gunshot wound victim is advisable. It may appear to some readers that this description of facilities and equipment represents the ideal. However, the life or liberty of an individual may depend upon the facts developed during the autopsy. This procedure is, after all, the core of all medicolegal investigative work in death cases where the body of the victim is available for examination.

The reasonable and proper facility for the conduct of an autopsy upon the victim of firearms injury can be evaluated in terms of place, personnel, and equipment.

PLACE

The autopsy area for the conduct of medicolegal autopsies may be provided by the public medicolegal system of the jurisdiction, or, in smaller communities, by the pathologist with the sanction of the hospital. In some geographic areas the preparation rooms of funeral homes are expected to serve as the facility. It must be stressed that the latter is not a satisfactory alternative to a centralized facility or the use of a hospital autopsy room, and such an arrangement should be condemned.

Location of the autopsy facility in the offices of the forensic pathologist is the ideal. This permits the examiner immediate access to the body without loss of time and energy in traveling to the body. Moreover, should questions arise after the autopsy, supplemental examination of the body is easy to accomplish. Separate the body and the pathologist, and the examination is likely to be limited to the autopsy itself with additional procedures virtually precluded because of the travel required.

Part of the requirement as to place is that there be adequate body storage facilities so that significant change in the appearance of the body due to decomposition will not take place after the arrival of the body and before the autopsy. Cold storage (at 2° to 6° C) is necessary. The security afforded the body must also be considered. The body, like all other items of physical evidence, must be kept from curious eyes and prying fingers. This is part of the chain of evidence necessary and provable in court.

Also of importance is the requirement of adequate lighting for visual examination and photography of the body. Some of the changes in body coloration brought about by exposure to carbon monoxide and by ingesting cyanide are subtle and may be overlooked if the lighting is inadequate. Examination of wounds by the use of a magnifying lens, a macroscope, or a dissecting microscope requires excellent and flexible lighting.

EQUIPMENT

X-ray equipment must be available. This may consist of fixed or portable x-ray equipment that can be moved to the autopsy area as needed. In some situations, the body can be moved to a radiology department. There are definite drawbacks to the latter course: movement of the body into an area utilized for patient care is esthetically repugnant, and if the body is decomposing and malodorous and is oozing fluids, a problem is posed regarding patient and staff acceptance of the procedure. This is one reason that x-ray examination of the gunshot wound victim is not infrequently omitted as part of the autopsy procedure.

Magnifying equipment must also be available. A dissecting microscope is a necessary and relatively inexpensive item of equipment still not found in many autopsy facilities. Lower-powered magnifying equipment ranging from magnifying lenses to mounted macroscopes should also be available. Mounted equipment may be provided on a wheeled cart which can then be positioned alongside any part of the body to make in situ examination of firearms wounds not only possible but practical.

PERSONNEL

It is impossible for the pathologist to examine adequately the victim of a fatal gunshot wound without the assistance of at least one other person. The positioning of the body for x-ray, the often time-consuming, prolonged, and exasperating search for the missile and the turning of the body require manual assistance. The days are gone when the forensic pathologist alone could undertake an adequate examination of a gunshot wound victim. Such investigations were often carried out without assistance, as a solitary endeavor, in the middle of the night. Small wonder that so many inadequate examinations took place. There is another, more subtle reason for seeking assistance: the presence of another person tends to encourage the pathologist to "go a little further." This may be due to the simple fact that the physical effort required is shared between two individuals, or perhaps the pathologist may, in effect, use the assistant as a sort of a "straight man," enhancing the quality and thoroughness of the work.

The person who serves as the assistant may be another pathologist, a pathology resident, a medical technologist, a nurse, or an autopsy room assistant especially trained for the task. The important consideration is that there be an adequate assistant and that he be available during the entire course of the autopsy of the gunshot wound victim.

Misconceptions in Gunshot Investigations

There are many misconceptions held by all manner of people concerning the trauma inflicted by firearms. Space does not permit the inclusion of an exhaustive catalogue of errors. Some, however, are encountered so frequently that special mention seems in order. Ten of the more significant misconceptions are discussed below.

MISCONCEPTION 1

The entrance or inshoot wound is always smaller than the exit or outshoot wound. There is a variant of this misconception which may be stated thus: The entrance wound is always circular and neat, the exit wound is irregular in shape, has a jagged margin, and just *looks* different. In actuality, the inshoot wound may be larger than the outshoot wound and may be irregular in shape in contrast to the outshoot wound which may be circular and may even have an abraded margin (Fig. 16-109). As an example, contrast a contact inshoot wound with a shored outshoot wound (Fig. 16-110). Also, consider a noncontact wound of entrance with a shored exit wound when the two wounds are similar in size and shape.

MISCONCEPTION 2

When the wound of entrance is higher on the body than the outshoot wound, it follows that the assailant was pointing the firearm slightly downward toward the victim at the moment of firing. This is nonsense. The course of the bullet through the body has nothing to do with the relative positions of the victim and assailant. For example, the victim may have been leaning forward at the time of being shot. He may have been lying on the floor. He may have been climbing over a fence. This misconception is one frequently entertained by the attorney who, in the course of prosecution or defense of the accused, is anxious to establish a relationship between the victim and assailant that will fit the theoretic actions of the two. The most positive derivation that can be made is that the course of the missile in the body is consistent with the firearm being pointed slightly downward toward the victim at the time of discharge. There are many other relationships between the victim and the assailant and manner in which the weapon was held and pointed that are equally consistent. The number and details of such are limited only by the imagination of those anxious to reconstruct the situation at the time of the shooting.

MISCONCEPTION 3

The bullet always travels in a straight line in the body, from the entrance to the exit wound, or wherever it came to rest in the body. This is not necessarily

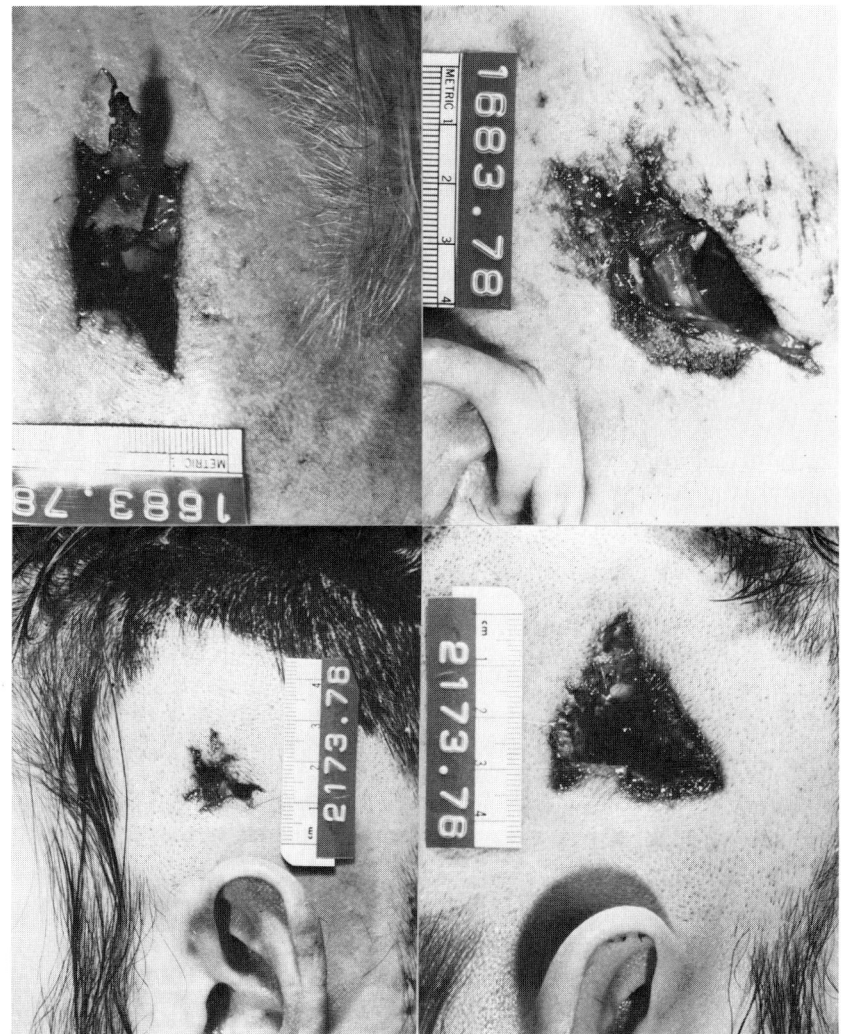

FIGURE 16-109. Explosive contact and outshoot wounds contrasted. Two pairs are shown. The two panels on the right are of the explosive contact type. The panels on the left represent the outshoot wounds on the opposite side of the head.

true. Internal ricochet can and does occur. When it occurs, it usually results from the bullet striking bone and being deflected from its initial course into a second or a third course. This happens with frequency when the bullet strikes the head, penetrating the skull, allowing the bullet access to the curved inner portion of the skull where it may easily be turned from its original intracalvarial trajectory (Fig. 16-111). In addition, it is not unheard of for a bullet to strike a fascial plane (as found between two muscles) and to follow the fascial plane gliding along it to its exit from the body or to its final resting place.

MISCONCEPTION 4

When the bullet emerges from the muzzle of the firearm, it is so hot that it will burn the skin. A variant of this misconception may be worded: The bullet

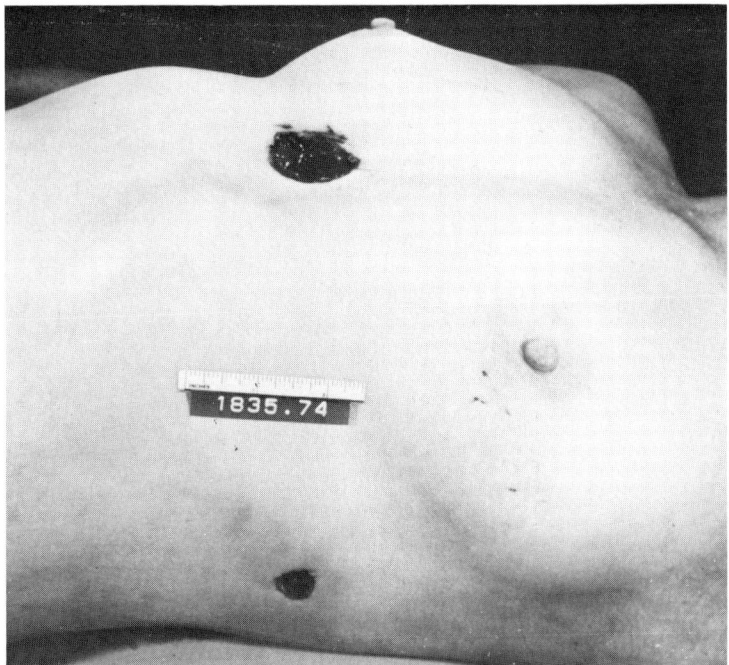

FIGURE 16-110. Explosive contact wound contrasted with shored outshoot wound. The firearm was held in contact with the skin over the sternum. The outshoot wound is of the shored type because the victim was lying on her left side at the time of shooting.

is so hot that all bacteria upon it are killed and the missile is really a sterile object. Neither statement is true. The heat generated by the burning of the powder is intense, but the bullet is exposed to the heat for a very short period of time; moreover, only the base of the bullet is exposed. In addition, the friction generated by the rubbing of the bullet against the bore creates further heat. However, the specific heat and density of lead, the principal material used in bullet construction, combine to require much heat to increase the bullet temperature. Firearms examiners who recover bullets immediately after firing from test boxes filled with cotton waste find warm, perhaps even hot bullets. Nevertheless, the cotton waste is never scorched or burned by the bullet itself. Also, experimental firing has shown that bullets are not sterile after being fired from a firearm.

MISCONCEPTION 5

The bullet shot from a rifled firearm, spinning at a very high rate of speed, essentially drills its way into and through the target. This spinning motion or drilling is responsible, at least in part, for the abrasion ring seen in wounds of entrance. This statement is a half truth. There is no question but that the bullet is spinning. However, the rate of forward motion is so great that during the passage of a bullet through the thickness of the human chest or abdomen, it will make only one or two complete revolutions. The bullet does *not* "drill" its way through the body.

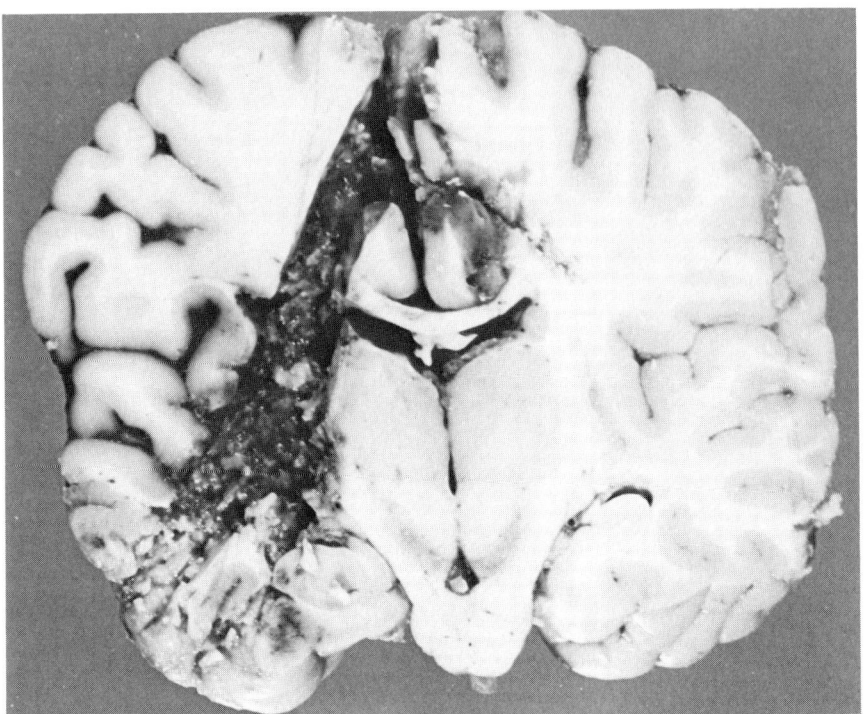

FIGURE 16-111. Internal ricochet. A cross section of the fixed brain is shown. The bullet entered the lower left, proceeding upward and slightly toward the right, impacting the skull and ricocheting to the right and downward, and somewhat to the back. The bone fragments carried into the brain by the bullet indicate the inshoot area.

MISCONCEPTION 6

Semijacketed or hollow-point pistol or revolver bullets make "hamburger" out of the organs of the chest or abdomen. This misconception appears to have arisen from ignorance of wound ballistics and from confusion of the effects of velocity and bullet design. Semijacketed bullets have long been available for high-velocity rifles. Since the physician or surgeon treating the victim of firearms injury rarely knows the type of weapon employed, but is aware that a semijacketed bullet was recovered (by the surgeon himself), it is logical for him to assume that the massive destruction is due to the bullet, when in fact it resulted from the high velocity of the rifle employed (Fig. 16-112). To obtain cavitation and marked release of energy directed radially, the velocity of the missile must be higher than the highest achieved with a pistol or revolver bullet that leaves the muzzle, perhaps as high as 1600 to 1800 feet per second.

Semijacketed or hollow-point bullets leave the muzzle at a lower velocity (at speeds of 1500 feet per second or lower), when fired from most handguns. These bullets are designed to expand or mushroom. This causes a more rapid slowing of the bullet in the body and a more rapid transfer of kinetic energy to the tissues. Moreover, such a bullet is not as apt to perforate the body, passing through it, and maintaining a part of its kinetic energy as it exits. It is the more rapid and more complete transfer of kinetic energy that causes the greater "striking power" or

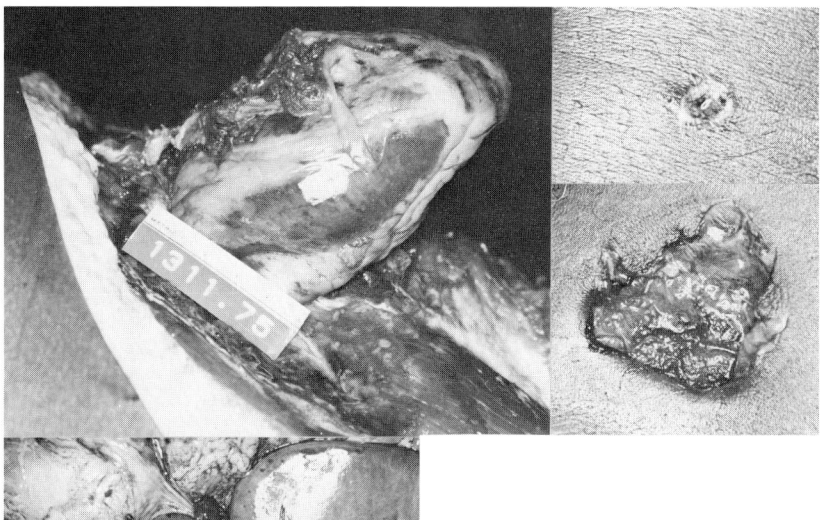

FIGURE 16-112. High-velocity rifle wounds. In the lower left is shown the liver (in situ) with a huge stellate-shaped wound made by a high-velocity rifle bullet. Another case is shown in the upper left with the heart protruding, blown partly out of the chest by a high-velocity rifle bullet; in the upper right is shown the inshoot wound, and immediately below it, the outshoot wound.

"knockdown" capability of semijacketed and hollow-point bullets. Despite the mushrooming effect of these bullets and more rapid transfer of kinetic energy to the body, the visible wounding of tissues and organs cannot be distinguished from that caused by other varieties of bullets, provided that the velocity is maintained below approximately 1500 feet per second.[35]

MISCONCEPTION 7

Many individuals die as a result of accidentally inflicted gunshot wounds sustained while cleaning a firearm. Actually, such accidents occur only rarely. Many times the gun-cleaning kit is at hand because the individual, bent on suicide, desires to make the investigating officials think that the wound was accidentally inflicted. Family members have been known to confuse the scene of death by the simple addition of a cleaning rod, oil, and patch. Sometimes the suicidal nature of the death is indicated by the contact type of wound in a position where accidental infliction would be nearly impossible.

MISCONCEPTION 8

Right-handed individuals commit suicide by holding the handgun in the right hand with the muzzle in contact with or close to the right temple. This is not the case. A moment's reflection will reveal the error. The handgun may be held with either hand, and any finger may be used to actuate the trigger, although the forefinger and thumb are most frequently so employed. Many individuals are not familiar with firearms; they are especially apt not to hold the weapon in the expected, normal, or "proper" fashion.

MISCONCEPTION 9

It is possible to determine how long the victim survived following fatal injury from an examination of the wound. Unfortunately, this cannot be done. There are many factors which modify the survival time following mortal wounding. Natural disease processes can combine with trauma to shorten life. Alcohol and drugs may certainly contribute to a decrease in the length of survival. The environmental temperature, humidity, and other factors may affect survival. The extent of the wounding is very important, of course, but it cannot always be determined from an external examination of the body. In fact, it may be difficult to determine, even with a thorough autopsy (see Figs. 16-117 and 16-118).

MISCONCEPTION 10

It is a simple procedure to perform an autopsy upon the victim of a firearm injury. All that is necessary is to find the wounds of entrance and exit, locate the bullet, and point out the traumatized tissues and organs. This statement is obviously untrue. It is the king of all misconceptions regarding firearms and the major reason this chapter was written.

SOME QUESTIONS AND ANSWERS ON TRAUMA

There are many ways of looking at trauma. Over 20 years ago, the noted forensic pathologist Alan Moritz authored a classic textbook that dealt with an overview of the pathology of trauma.[36] Despite the excellence of the book, it is now out of date, but no similar monograph has been produced to take its place. This chapter cannot hope to accomplish this task. By means of the questions and answers presented below, it is hoped that a maximum amount of information can be imparted with a minimum of verbiage.

1. *Can postmortem trauma be distinguished from that inflicted before death?*

Ordinarily, yes. The key is bleeding into the tissues. Postmortem wounding does not cause bleeding into the tissues. Of course, a defect in the wall of a properly situated blood vessel will permit the postmortem aggregation of blood in body cavities. A common example of this is the blood seen in the pericardial sac which surrounds the heart, resulting from the penetration of the heart with the needle used to instill drugs during resuscitation. The individual was dead when the puncture was made, yet blood leaked out of the heart and into the pericardial cavity. In examining Figure 16-113, note that one wound must have been made after death. There is no hemorrhage into the subcutaneous fat as is present in the other wounds. Figure 16-114, a close-up view of ice pick wounds, clearly shows hemorrhage into one wound and not the other. Death must have taken place after the one and before the other (see also Fig. 16-19).

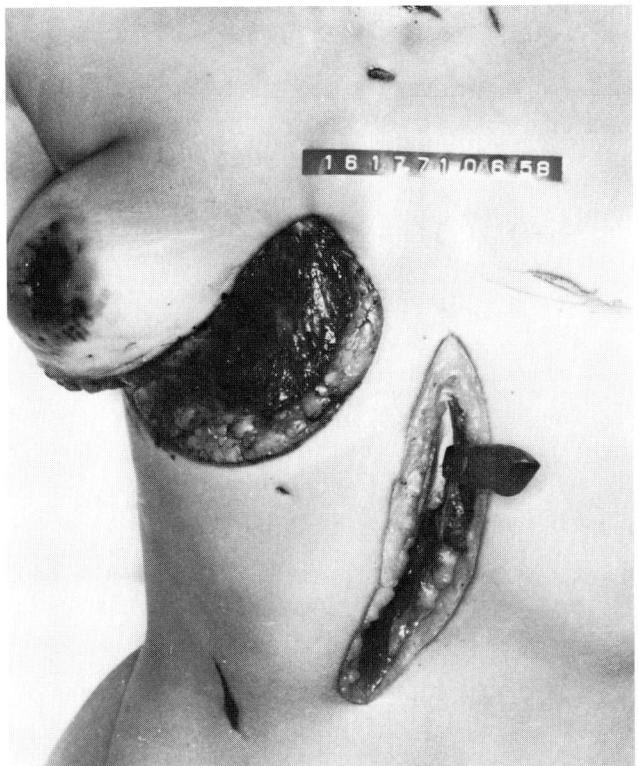

FIGURE 16-113. Pre- and postmortem knife wounds. The wound beneath the right breast of the victim was inflicted while she was alive. The central thoracic and abdominal wound was inflicted after death. There is hemorrhage into the subcutaneous fat of the former and not the latter.

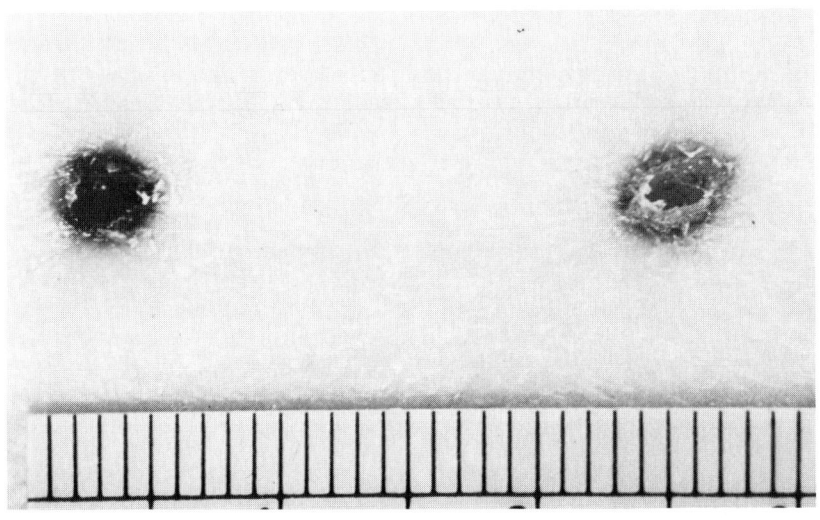

FIGURE 16-114. Pre- and postmortem ice pick wounds. Two of many ice pick wounds inflicted upon a man are shown. That on the left was inflicted before death, that on the right after death.

2. *Can a lethal degree of trauma be present with no external indication of the trauma being present?*

Yes. There are many common instances of this. A "wedging" type of blow to the lower chest and upper abdomen may tear the aorta within the victim, with no external manifestations of trauma whatsoever. This is seen in motor vehicle crashes. The weight of the individual who applies his knee to the upper abdomen of another may cause a rupture of the liver and death, without any overlying contusion of the abdominal wall. A gunshot wound of the head, inflicted with a small-caliber firearm, may be hidden in the scalp hair with no external bleeding to betray its presence (see Fig. 16-119). Manual strangulation can also be the cause of death with no external signs of trauma.

3. *Can resuscitative efforts, such as are applied by emergency medical technicians and hospital and other medical care personnel, cause trauma that cannot be differentiated from injury that was present before resuscitation was applied?*

Yes. This question actually deals with something of the same subject as question 1. Antemortem injuries are associated with bleeding into the tissues; postmortem injuries are not. However, in what has been termed perimortem injuries, those injuries that occur during the act of dying, hemorrhage may be seen involving the soft tissues. This may be due to the preservation of at least some pressure within the arterial system due to energetic external cardiac massage. The injuries that can be inflicted during resuscitative procedures are of many types and involve different organs and tissues of the body. Commonly the following tissues and organs are damaged during vigorous resuscitative efforts (these are listed in general order of frequency of occurrence): contusion-abrasion of chest wall (by the hand or a mechanical thumper), fractures of ribs, fractures of the sternum (breast bone), contusions of the heart, contusions and laceration of the liver (Fig. 16-115) and spleen, rupture of the heart and small intestine (usually duodenum), and other injuries too rare to warrant inclusion here. It is of great importance, therefore, to consider if the injury found could have been caused by resuscitation, and then to determine whether or not resuscitative procedures were actually employed before the interpretation of the injury is undertaken. It may be necessary to undertake a microscopic examination of the injured area to determine, if at all possible, whether the injury antedated the resuscitative effort.

4. *Can the time of infliction of the wound be determined?*

This is a variant of questions 1 and 3. As has been discussed in relationship to contusion, laceration, and blunt head injury, there is no precise timetable that can be followed to enable the time of infliction of the wound to be precisely fixed. An educated estimate is the best that can be expected from the pathologist. Actually, the most valuable use of the techniques of pathology is to be able to "rule in" as possible or to "rule out" as impossible a time of assault that is in question.

5. *Can death be much delayed following the infliction of trauma?*

Yes, of course. As has already been described, the rupture of liver, spleen, aorta, and sometimes of other organs may be delayed by hours, days, and sometimes weeks after the organ was weakened by the trau-

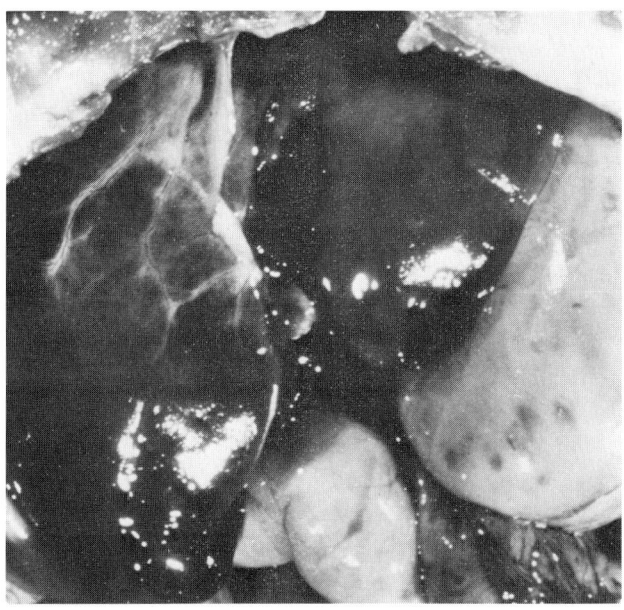

FIGURE 16-115. Laceration of liver. The laceration of the liver was caused by intensive cardiopulmonary resuscitative effort made by emergency medical personnel. The subject was a child.

matic episode. Delayed death due to fat or marrow embolism has also been described above. More commonly encountered are two other types of delayed death following trauma: pneumonia and deep leg vein thrombosis with pulmonary embolism. Both types are of substantial medicolegal importance, not so much because they occur, but because of the infrequency with which the proper cause and manner of death are entered upon the death certificate by physicians with little or no forensic scientific background. The fracture of the femur of the elderly subject treated initially by bed rest, and then by open reduction or pinning of the fracture of the neck of the femur, or even by near-immediate replacement of the entire head of the femur (so called joint replacement), places the patient in a difficult position: bed rest, anesthesia, and care in a facility where there may be bacteria in the environment that can (and do) cause pneumonia. Also true is the fact that many an older person does not possess the physical capability to prevent bacteria from establishing a foothold in the lung or airway with resulting fatal pneumonia. Despite the many advances in medical care, bedridden patients are still subject to thrombosis of the deep leg veins. Fragments of such clots may then break away and, riding in the venous blood, eventually enter the pulmonary artery there to cause both respiratory and circulatory dysfunction, and possibly death (Fig. 16-116). Such death may be sudden and unexpected in contrast to the "old man's friend," pneumonia, where the labored breathing, confusion, apathy, and dullness precede coma, unresponsiveness, and death. In both instances, however, the death certificate may indicate the cause of death as "pneumonia" or "pulmonary embolism" with no mention of the underlying and initiating trauma: the fall that caused the fracture of the femur. Such oversight causes serious problems for the surviving

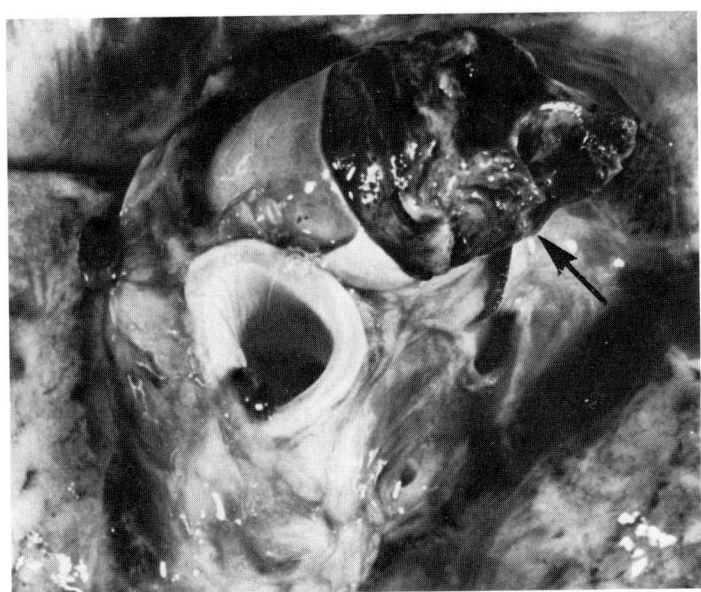

FIGURE 16-116. Pulmonary embolism. The pulmonary artery is clogged with blood clot (see arrow).

relatives with slow and improper estate settlements, and failure to properly claim insurance benefits. In some instances, an individual may be hospitalized for the treatment of a gunshot wound of the neck, with resulting paraplegia (loss of use of lower limbs) or quadriplegia (loss of use of all four extremities). In such instances the continuing hospital and nursing home care is fraught with hazard. The patient may well develop an infection of the urinary tract or the lungs months or even years after the assault. Even though the death is directly the result of the original wound, because of the interval in time between the injury and death, the death certificate may be incorrectly prepared. There are many possible variations upon this theme of trauma, delayed death, miscertification of the death, and subsequent problems in the settlement of the affairs of the deceased or failure of the criminal justice system to be aware of delayed deaths which are of a homicidal nature.

6. *How long did the victim live after the fatal wounding? Could the victim have carried out purposeful acts after the wounding?*

There is very little good information available to help answer these questions. Death does not occur instantly except under a few circumstances. Death obviously does not occur in the way many television programs would have us believe. Most of the information regarding the duration of life after fatal wounding comes from war, where the witnesses are under such stress as to be less than believable, and where wounding, at least in the armed forces, has been with high-velocity bullets and explosive shell fragments. The shock associated with the impact of bullets or shell or grenade fragments at high velocity is quite a different matter than the relative lack of shock encountered in wounding with low-velocity bullets and that suffered in motor vehicle crashes. Very little published information of value is available.[19] Every forensic pathologist has encountered instances when the death of the wounded individual apparently should have been quick, if not nearly instantaneous. Nevertheless, in these cases, the mortally wounded individual functioned well for many minutes before collapse. In the author's experience such situations are not rare, and the wounded individual may well exhibit much more than the expected ability to carry out intentional tasks before collapse. Death does not come instantly in the usual situation. The heart action may well continue for a short period following any sort of fatal injury. As long as the heart beats or respiratory effort continues, the individual cannot really be considered clinically dead. In more unusual instances, despite severe, obviously mortal wounding, the extinguishment of life does not follow quickly. Figure 16-117 depicts the extensive head injury resulting from a self-inflicted shotgun blast. The family insisted that no treatment be given, and none was. There was no intravenous support, no debridement of the wound, no treatment of any sort. The victim was unconcious, but survived for 45 hours. Figure 16-118 is a photograph of another person with a similar-appearing gunshot wound of the head; survival time was measured in minutes. It follows that the estimation of the duration of life after fatal wounding from examination of the wound and the general physical condition of the body is hazardous. So also is the estimate of physical capacity after fatal wounding.

7. *Can the degree of trauma be quantitated?*

Not really. At best the amount or degree of injury can only be roughly estimated as mild, moderate, severe, or extreme. There is much individual variation in the reaction to trauma. It should also be noted that the degree of natural disease process found at autopsy cannot really be quantitated.

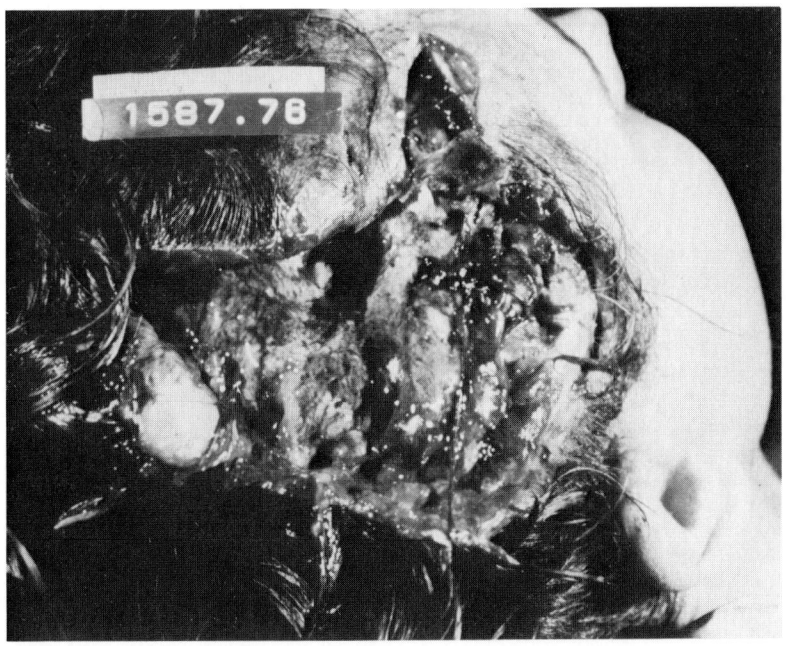

FIGURE 16-117. Survival with shotgun wound of head. The victim survived a self-inflicted shotgun wound for 45 hours. No treatment was given. Contrast this wound with that shown in Figure 16-118.

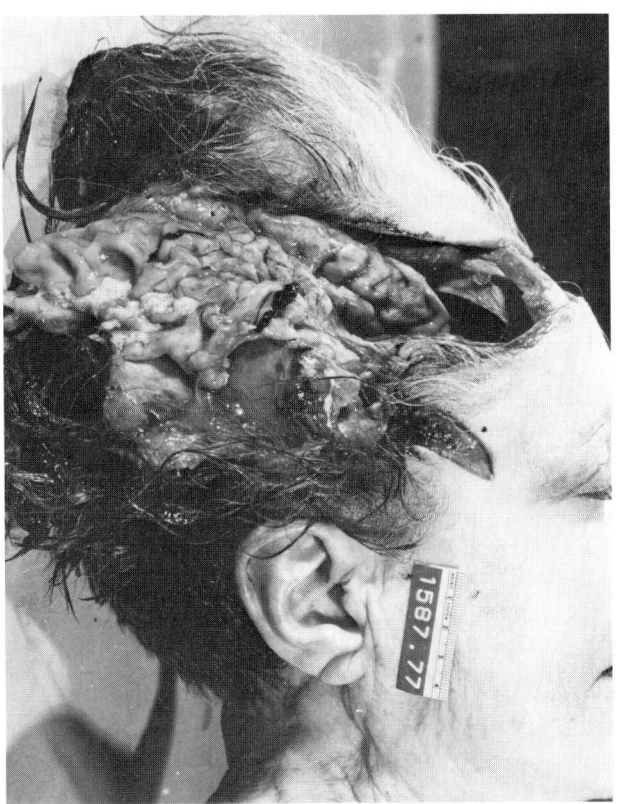

FIGURE 16-118. Nonsurvival with gunshot wound of head. The victim died within 5 minutes of wounding. No treatment could be given. In external appearance, the wound closely resembles that shown in Figure 16-117.

8. *What is the relationship of trauma and natural disease?*

This is an extremely complicated subject. Since neither trauma nor natural disease can truly be quantitated, the precise relationship between the two is also difficult to specify with precision. Obviously, a disease-ridden individual will generally withstand trauma less well than a healthy person. But the reserves of physical capability cannot really be determined at autopsy examination. In reality the autopsy taken alone is an inadequate device by which to evaluate the combination of trauma and disease. A better estimate may result from knowledge of the behavior and actions of the victim after sustaining the trauma and before death, rather than reliance on the autopsy findings alone.

9. *Would the victim have survived had he been given more prompt medical (or paramedical) assistance?*

This question arises with increasing frequency as emergency medical technical services are extended and popularized. It would appear that as such services are provided there will be more challanges regarding the alleged failure of the system to respond quickly enough to prevent death. A second source of the same question is the defense counsel who asks the autopsy pathologist if the victim would have survived if the emergency service had responded more rapidly to the case for help. The question is, of course, unanswerable. It should be obvious to anyone that the more prompt the treatment, the greater the opportunity for survival of the victim. However, who can predict what the vagaries of a more prompt response might be? How well can the emergency team be expected to perform necessary treatment? Could there be another highway accident involving the ambulance on the way to or from the scene of the accident itself? The possibilities are legion. Prediction is truly impossible.

10. *Can the wounds be altered from their original appearance?*

Yes, in many ways. In the event the victim survives for a time, healing is the natural way in which the wound is gradually altered from its original state. But there are many more "unnatural" ways in which the wound may be altered. An outline of these methods is given in Table 16-11. The possibilities are many and must be borne in mind by whomever examines the victim.

11. *Are situations where more than one type of weapon was employed actually encountered with any frequency?*

Yes. Such occurrences are not as rare as might be thought. Figure 16-119 illustrates the case of a homicidally inflicted throat cutting, in which a gunshot wound of the head was not predicted or found until the head, skull, and brain were examined at autopsy as part of the established routine. The gunshot wound was concealed by the thick, black scalp hair.

AUTOPSY RECORDS IN TRAUMA SITUATIONS

The importance of well-formed, reasonable autopsy records cannot be overemphasized. It is necessary that all injuries or wounds be detailed,

TABLE 16-11. ALTERATION OF WOUNDS

Living Victim
  Healing
  Treatment
    Emergency
      at scene of injury
      during transportation to hospital
      hospital
        emergency room
        operating room
    Hospitalization or nursing home existence

Dead Victim
  Resuscitative measures applied
    at scene
    during transportation
    emergency room
  No resuscitative measures applied
    by law enforcement officers
    by bystanders
    by coroner or medical examiner
    by funeral director
      "preparation" of body and embalming
    by accident or emergency room personnel
    by insects, animals, decomposition

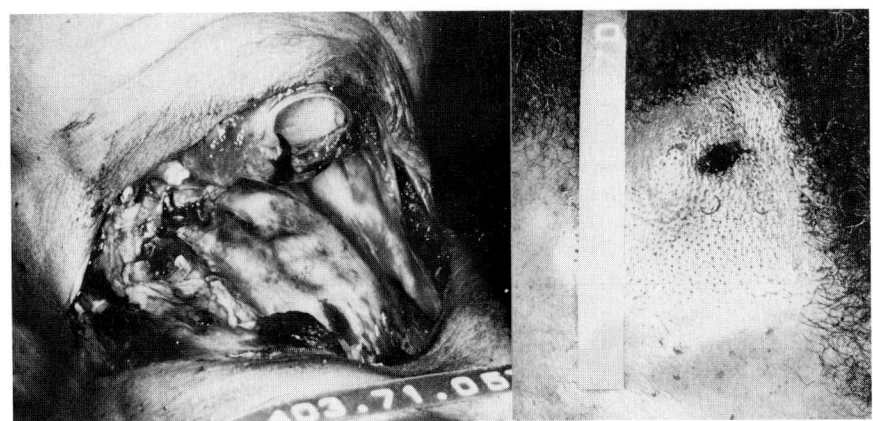

FIGURE 16-119. Throat cut and shot in head. The victim apparently died as a result of a cut throat, homicidally inflicted. Autopsy revealed a .22 caliber gunshot wound of the head, concealed by the heavy growth of scalp hair. The discovery of the gunshot wound explained the small amount of blood at the scene.

that their location be noted, and that any patterns of injury be recognized. The classic autopsy record, sometimes termed autopsy protocol, is a written description of what was done and what was found at the time of the autopsy. However, the reading of such a record does not necessarily suggest a visual concept of what was found. For this reason some pathologists make photographs part of the autopsy record. This is a logical and useful practice. Of equal importance is the use of diagrams upon which may be indicated the sites of trauma or other abnormality. Such diagrams are of particular importance in establishing patterns of injury.[17] Moreover, if preparations are made of body tissues and organs for examination under the microscope, descriptions of such examinations must be added to the autopsy record. If other examinations (chemical, x-ray, etc.) are undertaken, the results of these must also be included. Finally, some interpretation of findings, opinions, or conclusions linking the autopsy disclosures and the injury is needed. This should be expressed in nontechnical terms, so as to be understood by all.

Pathologists are traditionally trained to undertake the autopsy examination of the dead body in hospital surroundings. They become familiar with the hospital-oriented autopsy approach and with the preparation of a report or protocol especially designed to emphasize the hospital pathology facets of the findings, external and internal autopsy findings, provisional anatomic diagnoses, chemical and bacteriologic findings, microscopic examination, other special examinations, final diagnoses, and clinical correlation. In many ways the performance and recording of the specialized medicolegal autopsy of a victim of trauma parallel that of the medical or hospital type. However, there are significant differences. Table 16-12 compares the similarities and differences of the two types of autopsies. The differences in philosophy, orientation, content, and reporting can pose problems for the traditional pathologist who, trained and experienced in the carrying out of hospital autopsies, finds himself faced with the necessity of performing an autopsy on a victim of trauma. The major differences between the two types of autopsies are in examination of clothing, certain elements of the external examination, external and internal evidence of injury, provisional anatomic diagnoses, toxicologic exam-

TABLE 16-12. COMPARISON OF MEDICAL (HOSPITAL) AND FORENSIC AUTOPSY

Medical	Forensic
Clinical history	Circumstances surrounding death
Signs, symptoms	Emergency medical care
Laboratory findings	Hospital history
Diagnoses	Police and medicolegal reports
Hospital course	
No analogous phase	Clothing examination
	Inventory of garments
	Inventory of valuables
	Trace evidence
	Defects and patterns made by weapons
	Correlation with external and internal injuries
External examination	External examination
	Identification details
Details of hospitalization and therapy	Details of hospitalization and therapy
	Trace evidence
No analogous phase	External evidence of injury
	Details and patterns
No analogous phase	Internal evidence of injury
	Trace evidence
Internal examination	Internal examination
Body cavities	Body cavities
Systems	Systems
Organs and tissues	Organs and tissues
Provisional anatomic diagnoses	No analogous phase
Microscopic examination	Microscopic examination (may be omitted)
Chemical examination	Chemical examination
Bacteriologic examination	Bacteriologic examination
No analogous phase	Toxicologic examination
Diagnoses	Findings
Clinical correlation	Opinion (conclusion)

ination, and clinical correlation or opinion. Some further explanation of each of these procedures should be helpful at this point.

Examination of Clothing

The individual who dies during hospitalization is not wearing his clothing, but rather a hospital jacket or gown. The trauma victim who dies before admission to the hospital is usually wearing clothing which must be inventoried, inspected for trace evidence, examined for defects and patterns made by weapons and for correlation between the actual wounds on the body and the marks, patterns, and defects made by the wounding objects or weapons on the clothing. Moreover, the beginning of a chain of custody of the clothing must be made at the time the clothing is removed and examined.

External Examination Elements

Ordinarily, the patient who expires while in the hospital presents no problems in identification to the pathologist—not so in the instance of the body which arrives at the medicolegal official's laboratory. Indeed, identification may be one of the major problems needing solution in the latter situation. This requires skills and techniques quite different from those the hospital pathologist has available. In addition, the search for trace evidence and the associated recognition, preservation, transfer, and analysis may well be beyond the hospital pathologist's experience.

External and Internal Evidence of Injury

The details of all injuries, both external and internal, must be recorded. Location of injuries and the recognition of patterns of injury are additional points that must be included in the report of the autopsy. Trace or physical evidence may also be found during the search for internal injuries, and this must be properly cared for.

Provisional Anatomic Diagnoses

The hospital pathologist ordinarily prepares and distributes a report of provisional anatomic diagnoses immediately following the autopsy. This is a list of abnormal findings developed during the autopsy and reported to the physicians who cared for the person during life. It has value to the treating physicians who may then better communicate with the next of kin and may also serve as an input in the preparation of the death certificate. Such a list is of little value in the instance of the victim of trauma. Indeed, such findings may be confusing to the law enforcement officers, health officials, attorneys, and others who are the consumers of medicolegal information and reports. Until a final conclusion can be reached regarding a medicolegal case involving trauma, it may be best not to issue a report of provisional anatomic diagnoses.

Toxicologic Examination

In the medicolegal autopsy, specimens taken from victims of trauma are analyzed for toxic substances, the nature and extent of the toxicologic examination depending upon the nature of the case at hand. Alcohol, drugs, and other toxic substances, when present in sufficient quantity, singly or in combination, may explain the cause of the motor vehicle crash or the aberrant behavior of the victim of homicide. There is no counterpoint in the practice of autopsy pathology in the hospital.

Clinical Correlation or Opinion

The traditional hospital-oriented autopsy report ends with an attempt to correlate the clinical findings made by the physician, the hospital course, and response (or absence of response) to treatment with the pathologic abnormalities found at autopsy. This is expressed in highly technical medical terminology. In the instance of the autopsy of the victim of trauma, a final opinion needs to be expressed in lay language regarding the nature of the death.

Examples

Examples of important segments of medicolegal autopsy reports in instances of death due to trauma are given below. One autopsy report is provided in its entirety. It should be noted that each forensic pathologist has his own style of reporting. The examples that follow are not intended to propose either the best possible style or exclusive standards of quality or completeness.

STAB WOUND

External Evidence of Injury

1. Present in the left chest, level with the nipples and 3 cm to the left of the midline, there is a gaping stab wound, measuring 15 × 5 mm with the long axis in the vertical plane. On realignment of the edges, the wound is seen to measure 16 mm in length with the superior or upper end squared off and measuring 1 mm in width. The inferior or lower end has a "swallow-tail" appearance.

2. Present on the back of the left forearm, midway between the wrist and elbow, there is a 5 cm long, incised wound. The long axis of the wound is in the horizontal plane. The edges of the wound are sharp and neither abraded nor contused. The wound extends through the skin and subcutaneous tissue, but does not penetrate into the musculature.

3. Present on the palmar surface of the distal phalanx of the left thumb there is a 1 cm, superficial, incised wound, extending down into the musculature. The wound is in the vertical plane.

Internal Evidence of Injury

Subsequent examination reveals the knife to have perforated the left chest, passing through the fourth intercostal space, notching the superior edge of the fifth rib. The knife perforates the pericardial sac and the anterior wall of the left ventricle, midway between the apex and base. The stab wound in the left ventricle is 10 mm in length. The knife passes through the left ventriclar chamber, perforating the posterolateral wall of the left ventricle. The knife wound of exit in the posterolateral wall measures 2 mm in length.

There is 200 cc of clotted blood in the pericardial sac with 150 cc of blood in the left pleural cavity.

The length of the knife track is estimated to be 10 cm. The path of the knife is from front to back, from right to left and slightly downward.

Conclusion

It is my opinion that John L. Smith III, a 32-year-old white man, died as a result of a penetrating stab wound of the left chest. The knife perforated the left front chest wall, notching the fifth rib. The knife then perforated the heart. The length of the knife track is estimated at 10 cm. On the basis of the external examination of the wound, one can conclude that the weapon had a single cutting edge and that, when the deceased was stabbed, this cutting edge was directed downward. The maximum width of the knife blade is 1.5 cm.

The cutting wounds on the left thumb and back of the left forearm can be considered "defense wounds." These two wounds are located in areas frequently seen when wounds are incurred by an individual when he attempts to ward off the assailant and by grasping the blade itself.

BLUNT FORCE INJURY

External Examination

The body is that of an unclothed, normally developed, thin, white man, appearing approximately the stated age of 19 years, measuring 68 inches (173 cm) in length and weighing 118 lbs (54 kg). The irides are hazel. The scalp hair is brown and relatively long. An acneform eruption is present on the face. The teeth in the upper and lower jaws are natural and unremarkable. On the face, extending from the nostrils and mouth, streaking across both cheeks and over the angles of the jaw, there is a dried, apparently originally foamy material. A scar 2 cm in greatest dimension is present on the anterior aspect of the right forearm, at a point approximately 6 cm inferior to the central portion of the antecubital fossa. A linear scar, measuring approximately 6 cm in length, is present on the anterior abdominal wall in the right lower quadrant. This is situated in the transverse plane of the body and is in the central portion of that quadrant. Three small, irregularly shaped abrasions are present on the anterior aspect of the right knee and the adjacent superiormost portion of the right leg. A single abrasion is present on the anterolateral aspect of the left knee. None of these abrasions is more than 1.5 to 2 cm in greatest dimension.

Irregularly shaped, somewhat linear scars are noted in both antecubital

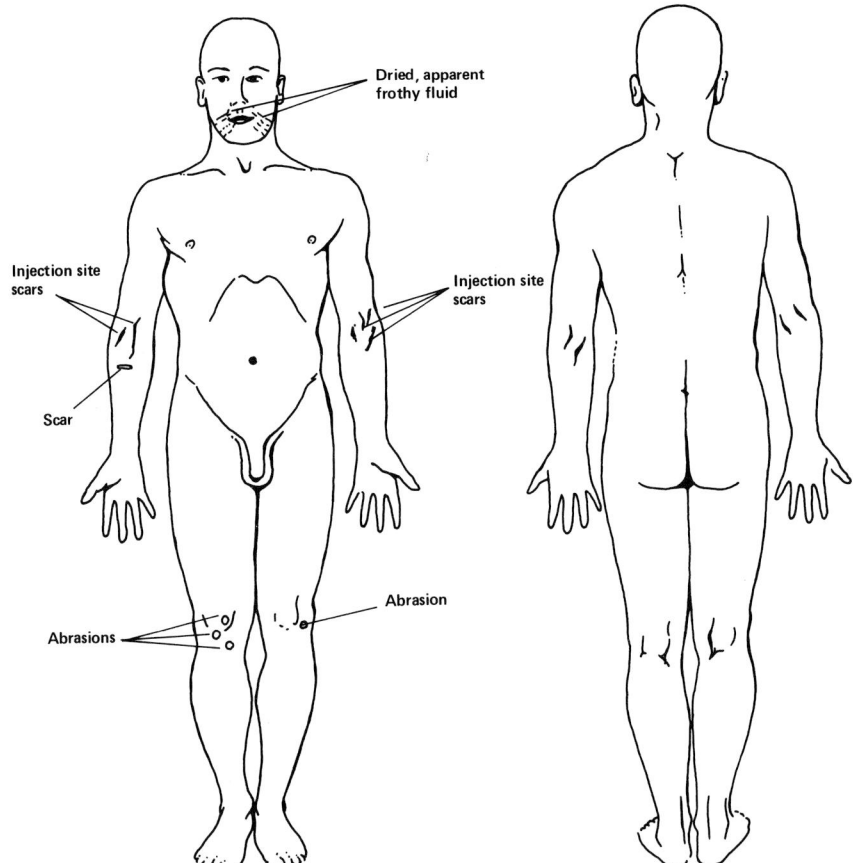

fossae. Two such scars are present in the right antecubital fossa and three in the left. The shortest of these measures approximately 1 cm in length and the longest approximately 5 cm in length. The linearity is generally in the longitudinal plane of the body, although those on the left course somewhat medially.

Internal Examination

HEAD. The scalp is intact externally; however, on reflecting the scalp anteriorly and posteriorly from a mastoid to mastoid incision, there is a remarkable amount of deep scalpine contusion over the vertex, extending over a distance of approximately 15 cm in the coronal plane and approximately 10 cm in the sagittal plane. Beneath this there is an irregular, 15 cm long fracture of the right and left parietal bones. This fracture is in the

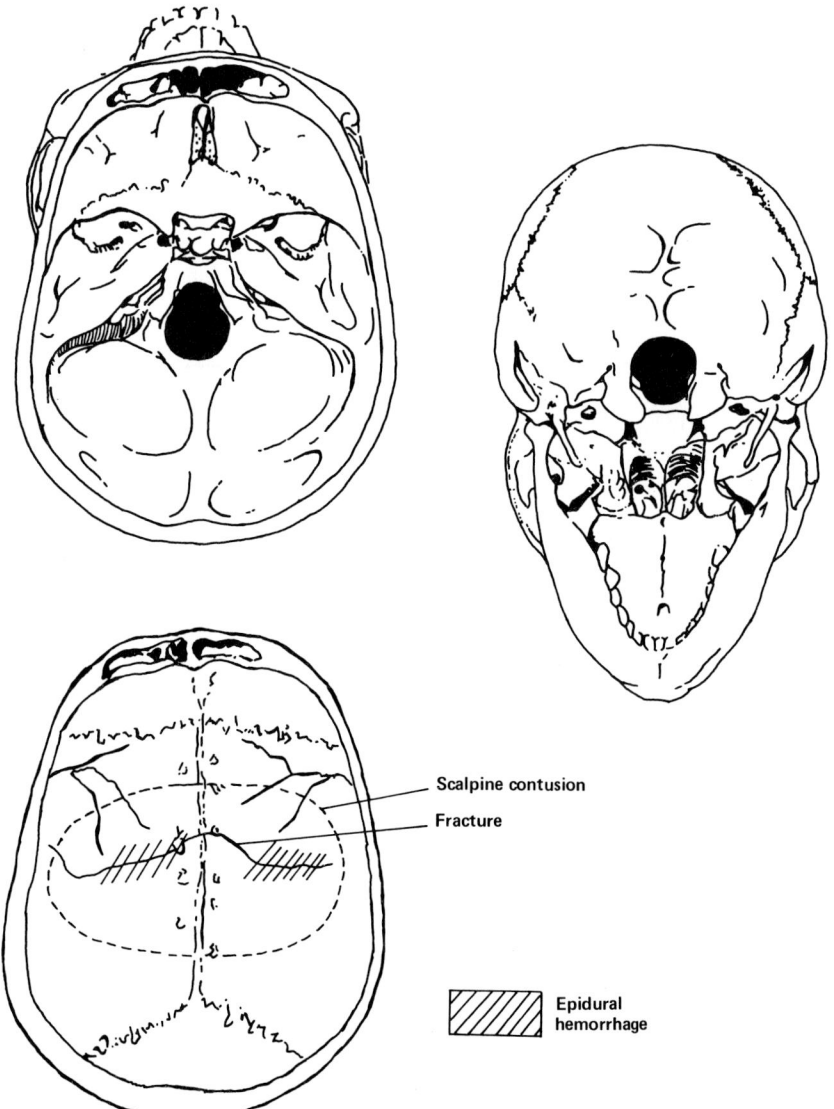

coronal plane of the body and is symmetrically placed so that each parietal bone is involved to the same extent as the other. No other fractures of the skull are noted. Bilateral small, epidural hemorrhages are noted in the region of the fracture line. Each of these measures approximately 6 to 7 cm in greatest dimension and aggregates not more than 20 to 25 cc of blood. The cerebrospinal fluid is bloody. There is an obvious intracerebral hemorrhage in the left parietotemporal area of the brain. Because of this the brain is preserved in formalin for further examination.

THORAX. It is symmetrical and the bony thoracic cage is intact. The lungs occupy nearly 100 percent of the available pleural volume bilaterally. The pleural cavities are dry. The mediastinal structures are in the midline and unremarkable in situ.

ABDOMINAL CAVITY. The organs occupy their usual locations and bear the usual relationships to one another. The peritoneal surfaces are smooth and glistening. No blood or an excessive amount of intraperitoneal fluid is present. The lymph nodes in the region of the gallbladder and surrounding structures are obviously enlarged.

LUNGS. They fail to collapse upon removal from the body. They are markedly subcrepitant. The external surfaces are smooth, glistening and dark red to nearly purple in color. On sectioning, they are found to have dark red to nearly purple, rather uniform-appearing parenchyma. Some frothy, pink fluid is present in the tracheobronchial system. The pulmonary arteries and veins are unremarkable, except for obvious red staining of the intima.

HEART. It is normal in size and shape. It is a right coronary preponderant type. The myocardium is softer than expected. There are no valvular abnormalities. The coronary arteries are the sites of a very mild degree of fatty streaking. The endocardium is stained pink. The myocardium is uniform in appearance throughout.

AORTA. It is the site of a mild degree of fatty streaking. The intima is stained pink.

GASTROINTESTINAL SYSTEM. The esophagus, stomach, large and small intestines are unremarkable. The stomach is empty.

PANCREAS. It is softer than expected and somewhat pink to red in color. It is otherwise unremarkable.

LIVER. The capsule is thin, smooth, and glistening. On cut section, a normal lobular architecture obtains. There are no focal abnormalities. The biliary outflow system is unremarkable.

SPLEEN. It is normal in size and shape. It is somewhat softer than expected. It is unremarkable on cut section.

ADRENALS. They are normal in size, shape, and location. On cut section, it is obvious that there is marked autolysis of the medulla bilaterally.

KIDNEYS. The capsules strip without difficulty, revealing completely smooth and unremarkable-appearing organs. On cut section, they are entirely unremarkable.

Microscopic Findings

LUNGS (2 H&E). Autolysis is the predominant feature. There is more than the usual and expected number of polymorphonuclear leukocytes in the larger blood vessels in some areas of the sections. Cross-polarizable material is easily demonstrated.

LIVER (1 H&E). There is a rather moderate degree of triaditis present.

KIDNEYS (3 H&E). Autolysis of the tubular cells is rather extreme. In other respects, the kidneys are unremarkable histologically.

SKIN (2 H&C). These sections have been taken from the antecubital fossae. There is some focal polymorphonuclear leukocyte reaction noted in the dermis in one section and in the other section there is a foreign body reaction with cross-polarizable material noted well within the superficial layers of the subcutaneous tissue.

Brain Note

After fixation, the brain shows extensive hemorrhage in the superficial portion of the central left temporal lobe. A large blood clot of approximately 50 cc protrudes from the macerated surface of the brain. Several superficial contusions are noted on the inferior surfaces of the frontal lobes bilaterally. A prominent cerebellar pressure cone and uncal grooving are noted. A few small, secondary hemorrhages are noted in the brainstem. Cut sections of the cerebrum reveal wedge-shaped, hemorrhagic lesions of the type expected in direct trauma over both cerebral convexities, the largest of these in the left temporal area measuring 8 cm in greatest extent. In the left parietal area, there is a second lesion, approximately 4 cm in greatest dimension. In the left frontal area there is a third lesion, approximately 2 cm in greatest dimension. These are all of the type expected of direct trauma.

Findings

1. Craniocerebral injuries
    a. Deep scalpine contusion of vertices
    b. Fractures of parietal bone, bilaterally
    c. Epidural hemorrhage, bilateral, parietal areas
    d. Multiple traumatic contusions of brain
2. Intravenous drug abuse
    a. History
    b. Paraphernalia found at scene
    c. Needle tracks found in both antecubital fossae
    d. Pulmonary edema
    e. Triaditis
    f. Enlarged portal lymph nodes
    g. Meperidine demonstrated in blood and urine
3. Early body decomposition, consistent with death 24 to 36 hours prior to time of discovery

Conclusion

In my opinion, (name), a 19-year-old white man, died as a result of head injury of the type expected from a direct blow to the top of the head. From history and from the examination of the body at the time of autopsy and subsequent toxicologic examination, the deceased is and has been a chronic intravenous drug abuser. No natural disease process of significance, other than that associated with intravenous drug abuse, was found at the time of autopsy.

Manner of Death

Homicide

Toxicology

Blood: Alcohol—trace amount of ethyl alcohol
ABN screen—negative
Alkaline drug screen—0.01 mg.% meperidine
0.26 mg.% demethylmeperidine*
Bile: Narcotics—negative
Urine: Alkaline drug screen—2.95 mg.% meperidine
6.60 mg.% demethylmeperidine*

REFERENCES

1. Robertson, I., and Hodge, P. R.: Histopathology of Healing Abrasions. *Forensic Sci.* 1:17–25, 1972.
2. Simpson, K.: *Taylor's Principles and Practice of Medical Jurisprudence.* Vol. 1. ed. 12. J. & A. Churchill, London, 1965, pp. 188–189.
3. Edwards, L. C., and Dunphy, J. E.: Wound Healing I. Injury and Normal Repair. *N. Engl. J. Med.* 259:224–233, 1958.
4. Russell, W. O.: Estimation of the Age of Wounds and Disease Processes. *Ann. Western Med. Surg.* 5:950–953, 1951.
5. Petty, C. S.: Soft Tissue Injuries: An Overview. *Am. J. Clin. Pathol.* 10:201–219, 1970.
6. Lindenberg, R., and Freytag, E.: Mechanism of Cerebral Contusions. *Arch. Pathol.* 69:440–469, 1960.
7. Parmley, L. F., Manion, W. C., and Mattingly, T. W.: Nonpenetrating Traumatic Injury of the Heart. *Circulation* 18:371–396, 1958.
8. Rockwood, C. A., and Green, D. P.: *Fractures.* Vol. 1. J. B. Lippincott, Philadelphia, 1975, pp. 1–118.
9. Munro, D., and Merritt, H. H.: Surgical Pathology of Subdural Hematoma Based on Study of 105 Cases. *Arch. Neurol. Psychiat.* 35:64–78, 1936.
10. Lindenberg, R.: Trauma of Meninges and Brain, in Minkler, J. (ed.): *Pathology of the Nervous System.* Vol. 2. McGraw-Hill, New York, 1971.
11. Contostavlos, D. L.: Massive Subarachnoid Hemorrhage due to Laceration of the Vertebral Artery Associated with Fracture of the Atlas. *J. Forensic Sci.* 16:40–56, 1971.
12. Ford, R.: Basal Subarachnoid Hemorrhage and Trauma. *J. Forensic Sci.* 1(2):117–126, 1956.
13. Freytag, E.: Autopsy Findings in Head Injuries from Blunt Force. *Arch. Pathol.* 75:402–413, 1963.

---

*Demethylmeperidine quantitation based on meperidine standard.

14. Lindenberg, R., and Freytag, E.: Morphology of Cortical Contusions. *Arch. Pathol.* 63:23–42, 1957.
15. Courville, C. B.: Forensic Neuropathology, II. Mechanisms of Craniocerebral Injury and their Medicolegal Significance. *J. Forensic Sci.* 7:1–28, 1962.
16. Courville, C. B.: Forensic Neuropathology, III. Intracranial Hemorrhage—Spontaneous versus Traumatic. *J. Forensic Sci.* 7:158–188, 1962.
17. Benz, J. A.: Injury Patterns. Paper presented at Basic Forensic Pathology I Workshop, American Society of Clinical Pathologists, Chicago, September 2–6, 1975.
18. Knight, B.: Some Mediolegal Aspects of Stab Wounds, in Wecht, C. H. (ed.): *Legal Medicine Annual, 1976.* Appleton-Century-Crofts, New York, 1977, pp. 95–105.
19. Spitz, W. U., Petty, C. S., and Fisher, R. S.: Physical Activity until Collapse following Fatal Injury by Firearms and Sharp Pointed Weapons. *J. Forensic Sci.* 6:290–300, 1961.
20. Hatcher, J. S., Jury, F. J., and Weller, J.: *Firearms Investigation, Identification and Evidence.* Stackpole, Harrisburg, Pa., 1957.
21. Coates, J. B., and Beyer, J. C.: *Wound Ballistics.* U. S. Government Printing Office, Washington, D.C., 1962.
22. Petty, C. S.: Firearms Injury Research. The Role of the Practicing Pathologist. *Am. J. Clin. Pathol.* 52:277–288, 1969.
23. U.S. Department of Justice, Law Enforcement Assistance Administration, National Institute of Law Enforcement and Criminal Justice: *An Evaluation of Police Handgun Ammunition: Summary Report.* U.S. Government Printing Office, Washington, D.C., 1975.
24. Petty, C. S., and Hauser, J. E.: Rifled Shotgun Slugs. Wounding and Forensic Ballistics. *J. Forensic Sci.* 13:114–123, 1968.
25. Wallack, B.: The Trouble with Slugs. *Am. Rifleman* 126:44–45, 97–98, 1978.
26. Cowan, M. E., and Purdon, P. L.: A Study of the "Paraffin Test." *J. Forensic Sci.* 12:19–36, 1967.
27. The Diphenylamine Test for Gunpowder. *F.B.I. Law Enforcement Bulletin* 4:5–7, 1935.
28. Further Observations on the Diphenylamine Test for Gunpowder Residue. *F.B.I. Law Enforcement Bulletin* 9:10–14, 1940.
29. Harrison, H. C., and Gilroy, R.: Firearms Discharge Residues. *J. Forensic Sci.* 4:184–199, 1959.
30. Guinn, V. P.: Recent Significant U.S. Court Cases involving Forensic Activation Analysis. *J. Radioanalytical Chem.* 15:389–398, 1973.
31. Rudzitis, E., and Wahlgren, M.: Firearm Residue Detection by Instrumental Neutron Activation Analysis. *J. Forensic Sci.* 20:119–124, 1975.
32. Wessel, J. E., et al.: Report on Gunshot Residue Detection. Prepared for the Law Enforcement Assistance Administration by the Aerospace Corporation. Report No. A.T.R.–75(7915)–1, September 1974, pp. 6–23 through 6–51.
33. Wolten, G. M., et al.: Final Report on Particle Analysis for Gunshot Residue Detection. Prepared for the Law Enforcement Assistance Administration by the Aerospace Corporation. Report No. A.T.R.–77(7915)–3, September 1977.
34. Stone, I. C., Di Maio, V. J. M., and Petty, C. S.: Gunshot Wounds: Visual and Analytical Procedures. *J. Forensic Sci.* 23:361–367, 1978.
35. DiMaio, V. J. M.: Personal communication, 1978.
36. Moritz, A. R.: *The Pathology of Trauma.* Lea & Febiger, Philadelphia, 1954.

CHAPTER 17

William J. Curran is Frances Glessner Lee Professor of Legal Medicine at Harvard University and Chairman of the State Medicolegal Investigation Committee of Massachusetts. Professor Curran writes regularly for the *New England Journal of Medicine* and teaches at the Medical School, Law School, and School of Public Health at Harvard. He was formerly Robert R. Utley Professor of Legal Medicine and Director of the Law-Medicine Institute of Boston University. He also served as Assistant Professor of Law and Government and Assistant Director of the Institute of Government at the University of North Carolina. Professor Curran is the author of several books in the medicolegal field including *Law, Medicine and Forensic Science* (with E. D. Shapiro); *Trauma and the Automobile; The Doctor as a Witness;* and *Medicolegal Proof in Litigation.* He is an Associate Editor of the *American Journal of Law and Medicine* and was formerly Medicolegal Editor of the *Massachusetts Law Quarterly.*

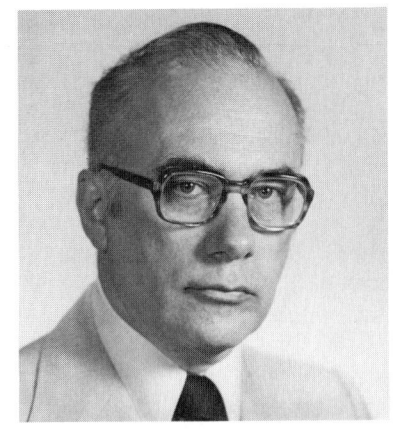

COURTROOM PRESENTATION OF EVIDENCE IN DEATH CASES

William J. Curran, J.D., LL.M., S.M.Hyg.

DISTINGUISHING CHARACTERISTICS OF DEATH CASES

Courtroom trials of death cases are like no other type of litigation. They are generally more emotional than other cases, especially if murder or manslaughter is charged. The atmosphere is always an uncomfortable one, with the pall of death hanging over the proceedings. The spectre of all human mortality sobers the participants and eliminates the touches of humor that might otherwise mitigate the solemnity, boredom, and routine of most trials.

The major difference, however, is the absence of the focal party in the case: the victim of the crime, or the plaintiff or testator in the civil action. In other cases the story of this party is the most important single portion of the evidence in the case. That person nearly always carries the burden of credibility of the crime or the civil suit. The degree of punishment or the amount of the money damages also very often depends upon the victim's or the plaintiff's story and the impression it makes on the trier of fact.

In death cases the interest of the judge and jury is shifted to a verbal reconstruction of the character of the dead person. They are curious about what the person was like, but no one really wants to say. There is a hesitation to speak disparagingly about the dead. In fact, there is a hesitation to speak of the dead at all, especially by name. He or she is called "the deceased," "the victim," or "the testator."

Death cases, especially criminal prosecutions, are usually taken quite seriously by all participants, including the higher authorities of the prosecutor's office and the judiciary. If the district attorney does try cases, he is apt to appear in the murder cases himself. Experienced judges are assigned to sit on death cases. Many jurisdictions require that defense attorneys be experienced (usually 10 years at the bar) before they can represent a defendant in court on a murder or manslaughter charge. The press and other media usually notice death cases more than most trials. In fact, they are probably the only kind of courtroom litigation where the charge matters as much as the prominence or newsworthiness of the parties. The emotional and mass media impact of murder trials is probably reduced significantly by the absence of a threat of the death penalty for the defendant, but the drama of death to the victim always kindles deeply felt fears and demands for punishment. The trial substitutes for more primitive retaliation. It is a necessary action of civilization. The French writer, Albert Camus, had one of his characters put it well, in *The Plague*, when he observed, "It is not the law that is important, it is the sentence."

PREPARATION FOR TRIAL

Several chapters in this section deal with the investigation of criminal death cases, and there is further coverage of investigational aspects and preparation of evidence for trial in later parts of this book. It is important to point out that all investigations should be conducted and all reports prepared as if they were to be used in court and be subject to challenge and cross examination. All investigative personnel and forensic pathologists should have courtroom exposure, if not as witnesses, at least as observers and backup consultants to those who do testify. Only with this experience can investigators and forensic scientists understand the legal significance of what they do, or don't do, and its full impact, for good or ill, on the administration of justice.

In this chapter, we will stress the preparation and presentation of evidence by the forensic pathologist, not only because attention is given to preparation and presentation by other forensic scientists in other chapters, but also because the forensic pathologist is often the key witness who gathers all of the evidence concerning the deceased and the cause and manner of death, and presents the full picture in court. The police and some on-scene investigators and any eyewitnesses to the crime may testify themselves, but laboratory-based scientists, even forensic toxicologists, are apt not to be called to testify if the forensic pathologist can effectively cover their contributions in his testimony. As will be noted later, there are legal evidentiary problems with this practice, but it is nevertheless quite common and is considered an efficient and expedient way of presenting the scientific medical evidence in a death case.

In the investigational-preparatory stages, the forensic pathologist should be concerned with the following:

1. *Gathering* and *marking* the pathologic evidence and other accompanying data;
2. *Preserving* the evidence for which he will be responsible;
3. *Recording* the evidence in a comprehensive report;
4. *Delivering* the report to proper authorities *promptly* after the investigation is completed and all consultant reports are received.

All of the above points are important. Failures in any of them can be crucial. They are overlapping and do not necessarily follow one after the other. For example, much of the evidence can be recorded at the same time it is gathered when the pathologist dictates findings during a medicolegal autopsy and also when photographs are taken at the scene and during the autopsy. All of these procedures will contribute to a prompt delivery of a report of the case.

If evidence is to be acceptable to the courts, it must be properly identified as to what it is and where it was found. The chain of possession of the evidence from the time it was found until it is delivered into the court must be secure and without doubt. The evidence must not be damaged, contaminated, or altered in any significant way. The clothes of the deceased are of particular importance to the pathologist. They should be removed carefully and only after their relation to the body and other factors, such as powder burns, bullet holes, and blood or other stains, has been noted and recorded, usually by color photographs. Knots in clothing or a rope should not be untied, but should be removed with as little disturbance as possible.

Other parties should not be allowed to disturb the evidence. If investigators or defense experts wish to examine the evidence prior to trial, it should be done under supervision of the medical examiner's office to assure continuity of possession and that the evidence is not thereby damaged, contaminated, or altered. In the series of deaths known as "the Boston Strangler cases," the author had the experience of having a State Attorney General demand that physical evidence from a number of different cases be turned over to a clairvoyant or spiritualist who had a reputation among certain gullible police groups for "solving" difficult cases. The Attorney General was then under severe political and mass media pressure to do something about the murders which were terrorizing the city. The forensic pathologists and the Law-Medicine Institute steadfastly refused to make any physical evidence available to the clairvoyant. Frustrated in his attempt to get a "feel for the murderer" through the clothes of victims and other materials, the clairvoyant was not to be denied; he offered his spiritual "solution" anyway and quickly left town.

We must encourage *promptness* in delivering the report, especially in cases where criminal conduct may be suspected. Nothing destroys a forensic pathology consultant's professional usefulness more than greatly delayed reports in important cases. Delays also encourage sloppy and incomplete reports as the pathologist attempts to put the material together in haste long after the event. As indicated above, the promptness of delivering a report is substantially aided by building in the recording of the material as the evidence is gathered.

Nevertheless we must caution against undue haste in arriving at conclusions due to pressure from investigators, prosecutors, family members, politicians, or the mass media. The investigation must be completed and consultant reports must be received and evaluated before a *final conclusion* is reached.

THE STORY TO BE TOLD

It was noted earlier that the personality of the missing party, the dead victim, is a matter of great curiosity in death-case litigation. There is a desire to reconstruct "the story" that the victim would tell on the witness stand in the ordinary case. In his excellent book, *The Pathology of Homicide*, Lester Adelson describes the postmortem investigation as a series of questions which could be asked of the victim.[1] The questions might be constructed as follows:

1. Who are you?
2. When did you become ill?
3. Where were you when you became ill or were struck violently?
4. Who struck you, or who tried to kill you?
5. Did you cause your own illness intentionally, or did you cause the violence to yourself intentionally or accidentally?
6. Was your illness, if any, related to your death?
7. When did you die?

The questions above are not entirely the same as those put by Adelson, and they are in somewhat different order. The first question is the foundation stone of most investigational techniques: it concerns personal identification. The second question is quite medical and does not occur in every case. The third question concerns the circumstances of the case or crime. Police investigators often confuse *where* a death occurred with *when* and *how* it occurred. These are all separate issues.

The fourth question is that favorite of the mystery writers: "Who done it?" Adelson saved this question for his sixth and last, rather because of its dramatic appeal and importance for the police and prosecutor. The list above attempts to maintain a chronological order, and so this question is raised earlier. The victim would know who struck him before he knew when he died.

The fifth question is actually an alternative to question four. It relates to a suicide or an accidental death. The sixth question relates back to earlier questions on pre-existing illness and asks if the illness caused the death or was related to it. This issue is of growing importance as more and more medicolegal cases are investigated where the deceased has evidence of pre-existing heart disease or cancer. (See the separate chapters in this section on these subjects.)

Question seven, as given above, is the issue of when the person died. This issue is related to the definition of death. The issue of time of death is one of the most difficult of all of the questions asked of the victims, even though many inexperienced attorneys and mystery writers seem to believe it is susceptible to very accurate determination.

Put differently, the forensic pathologist seeks to determine the cause, manner, mechanism, and approximate time of death of the individual under investigation. He will offer as much of an answer to these issues as he can with the material evidence available; with the help of other investigators, witnesses, and expert consultants; and within the confines of forensic pathologic science at its current stage of development.

PRETRIAL CONSULTATION

The forensic pathologist, like all expert witnesses, would prefer to have an adequate pretrial conference with the attorney who is going to call him. This can usually be assured in murder-homicide cases, but not always. It should occur in all litigation. In jurisdictions without readily available medicolegal investigation programs, trained forensic pathologists are often retained *only* where it is expected that the investigation relates to a homicide. The forensic pathologist is called because it is expected that he will handle the investigation, preserve the evidence, produce a report, and make a "good witness" at the trial. This approach by prosecuting attorneys usually means that only obvious homicides receive adequate investigation by forensic pathologists in their jurisdictions.

In the pretrial conference, the pathologist and the attorney should go over the previously prepared report, the certificate of death, and any demonstrative evidence, such as photographs and color slides, that the witness intends to show in court. If any contest is expected, such as by the testimony of other forensic pathologists, areas of possible disagreement should be reviewed. If the witness intends to change or modify any of his findings or conclusions, these should be pointed out to the attorney. As noted in our other chapters on courtroom presentation, there should be no unnecessary surprises on direct examination. These can be avoided with adequate pretrial consultation.

Where the witness is the official medical examiner or coroner's pathologist for the jurisdiction having conducted the postmortem investigation, his report will have been made available to the defense in most cases. Generally, there will be no pretrial conference with the defense attorney, unless the medical examiner or coroner's pathologist is not going to be called by the prosecutor, but is going to be called by the defense as their witness. In this situation, the same basic suggestions regarding pretrial preparation will prevail.

FORENSIC PATHOLOGISTS AS EXPERT WITNESSES

Forensic pathologists as a class are probably the best expert medical witnesses appearing in the courts today. They are the most traditional forensic scientific experts in the world. Even in the United States, that huge citadel of the advocacy system, forensic pathologists are the most commonly accepted impartial expert examiners in our court systems.

Various factors combine to guarantee forensic pathologists a uniquely secure and respected position as medicolegal witnesses:

1. They usually represent the public in a medicolegal investigative system as impartial experts rather than as paid representatives of the parties.
2. They are usually full-time specialists in medicolegal cases and have experience in police and judicial procedures.
3. They have usually gathered the evidence in the case and performed the medicolegal autopsy according to a well-conceived plan for gathering, preserving, and presenting medicolegal evidence.
4. The evidence they present has usually been fully evaluated by them and their staffs, aided by well-trained investigators and laboratory personnel.
5. In many cases, their evidence is not directly and professionally disputed; that is, by another forensic pathologist testifying for the other side. (This does not mean that parts of the evidence are not disputed by some witnesses, nor does it mean that the pathologist is not cross-examined.) Even in cases where opposing professional testimony is presented, the opposing expert is usually limited to examining the data gathered by the medical examiner-pathologist. A complete and independent evaluation is usually precluded by cremation or burial of the body. An order for exhumation is rare, especially when a full postmortem examination was performed by a competent forensic pathologist.

The above factors, of course, relate to the situation where the forensic pathologist is the impartial expert who was involved in the case from its inception, either as the medical examiner or coroner's physician, or as the retained consultant to the police and prosecutor on a regular basis. Moreover, these factors are enhanced by a high-quality medicolegal death investigation system with a well-equipped laboratory. Many of these factors will not apply when the forensic pathologist is called into a case by the defense in a criminal case, or when the litigation is noncriminal and requires only a general evaluation, such as testimony based upon hypothetical questions.

It may not be realized how important—and how unique—these factors are as compared to other medicolegal testimony, either in criminal or civil litigation. It is extremely rare for other medicolegal witnesses to be called regularly as *impartial experts*. Most other medicolegal consultants and witnesses are involved only after selection by one of the advocates, and, nearly all other medical "experts" are involved in forensic medicine only a relatively small part of their time. The only other frequently seen physicians in court are orthopedic surgeons and psychiatrists, neither of which are usually engaged solely or even predominantly in medicolegal cases.

Items 3, 4, and 5 above are also uncommon in other medicolegal areas. The party involved in these cases is dead. The body is usually available solely to the official medical examiner or coroner who conducts the only full, postmortem examination on the deceased. In litigation involving living persons, a medical examination can usually be arranged for the opposing party's medical expert. Further x-rays and laboratory tests can be ordered. Of course, these "opposition" medical examinations and tests may not be as valuable or as timely as the examinations and tests conducted by the attending physicians at the time of the original injury or illness, but they do constitute an independent medical evaluation.

We should note that a competent and ethical medical examiner or coroner's physician will take pains to record his findings fully and support them by laboratory tests, with ample tissue preserved, and will take color photographic slides in serial manner of all aspects of the case and the postmortem examination. This complete record will be made available to authorized, outside medicolegal experts for another party or government agency seeking an independent judgment of the findings and conclusions reached. It is ironic that the better the recording of the data, the more it can be evaluated by an independent expert and the findings and conclusions disputed. Less competent medicolegal findings, where the evidence is not retained and well recorded and where the protocol and reports are sketchy, brief, and filled with unsupported "conclusions," are clearly inadequate and suspect, but are often difficult to dispute because they provide little real data to examine.

COURTROOM TESTIMONY: SOME GENERAL SITUATIONS

As indicated above, the qualified forensic pathologist has a great deal "going for" him in courtroom testimony. The medicolegal system of coroner or medical examiner places the witness in the much-envied position of institutionally supported impartiality. This position and its appearance, or aura, must be preserved.

The greatest danger for the medical examiner or coroner's pathologist is to appear to speak as an arm of, or an agent for, the police and prosecutor. The independence of the office should be stressed in direct examination and defended in cross-examination. Various factors in the local administrative structure can be used to point out the independence. Moreover, the fact that the reports and evidence were made available to the defense, even if not utilized, should be noted and usually makes an important impression. The fact that the medical examiner is based at, or has a regular faculty appointment in, a university medical school also greatly enhances the independence of the position.

The forensic pathologist is not always in this desirable position of an impartial expert. He or she may be a private practitioner retained for this case by either party, or may be a medical examiner in another jurisdiction, but privately retained (and paid a personal fee) to offer an opinion in this case. In such situations, the forensic pathologist acts in a capacity similar to that of other medical expert witnesses. In direct examination, stress should be placed on the high level of professional medicolegal qualifications possessed by a forensic pathologist, especially board certification or board eligibility. If the witness is engaged full-time in medicolegal work, this should also be pointed out. The availability of a consultant forensic pathologist to both sides in criminal or civil cases should also be indicated. If the consultant only appears, or in recent years has only appeared, for prosecutors (or for particular defense attorneys), this can weaken his position and lead to allegations of partiality.

Returning to the medical examiner or coroner's pathologist, or to the coroner who is a physician and/or a forensic pathologist, the *appearance* of impartiality should be established and maintained out of the courtroom as well as within. This appearance should be maintained both as a general condition in the community and in regard to the particular case under investigation and prosecution. In public statements and speeches to local groups, the medical examiner or coroner should not "come on strong" as a law-enforcement official and crime fighter, even if the press loves to paint such a picture. The cloak of a medical detective, a modern-day Sherlock Holmes, is tossed over the shoulders of every "good-copy" medical examiner by the press. It is difficult to avoid. Nevertheless, effort must be made to create the real position and the believable appearance of professional, incorruptible impartiality. The press should be encouraged to publicize cases where the medical examiner and his office have aided in establishing innocence or have indicated that their findings were equivocal. In particular cases, premature releases of information should be avoided. Colorful descriptions of a murder as "heinous" or "fiendish" should also be avoided, since they characterize the case and encourage emotional responses and feelings of retaliation and revenge. The much-discussed murder case of Sam Sheppard, in Cleveland, contains many lessons on overly aggressive newspaper coverage and alleged prosecution bias on the part of the coroner's office.[2] The fact that much of the criticism may have been unjustified is somewhat beside the point; the appearance of bias was conveyed, often by slanted and distorted newspaper coverage. A reversal of the conviction was obtained in the Supreme Court of the United States, owing to the newspaper coverage and certain trial court errors, an unusual action by the Supreme Court, which rarely hears such appeals and even less often grants reversals on such grounds.[3]

DIRECT EXAMINATION: QUALIFICATIONS

The full professional qualifications of the forensic pathologist witness should be provided at the outset of direct testimony. These should not be "recited" in a dull monotone by the witness in response to a bored request to "state your qualifications." Credentials should be spaced out in answer to specific questions about basic medical education, pathology training, special medicolegal training and experience, and board certification or eligibility. University appointments should be noted. Some prosecutors like to move quickly and after establishing the fact that the witness is an official medical examiner, the chief medical examiner, or the coroner for the jurisdiction, they move directly to the case findings. In any contested case, this is a mistake.

Another common error is for the direct examiner to accede to the offer of opposition counsel to "stipulate" to the qualifications of the witness as "acceptable" or "well known" to the court and the attorneys. This supposed compliment to the witness and effort "to save time" should be seen for what it is: an attempt to avoid having the jury hear the witness' full professional credentials. Even experienced trial attorneys fall into this trap in important cases. In one of the most highly publicized murder trials in Boston history, where the police, prosecutor, and the medical examiner's office were divided about the case at various times, the defense called Dr. Milton Helpern, Chief Medical Examiner of the City of New York, as its star medical witness. Incredible as it may seem, the defense attorney agreed to a prosecution stipulation as to the qualifications of Dr. Helpern as soon as he was in the witness box and had given his name. Dr. Helpern went all through his testimony for an entire day before the defense realized its mistake and requested the indulgence of the court to go back and provide background on their witness, then the most renowned medicolegal practitioner in the country, president of dozens of medical societies and academies, and active on a worldwide basis in medicolegal work and scholarly writing. Could one expect that an ordinary jury of local citizens of the inner city of Boston and chosen (not excluded by their own action or by challenges of the parties) to serve on a murder case would know anything at all about this man? It is fortunate that the trial court judge did allow the attorney to provide the qualifications of Dr. Helpern.

PRESENTATION OF FINDINGS: DEMONSTRATIVE EVIDENCE

The medical examiner-pathologist should testify fully on direct examination concerning all of his significant findings as well as his conclusions. Usually the testimony should be presented in chronological order from the evidence gathered at the scene and on through the postmortem. A logical "story" of the circumstances of the death, as indicated earlier, should be provided. The cause, manner, mechanism, and approximate time of death should be described. Demonstrative evidence should be used, such as color photographic slides. A blackboard drawing can be used for indicating position of the body or trajectory of a bullet, but it must be quite accurate. At times, professional artists are retained to prepare line drawings for such issues. Color slides showing a steel bar passing through a gunshot wound and exit point were used on one occasion to demonstrate the angle of trajectory. The shiny, clean, steel bar was a very effective and clear demonstration of the point made by the witness.

The pathologist can also illustrate his testimony of how a killing took place or how the victim-deceased must have moved or struggled by demonstrating the action by his own movements or twists of his own body. This is a natural and effective method which can be employed as the witness responds to questions. One particularly impressive demonstration witnessed by the author was that of a pathologist who dramatized how an airline passenger might have struggled with his seat belt to get it off in a crash.

Care must be taken in these dramatic demonstrations by the pathologist witness to make them consistent with the evidence and developed from their own personal knowledge and experience. Keith Simpson, the well-known London forensic pathologist, notes a curious performance by a medical witness in the famous Bodkin Adams case. The witness demonstrated a "withdrawal fit" of a typical drug addict coming off morphine or heroin. The squirming and writhing was very compelling and was reported heavily in the evening press. The next day on cross-examination, the witness was forced to admit that he had never observed a single patient during drug withdrawal. Simpson reports, "The effect of the admission was catastrophic."[4]

"GRUESOME" PHOTOGRAPHY

Color slides and photographs are often objected to as likely to have an emotional effect upon the judge and jury.[5] Some trial courts have excluded photographs or slides as inflammatory or prejudicial, and the exclusions have been upheld as within the discretion of the judge.[6] At other times, photographs or slides are excluded as cumulative evidence or unnecessary detail to the witness' oral description. The better view, supported by most legal commentators, is that the gruesomeness or personally repellent quality of color photographs and slides is not proper grounds for exclusion when the pictures are a true representation of the facts and circumstances of the case. Jury members, sobered by the entire circumstances of a death case and their decisive role in it, seem to handle these aspects of the case quite well and value the objectiveness of the photography. It might be noted that the pictures, especially of the face and general appearance of the victim, also satisfy the jury's natural curiosity, mentioned earlier, about who the deceased was and what he or she was "really like" in life.

One particularly striking set of photographs seen by the author showed a headless body lying on one side of a railroad track and the head, neatly sliced off, lying nearby on the inside of the track. The case involved a mental patient who was alleged to have escaped from a state hospital and who went into a railroad yard at night and placed his neck over the track to commit suicide by being decapitated by a passing train. The photographs were submitted to show, by the neatness of the cut and absence of other injuries, that the deceased must have laid his neck firmly and directly on the track and that it was unlikely that he was merely struck down by a train as he tried to cross the track. The trial judge admitted the photographs as the best objective evidence to support the suicide allegation; he said he would have had great trouble believing that the deceased, even if mentally ill, could have done such a thing if he had not seen the pictures.

Where photographs or slides are particularly apt to raise issues of gruesomeness, it may be advisable to ask for a prior review of the pictures by the trial judge in his chambers or in the court with the jury excluded. The judge can then be "prepared" to see them rather than being confronted with them before the jury. A large series of pictures can be reviewed, allowing the judge to rule a few out without greatly hurting the demonstrative aspects of the whole set. At times a prosecutor will seem to be too willing to allow photographs to be excluded if objected to by the defense. This may occur because the prosecutor is so very confident that he can win his case without the pictures that he does not want to give the defense counsel any basis to appeal the case on grounds of trial court error in admitting evidence. For further discussion of the use of photographs at trial, see Chapter 6.

THE APPEARANCE OF NONPARTISANSHIP

The forensic pathologist expert witness should testify carefully and deliberately, always giving the appearance of nonpartisanship and respect for the court. Adelson suggests that he or she should testify "coolly" but never "coldly."[8] The expert witness should be understood by the judge and jury. This means providing technical information in technical language, but explaining and illustrating the key points. The witness must speak loudly and distinctly enough to be heard. The witness should not try constantly to "talk down" to the jury or to "over-explain" his answer. There is no need to ask the direct examiner, "Is that clear?" If the testimony is unclear, it is the lawyer's duty to ask further questions to provide clarification. The witness should not appear too eager to provide everything and to stay too long on the witness stand. A certain air of mystery and professional technicality should remain with the testimony; the jury must accept at least some of the findings and conclusions of the witness as his *expert* determination which can be appreciated fully only on the basis of proper education and training.

RANGE OF DIRECT INTERROGATION

The expert witness on direct examination should not volunteer further information beyond the questions asked. He should confine himself within the range of the interrogation, which is usually based on the prior reports of the pathologist and on the pretrial consultation. Staying within the questions reduces the surprises for the direct examiner and allows him to control the story being told and the order in which the findings are to be brought out. The witness who constantly volunteers unrequested information and "anticipates" lines of inquiry not yet posed will throw off the pace of the examination and give the appearance of eagerness, insecurity, and a lack of trust in the direct-examiner attorney to get the story out. Moreover, volunteered information is often not well prepared and is vulnerable to cross-examination as not a part of the report and unsupported by the findings.

CORRECTING THE EXAMINER

The witness should listen carefully to the questions and should pause before answering. If the direct examiner makes an obvious mistake in the question, or mixes up technical terms significantly, the witness should correct it before answering, such as by asking a leading question in return, "Did you mean to say . . . ?" and then going on quickly to respond to the proper area of inquiry. Sometimes the inadequacy in the question can be ignored and the witness can go on to answer the "correct question," if the one asked was not too far off the mark. From time to time, every experienced expert witness has had to "help out" counsel in this way.

Judges tolerate it well if it is not too blatant, even if the questioner's ego is somewhat deflated. Such corrections add to the relevance and usefulness of the testimony, which is, after all, the purpose of the interrogation. Sometimes, however, to the frustration of the witness, the direct examiner never does ask the most significant question, or misconstrues the line of inquiry. Very often there is nothing that can be done about this. Nevertheless the cross-examiner sometimes provides an opportunity to correct the situation when he does ask the key questions, expecting other responses. This is, in fact, one of the opportunities of cross-examination which inexperienced cross-examiners learn at their peril. It points out that when a cross-examiner says "No questions" at the end of a direct examination, it does not always imply a compliment to the expert as a fear of crossing verbal swords with him. It may well mean that the cross-examiner feels that his case was not damaged by the expert's testimony and he wants to leave it that way.

TESTIMONIAL STYLE

As far as the style of presenting forensic pathology evidence is concerned, it varies greatly with no set pattern which seems to fit all occasions. Experienced forensic pathologists who appear frequently in both informal hearings and more formal jury trials adopt a personal manner of testifying which is comfortable and successful for them. There are suggestions in Simpson,[9] Adelson,[10] and in the author's short text.[7] Specific suggestions and illustrative testimony can be found in trial practice manuals designed primarily for lawyers.[11] There is an interesting collection of observations by the well-known criminal defense lawyer, F. Lee Bailey,[12] and other examples provided by Lloyd Paul Stryker, a leading criminal lawyer of the 1920s and 1930s.[13]

Some forensic pathologists, such as George Burgess Magrath, the medical examiner in Boston in the earlier decades of this century, were quite flamboyant, both in and out of court. Some have adopted identifying affectations. Sir Bernard Spilsbury, the famous London forensic pathologist, wore a fresh flower in his buttonhole every day. New York City's first Chief Medical Examiner, Dr. Charles Norris, was an independently wealthy man who rode about New York on his investigations in his own chauffeur-driven limosine. Another American forensic pathologist took to wearing a ten-gallon hat and carrying a pistol with him at all times, though he was a Northerner born and bred, the son of a professor of Romance languages, and practiced his pathology in a northeastern urban area. Other practitioners, at least in their later years, have taken on the milder coloration of kindly, graying father-figures, quite disarming to the unwary cross-examiners who confront them.

MEDICAL CERTAINTY

In providing conclusions, the forensic pathologist is nearly always testifying on so-called "fact issues" such as cause and manner of death, rather than "ultimate issues" of guilt or innocence, so that opinion based upon reasonable medical certainty is adequate to support the testimony of the forensic pathologist. (This may be contrasted with higher degrees of certainty required in forensic psychiatry in some cases, as indicated in Chapter 43.)

Key questions, such as the cause of death, are usually put to the forensic pathologist in a deliberate manner, sometimes in hypothetical form ("Assume, doctor . . . .") if the pathologist cannot testify to all underlying questions, and ending with "Have you an opinion, based upon reasonable medical certainty, as to the cause of death?" The answer to this question is not to launch into an explanation. It is a simple *yes* or *no;* one either has an "opinion" or one hasn't. Only after one answers this question in the affirmative should he be asked, "And what *is* that opinion, doctor?"

Very often the opinion on a key question must be put in more qualified terms, such as that the findings are "consistent with" an alleged form of trauma, such as a fall against a hard object, or with the striking of the head with a blunt instrument of a particular type. This is often as far as the data will permit the witness to go in connecting up the findings of the postmortem examination, the physical evidence, and the theory of the case. This does, of course, mean that on cross-examination the witness must admit, if asked, that "consistent with" does not exclude other mechanisms which could reasonably or possibly have caused the same findings.

Some commentators have asserted that it is virtually impossible to convict a physician or other scientist of perjury for giving a false opinion in court. This is because proof would be required that the opinion was knowingly false when given, an admittedly difficult matter. Nevertheless, conviction for perjury is not out of the question. It has been found and sustained against a physician witness.[14]

CROSS-EXAMINATION

When cross-examination is on behalf of the defendant in a criminal case, the effort is usually not to prove a point, but to weaken a conclusion or finding favorable to the prosecution, to demonstrate bias, or to exclude "prejudicial" evidence. The witness may be asked if he is merely "speculating" about a finding or conclusion, or whether certain other "possibilities" less damaging to the defendant are not also persuasive of what happened in this case. Prior statements will usually have been examined and discrepancies in testimony will be questioned, if only to throw confusion into the minds of jurors concerning what the pathologist now asserts to be his or her position. It must be remembered that doubt in the minds of the jurors can defeat the prosecution's overall case. The witness should try to clear up confusion about the findings and conclusions and even minor points concerning the physical evidence and other factors. If the cross-examiner does not allow this, the witness can appeal to the judge, or can wait for direct re-examination when, hopefully, the prosecuting attorney will reopen the area and allow the witness to gather the loose ends into a logical framework and reinforce the testimony in chief.

The cross-examiner may also challenge the forensic pathologist's findings or conclusions by indirect attack on areas relied upon by the witness, such as consultant's reports, police reports, or hearsay of witnesses. At times, the cross-examiner will be able to force reopening of these issues. The strict application of the rules of evidence assert that an expert cannot build an opinion upon another opinion or base significant parts of his testimony upon the hearsay evidence he receives and relies on without knowing the facts himself.[15] The rule can be a serious stumbling block if followed literally. Most trial courts quietly ignore the rule in order to expedite the trial and save the time and effort of other personnel contributing to the overall evaluation offered by the expert on the witness stand.

More enlightened courts and the modern rules of evidence have completely abrogated the strict application of the rule.[16] In speaking of the rule in a medical diagnostic evaluation where the physician had relied on consultations and laboratory tests, the Wisconsin Supreme Court, as early as 1928, observed,

> In making a diagnosis for treatment, physicians must of necessity consider many things that do not appear in sworn proof . . . things that mean much to the trained eye and touch of the skilled medical practitioner. This court has held that it will not close the doors of the courts to the light which is given by a diagnosis that the rest of the world accepts and acts upon, even if the diagnosis is based in part upon facts which are not established by the sworn testimony in the case to be true.[17]

The strongest resistance of the courts to accepting hearsay or other opinions through the testifying expert is when the witness is not a treating doctor and is called by one of the parties as a consultant only for purposes of the trial. The statements received are then often considered self-serving and subjective.[18]

Objection can also be made to accepting expert opinions through death certificates and coroner's reports.[19] It is always best to have the responsible physician available to testify to opinions in such documents, but at times this is not possible, due to death or other incapacity or inavailability. Special rules of evidence allow admission of this type of document, but it is a weak form of evidence in a contested case.

There are excellent legal commentaries on the complexities of the rules of evidence concerning expert medical testimony.[20] We particularly recommend the paper by Rheingold,[21] which should be read along with the cases collected in the author's law school casebook to which the Rheingold paper is related.[22]

The defense in a homicide case can, of course, subpoena the other consultants or laboratory personnel and take their testimony directly, challenging them as "hostile witnesses," thus subject to leading questions and other aggressive tactics. If the pathologist relied on information from family members or friends of the deceased in forming his opinion, the defense counsel can explore these statements and challenge them directly with contrary evidence, thus weakening the forensic pathologist's underlying findings.

When the forensic pathologist is a defense witness, the cross-examination by the prosecution can be very aggressive. This is often due to the fact that the prosecutor is working closely with the medical examiner who testified on behalf of the prosecution. The medical examiner can usually provide suggestions to the prosecutor which can be used in cross-examination. Moreover, the forensic pathologist called by the defense is subject to challenge on a bias ground because he or she is "paid" by the defense. This is an unfair line of questioning and should be challenged. It is important, however, that the witness fee for testifying not be excessive in amount, and it is best that the fee be paid in advance of the testimony. It should be recalled that the defense-called forensic pathologist need not testify to a completely different theory than that of the prosecution. The defense witness need only create reasonable doubts about the accuracy of certain of the key findings or conclusions of the prosecution's evidence in chief. The defense witness should be careful not to "overreach" this standard, if what he or she has to work on will only allow such a limited position, or will only allow pointing out inconsistencies in the case for the prosecution. Defense counsel sometimes tries to "push" the expert witnesses to criticize the prosecution's witnesses or the local medical examiner in very severe fashion, or to take clearly opposing views which would virtually declare the defendant innocent. If this is the true position of the defense witness, it can be so asserted. However, caution should prevail if the facts will not support such an attack. It is enough for the defense witness to demonstrate the sloppiness of the investigation, the inadequacies of the work-up, and the opposing differential evaluation of the findings. The severe criticism and characterization can be left to the defense lawyer in his oral summation to the jury. The expert witness then continues to give the *appearance* as well as the substantive position of an impartial observer and reporter who states his findings and conclusions coolly, as Dr. Adelson advises, and lets the chips fall as they may. This is the best position for the forensic scientist, whether appearing for the prosecution, a civil-law plaintiff, or for the defense in any court of justice.

DIFFERENT TYPES OF JUDICIAL PROCEEDINGS

We have not felt it necessary to distinguish between types of judicial and quasijudicial proceedings where forensic pathology and other forensic science evidence may be presented concerning a human death. The evidence will differ very little from tribunal to tribunal, but the style of presentation may be less formal in preliminary hearings or before administrative agencies, such as retirement boards, than before felony courts. Some American coroners (and coroner-medical examiners, as in California) still exercise quasijudicial powers and preside over coroner's inquests, sometimes with impanelled juries to determine the facts of the inquest. There are some useful articles[23] and collections of appellate court cases[24] on inquests and inquest procedures. In Massachusetts, the first state to abolish the office of coroner, the responsibility for holding inquests in death cases was placed in the local district courts. A case involving an accidental drowning, but receiving prominence because of the involvement of a United States Senator, Edward M. Kennedy, resulted in important recommendations from the Supreme Judical Court for the reform of inquest proceedings.[25]

Forensic science witnesses may appear in preliminary proceedings such as inquests, "show-cause" hearings, administrative agencies, or grand jury investigations. Many of these are *ex parte;* that is, the tribunal hears only one party. The forensic pathologist in such cases is often presenting only the basic findings of the investigation and is not cross-examined. Nevertheless, the witness should not take the proceedings lightly. In grand jury hearings, the reputation of persons can often be greatly damaged due to indictments which clearly cannot stand up in later full-jury proceedings. The forensic pathologist should express his doubts about the case at this stage so that the prosecutor can evaluate whether or not the evidence will stand up in a later trial.

Another major caution worthy of note is that the forensic science expert should always review the testimony he or she has given at a preliminary hearing or lower court proceeding before giving evidence on the matter before a jury in a felony court or in a civil action. Inconsistencies and conflicts can be embarrassing to the witness unless good reason is presented for the change in findings or conclusions.

REFERENCES

1. Adelson, L.: *The Pathology of Homicide.* Charles C Thomas, Springfield, Ill., 1974, pp. 33–40.
2. Pollack, J. H.: *Dr. Sam, An American Tragedy.* Henry Regnery, Chicago, 1972; Holmes, P.: *The Sheppard Murder Case.* David McKay, New York, 1961.
3. *Sheppard v. Maxwell,* 384 U.S. 333, 1966.
4. Simpson, K.: *A Doctor's Guide to Court.* ed. 2. Butterworth, London, 1967, p. 52.
5. Conrad, P.: Evidentiary Aspects of Color Photography. *J. Forensic Sci.* 4:176–182, 1959; Ehrlich, P. J., and Jones, E. P.: *Photographic Evidence: The Preparation and Use of Photographs in Civil and Criminal Cases.* Anderson, Cleveland, 1967.
6. Scott, R.: Medicolegal Photography. *Rocky Mountain L. Rev.* 18:173–206, 1946; *State v. Morgan,* 211 La. 572, 20 So. 2d 545, 1947; Note, *Am. Law Reports,* 2d, 73:769 et seq., 1960.
7. Curran, W. J., and Shapiro, E. D. (eds.): *Law, Medicine, and Forensic Science.* ed. 2. Little, Brown, Boston, 1970; Supplement, 1974, pp. 396–406.
8. Adelson, op. cit., p. 31.
9. Simpson, op. cit.
10. Adelson, op. cit.
11. *Examination of Medical Experts.* Matthew Bender, New York, 1968; Sugarman, A. G. (ed.): *Examining the Medical Expert: Lectures and Trial Demonstrations.* Institute of Continuing Legal Education, University of Michigan, Ann Arbor, 1968.
12. Bailey, F. L.: The Pathologist: A Lawyer's Approach, in Sugarman, A. G. (ed.): *Examining the Medical Expert: Lectures and Trial Demonstrations.* Ann Arbor, 1968; Bailey, F. L.: *The Defense Never Rests.* Stein & Day, Briarcliff Manor, N.Y., 1971.
13. Stryker, L. P.: *Courts and Doctors,* Macmillan, New York, 1932.
14. *State v. Sullivan,* 24 N.J. 18, 130 A. 2d 610, 1957: Annotation, *Am. Law Reports,* 2d, 66:761 et seq., 1959; Curran and Shapiro, op. cit.
15. *Fidelity & Casualty Company of N.Y. v. Hendrix,* 440 p. 2d. 735 (Okla., 1968); *Wild v. Bass,* 252 Miss. 615, 173 So. 2d 647, 1965; *State v. David,* 222 N.C. 242, 22 W.E. 2d 633, 1942.
16. Cleary, E. W. (ed.): *McCormick's Handbook of the Law of Evidence,* ed. 2. West, St. Paul, Minn., 1972.
17. *Sundquist v. Madison Rys Company,* 197 Wis. 83, 221 N.W. 392, 1928.
18. *Brindley v. Williams,* 143 Ind. App. 691, 242 N.E. 2d 132, 168; Annotation, *Am. L. Reports,* 2d, 51:1051 et seq., 1970.
19. *Liberty National Life Insurance v. Power,* 145 S.E. 2d 801, (Ga. App. 1968); *Equitable Life Assurance Society v. Stinnett,* 13 F. 2d 820 (6th Cir 1965).
20. Ladd, M.: Expert Testimony. *Vanderbilt Law Rev.* 5:414–428, 1952; Voorris, A. H.; *N.Y. Law Forum* 13:651–660, 1967.
21. Rheingold, P.: The Basis of Medical Testimony. *Vanderbilt Law Rev.* 15:473–510, 1962.
22. Curran and Shapiro, op. cit., see also ed. 1, 1960.
23. *Inquests and Other Functions of the Coroner,* Illinois Legislative Council, Research Dept., Springfield, Ill., 1961; *The Role of the Inquest in Today's Litigation.* Law Society of Upper Canada, Toronto, 1975.
24. *Setting Aside or Quashing of Verdict at Coroner's Inquest. Am. Law Reports,* 2d, 78:1218–1220, 1961.
25. *Kennedy v. Justices of the District Court of Dukes County,* 356 Mass. 367, 252 N.E. 2d. 201, 1969.

ADDITIONAL READING

Belli, M.: *My Life on Trial.* Popular Library, New York, 1977.
Browne, D. G., and Tullett, D. V.: *The Scalpel of Scotland Yard.* E. P. Dutton, New York, 1952.

Camps, F. E.: *The Investigation of Murder.* Michall Joseph, London, 1966.

Havard, J. D. J.: *The Detection of Secret Homicide.* Macmillan, London, 1960.

Helpern, M., and Knight, B.: *Autopsy —The Memoirs of Milton Helpern.* St. Martin's Press, New York, 1978.

Langone, J. L.: *Vital Signs: The Way We Die in America.* Little, Brown, Boston, 1974.

Necessity and Effect in Homicide Prosecution of Expert Medical Evidence as to the Cause of Death. *Am. Law Reports* (3rd Series) 65:283–320, 1976.

Schreiber, F. (ed.): *Damages in Personal Injury and Wrongful Death Cases.* Practicing Law Institute, New York, 1965.

Smith, S.: *Mostly Murder.* Harrop, London, 1959.

PART 3 SPECIAL INVESTIGATIONS

CHAPTER 18

Carol Cooperman Nadelson is Associate Professor of Psychiatry at Harvard Medical School. She is on the staff of the Psychiatry Department at Beth Israel Hospital in Boston and is a member of the Boston Psychoanalytic Society and Institute. Dr. Nadelson graduated from Brooklyn College and earned her medical degree at the University of Rochester. She is a former consultant to the Peace Corps, and has been a fellow and faculty member of the Radcliffe Institute. Dr. Nadelson is also a fellow of the American Psychiatric Association and the American College of Psychiatry and is a member of the editorial board of *Psychiatric Opinion*.

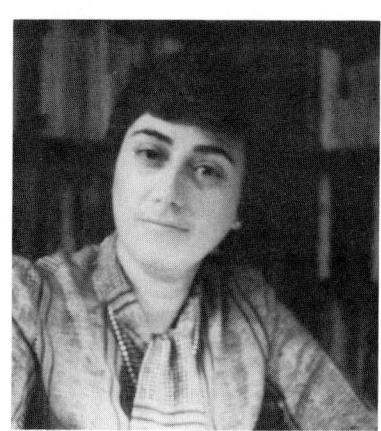

Malkah Tolpin Notman is Associate Clinical Professor of Psychiatry at Harvard Medical School and Beth Israel Hospital in Boston. She holds undergraduate degrees from the University of Chicago and is a graduate of Boston University School of Medicine and the Boston Psychoanalytic Institute. Dr. Notman is on the faculties of the Boston Psychoanalytic Institute and the Radcliffe Institute, and is a fellow of the American Psychiatric Association and the American College of Psychiatry. She is also a member of the editorial board of *Psychiatric Opinion*.

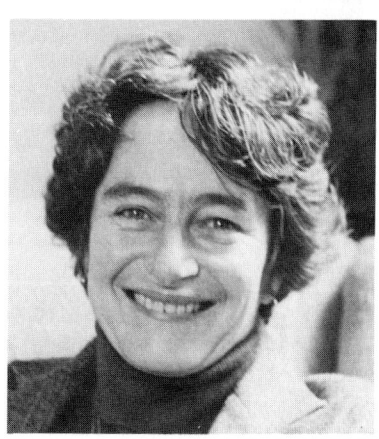

Elaine Hilberman is Associate Professor of Psychiatry and Assistant Director of Psychiatric Residency Training at the University of North Carolina School of Medicine at Chapel Hill. She is a graduate of City College of New York and of New York University School of Medicine. Dr. Hilberman is a fellow of the American Psychiatric Association and the author of *The Rape Victim*. She served on the Task Panel on Women of the President's Commission on Mental Health.

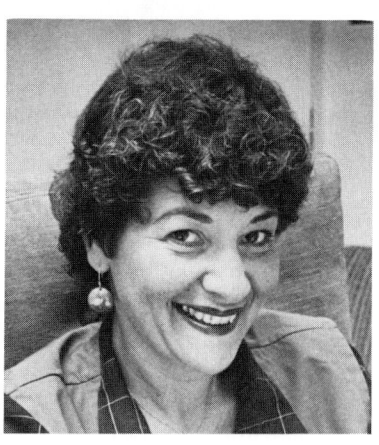

THE RAPE EXPERIENCE

Carol C. Nadelson, M.D.,
Malkah T. Notman, M.D., and
Elaine Hilberman, M.D.

DEFINITION OF THE CRIME

Rape has been defined as the act of taking anything by force.[1] Most statutes in the United States define rape as carnal knowledge of a person against the will of the person.[2] Two elements are necessary to constitute the crime: (1) sexual intercourse, and (2) failure to seek or to obtain the consent of the victim. Neither complete penetration of the vagina by the penis nor emission of seminal fluid is necessary. Most rapes include force or violence applied to the victim in order to accomplish the act, but acquiescence can be obtained by verbal threat or other circumstances indicating lack of consent.

The response of the rape victim is variable, depending on the circumstances, the setting where the action takes place, and her own personal response. She may fight back quickly when taken by surprise in an attack accompanied by threat of death or mutilation, or she may react more slowly and with disbelief in the forceful intentions of the man who continues to insist on sexual intercourse in the midst of a social encounter where sexual contact is unexpected and unagreed upon by the woman. In the latter situation, nonconsent is often overlooked or misinterpreted by assuming that certain social situations imply a willingness for a sexual relationship.[3]

The Uniform Crime Reports of the Federal Bureau of Investigation reveal an estimated total of 55,210 forcible rapes in 1974. This represented an 8 percent increase over the previous year, and a 49 percent increase over 1969.[4] Comparative statistics indicate that rape is the fastest growing of the violent crimes. While better reporting may account for part of the increase, the actual incidence of the crime appears to be increasing.

THE RAPE VICTIM'S EXPERIENCE

Burgess and Homstrom[5] have divided rape victims into three groups: (1) victims of forcible, completed or attempted rape; (2) victims who were an accessory due to their inability to consent; and (3) victims of sexually stressful situations where the encounter went beyond the expectations and ability of the victim to exercise control. In this chapter we will explore primarily the first category, recognizing that the lines drawn between the categories are often unclear. Despite differences in circumstances, the intrapsychic experiences of rape victims in all groups have features in common.

The rape victim has usually had an overwhelmingly frightening experience in which she feared for her life.[6] Generally the experience results in feelings of helplessness and intensifies conflicts about dependence and independence. It generates self-criticism and guilt which devalue her as a victim, and may interfere with trusting relationships, particularly with men. Other important consequences of the situation are a sense of shame, difficulty handling anger and aggression, and persistent feelings of vulnerability. Each rape victim responds in her own way, depending on her age, life situation, the circumstances of the rape, her specific personality style, and the responses of those from whom she seeks support.[7]

THE MYTHOLOGY OF RAPE

The mythology which surrounds rape has been developed, perpetuated, and reinforced by a number of attitudes and values which are reflected in both the medical and legal systems. Some of these myths are as follows:

1. Women can't be raped unless they want to be. A corollary of this might be that women enjoy rape, or that they at least unconsciously want it; therefore, there is no such thing as rape.
2. The rapist is a sexually unfulfilled and/or disturbed man carried away by a sudden, uncontrollable urge.
3. Rapists are always strangers to victims.
4. Rape occurs primarily on the street, and so as long as a woman stays home, she's safe.
5. Most rapes involve black men raping white women.
6. Women are raped because they ask for it by dressing seductively and walking provocatively; thus only "bad" women are raped.

The first of these myths represents a serious misperception of the situation, as well as of the concept of the unconscious. The prevalence of conscious or unconscious rape fantasies hardly makes every woman a willing victim and every man a rapist. The fantasy does not remotely capture the actual violence or degradation of the experience. While fantasies in which rape plays a part are frequent, the rape victim in a real situation knows that she is submitting because there is no choice without real danger to her person or to her life.

While definitive data are lacking, there are studies which shed light on some of the other myths involving rape. In 1971, Amir[8] published data which encompassed all cases of rape, not including incest or statutory rape, listed by the police in 1958 and 1960 in the city of Philadelphia. The data included 646 victims and 1292 offenders. Three-quarters of the rapes involved one or two assailants (single rape, 57%; pair rape, 16%); group rape (three or more assailants) was the pattern in 27 percent. Of the total number of incidents, 71 percent were planned in advance, and only 16 percent could be considered as resulting from an uncontrollable impulse. Group rapes were planned in 90 percent of cases, and single and two-assailant rapes in 58 percent of cases. Thus the "uncontrollable urge" theory of rape is challenged.

The myth that staying at home is safe fails to recognize that 56 percent of rapes in the Amir study occurred in the victim's residence, and the remainder were divided among automobiles, outside, and other indoor places. Moreover, in only half of the cases was the rapist a stranger to the victim, while the remainder included casual acquaintances, neighbors, boyfriends, family friends, and relatives. Husbands were not included in these statistics because, until quite recently, a sexual act between husband and wife was not considered rape under American law.

Hayman and Lanza[9] report on 1,223 cases in which the age of the victim ranged from 15 months to 82 years. Twelve percent were victims under 12, 25 percent were between 13 and 17, 32 percent were between 18 and 24, and 30 percent were over 25. The rapists were almost all less than 30 years of age. The overwhelming majority of reported rapes involved rapists and victims of the same race. Brownmiller[10] has suggested that this pattern may be changing. Most studies suggest a high proportion of intraracial rape, but the significance of this is unclear. It is possible that black rapists are more likely to be reported and apprehended, while white rape may be grossly underreported or less aggressively pursued when reported. A Denver study[11] is an exception in that the percentage of victims by race was similar to the at-large population; that is, 71 percent white, 15 percent black, 11 percent chicano.

In Amir's study, physical force was present in 86 percent of cases, the remainder involving various degrees of nonphysical force such as coercion or intimidation with or without weapons. Amir characterizes physical force in the following way:

Roughness (holding, pushing around)	29%
Nonbrutal beating (slapping)	25%
Brutal beating	20%
Choking and gagging	12%

These statistics do not include rape which ends in death. This group is reported in the homicide statistics rather than as rape. Thus, in one-third of the cases in which physical force occurred, extreme brutality was used.

In group rape there is evidently a higher frequency of both alcohol intake and prior criminal records, especially of sexual offenses. The assault is usually planned and is more brutal in terms of beatings and subjecting the victim to sexually humiliating practices in addition to the rape.

Victim behavior is described by Amir as submissive in 55 percent, with some degree of resistance in the remainder. At the time of the assault, the victim must decide whether she has a greater fear of the rape or of physical injury. Her actions will reflect her decision, usually without opportunity for thought. A dilemma is presented in that resistance increases the victim's chance of escape, but also increases the likelihood of violence toward her should she not escape.

Perhaps the most significant finding of Amir's study is that rape occurs in a context of violence rather than passion: "Rape is a deviant act, not because of the sexual act per se, but rather in the mode of the act, which implies aggression, whereby the sexual factor supplies the motive." While mythology has it that most rapists are sexually perverted, Amir suggests that rapists are a danger to the community not because they are necessarily sexually perverted, but because of their violence and aggression. They often may appear to be "normal," but they tend to have criminal records of offenses committed with brutality and violence. In his series, rapists tend to be young members of lower-class subcultures in which masculinity is expressed by displays of aggressiveness, which include sexual exploits against women. This is most evident in group rape, in which aggressive behavior is not the result of deviant sexuality, but of participation in a group which condones the use of force in attaining goals.

Clearly, as extensive as Amir's study is, the sample may be limited to specific subgroups because of the possibility that other cases are not reported to the police. The reported incidence greatly underreflects the actual incidence of rape. It is estimated that between 50 and 90 percent of rape cases go unreported. The Federal Bureau of Investigation attributes underreporting to fear and/or embarrassment on the part of the victims. The woman is often afraid of being accused of provocation or active participation in the rape. She is fearful of the reactions of husband, boyfriend, parents, or friends. In the case of a young victim, parents may wish to protect the child from the publicity and the legal ordeal. If the assailant is a close friend, relative, or employer, there are additional pressures not to report. Our own experience in Boston, working with the Beth Israel Hospital Rape Crisis Project, indicates that approximately 46 percent of women seeking medical aid reported the crime to the police.[12]

An examination of aspects of "victimhood" will help to explain this underreporting. Weis and Borges[13] describe in some detail the process by which a person becomes a victim, and specifically, the way in which our cultural norms determine that women are "legitimate" victims for rape. People are socialized to equate aggressiveness with masculinity, and passivity with femininity. The relations between the sexes are often seen "as an instrumental exchange whereby female servility is the price of male protection." Women have tended to internalize the psychological characteristics of the victim. They often do not know how to use techniques of physical self-defense. They fear male strength and often accept the mythology that the typical rape situation involves a stranger in a dark alley and that it is up to women to avoid both dangerous and compromising situations. In general, "nice girls" are believed not to get into trouble or to be raped. Males may perceive that aggressive conquest can be seen as an acceptable substitute for "masculine" failures in the economic and social spheres, so that aggressive and exploitative behavior toward women may become part of a mode of relating, and thus they may not conceive of such behavior as wrong or devious. The rapist may justify his behavior with the logic used for the legitimation of victims in general: she was in some way already inferior and she asked for and deserved it. Weis and Borges note that Amir himself uses this logic in his study. He characterizes a group of cases as "victim-precipitated rape," yet 92.7 percent of rapes in this group were accompanied by violence, while 45.9 percent of the victims were raped by more than one offender who humiliated the victim in 61.5 percent of cases. The victim's behavior was resistive in 48.7 percent of cases. One might similarly imply that attractive bank tellers precipitate bank robberies.

LEGAL CONSIDERATIONS

While we expect that hospitals and law enforcement agencies are legitimate places for reporting crime, many people trust neither of these institutions, especially with regard to rape. Hospitals suffer from lack of personnel trained to work with rape victims, both in the crisis period and in follow-up, and from lack of consistent and clear procedures for evidence collection. In the absence of a formal policy and sufficient information about the treatment of victims in crisis, personal attitudes and fears prevail. Clinicians are often in conflict about their role, especially with regard to confidentiality. In addition, the prospect of a court appearance is intimidating. The legal system also suffers from lack of personnel identified and trained to work with rape victims. The victim who reports does not receive consistent treatment because of high rates of police turnover, rotating shifts, and personal attitudes. People equate reporting with prosecution, and are fearful of harassment by law enforcement to prosecute. Finally, reporting and prosecution are both equated with the victim's life and past being made a matter of public record.

Unfortunately, there is considerable reality to the victim's fears, as reflected in the attitudes about the victim which prevail in the criminal justice system and in the statutes about rape. The report of the Center for Women Policy Studies comments that "the credibility of the rape victim is questioned more than that of any other victim of crime."[14] Forcible rape is the only crime for which an "unfounded" rate is calculated. It is also the only violent crime for which corroboration is frequently required.

One of the consequences of the corroboration requirement in unwitnessed rapes is that it is the victim who essentially stands trial. The assumption that women will make false accusations against men leads to a focus on the victim's credibility rather than on the crime. This assumption has been pervasive in the literature on the law, and raises serious questions about why these offenses are treated differently.

It is important to question this assumption from yet another perspective. What relevance does past behavior, social history, or mental make-up of a victim have in the determination of whether a crime was or was not committed? How accurate is a psychiatric report on predicting or deducing behavior?

Judge Hale's[15] statement that rape "is an accusation easily to be made and hard to be proved, and harder to be defended by the party accused" shows a lack of attention to the victim's experiences. The laws or court practices pertaining to rape trials may contribute to the unwillingness of the victim to report the crime to law enforcement agencies, much less agree to the ordeal of the trial. Wood[16] summarizes the complainant's ordeal and feels that the initial report becomes a traumatic event because of the requirement that an exquisitely detailed history of the rape be given and repeated to a variety of personnel connected with the subsequent investigation. Although attention has been focused recently on the importance of law enforcement sensitivity to the victim's mental state and the management of victims in crisis, this is not the first priority of law enforcement agencies. Thus victim interrogation may be impersonal and unsupportive if not frankly disbelieving and hostile. In some interrogations, the victim is asked questions about how many orgasms she had during the rape, what fantasies she had, and inquiry about past sexual encounters, all of which appear to be irrelevant to the establishment of the occurrence of rape. Wood points out that the police have considerable discretion as to whether or not any action is taken. They may refuse to accept the complainant's charges, or neglect to work on cases they feel are unsubstantiated. The acceptance of prevalent rape mythology makes it likely that these law enforcement personnel will often infer consent when none is given, or assume victim precipitation in many situations.

When the complaint reaches trial, there are three major elements of the legal defense in a rape case:[15]

1. Lack of identification—that the man accused is not the perpetrator of the crime.
2. Lack of penetration—that a sexual act did not take place.
3. Consent—that the intercourse was consented to or voluntary on the part of the woman.

Independent corroboration of the victim's story may be presented by an eyewitness, evidence acquired at the crime scene, and from the body of the victim or defendant. Since many rapes are not witnessed, circumstantial evidence is offered in most cases, including medical evidence and testimony, evidence of breaking and entering the complainant's residence, condition of clothing, bruises and scratches, emotional condition of the complainant, opportunity of the accused, conduct of the accused at the time of arrest, presence of semen or blood in the clothing of the accused or the victim, promptness of the victim's report to the police, and lack of motive to falsify. The complainant who attempts to restore a sense of control and cleanliness by bathing and changing clothes after the rape, or who is too frightened to report immediately, or who presents a calm exterior, may not be believed. The defense counsel can attack the case against the defendant by introducing evidence of the victim's mental illness, previous consensual intercourse with the same man, previous false accusations of rape, or an unchaste reputation. Supported by the myths about rape indicated earlier, many court cases seem to require evidence of a high degree of resistance by the victim, based on the belief that a healthy woman cannot be forcibly raped.

Recently, those studying victimology have recognized that resistance depends on the circumstances of the attack and the implications of continued resistance so that victim compliance is not a sign of consent but of futility.[17] The Report of the Center for Women Policy Studies comments on this issue:

> When and how a woman should resist a rapist are under hot debate. . . The few published studies of convicted rapists indicate that there are three or four different categories of offenders whose motives, methods, and reactions to resistance differ. Since rapists do not wear identifying labels, a woman cannot know which type she is confronting. . . .
>
> An important element of any program on defense against rape should be emphasis of the right of the woman to submit. Although some people successfully resist robbery, others are killed in the attempt, so no one is counseled to fight a robber. Although there are different values at stake, the choice should still be the victim's. Even a person who wants to resist and is trained to fight may be unable to do so when confronted with a situation which she or he perceives as dangerous.[18]

In the law of rape, consent is considered an affirmative defense which must be pleaded and proved by the defense. Otherwise, it is assumed that the woman did not consent to the intercourse. Nevertheless, after it is pleaded, the success of the consent defense depends practically on which version of the facts the jury believes. The defense must make its case believable and the victim's story unbelievable. This is often done through evidence of the complainant's general character or reputation for unchastity, the implication being that prior consensual intercourse, whether with the defendant or someone else, implies consent to intercourse in this instance, even though force, violence, and verbal threats may have been admitted by the defendant or proved conclusively by the victim.

Many women feel that the trauma of a court proceeding is too great, especially if there is little reason to hope that the assailant will be punished for his crime. Not only is rape the fastest growing of the *Index* crimes against the person, but among these it has the lowest proportion of cases closed by reason of arrest. In 1974, only half of the reported rapes led to an arrest, and 40 percent of men arrested were never prosecuted. Of the remaining 60 percent who were prosecuted, half were acquitted or had their cases dismissed.

Gates[19] cites a 1966 study of jury trials examining whether judges would have rendered the same verdicts as juries, and if not, what factors the judges thought influenced juries. In rape cases in which there was no extrinsic violence, one assailant, and no prior acquaintance of the victim and the assailant, the judge and jury would have reached the same conclusion in only 40 percent of cases. In the remaining 60 percent, the judge would have convicted where the jury acquitted. The judges concluded that in the absence of external evidence of violence, jurors ascribe to the complainant some contributory or precipitant behavior.

On the basis of jury decision, Hibey suggests:

> The jury's assessment of the credibility of the witnesses and their evidence is not always rational. This phenomenon stems in large part from certain ideas jurors have about the crime of rape, some of which are believed with such ferocity that jury verdicts are often examples of outright nullification—the ultimate and extreme exercise of the fact finder's prerogative.[20]

In addition to the complex social forces deterring reports of rape, the victim often has a set of internalized beliefs, stemming from her own socialization and self-perception, which decreases the likelihood of reporting. She often believes that the rapist is perverted or "sick." When the actual experience does not coincide with this view, since half of the assailants in rape cases are acquaintances if not trusted friends, she is left to wonder about her own complicity in the event. She "knows" that "nice girls" don't get raped and that it is not possible to rape a woman against her will. This false belief further contributes to her silence and her reluctance to report the attack to the police or to physicians or friends.

The Prince Georges County (Maryland) Task Force on Rape commented on the silence of the victim as follows:

> Rape and the investigation and treatment of the rape victim is a serious crime of assault on the body, but more grievously on the psyche of a woman. All too often, she is treated at best as an object, a piece of evidence, and is made to relive the experience, must face the incredul-

ity of the police, the impersonality of the hospital, and then must defend herself in court. Having been socialized to be passive, she is nevertheless expected to have put up a battle against her attacker. Her previous sexual experience can be used to impute her instability though the defendant's background often cannot be brought up against him. She does not have the benefit of a retained lawyer and sometimes the prosecutor does not have the time or perhaps the insight to prepare her beforehand for the ordeal of the trial. She suffers serious psychological stress afterward, largely due to the guilt and shame imposed by society. She may not recognize a need for professional help or she simply cannot afford it.[21]

Thus, as we have noted, there are multiple forces which act as deterrents to reporting, and it apears that it will be necessary to create a more sympathetic climate in order to allow the victim to identify herself as such to the hospital, law enforcement, and judicial systems. The House of Delegates of the American Bar Association has recently adopted a resolution[22] which would protect the victim from unnecessary invasion of privacy and the consequent psychological trauma. The proposed changes in law and practice include the elimination of corroboration requirements which exceed those applicable to other assaults, revision of the rules of evidence relating to cross-examination of the complaining witness, development of new procedures for police and prosecution in processing rape cases, and establishment of rape treatment and study centers to aid both the victim and the offender. Gates[23] and Wood[24] both recommend a redefinition of rape to include oral and anal intercourse and a delineation of varieties of rape to be contingent on the degree of force or violence used. They suggest that the resistance standard be dependent on "reasonable fear" and whether victim resistance was reasonable to expect under the circumstances of the assault. Reduced or graded penalties as with a system of degrees for rape, in line with comparable violent crimes, would increase the likelihood of jury convictions. The impact of such changes would eliminate the present distinction between victims of rape and victims of other crimes.

RAPE AS STRESS

The profound impact of the rape stress is best understood when rape is seen as a violent crime against the person, and not merely as a sexual encounter. Victims of violent crimes generally experience crises which may be unrecognized. Bard and Ellison[25] describe the stresses confronting the victim and emphasize the extent of the personal violation as an important factor. Burglary, for example, is experienced as a violation of the self in that one's home and possessions are symbolic extensions of the self. When armed robbery occurs, stress is intensified by the encounter between the victim and the criminal. The violation is compounded by a coercive deprivation of independence and autonomy in which the victim surrenders his or her controls under the threat of violence. An actual physical assault, in addition to the robbery, further stresses the victim because injury to the body serves as concrete evidence of the forced surrender of autonomy. Rape, then, is an ultimate violation of self short of homicide, with invasion of one's inner and most private space, as well as the loss of autonomy and control. Thus it is irrelevant to differentiate vaginal, anal, or oral intercourse when it is the self and not an orifice that has been invaded. The core meaning of rape would be the same, whether the victim were a virgin, a prostitute, a housewife, or a lesbian.

Rape can be viewed as a crisis situation in which a traumatic external event breaks the balance between internal adaptive capacity and the environment. It is similar to other situations described in the literature on stress, including community disasters,[26] war,[27] and surgical procedures.[28] The unexpected nature of the catastrophe and the variability of the resources of the victim in coping with an experience that may be viewed as life-threatening are critical factors in all crisis situations.

Although there are variations related to cultural and personality style, descriptions of stress reactions generally define four stages which vary in intensity and duration.[29] These responses are also found in rape victims:

1. An anticipatory or threat phase in which some anxiety facilitates perception of potentially dangerous situations so that they can be avoided. Most people protect themselves with a combination of internal psychological mechanisms which enable them to maintain an illusion of invulnerability, with enough reality perception to be protected from real danger. Thus, in situations where a potential stress is planned (i.e., elective surgery), individuals can protect themselves by strengthening those mechanisms which will ward off feelings of helplessness.
2. An impact phase in which varying degrees of disintegration may occur in a previously well-adapted person, depending on the degree of trauma and the adaptive capacity of the individual. During this phase, major physiologic reactions, including cardiovascular and sensorial shifts, may occur. The responses of people vary, from those who remain calm to those who respond with confusion, anxiety, and even hysterical outburst. Most victims show variable but less extreme responses. They demonstrate restricted attention span and automatic or stereotyped behavior. This clinical picture is seen in rape victims as well as in other crisis victims.
3. A post-traumatic or "recoil" phase in which emotional expression, self-awareness, memory, and behavioral control are gradually regained. Nevertheless, perspective may remain limited and dependency feelings may increase. Individuals perceive adaptive and maladaptive responses in themselves and may question their own reactions. A positive or negative view of one's ability to cope may affect the course of resolution of the particular trauma and future capacity to respond to stress. Self-esteem may be enhanced or damaged during this phase.
4. A post-traumatic, reconstitution phase in which victims try to put their lives back together again. At this time, the loss of self-reassuring mechanisms which had fostered a sense of invulnerability may result in a decrease in self-esteem. The victim then blames herself for lack of perception or attention to danger. When individuals begin to question themselves, and then the ability of the group or of society to be protective, a resulting traumatic neurosis may develop which is designed to protect the individual against further exposure to trauma, but which is psychologically costly, especially since it results in loss of self-esteem and of ability to take risks or to be innovative in other situations.[30]

Sutherland and Scherl[31] have reported on three phases of response to rape:

1. *The acute reaction.* This is characterized by signs of acute distress which include shock, disbelief, emotional breakdown, and disruption of normal patterns of behavior and function. The victim is often unable to talk about what has happened and may have difficulty telling family and friends, or reporting to the hospital or police. Guilt may be prominent, with fears that poor judgment may have precipitated the rape. During this phase, there are concrete concerns which demand fairly immediate attention. These include whether to tell family, husband, friends, children, or others what happened, as well as the implications of telling or not telling them. The victim is often concerned about publicity, about the likelihood of pregnancy or venereal disease, about her responsibility or ability to report the crime, about being able to identify the rapist, and about the impact of possibly seeing the assailant again.
2. *Outward adjustment.* This begins within several days to some weeks after the rape with an apparent temporary resolution of the immediate anxiety-provoking issues. The victim often returns to her usual life patterns and attempts to behave as if all is well, reassuring both herself and those close to her. Denial of difficulty and suppression of feelings are prominent during this period. The impact of what has happened is often ignored.
3. *Integration and resolution.* Depression frequently occurs, although it may be mild. The victim often needs to talk about what has happened in order to integrate the event with her self-image and to resolve her feelings about the rapist. The earlier attitude of tolerance and understanding of the rapist may be replaced by anger toward him. She may also wonder if she colluded in some unknown way with the rapist.

Burgess and Holmstrom[32] define a specific rape trauma syndrome in two stages: an immediate or acute response in which the victim's life style is disrupted by the rape, and a long-term process in which the victim reorganizes herself. In addition, they comment on two types of acute response: "the expressed style" in which the victim is emotional and visibly upset, in contrast with the "controlled style" in which the victim may appear to be calm to the casual observer. The authors also comment on the prevalence of guilt and self-blame in the initial phase. They discuss a reorganizational phase which has elements in common with other stress reactions, although it varies with each individual. The primary acute reaction is related to the fear of physical injury, mutilation, and death. Mood swings are common, as are feelings of humiliation, guilt, shame, self-blame, and fear of another assault by the assailant.

There is often surprisingly little clinical evidence of rage in rape victims, compared with the outrage stimulated in others upon hearing of the rape. Feelings of anger and desire for revenge often appear somewhat later. A primary defense may be an attempt to avoid thinking about the rape, although this is difficult to do. The wish to undo the event may appear in fantasies of how the victim might have handled the situation differently.

A wide variety of physical and psychological reactions may occur during this time period, depending, in part, on the location and extent of the injuries sustained. Specific symptoms occur, such as sleep disturbance and loss of appetite. These should be differentiated from similar symptoms caused by treatment, including hormones administered to prevent pregnancy.[33] Like Sutherland and Scherl, these authors report that the acute phase may last from a few days to some weeks and is generally followed by a reorganizational process. The manifestations of this second stage depend on the victim's personality style, available support system, and the treatment she encounters from others. Changes in life style are prominent, with impaired levels of function at work, home, and school. Some women may move to another residence, while others may be fearful of leaving their homes at all, or may give up autonomy by returning to their families. Sleep disruptions often continue with vivid dreams and nightmares. Early dreams with re-enactments of the actual rape are frequent. These later progress to a point where mastery of the rape may begin taking place, and the victim may apprehend the rapist or assailant of her dream. Phobias appear which seem specifically determined by the nature of the rape experience, such as fear of crowds or of being at home or outside, depending on the location of the assault. Sexual fears are common with a decline of interest as well as withdrawal from a previous partner.

There are specific situations which increase the complexity of the reaction. The victim who is raped by a friend or relative, an event more frequent with children and adolescents, has a greater psychological burden than would be true if the assailant were a stranger. She must also deal with issues of trust. The existence of psychological problems and/or maladaptive behavior patterns prior to the rape increases the likelihood of maladaptive coping patterns following the rape. Serious medical or psychiatric problems prior to, or as the result of, the rape may affect the outcome.

LIFE STAGE CONSIDERATIONS

Certain reactions relate directly to specific life stages. These reactions are described in the sections to follow.

The Single Young Woman

The single young woman between the ages of 17 and 24 is the most frequently reported rape victim. She is inexperienced and her relations with men have frequently been limited to family and friends. She has little sophistication, and she may easily become involved in an unwelcome sexual encounter. In this age group, rape victims frequently do have a prior acquaintance with the rapist. This may be the reason for a refusal to prosecute. She may reproach herself because she could have been more active in preventing the rape, and she experiences shame and guilt, regardless of the circumstances. These feelings, coupled with the victim's sense of vulnerability, may color her future relationships with men. This is especially true for the very young woman who may have had her first sexual experience in this context. The result can be a confusion of sexuality and violence.

The rape experience for a young single woman may revive concerns about separation and independence. She may feel inadequate to care for herself. Parents, friends, and relatives often respond by offering to take care of her again in an attempt to be supportive and reassuring. However, in doing this, they may foster regression and prevent mastery of the stress. Another problem for the younger rape victim is her perception of, and tolerance for, the gynecologic examination. Since she may have suffered physical trauma, is susceptible to venereal disease, and may become pregnant, a complete examination is indicated. It may be perceived, especially by an inexperienced or severely traumatized woman, as another rape. Thus, while she may be concerned about the intactness of her body, she will have difficulty with necessary procedures if they stimulate memories or reproduce in any way the original rape experience.

The Woman with Children

The woman with children must also deal with the problems of what, how, and when to tell them. If the event is known in the community, there are implications for her and her children. She is concerned about the trauma she may be inflicting as well as her image in their eyes. If she has a husband, she may be concerned about whether he can find her sexually attractive or even tolerate her. She may also have unexpected negative feelings toward her husband.

The Divorced or Separated Woman

The divorced or separated woman is in a particularly difficult position in that her credibility may be questioned because of her life style. She, in turn, may experience the rape as a confirmation of her feelings of inadequacy. She is especially likely to feel guilty and may fail to obtain aid or to report the crime. Her ability to function independently is challenged. If she has children, she may worry about her ability to protect and care for them. Questions may be raised about her adequacy as a mother.

The Middle-Aged Woman

The "middle-aged" woman is often in a period of reassessment of her life role, particularly in the face of changed relationships to her grown-up or already absent family members. Her husband may be in his own midlife crisis, and may be less responsive and supportive to her sexual and emotional needs. At this point the overwhelming experience of rape is particularly damaging. The myth that a middle-aged woman past her earlier, sexually most active period has less to lose than a younger woman is very much in error. It is difficult to quantify the self-devaluation and feelings of worthlessness and shame in any woman, especially such feelings in a woman who may be concerned about her sexual adequacy.

LONG-TERM CONSEQUENCES OF RAPE

There are no systematic data currently available about the long-term consequences of rape. In addition, it is difficult to predict all the long-term needs of the rape victim, since individual response patterns and circumstances differ so much. Some of the reactions which do appear clinically, often at a later date, are as follows:

1. Mistrust of men with consequent avoidance or hesitation to form relationships.
2. A variety of sexual disturbances, often presenting as sexual dysfunctions and marital conflicts.

3. Persistent phobic reactions.
4. Anxiety and depression which may be precipitated by seemingly unrelated events which in some way bring back the original trauma.
5. Persistent anxiety and avoidance of gynecologic examinations or procedures.
6. Suicide or suicide attempts. Preliminary studies of female suicide attempters suggest the possibility of a relationship between an earlier rape experience and suicide attempts.

There is clinical evidence of a silent rape reaction, one showing no signs of unusual disturbance. An earlier rape will often present problems later, and after some investigation it appears that the event is still very much alive and unresolved.

While it is apparent that a simple approach to the rape victim and her family cannot be provided, it is clear that crisis counseling, with follow-up for at least 1 to 2 years, may be necessary. In some circumstances the degree of trauma coupled with the previous developmental history of the victim may result in long-standing symptoms and even the development of a traumatic neurosis which requires intensive, long-term treatment.

COUNSELING ISSUES

There seems to be a consensus on three types of needs to be fulfilled in a counseling program: (1) crisis intervention to facilitate working through of the trauma and to diminish the likelihood of long-term psychopathologic consequences; (2) emotional support from whomever the victim comes in contact with during the crisis period; and (3) emotional support for family and friends of the victim.

There is some disagreement about the effectiveness of peer versus professional mental health counseling. Professionals often state that the trauma of rape is so serious that professional psychological help should immediately be made available. On the other hand, many feminists believe that it is detrimental to suggest to a victim that she needs professional help because it implies that her reaction is "sick," unless there is some indication that she cannot cope with the reality of the assault or its consequences. They believe that most victims need an empathetic listener and enough information to enable them to make realistic choices.

Rape crisis center counselors, who are generally volunteer lay people, usually state that they can assess their own limits and call upon professionals for advice and referral. Professionals often function in the training and supervision of lay counselors. The Center for Women Policy Studies recommends a coordinated and collaborative educational effort by physicians, hospitals, citizens, and criminal justice personnel as the most effective approach to training needs.[34] The psychiatrist or mental health professional can have both direct and consultative roles in all these educational endeavors.

The psychiatrist or mental health professional has many roles. In the emergency room setting, he or she functions in a consultative capacity with a variety of other specialty services such as gynecology, pediatrics, nursing, and social work. A collaborative alliance must be established in the emergency room which will facilitate medical treatment, enable the victims to make a decision about legal involvement, and help the victim work toward crisis resolution. Consultative/liaison skills are crucial to the development of integrated programs which depend on an interdisciplinary team approach as the primary treatment modality.

The mental health professional can assist other staff members in the acquisition of skills necessary for taking an adequate history and assessing the victim's emotional state and ego-functioning so that optimal treatment can be planned. It is useful to differentiate short-term crisis goals from long-term issues which may require a psychiatric referral. The perspective of the psychiatrist in evaluating which victims might appropriately benefit from long-term intervention can be extremely important. Adequate case supervision with a focus on family dynamics and the life context in which the rape occurs should be a major concern of every treatment program. Immediate or long-term supervision is especially important in hospital settings where counseling is often done by lay counselors or a variety of personnel functioning in training capacities.

Mental health professionals may be a referral resource for community agencies, crisis center, and other physicians. They can be consulted when there is a maladaptive or delayed response to the crisis. Women already suffering from other emotional problems can be rape victims, and this experience may well intensify pre-existing problems. The mental health professionals who are called upon must be knowledgeable not only in the special issues related to rape, but also in terms of the clinical skills necessary to serve as consultants to other therapists, treatment-team members, and cooperating community agencies.

The last decade has witnessed the spontaneous appearance of growing numbers of community-based rape crisis centers as part of a nationwide anti-rape movement.* These centers are largely staffed by volunteer, non-professional women, some of whom have been raped in the past, or who have been close to someone who was raped. Men are not usually accepted as volunteers in rape crisis programs. However, in some centers, men have been recruited to work with the significant men in the victim's life, or have organized themselves to support the crisis program and to provide services to male friends and relatives of rape victims.

Most community rape crisis centers have similar goals which include the following:

1. To provide supportive services to victims.
2. To reform the institutions which deal with victims.
3. To educate themselves and the public on rape-related issues.
4. To reform the law.

Direct services to victims are designed to meet the victim's needs for information, emotional support, and advocacy. Many centers have 24-hour telephone "hot-lines" which allow for immediate contact and support after a rape. Information is provided about local hospital and criminal justice procedure, and the victim is encouraged to make the necessary decisions about medical treatment, reporting to law enforcement, and communication with family and friends. Counseling services are usually limited to immediate temporary support and short-term follow-up through the use of peer counselors. The goal of counseling is the return of autonomous functioning and control, with prolonged dependency on the cen-

---

*A national directory of rape crisis centers is provided in Horos, C. V.: *Rape*. Tobey Publishing Co., New Canaan, Conn., 1974.

ter discouraged. Individual counseling is the rule, with group models reportedly less successful. Victim advocacy services include intervention with medical and law enforcement personnel when it is felt that the victim is receiving inappropriate or inadequate treatment and continuing contact by telephone and in person throughout the prosecutory phase. Anonymous reporting is often arranged for those victims who choose not to report the rape or rape attempt to law enforcement agencies. Additional services may include transportation, babysitting, and a place to sleep either when the victim fears returning home or when her home is judged to be unsafe.

Educational programs in the crisis centers have as aims self-education; the dissemination of information on rape prevention and resistance, as well as what to do if rape occurs; and community and personal attitudinal changes. There has been a focus on "demythologizing" the crime of rape, particularly with regard to the stereotypic assumptions about both the victim and the assailant. Public education programs have been conducted independently in cooperation with other groups, or with existing medical and criminal justice institutions. Educational efforts are viewed as a necessary precursor to reforms of the law enforcement and health care systems. Reform goals have been initiated in cooperation with these institutions, or by assuming a vocal, adversary position. Rape crisis centers have variously recommended or demanded an increase in women police officers, sensitivity to victim needs, and clarification of hospital and police protocols. Many centers have collaborative relationships with both hospitals and law enforcement agencies so that the counselor remains with the victim throughout the required procedures. Center advocates attend rape trials, and, on occasion, will "pack the court" as an additional method of public pressure to change courtroom behavior.

Despite the similarity of goals and services, each program has unique aspects which stem from the nature of the group itself as well as from the resources and attitudes of the community in which the center is located. Some centers remain alienated from professional institutions, while others work closely with existing medical and legal resources. Although most counseling is done by nonprofessional women, programs for training these women in the techniques of crisis intervention for rape victims have involved professionals in both medical and legal spheres. Despite the lack of psychological sophistication, counselors have been creative and innovative in providing support to victims and families. It is likely that psychiatric consultative and backup services would be welcomed by many centers.

Institutional-based rape crisis programs should not be considered an improved alternative which replaces the community rape crisis centers. Community groups may tend to attract younger and/or feminist women, while more traditional and/or older women will use institutional services. It is anticipated that community programs will continue to be necessary to provide support and to encourage referrals to appropriate medical and law enforcement facilities. Community programs also provide a wide spectrum of services not easily provided by traditional institutions, such as a safe place to sleep when the victim is fearful of returning home after the rape, or a companion to guide her through the time-consuming and traumatic experiences of the criminal justice procedure should she decide to prosecute. Finally, community groups continue to provide leadership for educating the public, and this will ultimately be reflected in changes in attitude on the part of the victim as well as the juror.[35]

Often the concerns of lay groups derive from their perception of the attitudes of professionals. Notman and Nadelson[36] have stated, "Until recently many psychiatrists have felt that rape was not a psychiatric issue, and further that psychiatrists had little to offer the rape victim. They often shared the view that the victim 'asked for it.' " The victim was then seen as acting out her unconscious fantasies, and, therefore, she was not "really" a victim. Thus the rape victim had not been offered the sympathetic understanding usually extended to people in crisis. Rape falls into a group of emotionally charged issues where prejudice prevents the objectivity which would be available if it were regarded as a traumatic experience. As noted, another manifestation of this prejudice has been the concern that a rape victim was making a false accusation, a concern that has not been supported by the evidence in the vast majority of cases.

Professionals have shared the mythology about the rape victim whom they perceive as a young, sexually attractive woman in some way exposing herself to a danger which could be avoided in the ordinary course of living, or, having initially agreed upon sexual intercourse, accusing her partner of rape in order to save herself from criticism. Holding these views fulfills several functions. It protects individuals who hold them from anxiety about their own vulnerability, and it states that "it can't happen here." This defensive position is further expressed by the focus on the sexual aspect of rape. If it is sexual, then the victim and the rapist could be seen as seeking sexual gratification together. The professional then can be protected from feelings of guilt or responsibility.

In our recent experience, concomitant with the development of a rape crisis program, changes have occurred in the attitudes of participating professionals with an increasing awareness of the crisis nature of the experience and an increased empathy for the individual victim.

The potential role of the psychiatrist or mental health professional is multifaceted, with clinical, administrative, teaching, supervisory, and research aspects. The role of the mental health professional with regard to the legal system is not entirely clear. It is not the function of the clinician to decide whether the victim has "really" been raped. Rape is a legal and not a medical term. The fact that the victim perceives herself as having been violated remains the significant event for purposes of the crisis center of any treatment program.

In the immediate aftermath of the rape, issues of personal safety and control emerge as primary concerns. The victim has just had an experience in which her very existence may have been threatened, with total loss of control of what was done to her. Her immediate needs are for a sense of physical safety as well as for assistance in assuming some control over what has happened to her and what will happen to her in her dealings with both individuals and institutions. The presence of an empathic and supportive individual, who may be a counselor, clinician, or friend, will enhance her sense of safety. She should not be left alone. She should be encouraged to talk and to ventilate her feelings with reassurance and validation of her responses. Whether this occurs in the police station, the physician's office, or the hospital emergency room, the issues are the same. In order to be effective, the counselor must have available information about medical and legal procedures so that the victim can be informed. Decisions about procedure, including reporting to the hospital or law enforcement agencies, must be made by the victim. While the counselor may have some opinions about what she ought to do, coercion has no place in the management of the rape victim.

Burgess and Holmstrom[37] summarize the assumptions they make in counseling victims. Their context is a short-term, issue-oriented crisis model with the goal of restoring the victim to her previous level of functioning as quickly as possible. Since the crisis disrupts the victim's life style in four areas—physical, emotional, social, and sexual—all of these issues are appropriate areas of scrutiny. The victim is assumed to be normal, that is, an individual who was managing her life adequately prior to the crisis. The rape is viewed as a crisis situation, and previous problems unassociated with the rape are not considered priority issues for discussion. When other issues of concern are identified which would require the use of a different approach, appropriate referrals are suggested to the victims.

An analysis of rape crisis requests[38] suggests that there are four major categories of need, namely for police intervention, medical intervention, psychological intervention, and emotional control (especially with victims who present in an incoherent state). There is an additional group who may not perceive that anyone can be of help to them, with ambivalence, if not hostility, about any intervention.

The following sections summarize appropriate areas for counseling intervention in the immediate phase.

The Assault

Considered here will be the circumstances and setting of the rape; the victim's details of conversation, including physical and verbal threats; details of behavior; amount and kind of resistance; the use of alcohol or drugs by either victim or assailant; and the victim's emotional and sexual reactions. The counselor's ability to learn about the details of the assault will clarify which of these concerns are most problematic. The focus may be on the rape as a first sexual encounter, or on intense guilt for not putting up a fiercer struggle. The victim who is beaten into senselessness may suffer far less emotional trauma than the woman who submits to rape when her life is threatened. The victim's coping strategy before and during the assault will become an issue after the assault.

Medical Concerns

Medical concerns include the quality of the victim's treatment in the hospital; interactions with medical and nursing staff; extent and type of physical injury; the possibilities of pregnancy and venereal disease; and the pelvic examination. The pelvic examination is a frequent focus for the victim's anger. Because many victims experience the pelvic examination as another rape, adequate preparation is important. Victims also are fearful that their bodies are irrevocably damaged.

Law Enforcement

Questions directly related to law enforcement include the following: Does the victim plan to report the rape; if she has reported, how was she treated; what kinds of questions was she asked; was she encouraged in, or dissuaded from, the pressing of charges against the assailant? Part of the counseling process is to help the victim vent her feelings about her treatment, as well as to validate her feelings.

Prosecution

The key prosecutory questions can be combined as follows: Does the victim plan to press charges, cooperate with the police investigation, and appear in court, and how does she feel about this? This is often an issue of high priority for the victim who must make this decision at a time when it is difficult to think rationally about anything. Concrete information is usually helpful. For example, some victims think they are breaking the law by not reporting and prosecuting. The victim's rationale for not wishing to prosecute may be quite realistic, given the treatment of victims by the courts, or may reflect her fears that she did indeed precipitate the rape. The counselor's role is to help the victim clarify for herself how she feels about these issues and to support the victim's decision, whatever it may be.

Social Support System

In terms of the social support system, the issues may be stated in three basic questions: Who are the important people in the victim's life? Whom does she plan to tell about the rape? What responses does she anticipate? How the rape may affect or change her relationship with significant others is invariably an issue in the immediate crisis period. An evaluation of the personnel support available will determine in part the extent to which continued counseling becomes necessary; that is, the availability of a strong social support network will diminish the need for ongoing counseling intervention. In contrast to most personal crisis where the counselor or therapist reinforces the importance of sharing the crisis with those who are significant in the person's life, no firm guidelines exist about communicating the event of the rape because of the real possibility that the revelation may disrupt the relationship. Thus a husband may perceive the rape as a deception by his wife, and the parents of an adolescent may project their own sense of guilt and become angry with the victim. At times, the counselor may have an important role to play in counseling the family. Family and friends must be sensitized to the meaning of the rape so that they are able to give honest support to the victim. Where there are pre-existing conflicts in relationships, the rape may aggravate the situation. In cases where the victim chooses not to tell close friends or family members, guilt or distancing may occur, for which the victim will need counseling assistance.

Physical Safety

If she lives alone, or was raped at home, the victim will likely be fearful of returning home. Moreover, the assailant (who most often has not been apprehended) may have threatened to return, or the victim may be fearful of this, even when a threat has not been made. A temporary resolution may involve identifying a friend with whom the victim can stay as well as available options for the future if it is necessary.

Preparation for Victim Responses

As previously described, there is a wide spectrum of immediate responses to rape. A victim may not wish to talk, or may show little overt emotional response. In any case, it is important for the counselor to prepare the victim for the range of reactions likely to occur, so that the victim becomes sensitized to her own feelings and has some awareness that the inevitable disruptions in life style are normal. Mild sedation for sleep is usually indicated as well. Knowledge that the victim can call upon the counselor throughout this period provides additional reassurance that she will not be left in isolation. Although the counselor's role with the victim in the later reorganization phase cannot be defined specifically because of the complexity of victim needs and responses, it is important to keep in mind the issues we have raised.

MEDICOLEGAL CONSIDERATIONS

The physician treating the rape victim has several tasks including immediate care of physical injuries, prevention of venereal disease, prevention of pregnancy, proper medicolegal examination with documentation by evidence collection for law-enforcement purposes, and prevention or alleviation of permanent psychological damage. These tasks are extremely complex since there are very different systems operating and producing conflicting demands.

The Report of the District of Columbia Task Force on Rape describes many of the problems which currently prevail in hospital treatment of victims.[39] The Task Force suggests that doctors resist seeing rape victims because they want to avoid court appearances. They also suggest that some doctors minimize or neglect signs of trauma in an attempt to avoid being called in to testify. This may be related to the lack of training in the treatment of the physical and emotional trauma resulting from the rape or in the methods of evidence collection. Hospital policies vary widely. In some institutions, examinations are performed by gynecologists, while at others, the lowest-ranking physician (without training in gynecology) sees the victim. Medical treatment is often inadequate and psychological treatment usually nonexistent. Victims have been known to wait for long periods of time to receive medical attention which is often perfunctory and impersonal. Issues concerning pregnancy and venereal disease may not be considered adequately. There may be no formal procedure for collection of evidence, and, even when such procedure exists, it may not be followed. Many hospital policies require that parents give consent before a minor is treated; some automatically call the police whether a victim wishes to report or not. Some victims choose to forgo treatment rather than have parents or police know of the rape. The problem of confidentiality in the doctor-patient relationship must be considered if testimony will be required of the physician or the counselor working with the physician.

There is currently a variety of formal reports and guidelines which make recommendations for improving hospital services to rape victims.[40-45] The major recommendations and considerations can be summarized as follows:

1. At least one medical facility in any given community should have a formal program for the comprehensive treatment of rape victims, with such services available on a 24-hour basis. Those hospital or clinic facilities which do not have comprehensive programs should have, as a minimum, a set of guidelines for treating rape victims.
2. Law enforcement agencies and the public should be made aware of the existence of comprehensive hospital services for rape victims.

3. Since treatment of the rape victim involves an interface between medical and legal issues, programs designed by medical facilities should operate within the context of their community and in cooperation with citizens' groups, law enforcement, and prosecutory agencies.
4. Treatment of the rape victim should be given high priority, second only to life-threatening illnesses or accidents, and should not be contingent on cooperation with the criminal justice system.
5. Adequate care of the victim is facilitated by a team treatment model. The team should include a support person, a nurse, a physician, and appropriate consultants, including a mental health professional. The support person should serve as an advocate/counselor/guide for the victim throughout the hospital process and should have familiarity with both crisis intervention techniques and criminal justice procedure. The nurse, usually a member of the regular emergency room staff, should coordinate the total treatment plan, assessing needs and explaining procedures. There are varying opinions about whether the physician should be a gynecologist, family practitioner, or specialist in trauma. Because the physician's medicolegal role makes it highly probable that the victim will perceive him/her as an investigator rather than an ally, counseling responsibilities are best handled by other team members. The role of the psychiatrist or other mental health professional as a consultant has been discussed earlier. Finally, while it is desirable to be able to offer the victim a choice regarding the sex of the team personnel, sensitivity and experience may be more important determinants of a successful intervention.
6. All hospital personnel who will have contact with the victim should be educated to the special problems of rape victims. The training program should include crisis intervention theory and practice, sensitization to the physical and emotional trauma of rape, and medicolegal issues. It is desirable that training efforts be accomplished in collaboration with citizens' groups and local criminal justice agencies.
7. Hospitals should have clear procedural guidelines for victim care and evidence collection with a specific and unambiguous description of the role and function of each member of the rape-crisis team. The medicolegal examination can be facilitated by prepackaged "rape kits" which contain all of the information and equipment necessary for examination and evidence collection.
8. Crisis intervention should be immediately available to all victims, their families, and significant other persons at the time of initial contact with the hospital.
9. The victim should be fully informed and consent obtained for all treatment procedures performed in the emergency room and afterward, with special emphasis on those steps taken to prevent pregnancy and venereal disease. The victim may be experiencing considerable confusion at the time of the hospital visit, and written information furnished to her at the hospital serves as reassurance that the appropriate preventive measures were taken. Otherwise, the patient may be uncertain about what further protection she may need after release from the hospital.
10. Follow-up treatment may be complicated by the profound denial which often follows in the immediate aftermath of the rape. The

victim may attempt to "forget" the assault, and may not keep subsequent appointments. For this reason, it becomes especially important to provide all available services during the initial crisis contact since this may be the only intervention for a given victim. Follow-up efforts may be more successful if they involve contact with the original treatment team members rather than new institutions and personnel. Thus the team physician should arrange to see the victim, with the support person maintaining continuing contact. When formal mental health referrals are indicated, the need for such services must be explained so that the victim does not assume that because she was raped, she must be mentally ill. All follow-up treatment plans must be contingent on the patient's informed choice, and all referral services should be suggested on the basis of their sensitivity to rape-crisis issues as well as their general professional capabilities.
11. The issue of financial responsibility for the rape victim's medicolegal examination has been the object of recent attention. While some states have statutes providing for financial compensation to victims of violent crimes, rape victims have not as yet been considered appropriate beneficiaries of such laws. Since the victim is expected to go through the ordeal of reporting to hospital and law enforcement personnel and then to face the trauma of the trial, it seems inappropriate that she also be expected to absorb the cost of the state's evidence. Payment for hospital services rendered should not be the responsibility of the victim, but should come from public funds.
12. While interagency collaboration is necessary to provide comprehensive services, all efforts should be made to protect the confidentiality of the victim. During the course of the examination, information about the victim may surface which is relevant to medical treatment, but irrelevant and potentially damaging in court (e.g., pre-existing venereal disease or contraceptive usage in a single woman). Team members must use caution in what is entered into the victim's medical record, and guidelines should be established to protect her confidentiality.
13. Although medical treatment cannot be made contingent on reporting to police, it is desirable for law enforcement agencies to know about the incidence of rape. An anonymous or "blind" report system might be instituted in which the location and modus operandi of the assailant are described, but the name of the victim withheld.

There are at present a growing number of hospital-based rape crisis programs which have incorporated these recommendations. While each program has unique features based on the nature of the area served, the availability of community resources, the state law, and the local criminal justice procedure, there are striking commonalities to all of these programs. Clear and unambiguous guidelines can be the basis for establishing and maintaining an effective and sensitive rape crisis intervention program in any community.

REFERENCES

1. *Random House Dictionary of the English Language.* Random House, New York, 1966, p. 1191.

2. Evard, J.: Rape: The Medical, Social and Legal Implications. *Am. J. Obstet. Gynecol.* 111:197–199.
3. Notman, M.T., and Nadelson, C.C.: The Rape Victim: Psychodynamic Considerations. *Am. J. Psychiatry* 133:4, 1976.
4. *Uniform Crime Reports for the United States.* Federal Bureau of Investigation, Washington, D.C., 1974.
5. Burgess, A.W., and Holmstrom, L.L.: Rape Trauma Syndrome. *Am. J. Psychiatry* 131:981–986, 1974.
6. Hilberman, E.: *The Rape Victim.* American Psychiatric Association, Garamond/Pridemark Press, Baltimore, 1976.
7. *Report of the District of Columbia Task Force on Rape.* Subcommittee of District of Columbia City Council, July 1973.
8. Amir, M.: *Patterns of Forcible Rape.* University of Chicago Press, Chicago, 1971.
9. Hayman, C., and Lanza, C.: Sexual Assault on Women and Girls. *Am. J. Obstet. Gynecol.* 103(3):480–486, 1971.
10. Brownmiller, S.: *Against Our Will: Men, Women and Rape.* Simon & Schuster, New York, 1975.
11. Giacinti, T.A., and Tjaden, C.: *The Crime of Rape in Denver.* Denver Anti-Crime Council, 1973.
12. Beth Israel Hospital Rape Crisis Intervention Project, Boston, 1975.
13. Weis, K., and Borges, S.S.: Victimology and Rape: The Case of the Legitimate Victim. *Issues in Criminology* 8(2):71–115, 1973.
14. Rape and its Victims: A Report for Citizens, Health Facilities and Criminal Justice Agencies, in *The Police Response: A Handbook.* Center for Women Policy Studies, Washington, D.C., 1975. (Copies available from Law Enforcement Assistance Administration, Washington, D.C.)
15. Hibey, R.A.: The Trial of a Rape Case: An Advocate's Analysis of Corroboration, Consent, and Character, in Schultz, L.G. (ed.): *Rape Victimology.* Charles C Thomas, Springfield, Ill., 1975.
16. Wood, P.L.: The Victim in a Forcible Rape Case: A Feminist View, in Schultz, L.G. (ed.): *Rape Victimology.* Charles C Thomas, Springfield, Ill., 1975.
17. Bard, M., and Ellison, K.: Crisis Intervention and Investigation of Forcible Rape. *The Police Chief,* May 1974.
18. Rape and its Victims, op. cit.
19. Gates, M.J.: The Rape Victim on Trial. Paper presented at Special Session on Rape, American Psychiatric Association, Anaheim, California, 1975.
20. Hibey, op. cit.
21. *Report of the Task Force to Study the Treatment of the Victims of Sexual Assault.* Task Force of the County Council of Prince Georges County, Maryland, March 1973.
22. *Am. Bar Assoc. J.* 61:464–65, 1975.
23. Wood, op. cit.
24. Gates, op. cit.
25. Bard and Ellison, op. cit.
26. Tyhurst, J.S.: Individual Reactions to Community Disaster: The Habitual History of Psychiatric Phenomena. *Am. J. Psychiatry* 107:764–769, 1951; Lendenmann, E.: Symptomatology and Management of Acute Grief. *Am. J. Psychiatry* 101:141–146, 1944.
27. Glover, E.: Notes on the Psychological Effects of War Conditions on the Civilian Population. Part I: The Munich Crisis. *Intern. J. Psychoanal.* 22: 132–146, 1941; Glover, E: Notes on the Psychological Effects of War Conditions on the Civilian Population, Part III: The Blitz. *Intern. J. Psychoanal.* 23:17–37, 1942; Schmideberg, M.: Some Observations on Individual Reactions to Air Raids. *Intern. J. Psychoanal.* 23:146–176, 1942; Rado, S.: Pathodynamics and Treatment of Traumatic War Neurosis (Traumatophobia). *Psychosomat. Med.* 4:362–369, 1942.
28. Deutsch, H.: Some Psychoanalytic Observations in Surgery. *Psychosomat. Med.* 4:105–115, 1942.
29. Janis, I.L.: *Psychological Stress.* John Wiley & Sons, New York, 1958.

30. Weiss, R.J., and Payson, H.E.: Gross Stress Reaction I, in Freedman, A.M., and Kaplan, H.J. (eds.): *Comprehensive Textbook of Psychiatry*. Williams & Wilkins, Baltimore, 1967.
31. Sutherland, S., and Scherl, D.: Patterns of Response Among Victims of Rape. *Am. J. Orthopsychiatry* 40(3):503–511, 1970.
32. Burgess, A.W., and Holmstrom, L.L.: The Rape Victim in the Emergency Ward. *Am. J. Nursing* 73(10):1740–45, 1973; Burgess, A.W., and Holmstrom, L.L.: *Rape; Victims of Crisis*, Robert J. Brady, Bowie, Md., 1974.
33. Massey, J.B., Carcia, C.R., and Emich, J.P.: Management of Sexually Assaulted Females. *Obstet. Gynecol.* 38(1):29–36, 1971.
34. Rape and its Victims, op. cit.
35. Hilberman, op. cit.
36. Notman and Nadelson, op. cit.
37. Burgess and Holmstrom, op. cit.
38. *Report of D.C. Task Force on Rape*, op. cit.
39. *Ibid.*
40. *Guidelines for the Treatment of Suspected Rape Victims*. Chicago Hospital Council, February 1974.
41. *Guidelines for Care of Victims of Rape and Sexual Assault*. Emergency Room Rape Crisis Program, North Carolina Memorial Hospital, Chapel Hill, N.C., 1975, Appendix II.
42. Talbert, L.M., and Warren, D.G.: *Guidelines for Management of Suspected Rape*. Chapel Hill, N.C., 1974, Appendix I.
43. Schmidt, P.: Rape Crisis Centers. *Ms.*, September 1973, pp. 14–18.
44. Wasserman, M.: Rape: Breaking the Silence. *The Progressive*, November 1973, pp. 19–23.
45. Horos, C.V.: *Rape*. Tobey Publishing Co., New Canaan, Conn., 1974. (Includes a national directory of rape crisis centers compiled by The Center for Women Policy Studies, Washington, D.C.)

CHAPTER 19

Theoharis K. Seghorn is Clinical Associate in the Psychology Department of Boston University and Director of Clinical Services at the Massachusetts Treatment Center. He completed his undergraduate and graduate studies at Boston University, receiving his doctorate in clinical psychology in 1970. Dr. Seghorn attended postdoctoral seminars at Boston Psychoanalytic Institute under Louis Chase and Norman Zinberg. He is a member of the American Psychological Association and the Society for the Psychological Study of Social Issues.

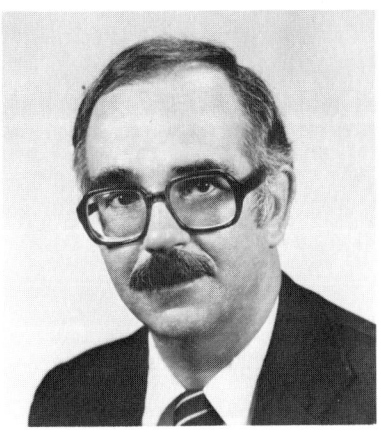

Murray L. Cohen is Professor of Psychology and Director of the Clinical Community Psychology Program at Boston University. He was educated at New York University, the University of Missouri, and Boston University, and is a graduate and Research Fellow of the Boston Psychoanalytic Society and Institute. The author of numerous papers and articles, Dr. Cohen is a member of the American Psychological Association and the American Association for the Advancement of Science.

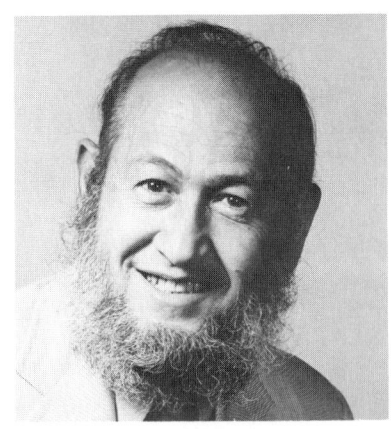

THE PSYCHOLOGY OF THE RAPE ASSAILANT

Theoharis K. Seghorn, Ph.D., and
Murray L. Cohen, Ph.D.

Since the early 1960s, there has been growing awareness that sexual assault is a multidetermined act and that rapists do not represent a homogeneous group in terms of background, psychological characteristics, or dangerousness. Throughout this period and up to the present there continue to be some reports, however, which fail to see this obvious heterogeneity and which attempt to define rape in some simply dynamic, sociological, or accidental terms.[1,2] Recent attempts to impose a single dynamic on what is a social rather than psychiatric or psychological entity are of limited worth in the clinical evaluation of the individual rapist. For example, Gebhard and associates[3] write that rapists are "criminally inclined men who take what they want, whether money, material, or women, and their sex offenses are by-products of their general criminality."

More recently, sociopolitical theories have gained attention. Brownmiller states that rape is an offense which is based on the sociological, historical, and economic fact that women are seen as chattel whose value is lessened by the violation.[4] Thus the act is not pathological, but the pathology resides in the sociocultural atmosphere and belief systems.

This chapter reports on extensive research with a group of rape offenders who have been studied, often for an extensive period of time, during their commitment for observation and treatment at the Bridgewater (Massachusetts) Treatment Center for Sexually Dangerous Persons. Most of this group of offenders committed the rape, or more than one rape, with force and violence. Our studies of this group clearly indicate that while the factors noted above, such as cultural and subcultural conditions, sociopolitical factors, and victim-related variables, play a role in understanding the offense, each individual act of rape is expressive of psychopathology in the rapist, at least among the types of rape offenders seen at the Bridgewater Treatment Center. The act is a living out, with both conscious and unconscious components, of early, unresolved life struggles in the developmental history of the offender which were reactivated in the immediate life situation.

Our clinical observations were made in the course of the 20-year history of the Treatment Center.[5,6,7] Over 1,500 rapists have been screened, more than 400 have been carefully evaluated during the course of a 60-day observation period, and 250 have been intensively studied for periods ranging from 2 to 15 years.

The studies we have conducted clearly indicate a lack of congruence between the psychology of the rapist and any specific psychiatric diagnostic category. Unlike the findings of Glueck and associates,[8] who concluded that most of the sexual offenders studied in New York in the 1950s could be diagnosed as pseudoneurotic schizophrenics, we have observed all types of character neuroses, character disorders, and more severe borderline personality and psychotic states. It is also evident in our experience that there are characteristics specifically involving experience with women, the meaning of sexuality, and the management of aggression which differentiate the rapist from other social offenders and other violent men. In addition, we have discovered that there are basic themes which appear in all studied rapists from the repetitive, frequently unsuccessful and relatively unaggressive rapist (usually charged with assault with intent to rape) to the most brutal psychotic-like rape-murderers. These rapists are differentiated from each other by the relative intensity of these themes and by their patterning.

The purpose of this chapter is to clarify the complex interaction of motivation themes and psychological characteristics of rapists in order to assist the forensic clinician in his or her contribution to the court.

BASIC ASSUMPTIONS

There are four basic assumptions which underlie the remaining discussion. They are as follows:

1. Rape is a meaningful act and its meaning can only be understood by a careful study of the situational context of the offense, the psychological characteristics of the offender, and the immediate and historical forces which act on these characteristics to produce the sexual assault.
2. Rapists are at differential risk to repeat the offense.
3. Although serious and undesirable errors do occur, with intensive study, the clinician can determine those rapists for whom changes in their internal states and external environments are essential in order to place them at minimal risk.
4. For some rapists the process of change must take place in a maximal security setting.

PSYCHOLOGICAL FUNCTIONING

The evaluation of the current psychological state of a rapist is no different from a complete diagnostic evaluation of any patient in clinical practice. We will focus here on those specific psychological features which contribute to the special psychology of the rapist.

The clinician's attention should be directed to a number of broad areas: (1) the offender's adaptation to reality which involves the sense of reality,

reality testing, and the acceptance of reality; (2) the quality, nature, and intensity of deviant sexual arousal which relates to the sexual aims and the degree to which aggressive feelings are connected to, or interwoven with, sexual arousal; (3) the social attitudes, moral responsibility, sense of right and wrong, and all belief systems which motivate the offender to guide, direct, delay, inhibit, or discharge these sexual and aggressive drives; (4) the quality of interpersonal attachments and the balance between the offender's self-directed needs and feelings (narcissism) and his other-directed feelings (object ties); (5) the quality of the offender's narcissism as reflected in appropriate self-esteem, realistic self-confidence, and the self-image, as well as feelings of the self being a meaningful part of a larger society (anomie); (6) related to this is the sense of self-involvement in life experiences which give meaning to existence whether this be in work, avocation, play, or nonutilitarian objects (art or possessions of personal meaning); (7) the availability (in a psychological sense) of alternative sources of gratification when the normal frustrations of life prevent direct fulfillment of important wishes and needs (sublimation and sublimation potential); (8) the ability to be attentive to, and to accurately perceive, the emotional and psychological state of others (empathy) and the ability to respond in terms of the awareness (tact, compassion, social sensitivity); and finally, (9) the management of aggression in adaptive ways as seen in assertiveness, active striving, and mastery.

It is clear that these factors may be differentiated conceptually, but in actuality they are interdependent and highly interrelated. Thus, in the following discussion, although the factors will be clearly identified and some effort will be made to discuss them separately, this separation will not always be possible in practice.

In the rapist, the gross ability to test reality and the reality sense is relatively intact, but there is a deficit in reality testing under stress and in general a marked disturbance in the relationship with, and acceptance of, reality. In addition, under situations of sexual or aggressive arousal, severe reality distortions occur in regard to how the offender sees himself and the victim. Other distortions occur as a result of the lack of a cohesive sense of the self which produces dramatic swings between negative self-evaluations and grandiose ideas and aspirations. The negative self-regard is most usually manifest, although there are instances of superficial masking of it, in a distorted self-confidence (cockiness) or an excessive preoccupation with physical features of the body. There is a constant need for support and approval from others, and the absence of approval is experienced as criticism. Feeling so vulnerable, the rapist tries to fend off further narcissistic injury by externalization of the difficulties experienced in life. Thus, although he is extremely sensitive to criticism, he experiences it as unjustified and further evidence that he is unloved. As part of the deficiencies in positive self-regard, there is a sense of magical entitlement which leads him to expect unexpressed needs to be satisfied, and when they are not, he experiences deprivation, frustration, and rage.

Of most significant diagnostic import are the rapist's feelings, thoughts, and fantasies regarding women; the degree to which these mental structures are sexualized; and the degree to which they contain aggressive or sadistic components. In every rapist there is a distortion of the mental representations of women having three characteristics, sometimes seen separately, but more often in some combination. These include negative images of women as ungiving, uncaring, hostile, controlling, and destroying; ambivalent images in which the ambivalence is split so that some women (especially the mother) are idealized and others are seen in the negative; and an excessive overidealization both of women and of sexual intercourse.

With rapists in whom the first two sets of images exist, women are at the most risk of physical injury or death. With rapists in whom the latter image predominates, the acts are most compulsive and repetitive, but the assaults are less violent.

When the evaluation discloses the overidealization, special attention should be given to defects in healthy narcissism (negative self-esteem) for, in these instances, the need for narcissistic support is fulfilled only by the sexual act within which the rapist seeks to experience the victim's response as the most satisfying sexual encounter in her life. It is only through this that the offender can defend, for a period of time, against the intense feelings brought on by the sense of nothingness.

The degree and level of sexualization of women must be considered in the context of aim-inhibited feelings (warmth, love, kindness, concern) and sublimations (the neutralization of infantile forms of sexuality). The act of rape, although it has the appearance of a genital sexual act, clearly does not involve important features of mature sexuality. Most frequently infantile forms of sexuality (sucking, licking, voyeurism, or exhibitionistic behaviors) are predominant interests, reflecting the rapist's arrested developmental level of sexuality. Alternatively, these interests are in the service of humiliating or degrading the women and reflect the aggressive component of infantile sadism. In many instances the sadistic component is expressed more explicitly in perverted acts of urinating or defecating on the victim or in the variety of forms of mutilation.

Any material indicative of the rapist's sexual preoccupation is of significance—excessive or compulsive masturbation, pornography, attraction to sadistic literature, perverted sexual interests, excessive sexual fantasy life—since they all refer to the relative absence of sublimation. To confirm this, we see an absence of alternative forms of gratification in the life of the dangerous rapist. There is no joy or pleasure in accomplishments, in skill development, in possessions; his life is devoid of active or passive enjoyment in sports, theatre, music, or learning. When we do see participation in some of these social forms, it is superficial and lacks deep attachment and meaning.

Defects in sublimation are mirrored in the absence of ties to social institutions as formal structures (churches or clubs) or as belief systems. There are severe deficiencies in moral values and responsibilities, and those values that are held are peculiarly idiosyncratic and excessively rigid. It is difficult to explain this peculiarity, and therefore a clinical example is offered:

> A young man who had committed a vicious sexual assault on a woman told us that the assault happened on a day when, filled with anger, he was looking for his cousin. She had been babysitting for one of his children, and he had heard from a friend of hers that she had sexually fondled his child. In addition, he was feeling despondent and hopeless because he had been out of a job for some time and there was no food, clothing, or money for electricity or heat. Also, he had sent his other, favorite, child to live with his father, an alcoholic man who had sexually abused our patient throughout his childhood years. We later learned that the severe financial difficulty was due to his refusal to accept unemployment compensation or any support from social agencies be-

cause of a conviction that it was immoral to take from others. Thus he permitted his sense of righteousness to result in the injury of his family and a helpless victim.

Although the rapist is narcissistic in the sense of being self-centered rather than object-centered, there is a serious impairment in healthy narcissism as it involves self-love or sense of an adequate self. This has been mentioned at a number of points in the previous discussion, but here two additional observations can be made. The absence of a sense of self-love prevents the rapist from feeling cared for and loved by others. It has been said that the greatest contribution to the virtuous life is the fear of getting caught. But we must add to this, "and having those who love us become aware of our lack of virtue." For the man who feels that no one truly cares, this external source of control is not available.

A second consequence of an impairment in healthy narcissism is the presence of grandiose ideas and a sense of omnipotence. Not unlike the bipolar depressive syndrome (manic-depressive psychosis), a defensive reaction against the pain of depression is the development of a grandiose self. The major unacceptable feeling of the dangerous rapist is depression related to a sense of helplessness, nothingness, and abandonment. It is a defensive reaction to these feelings that gives rise to the belief that the victim will not report him even though he may clearly identify himself (grandiosity), and that if reported, he will never be convicted (omnipotence).

Related, and contained in all of the above, is the lack of a development of empathy and of an empathic attitude toward others. As the rapist talks about the victim there is a gross lack of awareness of her horror and fear of injury and the sexual anxiety, shame, and disgust she must have felt. Such insensitivity is found as the offender talks about all significant persons in his life.

The clinical findings in the area of the management of aggression are quite clear. Every rapist has presented with a problem in the control or adaptive expression of aggression, but a number of different patterns of this problem appear. In one pattern there is a component that appears similar to Megargee's finding of overcontrol.[9] Such rapists have lived excessively passive, blocked, inhibited lives marked by an inability to achieve, attain, or progress in all spheres of life. The offender has no sense of active mastery, and frequently, as we will see below, the act of rape is dynamically related to mastery needs.

In a second pattern, aggressive attitudes and responses are a style of life in an individual who experiences the process of living as a Darwinian fight for survival. The aggression is not managed, directed, or controlled and is maladaptive in both its appropriateness as a response and its intensity. The objects of the aggression are not differentiated with regard to sex, age, or relationship to the offender. All human relationships are experienced with alertness to assault, and each encounter has a victor and a victim. Often there is no conscious experience of anger, and even brutal assaults can be affectless. In other instances a tone of anger is always present or imminent.

In a third pattern, angry and hostile feelings and aggressive behavior are specifically related to women. In some rapists, this is a characteristic feature of all relationships to women, and in others, it is specific to situations involving real or imagined sexual relations. In this latter instance the sexual arousal is accompanied by an anticipated sexual rejection or humiliation, and the aggressive response is reactive to this narcissistic insult.

In a fourth pattern, the disturbance in the management of aggression is due to the sexualization of the aggression. One rapist, after many years of therapy, described with some inner pain and distress how he could not prevent his sexual fantasies, which began with images of making love to a woman, from turning into thoughts of disemboweling her. Another could only have intercourse with his wife if she would permit him to tie her up and submit to somewhat muted sadistic acts.

FACTORS IN DEVELOPMENTAL HISTORY

No set of factors has been found which is in itself pathognomonic. For example, the frequently described triad of enuresis, fire-setting, and cruelty to animals is seen in the history of many rapists, but is not present in the most dangerous rape offenders. If the behavior has continued into adolescence, it should certainly be given serious weight. The same is true of a history of being used as a sexual object or being raised in a family where cruel, aggressive, and brutal behavior by the mother or father was present.

The psychological or physical absence of the father or of a significant male figure is of singular importance when the mother-child relationship is disordered. The dysfunctional relationship can take many forms such as emotional abandonment; harsh, cruel, and unloving mothering; explicit sexual behavior; or the prevention of separation and growth through reinforcement of regressive dependent behaviors.

In a large number of men found to be dangerous, the early childhood years were marked by "chaos"—sudden deaths in the family, automobile accidents or accidents within the home, frequent relocation of homes, sudden disappearance of a parent, emergency hospitalizations of the child or a family member, and interventions by social agencies (police, welfare, schools). It is as if some threat was always imminent.

Although we need much more careful study of these early years, it does appear that the rapist at most risk to repeat has had parenting which was poor and extremely unstable and an early childhood marked by difficulties with each of the basic tasks of development. However, as stated above, no specific pathogenic experiences have been discerned.

Developmental disturbances often continue through primary school years, the period of latency. He is unable to adapt to the generalized rules of the classroom, and two reactive patterns appear. Either he is disruptive, demanding of attention, and somewhat hyperkinetic, or he is passively aggressive in withdrawal and silent surliness. In either instance, peer relationships do not form, a sense of isolation and "being different" develops, basic learning skills are unnurtured, and, of great importance since most of the primary teachers are women, these negative experiences become associated with the inner representations of the "bad mother."

An important consequence is the reduction of resources for the development of sublimations. And since a major prognostic sign for dangerousness is the absence of sublimations and the defects in sublimation potentials, a careful study of the early childhood years and latency period is of great importance.

We must now raise a caution. We have seen a number of rapists who have committed particularly violent offenses, and whom we consider at risk to commit similar acts in the future, in whom this early and middle childhood pattern is not present. The underlying schizoid, acting-out, impulse disorder of borderline personality organization does not clearly manifest itself until adulthood. What is seen in its place is the excessively "good boy" who does not appear as a problem to parents, teachers, or social authorities. Peer relations are poor, but not obviously pathological. In these instances, under close examination, the good behavior is not a result of a coherent, internal set of attitudes and values of right and wrong, but arises from a defective sense of self and self-love. In other words, comfort does not come from carrying out or fulfilling a personal value (which would then lead to an enhanced "liking of oneself"); the motivation is instead to please the other so as to get the love and approval from the other. However, since there is a basic narcissistic deficit, the need for constant, unequivocal approval is so great that frustrations of the need must take place. Since here again the woman (mother, teacher) is frequently the agent of the frustration, particular negative, angry images are developed. The defect here is the failure of development of a self-esteem based on achievement and mastery.

An additional prognostic sign in the latency period is the presence of sexual behavior, sexual preoccupation, or sexual aggression. This is, of course, related to absence of the development of socialization as represented in sublimations. The infantile sexual life fails to become neutralized and internal resources for the expression of the child's impulse life fail to develop beyond direct or indirect sexual and sexual-aggressive forms. This failure also impacts on emotional development, and we see an absence of feelings of warmth, tenderness, love, compassion, sympathy, and empathy. In general, all altruistic feelings fail to mature.

Major attention must be paid to postpubertal development and to the adolescent years. In the dangerous rapist,* the increase in sexual drives that occur in puberty meets with no organized, internalized set of moral values (superego lacunae) and no altruistic feelings which could serve to modulate or delay their expression. The defect in sublimation prevents the neutralization of these drives, and we see the full range of sexual perversions surfacing. These may include voyeurism, sex play with animals, exhibitionism, frottage, obscene telephone calls, preoccupation with sexual sadistic fantasies, drawing pictures of girls in pornographic scenes, fetishisms, cross-dressing, excessive masturbation, coprophagia, and masochistic self-mutilation.

The tasks of adolescence are poorly negotiated by the dangerous rapist; these include separation from the parental ties and individuation of self, development of a realistic identity, seeking and establishing ties to peers without giving up a primary sense of self, further skill development for later life careers, establishment of heterosexual attachments, and re-establishment of moral and social attitudes at levels of self-integrity and self-esteem. The degree of failure in the management of these tasks is of critical importance for the clinical judgment, although when there is some degree of mismanagement in each of these spheres, this itself is indicative of a volatile, unstable character. The offender presenting such a picture in the context of having committed even one sexual assault should be considered at high risk.

---

*In our program, a "dangerous rapist" is one at high risk to commit further aggressive, assaultive rapes if not successfully treated. See further discussion in the upcoming section on prognosis and treatment.

THE DYNAMICS OF RAPE

Classification

The clinical and research literature contains many attempts at classifying rapists according to the motivational state of the offender during the sexual assault. Guttmacher and Weihofen found several discriminable classes among rapists based on motivation factors.

> Forced rape . . . has several basic motivational patterns. There is the rapist whose assault is the explosive expression of a pent-up sexual impulse. Or it may occur in individuals with strong latent homosexual components . . . These are the true sex offenders. Another type that is also sexual in origin, although not so manifestly so, is the sadistic rapist . . . Many of these individuals have their deep-seated hatred focused particularly on women. Then there is the third type of rapist who, paradoxically, is not primarily a sex offender. He is the aggressive, antisocial criminal who, like the soldier of a conquering army, is out to pillage and rob.[10]

Four groups are described by the authors, and although they do not present them in such terms, the following more dynamic statements seem to reflect their findings: (1) rape motivated by a sexual impulse which becomes so intense that defensive or controlling efforts were overwhelmed and the sexual desire was expressed; (2) rape that was not a breakdown of defense, but was itself a defense against strong homosexual wishes; (3) rape that was the expression not only of sexuality, but of a deep-seated hatred or aggressive feelings toward women; and (4) rape that did not so much express sexual or aggressive wishes, but rather a more general predatory disposition.

Gebhard and associates,[11] in their large-scale statistical study, described two major categories of rapists: (1) those for whom the aggression is the means to an end and who employ no more force than is necessary to achieve the end (usually coitus); and (2) those for whom violence is an end in itself or at least a secondary goal. In these cases the woman is either subjected to more force than is necessary or is mistreated after the sexual activity has ended.

Williams[12] eschews classification, but does show an appreciation for the complexity of rape, including the interaction of motivational and controlling forces. The latter forces involve both the developmental level of ties to the external object and the quality of the internalized restraining influences. Any given act of rape is a result of sexual and aggressive forces as they interact with control forces which are developmentally rooted in object relationships. The particularities of the act represent a point on a continuum.

Theme of Motivation

In studying the assaults and elaborating the findings by clinical data obtained from the treatment of rapists, we have found a broader range of motivations than described by others. We refer to them as themes in order to reflect the fact that they represent not only basic or derived needs, but include also the conscious and unconscious meanings of the needs and their emotional accompaniments.

A common theme is the rapist's desire to place the woman in a helpless, powerless, and submissive position. Some rapists describe this as the primary feeling and become more sexually aroused as they experience this sense of control and mastery of the woman. As this theme is analyzed by further clinical data, three separate, although interdependent, subthemes are found. First we see the need to place the woman in a passive position as an act of retribution through displacement. The offender feels helpless with women who he believes have made him powerless. An offender told us, "I feel helpless, very helpless in that I couldn't do anything about the satisfaction I wanted. Well, I'm going to put them in a position where they can't do anything about what I want to do."

A second subtheme, at a more unconscious level, is found in projective identification of the passive, helpless part of the rapist's personality which he is not able to accept. For a rapist in whom this theme is dominant, his own passive feelings are completely unacceptable and, in the victim's helplessness, he is able to deny his own sense of helplessness.

In the third subtheme, this mastery has the meaning of an identification with the woman the rapist has made helpless. The sexual pleasure derives from this identification which, in turn, is derived from the wish to be raped by a man or a phallic woman.

Within these themes, although the motivations are vicissitudes of aggression, there is relatively little physical injury to the victim.

In two related themes, the victim is at greater risk and frequently is verbally and physically assaulted. In the first, the primary feeling toward the victim is contempt, and the motivation is to degrade or defile her. An offender brutally forced a pregnant woman to engage in fellatio with him and then asked her if she would be able to look at her new child and if her husband would ever again want to kiss her. In the second theme, the feeling is not contempt but anger, and the sexuality serves not to degrade but to hurt in a more direct physical sense. A young man had just put his mother, who was in an alcoholic stupor, into her bed. As he turned away, he saw his mother's image in the mirror with her genitals exposed. He had an immediate thought to have intercourse with her and then the thought, in his words, "to eat her out." He was overwhelmed with a sense of rage, left the house, and ran through the street, smashing windows and breaking the antennas of automobiles. He then saw a woman on the street in front of him; he ran to her, grabbed her, pulled her off the street, and sexually assaulted her.

These feelings toward total strangers are understood in terms of a displacement from other significant figures as part of the process discussed earlier as a splitting of ambivalence. In these instances the displaced feelings of such offenders serve to maintain the positive and overidealized images of certain women, most usually the mother of their earliest years.

Although the victims in the two previous themes are at great risk, in two other themes the likelihood of severe injury is still greater. In the first, no positive images of women appear, but only images which serve as the object for the most intense rage. Women are seen as sexual opponents in a life and death struggle. Although women are at all times at some risk around such men (since the level of aggression is so high), the act of rape is realized when some sexual excitation occurs in the man. The excitation may be triggered by a memory, a fantasy, or the seeing of a woman. When the feeling occurs, it is believed to be provoked by the woman for hostile or destructive reasons, and the potential rapist feels under assault. He experiences his sexual attack, if there is any opportunity for one, as a counterattack, and the rage is destructive. In such cases, women are more often brutally assaulted and occasionally are murdered. As his rage increases, the offender's sexual feelings subside, he loses his erection, and he sees this as further proof that he has been sexually assaulted by the woman. A 16-year-old boy was asked by a summer resident of a vacation area to help her put away outdoor furniture. As they entered the house and the woman preceded him up the stairs, the boy had the thought that she was making a sexual invitation. This was followed by the thought that if he responded, she would reject and ridicule him. The boy became angry and felt that he hated her, and as they passed the fireplace, he picked up a poker and knocked her to the floor. As he was undressing her, he lost his erection. He had been astride her, but now he rolled her in the floor rug and beat her until he thought she was dead.

The second theme in which the woman's life is much endangered arises in those rapists in whom erotic and aggressive feelings are combined in what is known as sadism. In such offenders, the intensities of the two impulses serve to reinforce each other so that as aggressive feelings increase and are expressed, the offender becomes more sexually excited. As the excitation increases, the aggression becomes not only more intense, but of a more regressive, primitive, destructive quality. It is from this theme that the "lust murder" derives, and the victim's body shows the result of this sexual-aggressive frenzy.

In other themes, the aggression is more instrumental in the presence of intense sexual wishes. In one such theme, the rapist idealizes both women and the sexual act. Here the theme represents a sought for but never realized fantasy of a sexual experience with a sought for but never obtained, fantasied woman. It is in this theme that the clinical interpretation of rape as a living out of the Oedipal conflict is most supported. A rather dramatic example is a young man who admitted to over 200 sexual assaults, but in only two cases did he penetrate the woman. Prior to an attack, he would feel his body grow warm and he would feel it begin to swell. His fantasy was that the woman would yield to his approach, permit him to have intercourse, and then praise him for his adequacy.

Similar to this is the "machismo" theme, involving both individual and social factors. Here there is a self and peer definition of masculinity which not only gives license to rape, but also makes it a desideratum. "Scoring," and not the pleasurable response of the victim, is the major feature of this theme.

There are two additional themes in which the aggression is secondary to a component of sexuality. In both instances, the sexual assault results from an effort to fend off sexual anxiety. In the first, the source of the anxiety is a growing awareness of sexual interest in men, in male genitalia, and in sexual activities with men, namely fellatio and sodomy. The rape is the offender's shout to himself and to the world that he is not a homosexual. In the second instance, the source of anxiety is a sense of sexual inadequacy or of phallic incompetency, and the sexual assault is a psychological attempt to relieve this anxiety. In this instance, the offender asks the victim about his performance, yearning to hear that he "did well." Karpman[13] referred to the psychoanalytic concept of "castration anxiety" as an underlying feature of rape, and Hammer's study[14] found such anxiety in his sample of rapists.

Despite the fact that aggression is not the principal intent in these last two themes, the woman is at some risk to be injured if the offender's defensive efforts are not successful; that is, if the offender does not find relief from his homosexual feelings or his sense of inadequacy.

With regard to basic motivational factors, the act of rape descriptively involves both an aggressive and a sexual component, but in any particular assault, the relative importance of these impulses can vary. The primary aim may be hostile and destructive with the sexual factor in the service of this aggressive motivation. In other instances, the sexual motivation is primary and the aggressive aspects of the assault are instrumental for the fulfillment of the sexual aim. In a third pattern, the two basic motives are less differentiated and fused, and the resultant behavior can best be understood as fulfilling a sexual sadistic aim. Finally, in a fourth pattern, neither sexual nor aggressive motivation is in a heightened state, and the act is expressive of a general impairment of impulse control. This pattern is exhibited by men who are defined as social deviants, but they are not sexually or psychologically deviant.[15-18]

The Sexual Assault

It has become clear, and it is the major thesis of this chapter, that attention only to these or other motivational factors is an empty enterprise which may yield reliable classification but tells us very little for use in prognosis and treatment planning. In earlier sections the characteristics and developmental history of rapists were presented and the motivational themes were described. In the remainder of this section, attention will be turned to the specific organization of these components which produces the unique form and meaning of the assault. It is only when the clinician can determine, with some degree of completeness, why a particular man, at a particular time, carried out a given form of rape that a clinically sound recommendation for disposition can be made.

AGGRESSIVE AIM RAPE

In this pattern, the sexual assault is primarily an aggressive destructive act. The sexual behavior is not the expression of a sexual wish, but serves to humiliate, defile, hurt, or destroy the victim. The degree of violence may vary from simple assault to brutal, vicious attacks resulting in the victim's death. When aspects of sexuality are present, they enter the service of aggression, ranging from relatively benign verbal abuse, through biting and cutting, to the extreme of tearing of the genitals or breast, rupture of the anus through violent insertion of some object, or other sexually mutilating acts.

The women clearly appear to be victims of the offender's destructive wishes, and the rapist often readily describes his emotional state as one of anger. The anger that is experienced is clearly a displacement onto the substitute object, almost always a complete stranger. Most often a reconstruction of the circumstances leading up to the offense places the source of this rage in the mother or representations of her in a wife or girlfriend.

Rape occasionally occurs in the offender's automobile where the victim is brought either by physical force or by threat with a weapon. More likely the rape occurs in the victim's home with entrance gained by means of some ruse. The offense can often occur as a series of rapes committed within a relatively brief interval.

The offense appears often as an isolated behavioral loss of control in an otherwise superficially normal social and psychiatric history. The clinical interview reveals a long history of difficulty in heterosexual object relations despite a sexually active social life. For example, though many of these men are married, and those who are not are engaged or dating with regularity, there are difficulties in these relationships representing disturbances in warm and positive emotional feelings. The relationships are often marked by anger, mutual irritation, and at times, violence. This type of rapist tends to experience women negatively, as hostile, demanding, ungiving, and unfaithful. It is of interest that the women such men select as companions are often assertive and active, and by their manner and attitude, they place the offender in an intolerable, passive position. Thus the offender appears to create the very conflict in heterosexual relations that he then reacts to so inappropriately.

Most of these offenders have adequate occupational adjustments, showing not only a stability of work, but high-level skills and achievement with qualities of inventiveness and creativity. While able to enter into cooperative sharing relationships with men, they remain basically competitive, and the passive demands of mutuality lead to conflict and stress. In adolescence they often exhibit excessive, exaggerated masculine activity, often in partially controlled, socially acceptable, aggressive behavior, such as street brawls and high-speed driving. In nearly all of these men, there is an excessive body concern and a body narcissism. They are physically attractive and tend to be attentive to bodily health and hygiene.

There are moderate obsessive features, and the explosive outbursts can be seen to represent a regression as a response to different types of stress. While the outbursts may find socially acceptable outlets and allow feelings of warmth and kindness to be expressed, the dominant mode of relating is in a cool, detached, overcontrolled manner. As indicated, this type of offender is excessively counterdependent and intolerant of the passive aspects required of true mutuality in relationships. As a result, true friendships are rare, primarily because of the absence of depth and intensity in the formulation of object ties. It is this aspect which ultimately facilitates the release and expression of unneutralized aggression. What is noteworthy is that once control is re-established, feelings of concern appear, and efforts to undo or make some kind of restitution to the victim are evident above and beyond mere expressions of guilt. For example, the rapist will wash the victim, help her on with her clothes, or drive her to her home.

This reaction of concern is related to the underlying splitting and isolation of ambivalent feelings between the overidealized image of their mothers (or women in the abstract) as sources of all infantile and narcissistic needs and their experiencing, in their actual relationships with women, feelings of untrustworthiness, deprivation, and lack of faithfulness.

The splitting of ambivalence is only one feature of the defensive structure that includes displacement and isolation as primary mechanisms. Counterphobic attitudes prevail to assist in the defense against castration fears or more primitive anxiety, but it is the ineffectiveness of this defense that gives rise to the aggression when a woman is the source of the anxiety. The data seem to be best understood in terms of a decompensation often approaching psychotic proportions in men who have been otherwise able to deal with their intense rage toward women in relatively successful ways. The intense aggression appears to be both the result of splitting of ambivalence and a defense against experiencing the helplessness they fear in all object relationships, but most intensely with women.

SEXUAL AIM RAPE

A second pattern of characteristics that has been observed is quite different from that given above. Here the act of rape is clearly motivated by sexual wishes, and, though the degree of aggressive behavior varies, there is a relative absence of violence and brutality. The aggressive behavior is primarily in the service of the sexual aim.

The offense almost always takes place out of doors in isolated, darkened streets, parks, or wooded areas. Most frequently the offender approaches and embraces the women from behind, touching her breasts or genitals, holding on to her with some, but not excessive, force. If the victim should struggle, the offender will often release her and flee. Thus, in most instances, the actual charge will involve assault with intent to commit rape. At other times, the victim is so frightened that she passively submits, and the rape takes place without any additional force. It is often discovered that this pattern has been repeated many times in the past. An example in our experience was an offender who had assaulted over 200 women without ever having actually committed a rape.

The pattern is often similar: the victim is always a stranger, one who has been observed and followed until she enters an isolated area. The act itself is a living out of a fantasy with which the offender has been preoccupied and which he has employed in masturbation. In the fantasy the woman he attacks at first protests and then submits, more resignedly than willingly. During the sexual act, he performs with great skill, and she receives such intense pleasure that she falls in love with him and pleads with him to return. This is not an unusual fantasy of adolescent boys. But in these men the fantasy is given expression, and it is of such intensity that occasionally such a rapist approaches his victim after the offense with the belief that she will then accept his invitation for a continued relationship. Such men are preoccupied with sexual daydreams and fantasies and are compulsive masturbators. Aggression is not always present in the fantasies, and when it is, it appears in rather muted forms. There is no evidence from the offender's behavior, his conscious fantasies, or in the unconscious dynamics of the assaults that the aggression is eroticized to the degree of sadism seen in the third pattern of rape to be discussed below.

Sexual fantasies and assaults of this type are not the only indicators of a disturbed sexual life. From early in adolescence there is a marked inhibition in relations with female peers and an active involvement in perversions including sex play with animals, wearing women's underclothing, voyeurism, exhibitionism, frottage, and fetishisms. Relationships with male peers are similarly disturbed, in this instance, due to an inadequate sublimation or repression of homosexual feelings. In order to deal with the unacceptable homosexual wishes, the child is forced to avoid male companionship and thus becomes lonely and withdrawn. As he moves through his adolescent years, the sense of loneliness increases and he becomes increasingly shy and inept in social skills, which accentuates the passive features of his personality and intensifies the feelings of impotency and inadequacy. Passive gratification through his fantasies becomes the substitute for active mastery and further inhibits the development of a masculine identity. As such individuals approach the end of adolescence and enter young adult life, the passive solution intensifies underlying homosexual feelings which further threaten the repression. The acts of rape occur at this time and represent not only a defense against the homosexual wish, but also adaptive efforts to escape the implications of the passive-feminine resolution, to escape from the sense of the self as impotent and psychologically castrated. In addition, the offenses relieve the shame (and perhaps guilt) of the persistent pregenital perversions.

This type of rapist shows little or no antisocial behavior apart from the repetitive sexual offenses. He is, in fact, socially submissive and compliant, perceived by friends and neighbors as a quiet, shy, "good boy," more lonely than most, but nonetheless quite normal. In most areas of his life there is a general absence of even appropriate amounts of aggressive and assertive behavior. His approach to the tasks of life is tentative and has a phobic quality. This lack of assertiveness combines with a very negative self-esteem and a low level of aspiration, which prevents him from making significant attainments in either educational or occupational areas. There is a stable employment history, but the level of work is far below his aptitude and potential abilities. Despite a normal range of intelligence in this group, scholastic records show generally poor performance and frequent withdrawal from school prior to graduation.

The defensive structures, apart from the avoidance, repression, and inhibition described above include introjection mechanisms (reflecting the diffuseness in identity formation), projection of the severity of the superego (so that he feels despised and anticipates rejection), and a childlike denial (manifested by a naivete that permits him to be victimized and used by others).

A specific family pattern is noted in the histories of such rapists, which includes a weak father, not a passive, submissive man, but one who found the demands of family responsibility overwhelming and reneged in his role as father and husband. The mother tended to be nurturant, but very cold and hypercritical and an inconsistent but harsh disciplinarian who infantilized her son by overwhelming control and suppression. These mothers appear to have been preoccupied with sexual morality, and the most excessive control and rejection occurs in response to any expression of erotic interests or pleasure.

SEX-AGGRESSION DIFFUSION

A third pattern of characteristics we have observed reveals the presence of a strong sadistic component. There appears to be no ability to experience sexual acts without some degree of violence being present. The degree of sadism is quite variable with the extreme position seen in lust murders where excessive brutality and mutilation occur before, during, and even after the murder. This is relatively rare. The most usual behavioral pattern is forcible rape where the victim's defensive efforts and the offender's violence further excite the offender, the rape becoming a frenzied, sadistic act. After intercourse there is typically no further aggression. Such a offender is frequently impotent with women unless there is resistance. To become sexually excited, he will provoke in a teasing, playfully sexual manner, eliciting resistant behavior from his partner. Her resistance arouses in him aggressive feelings that become more intense and autonomous as his sexual arousal continues. The arousal and maintenance of the sexual desire appear to be a direct function of this initially mild arousal of aggression, but it should be noted that the emotion of anger is not present.

In most patients in this group, the sadistic quality of their sexuality is projected onto the victim. The victim's struggle and protestation are perceived as part of her own sexual excitation and not as a refusal: "Women like to get roughed up; they enjoy a good fight."

Although there is some neutralization of the aggression in relationships unrelated to sexual situations, the qualities of untamed aggression are still evident. Such individuals are assertive, overpowering, and somewhat hostile in all situations. Warmth and affection are completely absent. The most friendly meeting is punctuated by touching and pushing so that an encounter with such persons is a "bruising" one.

Such patients are usually married and in fact may have been married and divorced a number of times, always with a lack of true commitment to the relationship. The offender, and often his wife, are quite active in extramarital affairs. For him, this constant search and seduction is essential for his sexual excitement, not as a defense against feelings of inadequacy, but to satisfy the aggressive component of his sexual wishes. Intercourse with his wife is described as physically relieving but unsatisfactory; not infrequently he has difficulty in obtaining or maintaining an erection and normal connubial coitus is followed by feelings of revulsion. In some instances he can obtain satisfaction with aggression modulated by having his wife play a masochistic role. The wife, for example, permits herself to be tied up and verbally abused as she acts out a scene of being physically assaulted and raped by a stranger.

Persons exhibiting sex-aggression diffusion possess traits similar to those found in the psychopathic character. There is an extensive history of nonsexual, antisocial behavior, an absence of stable object ties, a lack of concern for others, difficulty in tolerating frustration, poorly structured control functions, and a relative absence of intrapsychic discomfort. These character defects in the organization and control of their instinctual life do not, however, prevent them from demonstrating industry and initiative in skill development, although this cannot be used for a socially successful occupational career. While the quest for manipulation and control of others is present to a great degree, gratification is also obtained through active mastery and personal accomplishment.

Developmentally there is an absence of the latency period. Sexual and aggressive behavior toward younger children, peers, and animals is prominent throughout the prepubertal years. Other indications of impulsive behavior and general lack of control are expressed in truancy, stealing, running away, and lying.

Such a behavior pattern is also found in the antisocial character disorder. In adolescence, significant differences appear in the organization of aggression which distinguish the sex-aggressive rapist from the antisocial individual. In the latter, the aggression comes under the control of the ego and serves it in its adaptive efforts. Aggression is relatively organized, controlled, and directed. In the sex-aggressive rapist, the aggression continues to be diffuse and unorganized; it maintains its primitive quality. The sexualization of the aggression so overwhelms the ego when the aggression is aroused that the control and discharge mechanisms fail to function. The antisocial individual may commit an assault or murder through the absence of concern for objects or to prevent the detection of his pillaging, but in such instances the aggressive behavior is organized in the service of survival.

In comparison with the other types of rapists, the sex-aggressive offender exhibits the clearest presence of paranoid features which, under certain conditions, are of a psychotic nature. Every human contact is approached with mistrust and suspicion and is experienced as a battle in which someone wins and someone loses; there is a total inability to experience interpersonal mutuality. Developmentally, the early lives of such persons are tempestuous times. Family life is marked by cruel and abusive behavior of the family members toward each other, except for the mother.

She is often described as the only member of the family with warm and compassionate feelings. Her pathologic need to give and to protect herself and her children from a typically sadistic father distorts her judgment of her children's behavior. She denies, rationalizes, and excuses the defective development of internal controls and actively supports a primitive oral demand pattern. The fathers of these patients are physically and psychologically cruel and sadistic, not only in their own behavior, but also in their incitement, support, and demands for similar behavior among the children.

IMPULSIVE RAPE

The final group we have observed is composed of rapists in whom neither sexual nor aggressive impulses play a dominant role in the act itself. This is the group which most closely fits the formulations of the antisocial character disorder. Such persons should not be considered sexually deviant in the ordinary sense of the term. The act of rape for this offender appears to be merely another manifestation of the inability to delay gratification of any impulse. In response to a transient sexual urge, he seeks gratification with the nearest available objects. In some instances the rape occurs as an incidental event in the course of another offense. A victim, accidentally discovered by the offender in the midst of a burglary, is raped because she is available and helpless. The degree of aggression is that consistent with the force necessary to gain control over the victim. In contrast with the sex-aggressive rapist, the aggression is goal-directed, under ego control, and serves the narcissistic sexual aim. The act is spontaneous rather than premeditated, and this impulsiveness characterizes the life-long adjustment problems of these men. The victim is raped because she is available and another object to be manipulated for the assailant's own narcissistic gratification. As others have noted, his stance pervades all of his relationships, and under normal circumstances he would have little difficulty in manipulating and seducing willing partners.

PROGNOSIS AND TREATMENT

Clinical evaluation of the rapist carries with it the task of making prognostic statements to the courts concerning the likelihood that the offender represents a continued threat to the community, his need for treatment and his treatability, and the setting where such treatment should occur.

The formulation that has been presented states that the evaluation must consider the state of the offender's ego functioning (reality testing, impulse control, attachments, etc.), the intensity and aim of his aggressive and sexual drives, and his environment (as a source of support and stress). We must note that the importance of the ultimate decision, involving as it does the potential deprivation of a person's liberty on the one hand and the danger to society on the other, demands the most comprehensive study. It is our experience that the assessment requires an extended period of time and a variety of clinical and behavioral data including those obtained from clinical interviews, an up-to-date probation report, psychological tests, and, when appropriate, interviews with the offender's family, employers, and victim.

The evaluation should also include a careful review of all official records and transcripts with a detailed study of the offense. Given the vicissitudes of plea-bargaining and other vagaries of the prosecutorial process, the actual charge may bear little relationship to the severity of the offense and the degree of pathology it indicates.

In the remainder of this section we will discuss the two major alternative dispositions: probation with outpatient treatment, and sentencing with residential treatment. It should be recognized that the clinician may be asked for a recommendation, but it is the court's ultimate responsibility in its role as an agent of the community to weigh retributive, protective, and rehabilitative needs in making a final decision concerning disposition.

Outpatient Management

The possibility of probation and outpatient treatment is likely to be entertained (1) when the offender has no prior court record or when the criminal history is relatively benign; (2) when the offense did not involve physical violence and the victim was uninjured; (3) where the adjustment prior to the offense shows significant strengths; (4) when the offense took place in the context of a clearly defined, unusual set of precipitating events; (5) when the offender truly feels guilt and remorse; (6) when the offender has social and occupational skills; (7) when there are supports available in the community such as a strong, intact family and employment opportunities; and finally (8) when the offender's current psychological status examination reveals no serious mental disorder.

We emphasize the need for clinical services to be augmented by probation supervision since experience has shown that the formation of a therapeutic alliance is extremely difficult. In the early stages of treatment, the offender appears to have re-established his premorbid level of adjustment. He appears to be working hard at understanding himself, his feelings, and the reasons for his behavior. The family or marital situation which may have been a contributing factor in the offense appears to function more smoothly than ever as the parents or wife unites with the offender against the external threat of prosecution and potential loss of freedom. Within a short period of time, however, as the immediate pressures are relieved, there is a re-emergence of characterologic defenses of avoidance and denial. The precipitating stresses, submerged under the greater threat of prosecution, surface with renewed intensity. Unresolved family problems intensify and are added to by the family's anger at the offender because of the public shame and embarrassment he has caused. The offender once again feels overwhelmed and may experience intense resistance to continuing a treatment which forces him to face these difficulties and to examine the underlying conflicts.

At such times it is only the authority of the court, maintained through probation supervision, which can insure continued cooperation in psychotherapy until these new hurdles are overcome.

Residential Treatment

At the other extreme are those persons whose offense is especially violent. The victim has been severely injured, and the offender has a history of similar assaults with or without a clear sexual intent. The aggression and rage characterizing the offense are characteristic of his interpersonal relationships, there is a lack of guilt or remorse, and there is a distortion in his perception of the victim and her role in the offense. The adjustment prior to the offense was poor, with minimal social and occupational skills, and the clinician concludes that there is a high probability of a recurrence of another dangerous offense within the environment to which the rapist is likely to return. Such "dangerous rapists" require extended inpatient treatment in a secure facility where the maximum therapeutic contribution of socialization and rehabilitation efforts found in a multidisciplinary, educational, vocational, and recreational program can be coordinated with intensive individual and group psychotherapy. Such a program is not feasible within a general correctional facility which, owing to its impersonality, ultimately reinforces adaptive mechanisms which are directly contrary to those necessary to effective extramural adjustment. Treatment for such dangerous rapists must encompass every aspect of their lives within the institution; even mundane aspects of daily life become the focus of therapy as patients learn to live together and accept increasing responsibility for their lives. The process is a protracted one and must provide for gradual reintegration into the community, with continuing long-term treatment and supportive services offered after the offender has returned to his home.

We view the minimum duration of treatment of the "dangerous rapist" in most cases as extending beyond 8 years (including inpatient and outpatient status) from the point of commitment to final termination of outpatient services. The reason for such an intensive long-term program is that for the patient, the task requires nothing short of a major restructuring of his adaptive functioning.

In formal group and individual psychotherapy, the patient works to understand the motivation for the offense and its origins in his life history. In group psychotherapy, interpersonal relationships are explored; perceptions of others and their perceptions of the patient are confirmed or reassessed and the distortion process understood. Guided groups within living quarters explore issues such as cooperation and shared responsibility in the maintenance of a stable microcommunity. The effort here is to develop a reflective rather than reactive orientation in dealing with conflict and stress. Finally, there is a strong emphasis on the development of conflict-free ego interests and skills as alternative, sublimated sources of gratification and as buttresses against regression in the face of potential assaults on ego integrity. Possibilities for reintegration into the community should be flexible and gradual, but definite. Of primary importance is the development of a working alliance with the therapist so that conflicts, wishes, and feelings are brought to treatment to be shared, understood, and worked through. Gradual access to the community enables the patient to test reality and his newly developing internal resources. Active treatment must continue well beyond the time a patient has been fully integrated into the community and achieves full outpatient status. Of crucial importance in such treatment is the recognition by therapists that new tasks and achievements signal not only progress, but also new sources of stress. Job promotions, plans to marry, or the birth of a child can foster a potential for regression as well as growth, and unless conflicts and feelings are addressed directly by the therapist there is a strong potential for pathologic reactions, such as acting out, during such periods. Treatment which may have been supportive in focus must reintensify toward active confrontation of the feelings about the life changes.

The percentage of rapists requiring such intensive court-ordered rehabilitation is small, on the order of 5 percent. For the majority of rapists who are likely to be incarcerated, the defects in functioning and distortions in interpersonal relationships, while present, are not sufficiently severe to warrant their commitment to a special facility for "sexually dangerous offenders." For such men a similar range of services and treatment should be available during the term of their incarceration, on a voluntary basis, either within existing correctional facilities or at special centers specifically intended for this purpose. While such persons are felt to be at lesser risk for a repetition of sexual assaults, the symptomatic pathology seen in the commission of the rape should be dealt with.

Finally, we turn to the unapprehended rapist who, according to most crime statistics, represents the majority of rapists who have committed such an offense. At the present time there is an overwhelming dearth of services available to these men who, often in crisis, recognize the need for treatment as they experience the fantasies or impulses to commit a sexual assault, or who, unapprehended, have already begun a pattern of such assaultive behavior. Utilizing even the limited current knowledge about rape and dangerous sexual assault, our communities could offer preventive treatment to such men who, because of fear, are unable to approach more traditional mental health delivery systems.

REFERENCES

1. Amir, M.: *Patterns in Forcible Rape*. University of Chicago Press, Chicago, 1971.
2. Gebhard, P., et al.: *Sex Offenders*. Harper & Row, New York, 1965.
3. Ibid., p. 205.
4. Brownmiller, S.: *Against Our Will*. Simon & Schuster, New York, 1975.
5. Cohen, M. L., Seghorn, T. K., and Calmas, W.: Sociometric Study of the Sex Offender. *J. Abnormal Psychol.* 74:249–255, 1969.
6. Cohen, M. L., et al.: The Psychology of the Rapist. *Semin. Psychiatry* 3:307–327, 1971.
7. Cohen, M. L., and Boucher, R. J.: *Clinical Prediction of Sexual Dangerousness*. American Correctional Association, Memphis, 1977.
8. Glueck, B.: *Final Report on Deviated Sex Offenders*. Department of Mental Hygiene, New York, 1956.
9. Magargee, E.: Undercontrolled and Overcontrolled Personality Types in Extreme Antisocial Aggression. *Psychological Monographs* 80(3), 1966.
10. Guttmacher, M., and Weihofen, H.: *Psychiatry and the Law*. W. W. Norton, New York, 1952, p. 116.
11. Gebhard, op. cit., p. 196.
12. Williams, A. H.: Rape-murder, in Slovenko, R. (ed.): *Sexual Behavior and the Law*. Charles C Thomas, Springfield, Ill., 1965.
13. Karpman, B.: *The Sexual Offender and His Offenses*. The Julian Press, New York, 1954.
14. Hammer, E.: A Comparison of H.T.P's of Rapists and Pedophiles. *J. Projective Techniques* 18:346–354, 1954.
15. Guttmacher and Weihofen, op. cit.
16. Allen, C.: *A Textbook of Psychosexual Disorders*. Oxford University Press, London, 1962.
17. Karpman, op. cit.
18. Gebhard, op. cit.

CHAPTER 20

Ross E. Zumwalt is currently Deputy Coroner for Cuyahoga County (Cleveland), Ohio. He is also Assistant Professor of Forensic Pathology at Case Western Reserve University in Cleveland. A graduate of Wabash College and the University of Illinois College of Medicine, Dr. Zumwalt is a former Instructor in Pathology at the Southwestern Medical School of the University of Texas Health Sciences Center at Dallas, and at the Southwestern Institute of Forensic Sciences. He is also former Assistant Medical Examiner for Dallas County, Texas. Dr. Zumwalt served in the U.S. Peace Corps between 1964 and 1966.

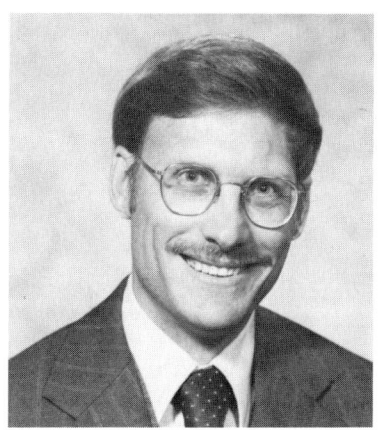

Charles S. Petty is Director of the Southwestern Institute of Forensic Sciences at Dallas, Chief Medical Examiner of Dallas County, Director of the Dallas County Criminal Investigation Laboratory, and Professor of Pathology and Forensic Sciences at the University of Texas Southwestern Medical School at Dallas. Dr. Petty holds degrees in pharmacy and physiology from the University of Washington and received his medical education at Harvard Medical School. He is a diplomate of the American Board of Pathology in pathologic anatomy, clinical pathology, and forensic pathology. Dr. Petty is former President of the American Academy of Forensic Sciences and is a Fellow of the American Association for the Advancement of Science, the American College of Physicians, the American Society of Clinical Pathologists, and the British Academy of Forensic Sciences.

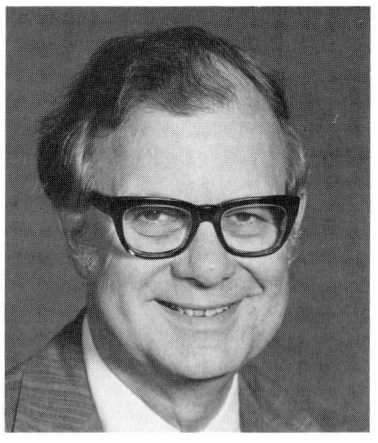

COMMUNITY INVESTIGATION OF RAPE AND SEXUAL ASSAULT

Ross E. Zumwalt, M.D., and
Charles S. Petty, M.D.

Successful investigation of sexual assault involves diverse public agencies and individuals. Cooperation between all the official agencies is essential; a breakdown in communication can result in improper processing of cases and eventual unsuccessful prosecution of the assailant or prosecution of an individual who was not the actual assailant. Since cases of sexual assault often arouse public indignation, news media and certain special interest groups are frequently involved. The cooperation of these unofficial agencies may also be important in the successful investigation of such cases.

The police officer or medical personnel first arriving at the scene of a sexual assault must initially provide for emergency medical care of the victim, summoning other medical aid if necessary. If the victim is severely injured, such medical care must receive priority over interviews or other investigation. When the victim has been removed to a medical facility or if the victim is dead, the scene should be secured and the necessary crime scene search initiated. Even if the victim is physically uninjured, she may still require immediate support for emotional trauma. The emotional distress related to the assault may make initial questioning less than satisfactory and, indeed, may so further emotionally traumatize the victim that even future cooperation may not be obtained. Therefore, the initial contact of the law enforcement officer with the victim poses a sensitive and delicate problem in interrelationships. It may be helpful for the victim to relate the details of the assault to a female law enforcement officer.*

---

*Woman-to-woman interview is said by some to be an effective way to deal with the sensitive nature of the reporting situation. However, it is the experience of some law enforcement agencies that the sex of the investigatory officer is really not a determining factor in the effectiveness of the investigation. Rape is really a crime of violence, not of sexual passion. (See Chapter 18 for further discussion.)

AGENCY INVESTIGATION OF SEXUAL ASSAULT

I. Law Enforcement
   A. Receiving of reports
   B. Emergency medical care
   C. Primary investigation
      1. Interrogation
      2. Scene investigation and physical evidence search
   D. Transfer of victim to medical care
   E. Secondary investigation
II. Medical Examination Facility
   A. Coroner, Medical Examiner
   B. Police surgeon
   C. "Contract" physician
   D. Examination of victim
      1. Pertinent medical history
      2. Examination of injuries
      3. Examination for procurement of physical evidence
      4. Motile sperm determination
   E. Treatment of victim
      1. Injuries (physical, psychic)
      2. Pregnancy, disease prevention
   F. Input to law enforcement investigation
   G. Input to prosecuting (defense) attorney
      1. Conference
      2. Deposition
      3. Testimony in court
III. Laboratory Facility
   A. Crime laboratory
      1. Local (police, county)
      2. State
      3. Federal (military C.I.D., F.B.I.)
   B. Physical evidence from victim
      1. Provision of kits, instructions for use
      2. Provision of refrigerated storage for specimens
      3. Establishment of chain of custody
      4. Instructions for transmittal
      5. Analysis
      6. Documentation and preparation of reports
   C. Physical evidence relating to incident but not directly obtained from victim (hair, stains, clothing, binding material, weapons)
      1. Maintenance of chain of custody
      2. Examination and analysis
      3. Documentation and preparation of reports
   D. Physical evidence from suspected assailant
      1. Provision of kits, instructions for use
      2. Provision of refrigerated storage
      3. Establishment of chain of custody
      4. Instructions for transmittal
      5. Analysis
      6. Documentation and preparation of reports
   E. Interaction with law enforcement agency
      1. Transmittal of reports
      2. Consultation and/or conference
   F. Interaction with prosecuting (defense) attorney
      1. Interpretation of reports
      2. Correlation with investigatory information
      3. Deposition
      4. Testimony in court

Since chances of recovering physical evidence from the victim decrease with time, prompt medical examination of any victim is important. Immediate transportation to the medical facility where examination will be conducted should be provided. Victims forced to find their own transportation often fail to go to the designated medical facility or delay the examination until valuable physical evidence is lost. Admittedly, not all charges of sexual assault are legitimate. In addition, in many cases there are contributing factors on the part of the victim. Nevertheless the initial investigating officer should not make a judgment on the merits of the case. Each case must be treated as a bona fide assault, and the victim should be advised not to change clothes, bathe, or douche prior to the medical examination.

Immediately after the proper medical examination, the law enforcement official may find it advantageous to interview the victim in greater detail. It may be helpful if the victim has a friend or relative present during the questioning.

After the initial medical examination there must be continuing communication between the police and the examining physician. The physician should have access to the initial police report as his comments correlating the report to his findings may be helpful. Alternatively, the law enforcement agency should have access to the physician to discuss his findings, and the physician's report should be readily available. The reports of police and physician should be otherwise regarded as confidential. If the physician is under contract to the police or another community agency, he should make his report to that agency and not to the victim. The physician has not established an ordinary patient-physician relationship and may elect not to follow the patient. He has no obligation to see or treat the patient again. However, if the victim herself contacted the physician for the examination and he intends to charge her a fee, then he has established a patient-physician relationship and is obligated to inform her of the results of the examination.

Follow-up investigation by the law enforcement agency is important. A second interview several days after the assualt may provide further information. Interviews with witnesses, friends, and relatives may be necessary and helpful to investigation of the case.

MEDICAL EXAMINATION

It is desirable in any jurisdiction to have a prearranged agreement for medical examination of rape victims. Since physical evidence deteriorates with time, it is not acceptable to wait for a prolonged period of time before the medical examination is undertaken. Only a prearranged agreement with a physician or group of physicians will avoid the difficulty of finding someone to conduct examinations around the clock. In many populous metropolitan jurisdictions there can be an agreement with a teaching hospital or a community hospital with large house staff to have the examinations conducted in the emergency room. In less populous areas a physician or group of physicians should accept responsibility for doing the examinations on a 24-hour basis. Occasionally a victim will desire to see her own physician for the examination. This may or may not be her privilege, but when it is, it can lead to difficulties. Most private physicians have no desire to do this type of examination, nor do they want the possible court involvement. In addition, they are unaccustomed to collecting physical evidence. Even if they consent to do the examination, it may be done incompletely, the proper specimens may not be collected and preserved, and the chain of custody may not be observed. In this instance it is imperative that the involved police official very carefully and tactfully inform the physician about the collection of physical evidence, its preservation, and chain of custody. These problems can be avoided when the examination is conducted by a physician who has agreed beforehand to examine victims of rape, who has the proper facilities and equipment to perform the examination, and who is experienced in collecting physical evidence.

The contract between the law enforcement agency and the physician or hospital should be written and specific. The individual role of the physician and the police officer should be clearly stated as to responsibility for transportation of the victim to the medical facility, treatment of any injuries, custody of specimens, notification of relatives or friends, relationships with the news media, compensation for services, and appearance in court.

Prompt and competent medical examination of the victim of sexual assault is essential for both medical and legal reasons. Injuries must be treated and proper collection of specimens must be made without delay. This medicolegal burden of the physician conducting the examination is compounded by the need for attention to emotional trauma and sequelae inherent in such an assault.

All aspects of the examination must be documented (in writing, diagrams, photographs, etc.). Attempts at recall several months, or even years, later in the courtroom can be embarrassing. The initial impression is important. Does the victim appear to be under the influence of alcohol or other drugs? What is her emotional state? What style of clothing is she wearing? Is the clothing torn, soiled, or stained?

All injuries should be described and, if possible, photographed. The entire body must be examined as injuries to the head, neck, and arms are frequently seen in victims of sexual assault. The absence of injuries of the perineum or vagina does not preclude assault or forced penetration.

The complete gynecologic examination has been described elsewhere.[1-3] However, in addition to the physical examination, the emotional condition of the victim should be evaluated. Ideally, professional counseling should be available and should be offered to the victim (see the following section describing rape crisis centers).

Proper collection of specimens is essential. It is best to have prepackaged kits available, containing those items essential for collecting, preserving, and storing all needed and available physical evidence. Detailed instructions and a checklist included with the kit are an invaluable asset. Having kits readily available avoids last-minute searches for containers and reduces the amount of time needed for the examination. A complete sexual assault kit should include:

1. Chain of custody form
2. Physician's examination form
3. Envelopes for trace evidence and hair collection
4. Comb for pubic hair combings
5. Scissors for pubic hair cuttings
6. Test tubes for blood collection
7. Filter paper for saliva collection
8. Cotton applicators and test tubes for vaginal, anal, and oral swabs

9. Culture tube
10. Microscope slides
11. Labels
12. Checklist

One part of the laboratory examination of substances removed at the time of the examination of the victim should be conducted promptly. This is the examination of the material from the vagina to determine whether the sperm present (if any) are motile or nonmotile. The presence of motile sperm is indication of very recent intercourse (perhaps within 4 to 6 hours of the time of removal of the specimen from the vaginal vault).* To save the specimens for later examination by laboratory personnel will allow time for the sperm motility to disappear. If a technologist is available or on call, the examination can be conducted by such a person on an emergency basis. In some systems, the examining physician conducts this brief check for motile sperm. All the equipment needed is a compound microscope and, of course, microscope slides and cover slips.

There are many difficulties in obtaining prompt and competent medical examination of sexual assault victims. Many physicians do not want to become involved in legal proceedings; they fear lawyers and courts in general. They have had little or no training or experience in testifying. There is little if any financial compensation for testifying, and in fact, a financial loss usually obtains due to time away from their practice. Most physicians, even gynecologists, have had little if any formal medical school or residency training in examination of victims of sexual assault and may be unsure of themselves in this situation. Physicians doing the examination often have no standardized protocol to follow and feel unfamiliar with this very practical forensic aspect of clinical medicine. Usually there is no feedback to the physician on adequacy of the specimens collected or results of laboratory analysis. Moreover, the examination is of necessity requested without scheduling, often at an inconvenient time for the physician. In addition to the above, some physicians apparently do not relate well with police personnel.

Because many physicians do not want to examine the victims of rape, sexual assault is often (by default) considered a nonmedical problem and thought of as a police matter. With this attitude it is no surprise that many examinations are improperly performed, the chain of custody incomplete, or the victim alienated by the physician's demeanor.

What is necessary then to improve the quality of medical evaluation of the assault victim? Basically, medical schools must become more involved in recognizing sexual assault as a medical emergency. Practical aspects of the care of victims of sexual assault must receive more attention in medical school lectures and residency training. The physician, as the professional with the knowledge necessary to do a competent sexual assault examiniation, must accept the moral obligation to do the examination. This attitude of service and obligation to the public must, of course, be reinforced in the medical schools.

---

*Specimens from the cervical canal may yield motile sperm for many hours up to several days after intercourse. Sampling of contents of the cervical canal rather than the vaginal vault may give rather unexpected results.[4,5]

CHAIN OF CUSTODY

Few physicians understand the legal requirements necessary for introduction of scientific information in court. One of the most misunderstood vital procedures for proper processing of evidence is the so-called chain of custody. The chain of custody is a method developed to verify the actual possession of an object from the time it was first identified (and collected) until it is offered into evidence in the courtroom.

Each specimen, when obtained, should be labeled with the victim's name, the time and date, the nature of the specimen, an identification number, and the physician's initials. Ideally, the specimen should be personally transferred to the investigating officer or laboratory supervisor. If this is inconvenient, it is acceptable to place the material in a locked container to which there is limited access. If the material is handled by an intermediary, that person must receipt the material and be included in the chain of custody.

The physician who is already reluctant to examine a case of sexual assault may subconsciously be careless with the material in such a way that the chain of custody may not be complete. It is difficult to believe that an examining physician would be deliberately careless with the chain of custody so as to be relieved of the burden of testifying in court. However, there have been instances of apparently overt refusal to conform even to the simplest chain of custody requirements. In such an instance the examining physician's actions may verge on culpable negligence.

LABORATORY ANALYSIS

The examination of the specimens from the vaginal vault for motile and nonmotile sperm, undertaken at the time of the medical examination of the victim, has already been mentioned. Identification of spermatozoa in vaginal swabs remains the best preservable evidence of recent intercourse. However, the absence of spermatozoa does not preclude recent intercourse. With the increasing number of vasectomies, aspermic seminal fluid is becoming common. Sperm may be discharged directly into the bladder in individuals who have had suprapubic prostatectomies. Seminal fluid from such persons may not contain sperm. Depending on numerous other variables, sperm may disappear rapidly from the vagina.[4-7]

Tests for the presence of prostatic acid phosphatase are most important. This enables one to identify seminal fluid even in the absence of sperm. The qualitative determination of acid phosphatase in vaginal washings or on vaginal swabs is a most useful procedure. Details of this technique may be found in the manual of a workshop given by Petty and Stone.[8] Quantitative determination of acid phosphatase has been advocated as an indicator of the span of time elasped between intercourse and collection of the specimen.[9-11] This may be useful, but the variables of sampling may militate against its accuracy. Refrigeration of the specimen for acid phosphatase examination from the time of collection until analysis must also be undertaken.

The examination of the material removed from the vaginal vault for blood group substances may be of use, particularly in the elimination of a person suspected of being the rapist. In such instances, the secretor status of the victim must be determined, for if she is a secretor, her own blood group substance will be found in the vaginal secretions.[12]

Combing of the pubic hair to find separate foreign hair is a most useful procedure. A specimen of the victim's own pubic hair should be procured. The preferred procedure is to cut the hairs at the skin surface. Occasionally, it may be necessary to have the hair roots available for examination and comparison. However, since plucking of the hair is an uncomfortable procedure, it is reasonable initially to procure hairs by cutting, and to resort to plucking hairs only when a need for the intact hair has been demonstrated. The victim can always be recalled for this purpose.

Scalp hair must be sampled and retained just as with pubic hair. This may be very useful to compare with hair found on the suspected rapist himself, or upon his clothing.

Fingernail scrapings and clippings may yield tissue (usually epidermis) which was raked off the assailant's skin surfaces as the victim attempted to defend herself. The victim may not even be aware of her actions. Broken fingernails are an indication of possible defense actions.

Medicolegal specimens must be handled somewhat differently in the laboratory than strictly medical specimens. Since it may be necessary to prove in court that there was no possibility of tampering with the evidence, locked refrigerators and other specimen storage areas must be available. If the specimens are receipted from the police or examining physician directly to the laboratory technician, that technician must enter the chain of custody and may have to testify in court as to his participation. If the specimen is removed from a locked specimen box and processed in the laboratory, it may only be necessary for the director or supervisor of the laboratory to enter the chain of custody, even though some of the laboratory technicians handled the specimen. In this case, only that supervisor (pathologist or director of laboratory) will have to testify in court. He can maintain the chain of custody in this manner if he can convince the court that the laboratory tests were done under his supervision and direction and that the specimens were handled so as to prevent any possibility of alteration. Such a system may be preferable to decrease the number of links in the chain of evidence as well as the amount of technician time devoted to court appearances. For the same reason, only the laboratory supervisor or director who anticipates testifying in court should sign the final report of analysis. The specific laboratory work sheets completed by the individual technicians should remain in the work folder, but should not accompany the official report.

ANAL AND ORAL INTERCOURSE

No mention has yet been made of possible penetration of the victim's anal and oral orifices by the rapist. The history related by the victim may indicate other than vaginal penetration or entry. However, fear, unconsciousness, or death may intervene, and oral and anal examination may be justified, even in the absence of history of such experiences.

Sperm and/or acid phosphatase may be detected in the mouth or rectum. Preservation of sperm is usually not as good as in the vagina. Salivation, drinking, and expectoration all tend to cleanse the oral cavity. Defecation may well rid the rectum of sperm and seminal fluid.

Contamination of the anal margin by the spilling of the seminal fluid from the vagina may well be the source of false-positive determinations. Such must be kept in mind when sampling the rectal contents.

VICTIMS OF SEXUAL ASSAULT OTHER THAN ADULT FEMALES

There are two classes of victims other than the adult female. Preadolescent females are sometimes subjected to sexual assault. In young girls, the element of incest is always to be considered. The practice of obstetrics and gynecology usually does not include patients who are very young. The practice of pediatrics, on the other hand, does not usually include the examination of victims of sexual assault. It may, therefore, be hard to find physicians willing to undertake examination of preadolescent female victims of sexual assault.[13]

The other class of sexual assault victim is the male. Here the point of penetration is either the anus (sodomy) or the mouth (fellatio). Again, there may be difficulty in finding an appropriate physician to undertake the necessary examination of such victims.

EXAMINATION OF THE SUSPECTED RAPIST

The examination of the suspected rapist may be part of the required sexual assault examination system. Penile washings to determine recent sexual activity may help in identifying possible suspects. In this test the suspect's penis is washed with saline, and the material is treated with Papanicolaou's stain. Cells consistent with vaginal and cervical cell populations and Barr body identification suggest recent intercourse.

Informed consent may be required of the suspect before he is subjected to examination. A court order may be obtained (in some jurisdictions) to effect an examination.

THE PROSECUTION OF THE SEXUAL ASSAULT SUSPECT

Prosecution of the sexual assault suspect is perhaps the most difficult part of the total public involvement in sexual assault. Historically, a small percentage of sexual assault cases have been successfully prosecuted. There are usually no witnesses; it is often the word of the victim against that of the suspect. The victim usually has to testify. She may be a poor witness and may be severely questioned. Historically, there has been a major reliance on circumstantial evidence—very little scientific evidence has been used. With the proper investigation and collection of scientific specimens, the emphasis is now shifting somewhat toward the better and more frequent use of scientific evidence. That does not, of course, discount the importance of eyewitness testimony.

The investigating police officer is valuable as a witness to describe the scene of the assault and the initial appearance of the victim. By accurately setting the scene, he can acquaint the jury with the circumstances of the crime. He must never appear judgmental on the stand. He should not volunteer information, nor should he attempt, if questioned, to conceal any unsavory aspects of the case.

The examining physician may be one of the most important witnesses. It is important, of course, for the physician to have a pretrial conference with the prosecuting attorney so that he will be aware of the questions the prosecutors will ask. In no way should he allow the prosecutor to guide him on how to answer the questions. The physician may take to the stand his personal notes concerning the case, but should take along no other information. The notes he takes to the stand are open to inspection by the attorneys representing either side of the case.

Photographs may be very effective in demonstrating injuries, and the physician should be given the opportunity to identify photographs of the victim and to introduce them into evidence.

It is particularly important to qualify the pathologist and laboratory technologist who serve as witnesses. Their testimony will be the most technical, and the jury must feel that they are qualified to give that testimony. Such expert witnesses must be able to communicate technical information in understandable language to the lay jury.

To the jury the victim is the most important witness. Jurors may disregard scientific evidence, particularly if it is questionable on the basis of subjective feelings from the victim's testimony. Because of the nature of the crime, the victim will almost surely have to testify. Before trial the prosecuting attorney should review the questions he intends to ask on the stand and also go over questions he expects the defense attorney to ask. During cross-examination the prosecuting attorney must be prepared to attempt to prevent the defense attorney from unnecessarily harsh questioning of the victim.

When the victim has been killed, the pathologist who performed the postmortem examination substitutes in a real sense for the victim on the stand. His description of the injuries and the results of laboratory analyses will inform the court as to the nature of the assault. His discussion of the age and physical condition of the victim and of toxicologic analyses will tell the court the condition of the victim at the time of the assault. If he was present at the crime scene, he may also be asked to describe his observations there.

The defense attorney has an important obligation to his client to provide the best possible defense under the circumstances. To do this the defense attorney should become familiar with the evidence in the case and the expert witnesses that the prosecution intends to employ. The witnesses should be willing to discuss their findings with the defense counsel before the trial. The prosecutor should know of any such pretrial conference with the defense and be given the opportunity to be present at that conference. Such pretrial openness will often prevent courtroom harassment and may even eliminate the need of the physician or technologist to appear in court.

RAPE CRISIS CENTER

Sometimes overlooked as a key component of an adequate system for the examination and support of victims of rape is the rape crisis center. Such centers may be official agencies, quasi-official agencies, or organizations supported by private funds with no official status. Many of the effective rape crisis centers were developed with the help of women's organizations. Others have been initially funded by federal grants (Law Enforcement Assistance Administration, usually through state planning agencies). There have been debates as to the merits of rape crisis centers, probably because of somewhat negative public and local governmental attitudes regarding support for the victims of crime and the popular opinion that the victim of rape is usually a "provocateur."

Professional counseling of victims of rape is the heart of the rape crisis center objective. Counseling is directed to the victim for several important reasons:

1. For reasons of the emotional (psychic) health of the victim:

a. to detect early emotional trauma originating from the rape;
   b. to prevent emotional trauma originating from the rape;
   c. to treat emotional trauma originating from the rape;
   d. to counsel with and treat recurrent (recrudescent) emotional trauma.
2. For reasons of criminal justice:
   a. to support the victim during the investigatory and pretrial phases, and during the courtroom procedures;
   b. to conduct educational programs directed toward prevention of rape;
   c. to help protect the victim from possible reprisals by the designated suspect prior to trial;
   d. to help educate law enforcement officers regarding emotional trauma ramifications of victims of rape.
3. For purposes of community education:
   a. to alter long-standing misconceptions of rape (the victim in the role of "provocateur"; rape as a source of sexual satisfaction to the rapist; etc.).[14]

There are many other possible reasons for the existence of a rape crisis center in any city, but the major foci of such a system are the victim, the criminal justice system, and the entire community, as indicated above.

Although many rape crisis centers depend to a great measure upon volunteer counselors, professional counseling capability, either directly available or by way of readily accessible consultants, is a very necessary component of a reasonable system. This permits the proper and necessary training of those volunteers who then may undertake the day-to-day task of responding rapidly to the urgent needs of victims of rape and who then provide the preliminary assessment of the victim for the use of the professional counselor.

The rape crisis center can be of great value in helping victims through the several very trying phases of the criminal justice system, particularly in supporting the sometimes ambivalent victim so that she may persevere through the prosecution and trial of the suspected rapist. Without such support some victims will withdraw charges, and the criminal justice system will have no alternative but to stop short of prosecution. Thus, although most crisis counselors do not really view themselves as part of the criminal justice system, a major part of their counseling activity may in fact relate directly to the criminal justice system.

Consider the victim of rape: should she become emotionally unable to bear the rigors of following the case through the twisted channels of the criminal justice system, unable to persevere and to continue to carry forward her desire to see the suspect stand trial, the interests of justice will not have been served. Furthermore, if emotional instability results, the victim may be forced to seek psychiatric help at state expense. The activities of the rape crisis center, from one point of view, may appear narrow and self-limited. Viewed in a different manner, the rape crisis center may appear as a signal component of the criminal justice system.

ASSESSMENT OF THE CRIMINAL JUSTICE SYSTEM

Assessment of the effectiveness of the criminal justice system in dealing with the victims of sexual assault is a difficult matter. Comparison of the efficiency of one local criminal justice system with another may be impossible. Many variables cause great differences between criminal justice systems. These will not be discussed here. Instead a brief analysis of those cases of sexual assault acted upon by the criminal justice system of a large metropolitan county (Dallas County, Texas) during one year (1977) is presented here in tabular form:

```
  805  Number sexual assault victims examined
 -137  False report or victim's refusal to press charges
  668
  -80  Not cases of rape, but incest, sodomy, etc.
  588
  -40  Juvenile assailant
  548
 -192  Not cleared; suspect not found
  356  Number of cases that potentially may go through entire crimi-
       nal justice system. These represent only 44 percent of those
       apparent victims of sexual assault who were examined in 1
       year.
```

The population of Dallas County is approximately 1.5 million. The incidence or rate of rape is, then, 54 per 100,000. Note that only those cases of rape or sexual assault which are reported to the law enforcement agencies, and where medical examination is requested, are included in this review.

What happens in these instances of sexual assault? A brief review indicates the manner in which the criminal justice system processes these cases:

on January 1, 1977	123 cases were pending action
	176 cases were filed upon
	3 cases did not fit the above categories
on December 31, 1977	128 cases went to conviction of the suspect
	10 cases resulted in acquittals
	66 cases were dismissed
	98 cases remained pending

Further details of convictions, acquittals, and dismissals follow:

```
Convictions
  No jury
    guilty plea         90
    not guilty plea     13
  Jury
    guilty plea          0
    not guilty plea     34
                       ---
                       137
```

It should be noted that there were 13 trials before the court and 34 trials before a jury. Thus in only 47 cases (6 percent) was there need for courtroom testimony from any member of the criminal justice system, including the examining physician.

Acquittals	
Nonjury trials	6
Jury trials	4
Directed verdict	0
	10
Dismissals	
Insufficient evidence	4
Defendant convicted in another type case	23
At request of complaining witness	13
Case refiled	16
Defendant could not be located for trial	3
Other	7
	66

An examination of the statistics above will help to explain why an *apparently* very low conviction rate results from a very large expenditure of time on the part of all elements of the criminal justice system: law enforcement agencies, examining physicians, rape crisis center counselors, and forensic laboratory workers, among others. What is interesting is that only ten defendants in 138 cases were acquitted! In other words, 7 percent of those defendants who progressed far enough into the criminal justice system to enter a plea of guilty or who stood trial were found not guilty.

The number of actual cases of sexual assault in a community will never be known with accuracy. Estimates of one to ten times the number of reported instances have been claimed. Only in recent years has sexual assault in its many different forms surfaced as other than a minor component of crimes of violence. Certainly much of the recognition of the sexual assault problem can be directly related to changes in sexual mores, the influence of the feminist movement, and the awakened interest of the federal government in law enforcement.

Given below are several forms developed for use in Dallas County, Texas. Included are:

1. An instruction sheet for rape examination (adult female victim)
2. A form for recording medical examination (adult female victim)
3. An instruction sheet for sexual assault examination (male victim)
4. A form for recording medical examination (male victim)

These particular forms have proved useful and have stood the test of time. Local practice will of necessity dictate variations in these sample forms.

INSTRUCTION SHEET FOR RAPE EXAMINATION

INSTRUCTIONS

1. With cotton-tipped applicator, make four slides of vaginal contents and spray immediately with fixative. *Allow to dry* about 2 to 3 minutes and place slides in slideholder (for spermatozoa examination).
2. Place this same applicator, wet with vaginal contents, in culture tube containing normal saline (for acid phosphatase).
3. Using disposable plastic pipet dropper, obtain a sample from the vaginal pool and place on a microscope slide. Cover with cover slip and

set aside for motile spermatozoa examination under the microscope. Discard the pipet dropper.
4. Using disposable comb, comb pubic hair region and place in labeled envelope. Discard comb.
5. Cut sample of pubic hair (about 10 to 12 hairs, cut close) and place in labeled envelope.
6. Obtain blood sample from patient (for comparison with semen type).
7. Label all containers, especially when additional samples such as fingernail scrapings are obtained.
8. Place all specimens in locked box marked for pickup.

SPECIAL NOTES

1. In cases involving oral-genital contact, swab the mouth (particularly the gums and pharynx) of the patient with a separate applicator and prepare a microscope slide smear; spray with fixative. Place the applicator in a separate culture tube for acid phosphatase detection.
2. Seminal fluid may be observed in the perianal area, especially in children. A separate cotton-tipped applicator moistened with saline can be used to swab this area for laboratory examination.

MEDICAL REPORT

Suspected Rape

Police Case Service No. _____   Police Jurisdiction _____

Name of Patient _____ EOR No. _____

Admitted Parkland Emergency Room: Date _____ Time _____

Name of Police Official with Patient _____ Badge No. _____

Authorization for Collection of Evidence and Release of Information
I hereby authorize Parkland Hospital and O.B. Associates to collect any blood, urine, tissue, or other specimen needed and to supply copies of ALL medical reports including any laboratory reports, immediately upon completion, to the Police Department and the Office of the District Attorney having jurisdiction.

Person Examined _____

Address _____

Date _____   Parent or Guardian _____

Witness _____   Address _____

CONSENT FORMS COMPLETED?
Physical examination (EOR Form)?   Yes[ ]   No[ ]

Collection of evidence and release of information? Yes[ ] No[ ]
Obtain photographs? Yes[ ] No[ ]

(Above information to be obtained by admitting nurse)

ASSAULT COMPLAINT   Date of Assault _____ Time _____

_____   _____ M.D.
Date   Examiner's Signature

HISTORY
1. Age:
2. Gravidity: Parity:
3. Date of termination of last pregnancy:
4. Age of menarche:
5. Date of last menses:
6. Last menses normal? Yes[ ] No[ ].
   If no, describe:
7. Patient known to be pregnant? Yes[ ] No[ ]
8. Symptoms of pregnancy? Yes[ ] No[ ].
   If yes, describe:
9. Most recent coitus prior to alleged assault:
   Date_____ Time_____ Condom used? Yes[ ] No[ ]
10. Current mode of contraception (prior to alleged assault):

11. Patient states she is (was) a virgin prior to assault? Yes[ ] No[ ]
12. Vaginal tampons used? Yes[ ] No[ ]. Age begun _____
13. Douching practiced? Yes[ ] No[ ]. Most recent _____
14. During alleged assault:
    Did penis penetrate vulva?   Yes[ ] No[ ]
    Did assailant experience orgasm?   Yes[ ] No[ ]
    Did assailant wear condom?   Yes[ ] No[ ]
15. Since alleged assault has patient:
    douched?   Yes[ ] No[ ]
    bathed or showered?   Yes[ ] No[ ]
    defecated?   Yes[ ] No[ ]
    urinated?   Yes[ ] No[ ]

_____   _____ M.D.
Date   Examiner's Signature

16. Has patient knowledge of:
    any present illness?   Yes[ ] No[ ]
    any present medication?   Yes[ ] No[ ]
    any drug allergy?   Yes[ ] No[ ]
17. Has patient had a venereal disease (past or present)?
    Yes[ ] No[ ]. Describe therapy.

SPECIAL INVESTIGATIONS

18. History of emotional illness? Yes[ ] No[ ]
    Describe.

19. Previous vaginal surgical procedures? Yes[ ] No[ ]
    Describe.

20. In 24 hours prior to alleged assault, did patient use alcohol or illicit drugs?
    Yes[ ] No[ ].
    Describe date, time, and amount of ingestion; frequency of use; duration of use; usual amount of intake.

_____   _____ M.D.
Date   Examiner's Signature

PHYSICAL EXAMINATION

1. B.P._____ Pulse_____ Temp. ___ °F Wt. _____ Ht. _____

2. General Appearance:

3. Emotional Status:

4. Clothing: stains? Yes[ ] No[ ]; foreign material? Yes[ ] No[ ].
   Describe.

5. Body Surface: bruises? Yes[ ] No[ ]; scratches? Yes[ ] No[lacerations? Yes[ ] No[ ].
   Describe.

6. Mouth:

7. Fingernails:

8. Pubic hair:

9. Vulva:

10. Hymen:

11. Vagina (no lubricant):

12. Cervix:

13. Uterus:

_____   _____ M.D.
Date   Examiner's Signature

14. Adnexa:

15. Rectovaginal:

16. Sketch of perineal findings (label all positive findings):

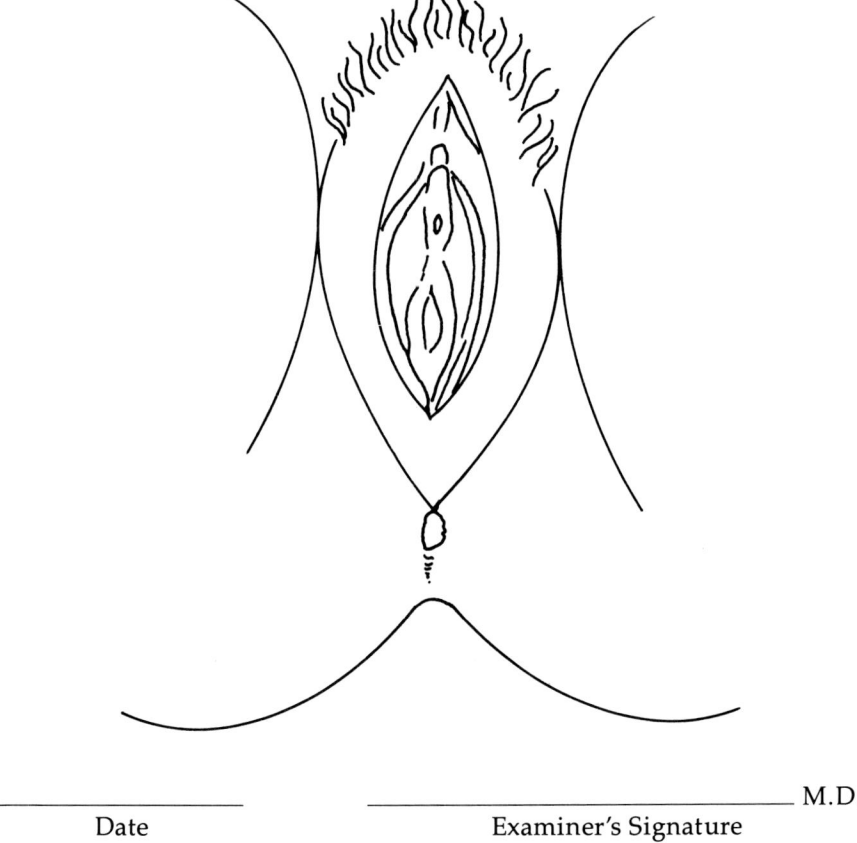

_____   _____ M.D.
        Date   Examiner's Signature

COLLECTION OF EVIDENCE

1. Two tubes of clotted blood—labeled (1, to Serology; 2, to Forensic Pathology Lab.).
2. Scrape and trim fingernails into envelope and label.
3. Comb and collect free pubic hair into envelope and label.
4. Cut off and label a few pubic hairs into separate envelope and label.
5. Collect any loose hair or dried blood and label (site collected).
6. Examine a saline wet mount for sperm: Present? Yes[ ] No[ ]; Motile? Yes[ ] No[ ].
7. Prepare two dry slides of vaginal contents or saline washing and spray with fixative. Allow to dry before placing in slide tray.
8. Do cervical culture for *N. gonorrhoea*.
9. Place wet cotton swab (wet with vaginal secretions) in dry test tube (semen typing). Place wet cotton swab in test tube containing saline (acid phosphatase).
10. If indicated:
    urine for pregnosticon? Yes[ ] No[ ]

wet and dry preps from mouth? Yes[ ] No[ ]
urine for urinalysis if bladder trauma? Yes[ ] No[ ]
X-rays obtained (indicated because of trauma)? Yes[ ] No[ ]
photographs? Yes[ ] No[ ]

Impression:

Recommendations
  Drugs:

  Appointments:

I hereby certify that this is a true and correct copy of the official office and/or hospital records concerning the examination of the above named patient.

_____ _____ _____ M.D.
   Date   Time   Examiner's Signature

Results of laboratory   Date   Results
procedures:

  1. Pregnancy test   _____   _____

  2. Serology   _____   _____

  3. *N. Gonorrhoea*   _____   _____
     culture

SEXUAL ASSAULT INSTRUCTION SHEET

(Male Patients)

INSTRUCTIONS

1. Using the cotton gauze pad provided, moisten this with a portion of the sterile saline in the culture tube labeled "acid phosphatase." Wipe the perianal area and place the gauze pad in the envelope provided.
2. Insert carefully cotton swab (1) into the anal canal without touching the perianal area. Prepare two slides with anal swab and spray immediately with fixative. *Allow to dry* about 2 to 3 minutes and place slides in slide tray (for spermatozoa search).
3. Place this same swab (1) in culture tube containing normal saline (for acid phosphatase).
4. Obtain blood sample from patient (for comparison with semen type).
5. *Oral-genital:* In these cases, carefully swab the mouth of the patient especially the gums and pharynx with swab (II) and smear on a microscope slide. Spray with fixative.
6. Place this swab (II) in separate culture tube containing normal saline (for acid phosphatase).

7. Label all containers, especially when additional samples such as fingernail scraping are obtained.
8. Place all specimens in locked drop box marked for pickup.

SEXUAL ASSAULT EXAMINATION—MALE PATIENTS

Police Case No. _____ Police Jurisdiction _____
Police Officer with Patient _____ Badge No. _____
Patient's Name _____ EOR No. _____
Admitted to PMH/EOR: Date _____ Time _____

Authorization for Examination, Collection of Evidence and Release of Information

I hereby authorize Parkland Memorial Hospital to collect specimens including blood, urine, tissue and clothing as needed. I understand that copies of all medical reports will be supplied to the police agency and office of the District Attorney. I authorize the police agency to obtain photographs for documentation of injuries.

Witnessed by _____ Patient _____

Date _____ Address _____

Parent/Guardian _____

Address _____

(Above information is to be obtained by admitting nurse)

BRIEF DESCRIPTION OF ASSAULT

Date of Assault _____ Time _____

PHYSICAL EXAMINATION

Name of Patient _____ Age _____

1. B/P _____ Pulse _____ Temp. _____ °F. Wt. _____ Ht. _____
2. Demeanor or emotional status of patient:
3. Describe any clothing stains or foreign matter:
4. Body bruises? Yes_____ No_____
   Scratches/lacerations? Yes_____ No_____
   Describe:
5. Mouth:
6. Genital area:
7. Anal examination:
8. During alleged assault:
   Did penis penetrate rectum? Yes_____ No_____

   Did assailant have orgasm? Yes_____ No_____

| | Did assailant wear condom? | Yes_____ No_____ |

9. Since alleged assault, has patient:
   - showered or bathed? Yes_____ No_____
   - urinated? Yes_____ No_____
   - defecated? Yes_____ No_____

10. Does patient know of:
    - any present medication? Yes_____ No_____
    - any present illness? Yes_____ No_____
    - any drug allergy? Yes_____ No_____

_____ M.D.
Physician's Signature

EVIDENCE COLLECTION

Name of Patient_____

1. Blood specimens obtained   Yes   No
   - Forensic Lab?   _____   _____
   - Serology?   _____   _____
2. Rectal swabs obtained?   _____   _____
3. Oral swabs obtained?   _____   _____
4. Items of clothing taken?   _____   _____
   Describe:
5. X-rays taken?   _____   _____
   Describe:

Physician's Impression:

Recommendations:

I hereby certify that this is a true and correct copy of the official examination of this patient.

_____ M.D.
Physician's Signature

_____   _____
Date   Time

REFERENCES

1. McCubbin, J. H., and Scott, D. E.: Management of Alleged Sexual Assault. *Texas Med.* 69:59, 1973.
2. Enos, W. F., Beyer, J. L., And Mann, G. T.: The Medical Examination of Cases of Rape. *J. Forensic Sci.* 17:50, 1972.
3. *ACOG Technical Bulletin Number 14.* July 1970, Revised April 1972. American College of Obstetrics and Gynecology, Chicago, 1970, 1972.
4. Wallace-Haagens, M. J., Duffy, B. J., and Holtrop, H. R.: Recovery of Spermatozoa from Human Vaginal Washings. *Fertil. Steril.* 26, 175, 1955.
5. Fredricsson, B., and Bjork, G.: Morphology of Postcoital Spermatozoa in the Cervical Secretion and Its Clinical Significance. *Fertil. Steril.* 28:841, 1977.
6. Davies, A., and Wilson, E.: The Persistence of Seminal Constituents in the Human Vagina. *Forensic Sci.* 3:45, 1974.
7. Rupp, J. D.: Sperm Survival and Prostatic Acid Phosphatase Activity in Victims of Sexual Assault. *J. Forensic Sci.* 14:177, 1969.
8. Petty, C. S., and Stone, I. C., Jr.: Workshop Syllabus: Medical and Forensic Investigation of Sexual Assault. Presented to the American Society of Clinical Pathologists, Miami Beach, March 9, 1977.
9. Gomez, R. R., Wunsch, C. D., Davis, J. H., et al.: Qualitative and Quantitative Determinations of Acid Phosphatase Activity in Vaginal Washings. *Am. J. Clin. Pathol.* 64:423, 1975.
10. Findley, T.P.: Quantitation of Vaginal Acid Phosphatase and Its Relationship to Time of Coitus. *Am. J. Clin. Pathol.* 68:238, 1977.
11. Schumann, G. B., Badawy, S., Peglow, A., et al.: Prostatic Acid Phosphatase. Current Assessment in Vaginal Fluid of Alleged Rape Victims. *Am. J. Clin. Pathol.* 66:944, 1976.
12. Dahlke, M. B., Cooke, C., Cunnane, M., et al.: Identification of Semen in 500 Patients Seen Because of Rape. *Am. J. Clin. Pathol.* 68:740, 1977.
13. Paul, D. M.: The Medical Examination in Sexual Offenses Against Children. *Med. Sci. Law.* 17:251, 1977.
14. Hilberman, E.: *The Rape Victim.* Basic Books, New York, 1976.
15. Field, H. S., and Barnett, N. J.: Forcible Rape: An Updated Bibliography. *J. Crim. Law Criminol.* 68:146, 1977.

CHAPTER 21

Joseph C. Rupp is Chief Medical Examiner for Nueces County (Corpus Christi), Texas. He received his undergraduate education at Muhlenberg College and studied biochemistry at Duke University, completing his doctorate in 1955, and receiving his medical degree from Western Reserve University Medical School in 1961. Dr. Rupp has served as Deputy Medical Examiner in Dade County, Florida, and in Hennepin County, Minnesota. For five years he was Associate Medical Examiner in Broward County, Florida. Dr. Rupp has served as a member of the Council on Forensic Pathology of the American Society of Clinical Pathologists and is a member of the Board of Directors of the National Association of Medical Examiners.

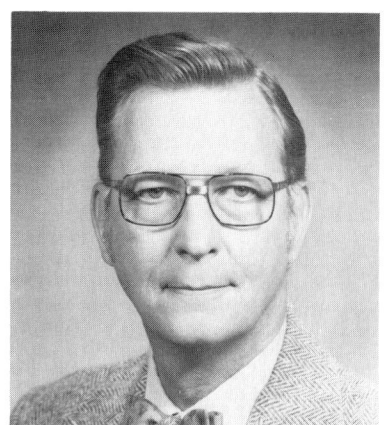

SEX-RELATED DEATHS

Joseph C. Rupp, M.D., Ph.D.

It is surprising that in our sex-oriented society, so little has been written concerning sex-related deaths. That there should be a significant number of sex-related deaths one can readily understand, for after all, sexual activity involves intimate personal contact, emotional excitement, physical activity, and in its more sophisticated forms, dexterity and coordination.

In a broad, general sense, a large number of routine barroom homicides, domestic homicides, and suicides may be considered as sex-related casualties in the "battle of the sexes," as it were. Within the home, fatal arguments concerning such sexual problems as infidelity are not uncommon. Barroom killings resulting from fights over women or other sex-related matters are almost a weekly occurrence. Not infrequently, suicide notes make it quite clear that the person has killed himself to teach a mate or lover a lesson that they will never forget. In this regard I think particularly of a married woman who checked into a motel and shot herself in the chest while lying in bed. The suicide note addressed to her husband was a classic of brevity and clarity, for it said only "you win." Such homicides and suicides occur under an infinite variety of circumstances, but because they present no particular problem to the investigator, the sexual nature of the death is often taken for granted or even overlooked.

A relatively large number of people are found dead in a partial or complete state of undress, usually within the privacy of the home. Perhaps we should not be surprised, because a majority of people are sick, in pain, or uncomfortable prior to death. Shedding restrictive clothing serves to provide some degree of comfort and relief. In the same vein it is surprising how many people die in the bathroom. Again, perhaps we should not be surprised, because sick people prior to death may experience nausea or diarrhea. They may feel the urge to defecate or urinate and be incontinent. The point to be made is that a nude or partially nude body does not necessarily indicate that one is dealing with a sex-related death. This type of finding is further complicated in the case of the alcoholic in which we see partial or complete nudity with the multiple bruises of the "falling-down drunk" in a house or apartment which is filthy or unkempt. These cases can be very difficult for the inexperienced investigator, and one must resist the puritanical impulse to equate nudity with deviant sexual conduct.

DEATHS DURING SEXUAL ACTIVITY

Men die not infrequently during sexual intercourse and almost invariably as the result of pre-existing cardiovascular disease, although an occasional death may occur as the result of a ruptured berry aneurysm with intracerebral and subarachnoid hemorrhage. Studies have shown that during sexual intercourse there is an increase in blood pressure, tachycardia, and hyperventilation due to emotional response and muscular exertion. In the presence of a significant degree of cardiovascular disease and an insufficient cardiac reserve, the increased demand on the cardiovascular system cannot be met, and the subject may die.

When death occurs, the subject is usually found nude in the bedroom of his home in the company of his wife. Under these circumstances, the investigator is reluctant to question the wife in detail concerning sexual activity at the time of death, and the wife will almost certainly not volunteer this kind of information. If, however, one overcomes his reticence and asks the proper questions, his suspicions will usually be confirmed.

When death occurs during sexual intercourse outside the deceased's home in the company of someone other than his wife, the case is generally referred to as a D.I.S., or "death in the saddle." Under these circumstances, we have superimposed upon the existing cardiovascular disease the added excitement of an illicit love affair with a strange woman in unfamiliar surroundings, usually after an evening out with a heavy meal and a significant amount of drinking, all of which add additional stress to the normal demands of sexual intercourse.

When a case of this type is investigated, it is not unusual to find that both the woman involved and the subject's wallet are missing from the scene, especially if the other party is a prostitute. Upon learning the circumstances of death, the family will invariably allege that the deceased has been drugged, poisoned, or otherwise "done in" and then robbed. In this way, they are able to avoid accepting the inevitable truth that "daddy" died in the arms of a "scarlet woman." One must be aware that no matter how obvious the D.I.S. may be to the investigator, it will never be obvious to or accepted by the deceased's family.

An autopsy is absolutely mandatory, not only to document the cardiovascular disease, but also to rule out the remote possibility of foul play. In addition to any natural disease, one should examine the gastric contents, obtain blood for alcohol analysis, and be sure to note lipstick marks on the body surfaces or clothing, as well as any clumsy attempts that have been made to dress the body after death, such as clothing worn backwards or inside out. Above all, in handling a case of this type, the investigator should be discreet for these cases present difficult problems in public relations, in spite of our recent, more liberal attitudes toward casual sex.

What applies to death during sexual intercourse also applies to death during masturbation. One will occasionally encounter a case where the findings at the scene and the position of the body leave no serious doubt that the subject involved died from cardiovascular disease or ruptured a berry aneurysm while masturbating.

The subject of natural death during sexual intercourse brings up another topic worthy of consideration. In the older literature on forensic pathology, one occasionally finds reference to seminal fluid staining on a dead body. The inference is made that when such staining is found, it indicates that the subject was engaged in sexual activity at or immediately prior to the time of death. Such an inference is unjustified. It is true that in a significant number of cases there is dribbling of seminal fluid from the penis and that fluid may even contain viable sperm, but the presence or absence of seminal fluid in no way reflects the type of activity engaged in at the time of death, for the experienced investigator often sees dribbling of seminal fluid where there is not even a remote possibility of sexual activity. The most important consideration is not the presence of the seminal fluid, but the location and the size of the stains. If the seminal fluid is present as the result of postmortem changes, then it will appear as a few small drops or stains on the penis, testicles, inguinal area, or on the underclothing. Only if the stain is large and of the order of magnitude of that produced by a normal emission is there reasonable evidence of sexual activity at the time of death. Each case must be evaluated on its own merits as to the findings at the scene, the background investigation, and the size and composition of the stain. Conclusions should be drawn only after analysis is made of all aspects of such a case.

TRAUMA AND MUTILATION OF THE GENITALS

The male genitalia, by virtue of their pendulent condition and easy vulnerability, are frequently traumatized, and such trauma may result in death. Self-mutilation of the genitalia is not unknown, and the circumstances surrounding such cases often show common features. In one case, after hearing a sermon on sin, the subject returned home, cut off his genitals and threw them on the fire in the fireplace. In another case, a subject upset by his homosexuality amputated his genitals after applying a tourniquet. Unfortunately, the tourniquet slipped from the amputation stump and the victim bled to death. In a third case, the subject became contrite after consorting with a prostitute, cut off his genitals and threw them on the kitchen table.

When one encounters a homicide involving mutilation of the male genitalia, a special set of circumstances usually applies. This type of crime does not involve a single male assailant, but rather is committed by two or more males in the presence of one or more female witnesses. Background investigation may reveal that the individuals involved are homosexual or bisexual. Killings by street gangs may also be of this type.

It should be pointed out that in any metropolitan area, rumors circulate with some regularity that a young boy has been found sexually mutilated in the restroom of a shopping center. Such rumors are invariably false, and where or how they originate or why they persist is unknown.

If one encounters a case of mutilation of the male genitalia and the genitalia are absent from the scene of death, then one should immediately suspect a household pet. Dogs and cats are carnivorous, and the genitalia are easily accessible, particularly if the person dies while nude or partially clothed. If there are no pets at the scene, and there is no good indication of a homicide, then a careful examination of the gastrointestinal tract of the deceased is in order, for there is a possibility that the penis will be found in the stomach of the deceased, as happened in a case of suicide in New York City. Under other circumstances, the penis may have been bitten off by a homosexual lover or a rape victim forced to perform fellatio.

When looking for suspects or assailants where there has been mutilation of the male genitalia, it is well to remember that women do not kill and sexually mutilate men; that men do not sexually mutilate other men, except under the circumstances described; and that while children may commit matricide or patricide, they do not sexually mutilate their parents in the process.

Another peculiar type of case which causes much misdirected investigative effort involves the gas station attendant who is found collapsed or dead on the floor of the gas station. If the subject survives, he may tell a story of being robbed by several men who, prior to leaving the station, inserted a grease gun into his rectum and pulled the trigger. If a death is involved, autopsy findings include a ruptured bowel, massive bleeding, and the presence of grease in the peritoneal cavity. Most often, however, these injuries are self-inflicted. Apparently these individuals have an irresistible urge to give themselves an enema with a grease gun. The grease used to lubricate automobiles is under about 30 psi of pressure, and when released into the rectum, the result may be fatal. If the subject survives, he is loath to tell the investigator exactly what has happened and concocts a story of robbery and sexual assault.

FEMALE DEATH RELATED TO SEXUAL ACTIVITY

Women almost never suffer a natural death during normal sexual intercourse. Perhaps they have greater control of tendencies to overexcitement, perhaps they take a more passive role, or perhaps they are less susceptible to cardiovascular disease, but for whatever reason, they tend not to die.

Nevertheless, the unnatural death of a female during sexual activity may occur under a variety of circumstances. For instance, death may result from aspiration of semen or impaction of the penis in the hypopharynx. With the increase of interest in oral sex within recent years, we will no doubt see more of these cases. The diagnosis is made by finding seminal fluid in the respiratory tree. Swabs should be taken routinely where the circumstances so indicate. Because ejaculate loses its opaque, gelatinous consistency with rapidity, the seminal fluid may look no different at autopsy than the normal secretions seen in the trachea and larynx.

The pregnant uterus is a very vascular structure, and if there is any sort of trauma to the venous sinuses, a fatal air embolism may result. This may happen during a self-induced abortion where a douche nozzle, rubber catheter, coat hanger, or other blunt instrument is introduced into the uterus. However, death from an air embolus may also occur if air is blown into the pregnant uterus during cunnilingus. Air enters the circulation and forms a mass of frothy bubbles which effectively block the flow of blood. Death under these circumstances is very rapid, and one victim described an intense tickling sensation from the air embolus just prior to death.

In order to detect an air embolus, one should first dissect the fat from the surface of the inferior vena cava and look for the frothy bubbles which will be visible through the vessel wall. One may also carefully elevate the tip of the right atrial appendage with a forceps and then open it in order to observe the frothy blood. Some authorities recommend opening the heart under water (i.e., filling the pericardial sac with water prior to severing the great vessels); however, this method is quite cumbersome and time-consuming.

A type of death which presents great difficulty for the investigator is the accidental strangulation or suffocation of a female during sexual intercourse. If intercourse is performed in a relatively confined space, such as the back seat of a car, it is possible for the male, during intercourse in the missionary position, to apply undue pressure to the thorax, neck, or face of his partner either with the weight of the body or by application of the forearm to the upper chest and neck. Under these circumstances, the female partner may be asphyxiated and her struggles go unnoticed in the heat of passion. The resolution of such a case is very difficult, for the manner of death must be determined by the scene and background investigation, rather than by the physical findings at autopsy.

"Burking," as this type of death is called, derives from William Burke, who, together with William Hare, killed 16 derelicts in Edinburgh during the years 1827 and 1828, and sold their bodies to Dr. Robert Knox for use as specimens in his anatomy classes. The method varied somewhat, but generally combined traumatic asphyxia with elements of suffocation. Burke would throw his whole body weight on top of the victim, sometimes sitting on the chest, then cover the mouth and nose with his hands while Hare pulled the victim around the room by the feet. Dr. Knox, who was an innocent party in the tragedy, had his career ruined in part by a piece of popular doggerel circulated at the time which went, "Burke's the butcher, Hare's the thief, Knox's the man that buys the beef." At autopsy there may be very few, if any, physical signs of a violent or asphyxial death. The presence of semen in the vagina is a great help in confirming the diagnosis. Not infrequently, the assailants in this type of case use almost identical words when describing the incident: "she gasped and suddenly went limp."

Sperm survival and prostatic acid phosphatase activity in the vagina of a dead woman are subject to a great deal of variation. Both sperm and prostatic acid phosphatase are extremely resistant to autolytic and decomposition changes and can persist under unsterile conditions for years. In the live female who has sexual intercourse and thereafter assumes an upright position, sperm and acid phosphatase are diluted with the natural secretions and drain from the vagina in a matter of hours. The situation is completely different in the female who has had sexual intercourse just prior to death, for there is no further secretion and no opportunity for drainage, and the sperm and acid phosphatase may remain in the vagina for a remarkable length of time. In any case where circumstances indicate, one should check for the presence of sperm and acid phosphatase activity, no matter how decomposed the body or how long since the time of death. In the Christie murders in London in 1953, the bodies of three young women who had been strangled and asphyxiated were found secreted in a kitchen cupboard. Two of them had been dead for approximately 8 weeks. Not only were identifiable sperm found in the vaginal fluid, but the sperm were so well preserved that the prosector always regretted that he had stained the preparations instead of examining wet mounts, for he felt that the sperm were in such good condition that they might have still been viable.

In our laboratory seminal fluid was kept in a test tube under nonsterile conditions, and a few well-preserved sperm were still recognizable after almost 200 days. Moreover, a strong positive acid phosphatase reaction was obtained after nearly 500 days.

SIMULTANEOUS SEX-RELATED DEATHS

Simultaneous sex-related deaths are almost exclusively confined to carbon monoxide intoxication during sexual intercourse in a motor vehicle. Under the usual circumstances, the car motor is left running to provide warmth for the occupants while in a state of partial or complete undress during sexual intercourse. Although these cases provide interesting lecture material, they are not difficult to diagnose with regard to cause and manner of death.

An interesting variant of this type of case was encountered a number of years ago. A student nurse and her boyfriend were seen to park in front of the nurse's dormitory 5 minutes before the 12 o'clock curfew. At midnight while locking the dormitory doors, the custodian noted the couple still seated in the front seat of the car. Upon investigation he found them both dead and the car motor still running. There was a defect in the exhaust system but not in the floor boards of the car. The carbon monoxide had entered the car through the passenger's window which was rolled down only about 4 inches. In 5 minutes, enough carbon monoxide had entered through this small opening to asphyxiate both occupants. Small wonder then that we see this type of death so frequently where two people are engaged in sexual activity, whose minds are many miles away from the possibility of a defective exhaust system and carbon monoxide intoxication.

SEX-RELATED HOMICIDE

Within our usual frame of reference, the sex murder is understood to involve the killing of an adult female by an adult male. Few of these crimes are premeditated in the sense that the assailant deliberately sets out to find a victim, then sexually assaults and kills her. The usual objective of an assailant is rape or sexual abuse, often with an element of sadism involved. The victim is generally unknown to the assailant and is selected at random from among women who happen to be easily accessible, not uncommonly a waitress, a bar girl, or a prostitute. Because the death is unplanned, the subject is usually killed by manual or ligature strangulation or by blunt trauma, not infrequently inflicted with a tire iron. In the sadistic killing, infliction of pain upon the victim is a direct source of sexual stimulation and gratification to the assailant. When the sadistic aspect of the crime is emphasized, one often finds mutilation, evisceration, or even evidence of cannibalism. The absence of sperm or acid phosphatase in or on the victim in no way detracts from the sexual nature of the crime, for the sadistic criminal obtains his gratification from the inflicting of pain, not necessarily from sexual contact with the victim. If the body has been mutilated, the disfigurement usually involves the breasts and genital area. If dismemberment is the only form of mutilation present, this does not mean that the crime was committed by a sadistic killer, for in the majority of cases, dismemberment by itself is a method of concealing the crime and preventing identification of the victim, or for allowing for easy disposal of the body.

The sex murder of this type is usually difficult to apprehend, not only because the victim is unknown or at best slightly known by the assailant, but also because such an individual tends to be emotionally unstable in all areas of activity and is likely to be a drifter who moves from one place to another without establishing permanent ties in a community. As with most sexual assaultive crimes, a sex murder is not an isolated incident in the life of the assailant, but is the culmination of previous aggressive sexual activity involving rape, physical assault, or perverted sex acts.

A variation is seen occasionally in the adult heterosexual murder which, if recognized, may significantly shorten the investigation. Occasionally, investigators find that the victim has a foreign object inserted in her vagina or rectum. This foreign object may be a bottle, table leg, broom handle, or stick, and there may or may not be injury to the genital organs. Death will occur as the result of manual or ligature strangulation, bearing witness once again to the spontaneity of the crime. In such a case, the assailant was usually known by the deceased. By this is meant that the subject has had some type of social contact or relationship with the deceased prior to the time of death, not simply a rapist-victim type of relationship. The situation which results in death and the insertion of a foreign object into the vagina follows a pattern. The assailant and victim have sexual relations, usually after a considerable amount of drinking. At the end of the intercourse, the victim may desire to continue the activity or may berate the assailant for his lack of stamina or the quality of his performance. At this point, an argument ensues and the assailant ends by strangling the victim and inserting the foreign object into the vagina. The thought behind this action is that since the assailant cannot fill the victim's vagina with what she desired, he will leave her with a substitute instead. This was graphically demonstrated in a case which occurred in Cleveland, in which an assailant got a sausage from the refrigerator and inserted it into the victim's vagina after she had been strangled. What is important is that when one recognizes this pattern, the first course of action should be interrogation of the victim's male friends and acquaintances, rather than the institution of a search for a random assailant.

CHILD MOLESTATION DEATHS

The deliberate killing of a child that does not involve the battered child syndrome may be considered to have an underlying sexual motive, whether or not there is physical evidence of rape or sexual molestation. The male assailant will kill male or female children, depending upon his particular aberration. However, it is outside the realm of our experience for an adult female to be involved in the sexual killing of a child except for a single case in which a possessive mother killed her adolescent son and then herself when he began to show an interest in girls.

The assailant who kills children not infrequently lives and works in the community where the crime is committed and may be a respectable member of the community with a wife and a family. Usually there is a history of previous deviant sexual behavior, and this is one of the reasons that files are kept of known sex offenders and their patterns of behavior.

Death at the hands of such an assailant is as the result of manual or ligature strangulation, blunt trauma to the head, or stabbing. One does not ordinarily encounter mutilation of the male or female genitalia, any sustained injury being associated with forcible rape, sodomy, or vigorous fondling or rubbing. Traumatic injury may be slight, and tears in the vaginal or rectal mucosa are not always easy to identify. A careful dissection must be carried out after removal of these structures.

The sexual nature of the crime must not be overlooked because of the presence of intact clothing or the absence of genital injury. The negative findings in this regard are as important as the positive, for along with the method of killing, a pattern of behavior is established which will not vary significantly with that found in other crimes perpetrated by the same assailant.

This type of assailant does not begin his criminal activities by committing murder. One will find a gradual progression, often commencing with window-peeping, flashing, or bestiality, and progressing to more aggressive forms of deviant behavior, such as fondling or sexual assault, and finally murder. The murder is incidental and occurs when the child resists the assailant, necrophilia not being part of the aberration, although the sexual assault may be carried out after the child has actually died.

It is difficult to obtain a conviction in the sex murder of a child, primarily because the crime is rarely witnessed and because juries are loath to believe that an individual could commit such a horrible crime. This situation is further complicated by the reluctance of the court to allow an accused's previous record of aberrant sexual behavior or previous sex crimes to be introduced into evidence in order that the prosecution can establish a pattern of behavior. Consequently, successful prosecutions are few, and punishment often involves no more than committal to a mental hospital. In a mental institution, this type of sexual deviate may not demonstrate a behavioral problem, because he is surrounded by adults, and is often certified sane and released after a few years of observation, or he may simply escape from the mental institution because of the lack of security. Once free, such an individual will invariably resume killing children. The only effective deterrent for this type of criminal is long-term incarceration with indepth therapy or judicial execution.

HOMOSEXUALLY RELATED DEATHS

Homosexuality is a sexual perversion, not an alternate life style. It must be placed in the same group of perversions which relate to other than normal sexual preference, such as bestiality (a sexual preference for animals), pedophilia (a sexual preference for children), gerontophilia (a sexual preference for the old), or necrophilia (a sexual preference for the dead). According to most estimates there are several million practicing homosexuals in the United States today. The "gay world" is a subculture with its own customs, meeting places, vocabulary, literature, and dangers. The homosexual is prone to a sudden, unexpected, and violent death with much greater frequency than the average citizen. The dangers stem from the general promiscuity of the homosexual, from the perverse sexual activity that is the common bond, and from the inordinate amount of time devoted to, and preoccupation with, the perversion.

Suicide is common in the "gay world." Many homosexuals are desperately unhappy, and they commit suicide for a number of reasons. The homosexual may be consumed by feelings of guilt about his way of life. He may be threatened with exposure, blackmail, or disgrace before family or friends. He may commit suicide because of unrequited love or a blighted romance.

In the investigation of the suicide of an adult male who has no history of a serious medical illness, who has not suffered a financial catastrophy, or who has not recently lost his wife or girlfriend, the possibility of a homosexually related death should be seriously considered. The general promiscuity of the male homosexual and his preoccupation with the perversion have far-reaching consequences beyond the high incidence of veneral disease in the "gay world."

The often fleeting attachments of the homosexual can lead to suspicion, jealousy, and murder. Such homicides are spontaneous, rather than planned, and usually involve blunt or sharp trauma rather than firearms. The use of excessive violence is a common finding attesting to the underlying anger and hostility. A homicide involving two adult males living together, who are neither students nor skid-row alcoholics, is often the result of a homosexual relationship.

Another large group of homicides peculiar to the "gay world" involves the "fag hustler." This individual is unique to the male sector of the "gay world" and makes his living by "hustling the faggots." He is a male prostitute, but because he is paid for his services and does not usually reciprocate in the sex act, he does not consider himself a homosexual. This is a feat of self-delusion, for in later life, when the "fag hustler" can no longer sell himself, he invariable ends up "buying it all back." The "fag hustler" begins his career by accepting money for his participation in a homosexual act, usually after having been seduced by an older homosexual. His role is that of anal or oral inserter. Not infrequently, the hustler will "roll a queer" and take his money and sometimes his car and clothes. If the victim offers any resistance, a fight and possibly death may be the result. In some instances, the violence ensues when the victim suggests that the hustler actively participate or reciprocate in the sex act. Such an invitation is a direct threat to the hustler's denied homosexuality, and he externalizes his fear and anger in physical violence. Again, this type of homicide usually contains the element of excessive violence.

When the assailant is apprehended, he will deny any knowledge of, or experience with, homosexuality and will claim that when sexual advances were made, he got angry but only meant "to punch the fairy in the nose." The investigator or police officer should not be misled, for a thorough background check will most often reveal the assailant to be a "fag hustler."

Finally to be considered is the accidental death of a male homosexual during the sex act. Sudden death may occur during fellatio as the result of aspiration of ejaculate with subsequent asphyxiation, or as the result of asphyxiation due to impaction of the penis in the hypopharynx. While this type of accidental death is rare, it is not unknown, and in a suspicious case it is important to check the trachea for the presence of sperm and prostatic acid phosphatase. Sudden accidental death may also occur during the act of sodomy. It is not unusual for the anal inserter to grasp the passive partner's neck in his hands, or to twist a towel or pillowcase around the neck, or to cover the head or upper part of the body with pillows or a mattress during the sex act. Occasionally, the result is that the receptor partner is strangled or smothered.

Investigation of this group of cases is simplified if the homosexual aspect is recognized early enough. One cannot make the diagnosis of homosexuality solely on the basis of physical findings at autopsy, although, in the confirmed sodomite, one may see epithelialization of the rectal mucosa, and in the confirmed "fist fucker" there may be a large, patulous anus. Such findings as butterfly or pansy tattoos may also be helpful if present.. One may also read the signs at the scene—an immaculate, well-cared-for, well-decorated bachelor apartment or house, the absence of female friends, black or dark color schemes, Greek or Roman statuary, fancy men's underwear, female clothing, and homosexual literature may all be helpful to the investigator.

The female homosexual does not meet a sudden, unexpected, and violent death with the same frequency as the male homosexual. This may be true for a number of reasons. In our society, the female is given greater latitude with regard to dress, occupation, and interpersonal relationships. Moreover, relationships between women tend to be more slowly established and to last for a longer period of time. Whatever the reason, the female homosexual often establishes a more permanent and meaningful relationship with her partner. However, one does occasionally see a lesbian homicide or suicide.

A male homosexual will sometimes become attached to, and often marry a wealthy older woman. She provides money, social status, and makes no sexual demands; he provides companionship and, quite often, care and genuine affection. In the "gay world" this is known as a "fag-hag" relationship. When the older woman dies and the young man inherits her money and property, the woman's family invariably claims that the death involved foul play. They will go to great lengths to prove this, for they want what they consider to be their rightful inheritance. I do not know of a single case of this type in which foul play was involved in the death.

Youth and good looks are at a premium in the "gay world" as nowhere else. To be 35 in the "gay world" is to be an "old auntie," and many male homosexuals are always on the lookout for young proselytes. Despite what some authorities would have us believe, sexual responses are, to a significant degree, learned and conditioned. When an inexperienced youth is wined and dined, flattered and fawned over, and finally seduced, the sex act may itself seem insignificant, and the act may be repeated until it is finally learned and conditioned. Once the aberration is fixed, cure is virtually impossible. Herein lies the pernicious and incidious evil of homosexuality.

AUTOEROTIC ASPHYXIA

There is a little-understood and quite unusual type of sexual death known as "sex hanging." This term, while in general use, does not provide a good description of the practice. Such a death should more accurately be referred to as autoerotic asphyxia, for while erotic and asphyxial elements are always present, the hanging element is not. Basically, the death involves asphyxiation by constriction of the neck in the course of a sexual fantasy or masturbation. In most cases, a rope or ligature is placed around the neck, and the free end of the rope is secured to a fixed object (hanging) or to one of the extremities of the body. Anoxia is produced by placing tension on the rope with resultant constriction of the veins of the neck and decreased blood flow to the brain. Death occurs when the anoxia is carried too far and the subject blacks out, at which time the weight of the body or the weight or tension of the extremity causes the ligature around the neck to tighten and the subject dies. It is thought that the production of partial anoxia during sexual activity heightens the feeling of sexual pleasure.

Autoerotic asphyxial death does not appear to be of recent origin, a few cases having been described in the older literature. However, these cases were usually interpreted as suicides. The real origins of this practice remain unknown; however, the first direct reference to it may be found in the novel, *Justine,* written by the Marquis de Sade in 1791. It is worthwhile to quote the pertinent paragraph, since de Sade's description is more graphic and poetic than our twentieth-century vocabulary permits.

> We take our stations; Roland is stimulated by a few of his usual caresses; he climbs upon the stool, I put the halter round his neck; he tells me he wants me to curse him during the process, I am to reproach him with all his life's horrors, I do so; his dart soon rises to menace Heaven, he himself gives me the sign to remove the stool, I obey; would you believe it, Madame? Nothing more true than what Roland had conjectured; nothing but symptoms of pleasure ornament his countenance and at practically the same instant rapid jets of semen spring nigh to the vault. When it is all shot out without any assistance whatsoever from me, I rush to cut him down, he falls, unconscious, but thanks to my ministrations he quickly recovers his senses.
> 'Oh Therese!' he exclaims upon opening his eyes, 'Oh, those sensations are not to be described; they transcend all one can possibly say: let them now do what they wish with me, I stand unflinching before Themis' sword!'

A footnote in the text attributes this practice to the Celts in pre-Christian Britain. If de Sade's claim is true, this may well account for the widespread use of the torque or thick, ropelike collar worn by Celtic warriors.

Within recent years, there has been general agreement that these deaths are accidental. However, as late as 1955, the few published articles on the subject still speculated as to whether the deaths might not, in reality, be suicides rather than accidents. Since these cases occur infrequently and at great distances from one another, no large, well-documented series has ever been compiled or thoroughly investigated. Because the scene of death and circumstances surrounding the death are invariably complicated and bizarre, and investigators are generally unaware of these details, findings are often misinterpreted. Even today, many such deaths are incorrectly ruled homicides or suicides, and much investigative time has been wasted by investigators searching for a nonexistent sexual psychopathic killer.

One of the most remarkable features of the autoerotic asphyxial death is that it occurs almost exclusively in males. To date there have been only two well-documented cases reported in females. These deaths involve males from the age of prepuberty onward, although more deaths are seen in the young adult age group. The distribution of cases is worldwide, occurring among many different races in both married and unmarried males. Some observers note that the individuals involved usually come from better than average economic circumstances and are of greater than average intelligence. However, the evidence in support of this claim is not convincing.

In the reported cases there is no known correlation between autoerotic asphyxia and other aberrant sexual activity, homosexuality, suicidal tendencies, or known mental illness. In short, the individuals who indulge in this practice appear to be otherwise normal heterosexuals with no known psychiatric problems.

Although the patterns seen in autoerotic asphyxia have similarities, each individual develops his own unique and peculiar technique. We may see many of the following features, singly or in combination, elaborated or emphasized to different degrees with the one common feature being the desire to produce a partial asphyxia while engaged in sexual or psychosexual activity. In addition to constriction of the neck, there may be binding of the head with a gag, mask, or blindfold; binding of the trunk and extremities with ropes, ligatures, tape, or chains; pinioning of the extremities with handcuffs, shackles, leg irons, belts, or leather thongs; binding of the genitals or suspension of heavy weights from the genitals; or insertion of foreign objects into the rectum. In many cases, the binding of the body is elaborate and intricate; however, detailed investigation always reveals that the restraints were self-applied. In some articles on the subject, the reference is made to some sort of escape mechanism which will allow the bound subject to release himself quickly should there be an impending disaster. This quick escape mechanism is the exception rather than the rule.

In addition to bonds and restraints, there is frequent evidence of self-mutilation, such as puncture wounds, cuts or burns, or one may find weights, clamps, or pincers attached to the genitalia or breasts. Not infrequently one finds pictures of nude females, bondage literature, or drawings surrounding the body where they may be easily viewed. In other cases the act is performed in front of a mirror. Transvestism often plays a part, and the subject is found wearing female apparel. However, the element of transvestism is seldom carried beyond the use of female underclothing, such as panties, tight girdles, garter belts, and brassieres. In addition, gloves, high-heeled shoes, or boots tend to be a favorite item of clothing.

There is no doubt that self-induced erotic asphyxia is a habitual practice and over a period of time is elaborated and embellished. The variety and quality of equipment used indicates a preoccupation with the act and an overwhelming compulsion to produce it. In many cases, the accouterments show a significant amount of wear and much care in construction. The restraints are not uncommonly custom made with evident craftsmanship, indicating the importance of the practice to the individual.

If we examine autoerotic asphyxia in its varying forms, we come to realize that there is a rather systematic progression as the practice is repeated and the practitioner becomes older. In the youngest individuals, we see no overt signs of sex play or masturbation at the scene of death. The body is usally suspended by a noose with the clothing intact and the genitals not exposed. Determination of the true nature of the case depends upon a detailed and thorough background investigation and elimination of the possibility of suicide. Some of these cases are undoubtedly accidents while at play, but an appreciable number are sex hangings in their preadolescent form.

In the early adolescent stage, we find the individual suspended with the body fully clad, but with the penis or genitals exposed and frank evidence of masturbation. In this type of case, if the body is first discovered by the family, the clothing will be adjusted before the authorities are called. After suicide has been eliminated as a possbility, the family must be questioned in detail at an appropriate time.

In the next stage, usually involving the older teenager or young adult, we see complete nudity, usually with suggestive pictures or a mirror near the body and with a fair degree of frequency some evidence of bondage or transvestism.

In the final stage, we see the act embellished with all the elements previously described—bondage, mutilation, transvestism, etc. From the well-worn equipment often found at the scene there is no doubt that this act is repeated with a much greater frequency than one would like to believe. After investigating these cases, one also comes to the realization that in the older individual there must definitely be an awareness of the great risks involved in this practice, and perhaps the risk of a potentially fatal outcome ultimately heightens the excitement.

What is the origin of this behavior? It has more or less been assumed that some type of salacious literature exists which describes the practice. However, many years of investigation have failed to yield evidence to support this supposition. On the contrary, the evidence indicates that the practice of producing partial anoxia while engaged in sexual activity is not learned from any printed source or by word of mouth. It is true that occasionally one finds bondage literature at the death scene or among the possessions of the deceased, but this is always of the sadomasochistic type involving pictures and stories of women bound and tortured. It is never directly related to autoerotic asphyxia. In the absence of any evidence to the contrary, one must accept the idea that each of the persons involved comes to this practice by individual experimentation at a very early age and that the idea of constricting the neck with the production of partial anoxia while engaged in sexual activity is instinctual. In support of this, I would refer to a recent case brought to my attention in which a young man committed suicide by shooting himself. His suicide note and possessions indicated that he was a practitioner of autoerotic asphyxia which he embellished with elements of transvestism. His suicide note stated that he thought he was going mad. Because he had never heard of the practice of autoerotic asphyxia, he thought his behavior was unique. Filled with alarm, he decided to kill himself.

The implications of autoerotic asphyxia extend far beyond the simple concept of heightened sexual gratification by production of partial anoxia. In the sex hanging we see manifestations of sadism, mashochism, transvestism, fetishism, and narcissism. One cannot help but speculate as to the greater meaning of autoerotic asphyxia, perhaps representing some as yet unrecognized primeval instinct. Might it not be that the blindfolds, gags, ligatures, and anoxia are merely the acting out of the fetal memory, for certainly there are parallels in uterine life. Speculation is unlimited, but the only remaining fact is that we know far too little about this form of human behavior. Autoerotic asphyxia is carried on by thousands of individuals who arrive at this practice independently of one another. It represents an as yet unexplored, almost unknown, aspect of human behavior. There is every indication that what might be learned from a thorough scientific study of autoerotic asphyxia might prove a significant contribution to our understanding of human sexuality.

ADDITIONAL READING

Barzun, J. (ed.): *Burke & Hare: The Resurrection Men: A Collection of Contemporary Documents Including Broadsides, Occasional Verses, Illustrations, Polemics, and a Complete Transcript of the Testimony at the Trial.* (History of Medicine Series, No. 43) Scarecrow Press, Metuchen, N.J., 1974.

Marquis de Sade: *Justine, or the Misfortunes of Virtue.* Putnam, New York, 1966.

CHAPTER 22

Earl F. Rose is Professor of Pathology at the University of Iowa. He is a member of the National Association of Medical Examiners and a Fellow of the American Academy of Forensic Medicine. Dr. Rose was educated at Yankton College, the University of South Dakota, the University of Nebraska College of Medicine, and Southern Methodist University. He is former Professor of Pathology at Southwestern Medical School of the University of Texas Health Sciences Center at Dallas. Dr. Rose is a diplomate in anatomic, clinical, and forensic pathology of the American Board of Pathology.

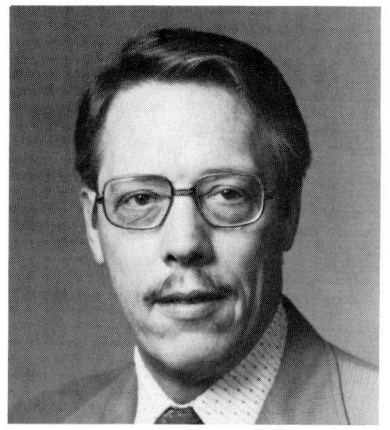

DEATHS RELATED TO MEDICAL CARE

Earl F. Rose, M.D., LL.B.

All diagnostic and therapeutic procedures used in medical practice have the potential to injure a patient; thus it is theoretically possible for any type of medical care to contribute to, or be directly responsible for, the death of a patient. Death while under medical care does not necessarily mean unsatisfactory or negligent medical care, but our interest is in those patients whose deaths are unexpected and ordinarily do not result from diagnostic or therapeutic procedures. When death does occur, it is the legitimate subject of inquiry, and the first item is to identify those factors in the medical care which *could* have resulted in the death. The object of this chapter is to assist those interested in identifying this problem and to aid them in sorting out, understanding, evaluating, and utilizing the scientific evidence when the issue is that of death related to medical care.

Medical progress has brought dramatic advances in the diagnosis and treatment of diseases, but with each advance there have been adverse reactions and occasional deaths. When a patient dies while under medical care, the determination of a causal effect between the medical care and the death may tax one's ingenuity. New facts regarding iatrogenic diseases and deaths are constantly being discovered and reported in the medical literature; it may be years after a drug or treatment procedure is introduced before the untoward side effects are appreciated. The reason for a person's death while under medical care, and whether or not the medical care contributed to or caused the death, is of immediate importance to the relatives, but it is also of immense value to all who are involved in medical care, to those manufacturing and selling devices and drugs, and to persons pursuing litigation.

APPROACH AND ANALYSIS

An analytical design is necessary in dealing with the complex issue of death resulting from medical care. Classification of patient injuries, a format designed by Mills[1] for the development of an injury prevention program, is adapted as a starting point in determining whether a death *could* be related to medical care. If there are deficiencies in the medical care, these should be determined without respect to legal negligence, but as a fact issue. The steps that should be taken in the investigation are discussed below.

The medical history should be reviewed with attention to the disease(s) that the patient had, the diagnoses and the bases for the diagnoses, and the care and treatment the patient received. This requires meticulous examination of all medical records to include the medical history of the patient, the findings while under medical care, and conclusions drawn from the findings, diagnostic and therapeutic maneuvers employed, and the general care the patient received, including the handling of any emergencies or complications of the primary diseases, as well as those involving diagnostic or therapeutic procedures.

Categories where suspicious iatrogenic injuries may occur will include the following:

1. Delay in diagnosis:
   a. inadequate medical history taken from the patient;
   b. inadequate physical examination;
   c. inadequate selection of diagnostic tests (e.g., cervical cytology for carcinoma);
   d. inadequate selection of diagnostic x-rays;
   e. failure to perform diagnostic procedure (e.g., failure to biopsy slowly growing breast carcinoma until the malignancy is widespread);
   f. improperly performed diagnostic tests or x-rays.
2. Diagnostic errors:
   a. misinterpretation of information acquired by history;
   b. misinterpretation of information acquired by physical examination;
   c. misinterpretation of diagnostic tests or x-rays;
   d. mistake in the interpretation of tissue biopsy (e.g., pathologist interprets malignant melanoma as benign nevus).
3. Performing unnecessary diagnostic or therapeutic procedures with fatal consequences.
4. Therapeutic misadventure. The creation or occurrence of a new disease or abnormal condition arising out of diagnostic procedures or therapeutic modalities (e.g., drug reactions, massive hemorrhage following a biopsy or operation, perforation of the esophagus during endoscopy, etc.).
5. Delay in recognition and/or improper treatment of medical and/or surgical complications which aggravate the primary disease condition (e.g., cardiac arrest, drug reactions, internal hemorrhage).
6. Incomplete removal of an abnormal condition or the improper use of available therapy, including drugs.
7. Inadequate or inappropriate care and follow-up by the medical and hospital personnel, including nurses.

The determination of the medical care personnel or others who might be responsible for a death occurring under medical care requires an analysis of the duties of these various people. As drugs are frequently involved in patient complications, their administration demands detailed documentation. It should not be overlooked that most often it is the patient whose errors in judgment lead to fatal consequences, for he or she may delay in seeking medical attention or may not follow instructions. In addition, the fatal consequence may not be anyone's fault, but rather the natural progression of the disease. Notwithstanding, when the question of death related to medical care is raised, a careful analysis is indicated.

When the activities of the physician are considered, the following should be examined:[2]

1. Delayed diagnosis or therapy.
2. Indicated procedures not performed.
3. Procedure or therapy occasioned by a misdiagnosis.
4. Improperly performed procedure.
5. More appropriate alternative available but not employed.
6. Operation or therapy not indicated from diagnosis made (e.g., drugs).

When injury may be related to a drug, the following list of factors by which the injury might have occurred should be checked:

1. Overdose;
2. Inadequate dose;
3. Improper route of administration;
4. Adverse interaction with another drug;
5. Allergic reaction;
6. Wrong drug;
7. Wrong patient.

When medical and hospital personnel, including nurses, are being considered, the following causative factors may be involved:

1. Professional conduct:
   a. improper performance of duties;
   b. delay in performance of duties;
   c. inadequate assessment of patient;
   d. misidentification of patient;
   e. delay in notifying physician of development of complications;
   f. failure to notice improper order or to obtain proper order;
   g. failure to instruct patient.
2. Monitoring patient:
   a. improper protection of patient (e.g., side rails or restraints as necessary);
   b. failure to monitor vital signs including cardiac, respiratory, renal, and neurologic.
3. Maintenance of proper environment (e.g., hospital "nosocomial" infections).

At this point the investigator should be ready to summarize the medical information that has been gathered. The summary can be outlined as follows:

1. The name of the disease or condition in medical terminology.
2. the name(s) of all diagnostic or therapeutic procedures from which

the injury may have arisen. This should include diagnostic procedures and drug dosage, as well as how the drugs were administered, nursing management, anesthetic procedures, etc.
3. The names of all abnormal conditions or diseases in medical terminology.
4. The tentative cause or reason for the abnormal condition or disease.
5. The identity and activities of medical personnel or others who had access to the patient, either directly or indirectly, and who could have caused or contributed to the patient's death while under medical care.

RESEARCHING THE MEDICAL LITERATURE

The ability to find authoritative current medical information rapidly and efficiently is paramount to the evaluation of the fact issues raised when death is possibly related to medical care. The medical literature can be searched quickly and efficiently if appropriate guides and suitable methods are utilized.

Medical textbooks are unequaled for lucid explanations of well-recognized conditions, syndromes, or diseases; however, they treat subjects in a somewhat superficial manner and may be out of date, in rapidly evolving areas of medicine, by the time they go through the publication progress from manuscript to printer. Textbooks do, however, provide a background for further investigation of a particular medical topic. The most current developments in medicine, as in other sciences, are found in the professional journals.

With a summary of the medical information derived from the review of the patient's medical history and records, the researcher is prepared to begin researching the medical literature. However, to find the pertinent medical references, the medical information must be translated into the correct form. Thus the correct *subject heading*, in order to find the references, is a necessity. Found in the *Medical Subject Headings* or the *Key Word Index*, the subject (e.g., drug, disease, complication) is checked against the alphabetical list of medical subject headings. In these references, the noun is customarily listed first and the modifier follows:

> Shock, cardiogenic
> Shock, endotoxic
> Shock, hemorrhagic
> Shock, surgical

Specific references are given under the article title, the author, and the journal in which they appear. The title of the publication often gives a clue to its usefulness, but the reading and evaluation of each published paper on the topic is the rule.

A rapid way to accomplish a search of the medical literature is through a computer-assisted literature search. While the library user had a choice of using either machine-searching or standard hand-searching of the indexes, the advantages of machine-searching often outweigh those of hand-searching, especially if the search involves a combination of search terms. A computer search takes only a fraction of the time involved in a manual search, and one can be more confident in computer-searching that important citations have not been overlooked. Additionally, indexing for machine-readable bases is often more comprehensive, in greater depth, and always more quickly updated than the printed counterpart. Through the computer terminal, one can take advantage of "Medline" and its on-line capabilities. All regional medical libraries, most libraries in medical schools, and some libraries of large medical societies, research institutes, and hospitals have this service. "Medline" derives its name from "Medlars" plus "on-line." Medlars is an acronym for Medical Literature Analysis and Retrieval System, and the automated searching and printing program of the National Library of Medicine in Bethesda, Maryland. A Medline provides direct access to the articles in 1,100 high-priority medical publications and contains from 350,000 to 450,000 references. It has the complete collection of references for the 3 years prior to the current year, and to this foundation are added, month by month, new references. At the end of the current year the references for the earliest year are dropped from the data base. The files in this data base correspond to *Index Medicus,* a printed index which covers, in addition to clinical medicine, all areas of medical research, biochemistry, virology, nutrition, and bioengineering. A medical librarian is needed to work out the searching strategy. The search with the computer usually requires up to half an hour, and the references are printed out at this time. If there is a large number of references, these may be printed off-line by the computer in Bethesda and mailed directly to the searcher. The expense of the search is really quite modest.

Another approach that does not use the computer is a perusal of the current issue of *Index Medicus.* Provided with a valid subject heading, the researcher reviews *Index Medicus* with a reference slip to record all vital elements of the citation and to make notes when the article is read. The *Index Medicus* covers both English and foreign-language journals with the English articles listed first under main headings and subheadings. *Index Medicus* provides the most complete listing, for it references 2,400 of the most used and best known medical journals published throughout the world. For those desiring rapid access to the titles and authors of a majority of published articles in the English language, the National Library of Medicine has published the *Abridged Index Medicus,* a monthly issue first appearing in January 1970. This can be found in practically all hospital libraries.

ADVERSE DRUG REACTIONS AND DRUG-RELATED DEATHS

Magnitude of the Problem

Adverse drug reactions and drug-related deaths are well known, receiving extensive publicity in both the lay press and professional publications. There has been a marked increase in the diagnostic, therapeutic, and prophylactic agents now available to the practicing physician. To compound the problem, there are many over-the-counter drugs for direct purchase and self-medication and a marked rise in the use of illicit drugs and their various vehicles. Industrial and occupational hazards have also been on the increase. Though this section is concerned with adverse drug reactions and drug-related deaths while under a physician's care, the principles of investigating reactions and deaths due to illicit drugs, self-medication, and occupational and industrial chemicals lend themselves to the principles of investigation to determine causal effect. The hazards and regulation of consumer products are eloquently discussed in the two-volume study, *Consumer Health and Product Hazards* (cosmetics and drugs, pesticides, food additives, chemicals, electronic products, and radiation), edited by Epstein and Grundy.[3]

It is estimated that as many as 5 percent of medical hospital admissions are due to adverse drug reactions and that a minimum of 15 percent of hospitalized patients experience at least one adverse drug reaction.[4] However, if this is correct, then the incidence of reported deaths from adverse drug reactions is remarkably low. One such report presents an incidence of only 0.22 percent (16 deaths in 7,423 hospitalized patients); 11 of these 16 patients were terminally ill with heroic therapeutic efforts employed.[5] A paper published by the Armed Forces Institute of Pathology, *Registry of Tissue Reactions to Drugs*,[6] classified 827 autopsies of adverse drug reactions and found that 3 percent (25) were due to therapeutic error, thus being deaths that were drug-related. Anti-infective and anesthetic agents accounted for more than half of these deaths. Others "conjecture" that an estimate of 60,000 to 140,000 adverse drug-related deaths each year is extremely conservative, and even suggest that this figure probably does not include drug-induced deaths in the ambulatory and extended care populations.[7] Indeed this seemingly inflated figure may be correct, as a high index of suspicion is required to make the diagnosis of a drug-related death. The tissue or autopsy diagnosis is very difficult, for rarely are there incriminating pathognomonic organ changes. The tissue reactions may be those of nonspecific inflammation, degeneration and necrosis, hyperplasia (and perhaps neoplasia), and drugs may be associated with teratogenesis and metagenesis (see section on drug-induced congenital abnormalities). In addition, there may be a well-recognized disease process for which the drug may have had extensive usage and not be recognized as having a hazardous effect. Thus the role of the drug in causing the death is not appreciated. An example is the special rule of the Department of Health, Education and Welfare barring the drug Phenformin as an imminent hazard to the public health, as the death rate among its users for diabetes mellitus was far higher than was regarded as acceptable for any other drug approved.[8] Many drugs present unique problems that either are not recognized by the entire medical profession, or are not perceived by the individual physician. The widely used drug acetaminophen, for example, is available without prescription and is used as an analgesic, antipyretic, and anti-inflammatory drug under the trade names of Tylenol, Apamide, Conacetol, Bebralin, Nebs, and Tempra. The usual tablet contains 325 mg of the drug, and 15 gm ingested will cause severe liver toxicity and probably death if the half-life of the ingested dose is over 12 hours.[9] Although it is imperative that therapy be instituted as early as possible, the blood levels may not reflect the amount of drug ingested, and toxic symptoms preceding liver necrosis and death may be delayed for as long as a week.[10] To complicate the matter further, the antidotes have untoward side effects and are of unproved safety. Still, this is a drug-related death while under medical care.

Analysis of the Problem

In spite of the prolific extant literature, there is no panacea for easily determining causal relationship between particular drug(s) and adverse drug reactions and death. Initially there should be an analysis and determination of (1) the drugs and chemicals to which the patient was exposed, and (2) the medical conditions and diseases from which the patient suffered. This analysis includes all parts of the medical records with listing of all drugs received and the doses, as well as the symptoms, signs, and diagnoses. When a particular drug or chemical is suspected, the subject should be researched in the medical literature. In addition, the *Physician's Desk Reference* provides current information, including contraindications and adverse reactions to drugs, with pertinent references. Working from a particular disease condition, in an effort to determine if this could have been caused by a drug or chemical, is facilitated by use of a text such as *Iatrogenic Diseases*.[11] Quite inclusive, this book is well-referenced and has an index of organ systems in which drugs have caused disease, including skin disease, blood dyscrasias, cardiac dysfunction, intravascular clotting, lung disease, disorders of hepatic function, disturbances of porphyrin, carbohydrate and fat metabolism, disturbances of water and mineral balance, endocrine dysfunction, renal disease, disease of the nervous system, disorders of the eye and ear, and drug-induced or aggravated infective conditions. Irey[12] has referenced a study of 2,700 cases of adverse drug reactions, including anaphylactic deaths, liver damage from phenothiazines, drug-overdose deaths, hexachlorophene toxicity, pediatric drug reactions, myocardial lesions in anaphylaxis, vascular lesions due to oral contraceptives, drug-associated sickle cell crisis, intimal vascular lesions due to female reproductive steroids, and atypical endocervical hyperplasia.

Drug Interaction and Bioavailability

With the increasing use of multiple therapeutic agents, it has become evident that the pharmacologic action of a drug may be greatly altered in patients receiving other drugs. It has been estimated that only 9 percent of hospitalized patients receive no drugs, while 70 percent receive one to four drugs regularly, and 21 percent five or more.[13] The problem is complicated in the ambulant patient who has access to over-the-counter drugs. Although the FDA (Public Law 87-731, 1962) has control over research, clinical testing, and marketing of drugs, it is impossible to determine experimentally the interactions of all drugs before they are placed on the market, for the combinations are endless. The interaction of antibiotics with other drugs[14] and the interactions of sedatives, hypnotics, and antianxiety agents[15] are of particular clinical significance. In addition, drugs may affect clinical laboratory results, misleading the unwary physician.[16]

Modern therapy is limited by the problem of drug specificity, for drug therapy is often empiric with excellent results in one instance, but with harmful or even fatal consequences in another patient with the same condition. There are general rules regarding drug therapy, yet sporadically patients seem to assert their own individuality. Thus the physician, in addition to general rules and established procedures of drug therapy, must "titer" each patient's response to treatment, ever aware that each has the potential of a therapeutic misadventure. The reasons for this variability are many and include altered absorption into the body so that the drug does not get to the specific target-disease area in sufficient concentration; otherwise the drug may have an untoward effect on other organ systems or may interact with another drug to alter the therapeutic effectiveness of both. This section attempts to provide the reader with a brief overview of the problems of drug therapy, most particularly when multiple drugs are used.

ABSORPTION

Bioavailability is but the first of many factors influencing the effect of a drug or chemical, for it is necessary for a drug to reach the general circulation in order to produce a therapeutic effect. Drugs are of course much more readily available when administered parenterally, particularly into the veins. However, the site of injection, the circulation to the area, and the solubility of the drug in tissue influence the bioavailability. When given orally, the absorption from the intestinal tract may not be predictable, for the drug may be inactivated in the intestines, there may be incomplete absorption, or, in case of hyperperistalsis, there may not be time for the drug to be absorbed. Moreover, the drug may interact in the gastrointestinal tract with food and other drugs. An example of this is the formation of insoluble complexes when the antibiotic tetracycline is combined with minerals and cannot be absorbed.[17] Other variables influencing bioavailability of orally administered products include gastrointestinal pH, the function of the liver and pancreas, and diseases of the stomach.[18] Even the same person may show variation at times in adequacy of absorption from the intestine.

DISPLACEMENT FROM ALBUMIN CARRIER SITES

Drugs are usually both free in the plasma and loosely bound to the plasma protein albumin. There are several binding sites on each albumin molecule with the albumin-bound portion of the drug being metabolically inactive, while the free portion is active. The drug is freed from the albumin bond as the free portion is metabolized in conformity with the law of mass action maintaining an equilibrium. Consequently, the protein-bound portion acts as a reservoir and prevents wide fluctuation between ineffective levels and toxic levels. Drugs may compete for similar binding sites, one having the greater affinity displacing another. The therapeutic or toxic effect of the displaced drug is increased, for the effective concentration is higher. But the duration of action is shortened because a greater quantity of the unbound drug is available for metabolism and excretion. For example, the anticoagulant coumadin is quite easily displaced from its bond to albumin. This displacement leads to fluctuations in the effective concentration in the blood. There is then delivery of excessive quantity of the drug to its site of action immediately after administration of the drug, but with inadequate concentrations between doses.

LIVER ENZYME INDUCTION

The simultaneous administration of two or more drugs may result in interactions that increase or decrease the intended effects of one or every drug. These interactions result from metabolic alterations that are "induced" in the liver's microsomal enzymes responsible for the metabolism of the drugs—hence the term "enzyme induction." Several hundred chemicals found in drugs and the environment are known to affect the activity of these drug-metabolizing enzymes of the liver.[19-21] Examples of inducers include insecticides, herbicides, dyes, food preservatives, nicotine, and alcohol in addition to drugs. It is of interest that cigarette smoke contains the inducer benzo(a)-pyrene and other polycyclic hydrocarbons implicated in lung cancer.[22] There does not appear to be any relationship between the structure or activity of these drugs and chemicals and their ability to induce increased activity of these liver enzymes.

Illustrative examples of enzyme induction involving commonly used substances are those of phenobarbital and ethyl alcohol ingestion. When phenobarbital is prescribed with anticoagulant drugs (e.g., coumadin), the phenobarbital induces enzyme action in the liver, resulting in an increased rate of metabolism and destruction of the anticoagulant, leading to a decreased effectiveness of the anticoagulant. If the phenobarbital is then discontinued, the enzyme induction effect of the phenobarbital decreases over a week or more, and the anticoagulant is not as efficiently destroyed. The net effect is an increased effectiveness of the anticoagulant, resulting in a predisposition to severe hemorrhagic problems. It is easy to see that the patient could bleed from a chronic peptic ulcer. Likewise, the risk of a cerebral hemorrhage in the hypertensive patient would be enhanced. When there is chronic ethyl alcohol consumption, the metabolism is enhanced in a variety of drugs, including those used for the control of epileptic seizures, diabetes, the anticoagulation of blood, and for sedation (e.g., dilantin, tolbutamide, coumadin, barbiturates). The chronic consumption of ethanol also increases its own metabolism as well as a variety of other drugs. However, a single large dose of ethyl alcohol inhibits drug metabolism, which accounts for the enhanced sensitivity to barbiturates and other sedatives that is seen in intoxicated persons.[23]

Drug Allergy

Allergic reactions to drugs occur when a drug combines with a large molecule in the body, usually a protein, in essence forming a new substance which the body recognizes as "foreign" and attempts to destroy by forming antibodies against it. In the course of destroying the drug-protein complex, the body injures itself. As a rule, drugs do not cause allergic reactions until they have conjugated with large molecules of the body. There is a low overall incidence of allergic drug reactions, and there is also a marked variation with different drugs in frequency of reactions and their occurrence in specific organ systems.[24] Unfortunately there is no single, universally applicable test for predicting drug allergies.[25] In vitro laboratory assays for the detection of serum antibodies to drug hypersensitivity have been developed, but are not generally available. Direct skin testing for antibodies is particularly useful in penicillin allergy, and the dangerous anaphylactic sensitivity is indicated by the development of a marked skin response within 15 to 20 minutes. Skin testing is also useful when local anesthetics are to be used, but in other forms of drug hypersensitivity, it is probably of little or no value unless there is a well-established history of prior reactions to the drug. The clinical manifestations of drug allergy are discussed below.

ANAPHYLAXIS

Systemic anaphylaxis is an acute, life-threatening allergic reaction which may include shock, cardiac arrhythmias, and laryngeal edema with choking. Occurring most frequently with intravenous or intramuscular administration in a highly sensitive person, it can also occur in highly sensitive persons after ingestion or even respiratory exposure. Penicillin has been often incriminated, but with improvement in penicillin preparations and awareness of the problem by the medical profession, the mortality has been substantially lowered. A wide variety of diagnostic agents, local anesthetics, and therapeutic drugs have been implicated in severe or fatal anaphylactic reactions.[26,27]

SERUM SICKNESS

Serum sickness is an allergic reaction to drugs which is characterized by fever, rash, enlarged lymph nodes, edema, arthritis, and occasionally by nerve and kidney inflammation. This condition may develop with the first exposure to a drug when the drug attaches to a circulating body protein, and antibodies are consequently produced. There is usually a latent period from the initial administration of the drug to the clinical reaction of at least a week, the period required for the body to synthesize sufficient antibodies against the drug-protein complex.[28]

CYTOTOXIC REACTIONS DIRECTED AGAINST INDIVIDUAL ORGANS

These are immunologic reactions in which a drug reacts or interacts with an organ, resulting in damage to the organ. Unfortunately, these are not rare and may be either acute or chronic. The commonest forms encountered clinically are immune hemolytic anemia, thrombocytopenia, and granulocytopenia. In hemolytic anemia, the red cells are altered and are susceptible to accelerated destruction. Patients suffering from thrombocytopenia have reduced platelets and increased bleeding, while those with agranulocytosis have reduced white blood cells and are most vulnerable to infections. Death can occur from anemia, bleeding, or infection which is directly caused by drugs.

Drugs and Congenital Malformations

Irrespective of the cause, defects existing at the birth of a child create problems and generate questions. Nearly 3 percent of all newborns have congenital malformations, most of these limited to one site in the body, and malformations are the most common cause of childhood hospitalization in North America.[29] Although about one-third of congenital abnormalities are life-threatening, in many instances they are not lethal, as witnessed by the malformed limbs of children whose mothers were exposed to thalidomide[30] or haloperidol[31] during the first trimester of pregnancy. Not only is the teratogenicity of these particular drugs quite firmly established, but it is recognized that chemically reactive metabolites of drugs and chemicals may mediate many serious reactions, including mutagenesis.[32] Unfortunately, scientific information regarding the cause and prevention of congenital abnormalities remains limited. It is estimated that of the 3 percent of children born with congenital abnormalities, the cause is established in less than 20 percent. In about 10 percent there are associated gene mutations, while 5 percent are *known* to be due to a teratogenic agent.[33]

Malformations may be multiple in the same child, or they may be a single localized malformation. Localized malformations such as cardiac anomalies, cleft lip and palate, and clubfoot deformities may be due to the additive effect of minor gene abnormalities and environmental factors.[34] To recognize whether a malformation is due to a gene mutation or to environmental factors such as drugs or chemicals is difficult indeed, for it is based in part on clinical evaluation. A malformation occurring in more than one member of the same family can have at least four causes. Malformations due to teratogens such as maternal alcoholism[35] or trimethadion[36] can only be established by a carefully taken history of the pregnancy coupled with a review of the medical literature, heritable chromosome abnormalities diagnosed by chromosome analysis, and multifactorial or mendelian inheritance. The diagnosis of the latter is established by systematically collecting data from large numbers of families to determine whether the affected siblings or parents and the child reflect multifactorial or mendelian inheritance. Modern geneticists label any characteristic, normal or abnormal, that segregates in a manner described by Mendel as exhibiting a mendelian pattern of inheritance. About 1,000 diseases are currently suspected of being inherited in a mendelian fashion. Occurring in clinical practice are nearly 600 disorders known to show genetic dominant expression and about 450 that are recessive. Of these, over 90 are X-linked.[37]

DEATHS RELATED TO SURGICAL CARE

Surgery involves numerous medical personnel acting individually and in concert to provide a type of patient care. Untoward events occasionally leading to the death of a patient can occur prior to, during, or following the actual operative procedure. These events are grouped under the heading of death related to surgical care. The bulk of malpractice cases brought to litigation have been surgical in nature or at least related to operative procedures. The American Surgical Association formally acknowledges that when unforeseen and undesirable injury to a patient occurs while under surgical care, the patients so injured are entitled to appropriate reparations.[38]

Deaths related to surgical care include delay and error in the diagnosis of an illness in which surgery is the treatment of choice; deaths from premedication errors prior to an operation; anesthetic events during surgery; hemorrhage, shock, or cardiac arrest while under anesthesia; events during surgery including severe burns from electrosurgery; explosions from electrocautery of the poorly prepared bowel;[39] and incomplete surgery when in the course of an operation the surgeon fails to perform some or all of the procedures indicated. Postoperative events such as delayed hemorrhage, pulmonary emboli, and nosocomial infections are related to surgical care. In addition, surgical complications may be delayed for weeks, months, or even years. Surgical injury to a ureter during operations in the lower abdomen, such as hysterectomy, may not be immediately apparent but may lead to delayed kidney damage and perhaps death. Artificial plastic and metallic devices implanted in the body may fail to function properly after many years of good service. A prime example of this delayed surgical complication is the prosthetic or artificial heart valve. This may become thrombosed or worn and malfunction years after placement. Even surgically implanted cardiac pacemakers may fail to perform properly when other later surgical procedures are performed,[40] or through no fault of the device or of the surgeon. Electromagnetic potentials in the patient-environment such as television transmission or a microwave oven may lead to cardiac arrhythmias.[41] Such dangers are slight, but they are real, though it may be stretching credulity to assign such deaths to complications of surgery.

There are a number of situations where surgical inaction may lead to the death of a patient. Appendicitis, being one of the more common complaints with which mankind is afflicted, can result in tragic consequences if not promptly diagnosed and adequately treated. Commonest among the surgical inactions leading to patient death is the failure to diagnose an ectopic pregnancy with resulting rupture of the fallopian tube with massive and often fatal intra-abdominal hemorrhage. The rather common tonsillectomy may also be complicated by massive hemorrhage, cardiac arrest, and death. Each individual situation must be evaluated on its own merits, for there are rare *prima facie* instances where death can be attributed to the surgical team.

Surgery has inherent risks for the patient, but there are also risks for the people working in the surgical suite. Those working in the operating room area are subject to serious occupational health hazards including an increase in rate of spontaneous abortions, higher incidence of congenital abnormalities in their children, and more liver disease and cancer.[42]

DEATHS RELATED TO ANESTHESIA

Death directly attributable to anesthesia may not be preventable since this procedure always involves an inherent risk. Equipment failure, cardiac arrest, liver or kidney damage, and malignant hyperthermia are the major dangers when general anesthesia is used, but anesthetic procedures on ambulatory patients or outpatients may be also hazardous in the individual patient.[43]

Equipment failure or mislabeling of oxygen and anesthetic gases may go undetected for months and may not be identified as a cause of resulting deaths. A number of anesthetic agents, including cyclopropane, diethyl ether, divinyl ether, and ethylene will burn if mixed with air, and generally will explode violently if mixed with oxygen. Therefore, fire and electrical safety problems are most important in operating room safety.

Cardiac arrest during the induction of anesthesia or while the surgical procedure is in progress may be due to inadequate preanesthetic medication, obstruction of the airway from aspiration of food, vomitus or instruments, insufficient oxygenation, excessive carbon dioxide in the inspired air, too rapid induction of the anesthesia, an overdose of the anesthetic agent, hypersensitivity of the individual to the anesthetic agent employed, or neurogenic vagal stimulation initiated by the endotracheal intubation or other anesthetic maneuver.

Halothane is an anesthetic agent introduced into clinical practice in 1956. It was widely used, being nonflammable, potent, not unpleasant to breathe, and capable of producing rapid anesthesia induction and rapid recovery from anesthesia. However, there are many published reports of hepatitis following the use of halothane.[44] The incidence of liver damage is said by other authors to be quite small and not appreciably different from that following the use of other agents. Thus there is an unresolved issue of the liver toxicity of halothane. Those believing that halothane is hepatotoxic relate this to a body defense mechanism similar to the antigen-antibody response. The first exposure to the anesthetic agent builds up antibodies, and with subsequent exposure an antigen-antibody reaction occurs, resulting in liver injury and frequently death. Methoxyflurane is another noninflammable, volatile liquid which produces an excellent general anesthesia. However, instances of nephrotoxicity and fatalities have been reported.

Malignant hyperthermia, as the name implies, is a condition of unknown cause in which the body temperature increases to a range of 104 to 112° F with mortality ranging from 64 to 83 percent, hence the designation of "malignant." Fortunately it is very rare, occurring in approximately 1:14,000 general anesthetics.[45] The hyperthermia may be fulminant with a rapid rise in body temperature with rigidity of the skeletal muscles shortly after the induction of anesthesia; or it may be delayed and skeletal muscle rigidity may or may not be present.[46] The condition appears to be familial, and CPK elevations in the blood noted on preanesthetic testing may indicate a predisposition or susceptibility to malignant hyperthermia during the general anesthesia. Prediction of its occurrence, however, is extremely difficult or impossible, and a history of an unusual anesthetic episode in the family may be the only indicator. The treatment includes discontinuance of the anesthesia and surgery when possible, 100 percent oxygen, and hypothermic measures. Later complications include muscle and liver damage, renal damage from myoglobinuria, fluid and electrolyte imbalances, and disseminated intravascular coagulation.

CARDIAC ARREST

When death while under medical care is attributed to cardiac arrest, two questions immediately come to mind: What caused the cardiac arrest, and was prompt diagnosis with immediate resuscitative attempts instituted by those entrusted with the medical care of the patient?[47,48] Cardiac arrest is the sudden, unexpected, inadequate, or ineffective cardiac output of blood with resultant inadequate supply of blood to meet the needs of the body. The brain is particularly susceptible to hypoxia, and inadequate supply of blood with oxygen and permanent brain injury or death may occur if immediate corrective steps are not taken. It is generally agreed that there is a 3- to 4-minute critical period after cardiac arrest beyond which some of the brain cells, deprived of the required oxygen, cannot survive. Cardiac arrest occasionally complicates procedures commonly employed in the diagnosis and treatment of disease and is an inherent risk during surgery and anesthesia. Cardiac arrest is not necessarily fatal, nor need there be residual brain damage if the diagnosis is promptly established and cardiopulmonary resuscitative procedures are successful.

The term "cardiac arrest" is not entirely accurate, for "arrest" implies standstill of the heart. A better expression would be "cardiac rhythm disturbances with failure of the heart as a pump." However, this form is obviously too cumbersome, and the term cardiac arrest has come to include sudden life-threatening rhythm disturbances of heart action where there is inadequate or ineffective pumping of the blood by the heart. These include ventricular standstill, where the action of the heart is totally arrested; ventricular bradycardia, in which the heart pumps so slowly and infrequently (less than 20 per minute) that adequate circulation cannot be maintained; ventricular fibrillation; and ventricular tachycardia, where the ventricular chambers contract over 200 beats per minute, and the heart is ineffective as a pump, for insufficient blood leaves the heart to support the brain. Cardiac arrest, including these various disturbances of heart rhythm, may be due to a number of causes; however, the cause may not be identified in some instances. The following factors should be considered either alone or in combination as predisposing a patient to cardiac rhythm disturbances:

1. Inadequate oxygen to the heart muscle as occurs with sudden occlusion of a coronary artery.
2. Surgery of any type imposes a strain on the heart which may precipitate cardiac arrhythmias, myocardial infarcts, or heart failure. Patients with heart disease are particularly prone to arrest during surgery; however, arrest may occur in the normal heart even during minor procedures that are of short duration. Viscerocardiac reflexes with cardiac arrest may be due to handling of the internal organs at the time of operation.
3. Medications which have a specific toxic action on the heart may cause arrest, and other drugs may result in an allergic reaction or cause vomiting with aspiration of gastric materials with arrest of the heart.[49] Quite a number of drugs either depress or heighten the irritability of the heart and conduction system, thus predisposing to cardiac arrhythmias.
4. Blood chemistry imbalance of any cause. This is frequent in burn patients, perhaps because intravenous blood and fluid infusions can aggravate or precipitate heart failure, pulmonary edema, or cardiac arrest.
5. Shock from massive hemorrhage or allergic reaction to drugs or other substances.
6. During anesthesia, cardiac arrest may be traced to inadequate preanesthetic medication, inadequate ventilation of air into the lungs, obstruction of the airway due to instruments or the aspiration of vomitus, excessive carbon dioxide in the inspired air, too rapid induction of anesthesia, an overdose of the anesthetic agent, hypersensitivity of the individual to the anesthetic agent employed, or reflex viscerocardiac stimulation resulting from endotracheal intubation or other anesthetic maneuvers.
7. In blacks who carry a genetic trait resulting in sickling or destruction of red blood cells.

The diagnosis of cardiac arrest is based on the absence of pulses, no obtainable blood pressure, dilated pupils, loss of consciousness if the patient was awake, and failure to bleed from cut vessels at the time of surgery. The treatment includes resuscitative efforts. Cardiopulmonary resuscitative techniques are well recognized, and proficiency in these procedures is expected of persons working with patients exposed to this risk.[50] There are dangers inherent in the resuscitative efforts, including rib fractures, heart and lung injury, pneumothorax, marrow emboli, and defibrillation injuries to the heart with residual compromised heart function.[51]

INCIDENTS IN INTENSIVE CARE UNITS

The intensive care units of hospitals are possessed of a certain glamour for they connote life-saving procedures, and admittedly these facilities have very often sustained the lives of those in extremis. Yet, if the intensive care unit is evidence of medical progress, it may also create diseases of medical progress.[52] The question one struggles with is whether an individual, who would have died without the intensive care and dies somewhat later, has in fact died as a complication of the intensive care.

Concentrated in the intensive care unit (ICU) of a hospital are sophisticated therapeutic devices and emergency procedures with equipment and personnel to constantly monitor and evaluate the critically ill patient, both clinically and bioelectronically. Customarily, these include precise studies and monitoring of cardiorespiratory function, the cerebral state, and hepatic and renal functions. These are coupled with artificially supported respiration and heart rhythm control. Precise electrolyte, pulmonary gas, and arterial gas studies are immediately available. Patients found in the ICU include those with strokes, acute pulmonary insufficiency, cardiac arrhythmia and arrest, severe heart failure, myocardial infarction, renal failure, drug overdose, diabetic coma, and hypoglycemic shock.

Respiratory derangements as complications of the ICU occur with some frequency. Laryngeal and tracheal injury from passing artificial ventilatory tubes may lead to ulcerations, necrosis, and tracheal stenosis if the patient survives. The "solid lung syndrome" or "respirator lung" is often found in the patient who dies in the ICU. The determination of whether this is an iatrogenic disease or a result of pre-existing disease of the lung is not always possible. Disease conditions such as shock, severe trauma, sepsis, and extensive burns may lead to solid lungs. On the other hand, the use of oxygen, narcotics, curare, and airway obstruction of any cause, including ventilatory tubes, are iatrogenic factors leading to respiratory depression and ultimately the respirator lung. The lung becomes solid with the development of bronchial breathing and appears frothy on X-ray. There is a normal Pco_2 with a decrease in arterial oxygen saturation during the terminal day, and the patients will have received ventilatory assistance and oxygen prior to death.

The introduction of intravenous and intra-arterial tubes into the vessels and heart is an integral part of the ICU. In the smaller vessels, complications of hemorrhages, thrombosis, and infection occur. Deep vein thrombosis may develop, and should these embolize, pulmonary infarction and death may result. The use of the central venous pressure catheter or pacemakers introduced into the superior vena cava may on occasion lead to death. The superior vena cava may thrombose with subsequent embolization, or a thrombus may become infected with showering of septic emboli to the lungs and other organs with resulting infections. Pacemakers introduced into the heart may, on rare occasions, perforate the heart with massive internal hemorrhage resulting.

DIAGNOSTIC X-RAY PROCEDURES

Diagnostic x-ray procedures carry a degree of calculated risk, and while complications are rare in comparison to the number performed, an occasional death may occur. Generally, deaths are due to idiosyncratic reactions to the radiologic contrast media which cannot be reasonably determined beforehand. However, those using radiologic contrast materials for diagnostic purposes are expected to be aware of the dangers, contraindications, and adverse reactions incidental to their use. They should be prepared with both facilities and knowledge for the treatment of such reactions.

Barium sulfate is the most commonly used radiologic contrast medium. The barium enema and the upper GI series are familiar diagnostic procedures. There are many other procedures and substances widely used in radiologic diagnoses that incorporate material which, like barium, are visible, or "radiopaque," when the body is x-rayed. They are visible because they "contrast," due to their specific properties, with the surrounding tissues when viewed with a fluoroscope or with films. Contrast media may be either radionuclides (radioactive isotopes) which emit radiation which is then imaged on the film, or radiopaques which, because of their density, result in opacification. The radiopaque media may be either soluble or insoluble. Barium sulfate is the major insoluble radiopaque material and rarely results in complications, although transmission of viruses,[53] penetration or perforation of the bowel wall with a barium granuloma,[54] or even death from barium intravasation into the portal system with death[55] may result from an improperly placed enema tip. Iodine-containing material is the most significant soluble radiopaque media, for while it has a high atomic number with high absorption characteristics, it is also associated with significant severe reactions and occasionally with patient death. Iodine-containing material may be given by mouth for visualization of the gallbladder, in which case the iodine is absorbed from the bowel to be secreted by the liver and concentrated in the gallbladder. Soluble iodine-containing contrast media is widely used to visualize the urinary tract. Here it is given intravenously and is concentrated in and excreted by the kidney. Consequently, its value in diagnosing diseases of the kidney and urinary tract is widely appreciated and applied, and failure to use this form of diagnostic procedure may constitute negligent medical practice. Iodine-containing media are also given intravenously or intra-arterially for the demonstration of blood vessels. With the development of vascular surgery, this procedure is used, prior to coronary bypass grafts, to demonstrate arteries of the extremities, brain, kidneys, adrenal, liver, pancreas, and mesentery. Complications associated with soluble iodine-containing contrast media vary from insignificant nausea and flushing to shock, convulsions, respiratory and cardiac arrest, and death. The mechanism of toxicity is not fully established, but it is believed that inhibition of the enzyme cholinesterase may lead to altered capillary permeability and cardiac conduction abnormalities.

Friedman[56] has prepared a clear discussion of the precautions and the relative and absolute contraindications to intravenous use of iodine-containing substances, as well as the drugs and equipment that should be in the emergency cart to treat untoward reactions.

TRANSFUSION REACTIONS AND SERUM HEPATITIS

The administration of blood may be fatal if a patient suffers a transfusion reaction from incompatible blood or develops a disease such as serum hepatitis transmitted via the blood. The transfusion of blood depends on a number of technical steps with attendant safeguards. The technical steps include the collection of blood from the donor, the typing and testing of the donor's blood, the typing of the recipient's blood, the crossmatching of the blood of the donor with that of the recipient to assure compatibility, and the transfusion of the donor blood into the recipient patient. The transfusion of incompatible blood can result when a member of the laboratory staff makes a mistake in the typing of the blood, and the recipient of the blood has a transfusion reaction. Mislabeled blood, clerical errors, and the administrative error of transfusing the wrong persons are instances of mistakes that can lead to transfusion reactions which may be fatal. The courts have indicated that the liability of the blood bank staff exists in taking, typing, crossmatching, and, to a lesser degree, administering blood to the recipient.[57]

Viral hepatitis, which may be fatal, is transmissible by whole blood or frozen blood,[58] or from blood products such as Konyne.[59] Konyne is a concentrate of Factors II, VII, IX, and X, given intravenously for bleeding disorders. Fatal viral hepatitis can also be transmitted by contaminated needles and other hospital equipment, and hepatitis is a serious threat to both patients and staff members in renal hemodialysis units.[60,61]

CANCER DEATHS RELATED TO MEDICAL CARE

Neoplasia Induced by Medical Treatment

Reported instances of cancer induced by medical treatment are rare since the manifestations of neoplasia occur many years after the completion of the course of treatment. It is difficult to establish a cause and effect relationship between the therapy and the tumor. The classic example is the liver neoplasia (hemangioendothelioma) induced by thorium dioxide (Thorotrast), in which the latent period may be decades. In 1965, Da Silva Horta and coworkers[62] checked the records of 2,377 patients who had received thorium dioxide injections as a radiographic contrast media between 1930 and 1952. They found 22 cases of thorium dioxide-induced liver hemangioendothelioma in which the latent period was 20 years or more. In addition, there were 16 cases of fatal blood dyscrasias, six acute and two chronic leukemias, and six aplastic anemias. These studies were confirmed by other authors. Although thorium dioxide is no longer used, tumors caused by its use in the past still sporadically appear and go unreported in the medical literature as this is a well-recognized entity.

Drug-induced neoplasia tends to develop at the sites where there is maximum concentration of the drug. Thus thorium dioxide is carcinogenic in the liver because it is stored, metabolized, and excreted by the liver. Bladder carcinoma due to drugs and chemicals is to be expected, for the bladder is exposed to concentrated urine for periods of time. Examples of drugs incriminated in urinary tract carcinoma include chlornaphazine[63] and the analgesic phenacetin.[64] The arsenicals are also carcinogenic, and although they are not part of the current medical armamentarium, they are widely distributed in the environment. Skin and vulvar carcinoma from exposure to pesticides is well recognized.[65]

The widespread use of therapeutic and contraceptive steroids has led to a number of neoplastic complications. Diethylstilbestrol was widely used at one time as a way of preserving the pregnancy when maternal bleeding was present.[66] Many years later, vaginal adenosis and clear cell carcinoma of the vagina developed in a significant number of the female children of these mothers.[67,68] These tumors continue to appear sporadically, a grim reminder that the long-term effects of many drugs used in medical therapy are unknown. Contraceptive steroids can lead to adenomas of the liver in females who take them for birth control, and although these adenomas are considered benign tumors, they may grow to a large size and rupture, resulting in death from massive hemorrhage into the abdomen.[69] It is also reported that if a mother inadvertently continues to use oral contraceptives into pregnancy, the infant may develop a benign liver tumor.[70] Drugs may also be implicated in the induction of neoplasia by interfering with the patient's immune mechanisms.[71] Drugs such as prednisone and azothioprine, used in renal transplant patients to prevent rejection of the kidney, may alter the body defenses to tumors and thus lead to death related to medical therapy.[72]

Ionizing radiation, used medically for diagnosis (X-rays) and treatment, is a well-documented carcinogen. Radiologists who are occupationally exposed to radiation have a significantly higher death rate from leukemia than do other physicians and the general population. Patients irradiated for the treatment of ankylosing spondylitis have a greater incidence of leukemia, and children who have been irradiated before birth also have a greater risk of developing leukemia in the first decade of life.[73] It is now recognized that individuals who received therapeutic doses of X-radiation or radium application to the head, neck, or upper thorax for various nonmalignant conditions during infancy or childhood have an increased risk of developing cancer of the thyroid gland and, to a lesser extent, of the salivary glands and other structures of the head and neck.[74] Fortunately, these tumors are generally slow-growing, but efforts must be made to identify (from the medical records of therapy) those individuals at risk so that they can be examined and treated if necessary.

Delay in Diagnosis

Early detection of cancer is often an important factor in improving the chances for a cure or prevention of further spread of the disease. There has been a great deal of publicity and information about the incidence and risks of cancer, and delay factors in making the diagnosis and instituting treatment may be either from procrastination by the patient or the physician. Failing to perform or order a biopsy, diagnostic test, or X-ray may be the cause of the delayed diagnosis. When a reasonably careful physician or surgeon would conclude, on the basis of the patient's symptoms, that a biopsy or other diagnostic test or X-ray is indicated, failure to advise or perform the procedure may constitute negligent medical practice. As a matter of fact, Section 405.1028(h) of the Medicare law requires that all tissues removed surgically be examined by a pathologist, at least macroscopically. There is little difficulty in finding expert medical testimony to show that the patient's chances of survival are appreciably better if indicated diagnostic procedures are performed. Mittelmann and Scholhamer,[75] in an analysis of 36 medical malpractice claims related to the diagnosis of cancer, have reviewed the literature and made suggestions for claims prevention.

A delay in diagnosis can also result from incorrect interpretation of an x-ray film by the radiologist or incorrect diagnosis by the pathologist examining biopsied tissue. The delay in diagnosis persists until the films or slides are reviewed, or the tumor is widespread and the nature of the disease is clinically obvious. Failure to recognize a malignant neoplasm when one is in fact present can, of course, result in the patient's death. On occasion it is most difficult to distinguish histologically benign, premalignant, and malignant lesions, particularly of the breast. The distinction between benign nevi (moles) of the skin and the malignant melanoma (black cancer) can be most troublesome. It is the practice in our hospital to have consultation if there is any question regarding the distinction between benign and malignant lesions. Consultation may not resolve the question, but providing the patient with the optimal diagnostic skills available is, we believe, a reasonable standard of medical care.

The Supreme Court of Illinois held that the statute of limitations does not begin to run until the mistaken diagnosis was, or should have been, discovered.[76]

Complications of Therapy

The complications of cancer therapy are as numerous as the therapies employed. The complications of surgery for cancer are, as with other surgical procedures for other diseases, numerous and include hemorrhage and shock, cardiac arrest, and anesthetic difficulties, among many others. Surgery for carcinoma, by necessity, must be extensive to eradicate the disease, and complications are inherent risks of the procedures. Radiation is an effective means of combating some forms of cancers, but the characteristics that endow ionizing radiation with its remarkable tumoricidal properties at the same time cause damage to nontumorous tissues within the radiation field. This can result in severe patient distress, disability, and occasionally death. Complications which may be fatal include acute exudative radiation pneumonitis, ulcerative gastritis or enteritis, ulcerative dermatitis and mucositis, and radiation nephritis.[77,78] Chemotherapeutic antineoplastic drugs and chemicals have frequent and severe side effects that may lead to fatal complications. The most serious and frequent toxicity encountered with antineoplastic compounds is depression of the bone marrow. Anemia, a propensity to hemorrhage, and susceptibility to "opportunistic" infection with microorganisms such as *Candida albicans* or Staphylococcus may follow bone marrow depression.[79] Chemical antineoplastic agents may be responsible for a variety of clinical problems in the lungs, by direct or secondary mechanisms. These include infections, pulmonary emboli, adult respiratory distress syndrome,[80] and drug-induced pneumonitis.[81,82]

DEATHS RELATED TO HOSPITAL CARE AND NOSOCOMIAL INFECTIONS

A hospital is not a cocoon of safety insulating a patient from a hostile world, and when a death results from some aspect of hospital care it is customary to attribute death to the condition leading to the hospitalization. Thus it is no more possible to catalogue the specific aspects of hospital care that can be fatal than it is to obtain statistics indicating the incidence of such fatalities. Cardiac arrest and misadventures involving hospital-dispensed drugs are exceptions that may be recognized and documented in hospital records, and because of their frequency, they are separately discussed. Suicide while under care in a hospital and falls on hospital premises which lead to death are not within the scope of this chapter, for they raise different issues of cause and responsibility.

Practically every aspect of hospital care could conceivably contribute, or directly lead, to the death of a patient. The extremely rare death from orthopedic traction,[83] and the relatively common hospital-related infection and pulmonary emboli are but examples. The sudden collapse and death of a patient, due to a lethal pulmonary emboli, is a specter which haunts every physician who has practiced clinical medicine. A thrombus from which the embolus originates is nearly always formed in the leg veins, particularly the calf; in gynecologic and obstetric patients, the offending site is likely to be the pelvic veins. The dominant factor in the formation of the thrombus in the leg seems to be a slowing of circulation. It is predisposed to by cardiac disease, debility, obesity, and abdominal operations which interfere with movement and breathing. Prolonged immobilization in bed also predisposes the patient, and the pressure of hard hospital mattresses on the calf of the leg may empty veins, bringing the internal vein surfaces into contact, resulting in injury to the lining and the subsequent formation of a clot. In the surgical patient, the sudden occurrence of the pulmonary emboli customarily takes place 2 to 3 weeks after the operation when the patient is in the recovery phase. There is a sudden restlessness, shock with substernal distress, and collapse, sometimes followed by death after a few minutes. The horror of the family and the distress of the nurses and physicians is too obvious to warrant discussion. Unfortunately, the prevention of pulmonary emboli is difficult. In fact, recognition of the leg vein thrombus in the prodromal period is difficult or impossible. Prevention may include early ambulation of the patient, prevention of injury to the legs, elastic wrappings of the legs when possible, and in some instances the use of anticoagulants. If there are small emboli to the lung, this may alert the medical staff of the possibility of a later-occurring, larger and potentially fatal embolism.

A fluid overload may not be significant in patients with adequate circulatory and renal function, yet fluid overload resulting from too vigorous intravenous fluid therapy may be fatal in the individual patient. The compromised heart and the failing kidney may not be able to compensate for the accumulations of fluid. The lung, with its unique circulatory pressures, is particularly vulnerable to fluid overload with the fluid accumulations interfering with respiration. The edematous lung is also susceptible to bacterial infections, for edema fluid provides excellent media for the growth of microorganisms. Fluid overload has been observed in patients with facial burns or in intubated patients in which the fluid overload has been the immediate cause of death. The respiratory passages are narrowest in the vocal cord area, and both burns to the face and plastic or rubber tubes that have been in the larynx may injure the larynx and the vocal cords. With fluid overload, the already injured laryngeal area may become edematous and the small passage may become obstructed. The burned patient is frequently given opiates for the control of pain, and the patient who has had tubes in the larynx may be immediately postoperative and under sedation; therefore, these patients cannot easily call attention to their respiratory difficulties. If an autopsy is performed, the appearance of the swollen vocal cords is awesome. Is the death of a burned patient dying of asphyxia from swelling of the vocal cords resulting from fluid overload a medically related death, or is this a death related to the incident causing the burns?

No less dramatic is the patient dying in the hospital from food asphyxia. Suffocation due to the inhalation of food is reported to account for 1.3 percent of all deaths of patients who come to autopsy at a hospital for chronic diseases.[84] These patients die suddenly, during or shortly after meals, and myocardial infarction is frequently misdiagnosed. Sedation, old age, and poor dentition predispose to the aspiration of food. The danger of food asphyxiation in hospitalized patients would be minimized by appropriate diets, the judicious use of sedation, observation of patients during meal time, and hospital personnel trained in methods of extracting food.

Nosocomial infections are hospital-based infections as contrasted to community-acquired infections. A nosocomial infection is defined as one not present or incubating in the patient at the time of admission to a hospital. Nosocomial bacteremias are demonstrated by positive blood cultures in approximately four per 1,000 hospital admissions,[85] and the added hospital costs in a single large city hospital were estimated at $5 million per year.[86]

Nosocomial infections are encountered more frequently in surgical patients, but the incidence is also significant among medical, obstetric, and pediatric patients, and in the newborn nursery.[87] The use and/or misuse of urinary catheters as well as techniques and equipment employed in intravenous therapy, hyperalimentation, and respiratory therapy account for most of these infections. An indwelling urinary or intravenous catheter in place for 48 to 72 hours significantly increases the likelihood of a bacteremia which may lead to a fatal infection. Patients who are immunosuppressed, as in the kidney transplant recipient, or those on chemotherapeutic drugs for cancer, may die as a result of the infection.[88] Therefore, methods must be instituted and procedures monitored in a hospital to decrease the likelihood that patients placed in contact with pathogenic organisms will contract a disease.[89] There is an extensive body of information regarding the substantial reduction in hospital-associated infections through the use of correct procedures and methods.[90]

INCIDENTS INVOLVING INSTITUTIONALIZED AND ELDERLY PATIENTS

The physically and mentally handicapped and the elderly not only experience acute conditions requiring medical care, but often have additional problems. Unfortunately, custodial institutions and those caring for the chronically ill may serve purely as human warehouses, offering little or no medical care. Regrettably, this type of care, or lack of care, must be included under the aegis of "death related to medical care." Physicians may avoid caring for these patients for many reasons, personal as well as economic, for cures are infrequent and professional gratifications may be limited. Physicians' major criticisms of nursing homes include lack of adequate medical personnel, lack of adequate medical supervision, shortcomings in physical plant amenities, and poor attitudes on the part of the employees.[91] It is hardly necessary to catalogue specifics regarding medical supervision, plant facilities, and employee attitudes since these are revealed only when the individual institution is evaluated.

When death occurs in the chronically ill or debilitated patient who is institutionalized or in a nursing home, there is a tendency to certify the death as "natural" and due to the chronic condition that led to the person's being placed in the facility, or due to a stroke, myocardial infarct, or "the friend of the old man"—pneumonia. A lack of concerted and appropriate care can lead in a subtle way to the complications which are the immediate cause of death. Examples include a delay in the diagnosis of cancer, urinary retention with resultant bladder and kidney infection, poor nutrition, and osteomalacia with a hip fracture from minor trauma, with pulmonary emboli or pneumonia as the terminal event. Moreover, the elderly may quickly forget instructions and fail to take their medication, with resulting complications. The problem, however, is not limited to the elderly, for even children who require long-term medication or care can be inadvertently injured by the medical care. An example of this is the long-term administration of anticonvulsant drugs. These drugs can accelerate the metabolism of vitamin D and overt abnormalities of serum calcium and alkaline phosphate, or rickets can develop.[92] This same complication can develop in institutionalized patients who are nonambulatory, or kept indoors.

Individualization of the medical needs of each patient in a nursing home or institution is the first priority, not only to prevent deaths related to their medical care, but also to promote more humane institutions. The individual needs of the elderly patient may appear trivial to the healthy person, but such matters as a bent spoon to facilitate nutrition in the arthritic patient are significant measures in medical care. Publications devoted to these seemingly mundane subjects in reality establish a "standard of medical care"[93] which should be followed and respected.

REFERENCES

1. Mills, D. H.: Medical Injury Information: A Preparation for Analysis and Implementation of Prevention Programs. *J.A.M.A.* 236:379–381, 1976.
2. Ibid.
3. Epstein, S. S., and Grundy, R. D. (eds.): *Consumer Health and Product Hazards.* The MIT Press, Cambridge, Mass., 1974.
4. *Report of the International Conference on Adverse Reactions Reporting Systems.* National Academy of Sciences, Washington, D.C., 1971.
5. Caranascos, G. J., et al.: Drug-associated Deaths of Medical Inpatients. *Arch. Intern. Med.* 136:872–875, 1976.
6. Irey, N. S.: Adverse Drug Reactions and Deaths: A Review of 827 Cases. *J.A.M.A.* 236:575–578, 1976.
7. Taller, R. B.: Drug-induced Illness. *J.A.M.A.* 229:1043, 1974.
8. Phenformin: Removal from General Market. *FDA Drug Bull.* 7:14–16, 1977.
9. Prescott, L. F., et al.: Plasma-Paracetamol Half-life and Hepatic Necrosis in Patients with Paracetamol Overdose. *Lancet* 1:519–522, 1971.
10. Ambre, J., and Alexander, M.: Liver Toxicity After Acetaminophen Ingestion: Inadequacy of the Dose Estimate as an Index of Risk. *J.A.M.A.* 238:500–501, 1977.
11. D'Arcy, P. F., and Griffin, J. P.: *Iatrogenic Diseases.* Oxford University Press, New York, 1972.
12. Irey, N. S.: Adverse Reactions to Drug and Chemicals: A Resume and Progress Report. *J.A.M.A.* 230:596–98, 1974.
13. Sotaniemi, E., and Palva, I. P.: The Use of Polypharmaceutical Drug Therapy in a Medical Ward. *Ann. Clin. Res.* 4:158–164, 1972.
14. Kabins, S. A.: Interactions Among Antibiotics and Other Drugs. *J.A.M.A.* 219:206–212, 1972.
15. Kosman, M. E.: Pharmokinetic Drug Interactions: Sedative, Hypnotic and Antianxiety Agents. *J.A.M.A.* 229:1485-1488, 1974.
16. Hansten, P. D.: *Drug Interactions: Clinical Significance of Drug-Drug Interaction and Drug Effects on Clinical Laboratory Results.* ed. 2. Lea & Febiger, Philadelphia, 1973.
17. Prescott, L. F.: Pharmokinetic Drug Interactions. *Lancet* 2:1239–1243, 1969.
18. Koch-Weser, J.: Bioavailability of Drugs. *N. Engl. J. Med.* 291:233–237, 1974.
19. Conney, A. H.: Pharmacological Implications of Microsomal Enzyme Induction. *Pharmacol. Rev.* 19:317–366, 1967.
20. Conney, A. H., and Burns, J. J.: Metabolic Interactions Among Environmental Chemicals and Drugs. *Science* 178:576–586, 1972.
21. Gelehrter, T. D.: Enzyme Induction. *N. Engl. J. Med.* 294:589–595, 1976.
22. Kellerman, G., Shar, C. R., and Luyten-Kellerman, M.: Aryl Hydrocarbon Hydroxylase Inducibility and Bronchogenic Carcinoma. *N. Engl. J. Med.* 289:934–937, 1973.
23. Adverse Interactions of Drugs. *Med. Letter* 17:17–24, 1975.

24. *Report of the International Conference on Adverse Reactions Reporting Systems.* National Academy of Sciences, Washington, D.C., 1971.
25. Parker, C. W.: Drug Allergy. *N. Engl. J. Med.* 292:957–960, 1975.
26. Parker, C. S.: Drug Reactions, in Samter, M., and Alexander, H. H. (eds.): *Immunological Diseases.* Little, Brown, Boston, 1965.
27. DeWarte, R. D.: Drug Allergy, in Patterson, R. (ed.): *Allergic Diseases, Diagnosis and Management.* J.B. Lippincott, Philadelphia, 1972.
28. Kniker, W. T., and Cochrane, C. G.: The Localization of Circulating Immune Complexes in Experimental Serum Sickness. *J. Exp. Med.* 127:119–136, 1968.
29. Holmes, L. B.: Inborn Errors of Morphogenesis: A Review of Localized Hereditary Malformations. *N. Engl. J. Med.* 291:763–773, 1974.
30. Somer, G. F.: The Foetal Toxicity of Thalidomide. *Proc. Eur. Soc. Study Drug Toxic.* 1:49–58, 1965 (Bertilli, A. (ed.): *Teratology.* Amsterdam, Excerpta Medica, 1969).
31. Kopelman, A. E., McCullar, F. W., and Heggeness, L.: Limb Malformations Following Maternal Use of Haloperidol. *J.A.M.A.* 231:62–64, 1975.
32. Gillette, J. R., Michell, J. R., and Brodie, B. B.: Biochemical Mechanisms of Drug Toxicity. *Ann. Rev. Pharmacol.* 14:271–288, 1974.
33. Shepart, T. H.: *Catalog of Teratogenic Agents.* ed. 2. The John Hopkins University Press, Baltimore, 1976.
34. Carter, C. O.: Genetics of Common Disorders. *Br. Med. Bull.* 25:52–57, 1969.
35. Jones, K. L., et al.: Pattern of Malformation in Offspring of Chronic Alcoholic Mothers. *Lancet* 1:1267–1271, 1973.
36. German J., Knwal A., and Ehlers, K. H.: Trimethadione and Human Teratogenesis. *Teratology* 3:349–361, 1970.
37. McKusick, V.A.: *Mendelian Inheritance in Man.* ed. 4. The Johns Hopkins University Press, Baltimore, 1975.
38. American Surgical Association Statement on Professional Liability, September, 1976. *N. Engl. J. Med.* 295:1292–1296, 1976.
39. Ragins, H., Shinya, H., and Wolff, W. I.: The Explosive Potential of Colonic Gas During Colonoscopic Electrosurgical Polypectomy. *Surg. Gynecol. Obstet.* 138:554–556, 1974.
40. Smyth, N. P. D., Parsonnet, V., Escher, D. J. W., and Furman, S.: The Pacemaker Patient and the Electromagnetic Environment. *J.A.M.A.* 227:1412, 1974.
41. Switz, D. M., Clarks, A. M., and Longacher, J. W., Jr.: Electrical Malfunction at Endoscopy: Possible Cause of Arrhythmia and Death. *J.A.M.A.* 235:273–274, 1976.
42. Spence, A. A., et al: Occupational Hazards for Operating Room-based Physicians: Analysis of Data from the United States and the United Kingdom. *J.A.M.A.* 238:955–959, 1977.
43. Putman, L. P.: Pseudocholinesterase Deficiency: An Additional Preoperative Consideration in Outpatient Diagnostic Procedures. *South. Med. J.* 70:831–832, 1977.
44. Walton B., et al: Unexplained Hepatitis Following Halothane. *Br. Med. J.* 1:1171–1176, 1976.
45. Jones, E. W., and Burnap, T. K.: International Symposium on Malignant Hyperthermia. *Anesthesiology* 36:192–193, 1972.
46. Stephen, C. R.: Typical Cases of Malignant Hyperthermia, in Gordon, R. A., Britt, B. A., and Kalow, W. (eds.): *International Symposium on Malignant Hyperthermia.* Charles C Thomas, Springfield, Ill., 1973, pp. 11–15.
47. Sagall, E. L.: The Prevention of Cardiac Arrest—A Medical-Legal Problem, in Wecht, C. (ed.): *Legal Medicine Annual 1970.* Appleton-Century-Crofts, New York, 1970, pp. 195–211.
48. Sagall, E. L., and Reed, B. C.: *The Heart and the Law—A Practical Guide to Medicolegal Cardiology.* Macmillan, New York, 1968.
49. Alexander, C. S., and Niño, A.: Cardiovascular Complications in Young Patients Taking Psychotropic Drugs. *Am. Heart J.* 78:757–769, 1969.
50. Eliot, R. S., Wolf, G. L., and Foraker, A. D. (eds.): *Contemporary Problems in Cardiology.* Vol. 3: Cardiac Emergencies. Futura Publishing Co., Mount Kisco, N.Y., 1977.

51. Dahl, D. F., Ewy, G. A., and Warner, E. P.: Myocardial Necrosis from Direct Current Countershock. Effect of Paddle Electrode Size and Time Interval Between Discharges. *Circulation* 50:956–961, 1974.
52. Fattal, G. A., and Wyatt, J. P.: The Intensive Care Unit and the Pathology of Progress, in Sommers, S. C. (ed.): *Cardiovascular Pathology Decennial*. Appleton-Century-Crofts, New York, 1975, pp. 343–369.
53. Classen, J. N., Martin, R. E., and Sabagal, J.: Iatrogenic Lesions of the Colon and Rectum. *South. Med. J.* 68:1417–1428, 1975.
54. Lull, G. F., Bryne, J. P., and Sanowski, R. T.: Barium Enema Granulomas of the Rectum. *J.A.M.A.* 217:1102–1103, 1971.
55. Salve, A. F., Caprin, C. W., Leigh, K. E., and Dillihut, R. C.: Barium Intravasation into Portal Venous System During Barium Enema Examination. *J.A.M.A.* 235:749–751, 1976.
56. Friedman, P. A.: Legal Implications of the Use of Radiologic Contrast Media, in Wecht, C. (ed.): *Legal Medicine Annual: 1975*. Appleton-Century-Crofts, New York, 1976, pp. 249–260.
57. *Joseph v. W. H. Groves Latter-Day Saints Hospital*, 10 Utah 2d 94, 348, P 2d 935 (1960).
58. Tullis, J. L.: Incidence of Post-transfusion Hepatitis in Previously Frozen Blood. *J.A.M.A.* 214:719–723, 1970.
59. Erwin, W. S., and Nuckols, W. A.: Serum Hepatitis After Konyne Administration. *Va. Med. Monthly* 99:396–397, 1972.
60. Hemodialysis-associated Hepatitis, in *Hepatitis Surveillance Report 33*, Center for Disease Control, Atlanta, 1971, pp. 6–17.
61. Garibaldi, R. A., et al.: Hemodialysis-associated Hepatitis. *J.A.M.A.* 225:384–389, 1973.
62. Da Silva Horta, J., DaMotta, L. C., Abbatt, J. D., and Roriz, M. L.: Malignancy and Other Latent Effects Following Administration of Thorotrast. *Lancet* 2:211–215, 1965.
63. Mayler, L. (ed.): *Side Effects of Drugs*. Vol. 5. Excerpta Medica Foundation, Amsterdam, 1966, pp. 475–476.
64. Bengtsson, U., Angervall, L., Ekman, H., and Lehmann, L.: Transitional Cell Tumors of the Renal Pelvis in Analgesic Abusers. *Scand. J. Urol. Nephrol.* 2:145–150, 1968.
65. Friedrich, E. G., Jr.: Vulvar Carcinoma in situ in Identical Twins—An Occupational Hazard. *Obstet. Gynecol.* 39:837–841, 1972.
66. Noller, K. L., and Fish, C. P.: Diethylstilbestrol Usage: Its Interesting Past, Important Present, and Questionable Future. *Med. Clin. North Am.* 58:793–810, 1974.
67. Robboy, S. J., Scully, R. E., Welch, W. R., and Herbst, A. L.: Intrauterine Diethylstilbestrol Exposure and Its Consequences. *Arch. Pathol. Lab. Med.* 101:1–5, 1977.
68. Exposure in utero to Diethylstilbestrol and Related Synthetic Hormones (Contribution from National Cancer Institute). *J.A.M.A.* 236:1107–1109, 1976.
69. Edmonson, H. A., Benton, B., and Henderson, B. E.: Liver-cell Adenomas Associated with Use of Oral Contraceptives. *N. Engl. J. Med.* 294:470–472, 1976.
70. Otten, J., et al.: Hepatoblastoma in an Infant After Contraceptive Intake During Pregnancy. *N. Engl. J. Med.* 297:222, 1977.
71. Hyun-Hahk Kim, and Williams, T. J.: Endometroid Carcinoma of the Uterus and Ovaries Associated with Immunosuppressive Therapy and Anticoagulation. *Mayo Clin. Proc.* 47:39–41, 1972.
72. Doak, P. B., Montgomerie, J. Z., North, J. D., and Smith, F.: Reticulum Cell Sarcoma After Renal Homotransplantation and Azothioprine and Prednisone Therapy. *Br. Med. J.* 4:746–748, 1968.
73. Stewart, A., Webb, J., Gioes, D., and Hewitt, D.: Malignant Disease in Childhood and Diagnostic Irradiation in utero. *Lancet* 2:447, 1956.
74. *Irradiation Related Thyroid Cancer: Information for Physicians*. DHEW Publication No. (NIH) 77-1120, Washington, D.C.

75. Mittelmann, M., and Scholhamer, C. F.: Cancer and Malpractice Claims. *Cancer* 39:2573–2578, 1977.
76. *Lipsey v. Michael Reese Hospital* 46 Ill. 2d 32, 262 NE 2d 450 (1970).
77. Berdjis, C. C. (ed.): *Pathology of Irradiation*. Williams & Wilkins, Baltimore, 1971.
78. White, D. C.: *An Atlas of Radiation Histopathology*. National Technical Information Service, U.S. Department of Commerce, Springfield, W. Va., 1975.
79. Armstrong, D., Young, L. S., Meyer, R. D., and Blevins, A. L.: Infections Complications of Neoplastic Disease. *Med. Clin. North Am.* 55:729–746, 1971.
80. Hewlett, R. I., and Wilson, A. F.: Adult Respiratory Distress Syndrome Following Aggressive Management of Extensive Acute Lymphoblastic Leukemia. *Cancer* 39:2422–2425, 1977.
81. Rodin, A. E., Haggard, M. E., and Travis, L. B.: Lung Changes and Chemotherapeutic Agents in Childhood. *Am. J. Dis. Child.* 120:337–340, 1970.
82. Sostman, H. D., Matthay, R. A., Putman, C. E., and Walker, C. J.: Methotrexate-induced Pneumonitis. *Medicine* 55:371–388, 1976.
83. Coppola, A. R.: Stryker-Frame Death. *Va. Med. Monthly* 104:475–476, 1977.
84. Irwin, R. S., et al.: Food Asphyxiation in Hospitalized Patients. *J.A.M.A.* 237:2744–2746, 1977.
85. Spengler, R. S., Greenough, W. B., and Stolley, P. D.: Characteristics of Nosocomial Bacteremias and Associated Risk Factors. *Am. J. Epidemiol.* 104:322, 1972.
86. Hospital-based Infections Cost Patients Many Days. *J.A.M.A.* 237:2459–2460, 1977.
87. Paredes, A., et al.: Nosocomial Transmission of Group B Streptococci in a Newborn Nursery. *Pediatrics* 49:679–682, 1977.
88. McDougal, B. A., et al.: Nosocomial Influenza A Infection. *South. Med. J.* 70:1023–1024, 1977.
89. McGowan, J. E., Jr., Parrott, P. L., and Duty, V. P.: Nosocomial Bacteremia: Potential for Prevention of Procedure-related Cases. *J.A.M.A.* 237:2727–2729, 1977.
90. Hewitt, W. L., and Sanford, J. D. (eds.): Workshop on Hospital-associated Infections. *J. Infect. Dis.* 130:680–686, 1974.
91. Golin, C. B.: The Trouble with Nursing Homes. *Am. Med. News,* September 24, 1976, pp. 1–5.
92. Anst, C. S.: Anticonvulsant Drugs and Calcium Metabolism. *N. Engl. J. Med.* 292:587–588, 1975.
93. Hooker, S.: *Caring for the Elderly People*. Routledge & Kegan Paul, Boston, 1976.

CHAPTER 23

Marvin E. Aronson is Medical Examiner of the City of Philadelphia. He is also Adjunct Associate Professor of Pathology at the University of Pennsylvania and holds clinical academic appointments at Hahnemann Medical College, Jefferson Medical College, and Temple University. Dr. Aronson is a member of the Board of Directors of the National Association of Medical Examiners, and is a diplomate in forensic pathology of the American Board of Pathology. He is also a member of the Editorial Board of the *Journal of Forensic Sciences*.

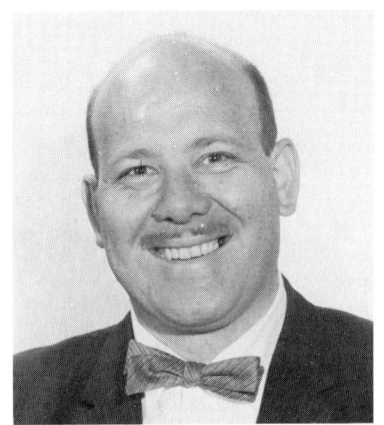

PUBLIC HEALTH ASPECTS OF MEDICOLEGAL DEATH INVESTIGATION

Marvin E. Aronson, M.D.

PUBLIC HEALTH DEATHS

Medicolegal death investigation is usually defined as the investigation of any death which is either obviously due to unnatural causes or is suspected of being other than completely natural in its cause. Also included are deaths where there is no evidence of cause at all, as when an apparently healthy person drops dead on the street and was not under regular medical care for a particular ailment. An important part of medicolegal death investigation in every community is the detection of unsuspected disease which has the potential for becoming, or which is, of epidemic proportions. Medicolegal death investigation also helps to establish the cause of deaths in situations of community danger such as accidental or deliberate contamination of water supplies, food, or air which affects numbers of people. The medicolegal death investigator is the only public official who can investigate these types of cases in an effective manner. He can consider clusters of cases arising at the same time or from the same geographic area merely by being alert as to the types of cases which appear in the daily or weekly workload as well as by the monthly and semiannual appraisal of the statistics which are generated by his office. For example, in the early sixties, a sudden increase in deaths in the "skid row" district of a metropolitan area was detected over a weekend and traced to a new formulation of a wax-alcohol product, *Sterno*, containing a much higher concentration of methyl alcohol than previously used. The product was being eaten by chronic alcoholics as a cheap method of obtaining alcohol. The "epidemic" was limited to about 30 individuals, and only eight deaths resulted.

Historically speaking the first death investigations in the modern era were usually performed under the public health authority of the government. The first autopsy recorded in the City of Philadelphia was done in pre-Revolutionary days on a seaman who died on board ship en route from the entrance of Delaware Bay to Philadelphia. An autopsy was ordered by the city to be conducted on the ship by a local physician. The ship was allowed to come to dock only after it was determined that the death was not due to contagious disease.

HEALTH DEPARTMENTS AND DEATH INVESTIGATIONS

The authority to perform autopsies without the consent of the next of kin is an intrinsic prerogative of government. It is an important function of public authority to control contagion in its geographic area. The responsibility is usually delegated to officials at county levels. It may be delegated directly to the death investigator or indirectly through the health official of the government.

The location of the medicolegal office within the administrative framework of the health department makes for an easy cooperation and exchange of information. The information can be on an individual basis where the local health office supplies data concerning the previous health status of the deceased person, or more generalized, as where health department statistics of diseases and causes of death provide clues and background to the death investigator. The reverse flow of information is also important. During the drug-abuse death peak period of the late sixties and early seventies, the medicolegal offices all over the country were the most reliable, and sometimes the only, source of statistics as to the prevalence of drug abuse. The observations of the medicolegal offices were used to plan programs and to obtain support and funding for multiple aspects of public health activities in the field of drug-abuse control. During the episode of infection which occurred among visitors to Philadelphia in 1976, and which acquired the misleading name of "Legionnaire's disease," the Medical Examiner's Office was the principal source of information, both positive and negative, which was used by the Public Health Department to make decisions as to what, if any, measures should be taken to control the contagion during the early stages. The Medical Examiner's Office was also the principal source of biological material which was analyzed elsewhere to clarify the organism involved in the disease. The Public Health Department, and later the Federal Center for Disease Control, supplied the Medical Examiner's Office with valuable epidemiologic data which assisted in the clarification of the nature of the outbreak.

Other chapters of this text provide clinical detail on the medicolegal investigation of deaths related to disease and other public health matters, especially Chapters 8, 9, and 10, which discuss suicide, heart disease, and neoplastic diseases.

DEATHS IN HOSPITALS AND NURSING HOMES

An important extension of the medicolegal death investigator's function is with reference to deaths occurring in hospitals. Here are considered not only the obvious cases where the original admission to the hospital was for treatment of trauma, but also where the death may have been related to a therapeutic or diagnostic procedure. Not all jurisdictions have the legal power, the budget, or the desire to review all such cases, but they are probably the most significant investigations so far as the professional medical community is concerned. In cases where a person sustains obvious injury outside of the hospital, and the physicians try to save his life and fail, there is usually little question as to the sequence of events and their significance. On the other hand, when a person sustains an injury in a hospital, there are usually more questions than there are answers. Furthermore, an internal investigation by pathologists employed by the hospital may be suspect. Thus it is very important to document all of the available facts as soon and as objectively as possible. Such prompt investigations often suffice to clarify the circumstances of the death and frequently forestall medical malpractice litigation. They may also uncover and preserve evidence of definite failure to meet the usual standards of medical care.

A further extension of the interest of medicolegal death investigators is in the field of deaths which occur in nursing homes, extended-care facilities, and boarding houses. As the population of the country grows older, these institutions will become even more important in the housing of older citizens. Many of these facilities are informally organized and unlicensed, and avoid coming to the attention of the public authority until there is a death. A small minority of these institutions are operating on an extremely shaky financial and moral basis. The number of profitable irregularities can be mind-boggling when exposed. Such marginal operations may become involved in deaths of residents who were starved, neglected, or beaten. The mistreatment is usually superimposed upon some underlying natural disease or aging process, making the death investigation very difficult. Location of the medicolegal death investigators within the health department provides an easy means for the exchange of information by the medicolegal officials with those responsible for the regulation and licensure of such institutions.

HEALTH DEPARTMENT LOCATION: ADVANTAGES AND DISADVANTAGES

There are advantages and disadvantages to having a death investigation unit located within a health department (Table 23-1). In favor of this location is the possibility that the death investigator may be poorly prepared or personally disinterested in handling administrative and financial aspects of government bureaucracy. The health department administrators can handle most of these duties very well, leaving the death investigator to his clinical work and, hopefully, to some research efforts. A second factor in favor of this location, as noted earlier, is the ease of cooperation with other public health units. Moreover, educational programs can be implemented, supplemented, and initiated within the health department which are beneficial to the activities of the death investigator. These include professional programs covering suicide, mental health, drug abuse, alcohol abuse, and problems in nursing homes and hospitals. Another benefit is the fact that the death investigator is freed from implications of bias which might plague him in being an arm of the police department or prosecutor's office. Location within law-enforcement agencies can have the further effect of limiting the death investigator's jurisdiction to criminally related cases.

There are several factors which can be cited against the placing of the medicolegal unit within the health department. The most significant is the fact that when the unit asks for its annual budget, the presentation format is such that the medicolegal program may be lost among the re-

TABLE 23-1. THE MEDICOLEGAL DEATH INVESTIGATION SYSTEM LOCATED WITHIN THE HEALTH DEPARTMENT

Advantages	Disadvantages
1. Administrative support in personnel organization and budget preparation.	1. Cannot appeal directly to the public for increases in funding or sustained funding.
2. Communication and cooperation with other units in health departments.	2. Cannot take advantage of contact directly with executive and legislative branches of government.
3. Educational programs integrated with health department.	3. Cannot be seen to be independent of the health department; possible influence where investigations involve other health departments, operated or licensed facilities for health care.
4. Independence from police department or prosecutor's office in the investigation of criminal deaths.	
5. Independence from elective office (as with coroners and district attorneys).	

maining, much larger budget items of the health department. This is exceedingly important when there is a fiscal difficulty resulting in the overall slashing of budgets. The health officer may not place the medicolegal unit within his highest priorities because of lack of understanding of its value, or because of its essential independence of functions. Owing to their location within the health department, there is necessarily less opportunity for death investigators to go directly to the public to appeal for additional funds, such as is the case when a coroner runs for re-election. Lastly, there is the corollary of my comment on location in a law enforcement agency: When the medicolegal investigator works within a health department which operates health care facilities, or even licenses them, he could be suspected of bias when he reviews a death which takes place in such a facility.

It should be clear from the above that there are no easy answers to location of any public responsibility. The social, geographic, and economic nature of the jurisdiction must be considered in each case. The single most important factor, however, in the success or failure of a given medicolegal death investigation system remains the personality of the people involved. Any medicolegal system can succeed with dedication, interest, and objectivity, and none will succeed without enthusiasm and fairness on the part of those who actually operate the system.

CHAPTER 24

Charles R. Baxter is Professor of Surgery at the University of Texas Southwestern Medical School at Dallas and is Medical Director of the Skin Transplant Center for Burns. Dr. Baxter received his undergraduate and medical education at the University of Texas. He served as President of the American Burn Association in 1972 and 1973, and has chaired the Research Development Committee of the International Society of Burn Injuries. Dr. Baxter currently serves on the Executive Board of the American Association of Tissue Banks.

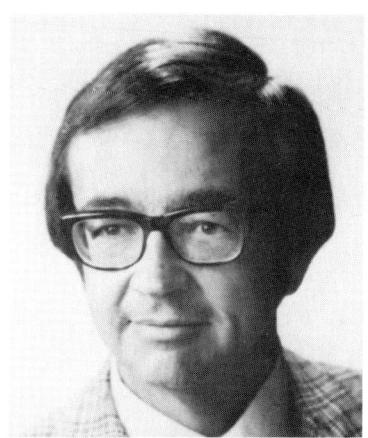

Ellen L. Heck is a Faculty Associate in the Department of Surgery of the University of Texas Southwestern Medical School at Dallas, as well as Director of the Skin Transplant Center for Burns and University Coordinator of the Lions Sight and Tissue Foundation. Ms. Heck is an alumna of Texas Women's University and has pursued graduate studies at Central Michigan University and the School of Medical Technology of Parkland Memorial Hospital in Dallas.

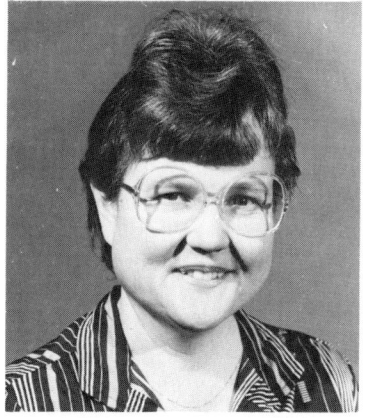

Charles S. Petty is Director of the Southwestern Institute of Forensic Sciences at Dallas, Chief Medical Examiner of Dallas County, Director of the Dallas County Criminal Investigation Laboratory, and Professor of Pathology and Forensic Sciences at the University of Texas Southwestern Medical School at Dallas. Dr. Petty holds degrees in pharmacy and physiology from the University of Washington and received his medical education at Harvard Medical School. He is a diplomate of the American Board of Pathology in pathologic anatomy, clinical pathology, and forensic pathology. Dr. Petty is former President of the American Academy of Forensic Sciences and is a Fellow of the American Association for the Advancement of Science, the American College of Physicians, the American Society of Clinical Pathologists, and the British Academy of Forensic Sciences.

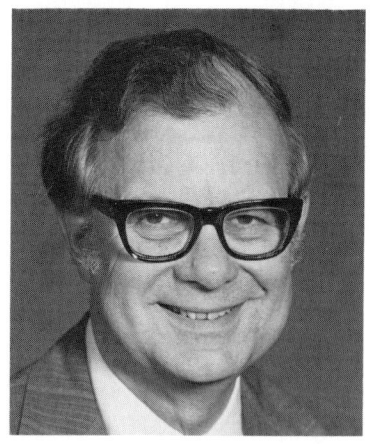

TRANSPLANTATION PROGRAMS AND MEDICOLEGAL INVESTIGATION

Charles R. Baxter, M.D.,
Ellen L. Heck, B.S., M.T., and
Charles S. Petty, M.D.

Transplantation of organs and tissues can proceed only when the organ or tissue needed by the recipient is made available by a donor. The procedure of transplantation is not new or unique: several million units of blood (a tissue) are made available in the United States each year by donors who for altruistic or profit motives provide several million recipients with the much needed tissue. This type of donor activity is representative of one form of donation. There are others, and a more complete list might be as follows:

1. *Living Donor.* Organs or tissue donated by express permission of the donor who survives the donation, as of a single kidney.
2. *Living Donor.* Organs or tissue donated by express permission of next of kin of the person who is in coma and expected to die. The donation is effective:
   a. At death, when it comes.
   b. At death, with time of donation prearranged and controlled by physiologic support systems discontinued after the donation is complete.
3. *Dead Donor.* There are at least three methods:
   a. Organs or tissues donated by express permission of next of kin.
   b. Donation arranged prior to death by the subject himself.
   c. Other donation authorized by statute, as by a medical examiner.

There are various possible permutations among the foregoing, and one addition might be made. The "sale" of blood by individuals has set a precedent that might be followed in making available certain organs for transplantation by "selling" them, such organs to be removed immediately or upon the death of the profit-oriented donor. A recent article by

Brams[1] discusses in detail this philosophy of providing organs for transplantation and authorizing such sales by state statute.

Even excluding from consideration the millions of units of blood donated and used each year in the United States, transplantation of other tissues and organs has become very important in several areas of modern medicine. This chapter will not include discussion of donations from the living who survive (type 1 above), but will be concerned with the other groups of "living donors" (types 2a and 2b) and the dead donor (type 3). Regardless of the designation "living" or "dead," these classes of transplantation donors provide what are usually known as cadaver organs or tissues. This type of donor, providing organs or tissues at death, is responsible for the provision of most transplantable organs and tissues (excepting, of course, blood). Eyes (corneae), skin, kidneys, hearts, livers, lungs, and pancreases, among others, are all provided by dead donors and as such the transplants are of cadaveric origin.

Transplantation of cadaveric organs to living recipients has now assumed such a major role in the practice of clinical medicine that interested groups in almost all metropolitan areas or medical centers are now in the process of rapidly developing transplant programs. Increasing acceptability of organ donation by the public and improved clinical results of transplants ensure the continued growth of many of the established programs, the creation of new programs, and a new era of research in organ utilization and banking.

Because the best cadaveric transplants come from young, nondiseased individuals, the largest group of donors consists of victims of fatal accidents, suicide, homicide, or sudden death resulting from natural causes. The medicolegal officer generally exercises jurisdiction over these deaths. This nonhospitalized population could account for donations of most organ transplants. Tissues such as skin and eyes as potential transplants are subject to lenient limitations on age, time after death, and concomitant disease. Hospitalized donors will, of course, continue to account for most donations of organs such as kidneys, which thrive best after transplantation when the donor's physiologic support systems are discontinued only after donation.

In the early days of transplantation, the role of the pathologist was generally very limited and dealt primarily with the legality of the specific transplantation proposed. Today the pathologist's role is expanding to embrace a more active partnership concerned with permission, procurement, autopsy verification of disease states limiting tissue use, coordination of transplant groups, and even influencing favorable legislation and attitudes of government at all levels toward transplantation programs.

The increasing use of organs and tissues for transplantation has changed the role of forensic medicine from a passive one to one of pivotal importance and responsibility. Indeed, a whole new area of cooperation and interdependence exists between forensic medicine and clinical medicine. An active transplant program depends on cooperative efforts involving a wide range of persons, both lay and professional. When a medical need exists for donations of organs and tissues, this need must be made known to all those who may be concerned directly or indirectly with its fulfillment. Hospital administrators, medicolegal officers, physicians at all levels, nurses and chaplains must all give more than merely tacit approval to the program. Awareness and support of the local clergy is a major asset in public acceptance of any transplant program, even though ministerial participation may be only of a passive type.

Another group or profession whose role in the transplant program is of great importance is that of morticians or funeral directors. Medical personnel are often totally unaware of the intricacies and the art involved in the mortician's specialty. The cosmetic acceptability of the dead body, as well as the effectiveness of embalming, is of great importance in a society with social mores which dictate an "open casket" viewing in many funeral services. From consultations and our own experience with funeral directors we have identified certain areas of mutual concern and interest. Minimal delay in releasing the body to the funeral director is always an important consideration. Also of great importance is the proper ligation of blood vessels when organs have been removed so as to aid in the efficiency of embalming and the prevention of fluid leakage. A special problem for the funeral director is the removal of organs or tissue from the surface of the body. For example, when skin is removed, plastic covering is needed to prevent leakage of embalming solution from donor sites. Skin is removed using an air- or electric-powered dermatome following preparation of the donor site with an iodophor solution. The depth of removal is approximately 0.0016 inch, exactly the same as the removal of skin from a living person for grafting. In our experience the best areas from which to remove skin are the back below the shoulder blades and the lower extremities. These areas have proven to be of least inconvenience to funeral directors and still yield a reasonable amount of skin for transplantation purposes. In instances where bodies have been donated to medical science or when there will be no viewing of the body at the funeral, additional broad skin surfaces may be used as donor sites. When the eye is to be removed, it is first cleansed with normal saline to remove any debris. The conjunctiva is separated from the eyeball 3 mm from the edge of the cornea. The four main muscles attached to the eyeball are looped with muscle hooks and cut close to the eyeball. The remaining muscles and optic nerve are then cut, and the eye is placed immediately in a sterile bottle and saturated with normal saline, but not immersed. The empty socket may be filled with a suitable padding, and a plastic cap may then be placed over it. This will aid in a more lifelike appearance of the face when the eyelids are closed.

The cornea may be removed by using a corneal trephine. With this device only the cornea and a small amount of adjacent tissue are removed from the globe—quite a different procedure than is involved with the enucleation technique.

Publicity has generally been avoided by members of the medical profession, but it is important to the transplantation service. An awareness and understanding of the benefits and needs of any organ transplantation service cannot be adequately communicated without extensive and ongoing publicity utilizing all forms of mass media. "Transplant, don't bury" bumper stickers as well as billboard advertising and Sunday supplement articles are now seen in many parts of the country. Information news stories and reports of successful transplant procedures provide valuable publicity. Of course, careful observation of the confidentiality of both donor and recipient should be a part of any such reporting. Civic groups and church organizations are another forum which may be used to interest the public in transplantation. Not infrequently civic groups become interested in the programs and help generate interest among other groups, and may even provide support. Proper publicity is an immeasurable asset; improper publicity may result in destruction of a vital program.

Transplantation programs must act within professional and legal boundaries. Legal consent for organ donation is of prime importance (Table 24-1). Consent to procure organs or tissues for transplantation varies from one state to another but usually includes uniform donor card laws and consent of next of kin: husband/wife, eldest child, father/mother, brother/sister, legal guardian, or legal representative-executor. All 50 states have adopted the Uniform Anatomical Gift Act. The benefits of this legislation may not yet have come to full fruition since in many states the Uniform Act has not been highly publicized. Drivers' handbooks or manuals which are available through some state Departments of Safety now include information on the various donation programs available within the state and the addresses and telephone numbers of their representatives.

TABLE 24-1. LEGAL CONSENT FOR CADAVER ORGAN DONATION

By the donor himself:
 1. By willing organs, tissues, or his entire body.
 2. By other written instruments:
    a. Desire expressed on a card carried by the donor. (Cards are furnished by local eye banks, kidney banks, kidney disease societies, or other groups.)
    b. Desire expressed on a driver's license carried by the donor.
    c. Desire expressed on a bracelet or necklace worn by the donor.
    d. Predesignation of desire with the funeral director as part of the prearrangements for funeral services.

By the next of kin:
 1. Direct written permission.
 2. Telephoned permission with a listening witness or with supplemental written authority.

By other donor under statutory authorization:
 A medicolegal official may be authorized at his discretion to provide specified anatomical parts, organs, or tissues to a transplantation agency.

By court order:
 An order may be issued by a court for the use in transplantation of certain tissues or organs occasionally encountered when the donor is a ward of the state.

By sale:
 Arranged prior to death with payment effected during the life of the donor and with transplantation to take place upon the death of the donor.

Insofar as the above table is concerned, two points deserve comment. There is a newly authorized method of providing space on the driver's license so the driver may indicate his desire regarding organ or tissue donations. Several states have adopted this method. As an example, the Texas statute is given here.* As most people carry with them their driver's licenses, it is apt to be present at the time of death. Thus delay between death and discovery of intent of donation is minimized.

---

*Article 6687b, Vernon's Texas Civil Statutes (Anatomical gifts; execution on reverse side of driver's license).

Section 11B. (a) A gift of any needed parts of the body may be made by executing a statement of gift printed on the reverse side of the donor's operator's, commercial operator's, or chauffeur's license. A signed and witnessed statement of gift thereon shall be deemed to comply with the Texas Anatomical Gift Act (Article 4590-2, *Vernon's Texas Civil Statutes*). The gift is invalid on expiration, cancellation, revocation, or suspension of the operator's, commercial operator's, or chauffeur's licence. To be valid, the statement must be executed each time the operator's, commercial operator's, or chauffeur's license is replaced, reinstated, or renewed.

(b) The Department shall print a statement certifying the willingness to make an anatomical gift on the reverse side of each operator's, commercial operator's, and chauffeur's license.

Recently enacted laws in some states permit coroners or medical examiners or their designated agents to remove certain organs for transplant if no objection to this removal is known to the official. Again, we reprint the Texas law on the subject.† This law places the burden of notification of objection on the next of kin. Some medicolegal officers may be reluctant to proceed on the strength of this law alone, perhaps because of the novelty and insufficient public awareness of the goals sought by the lawmakers.

Although in most cases organ donation and medicolegal investigations proceed smoothly, there are areas where difficulty can arise. In all cases under the jurisdiction of a medicolegal officer, his permission must be obtained prior to removal of organs. In cases which require physiologic support systems such as heart, kidney, or liver transplant, consent to proceed is often granted without inspection by the official prior to removal of the organ. Prior autopsy of the donor does not interfere with eye donation (unless vitreous fluid is removed) or skin donation under usual circumstances. It may, in fact, be of value to have the pathologist's observations as to evidence of disease. Removal of bone and dura and certain other tissues and organs may require special cooperation between the medicolegal official and the physician. In many cases where time after death is not the limiting factor, avoidance of bacterial contamination is.

Operating rooms need not always be used as the site for procurement of organs for transplantation. When physiologic support systems are necessary, the use of the operating theater may be required. When physiologic support systems are not necessary and avoidance of bacterial contamination is of great importance, the operating room may not necessarily be required. The increasing cost of operating room use and the scheduling

---

†*Vernon's Texas Annotated Statutes: Code of Criminal Procedure*, Article 4590-4 (Justice of the peace or medical examiner; permitting removal of corneal tissue).

Section 1 (Permission to Take Tissue). On a request from an authorized official of a nonprofit corporation chartered under the laws of Texas, to obtain, store, and distribute donor eyes to be used by those licensed to practice medicine for corneal transplants, for research, or for other medical purposes and whose medical activities are directed by one licensed to practice medicine in Texas, for corneal tissue, the justice of the peace or the medical examiner may permit the taking of corneal tissue if:
(1) the decedent from whom the tissue is to be taken died under circumstances requiring an inquest by the justice of the peace or the medical examiner; and
(2) no objection by a person listed in Section 2 of this Act is known by the justice of the peace or the medical examiner; and
(3) the removal of corneal tissue will not interfere with the subsequent course of an investigation or autopsy, or alter the postmortem facial appearance.

Section 2 (Objection to Taking Tissue). Objection may be made known to the justice of the peace or the medical examiner by the following person:
(1) the decedent's spouse;
(2) if no spouse, the decedent's adult children;
(3) if no adult children or spouse, the decedent's parents; or
(4) if no parents, adult children, or spouse, the decedent's brothers or sisters.

Section 3 (Liability for Damages). The justice of the peace, the medical examiner, and the eye bank official are not liable for damages in a civil action brought by a person listed in Section 2 of this Act who has not objected prior to the removal of the corneal tissue on any theory of civil recovery based on a contention that the consent of plaintiff was required prior to the removal of corneal tissue as authorized by this Act.

(Acts 1977, 65th Leg., p. 16, ch. 11, eff. March 10, 1977.)

problems make it less than optimal to expect to use the operating room for removal of all organs and tissues. In our experience and that of several other institutions, the use of the autopsy area (which can be used for aseptic procedures) has proven quite satisfactory. Such an area is more readily available than operating suites, and there is no competition with an operative schedule or delay in releasing the body to a funeral director. In cases which require strictest sterility, a cooperative program could provide space in a forensic department and be equipped by the transplant services to enable both autopsy and transplant procurement to proceed simultaneously. The benefits of such a program to the patients are obvious. Costs are reduced, and the pathologist has available a mini-operating suite for any needed special procedures. At present many transplant programs are still endeavoring to use hospital operating rooms, but because of the reasons stated above, the use of a combined pathology-surgery room is anticipated to become more popular.*

As an example, the program that has been functioning for several years in the Department of Surgery at the University of Texas Southwestern Medical School is based on a high degree of cooperation with the Southwestern Institute of Forensic Sciences at Dallas. The Institute and the Medical School are conveniently adjacent. Each morning the medical examiner provides personnel of the surgery department with the names and numbers of the next of kin of those who have died under circumstances such that the medical examiner has obligatory jurisdiction for the investigation of death. The Department of Surgery coordinator then calls the next of kin and requests permission to remove skin from the body for transplantation purposes. At the same time permission is sought for removal of the eyes to serve as corneal tissue transplants.

Despite the fact that Dallas is considered to be a socially conservative community, the results of this program have been outstanding. In 39 months, 54 percent of the next of kin who were contacted (460 instances of 847 contacted) gave permission for removal of skin. Perhaps this success is related to the large amount of very positive publicity given the Burn Unit at Parkland Memorial Hospital, which serves the Dallas County area, the prime user of the banked skin. The response to the request for donation of eyes has been just as enthusiastic; the program is new and the publicity afforded it has not been extensive. Even better results may eventually be achieved.

The individual chosen to contact the next of kin for permission to remove organs or tissues for transplantation purposes is an all-important factor. Upon that person rests the success or failure of the entire procurement system. The contact person must be aggressive but understanding and sympathetic, technically knowledgeable but in harmony with the death and funeral mores of society. Because of the essential characteristics of the very personal, intimate type of communication between the representative of the transplant center and the family member, it would seem

---

*It is important to keep in mind that the provision of a special room in the forensic laboratory is costly as measured in capital expenditure and maintenance costs. The transplantation service may help to defray the costs of the area provided. However, it might be useful to examine the potential number of donations. Obviously, the cost of the provision of a special room with the needed equipment must be balanced against a reasonable number of expected organ or tissue donations.

that a very small, dedicated staff, rather than a large, impersonal bureaucracy, would be best fitted for the task.

Increasing interest in the use of transplantation techniques led to the formation of the American Association of Tissue Banks. This group has taken on the task of proposing transplant standards for all transplantation specialties. These standards may soon become a guide for government regulations. The day of the unregulated, "under the table" or "operating room refrigerator" transplants is rapidly drawing to a close. Quality control of procurement and storage and well-defined acceptability criteria will benefit all involved with transplantation. It will stimulate new research to improve transplantation success rates and to find alternative means for achieving successful results. Certainly patients will benefit from improvements in the quality of donor organs; physicians will be assured of greater acceptability of the transplants, both medically and legally; and the medicolegal investigator will have confidence in releasing organs only to those banks that he knows can meet these standards.

With expansion of organ and tissue banking programs, we can anticipate a substantial reduction in the number of patients who are waiting for donor organs. In addition, the expansion of transplantation and organ banking will stimulate cooperation between basic and clinical scientists as well as forensic scientists. Medicolegal officials who deal not only with death and the law, but also with death as it advances knowledge to benefit the living, are logical partners in this expansion. Here, too, through the transplantation programs, medical advancements through death are achieved for the living.

Very few articles have been written about the actual ongoing activities involved in the procurement of tissues and organs suitable for transplantation. The criteria for suitability; the satisfaction of legal requirements to permit collection of organs; and, of course, the surgical selection of patients, the transplantation procedure, followup of patients, and a variety of clinical aspects have been documented in medical and lay publications alike. Only four articles, in addition to the one cited earlier in this chapter, are deemed of direct pertinence, and these are included below in the list of references.[2-5]

REFERENCES

1. Brams, M.: Transplantable Human Organs: Should Their Sale be Authorized by State Statutes? *Am. J. Law Med.* 3:183–195, 1977.
2. Davis, J. H., and Wright, R. K.: Influence of the Medical Examiner on Cadaver Organ Procurement. *J. Forensic Sci.* 22:824–826, 1977.
3. Knight, B.: Forensic Problems in Practice—Law and Ethics in Transplantation. *Practitioner* 216:471–474, 1976.
4. Louisell, D. W.: The Procurement of Organs for Transplantation. *Northwestern U. Law Rev.* 64:607–627, 1970.
5. Pliskin, J. S.: Cadaveric Kidneys for Transplantation: Is There a Need for More? *J. Forensic Sci.* 21:83–97, 1976.

CHAPTER 25

Vincent J. M. Di Maio is a Medical Examiner for Dallas County and is Associate Professor of Pathology at the University of Texas Southwestern Medical School, as well as Editor of the *Forensic Science Gazette*. A graduate of St. John's University and the Downstate Medical Center of the State University of New York, Dr. Di Maio is Chairman of the Council on Forensic Pathology of the American Society of Clinical Pathologists and is a Fellow of the American Academy of Forensic Sciences and the College of American Pathologists.

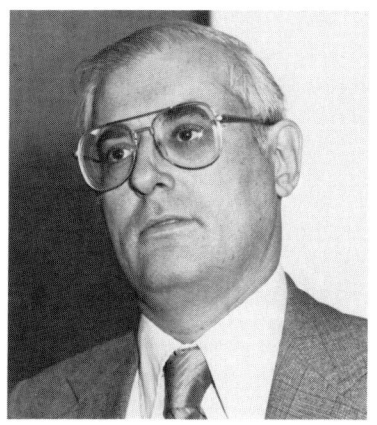

Charles S. Petty is Director of the Southwestern Institute of Forensic Sciences at Dallas, Chief Medical Examiner of Dallas County, Director of the Dallas County Criminal Investigation Laboratory, and Professor of Pathology and Forensic Sciences at the University of Texas Southwestern Medical School at Dallas. Dr. Petty holds degrees in pharmacy and physiology from the University of Washington and received his medical education at Harvard Medical School. He is a diplomate of the American Board of Pathology in pathologic anatomy, clinical pathology, and forensic pathology. Dr. Petty is former President of the American Academy of Forensic Sciences and is a Fellow of the American Association for the Advancement of Science, the American College of Physicians, the American Society of Clinical Pathologists, and the British Academy of Forensic Sciences.

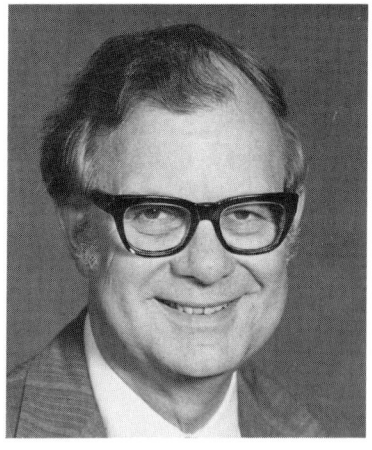

MULTIPLE DEATH INVESTIGATIONS

Vincent J. M. Di Maio, M.D., and
Charles S. Petty, M.D.

Both the forensic pathologist and the police officer are oriented to death investigation in which there is but a single death. Multiple deaths, when encountered, are generally of the motor vehicle or mass disaster types. There are, of course, occasional multiple homicides during a domestic quarrel, barroom brawl, or hold-up. These cases are usually very obvious to the investigator. Witnesses are common and when the police arrive on the scene, they immediately know with what they are dealing.

Cases of simultaneous multiple deaths of obscure origin or unusual multiple homicides are special situations to be handled with more than the usual care. Such deaths are rarely encountered. Unfortunately, when they do occur, they often are mishandled. Not uncommonly, the first investigators at the scene make hasty and sometimes false assumptions which lead to erroneous conclusions. The inept investigation of the scene may lead to destruction of evidence and eventual inability to prosecute a criminal case successfully or to solve civil problems arising from the deaths. The errors committed usually result from ignorance as to the causes of obscure multiple deaths, coupled with a failure to follow standard investigative procedures. If the primary investigator has some basic knowledge of the causes of multiple deaths and takes some simple steps to preserve the scene, such cases may be no more difficult to investigate than those involving a single death.

Obscure multiple deaths can be grouped into four main categories, depending somewhat on the manner of death. A fifth category might be termed "common grave discovery." The manner of death in this situation is variable. Table 25-1 summarizes this classification.

MULTIPLE NATURAL DEATH

Multiple natural death is extremely rare. The assumption is that such deaths are not due to natural disease processes. Occasionally, multiple

TABLE 25-1. CLASSIFICATION OF OBSCURE MULTIPLE DEATHS

I. Natural Death
   A. Coincidence
   B. Death of one, excitement precipitates death of second
   C. Death of one, body retained, then death of second
   D. Food poisoning
   E. Common infection—pestilence

II. Accidental Death
   A. Mass disaster
      1. motor vehicles
      2. drowning
      3. aircraft, train
      4. fire, explosion
   B. Carbon monoxide
      1. residences
      2. motor vehicles
   C. Asphyxiating gases
      1. natural gas
      2. carbon dioxide

III. Homicidal Death
   A. Witnessed
      1. "barroom brawl," domestic
      2. sniper, terrorist, hostage holding
   B. Unwitnessed
      1. family homicides
      2. family suicide pacts

IV. Homicidal Death with Suicide

V. Common Grave Discovery
   A. Multiple homicides
   B. Forgotten graveyard

deaths due to carbon monoxide poisoning, in which there had been vomiting prior to loss of consciousness, are initially ascribed to food poisoning. Food poisoning, however, will virtually never cause multiple death within a short enough time period so as to present to an investigator multiple bodies at a scene. Death from food poisoning usually takes many hours, if not days, and is associated with violent symptoms (e.g., vomiting and diarrhea), thus providing ample time and desire for the victims to seek some medical aid. Botulism is a rare form of food poisoning. The symptoms are initially relatively benign and gradual in onset. It is unlikely, however, that a number of individuals will die of botulism poisoning at the same time and place without any of them seeking medical therapy. In all the more common forms of food poisoning there is usually more than ample time for the individual to realize that he is seriously ill and to seek medical attention.

Infectious (contagious) disease such as plague and cholera may cause multiple deaths within a short time span. These diseases, however, are rarely encountered in this country, due to widely applied immunization techniques and public health control measures. As in cases of food poisoning, the symptoms will be of sufficiently severe nature and duration for the afflicted individuals to realize that they are sick and to seek medical attention. Only in an epidemic situation would one encounter several bodies at a single scene, due to an infectious disease. In such a situation, however, the medicolegal investigator in all probability would be aware of the existence of the epidemic, whatever it might be.

The most common cause of multiple death due to natural disease found at a single scene is coincidence. Thus, in a large building in an older section of the community, there may be a number of elderly residents. By pure chance, two or more may die on the same day in the same building.

There is another less common explanation. This involves elderly couples living together. One may die and the excitement of the death may in turn precipitate a sudden, fatal heart attack in the other, thus resulting in two bodies at a scene.

Rarely encountered are cases involving reclusive elderly couples in which, when one dies, the other, because of senility or mental disease, does not report the death, but preserves the body. The first body is often not found until the second individual dies. The original body may have been kept for weeks, months, or even years, despite odors and contamination of surroundings with the body fluids.

MULTIPLE ACCIDENTAL DEATH

The second major category of obscure deaths is that in which the manner of death is accidental. Transportation accidents and "Acts of God" are not discussed in this section on accidental deaths as they are almost never of the obscure type.

As a general rule, if two or more individuals are found dead in a house, motor vehicle, or any type of enclosure and there is no external evidence of trauma, the most probable cause of death is an asphyxiating gas. In houses and motor vehicles the gas is almost invariably carbon monoxide. In houses, the source of carbon monoxide is usually a defective gas heater or gas furnace, which uses natural gas. Carbon monoxide is not a constituent of natural gas, but is produced by incomplete combustion of methane, the principal constituent of natural gas.* The incomplete combustion may be due to the deposition and accumulation of carbon at the flame source. Carbon monoxide may also be formed if a metal pot is inadvertently left on a gas range over an open flame. The flame deposits ever-increasing quantities of carbon on the bottom of the pot. After a while, the flame, acting on the incandescent carbon, produces carbon monoxide.

Carbon monoxide deaths occurring in vehicles may be due either to defects in the vehicle or to environmental peculiarities. Deaths from carbon monoxide in a vehicle frequently occur in winter, when the motor is left on to run the heater. Because of a defect in the exhaust system, carbon monoxide accumulates in the vehicle, poisoning the passengers. Such deaths are common along "lovers' lanes," and are sometimes encountered in parked police patrol cars. A partially open window is no guarantee of protection as the carbon monoxide may be produced faster than the vented air can escape.

An automobile does not have to be defective for carbon monoxide to accumulate in the passenger compartment. Thus, in one case, an individual was caught in a traffic jam in a sunken area of the road on a hot, muggy day. All the involved vehicles were producing large quantities of carbon monoxide. This accumulated in the depressed roadway area, producing a very high level of carbon monoxide in the atmosphere and thus in the victim's blood. This aggravated a severe heart condition, precipitating his death.

---

*Illuminating or coal gas was widely used at one time in certain areas of the United States. This was produced by the incomplete combustion of coal or coke and contained a large percentage of carbon monoxide. As such, illuminating gas itself was lethal upon even short periods of inhalation. Illuminating gas may be utilized again as natural gas supplies dwindle, and carbon monoxide intoxication from leaking gas may once again be a frequently encountered problem.

Deaths from carbon monoxide also occur in individuals using unvented fires of charcoal briquettes to keep warm. Such deaths have occurred in hunting cabins or in the rear of vans utilized by campers. The use of charcoal briquettes in any confined space will result in the production of large quantities of carbon monoxide and a lethal environment.

The symptoms of carbon monoxide poisoning are insidious. Individuals may experience dizziness, headaches, nausea, and vomiting, followed by loss of consciousness and sometimes death. Because of the vomitus present, the investigators may misinterpret the cause of death as food poisoning. The insidious nature of the symptoms is illustrated by the fact that the victims may misinterpret their significance. Thus a young lady confided to her obstetrician-gynecologist that she had found a man with whom she was deeply in love. She knew that she was really in love because whenever they parked and he kissed her, she would "get faint and light-headed." She would then have to leave the car to get some fresh air before coming back to her boyfriend. Shortly after this disclosure was made, the boyfriend returned home one evening, parked his car in the driveway, and left the motor running while he sat in it. A few hours later he was found dead of carbon monoxide poisoning. Examination of the car revealed a defect of the exhaust system. The woman's amorous feelings were obviously due to carbon monoxide!

People dying of carbon monoxide poisoning usually have a cherry red color of the skin. In contrast to the sallow appearance of most dead bodies, these individuals look "healthy." However, no diagnosis of carbon monoxide poisoning can be made solely on the basis of coloration. Cyanide and some other poisons, and exposure to cold may also produce a cherry red color. In other instances, people may die with relatively high levels of carbon monoxide without any noticeably unusual coloration. The only certain method for determining whether a death is due to carbon monoxide poisoning is to obtain a sample of blood and analyze it for the presence of carboxyhemoglobin. This analysis is easy to perform, and most clinical laboratories have some capability to determine whether or not carbon monoxide has joined with the hemoglobin of the blood so as to form carboxyhemoglobin.

Most individuals who die from carbon monoxide poisoning in situations other than fires (where carbon monoxide is always present) have carboxyhemoglobin levels above 55 percent. However, lower levels can also cause death.

When a natural disease process exists prior to the carbon monoxide intoxication, the lethal level of carboxyhemoglobin may be well below 55 percent. Arteriosclerotic heart disease, interacting with carbon monoxide, may result in death with the carboxyhemoglobin level at 25 to 45 percent. Autopsy examination of the victim (to establish the heart disease) and laboratory analysis of the blood (to prove the presence of carboxyhemoglobin) are both necessary to establish the cause of death.

Interpretation of carboxyhemoglobin levels is rendered somewhat difficult because of smoking habits. "Normal" levels of carbon monoxide in heavy smokers have been as high as 13 percent, although the level is usually lower (3 to 6 percent).

Less frequently, other gases, such as methane (the principal ingredient of natural gas) or carbon dioxide, cause death. Both methane and carbon dioxide are not toxic in themselves. They cause death by exclusion of oxygen. Both gases are odorless. The odor detected when a gas range is turned on is usually due to methyl mercaptan, added to the natural gas to make it easily detectable. Methane and carbon dioxide cause rapid death by suffocation when they dispace the bulk of the available oxygen. Loss of consciousness may occur in seconds when the level of oxygen is reduced to 25 percent below normal. Death will follow in minutes[1] unless the individual is removed from the area or resuscitative measures are applied.

Deaths from methane and carbon dioxide occur in sewers, mines, and distillery vats. In such deaths, no attempt to retrieve the bodies should be made until an individual is available with a self-contained life-support system. Gas masks (of the cannister or filter type) are not effective because these gases cause death by displacement of oxygen only.

In sealed chambers in which there are large quantities of fungi, the organisms may have so depleted the atmosphere of oxygen that individuals entering these chambers will immediately collapse and die.[2] Again, death is not due to a toxic gas, but rather to the lack of oxygen.

The police officer or medicolegal investigator, by determining that a gas has caused multiple deaths, may prevent other deaths as a form of "preventive forensic medicine." Thus police were summoned to a scene where a number of individuals were found either unconscious or dead. The living victims were transported to a hospital where they immediately began to improve. They all described nausea, vomiting, and headache prior to loss of consciousness. The physicians at the hospital, who were not aware of the possibility of carbon monoxide poisoning, ascribed all the symptoms to severe food poisoning. While preparations were being made to discharge the individuals, the medical examiner who autopsied the dead victims found the cause of death to be carbon monoxide poisoning. He contacted the police in time to prevent the recovered victims from returning to the potentially lethal environment.

MULTIPLE HOMICIDE

The third of the four main categories is that of multiple homicide. This does not include the typical domestic quarrel or barroom brawl, but rather the "different" or "unusual" multiple homicide. The cause of death is usually fairly obvious. There may be multiple gunshot or stab wounds. The bodies may have been bound or may have been piled in one area. The important part, however, of the investigation of multiple homicidal deaths is the proper handling of both the scene and the bodies. The scene processing from the point of view of the police investigator and the medicolegal investigation is described below.

Case 1: Improper Investigation at Scene

A young boy stated that on returning home he found both parents and a brother dead of gunshot wounds. He claimed that he heard someone moving in the back of the house, picked up a weapon, and shot the intruder who had killed his parents and brother. Subsequent police investigation was very superficial. The murder weapon (a rifle) was extensively handled by the investigators at the scene. Within a few days doubts arose as to whether the alleged murderer killed by the son was the actual perpetrator of the crime. Examination of the rifle for latent prints was now productive only of the fingerprints of the several investigating officers. Extensive handling of the weapon prior to its examination for fingerprints had obliterated the much-needed evidence. A grand jury investigation was then conducted. The son refused to testify, and although there was some suspicion as to his involvement in the deaths, no firm conclusions could be reached. The case is still unresolved.

Case 2: Good Investigation at Scene

A married couple were found dead in their house with a .45 caliber automatic pistol on the floor between the bodies. The wife had multiple gunshot wounds of the front of her body, and the husband had an apparent entrance wound in the middle of the forehead. The police investigation was casual with the case written off as a homicide by the husband followed by his own suicide. Subsequent autopsy, however, revealed that the bullet that killed the husband was fired into the back of his head and not at close range. The gunshot wounds of the wife were three in number and were all fired at a long range as well. Subsequent reinvestigation of the scene by the medical examiner with correlation of the wounds with bullet holes in the furniture and wall revealed that the wife had been shot three times while sitting on the sofa. Deduction based upon bloodstains and the position of the bodies indicates that she stood up and struggled with her husband, apparently knocking his glasses off. (Because of severe eye disease, he had "tunnel vision" and was nearly blind without his glasses.) The wife then gained control of the weapon and fired it twice, one bullet striking him in the back of the head and the other entering the ceiling. She dropped the weapon, staggered over to the telephone, and died shortly after placing a call for help. This is actually a case of double homicide, rather than a homicide and suicide as originally interpreted.

Multiple Homicide with Suicide

Occasionally a scene of multiple violent death is encountered in which a preliminary investigation leads to the conclusion of multiple homicide followed by suicide of the murderer. Based on this assumption, the case may then receive only superficial investigation and documentation. However, the initial data and assumptions about the individuals involved may have been incorrect. The law enforcement investigator and/or the representative of the medical examiner's or coroner's office may have misinterpreted the medical evidence at the scene. The improperly interpreted investigation may then lead to misinterpretation of the autopsy findings. Thus an error or omission may be compounded and disastrous consequences may ensue.

Most multiple homicides followed by the suicide of the murderer involve entire families. Because of this, the case may appear to the investigating officer to be "routine" or "open and shut," and a thorough investigation may not be undertaken. However, the sudden violent death of an entire family may easily be mistaken by members of the community as the action of a demented murderer who is still at large. Pleas for protection from, and arrest of, the nonexistent assailant may excite both police and public and may be exaggerated by newspaper, television, and radio reports.

Most families are considered by others to be more or less normal and stable. It is difficult for anyone to accept as fact the murder of all other members of a family by the remaining one. Strong community service activities and church affiliations are stressed by friends and neighbors who may refuse to realize that the "good" family member was driven to murder and suicide by pressures unrecognized by his peers. This is a commonly encountered reaction of friends, neighbors, and other members of the community. To counter this expected, somewhat emotional reaction, a complete investigation and thorough documentation of the entire case of multiple death is absolutely essential.

It should also be noted that the settlement of insurance claims and perhaps even the proper partition of the estate will depend upon the investigation of the multiple homicide-suicide case. It may be necessary to determine in what order the several victims died as well as the actual victim of a self-inflicted wound.

Case 3

This case involved the deaths of all members of a model, church-going family who had not been seen for a number of days. On entering the house, police found four bodies in an early state of decomposition. All were wearing night clothes. The father was found at one end of the house with a gunshot wound of the head. At the other end of the house, the mother was found dead in bed with three gunshot wounds. In an adjacent bedroom two children were found, each with a close range gunshot wound of the forehead. Lying between the two bodies was a revolver. The house was locked and there was no evidence of robbery. Money was open to view and had apparently not been disturbed. It was fairly obvious to the police and to the investigative members of the medical examiner's office that a multiple homicide-suicide had taken place. However, many members of the local community believed that the tragedy was a mass murder by an unknown assailant, and some were fearful for their lives. Statements from the police department and the medical examiner's office confirming the multiple murder-suicide nature of the deaths eventually calmed the excited community members.

The immediate problem was to determine who was the murderer and in what sequence the killings had occurred. (In many states, the last survivor of such a murder-suicide incident, excluding the perpetrator, would be considered the heir to any property.) The father had been shot in the forehead at close range, apparently while asleep on the couch. A trail of blood indicated that he tried to reach a telephone after being shot, but collapsed and died. The mother was shot three times. Lying at the foot of her bed was a pillow case. This had obviously been wrapped around a firearm at the time of discharge. That the weapon was a revolver was indicated by the flare from the cylinder-barrel gap. Blood on the pillow was not that of the mother, but rather the father's. Therefore, it was deduced that this pillow case had been wrapped around the weapon at the time the father was shot (possible in an attempt to silence it). The pillow case had been carried to the mother's bedroom where it was dropped.

The mother had been shot twice in the head and once in the trunk. The wound of the trunk and one wound of the head were not fatal. The nonfatal wound of the head was caused when the bullet struck the skull in a tangential manner and slid along the scalp. The fatal wound in the forehead was caused by a bullet fired at close range.

Across the hall was the girl's bedroom. It was in this room that the bodies of the girl and boy, with the revolver between them, were found. Both had died of short-range gunshot wounds of the forehead. No primer trace metals were found on the children's hands. Testing of the weapon showed that it would not deposit primer trace metals on the hand when it was discharged. Thus it could not be determined by this method alone which child had fired the weapon.

The firearm was a seven-shot .22 caliber revolver. It was not unloaded at the scene but was transported as found to the criminal investigation laboratory where the seven chambers were found to have been loaded with six rounds of Remington ammunition and one round of Winchester ammunition. Six of the seven rounds had been fired, the last fired being a Remington cartridge. The round fired prior to the Remington was also a Remington cartridge. The round fired prior to this was the Winchester cartridge. Examination of the entrance wounds on the foreheads of the children with a dissecting microscope revealed that the wound in the forehead of the girl contained unburnt grains of flattened powder. The unburnt powder in the boy's wound was flake powder. The Remington .22 rimfire ammunition was loaded with flake powder, while the Winchester .22 rimfire ammunition was loaded with flattened ball powder. Therefore, the girl must have been shot with the Winchester cartridge. After she had been shot, two rounds of Remington ammunition were fired. We can, therefore, conclude that the girl could not have been the murderer, because it would have been impossible for her to have fired two shots after she received the fatal wound in the head.

Based on data from the autopsy and the scene investigation, the crime was reconstructed as follows:

The boy took the revolver and shot his father, who was sleeping on the couch. The shot was fired at close range with a pillow case wrapped about the weapon. He then went to his mother's room where he dropped the pillow case and shot her twice, once in the trunk and once in the head. Neither of these wounds was fatal. However, the wound in the head rendered her unconscious. By this time, his sister had been awakened by the noise. He then went into her room and shot her once in the forehead, using the Winchester cartridge which was the next cartridge to be fired in sequence. After shooting his sister, the boy apparently heard his mother moving about in her bed, possibly calling for help or moaning. He then went back to her and shot her in the forehead at close range. Finally, he returned to his sister's bedroom, stood over her body, and shot himself in the forehead.

POLICE INVESTIGATION OF MULTIPLE DEATH

The police investigator may not be aware of the nature of the deaths until the investigation is well underway. Therefore, the same principles of investigation apply to all three categories of death described above, based solely upon manner of death.

One of the essential points to be remembered in the investigation of multiple death scenes, or of any death scene, is that the first officer to arrive should leave the scene undisturbed and protect it from unwarranted intervention. He is, of course, justified in "walking through" the scene to see if anyone is alive and in need of medical attention, and, in the instance of an apparent homicidal death, to see if the assailant is still present. It should be emphasized that the action of "walking through" should be limited to just that.

It may be quite obvious that a given individual is dead. In such an instance, there is no need for the first officer to disturb the body. If there is the slightest hope that the individual is alive, however, that officer should immediately call for medical help. When he realizes that there is more than one body, he should recognize that this is an unusual death scene and call for help. The first officer should not have disturbed anything. However, if he has, he must be certain to inform those officers assigned to the case.

All death scenes appear to draw a curious crowd, which should be kept away because of the propensity to loot. Spectacular cases, especially those in which there are multiple deaths, attract not only the usual spectators, but also curious police officers, including higher ranking police officials and sometimes other public officials. These individuals can contaminate and destroy a scene just as can ordinary citizens. To deny such persons access to the scene tactfully and effectively may be very difficult but must be accomplished.

The members of the investigating team should keep in mind the many possible ramifications of a multiple death case. They must not conduct a simplified, superficial, or perfunctory investigation. If anything, the investigation must be more detailed and better documented than that undertaken in the much more frequently encountered single-death case.

PROPER MEDICOLEGAL INVESTIGATION OF SCENES OF MULTIPLE DEATH

Police agencies have overall control of, and responsibility for, a crime scene investigation. In death investigations, however, the medical examiner or coroner has jurisdiction of the body. After preliminary examination of the scene, the police should allow the representative of the medical examiner's or coroner's office to examine the body. The officers themselves should have neither touched nor moved the body, for once moved, a body can never be placed in the same position. Therefore photographs must be taken before the body is examined. Moreover, the very act of moving the body may result in the loss of trace evidence and the introduction of misleading contaminants.

The examination of a body at the scene by the representatives of the medical examiner's or coroner's office should be limited. It is impossible to examine a body adequately at a scene, no matter how experienced the physician or lay medical investigator may be. There may be inadequate lighting, distraction caused by investigators and spectators, and a lack of specialized equipment and assistance for examination of the body. In addition there is usually an urgent desire to remove the body from the scene.

At all scenes of death the medical examiner or his investigator should manipulate the body or bodies as little as possible. In homicidal deaths in which there is close contact between the assailant and the victim, trace evidence may be transferred from the former to the latter. It is for this reason that the body must be protected so that such trace evidence will not be lost during transportation and subsequent examination of the body. Bags should be placed on the hands. Paper bags should be used instead of plastic bags because the paper will not cause as much moisture to be retained when the body is taken from a warm environment and placed in the refrigerated storage area to await autopsy. This fluid condensation may wash away, dilute, or smear trace evidence and may also initiate early decomposition of the plastic-covered fingers, hands, and wrists. The body should be wrapped in a clean, white sheet. The use of the sheet is to prevent loss of physical evidence as well as to prevent extraneous material from being deposited on the body and clothing during the process of removal, transportation, and storage. Such material might be mistakenly assumed to be related to the assailant or the place of death. Bodies should not be fingerprinted at the scene or prior to examination of the hands by the pathologist since, in the process of manipulating the fingers, trace evidence can be lost. Furthermore, the use of fingerprint ink may make subsequent analyses for trace metals to detect gunshot residues difficult, if not impossible, to interpret.

The body should then be transported directly to the morgue. It should not be undressed prior to examination by the pathologist. In many instances of death by violence, examination of the clothing may be just as important as the autopsy itself. The body should not be embalmed prior to autopsy. Embalming causes fixation of tissue with changes in the hardness, pliability, and color of tissue and organs. In addition, the embalmer closes and masks those defects caused by trauma and also usually cleanses the body. So it is that the trace evidence on the clothing and body is apt to be removed, lost, and altered by the embalmer. It should also be noted that the removal of blood and its replacement with embalming fluid will pose problems for the toxicologist when he is asked to analyze the tissues so as to detect and quantitate toxic substances.

Any investigation involves the gathering of information of which some (if not much) is used. This is also true of laboratory analyses and autopsy examination: much of the work undertaken will never be used by the investigating officers or the courts. The undertaking of unnecessary work is always discouraging to those who must do it. This is an inescapable burden as there is no known way to limit the gathering of information to just the needed and useful evidence.

The unnecessary investigation report can always be filed, the order for a laboratory analysis can be cancelled, useless physical evidence can be discarded, and even the information gathered from the autopsy can be disregarded. However, if the investigational information was never gathered, the evidence not collected, the laboratory analysis not ordered, and the autopsy not conducted, a full and proper examination into the multiple deaths can never be undertaken, either at the time of the initial investigation, or at a later date.

Some routine analyses and tests may be performed over and over again in the investigation of different death situations, seemingly always with negative results. This may lead to a temptation to abandon these tests as "unproductive and unnecessary." However, when one of these tests is productive of positive results, all the work long felt to be needless will suddenly become justified. A good example of t..is is the examination of material removed from beneath fingernails of those dead of homicidal violence. In our Dallas office, over a period of 4 years, fingernail scrapings were examined without useful results. Eventually, however, a fragment of skin was found underneath the fingernail of a rape-homicide victim. On examination, the skin was identified to be that of a black male with blood group substance B present. These analytical results were of great use in characterizing the assailant as a black male with type B blood. In addition, this information was most useful in the better understanding of blood stains in the apartment where the murder took place, and was corroboratively used in interpreting the blood group substance found in the vaginal fluid. This one positive finding justified the 4 years of fruitless and somewhat frustrating examinations of fingernail scrapings.

COMMON GRAVE DISCOVERY

Common grave discoveries occur infrequently. The unexpected discovery of a burial site of victims of murder does, however, occur, as happened during the past decade in two spectacular cases in Texas and California with each burial site yielding many bodies. However, the usual reason for the presence of more than one body in a single burial site is not homicide, but rather that road or building contractors have uncovered a forgotten cemetery. The site may prove to have been an Indian burial ground, a slave cemetery, an unmarked churchyard, or perhaps a private family cemetery.

Among the many perplexing aspects of the discovery of multiple graves are the problems of identification of decomposed bodies or skeletonized remains, the length of time that the bodies have been buried, and the cause and manner of death. The practical (and puzzling) questions involve how many bodies are buried at the site, what land area the burial ground covers, whether all the burials were undertaken at the same time, and, if not, how much time elapsed between the separate burials.

No protocol, checklist, or guidelines will suffice for all possible variations of the common grave situation. A survey of the area, utilizing aircraft and cameras loaded with infrared film as well as black and white and the usual color film, may be of great help in the location of the graves. There is always the tendency for the investigators to call immediately for earth-moving equipment. Even when under the control of highly skilled operators, these heavy machines may destroy or cover up parts of bodies or skeletons. In a very real degree, the site should be considered an archeologic "find" and should be treated in a manner similar to an archeologic "dig."

Many universities have competent departments of archeology, and their faculties may be solicited for help. The finding of coffin hardware and other artifacts may help to distinguish a true cemetery site from a mass burial area. The examination of bones by a well-qualified physical anthropologist will be of great help in the determination of the sex, age, race, and stature of the skeletonized bodies. It must be obvious that a slow and cautious approach, using a team of qualified individuals of different scientific disciplines, is the basic requirement for the successful investigation of a common grave site.

Very little information is to be found in the literature regarding the investigation of multiple death situations. Possibly this is because they do not occur with frequency, and no great distinction has been made between multiple-death and single-death scenes. Those multiple deaths that are reported usually involve psychotic killers.[3,4] The foregoing discussion of multiple death investigation is offered to help the investigator of such events, whether he be a pathologist or a law enforcement officer, to conduct such investigations properly and efficiently in the public interest.

REFERENCES

1. Sax, N. I.: *Dangerous Properties of Industrial Materials.* ed. 3. Van Nostrand Reinhold, New York, 1968.
2. Di Maio, D. J., and Di Maio, V. J. M.: Two Deaths Caused by a Lack of Oxygen in an Underground Chamber. *J. Forensic Sci.* 19:398–401, 1974.
3. Banay, R. S.: Psychology of a Mass Murderer. *J. Forensic Sci.* 1(4):1–6, 1956.
4. Evseeff, G. S., and Wisniewski, E. M.: A Psychiatric Study of a Violent Mass Murderer. *J. Forensic Sci.* 17:371–376, 1972.

PART 4 FORENSIC PSYCHIATRY AND PSYCHOLOGY

CHAPTER 26

A. Louis McGarry is Professor of Clinical Psychiatry at the State University of New York at Stony Brook and Director of the Division of Forensic Services at the Nassau County Medical Center in East Meadow, New York. A graduate of Harvard College and Boston University Medical School, he is a Fellow of the American Psychiatric Association and a member of the Committee on Psychiatry and Law of the Group for the Advancement of Psychiatry. Dr. McGarry is a former Associate Clinical Professor of Psychiatry at Harvard Medical School. He has also served as Assistant Commissioner of Mental Health for Legal Medicine in the Massachusetts Department of Mental Health and as Associate Professor of Legal Psychiatry in the Law-Medicine Institute at Boston University. The author of numerous professional papers and monographs, Dr. McGarry is former Chairman of the Editorial Board of the *Massachusetts Journal of Mental Health* and is currently a member of the Editorial Board of *Psychiatric Opinion*.

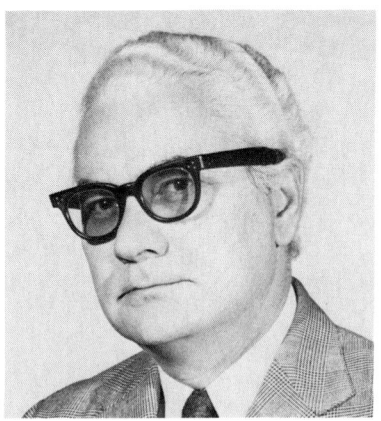

OPERATIONAL ASPECTS, TRAINING, AND QUALIFICATIONS IN FORENSIC PSYCHIATRY

A. Louis McGarry, M.D.

In this chapter we will examine operational and structural problems in forensic psychiatry programs, and we will also propose certain standards for training and professional qualifications in the field. We feel that a combined approach is preferable to separate chapters, largely because these issues are closely interrelated in most programs. Unlike the medicolegal death investigational field, forensic psychiatry is still dominated by individual professional consultants without large staffs or organizations. Even where public agencies do exist, such as psychiatric court clinics, the professional staffs are usually quite small. In some programs the forensic service includes psychiatrists, psychologists, and psychiatric social workers associated together in effective team efforts. The psychiatrist may, however, be found working alone, dependent upon the probation staff for investigation or patient records. In view of these conditions, we will place considerable stress on professional quality standards and the practices and procedures of individual forensic psychiatrists in conducting psycholegal examinations and evaluations.

PSYCHIATRIC INVOLVEMENT IN LEGAL SETTINGS

Some years ago, one of the pioneers in the field of behavioral science and law, Professor Sheldon Glueck, reviewed the relations between psychiatry and law in a series of lectures, and later a book with the engaging title, *Psychiatry and the Law: Cold War or Entente Cordiale?*[1] In more recent years these relations have been characterized by a negative response to the question posed by Dr. Glueck's title. A growing, zealous, and activist "mental health bar" has developed which increasingly has challenged psychiatric practice and competence, particularly in state mental hospital settings and in the legal process.[2] If this can be called a war, it can hardly be characterized as "cold," and it is certainly not an *entente cordiale*.

It is curious that this growing legal attack on the mental health disciplines comes after modern psychiatry has made more significant progress in the treatment of the mentally ill in the past 20 years than at any earlier period in history. It comes, as well, after the community mental health movement has dramatically decreased the census of public mental health facilities, substantially shortened the average length of mental hospitalization, seen the decreasing stigmatization of psychiatric illness, and brought about the substantial growth of psychiatric care in community general hospitals. Those of us old enough to have witnessed the progress in the care and treatment of the mentally ill in the past two decades and who can compare the "human warehouses" that passed for public mental hospitals 20 or more years ago to the small, open, active community mental health centers of the 1970s can attest to the progress that has been made. This progress, to be sure, is not uniform, and many of our mental health facilities continue to have inadequate resources.

The involvement of mental health disciplines in the operation of the law has been subject to the harshest criticisms. Leading psychiatrists such as Seymour Halleck[3] have spoken out against the involvement of psychiatrists in the law except in a therapeutic role. Too often forensic psychiatry has been judged in the context of the vexing assessment of criminal responsibility, which is more a question of morality and social policy than a matter of science or law, and in the prediction of dangerous behavior, a challenge to which no discipline has adequately risen. Among the difficulties in the relationship between mental health disciplines and the law are differing role models and values—the healer versus the concept of deterrence, and rehabilitation versus preventive detention. Norval Morris has observed that whenever mental health power and criminal justice power are combined, as in the indeterminate, ostensibly civil commitment of the sex offender, the two powers are mutually corrupted.

Despite the criticism, despite the attacks, it continues to be true that the mental health disciplines are called upon frequently in the legal process. Pollack has estimated that there are one to two million mental health examinations annually in the United States in connection with legal proceedings.[4] There is every indication that these activities will not only continue but will expand. In recent years, statutorily mandated psychiatric examinations of drug offenders and pre-hospital screening psychiatric examinations of criminal defendants have increased psychiatric input into the criminal justice system. It follows that the forced marriage of psychiatry and the law will continue apace in the foreseeable future.

Much of the literature produced by mental health authorities in the legal-behavioral science field has been devoted to the law itself. Some of us have even had the audacity to write laws. This has been characterized as a kind of identification with the aggressor or an "out-lawing" of the lawyers. Little of what mental health authorities have published has been devoted to clinical approaches to the many and varied involvements of clinicians in relation to the legal system. This book is committed to an attempt to fill a void in describing not only how to approach and deliver mental health clinical services to the legal system, but also how to do it efficiently and well.

CLEARER QUESTIONS AND MORE RELEVANT ANSWERS

The single greatest source of confusion and dissatisfaction in the involvement of psychiatrists in the legal process is that they are asked to give answers to questions which are not clearly articulated. It should be a basic principle that any psychiatric report to a court begin with a statement of the question or questions that the examiner understands to have been posed by the court or by counsel.

Of course, the manifest questions in these encounters often serve latent purposes in psycholegal exercises which may be conscious or unconscious. This must be understood in the realistic context of courts which are flooded with litigation and must seek assiduously the disposition of cases which spare the overtaxed time, energy, and resources of both the criminal justice and civil justice systems. Nothing is more exemplary of this reality than the fact that by plea-bargaining and negotiation between the parties, the great majority of criminal and civil actions are settled out of court. The prevailing practice is the settling of disputes short of the full procedural panoply of the legal process in the interest of efficiency. It is not surprising that the courts have been willing, in such a context, to abrogate their authority to psychiatrist-mediated alternatives, notably in the area of competency to stand trial. Thus, when a court orders a mental examination of a pretrial defendant, it presumably is posing, although rarely articulating, the common-law questions of whether the defendant understands the nature of the proceedings against him and whether he can rationally assist his counsel in his defense. If the court accepts the answer that "the defendant is schizophrenic" as dispositive of these questions, we witness the worst in both the psychiatric and judicial fields in the exercise of their responsibilities. A resulting mental hospital commitment may or may not be clinically appropriate.[5] Most importantly, however, the court docket then is cleared of the case due to the defendant's hospitalization. He is then merely a forgotten statistic in the crush toward disposition.

THE MENTAL STATUS EXAMINATION

Whatever the psycholegal context, the basis for an adequate psychiatric response to the questions asked or implied by the court or other tribunal should be an adequate mental-status assessment of the examined person. Those areas of abnormality or disability uncovered in the mental status examination can and should be applied to the particular legal question or questions asked of the clinician which are relevant to the legal inquiry. Lay persons, including lawyers, judges, and jurors, can understand, if they choose to, the parameters of the standard mental status examination. This is particularly true if the clinician documents his mental status examination with direct quotations from the examinee's responses and with factual data describing his appearance and behavior. The clinician need not sacrifice the relative precision of professional concepts or terminology in communicating to the courts. Such terminology, with added effort, can be translated into terms of common human experience which render them comprehensible.

PROBATIVE VALUE

The concept of probative value in the law is an important one for the clinician to understand. In the hierarchy of clinical probabilities in ascending order of likelihood, physicians generally follow the level first of a differential diagnosis, then a diagnostic impression, and finally an established diagnosis. It must be stressed that only the latter is of probative value in a court of law. When relying on expert opinion, the legal process generally suspends evidentiary rigor, particularly for the behavioral expert. This permits the expert, by virtue of his unique experience and competence, to sift the wheat from the chaff, even in hearsay data, in arriving at his opinion. Such status and authority conferred on the expert in a court of law should not be assumed lightly. Thus, when the expert witness is asked, as he must first be asked, whether or not he has an opinion, his answer should be "no" unless that opinion is within reasonable scientific certainty. In the field of psychiatry, the required support for certain types of psycholegal opinions has become more stringent in recent years, both in statutory law[6] and in court decision.[7] In civil commitment, for example, the psychiatric witness or certifier (on commitment papers) must support his conclusion by citing actual instances where the person has committed or attempted dangerous acts of physical aggression against himself or others. The courts may also require testimony of witnesses who directly observed the violent or destructive behavior.

STRUCTURE AND OPERATION

The last national survey of fields of specialization for psychiatrists was published in 1969 by the National Institute of Mental Health.[8] It reported that of the 16,449 members of the American Psychiatric Association, 211 (1.3 percent) had indicated forensic or correctional psychiatry as their primary fields, while 407 (2.5 percent) indicated these as their secondary fields. Whether or not these data are accurate, it is very likely that the number involved is substantially larger today. The membership of the American Academy of Psychiatry and the Law, founded in 1969, is limited to psychiatrists who devote a substantial portion of their professional activity to forensic psychiatry. Current membership is approximately 700. In addition, there are probably hundreds of physicians not formally trained in psychiatry who are active in the legal system in clinical areas of prison medicine and in evaluation functions in courts on such matters as civil commitment, competency to stand trial, and criminal responsibility. In recent years, many physicians have functioned for courts in activities related to the epidemic of drug abuse in the late 1960s and 1970s.

The characteristic settings where forensic psychiatry is practiced are psychiatric court clinics; inpatient mental hospitals, usually with security facilities; in jails or places of detention; and in a very few general hospitals with forensic psychiatry wards.

The psychiatric court clinic model, developed in the early part of this century by Healy and Broner, proved to be the forerunner of the child guidance clinic.[9] Court clinics are usually located in the courthouses themselves. Those clinicians who have been active in court clinic work stress the importance of the courthouse location, since much is accomplished with court personnel, particularly probation officers, by informal "corridor consultation." Most court clinics in the United States restrict their activities to examinations and consultations for court personnel and do not attempt a treatment role. This restrictive approach has its risks in that it can quickly become routinized, unrewarding, and even stultifying. In New York City, where much of the work of the court clinics is concerned with examinations on the question of competency or fitness to stand trial, these clinics have been dubbed "fitness factories." With the exception of those in Massachusetts, most court clinics across the United States are located in the largest cities and are associated with a felony court. Their activities usually include examinations on competency to stand trial, criminal responsibility, and dispositional recommendations. Although much less in number, some domestic relations, juvenile, and family courts are also served by court clinics and deal, in substantial measure, with the difficult challenges of marital counseling, child custody, and juvenile delinquency.

As part of a survey taken in 1970 of community mental health clinics in the United States, the National Institute of Mental Health inquired about the operation of court clinics.[10] The responses indicated the existence of 53 court clinics in ten states and the District of Columbia. (There were 21 clinics in Massachusetts; 12 in New York; five in California; three each in Maryland, Missouri, and Ohio; two in Pennsylvania; and one each in Florida, Hawaii, Utah, and the District of Columbia.) Although the 1970 survey is probably underreported, there are no data available that indicate further substantial growth except in Massachusetts. It is likely that there is a great deal more forensic psychiatric activity in a less formal, less structured fashion occurring between courts and local mental health centers than in the structured court clinic settings.

In his assessment of the relations between psychiatry and the law, Glueck closed his treatise by citing some events in Massachusetts which suggested something of a thaw in the heretofore rather chilly relations between the two disciplines. That state had established a series of court clinics of a different model than described above. To begin with, the focus was not on the large county superior courts with felony jurisdiction, but rather on the neighborhood courts with misdemeanor jurisdiction covering geographic areas with populations of roughly 50,000 to 75,000. In addition, from the beginning there was a commitment to treatment (often as an alternative to institutionalization), especially for juveniles.[11] In later years, the legislature of Massachusetts added drug abuse screening and competency to stand trial evaluations to the responsibilities of the court clinics. By 1977 there were 32 court clinics in the Commonwealth, constituting the only statewide system of its kind in the United States.[12]

SECURITY FACILITIES

Security mental hospitals or security parts of large state hospitals are the usual settings for inpatient psychiatric care and treatment for defendants or prisoners in the criminal justice system and for patients civilly committed who require strict security. Characteristically, there is a single such secure facility in each state. In the past decade, these institutions have been under legal attack on various grounds. Their patients may be regarded as the relatively neglected stepchildren of the open-door, relaxed security of the community mental health facilities of more recent years. Patients with the taint of alleged criminality, or who are regarded as too dangerous (accurately or, for the most part, inaccurately) are relegated to security facilities. Recent studies[13] have revealed extreme clinical conservatism in decisions to release such patients or to return them to open facilities.

Security institutions are usually located in geographically isolated, rural areas. It is generally difficult to attract professional staff to such remote and onerous institutions. Alternatives have been proposed,[14] and at least one state, Tennessee,[15] has implemented a plan to replace the single statewide security facility with multiple, smaller, regional facilities.

Psychiatry in correctional settings is dealt with elsewhere in this book, particularly relating to mental health services for prisoners after conviction and sentencing. A major area neglected by mental health workers has been the servicing of the needs of persons detained in jails prior to trial and during criminal proceedings against them. For many such detainees, particularly those incarcerated for the first time, such an experience constitutes a severe personal crisis. It is a time when suicide is a serious threat.[16] The usual pattern is for such places of detention to have their medical needs covered by a general practitioner with little or no psychiatric training. Insofar as psychiatrists are involved in such settings, their activities are usually of a ministerial nature; for example, certifying as to mental illness when a prisoner is to be transferred to security mental hospitalization. A treatment role for the psychiatrist in places of detention is very much the exception, if it exists at all.

During the 1960s and 1970s there has been a shift in the delivery of mental health services away from large public and private mental hospitals to psychiatric units in general hospitals with smaller geographic coverage. At this time there are more psychiatric patients being treated in general hospitals across the country than in facilities devoted exclusively to mental patients. More successful methods of treatment, including the application of psychotropic drugs, have made this approach actuarially sound from the point of view of third-party insurance. Basic, however, to such operations is the fact that psychiatric patients in general hospitals are expected to be able to adapt to unrestricted, open settings. Despite anxiety to the contrary, the great majority of psychiatric inpatients have demonstrated that they can so adapt. The criminal offender, however, is rarely offered the benefits of such a choice.

As discussed in a number of other chapters in this text, mental health professionals face many ethical dilemmas when serving in correctional institutions.[17] Are they primarily agents of the state helping to protect society from dangerous human elements, or are they clinicians offering treatment to patients in need? In the author's experience, the most successful delivery of mental health services in such settings is accomplished when the mental health professional staff has an independent status from the correctional authority. This can be achieved operationally when the staff is hired and paid by, and accountable to, a department of health or mental health under professional medical direction.

QUALIFICATIONS AND TRAINING

After a number of years of planning, an accreditation system has now been established for certifying forensic psychiatrists in the United States. In 1979, the first 29 psychiatrists were certified by the American Board of Forensic Psychiatry. The Board was formed by the American Academy of Forensic Sciences, the Forensic Sciences Foundation, and the American Academy of Psychiatry and Law.[18] As yet there is no formal accreditation system for training programs in forensic or legal psychiatry.

Basic to the subspecialty accreditation, of course, is the prior certification by the American Board of Psychiatry and Neurology, the body recognized by organized medicine as competent to confer specialty status in general psychiatry, neurology, and child psychiatry.[19] The Forensic Board requires prior certification in general psychiatry, licensure to practice in the jurisdiction in which the applicant resides, and citizenship in either the United States or Canada. It also requires 5 years of residency training and "substantial experience" in forensic psychiatry.

At the present time there are 13 formal training programs in forensic psychiatry in the United States. These are conducted in a variety of clinical and academic settings. Despite the activity of many psychiatrists and psychologists in the legal and correctional systems, there has been only limited governmental and private support for research and training. An exception has been the funding of some forensic psychiatric research by the Center for Crime and Delinquency of the National Institute of Mental Health.

How does a judge, an attorney, or a member of a jury accurately gauge the technical forensic qualifications of a psychiatrist? One criterion commonly offered is the number of clinical medicolegal examinations the psychiatrist has conducted in a particular medicolegal area. In the author's experience, this is the least persuasive credential of them all. The psychiatrist who has been wrong a thousand times ought not to be accorded status on his one thousand and first examination.

Academic appointment is frequently offered as evidence of competency and, on balance, is probably worthy of significant weight. Of course, the level of the appointment and the academic institution should be a part of the weighing.

Publications as evidence of competence are problematic. Usually the number of publications is offered and not challenged. The nature of the publications is of primary importance. News-media coverage and letters to the editor of a medical journal have actually been cited as publications. Book reviews and editorials, although respectable, especially if they appear in prestigious journals, can only be regarded as padding if offered in the numbers game of publications.

Training in approved programs is an essential qualification. However, it should be noted that once enrolled in an approved psychiatric residency program, or even in a fellowship in legal psychiatry, a trainee is very rarely dropped for incompetence if he or she chooses to endure. While it is true that such training is essential, it is no guarantee of quality in the individual practitioner.

Membership in professional societies and honorary fellowships are of limited value in establishing the credibility of an expert forensic psychiatrst. Such honors too often derive from committee work and paying one's bureaucratic dues in the organization without necessarily showing any real distinction or making a significant contribution.

If this commentary appears to be rather severe with respect to the qualifications and credibility of psychiatrists in the legal forum, the reader should remember that a textbook that purports to be authoritative must describe not only what can be established with credibility in the legal system by behavioral scientists, but also what cannot. The expertise of psychiatry has been oversold in the past. Expectations have been exaggerated and magical solutions to currently insoluble sociolegal problems have been expected, but not delivered, given the state of the profession's science and art.

STATUTORY ATTEMPTS TO ESTABLISH FORENSICALLY QUALIFIED PSYCHIATRISTS

At least two states have attempted to provide for specific designation of particular psychiatrists as qualified in forensic psychiatry. Until recently,

New York required the filing of qualifications with the Department of Mental Hygiene. However, no experience or training in the forensic area was required, and designation was conferred if the psychiatrist was eligible for general psychiatry board certification[20] or had "equivalent" experience (five years of clinical practice). This paper exercise was abandoned by statute[21] in 1976, and all general board-eligible psychiatrists were declared qualified without specific designation.

In 1971, Massachusetts implemented a new statute which was more ambitious than New York's with regard to forensic qualifications. Several sections of the statute specified that only psychiatrists qualified in the asessments of competency to stand trial and criminal responsibility,[22] qualified to certify those prisoners who require mental hospital commitment,[23] and qualified to certify as to the necessity for the involuntary commitment may legally be sworn in as expert forensic psychiatrists for the several areas noted.[24] The establishment of procedures and standards for these designations was left for the rules and regulations of the Massachusetts Department of Mental Health. These regulations required that psychiatrists be specifically designated as qualified in the several forensic areas above by one of seven Regional Directors of Legal Medicine of the Massachusetts Department of Mental Health, each of whom were experienced in forensic psychiatry. These designations were usually based on an interview in which the applicant psychiatrist satisfied the Regional Director that he or she was familiar with the relevant legal standards and procedure in the various forensic determinations, and, if not, instruction was given to insure such familiarity. Board certification or at least eligibility in general psychiatry was also required. It is difficult to evaluate the effects of this system on the quality of forensic psychiatric service resulting from these procedures. The Massachusetts courts were far less than uniform or consistent in requiring these qualifications during the short time the program was in existence. It was a casualty of the severe budget cuts in 1975 in the Department of Mental Health, passing out of existence along with all seven positions of Regional Director of Legal Medicine.

TOWARD A STANDARD FOR FORENSIC PSYCHIATRY

Given the paucity of organized and recognized programs in forensic or legal psychiatry, the newly established certification board will face no easy task in setting standards. After an initial "grandfather phase" when only experience in the field will be expected, the board must define specialized training requirements.

As noted earlier, the Forensic Board now requires only an undefined "substantial experience" in forensic psychiatry. The candidate must report his prior experience in some detail, but no mix is required of formal residency training in the forensic specialties along with "experience." Furthermore there is as yet no definition of the types of clinical experience which might or should be included in a well-rounded clinical background, such as service in a regular or consultative role to a criminal or civil court, service in a correctional institution or with a parole board, or service in an academic setting such as a law school or a criminology department.

In all likelihood we can expect the Forensic Board to sharpen its eligibility standards in the future. We can expect that forensic psychiatric residencies of from 1 to 2 years may be required after a 3-year general residency. A full 5-year program could be provided, based upon a 3-year general psychiatry placement, followed by 2 years of formal academic and clinical training. Such a program, funded by a Federal grant, was in operation at the Boston University Law-Medicine Institute during the 1960s.[25]

Certain basic legal training should be provided in the program, including an introduction to jurisprudence, the structure of the legal system, criminal law and procedure, the law of evidence, and civil and probate procedure. Moreover, it is not unreasonable to expect certified forensic psychiatrists to know their way around a law library. Emphasis has been placed here on the legal dimensions of the curriculum, since such training enables the psychiatrist to communicate effectively within the legal system.

On the side of clinical approaches to forensic psychiatry, the training content might follow something along the lines of the main discussions in the forensic psychiatry section of this text, including the relevant chapters in other sections, such as those on suicide investigation and rape. There could, of course, be other curricular areas, such as a review of the sociological theories of crime and delinquency.

The new certifying body has chosen the term "forensic psychiatry" to cover the entire field. In its proper sense, the word "forensic" relates only to the areas of psycholegal evaluation, reporting, and testimony. This is too narrow a definition to cover the full involvement of psychiatrists in the administration of justice. Psychiatrists treat patients who are involved in the parole, probation, and correctional systems. Moreover, psychiatrists, as behavioral scientists, can contribute valuable insight to the basic philosophy of law. Curran has proposed the broader term "legal psychiatry" to include both the forensic and treatment functions.[26] His term is similar in usage to the general description of "legal medicine" which covers all aspects of medical specialization related to legal settings. Robitscher has suggested the term "social legal psychiatry."[27] In his chapter in this text, Roth uses the term "correctional psychiatry" to cover both the forensic and treatment aspects of psychiatry in the correctional system.

No matter which terms are selected, the training programs themselves should not be narrow in scope. They should include both court-related activities and clinical experiences. There is a wide variety of judicial opportunities in criminal courts, juvenile courts, family and probate settings, and civil jurisdictional systems. Clinical placements can be obtained in correctional settings, drug abuse treatment programs, psychiatric court clinics, and the forensic psychiatry departments of mental hospitals and general hospitals. There could also be placements with the staffs of government commissions revising the mental health laws and as fellows with the Committee on Law and Psychiatry of the Group for the Advancement of Psychiatry.

If qualifications and standards can be developed in the subspecialty of forensic or legal (and correctional) psychiatry within the broad outlines suggested above, and if these standards can be installed and monitored effectively, a giant step will have been taken toward insuring high-quality, creditable services in psychiatry for the American judicial, law-enforcement, and correctional systems.

REFERENCES

1. Glueck, S.: *Law and Psychiatry: Cold War or Entente Cordiale?* Johns Hopkins University Press, Baltimore, 1962.
2. McGarry, A. L.: The Holy Legal War Against State Hospital Psychiatry. *N. Engl. J. Med.* 294:318–320, 1976.

3. Halleck, S.: Introductory Remarks. *Psychiatric Ann.* 4:3–6, 1974.
4. Pollack, S.: Psychiatric Consultation for the Court, in Mendel, W., and Solmon, P. (eds.): *The Psychiatric Consultation.* Grune & Stratton, New York, 1968.
5. McGarry, A. L., et al.: Competency to Stand Trial and Mental Illness, Crime and Delinquency Issues. Monograph Series, DHEW Publication No. (HSM) 73-9105, Washington, D.C., 1973.
6. Massachusetts General Laws, Chapter 123, Section 1; Arizona General Laws, Chapter 5, Section 36-501.
7. *Suzuki v. Quisenberry,* 411 F. Supp. 1113 (D. Hawaii 1976); *Comm. v. Lamb,* Mass. 1973.
8. The Nation's Psychiatrists: National Institute of Mental Health. Public Health Service Publication No. 1889, Chevy Chase, Md., 1969.
9. Halleck, S. L.: American Psychiatry and the Criminal: A Historical Review. *Am. J. Psychiatry* 121 (Suppl.), 1965.
10. Personal communication to W. J. Curran from Carl A. Taube, Chief, Survey and Reports Section, Biometry Branch of the National Institute of Mental Health, February 25, 1971.
11. Russell, D. H., and Devlin, J. H.: The Massachusetts Court Clinic Program. *Juvenile Court Judge's J.* 3:3–5, 1962.
12. Friel, L.: Annual Report, Division of Legal Medicine, Massachusetts Department of Mental Health, 1976.
13. Steadman, J. H., and Halfon, A.: the Baxstrom Patients: Background and Outcomes. *Semin. Psychiatry* 3:376–385, 1971; McGarry, A. L., and Parker, L. L.: Massachusetts Operation Baxstrom: A Follow-up. *Mass. J. Mental Health* 4:27–41, 1974.
14. Greenland, C.: The Three Special Hospitals in England and Patients with Dangerous, Violent or Criminal Propensities. *Med. Sci. Law* 18:253, 1969; Morris, N.: Psychiatry and the Dangerous Criminal. *S. Cal. Law Rev.* 41:514, 1968; McGarry, A. L.: Titicut Follies Revisited: A Long-range Plan for the Mentally Disordered Offender in Massachusetts. *Mental Hygiene* 54:20–27, 1970
15. Laben, J. K., et al.: Reform from the Inside: Mental Health Center Evaluation of Competency to Stand Trial. *J. Community Psychiatry* 5:52–62, 1977.
16. Danto, B. L. (ed.): *Jailhouse Blues, Studies of Suicidal Behaviors in Jail and Prison.* Epic Publications, Orchard Lake, Michigan, 1976.
17. Miller, J. G.: Professional Dilemmas in Corrections. *Semin. Psychiatry* 3:357–362, 1971.
18. Forensic Certification Begins. *Psychiatric News* 11:1, 16, 1976.
19. Robitscher, J. B., *Pursuit of Agreement: Psychiatry and the Law.* J. B. Lippincott, Philadelphia, 1966.
20. The Mental Hygiene Law, Consolidated Law of New York, Book 24A, Section 13.45
21. New York Laws of 1976, Chapter 435.
22. Massachusetts General Laws, Chapter 123, Section 15.
23. Massachusetts General Laws, Chapter 123, Section 18.
24. Massachusetts General Laws, Chapter 123, Section 35.
25. Curran, W. J., and Russell, D. H.: The Law-Medicine Institute After Ten Years. *Boston U. Law Rev.* 49:1–13, 1969.
26. Curran, W. J.: The Confusion of Titles in the Medicolegal Field: An Historical Analysis and a Proposal for Reform. *Med. Sci. Law* 15:270–275, 1975.
27. Robitscher, J. B.: The New Face of Legal Psychiatry. *Am. J. Psychiatry* 129:315–321, 1972.

ADDITIONAL READING

Bonnie, R. J. (ed.): Psychiatrists and the Legal Process: Diagnosis and Debate, in *Psychiatric Annual.* Insight Communications, 1977.

Danto, B. L.: Writing Psychiatric Reports for the Court. *Int. J. Offender Ther. Comparative Criminol.* 17:123–128, 1973.

Houts, M. (ed.): Mental Status Examination, in *Lawyers' Guide to Medical Proof.* Matthew Bender, New York, 1966.

Meyers, A.: The Psychiatric Examination. *J. Criminal Law Police Sci.* 54:20–35, 1963.

Rubin, J. B.: The Psychiatric Report, in Allan, R. C., Ferster, E. Z., and Rubin, J. B. (eds.): *Readings in Law and Psychiatry.* Johns Hopkins University Press, Baltimore, 1975.

Strub, R. L., and Black, F. W.: *The Mental Status Examination in Neurology.* F. A. Davis, Philadelphia, 1977.

CHAPTER 27

Seymour Pollack is Professor of Psychiatry and Director of the Institute of Psychiatry, Law and Behavioral Science at the University of Southern California. He also holds a professorship in the University's School of Public Administration. Dr. Pollack received his B.A. in zoology and psychology from the University of California at Berkeley, his M.A. in psychology from the University of California at Los Angeles, and his medical degree from the University of California at San Francisco. The author of numerous professional articles and papers, Dr. Pollack is a member of the American Academy of Forensic Sciences, the Group for the Advancement of Psychiatry, and the American Academy of Psychiatry and Law.

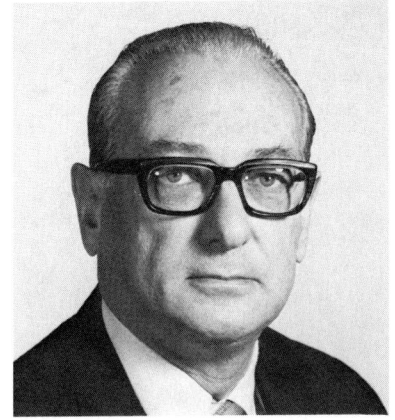

PSYCHIATRY AND THE ADMINISTRATION OF JUSTICE*

Seymour Pollack, M.A., M.D.

Almost ten years ago at an annual meeting of the American Academy of Forensic Sciences, Professor Henry Weihofen† discussed the definition of forensic psychiatry and the principles of forensic psychiatry for psychiatric legal opinion-making that I had proposed.‡ His critique was simple and blunt. He agreed with my definition and believed that the principles were operationally sound, but he doubted that psychiatry and psychiatrists, including forensic psychiatrists, would openly accept them. He

---

*I am indebted for many of the legal concepts in this chapter to Professor Harry W. Jones, Cardozo Professor of Jurisprudence at Columbia University, whose article, "The Practice of Justice" in the *Washington University Law Quarterly* (1966, pp. 133–146), provided a basis for my title and also the grist of jurisprudence to which I have applied my concepts of forensic psychiatry.

†Professor Henry Weihofen, Emeritus Professor of Law and Dean at the University of New Mexico School of Law, could aptly be described as the legal dean of American forensic psychiatry. Among his many contributions to this field is a text he co-authored with Dr. Manfred Guttmacher, pioneer forensic psychiatrist and chief medical officer of the Supreme Bench of Baltimore (*Psychiatry and the Law*, W. W. Norton, New York, 1952).

‡Forensic psychiatry was defined as the application of psychiatry to legal issues for legal ends, and the psychiatric-legal consultation one in which the legal ends directed the psychiatric inquiry. Guiding principles were then detailed and outlined in order to help the forensic psychiatrist to relate his clinical material more adequately and reliably to the legal issue for the legal purpose. These concepts were more fully presented in papers published in 1967 and 1968 (Pollack, S.: Psychiatric Consultation for the Court, in Mendel, W., and Solomon, P. (eds.): *Psychiatric Consultation*. Grune & Stratton, New York, 1967; and Pollack, S.: Principles of Forensic Psychiatry for Psychiatric-Legal Opinion-Making, in Wecht, C.: *Legal Medicine Annual: 1971*. Appleton-Century-Crofts, New York, 1972).

predicted that psychiatrists would be especially negative in their reaction to the first major guiding principle I had propounded, that forensic psychiatry is directed to legal ends and is thereby dominated by the values of the legal system. My limited success, during subsequent years, in popularizing this definition and these principles has amply demonstrated the correctness of Professor Weihofen's forecast. This chapter further describes my "unregenerate" efforts to make palatable to psychiatrists the definition of forensic psychiatry to which I adhere.

A few years ago, in a further attempt to clarify this role of the forensic psychiatrist, I described forensic psychiatry as the instrumental use of psychiatry for legal purposes, its goal being to augment and support the rule of law. In that article[1] I addressed the question of the ends of law as those directed by the rule of law bottomed on the legal value of justice. Within this frame of reference, the forensic psychiatrist is perceived as an agent of the law, promoting legal justice. For forensic psychiatrists, however, the appellation of "agents of the law" carries a pejorative, if not a prostituting, connotation.

The rejection by many psychiatrists of the legal agency role does not necessarily mean that they are unwilling to serve the law by applying their knowledge to legal issues. Forensic psychiatrists resent being perceived as physicians who are directing themselves to the ends of the legal, rather than the medical, system. They object to the idea that they have become agents or "tools" of the law. Their most frequently expressed criticism of their participation in the legal system is that they feel themselves to be misused and abused by its hierarchy.[2]

By contrast the legalists, whether judges or attorneys, government executives or legislators, look favorably upon their being pictured as agents of the law. The term "agent" connotes for them a positive ideal in the sense that law supports order and harmony in our society by promoting the goals of civil and criminal justice. The ends of law are colored by the value system of justice, and legalists perceive themselves ideally as agents of justice. They call upon the forensic psychiatrist to accept this role in the application of his expertise to legal issues.*

---

*At a recent meeting of the American Academy of Psychiatry and Law (New Orleans, October 1977), a panel of judges and attorneys were criticizing forensic psychiatrists for their refusal to address legal issues for the purposes of the law. In reply to a direct question as to whether legalists accept the concept of the forensic psychiatrist as the agent of the law, a judge replied strongly in the affirmative, but he stated that the psychiatrist was not the agent of the (specific) lawyer or judge. This distinction was not pursued, but it does highlight the legalists' concern that the forensic psychiatrist apply himself to the ends of the law while hopefully being able to avoid being misused. Legalists most frequently criticize the forensic psychiatrist for not directing himself to the legal issue, as this issue carries significance for legal purposes. Instead the forensic psychiatrist may present an educational treatise in order to change the legal issue to one more acceptable to (the psychiatrist's) medical ethics and values. The psychiatrist may introduce a psychiatric or psychological dimension to the legal issue, a dimension in which the law is not interested in the instant case at the particular time and circumstances. Alternatively, the psychiatrist may direct attention to the nullity or absurdity of the legal issue as he sees it, with the belief and suggestion that society would benefit, if not the instant party, if this legal issue were translated into or approached as a mental health matter. In other words, too often the forensic psychiatrist's contribution is considered useless, if not destructive, to legal justice because it does not address the legal issue for the ends of the law. The basic conflict between psychiatry and law, sometimes referred to as an in-

A major question in dispute among medical practitioners is whether the psychiatrist should ever direct himself to ends other than medical ones. As noted in a previous article,[3] I believe that psychiatry, as a branch of medicine, does carry the responsibility to direct itself to the ends of other systems that go to make up and support our society. Nevertheless, major ethical issues are present in the instrumental use of psychiatry. Some of these will be addressed in the body of this chapter.

Returning to my thesis that forensic psychiatry is the application of our field to the ends of law, I conceive of justice as the chief end, the embodied ideal of the system of law. It is my firm belief that the ends of justice are supported and enhanced by contributions from forensic psychiatry to the legal system and legal practice. It is the presumptive correctness of this belief that, in my opinion, justifies the field of forensic psychiatry in (1) its support by society at large and by the legal and medical professions in particular, (2) its continued growth and development, and (3) its validation as a subspecialty of psychiatry.†

My definition of forensic psychiatry and my model of role/function for the forensic psychiatrist are unacceptable to many colleagues who reject any and all agency roles, ends, and values outside those of the institution of medicine. Nevertheless, both the concept of the instrumental use of psychiatry for the ends of law, exemplified by justice, and the role/concept

---

herent impasse in communication, is in this area of thrust and purpose. The law calls upon the psychiatrist to apply his expertise in the legal direction for the purpose of the law, whereas the psychiatrist replies by applying his expertise in the medical direction (i.e., applying his material to the legal issue as he interprets this issue through the medical value system of health rather than the legal value system of justice).

†Cf. Pollack, S.: Forensic Psychiatry—A Specialty. *Bull. Am. Acad. Psychiatry Law* 2(2), April 1974; Pollack, S.: The Role of Psychiatry in the Rule of Law. *Psychiatric Annals* 4(8), August 1974. The characterization of forensic psychiatry as a *de facto* specialty appears warranted on the basis of the number of psychiatrists who are practicing what they and others call forensic psychiatry. In recent years we have witnessed the rise of professional groups and societies especially concerned with furthering the development of this field, notably the American Academy of Psychiatry and the Law, and standing subcommittees of psychiatry and law in the American Psychiatric Association and the Group for the Advancement of Psychiatry. Moreover, professional journals devoted to the topical subject matter of psychiatry and law have appeared, such as the *Bulletin of the American Academy of Psychiatry and the Law* and the *Journal of Psychiatry and Law*. A few formal postgraduate advanced education and training programs in forensic psychiatry have been developed throughout the country to augment specialized experience in forensic psychiatry by course work and preceptor supervision. These have been promoted by universities, hospitals, clinics, and court agencies. A formally organized and academically structured specialty training program in forensic psychiatry was established in 1961 at the University of Southern California Institute of Psychiatry, Law and Behavioral Science in Los Angeles, sponsored by the Crime and Delinquency Section of the National Institute of Mental Health. Here a full-time one- to two-year fellowship program was offered to psychiatrists upon completion of their formal three-year residency training program in psychiatry. Postdoctoral psychologists have also been accepted in this program which continues to support five to ten fellows per year. Earlier programs had been short-lived at the Menninger Clinic at Topeka, Kansas, and the Law-Medicine Institute of Boston University. Nevertheless, increasing interest in the field subsequently stimulated the development of new university, court clinic, and hospital programs so that by the 1970s a number of centers were offering different kinds of advanced specialty programs for postgraduate training in psychiatry.

of the forensic psychiatrist as an agent of justice may become more palatable to practitioners of forensic psychiatry if they were more fully to understand and more clearly to perceive the question of how forensic psychiatry serves the law by augmenting the practice of justice. The present chapter addresses this question and is thus entitled "Psychiatry and the Administration of Justice."

FORENSIC PSYCHIATRY AS FORENSIC FACT-FINDING FOR LEGAL PURPOSES

I have defined forensic psychiatry as an interface specialty concerned with the instrumental use of psychiatry, the application of psychiatric theory, principles, and practice to legal issues for legal ends.[4] It is psychiatric fact-finding for legal purposes.

A basic difference exists between the institutional and instrumental uses of a discipline or system. The former, institutional use refers to the discipline's use in a primary sense, directed to its original basic purpose, goals, and values. The latter, instrumental use refers to the discipline's use as a tool for a purpose other than its original purpose. Thus the institutional use of medicine is directed to the ends and values of *health* by means of diagnosis of illness, treatment, prevention, and rehabilitation, whereas its instrumental use is directed to *nonhealth* ends (i.e., other societal ends not related to health, such as its use for the ends of the legal system).

It should be recognized that the instrumental use of medicine is widespread and that the practice of medicine is frequently applied to nonhealth ends. The instrumental application of medicine is demanded by society in order to obtain necessary medical opinions about a variety of social issues. Thus forensic psychiatry, as I define it, is only one area of a much broader field of forensic medicine in this instrumental sense.

In addition, forensic psychiatry is only one of many different forensic sciences, each of which is a scientific adjunct to the legal fact-finding process for legal purposes. Thus forensic psychiatry shares its legal thrust with forensic pathology, toxicology, anthropology, immunology, chemistry, dentistry, and other physical, medical, and social sciences, as well as the fields of criminalistics and questioned documents. Society calls on all of these disciplines to help in the resolution of legal disputes. Although many include in the field of forensic psychiatry a variety of instrumental applications of psychiatry for social purposes in addition to the specific ends of law, technically and puristically, forensic psychiatry limits its fact-finding to legal issues for legal ends.

Ends of law are expressed in both law-making and law-applying. Laws may relate, on the one hand, narrowly to issues and regulations that are significant for the ends of the mental health system, and, on the other, to issues and regulations significant to the ends of a wide variety of other systems in our society (e.g., those of the educational, transportation, and criminal justice systems). The instrumental use of psychiatry is demonstrated when psychiatry directs itself to ends of systems other than mental health in both law-making and law-applying.

Forensic psychiatry is thus an aspect of consultation psychiatry (i.e., psychiatric fact-finding for legal consultation purposes). For law-making, such psychiatric fact-finding may be broad and may include consideration of, and involvement with, policy-making, but in law-applying, fact-finding has a narrower thrust and is limited to the legal issue as defined and set by the law.

Although forensic psychiatry is actually related to both law-making and law-applying, in operation psychiatric fact-finding is most frequently involved with, and is most visible in, the law-applying arena of the legal system (i.e., as psychiatric fact-finding for legal litigation purposes), and it is in this law-applying sense that the phrase *forensic fact-finding* is used in this chapter. The forensic psychiatrist thus conducts his forensic fact-finding for the evidentiary process of litigation (i.e., for the ends of the law as these are obtained through the evaluation of psychiatric evidence in the legal litigation process).

The instrumental use of psychiatry in law is widespread and most visible. It includes the application of psychiatry for such diverse purposes as assessing possible mental disability for work, insurance, or pension eligibility; local, state, and federal licensure; regulated privileges such as driving a car or piloting an airplane; family law issues such as annulment, divorce, and custody; immigration status; competency in criminal trials; and criminal responsibility. In all of these the field of psychiatry is applied to the evaluation of patients involved with legal issues, not for their health, but rather for the purpose of helping the legal system to settle their disputes.

I would like to stress that forensic psychiatry, as I define it, is solely the instrumental use of psychiatry for forensic fact-finding purposes. It is an exploratory, *not* a treatment, tool. It does *not* include the psychiatrist's instrumental role as one who treats the individual for the ends of the law. The role/function of the forensic psychiatrist is only that of an agent of the law as a legal fact-finder, *not* a treatment-giver. In this role the forensic psychiatrist is a consultant to the legal system. As a consultant to law-making or law-applying processes of the legal system, he is an opinion-giver and never a decision-maker. He is most visible as the psychiatric expert witness in the courtroom arena. Thus the forensic psychiatrist does *not* treat for legal ends.

If the psychiatrist assumes a treatment role/function for legal ends, rather than for health, additional ethical questions are raised about his acting as an agent of the law in his "treatment" of a "patient" for such nonhealth purposes. These ethical questions will also be addressed in the body of this chapter.

ETHICAL ISSUES OF PSYCHIATRIC FACT-FINDING FOR LEGAL PURPOSES

Even though the forensic psychiatrist accepts the ethicality and responsibility of psychiatric fact-finding for the ends of justice, the instrumental use of psychiatry for the ends of the law may still create problems. These arise in two areas: (1) problems the psychiatrist has in accepting the value system of justice in the law; and (2) problems developing when the ends of the law are unacceptable to the psychiatrist.

I have mentioned that forensic psychiatry is an adjunct to fact-finding in our legal system; in this sense the forensic psychiatrist is an agent of the legal, and not the mental health, system. He operates under the aegis of the legal system, and his functions are subject to all of the circumscriptions and constitutional due process guidelines related to legal fact-finding. In other words, under our form of democratic government and in our liberty-seeking, privacy-insuring society, the application of forensic psychiatry is bound by the same legal rules that regulate the exploring and procuring of all facts as legal evidence.

In the instrumental use of psychiatry for legal purposes there are ethical principles that inhere in the psychiatrist's attempts to explore and define the individual litigant's behavior and mental state. The application of forensic psychiatry is bound by the values of the legal system.[5] These ethical principles derive from the field of law and the practice of justice. Thus the forensic psychiatrist should pursue his fact-finding with scientific integrity, intellectual honesty, and vigor, but only with an approach consistent with the legal values of justice.

The psychiatrist should enter into an interview of a party only with that party's knowledge and consent. The psychiatrist should make his role/function known. The patient should understand the psychiatrist's relationship to him and the relationship of the examination to his legal issue. He should know that he is being examined for legal, and not treatment, purposes. In this sense the forensic psychiatric examination is conducted in a setting of informed consent. In those instances in which a judicial order has legally imposed the examination upon the party, the patient should still be informed that the psychiatric examination may be refused by him, subject to legal conditions and possible sanctions. For example, in some jurisdictions, if the patient refuses to be examined by the court-ordered psychiatrist, he may be foreclosed from introducing into evidence any private psychiatrist's opinion about his mental state, or he thereby may be foreclosed from using any mental-state issue in his legal action. In such instances the patient's counsel is knowledgeable about the legal conditions related to the examination and should be informed about the examination problems by the psychiatrist in order to promote the ends of justice.

The psychiatrist should be assured that the patient is one who voluntarily and understandingly subscribes to the examination in the sense that his constitutional due process rights are safeguarded. The patient may not necessarily subscribe to the purpose of the examination, but he is, at least, voluntarily accepting the examination at both the request and knowledge of his counsel. If the patient is psychotically disturbed or is otherwise mentally disabled so that he is incapable of rational understanding or cooperation, this forensic psychiatric examination is also conducted with the knowledge and consent of the patient's attorney for the specific legal purpose of the examination.

Questions have been raised about the ethical aspects of forensic psychiatry examinations of apprehended criminal suspects prior to their obtaining legal counsel. In my opinion, such examinations are as ethical as any other examinations conducted by agencies of law enforcement and prosecution during this initial phase of the criminal justice process. The psychiatrist who is participating in such an examination is obviously a functionary of these agencies and must make his role perfectly clear to the suspect. He must provide the accused with all of his applicable due process safeguards (e.g., those protecting against self-incrimination and unwitting confessions).

The forensic psychiatrist must abide by the legal precepts of confidentiality and privilege that prevail in his jurisdiction and apply to his specific case. During his exploration he should not subject the party to potentially harmful exploratory techniques, such as those involving drugs or potentially dangerous physical procedures, without consent of counsel, and possibly court action should precede any significant modification of the standard psychiatric examination. In conclusion, the thrust of all of the above is to underscore that psychiatric fact-finding for legal purposes is intimately tied to the values and ends of the legal system of justice.

Problems arise for the forensic psychiatrist when his involvement is requested with legal issue or ends which are ethically unacceptable to him. Under such circumstances, the ethical position of the forensic psychiatrist should be to refuse to participate in, or withdraw from, the consultative role when this comes to his attention.

Issues and ends of civil justice do not generally arouse strong negative attitudes and feelings among psychiatrists; consequently, few psychiatrists experience ethical conflicts in their application of forensic psychiatry to civil issues such as workers' compensation, social security and insurance benefits, civil competency issues, and family law matters of divorce and child custody. Nevertheless, the ends of criminal law and the values of criminal justice are especially odious to many psychiatrists; many, therefore, refuse to participate as forensic psychiatrists in criminal-legal matters, especially on issues of criminal responsibility.

When they do participate in criminal-legal matters, many psychiatrists are more acceptant of their role as consultants for the court than for advocate counsel. Even when psychiatrists do consult for advocate counsel, many are more comfortable as consultants for criminal defense than for criminal prosecution because this role/function is more compatible with their therapeutic philosophy of helping the individual. This same therapeutic philosophy influences many psychiatrists to be more favorable to an individual civil plaintiff than to defense counsel representing an insurance company or a government agency.

Some psychiatrists feel so negatively about the ends of the criminal justice system that their opinions become biased. Some use their forensic involvement as an opportunity to disseminate their negative views about criminal justice. Others, unless challenged, do not disclose the strong underlying biases that have substantially influenced their opinions. It is my view that the forensic psychiatrist should always reveal his own attitudes.

In conclusion, the ethical approach for the forensic psychiatrist is to avoid consultative participation in those legal issues and for those ends about which he holds such strong feelings and attitudes that it would be difficult, if not impossible, for him to be neutral, objective, and impartial in his forensic fact-finding.

The issue of capital punishment arouses the most intense emotional and ethical conflict. Many psychiatrists hold that it is unethical for the forensic psychiatrist to participate in a capital case in which his evidence could lead to the defendant's execution. They hold similar views about the psychiatrist's examination of a condemned felon awaiting execution. Psychiatrists are against such participation for moral, ethical, or emotional reasons.

Following my testimony in the trial of Sirhan Sirhan for the murder of Senator Robert F. Kennedy, I have regularly refused requests from the courts and prosecuting attorneys for psychiatric opinions on criminal responsibility in capital cases. Earlier, although personally opposed to capital punishment, I had recognized it as an accepted part of the criminal law, and thus I felt that it was not unethical for forensic psychiatrists to participate in capital cases for the prosecution if they were able to accept this principle of criminal justice. I no longer can do so, and therefore I curtail my involvement.

When the forensic psychiatrist curtails his psychiatric-legal participation either by excluding himself from certain legal issues or by limiting himself to one or the other side in the adversary system, he poses additional ethical questions. For example, should a forensic psychiatrist limit his participation solely to criminal prosecution or defense? In my opinion, either limitation is ethical, although each creates other problems.

The forensic psychiatrist's differential involvement with legal issues and legal advocates creates additional problems in that, in the practice of forensic psychiatry, the appearance and projected image of neutrality, impartiality, and objectivity are as important as the authentic characteristics. Credibility and related persuasiveness are dependant upon the image. Thus the forensic psychiatrist who restricts his involvement to one or another category of advocate is always suspected of advocate bias, and his credibility is accordingly impugned.

For this reason the forensic psychiatrist should try to avoid participation with only one of the adversary positions in litigation. Thus it would be preferable if he were available to consult for either side in order to reduce the challenge of alleged advocacy bias. Unfortunately, the ethical constraints on the forensic psychiatrist in restricting his involvement with certain legal issues and preventing him from participating in issues whose ends are unacceptable to him place him at risk. The realities of the adversary system too often act to prevent the forensic psychiatrist's involvement as a middle of the road expert witness. Soon after entry into the practice of forensic psychiatry, most expert witnesses are "tagged" as (civil) plaintiff or defense psychiatrists, or as being for prosecution or defense in criminal actions, because of their identification with one or the other adversary positions.

Challenge to the use of psychiatric data as legal fact-finding also comes from many who believe that psychiatrists cannot reliably identify features of dangerousness to support the application of such data to legal ends. Research studies clearly indicate that the ability of psychiatrists to identify features predictive of dangerous conduct in the distant future is generally poor. Nevertheless, on a clinical level, psychiatrists continue to offer judgments, on the dangerousness to self and others, of their mentally ill patients, especially as predictions of such dangerousness are related to conduct in the more immediate future. Appellate courts have tended to uphold the legal obligations of psychiatrists to predict dangerousness of their patients under special circumstances.[6]

The "treatment" of patients for nonhealth purposes has promoted heated controversy and ethical conflict among psychiatrists. I have stressed that the field of forensic psychiatry is limited to psychiatric *fact-finding* for legal purposes and that it does *not* include "treatment" for legal ends. At the 1977 World Congress of Psychiatry, the Hawaiian Declaration of Human Rights supported the position that the psychiatric "treatment" of patients for nonhealth purposes is unethical. Soviet psychiatrists, using psychiatric treatment modalities, who have brainwashed political prisoners for the ends of their government were singled out for special criticism.

In the United States it was learned that psychiatrists working for the CIA and the military establishment, either directly or by contract, for many years had "treated" unknowing citizens with hallucinogenic drugs for military purposes. Visibility of these programs led to a dramatic outcry and scathing criticism, with the result that such "treatment" was discontinued. When programs for psychiatric "treatment" of prison inmates who were having "adjustment problems" reached public visibility, these "treatment" programs also received severe criticism and were discontinued.

Today, controversy rages over the question of how much involvement the mental health system should have in promoting and augmenting social control of the mentally ill persons (i.e., the question of involuntary detention and treatment of the mentally ill for social control purposes). Most frequently these questions are posed in the context of challenge to the right of the mentally ill person to freedom and his right to reject involuntary treatment.

The same challenges are directed to the involuntary treatment of the mentally ill offender who is either in custody or under some other form of social control imposed by the criminal justice system (e.g., the offender on probation who "accepts" psychiatric treatment as a condition of probation in lieu of sentence, or the offender on parole whose condition of parole includes psychiatric treatment).

Challenge to the use of forensic psychiatry for social control purposes also comes from the many studies that indicate the low levels of accuracy and reliability in psychiatric skills for the identification of dangerousness of both criminal and mentally ill offenders.

In contemporary society, social control is one of the purposes of criminal, quasicriminal, and civil law. Social control, under certain conditions and with adequate legal safeguards, is a legal measure that is imposed upon some parties for either their own protection or for the safety of others. Critics of the use of the mental health system for the ends of social control maintain that social control should be solely a function of the criminal justice system. Because forensic psychiatry data often serve as legal evidence directed to issues of social control with involuntary detention and/or involuntary treatment, forensic psychiatry has been challenged by civil libertarians and by civil rights-oriented psychiatrists. They hold that forensic psychiatry is a frightening tool that is being used to subvert and destroy our democratic institutions and civil freedoms.[7]

Those who see forensic psychiatry as a tool of the establishment conceive of this field as a covert, insidious weapon of the ruling class, used to maintain the status quo of conservative middle-class values and the prevailing sociopolitical system. They urge that forensic psychiatry be eliminated as a fact-finding tool for legal evidence directed to social control.[8]

As mentioned previously, social control is one of the accepted ends of law and reflects both civil and criminal justice. In my opinion, it is not unethical for the forensic psychiatrist to apply his material to civil aspects of social control. Nevertheless, opponents of the use of the mental health system for social control purposes feel as strongly about their position as I do about capital punishment. Obviously, psychiatrists holding this attitude should not participate in psychiatric-legal fact-finding leading to this end.

The application of psychiatry to social control issues is acceptable to most psychiatrists. Civil social control, to most, is an acceptable legal purpose, and criminal social control is a necessary legal end and a socially desirable one. Most forensic psychiatrists, therefore, experience little conflict in fact-finding for either purpose.

In conclusion, forensic psychiatry, as a fact-finding tool for legal purposes, can unquestioningly be abused and misused by the legal system. Concern about this possibility should promote constant supervision, monitoring, and review of the use of forensic psychiatry as a legal tool. Moreover, efforts should be directed by the fields of psychiatry and law to develop and utilize guidelines for forensic psychiatry to reduce the risk of such abuse. By the application of guidelines for psychiatric-legal opinion-making, the abuse of forensic psychiatry can be further reduced as forensic psychiatric opinions become more reliable. Thus, as I see it, the possibility of abuse or misuse of forensic psychiatry is not an adequate reason for discarding or restricting the use of psychiatry for legal purposes. On balance, forensic psychiatry appears to be a significant adjunct to the legal fact-finding process in that its benefits to the cause of justice far outweigh the risks of its abuse.

PSYCHIATRY IN THE CAUSE OF JUSTICE

What I am suggesting in this chapter on the benefits of psychiatry to the cause of justice follows the thinking of Judge Jerome M. Frank, leading American jurist and legal realist, who pictured the practice of law as balanced between two concepts. On the one hand are general legal principles which promote the illusion of law as an inflexible body of rules, administered dispassionately with impartiality, neutrality, and objectivity, that lead inevitably to fixed and certain results. Judge Frank called this the myth of law. On the other hand, this concept was balanced by the operation of legal processes in our system of law, processes that allow the expression of social and legal fairness and satisfy our desire for justice. The thrust of Judge Frank's exposition was directed mostly to the ways in which our jury-trial system functions to circumvent the apparent fixity and certainty of the law and to serve the demands of legal justice, while at times not even applying the law.[9]

Forensic psychiatry, in my opinion, also functions as a significant instrument of the law to promote the fairness concept of legal justice. Contributions from the forensic psychiatrist serve the trier of fact in his attempts to reconcile rules of law with the concept of justice, as fairness, in the individual case. Forensic psychiatry performs this function by providing material to the legal system that promotes the individualizing and humanizing thrust in our legal search for fairness in civil and criminal justice.

For centuries legal philosophers have described justice as an elusive and protean concept. Aristotle observed that justice was vague and ambiguous, and, at times, even difficult to distinguish from injustice.[10] Nevertheless, to modern man it is the value of justice as fairness that the law is all about. Although the concept of justice reflects different kinds of social organizations and political governments, and changes from generation to generation or era to era, the value of justice to modern man has historically retained its underlying tie to the substantive concept of basic fairness. It is to this concept of legal justice, as basic fairness in law, that forensic psychiatry addresses itself, in that for modern law, fairness in the resolution of many legal disputes requires consideration of psychological and mentalistic elements in the use of subjective standards. Thus fairness for legal justice calls upon facts adduced by forensic psychiatry for demonstration of relevant evidence that is material to psychological issues in law.

INDIVIDUALIZATION IN LAW AS JUSTICE

Two features of contemporary American law distinguish it from its historical derivatives and serve as a fountainhead for our current concept of fairness in legal justice. One is the feature of individualization; the other is the humanistic quality of modern law.

As Anglo-American law has matured, a greater emphasis has been placed on the individual and the individual case. This emphasis on the merits of the individual case is a distinctive feature of our case-law approach to law. Contemporary legal scholars look upon our laws not only as a body of explicit rules, but also as a system for individualization in the application of justice. Sophisticated contemporary justice demonstrates a movement away from the "slot-machine" theory of justice to the individualization of justice colored by the sensitivities of human experience.

Forensic psychiatry, in its concern for the uniqueness of the individual and the singularity of the case and in its interest in clarifying how this individual's mental state relates to the legal issue, contributes significantly to the contemporary legal emphasis on individualization. In this sense forensic psychiatry can be looked upon as a tool to be used by the trier of fact for finding justice in the individual case, a tool for individualization in the rules of law. As was mentioned above, Judge Frank held that such individualization of law is not allowed to operate in the open, but rather functions by surreptitious methods, notably through the use of the jury.[11] I believe similarly that forensic psychiatric data serve to promote individualization of law to augment justice. Society seeks such data to satisfy its desire for fairness, but hesitates to accept and admit them too openly. Nevertheless, the trier of fact, through forensic psychiatry, obtains additional evidence which he may use to mitigate and circumvent the harshness and inflexibility of the rule of law.

Of importance is a point which cannot be too strongly underscored: forensic psychiatric data, as fact and opinion evidence about the individual's mental state, must *not* be colored by the forensic psychiatrist's concern about justice; these facts must be applied to the rule of law as it exists. They should *not* be biased by the forensic psychiatrist's own concept of fairness. The trier of fact has the privilege and duty of dispensing justice in the particular case, *not* the psychiatric expert witness. If the forensic psychiatrist were to allow his opinions to be colored by his own concept of fairness, he would be usurping the function of the trier of fact, and his biased opinion, recognized as such, should be accorded little probative weight. In this sense, forensic psychiatry, like all other forensic sciences, must assume the position of fact-finding, undiluted by the value of justice but presented for the administration of justice. The evidence of forensic psychiatry provides the trier of fact with a basis for understanding the individual's mental state and supplies individualistic elements relevant to the legal issue. It is for the trier of fact, judge or juror, *not* the psychiatrist, to weigh this evidence and determine how the elasticity of justice will balance the rigidity of the law.

Today an increasing amount of legal decision-making turns on the decision-maker's impression as to the essential justice of an individual matter. In our adversary system of justice this means that more and more legal decisions are not made in courts by judges, but in offices of public and private civil and criminal attorneys. Here forensic psychiatric reports, highlighting the individual characteristics of the case, may greatly influence the decision-making. In civil issues, the medical-legal report carries considerable weight in determining out-of-court compromise settlements. Psychiatric-legal reports constitute a significant percentage of such medical-legal reports. In criminal-legal issues, the number of psychiatric reports, compared to other medical-legal reports, is even more frequently encountered.

THE HUMANISTIC ASPECT OF LAW AS JUSTICE

I would like now to turn to the second attribute of modern law which directs itself to our contemporary concept of justice—the humanistic aspect of law. In recent years the law has become increasingly concerned with the psychological, mentalistic, and subjective features of human conduct, considering these as features that singularly characterize mankind and make man the unique being he is. Our modern concept of law for the ordering of human society, and especially the concept of justice in law in the exercise of justice, is based on recognition of the humanness of mankind and the attribution to man of sophisticated mentalistic functions that universally underlie human conduct and behavior.

Increasingly over time these mentalistic or subjective elements of human conduct have been accorded greater weight for legal definition of a growing number of legal issues. It is this feature that I refer to as the humanistic aspect of contemporary law, and it is this humanistic aspect of law that today carries a significant quantum of justice. In other words, the concept of justice, as fairness, requires that humanistic elements be taken into account in assessing and judging many legal actions. Forensic psychiatry, I believe, contributes to this humanistic aspect of law by exploring these subjective features in the individual case and in their relationship to the legal issue, and by presenting them for consideration to the trier of fact in his quest for justice under law.

Over the past two hundred years, Anglo-American law has witnessed a shift from sole or primary emphasis on objective theories to include subjective theories of legal approach and subjective definitions of terms and proof of facts. In recent years an increasing number of criminal and civil issues have been defined by *both* objective and subjective theories.

By the objective theory in law is meant that the legal meaning of a term, for its proof, is limited to the particular physical fact demonstrating that term (i.e., the legal meaning of the term is derived from objective physical evidence of the actual conduct). By objective standard of proof is meant that evidentiary proof relies upon an objective determination of fact. Proof of the alleged act is adduced through objective data. The act is accepted as such in the objective sense, in that a judgment as to its validity is established through the eyes of the actual or hypothetical observer of the act.

The subjective theory in law holds that the meaning of the term resides in the state of mind, the mentalistic features characterizing the individual's state of mind. The subjective standard of evidentiary proof utilizes psychological data and subjective features, the mentalistic elements of the act, as evidence, and takes these into account in probative fact-finding. Thus a subjective theory relies on the individual's subjective narration and description of his mental state; the act is viewed through the eyes of this individual rather than through the eyes of the beholder.

Phrasing it simplistically, under the objective theory or standard, the term in question is defined by a particular kind of conduct (i.e., the act, as a physical, objectively demonstrable form of behavior, speaks for itself). The subjective theory defining that same act would not use the objective evidence, but rather would rely on subjective data. To obtain these data one would have to raise certain questions: What did the individual mean by the act? What were his motives? Did he intend the act? Did he intend to engage in this specific civil transaction or in this particular criminal action? And, did mental dysfunction or mental impairment prevent him from exercising this specific purpose? Answers to these questions can come, in part, from psychiatric evidence.

An example from tort law may further clarify the difference between the objective and the subjective theory in law. For example, one can define negligence legally by using an objective theory of negligence, one in which evidence of negligence is adduced from an individual's particular kind of conduct, from the objective acts themselves as they were physically demonstrated, and as society accords to these demonstrated acts the appellation of negligence. One can also legally define negligence by a rival subjective theory in which negligence is defined by the individual's state of mind (e.g., as a mental attitude of undue indifference with respect to one's conduct and its consequences). For evidence of this latter theory one can call upon the individual to describe his state of mind at the time, its mentalistic features, and its psychological functions as these related to the legal issue.[12] This latter approach defines the term from a subjective point of view, or from a particular mental state, as against a particular kind of conduct; it is this latter approach, of course, that calls upon the forensic psychiatrist for this special kind of evidence.

Increasing emphasis on the humanistic aspect of the law thus accords weight to significant human values inherent in the purpose and meaning of the act, in its import to the actor, and in his motivation for the act. The trier of fact is concerned with these humanistic elements of the act, and not merely with the act alone. These mental elements and their values are believed worthy of consideration in the law's concern for justice, in spite of the fact that their introduction substantially increases the complexity, and even the prolixity, of the law. These elements introduce flexibility into the legal system and provide additional materials to balance the concept of the fairness of justice against the rigidity of the rule of law.

In recent years subjective theories have been introduced for a number of legal issues, so that both objective and subjective theories may be used in proof (i.e., both physical data and subjective data are admissible as evidence for probative purposes). For example, we have witnessed increasing accent on subjective standards for proof of causation in tort law and worker's compensation issues, as well as in areas of property ownership, contracts, tax issues, and family law matters of custody. Nevertheless, it is in criminal law that subjective theories have been most emphasized.

In criminal law the individual's mental state, in the concept of *mens rea*, has traditionally been of legal concern, and evidence of the accused's mental state is admissible to prove his culpability. The defendant's mental state is assumed to be unimpaired unless significant evidence is adduced to demonstrate the contrary. In other words, there is a rebuttable presumption that the defendant had a sound mind when he committed the illegal act. Both objective and subjective theories of defense are available. Psychiatric evidence is admissible to support theories of mental nonresponsibility. A number of mental-responsibility theories of defense have been developed, such as the defense of unconsciousness, the insanity defense, and the theory of diminished capacity.

In recent years we have seen a progressive drop in the threshold level of mental impairment that could overturn the presumption of sound mind in the defendant. This drop is most dramatically evidenced in the recently developed concept of diminished capacity. One jurisdiction after another has experienced a reduction in the threshold level of mental impairment defining criminal nonresponsibility, in the changes from the M'Naughton rule of insanity to that of the American Law Institute Model Penal Code. In addition, in recent years, subjective theories have been introduced for such criminal-legal concepts as duress and entrapment.

In this movement from objective to subjective theory there is growing emphasis on the mentalistic aspects of law and an increasing recognition of the humanistic element of justice. I believe that the use of forensic psychiatry for this purpose fulfills deep psychological needs for such justice in our democratic, freedom-loving, individualistically oriented society.

If the central objective of our legal system is the satisfactory administration of justice, one which will keep society reasonably at peace, then forensic psychiatry serves admirably to provide data to the fact-finder for his consideration in the administration of such justice. Thus I perceive forensic psychiatry as a humanistic tool which the trier uses to reconcile the universal rules of law with justice in the individual case.

This use of forensic psychiatry is most visible in the types of criminal-legal actions that arouse strong and intense emotional reactions, such as in highly publicized criminal cases. The criminal trial of Sirhan Sirhan for the assassination of Senator Robert F. Kennedy provides such an example. Many probably recall the emotional intensity surrounding this trial and the negative reactions to the psychiatric testimony introduced by the defense on the issue of the defendant's diminished capacity. Consider how loud an outcry would have arisen, however, if no evidence had been allowed in the trial to explain to the jury, and to the public at large, what Sirhan's mental state was at the time of the assassination. I believe that our system of justice would have demanded an accounting of the defendant's mental state, even if the trier of fact had concluded, as he did, that Sirhan's mental state was not adequately impaired to excuse him on the defense's theory of diminished capacity.

After the culmination of this trial, I obtained interviews from each juror who had heard the extensive psychiatric and psychological evidence in this case and had deliberated about Sirhan's guilt. Interestingly, almost all of the jurors had entered this trial believing that Sirhan must have been seriously mentally ill and very mentally impaired in order to have carried out the act as he did. Nevertheless, as defense psychologists and psychiatrists presented their evidence, these jurors became increasingly convinced of the probability that Sirhan's mental state was not sufficiently impaired to excuse him from criminal responsibility for first-degree murder, and that his mental impairment did not satisfy the defense theory of diminished capacity. The important point I would like to stress, however, is that the psychological and psychiatric evidence adduced in this case and presented at trial fulfilled an important function for the administration of criminal justice. Our contemporary concept of fairness in this matter made it desirable that the subjective, mentalistic elements of Sirhan's mental state be presented for consideration by the trier of fact.

It is largely because of the movement of criminal law toward the individualistic and humanistic features of justice, and the corresponding concern in the law about psychological and mentalistic elements in the definition of crime, that, in my opinion, criminal law is eager to accept forensic psychiatry as a field which supports these trends.

CRITICISMS OF PSYCHIATRIC EVIDENCE

It is likely that the law has been too uncritical in accepting forensic psychiatry as a forensic science and, in science's name, has justified the dispositive effects that are judicially accorded to forensic psychiatry. Today, in many ways, psychiatry is more of an art that a science, and forensic psychiatry is no more of a science than is psychiatry in its application of psychiatry to legal issues for legal ends. This does not mean that forensic psychiatry need be discarded and that psychiatric opinion evidence should be legally inadmissible; it means only that such evidence should be considered with caution and circumspection.

Many legal commentators are critical of the trend toward acceptance of forensic psychiatric opinions, believing that forensic psychiatry has too controlling an influence on the legal outcome in many civil issues, such as child custody matters, and in criminal-legal issues, such as mental incompetency to stand trial and criminal responsibility. They see the forensic psychiatrist as replacing the legal tribunal. Such a corruption of the legal system may actually develop if the forensic psychiatrist is removed from the challenge of the adversary system, as is recommended by some psychiatrists and legalists. For example, *in camera* opinions by the psychiatric expert witness may, in fact, control the legal outcome; similarly, an uncritical prosecuting attorney may give undue weight to a psychiatrist's expert opinion and drop prosecution of an otherwise deserving, prosecutable case, or an inept defense attorney may fail to raise a plea of insanity because he uncritically accepts a psychiatrist's opinion which fails to support the insanity defense.

I believe it necessary that forensic psychiatry remain in the forum of the adversary system and be subject to the challenges of cross-examination. Forensic psychiatric data are "too soft" and idiosyncratic. They are too unstandardized. Vagueness in the concepts of mental illness and the multiplicity of theories about mental illness make it relatively easy for psychiatric practitioners to describe mental impairment primarily, if not solely, on the basis of their philosophy or bias. Most frequently the psychiatric expert witness's assumptions are not articulated, and little or no reasoning is demonstrated to support conclusory opinions. Under these circumstances, adversary challenge to psychiatric opinions is absolutely necessary. Moreover, cross-examination of the expert witness acts to safeguard against the potential arbitrariness of so-called experts and guarantees against the cloaking of psychiatric expert witness evidence in the trappings of hard science.

Furthermore, legal caution holds that the *ipse dixit* of experts should not be substituted for the judicial process in our democratic society and that legal decision-making should remain in the domain of the layman. At times psychiatric expert-witness opinions appear to replace the decision-making of the trier of fact, but when this occurs it most frequently results from derelictions in the legal process and is not the fault of opinion-making by the forensic psychiatrist.

Courts have struggled for years with the question of whether the psychiatric expert witness should be allowed to express an opinion on the ultimate question of fact to be decided by the trier of fact. Many jurisdictions specifically prevent the expert witness from applying his opinion to the ultimate legal question. In federal jurisdictions and in California and some other states, this is not only allowed but is encouraged in order to force the expert witness to apply his material more relevantly to the legal issue. In spite of the problems it raises, it is my opinion that the latter approach is preferable. By applying the breadth of psychiatric data and reasoning to explain his opinion on the ultimate question, the psychiatric expert witness contributes more significantly to the administration of justice.

Psychiatric evidence is frequently important at trial for the purpose of developing the record for possible appeal. In especially inflammatory cases, psychiatric evidence is often rejected by the trial tribunal. Under less public pressure and scrutiny, however, a more objective tribunal may perceive such evidence as credible and persuasive. Although in our system of law appellate courts do not retry cases in the sense of accepting new evidence for consideration, an appellate court may give significantly more weight to psychiatric expert-witness evidence than the jury. As a result the appellate court may substantially modify a prior judgment. In a number of instances in California, trial judgments have been modified or even reversed on the basis of psychiatric evidence in the record. Even when a judgment is affirmed, the appellate court may rely substantially on the psychiatric evidence in the record. For example, in its review of the Sirhan appeal, the California Supreme Court devoted much of its opinion to a differential analysis of psychiatric testimony by the prosecution as against testimony by the defense, and thereby affirmed the conviction and sentence. It is apparent, therefore, that in this way forensic psychiatric material provides additional balance to the scales of justice.

The challenge to forensic psychiatry from legalists and laymen has been largely directed to the use of forensic psychiatry in criminal litigation. Attacks upon the use of psychiatric evidence in criminal law are often subtle and covert attacks by legal conservatives upon the concepts of individualization of law and on the humanistic aspects of law which characterize the modern concept of criminal justice. These critics would hew to the rigid, inflexible rules of general law and negate the concept of flexible, individualized justice in order to give greater emphasis to their interest in stronger and more successful prosecution and heavier, more severe criminal sanctions.

COST-BENEFITS OF FORENSIC PSYCHIATRY FOR THE CRIMINAL JUSTICE SYSTEM

The question can be raised as to whether forensic psychiatry is a luxury that modern society may possibly be unable to afford. The increasing use of psychiatric expert witnesses and the mushrooming of psychiatric evidence in an already overburdened legal system have led some to recommend that psychiatric evidence be entirely eliminated from the trial system. Others hold that its use should be markedly circumscribed (e.g., limited to a few selected trial issues or restricted to a few special phases of the legal process, such as sentencing of the criminal offender. It is self-evident that only those contributions of forensic psychiatry should be admissible that are relevant to a legal issue, and only that evidence should be admissible that is sufficiently reliable for legal purposes.

The low reliability of forensic psychiatry has been increasingly pointed to by vocal critics of psychiatry. It is possible that challenge to forensic psychiatry on the basis of its low reliability may significantly reduce forensic psychiatry's contributions to the law in the foreseeable future, that is, until its level of reliability rises to a more acceptable threshold.

On the other hand, any limitation of forensic psychiatry will serve markedly to constrain and reduce the concept of fairness in justice that has developed in modern law. I doubt that the answer to the above question is wholesale abandonment of forensic psychiatry in the trial process. Possibly there are some issues for which psychiatric evidentiary data may reasonably be set aside or reduced with a consequence of more economical, reliable, and efficient administration of justice. If society wishes to pay the price of altering the balance of justice in this direction, it may do so. I, for one, hope that society will continue to recognize that the price paid for supporting the concept of fairness in justice, although substantial, is necessary for the maintenance of our ideal of a just, democratic society.

The attack upon forensic psychiatry by both mental health practitioners and legalists is justified on the basis of the poor quality of some psychiatric expert-witness testimony and reports. The poor quality of these contributions raises questions about the credibility of forensic psychiatry. Some judges have held that forensic psychiatric evidence is more obfuscating than enlightening to the administration of justice.

These criticisms can be answered by improving the quality of forensic psychiatry. Qualifications for practitioners in forensic psychiatry should be established, and a move in this direction has already taken place with the creation of the American Board of Forensic Psychiatry. Advanced education and training in forensic psychiatry should be promoted in departments of psychiatry and hospitals throughout the country. Finally, the reliability of psychiatric evidence can be upgraded and its credibility enhanced by formulating guidelines for psychiatric opinion-making for legal purposes; some such guidelines have already been formulated and articulated.

In conclusion, the application of forensic psychiatry to legal issues can be considered to be intimately related to positive values inherent in the fairness concept of legal justice and also to a number of other value concepts significant to democratic society, such as those of individual autonomy, liberty, freedom, and equality under law. Forensic psychiatry in the form of psychiatric fact-finding for legal purposes supports these basic value concepts. In my opinion, any substantial modification in the application of forensic psychiatry to law is premature at this time. It would result in significant changes in law, both in substance and procedure, with interacting repercussions to the legal and mental health systems that are difficult to comprehend. It would have a negative rather than positive impact upon our society. Although the cost of forensic psychiatry fact-finding is significant, in my opinion, the benefits far outweigh the costs. It is therefore doubtful that, on balance, society would benefit if the use of forensic psychiatry for trial purposes were abandoned.

CONFLICT OF VALUES IN PSYCHIATRY WITH THOSE OF LAW

The major challenge to forensic psychiatry emanates from the field of psychiatry itself. It stems from the instrumental aspects of forensic psychiatry and from the need, in this instrumental application, to substitute the values and goals of law for those of medicine and psychiatry. Obviously the values of mental health often do conflict with those of legal justice. This conflict in values is primarily responsible for the hostility of psychiatrists to forensic psychiatric practice.

A recent experience vividly demonstrates the conflict in values between those of psychiatry and those of law. It shows how psychiatrists adhere fixedly to their therapeutic philosophy and values (associated with health and treatment) in the face of opposing legal forces that attempt to promote the values of legal justice as a higher and more socially significant value than health.

At a recent meeting of the National College of District Attorneys in Denver, Colorado, a deputy district attorney discussed legal problems in the prosecution of rapists and sexual child-abuse offenders. Many rape and child-abuse centers have recently developed throughout the country. These direct themselves primarily to treatment of the rape and child-abuse victims.

The speaker noted that victims of child molestation are being treated with increasing frequency in these centers. Prosecutors have found, he observed, that mental health workers involved with these victims are often antagonistic to prosecution in that they believe that subjecting the child victim to the trial process will cause more emotional trauma to the child than that caused by the sexual molestation or assault. Therefore, in their concern for the child's mental health, they steadfastly resist the prosecutor's efforts to have the child victim testify as the prosecuting witness.

Frequently, directed by their therapeutic philosophy, psychiatrists have also been successful in influencing the victim's parents both to avoid involvement in the criminal action itself and to promote and support the child victim's rejection of the prosecution-witness role. The child victim is helped to "forget" what has happened, so that the prosecution's case against the offender must be dropped. Here we see frank and open conflict between the goals of mental health, as viewed by the treating psychiatrist, and the ends of law and criminal justice, as viewed by the prosecutor.

The "vision" of the treating psychiatrist has been described as monocular. In a metaphorical sense, he sees the psychiatric data solely through the eyes of his therapeutic posture. The "vision" of the forensic psychiatrist, in this same sense, should be binocular in that it should promote his "seeing" the material of psychiatry through the eyes of the law as well as those of the clinician. With such binocular "vision" the forensic psychiatrist can most effectively apply his clinical material to legal issues for legal purposes. Nevertheless, the therapeutic philosophy which is basic to psychiatry frequently serves to promote errors in psychiatric-legal judgment-making.

The major errors committed by psychiatrists in the practice of forensic psychiatry result from their inability to comprehend the need to curb or abort their therapeutic philosophy in their application of psychiatry to legal purposes. That is, they apply themselves to the legal issues, but unwittingly, though sometimes consciously, they direct their opinions to therapeutic goals rather than legal ends and thus pervert the aims of justice.

This difficulty in comprehension was satirized by columnist Art Buchwald in a story about a student who was interviewed by Buchwald at the former's graduation. Buchwald asked the student, "Suppose you were the Prince of Denmark. You came home from school to find that your uncle had murdered your father and had married your mother. You fell in love with a beautiful girl and mistakenly murdered her father. The beautiful girl went crazy and drowned herself. What would you do?" Buchwald had asked the student this question because he was an English major, although the question could just as appropriately have been directed to a psychoanalyst. There was a long pause as the student pondered the question. Then the student answered, "I think I would go for my master's degree."

The significance of the tragedy was curiously beyond the student's comprehension, and he gave the response most familiar to him, albeit inappropriately, that he would continue with school. In the same way I believe that the forensic psychiatrist often is unable to comprehend the need to move from his traditional and familiar therapeutic philosophy to the less familiar philosophy of law. He has an even more difficult time in comprehending the legal values and often rejects them out of hand because they appear antitherapeutic and conflict with his basic professional values.

It is possible that I err in equating the young English major's inability to comprehend the significance of the tragedy presented to him with the psychiatrist's inability to comprehend and accept the legal philosophy and values of law; it is even possible that it is unfair for me to do so. After all, the credo of the psychiatrist is his therapeutic philosophy. I cannot fault him for refusing to give it up. Nonetheless, if my definition of forensic psychiatry is correct, and forensic psychiatry requires that the examiner apply himself to legal issues, and if his involvement in forensic psychiatry is permeated and controlled by legal values rather than those of psychiatry, then there is a conflict and dilemma for the forensic psychiatrist.

For forensic psychiatric purposes I have denominated the therapeutic philosophy of psychiatry as a *therapeutic bias* and believe it to be the major problem area experienced in the forensic psychiatrist's role/functions. It influences him insidiously, disguising itself in many different ways, and crops up unexpectedly again and again without warning. Throughout my years of practice in forensic psychiatry, I have recognized it only in hindsight as having repetitively influenced my role and function in forensic psychiatry. In spite of my constant concern and awareness, it continues to manifest itself. I have almost been ready to conclude that in spite of my caveats, I may not truly want to give up my therapeutic bias. I do know that it causes major conflict for me, as it does for many others, in the practice of forensic psychiatry.

In our contemporary democratic society, the concept of fairness in the application of legal justice is a major value. In the administration of justice, such a concept of fairness acts as a balance to the rigidity and inflexibility of legal rules of law. This concept of fairness is based upon individualization of law and humanistic elements in the law. These humanistic elements stem from the unique psychological and mentalistic aspects of man. It is these psychological and psychiatric features that are the significant evidentiary substrate of forensic psychiatry. Forensic psychiatry serves as a substantial adjunct to evidentiary fact-finding and thus acts to promote the concept of fairness in justice through law.

REFERENCES

1. Pollack, S.: The Role of Psychiatry in the Rule of Law. *Psychiatric Annals* 4(8), 1974.
2. Cf. *Misuse of Psychiatry in the Criminal Courts: Competency to Stand Trial.* Publication No. 89, Group for the Advancement of Psychiatry, New York, 1974.
3. Pollack, op. cit.
4. Pollack, S.: Psychiatric Consultation for the Court, in Mendel, W., and Solo-

mon, P. (eds.): *Psychiatric Consultation*. Grune & Stratton, New York, 1967; Pollack, S.: Principles of Forensic Psychiatry for Psychiatric-Legal Opinion-Making, in Wecht, C. (ed.): *Legal Medicine Annual: 1971*. Appleton-Century-Crofts, New York, 1972.
5. Pollack, op. cit. See especially "Principle of Legal Dominance" in this set of forensic psychiatric guidelines.
6. Cf. *Tarasoff v. The Regents of the University of California*, 17 C.3d 425, 1976.
7. Cf. Szasz, T.: *Law, Liberty and Psychiatry*. Macmillan, New York, 1963; Szasz, T.: *Psychiatric Justice*. Macmillan, New York, 1965.
8. Ibid.
9. Frank, J. N.: *Law and the Modern Mind*. Brentano's, New York, 1930.
10. Justice, in *The Nichomachean Ethics of Aristotle*. (W. D. Ross, tr.) Clarendon Press, Oxford, 1954.
11. Frank, op. cit.
12. For further exposition of the difference between objective and subjective theories in law, see Fitzgerald, M.A. (ed.): *Jurisprudence*. Sweet & Maxwell, London, 1966.

CHAPTER 28

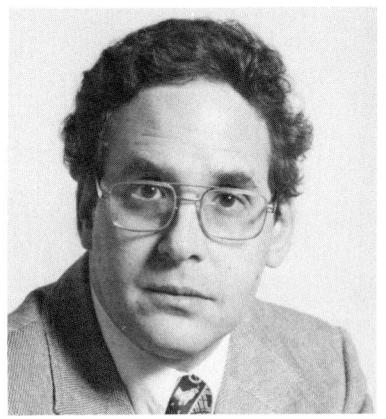

Loren H. Roth is Director of the Law and Psychiatry Program of the Western Psychiatric Institute and Clinic at the University of Pittsburgh. He served as a staff psychiatrist at the Center for Studies of Crime and Delinquency of the National Institute of Mental Health in Rockville, Maryland, and as the General Medical Director of the U.S. Federal Penitentiary at Lewisburg, Pennsylvania. Dr. Roth is a member of the Psychiatry and Law Section of the Group for the Advancement of Psychiatry. He is also the Editor of the *Newsletter* of the American Academy of Psychiatry and Law.

CORRECTIONAL PSYCHIATRY

Loren H. Roth, M.D., M.P.H.

The title of this chapter may well be a misnomer. Despite noteworthy but sporadic accomplishments,[1-5] few psychiatrists can assert that theirs has been either a very comprehensive or well-received contribution to American prisons and their inmates. Some would suggest that the peak period of correctional psychiatry has been passed, its conceptual thrust lost. A more realistic assessment should note that a confusion of roles[6-8] and an unsatisfactory volume and quality of needed mental health and general health services[9-13] (with such insufficiencies suffused with overblown rhetoric)[14] have too often characterized medical input and thought concerning prisons and jails. Of late, and perhaps paradoxically, considering the continuing evidences of the ineffectiveness of most correctional treatments,[15,16] the fear of some is that psychiatry and the behavioral sciences are too efficient and too effective, rather than ineffective, as change agents for the prisoner population.[17,18]

Although sympathetic in part to the considerable body of opinion now questioning aspects of the so-called medical model in corrections,[19-21] this discussion of correctional psychiatry will nevertheless indicate why more, rather than less, genuine psychiatric and medical services are needed in prisons and jails. Also proposed is the thesis that correctional psychiatry cannot simultaneously be the handmaiden of the correctional bureaucracy and also serve its traditional therapeutic aims. Correctional psychiatry will hardly be even a possibility until psychiatrists and those who look to psychiatrists for guidance and service in prisons recognize that the majority of inmates, both violent and nonviolent, are not mentally ill.[22-24] It must be further acknowledged that reliable psychiatric treatment for most repetitively antisocial or dangerous persons simply does not exist[25,26] and that the institutional psychiatrists can only with great difficulty serve two masters—the correctional establishment and their own patients.[27] Prisons, jails, and quasiprisons are hardly the optimal environment for rehabilitation,[28,29] and with notable exceptions, few psychiatrists are presently enthusiastic about the likelihood of coercive cure for antisocial behavior.[30] Nevertheless, viable models for a future correctional psychiatry do currently exist, models which would afford inmates the opportunity to receive conventional mental health and general health services while incarcerated, and which would allow the correctional psychiatrist to serve certain consultative functions.

Psychiatry practiced in prisons and jails must at all times strive to duplicate the best of psychiatry practiced in other settings, sharing its essential aims.[4] A useful correctional psychiatry would be one that is knowledgeable concerning the special aspects of health services delivery within the prison environment, inmate- rather than societally oriented, and wherever possible, divorced from the preoccupation with whether inmates, either because of the direct efforts of the psychiatrist or in agreement with his "prediction" will recidivate. The purpose of this chapter is therefore to acquaint the practitioner with the practical information necessary to achieve these aims so that, hopefully, he may maintain his professional skills, his interest, and his empathy for his prisoner-patients, rather than retreating from the institutional scene in haste, depression, and anger.

DEFINITION OF THE FIELD

Historical Review

The construction of prisons was a Quaker-inspired reform movement of the late eighteenth and the early nineteenth centuries.[31] Prisons were intended to allow the offender to reflect on his crimes and to repent in order that he might regain his freedom. Rather than promoting reform, the deleterious effects, on the physical and mental health of inmates, of certain prison practices consistent with this movement were soon noted.

> In the early years of the Auburn Prison, administrators tried an experiment to test the efficiency of the Pennsylvania system. They selected eighty of the most hardened convicts and placed them in solitary confinement and enforced idleness from Christmas 1821 through Christmas 1823. So many of these men succumbed to sickness and insanity that the experiment was scrapped in 1823.[32]

A somewhat similar nineteenth-century report came from William Farr in England. Farr, considered one of the fathers of epidemiology, noted that "prisoners rarely labour under any serious disease at the time of their committal." However, while "8 inmates were executed [in] 1837 . . . the average annual number of deaths due to imprisonment was 51."[33] The inhumanity of the prison system was thus apparent at an early point. The subsequent conceptual problem for psychiatry has been whether, in modesty, it might assist in rendering a too frequently inhumane system of punishment and incapacitation (albeit labeled reform) to become generally more humane, more solicitous of the person, or alternatively, whether psychiatry would do better to advocate a more scientific penology, one oriented more toward treating illness and correcting individual deficiencies so as to decrease inmate recidivism.

Halleck[2] and Fitzpatrick[34] have summarized the contributions of nineteenth- and twentieth-century psychiatry and psychoanalysis to corrections and criminology. These sources delineate the main figures, their theories regarding criminality, the psychological evaluation of offenders, and the provision of mental health services. The details will not be repeated here. Suffice it to note that of the 100 milestones given by Halleck in the history of American psychiatry and the criminal (1800 to 1960), many seeming advances have proved themselves as much problems as solutions[35,36] (e.g., the creation of special institutions for the "criminally insane," or sexual psychopathic legislation which mandated medical rather than penological treatment for sex offenders).[37]

In the nineteenth century, physicians led the way in encouraging the examination of the criminal offender as an individual. Psychiatry "attempted to discover scientific explanations for the behavior of criminals rather than relegating them completely to moral condemnation or to pessimistic theories of social inevitability."[2] Although the biological approach of the late nineteenth and early twentieth centuries was naive at best, and calamitous at worst (i.e., sterilization of criminals during the early twentieth century), medical and psychiatric interest in the biology of antisocial and aggressive behavior has continued to be strong until the present day (e.g., recent medical studies of the neurophysiology, endocrinology, and genetics of aggressive and violent behavior).[38] Nevertheless, a serious question can be raised today as to whether the general subject matter of the biology of crime lies at all within the province of correctional psychiatry. Unitary theories linking one or another biological entity to criminal behavior have had a characteristic and disappointing history, namely, early enthusiasm and later rejection as more scientific data become available. This dictum, for example, seems to apply to the findings and discussions over the last ten years regarding the contribution of the XYY chromosomal variant to aggressive behavior.[39] Furthermore, some psychiatrists have taken the position that to the extent that biological interventions for offenders involve great risk to them, and to the extent that there is some question about the "voluntariness" of the inmates' request for such intervention, these modalities, in fairness, should be made available to offenders only during periods of freedom and when they are no longer under legal control.[40]

During the early twentieth century, psychiatrists working in both court clinics and prisons devoted considerable effort to examining inmates in order to determine how many were mentally ill. Throughout the 1920s and 1930s, the psychiatrist who worked with the criminal held a relatively esteemed position.[2] From the 1930s until the 1960s, however, the amount of psychiatric services provided to prisoners failed to keep pace with the prison population. Numerous surveys, over many decades, have discovered a paucity of psychiatrists actively involved in prisons and jails.[2,10,41] In 1976, the United States Bureau of Prisons employed 14 full-time psychiatrists for some 27,000 inmates. Six additional positions were unfilled. The Alabama penal system recently employed virtually no mental health professional employees or consultants for its 3,800 inmates.[41] Within the psychiatric profession the prestige of correctional psychiatry declined. Psychoanalytic theories of criminality gained prominence during the 1940s[2,34] but failed to furnish a practical rationale for the treatment of the offender. The 1950s were characterized by the growth of special medical-penological programs for the handling of the recalcitrant offenders (e.g., the opening by the State of Maryland in 1955 of the Patuxent Institution for the treatment of "defective delinquents").[30,42] Small groups of interested psychiatrists met together and began to publish specialized journals devoted to offender treatment (e.g., the Association for Psychiatric Treatment of Offenders [APTO] which publishes the *International Journal of Offender Therapy and Comparative Criminology,* formerly the *Journal of Offender Therapy*). Other specialty journals in the area of correctional psychiatry, past and present, include the *Journal of Criminal Psychopathology, The Prison Journal, Corrective and Social Psychiatry,* and the *Journal of Behavior Technology Methods and Therapy* (formerly *Corrective Psychiatry and Journal of Social Therapy*).

It is probable, however, that neither the formulation of specific psychiatric theories of offender pathology and treatment, nor the provision of conventional or special mental health services to the prisoner population has been the most influential contribution of correctional psychiatry (and the other behavioral and helping sciences). Throughout the 1940s and 1950s, but especially in the 1960s, the discipline helped to promote a view of corrections and the prison system which re-emphasized its potential for habilitation and also made the contribution that individualized rather than mass handling of offenders would more likely promote their "rehabilitation." During the 1940s and 1950s, the Federal Bureau of Prisons gradually emerged as the national pacesetter in corrections, introducing new concepts such as "diagnosis," "classification," and the use of professional personnel such as psychiatrists and psychologists to help rehabilitate inmates.[31] The innovations of the Federal Bureau of Prisons were incorporated into many state systems. A wide variety of programs, albeit piecemeal but educational and vocational in nature, were also introduced into prisons with a hope not only that inmates would be less idle, but also that through the inmate's participation in such programs, he would be rehabilitated. Though Karl Menninger's advice, given in 1927, that psychiatric reports should influence all sentencing, release, and transfer of inmates was never operationalized,[2] the dictum that "the object so sublime" is to "make the punishment fit the crime," was replaced (at least in rhetoric if not in fact) by a correctional notion that "the object so sublime" is to "make the punishment fit the criminal." Under such a conception, when they were available, psychiatrists during the 1960s and 1970s became involved in a wide variety of correctional roles, including evaluation of offenders for purposes of sentencing and classification, in-prison treatment of offenders, pre-parole assessment, and program development and training of other correctional workers. Some psychiatrists were even destined to function as "wardens" within specialized settings.[3,43–48]

A representative statement was made in 1971 concerning one generally accepted role for psychiatry and corrections. "In the quest of individualized treatment psychiatry becomes a valuable ally to the law in its efforts to identify and diagnose those offenders who can benefit from something more than simply punitive incapacitation."[44] This quotation is by no means an isolated one. There has been a tendency for many psychiatrists interested in law and corrections to formulate a medical-type approach with respect to the offender. Benjamin Karpman observed in 1949 that "[we] have no more reason to punish them for behavior over which they have no control than [we have] to punish an individual for breathing through his mouth because of large adenoids. . . ."[49] Sheldon Glueck predicted, "There will be no prisons—only hospitals."[50] Arthur Zitrin noted that "modern psychoanalytic concepts will not make very much of a distinction between those who are evil and those who are sick. I think they're all sick in different kinds of ways. That's my point, and I think the prescription for the different kinds of sicknesses is what the psychiatrist can help with."[51] Of course, psychiatrists are not the only ones to have struggled with these issues: "It is time to admit that the sick and the wicked are not scientifically distinguishable: time to scrub this distinction out of our laws and to do away with the consequential rigid classification of custodial institutions into the medical and the penal; and time to replace the once-for-all sentencing decision by a more flexible system under which the treatment of offenders, whether medical or nonmedical, is continuously adjusted to the results achieved."[52] The language and logic of medicine, although most likely appropriate for only a small number of offenders, were in the midst of being extended to great numbers of them.

The Present Scene

Both corrections and psychiatry have changed since 1971. Even if there were no consensus as to who was responsible for the mass violence and deaths at Attica Prison, there was general agreement that rehabilitation of inmates would never be achieved within the usual milieu of the large and closed institution.

Following Attica, correctional philosophies diverged. One school maintained, despite past rhetoric and seeming failures,[15,16] that the truth was that the corrections model "has never been tried."[53-55] This school hoped that individual handling, the correct matching of the offender with the proper treatment modality, and the development of smaller, more personalized, community-based institutions would promote offender rehabilitation.

In the early 1970s, other national groups, convinced that institutions have harmed more than helped their inmates, called for both increased community handling of offenders and for a moratorium on the construction of new jails and prisons. It was argued that only the dangerous offender should be confined.[56,57] Finally, prominent critics of corrections, convinced that in fairness and in fact rehabilitation cannot be the primary justification for incarceration, called for an end to hypocrisy.[58] Prisons serve multiple functions including punishment, incapacitation of offenders, and deterrence to other offenders. It is unlikely that these objectives will ever be subservient to that of "rehabilitation." In part, the point of these critics has been that the tools of individual offender rehabilitation, namely, the disparate sentence, the contingent parole,[59] and the indeterminate sentence,[60] are not only unfair, but also compound rather than ameliorate the destructiveness of the prison experience.

The new trends of corrections thus emphasize both a decrease in discretionary handling of offenders and an improvement in the prison milieu, more as a matter of human decency and in order to do the "least harm," rather than necessarily to "treat the inmate." Rehabilitation is hoped for but not necessarily expected. Participation by inmates in programs of self-improvement is to be encouraged but is to be voluntary and optional. Neither is the inmate's release to be contingent on such participation.[61,62] As noted by Norval Morris, the rehabilitative model of corrections "suffers fundamentally from a belief that psychological change can be coerced."[58] But whether the new corrections of the seventies and eighties will be only an excuse for continuing neglect of inmates and for more severe and more lengthy, rather than more certain, punishments remains to be seen. If anything, the prison and jail milieu as it exists today is as bad as, or worse than, the milieu of the previous decade.

If the corrections approach is now at a point of some consternation both with itself and its clients, what can be said of psychiatry? In truth, there is also a ferment undermining some of the traditional concerns of correctional psychiatry. It is questioned whether the terms "psychopathy" and "sociopathy" do not conceal more than they convey,[63,64] and whether psychiatry has not in the past clearly oversold itself as a predictor of both dangerousness and recidivism.[65,66] As with others in corrections, psychiatrists have become more modest concerning their ability both to intervene successfully and to predict the future behavior of antisocial persons. If psychiatrists traditionally have criticized the operation of prisons and jails, a similar questioning by corrections of the proper role of psychiatry is not now out of place.

Future Directions: The Psychiatrist and the Normal Offender

As might be anticipated from the previous discussion, this author advocates no pivotal role for psychiatry in the long-term direct treatment and handling of the "normal offender." The psychiatrist's track record here is unproved and his skills are not unique. Without the incentive of release, it remains to be seen whether inmates will voluntarily seek such treatments as group psychotherapy, still the mainstay of correctional psychiatric treatment.[67,68] When release is an incentive, the ensuing consequence is often "game-playing" by the inmate and role diffusion for the psychiatrist. These reservations regarding the role of psychiatry vis-à-vis the direct treatment of the normal inmate, however, by no means belittle the role the psychiatrist can and should play in crisis intervention for even the "normal" incarcerated inmate, nor do they limit the importance that psychiatry ought to attach to promoting "normalization" of the prison environment, helping to decrease wherever possible its harshness, and helping to increase its opportunities for individual growth.

Future Directions: Psychiatry and the Mentally Ill Offender

Here there is a problem of definitions. Only a small percentage of inmates suffer from well-defined severe psychiatric disorders (i.e., the psychoses). The clearly mentally ill offender is wanted by no one—neither the prison, the prison-hospital, the hospital-prison, nor the hospital. The disruptive, aggressive, but nonpsychotic prisoner becomes administratively defined as "mentally ill" in order to facilitate recurring geographical cures. The trained psychiatrist is seldom available to treat or help manage either of these groups. Considering the small number of psychiatrists who have actually been available in the past to prison and jail systems (and in all likelihood will be available in the future), psychiatry would do well if it could attempt to meet the genuine mental health needs of these persons, let alone attend to the problems of "normal" offenders.

In summary of this introductory section, future correctional psychiatry would do well to be more modest in its aims. At least for the foreseeable future, prisons and jails are here to stay, and its seems unlikely that "rehabilitation" will ever constitute the primary function of these institutions. Curious and motivated psychiatrists now have an opportunity to offer their services voluntarily to those inmates who genuinely seek them. In addition they can play a helpful role in providing consultation to the prison community. In my view it is in the area of direct services to the mentally ill inmate and in crisis intervention, however, that the psychiatrist's future role in corrections most clearly lies.

THE INMATE EXPERIENCE

Overcrowding exacerbates the stresses of institutional life and compounds the endemic problems of prisons and jails, including poor living conditions, lack of meaningful work, inter-inmate violence, sexual exploitation, and weakening of the inmate's usual affectional ties. Unfortunately, however the prison population of the United States, now about 250,000 inmates, constitutes an all-time high.[69] Depending upon their crime, most of these inmates will serve from two to five years behind bars. In addition, approximately 160,000 persons are daily residents in local jails.[70] These figures do not include some 25,000 juvenile offenders resident in closed facilities.[71]

With rare exceptions these offenders are seldom provided custody in surroundings which approximate the "free world." In numerous states during the 1970s, prison and jail conditions have been declared in violation of constitutional guarantees respecting both the physical and psychological needs of their inmates.[29,70,72-75] Consider, for example, the recent litigation in Alabama in which sweeping court orders have mandated widespread reform in all areas of prison life, the implementation of such reform to be monitored by a court-appointed Human Rights Committee:

> The living conditions in Alabama prisons constitute cruel and unusual punishment. Specifically, lack of sanitation throughout the institutions—in living areas, infirmaries, and food service—presents an imminent danger to the health of each and every inmate. Prisoners suffer from further physical deterioration because there are no opportunities for exercise and recreation. Treatment for prisoners with physical or emotional problems is totally inadequate.[76]

Moreover, the jail milieu is usually worse, not better, than the customary prison setting.[29,70]

Of importance to the correctional psychiatrist then is that he or she gain some acquaintance with the prison or jail setting, the manner in which incarceration provokes stress for the inmate, and the ways in which the inmate characteristically adapts to this stress. Extremely useful sources of information, not frequently enough consulted by either correctional officials or correctional psychiatrists, are the inmates' own accounts of the prison or jail experience.[77,78]

The Jail Experience

Save for the clearly inadequate inmate relieved to be back in custody, to be jailed is to be uncertain, frightened, or angry:

> 'Why did I do it?' 'If only I hadn't done that.' 'Why did I get into this mess?' . . . Regret and remorse probably reach the greatest intensity in the first few days when the impact of the disjointed experience is the greatest, but this type of reflection on the offender's past continues throughout the presentencing phase.[77]

Only about 10 percent of jail inmates are charged with felony offenses. Nationally, on a given day, some 42 percent of jail inmates have been convicted and are serving brief sentences, usually of less than one year.[70] The remainder of jailees await arraignment, trial, or transfer. A significant portion of jailees have alcoholic or drug problems.[29] Problems of substance withdrawal are frequent. Increasingly, the chronically mentally ill, no longer able to be treated in state mental institutions or anywhere else, are jailed for minor misbehavior.[79] In some jurisdictions other mentally ill persons may be temporarily held, awaiting eventual transfer to mental institutions.[29] "Many jail inmates are really disguised health and welfare cases that require some other mode of help or treatment."[70] The petty offender and the jail repeater know that their stay will be a short if nonproductive one. The offender charged with a more serious crime faces the uncertainty of bail, plea bargaining, and eventual sentence or return to prison. Usually there is nothing to do to cope with this uncertainty, only idle time to be spent.

> The hours are spent crowded with other prisoners in narrow aisles in front of the cells or in small day rooms. [The offender] plays cards, dominoes, reads, and sleeps. . . .[77]

It should not be surprising then that the jail experience, albeit briefer, is for the inmate frequently as stressful as, or even more stressful than, longer term imprisonment. Suicide, self-mutilation, displaced violence toward other inmates in the form of sexual and other types of violent outbursts, panic and/or social withdrawal are the potential outcomes of such stress. These are the outcomes that the correctional psychiatrist hopes to help avert.[80]

The Prison Experience

Generalization is dangerous when attempting to characterize the impact of somewhat disparate institutions upon disparate persons for variable lengths of time. For example, in spite of oppressive surroundings and punitive handling, the occasional inmate, finding within himself both courage and individuality, may grow, seek opportunity, or otherwise mature in prison,[81] even if such growth need not always lead to a happy conclusion.[82] For others, either habituated by many years of dependency and regimentation, or otherwise psychologically so disposed, "free-world" skills atrophy, and the prison becomes their only home.[83] Neither of the above adaptations to prison is perhaps so frequent as the inmate's tendency of learning "to do time," to make accommodations with both the inmate subculture and the prison staff so as to live as comfortably as is possible in prison and to secure release at the earliest possible time. Nonconformity with prison norms and even rebellion are, of course, also seen. This has become a particular problem in the 1970s as the prisons have been clogged with younger, more dangerous, and more repetitively violent inmates,[84] inmates not so inclined to accept the solidarity aspects of the old-time "convict code" and to join the inmate subculture. Perhaps the fairest summary statement, though, would be that for most inmates, what they most want from prisons (understandably) is that their time go as smoothly and as quickly as possible.

Surprisingly few quantitative studies have systematically assessed the impact of the prison experience upon inmate psychology or performance.[78,85-87] There are, however, many sensitive accounts of prison life and the psychology of incarceration.[1,3,78] Of direct relevance to correctional psychiatry are some of the following themes and features of ordinary prison life.

AUTHORITY AND CONTROL

A powerful dynamic in prison settings which affects the equilibrium of both inmates and staff revolves around authority relationships. In the closed prison society, this issue of control[88] profoundly affects multiple behaviors of the dyads and triads of prison life: individual inmates or inmate groups vis-à-vis each other, inmates versus custodial staff, and either or both of these groups versus "treatment staff." For example, homosexual contacts in prison, though at times a reflection of otherwise unachievable intimacy or a matter of simple sexual release per se, even more frequently reflect issues of control (i.e., who is to have status and power among the inmate group). It will be rather quickly established whether the new inmate will be labeled a "punk" and exploited or instead fight back. In fact, the aggressor or active partner who engages in homosexual acts in prison often does not regard himself as homosexual. To take another example, prison practices which might possibly promote better mental health of inmates (e.g., privacy of visits, absence of strip searches, freedom for inmates to form friendships at varying levels of the prison community) seemingly cannot be instituted or maintained because of custodial concerns that "operational control" of the prison be at all times maintained. Other themes relating to control may more directly confront the psychiatrist when he wishes to institute treatment of a clearly mentally ill inmate (e.g., rumor among the inmate population), or the inmate himself may question the rationale for the treatment. Meanwhile the psychiatrist knows that if he fails to help the prisoner and to modulate the inmate's erratic behavior, the prison system has at its disposal, and will employ, alternative means of control which the psychiatrist may abhor, such as isolation or segregation. Throughout incarceration, then, the inmate fears and resists further control or restriction, the custodial staff fears its absence, and the psychiatrist or other treatment staff easily becomes caught in the same dilemma.

THE TEMPORAL PROFILE OF INCARCERATION

In order to understand the stress for the inmate of the prison experience, and the inmate's subsequent coping behavior, it is useful, if somewhat arbitrary, to divide the prison experience into temporal phases—early, middle, and late (prerelease).

The early phase of incarceration bears some similarity to reception into jail. There is further wrenching of the inmate's community ties as contacts with wives, families, or girlfriends diminish. An initial data-gathering phase, "classification," may ensue during which the offender is in limbo regarding what is to be expected of him during his prison stay and what will be his prerogatives within the prison.[89] For some inmates the length of their sentence hangs heavy, and there is accompanying denial of their probable future and much fantasy concerning early release. The inmate may pursue continued legal activity. Meanwhile adjustments must begin to be made with fellow inmates as the new inmate's reputation is established with his peers. Epidemiologic studies give some testimony to the relative difficulties of adjustment during this early period of incarceration. For example, suicides in prison, perhaps not so frequent nor as great a risk as in jails, are more apt to occur during the early period of incarceration,[90] as are episodes of inmate violence against one another or against prison staff.[91] In another study, the proportion of inmates appearing at sick call was found to be highest during the first year of imprisonment.[92] In various ways during this initial period, the inmate must learn to do his time "a day at a time," otherwise he may be "broken" by the prison.

The temporal profile of incarceration is U-shaped, the middle phase of imprisonment representing a period of somewhat greater psychological stability, albeit frequently at the expense of inmate autonomy, and with some accompanying deadening of routine.

> Symptoms of anxiety and depression as well as self-destructive impulses rapidly diminish during incarceration as group acceptance and assimilation take place.[87]

The above observation, however, should not deceive. The time spent in prison is seldom constructive. The inmate's identification with the prison subculture and his preoccupation with its diversions and currency (e.g., gambling, cigarettes, contraband drugs, and liquor) both impede any constructive psychological change within him, as well as making him susceptible to the pressures of the other inmates.[87] Disappointing news from home, missed visits, periods of time spent in isolation-segregation secondary to minor misbehavior, victimization secondary to quarrels with other inmates, and dashed parole hopes may all provoke breakdowns, occurring in different groups of inmates with varying frequencies.[78]

> Indeterminate sentences also may contribute to denial by encouraging false hopes. For inmates having such sentences there is a formalized, unwritten minimum time which must be served which varies with the nature of the offense. Inmates, who are not made aware of this or cannot accept it, may very early become intensely involved in institution programs and then react to a denial at their first parole hearing with depression, anger, or abandonment of behavior that would ultimately lead to release.[3]

Coping with anger is particularly difficult as the inmate attempts to build a record of institutional adjustment which will not preclude release. Though this observation may seem a bit dated, and prison practices regarding parole and indeterminacy are changing,[93,94] the sentiment expressed is nevertheless still highly relevant. Inmates are seldom honestly apprised by correctional officials of their realistic chances for release, and accepting the time to be served is a psychological hurdle contributing to bitterness and resentment of inmates concerning their prison handling. To control his impulses, or for purposes of self-protection, the inmate may himself seek segregation status or isolation from other inmates.[3] Though during the earliest phase of incarceration the occasional inmate may express the view that he is getting what he deserves or that he "got off light," for most inmates, as the time passes, the ongoing punishment and the deprivation seem to him progressively more unjust and excessive. Numerous commentators have, of course, criticized the excessive lengths of American prison sentences, sentences that if anything will probably increase rather than decrease in length during the next decade.

The final phase of incarceration, that of prerelease, is again a period of relative disequilibrium for the inmate. Similar to the experiences of others in the "free world" (e.g., the terminal phases of a military or even a school career), the inmate is "short-term." "Being short" may be a period of weeks, months, or even years for the inmate who is serving a very lengthy sentence. "Being short" is essentially a psychological perception that the prison stay is going to end. There are new realities to be faced upon release, realities which the inmate is ill-equipped to meet. These burdens are also compounded by the inmate's first-hand knowledge of societal opportunity structures, such as the nonavailability of jobs upon release. During this late phase there may be frequent visits to the prison hospital, requests for sleeping medication, irritability, and excessive caution taken by the inmate so that his ongoing behavior will not otherwise jeopardize the expected release. On the other hand, some men will engage in behaviors that delay release (e.g., the inmate who runs away from a minimum-security setting shortly prior to expected discharge). Prison staff speculate that the inmate "knew he wouldn't make it anyway," and so he sabotaged his release. Because release will occur, clearly any psychological growth that the inmate might achieve during the prerelease period is relevant to nonprison adjustment. The release period seems therefore a particularly relevant one in terms of crisis intervention.

PSYCHIATRIC PROBLEMS OF PRISONERS

A range of psychiatric pathologies, both traditional and somewhat special, may be exhibited by prisoners. Surveys that have quantified the number of inmates who are mentally ill, or the percentage of all offenders who are mentally ill (whatever their legal status), have reached varying conclusions, depending upon the definitions used, the methods employed, and the nature of the population surveyed.[23,95] Inmates who are clearly disturbed may be diverted or transferred from regular prisons or jails into special facilities for mentally ill offenders. These offenders include those being evaluated for competency to stand trial, those previously adjudged incompetent who were found not guilty by reason of insanity, those who were mentally ill at the time of sentencing, and those who became mentally ill while serving prison terms.[96-98] Such diversion from prison or jail may reflect as much the vagaries of legal and administrative processing as the mental state of the inmate per se.[99] Presently, however, there is increasing judicial and administrative criticism of the nature of treatment actually provided to mentally ill offenders in the traditional "hybrid institutions," mixed medical-penal fortress-type settings, as well as growing judicial recognition that due process protections must be afforded mentally ill inmates prior to transfer to a hospital setting.[100,101] Examples of such changes are the indictments on the nature of care and handling afforded mentally ill inmates at the Matteawan State Hospital for the Criminally Insane in New York,[102,103] and the improvements recommended for Lima State Hospital, a special security mental facility in Ohio.[104] These developments anticipate a future wherein psychiatric services will need to be available for inmates, even those who are seriously ill, within the traditional prison environment or within special psychiatric units to be established within prisons.

The experienced correctional psychiatrist is never surprised to encounter mentally sound inmates detained within special facilities for the mentally ill and psychiatrically untreated inmates within prisons and jails.

Labels are highly misleading when attempting to understand the careers of mentally ill offenders.

The Mentally Ill Prisoner

It may be stated that at various times approximately 15 to 20 percent of prison inmates manifest sufficient psychiatric pathology to warrant medical attention or intervention.[23,44,48] A 1976 court-ordered reclassification of Alabama prisoners arrived at a figure of 20 percent in "bad need of psychological therapy."[105] The number of prisoners manifesting psychoses or otherwise severe psychiatric disturbances is, however, considerably less than 20 percent, probably on the order of 5 percent or less of the total prison population.[23,48,106] Other surveys have revealed an even smaller percentage of offenders who are severely mentally ill (i.e., those diagnosed schizophrenic).[25] The work of the St. Louis group led by Dr. Samuel B. Guze is perhaps the best known in this area because of its systematic approach and precise diagnostic formulations. Only 1 percent of released male felons were diagnosed as schizophrenic. A high percentage of male felons (78%) were, however, diagnosed as sociopathic or exhibiting an "antisocial personality," a behavioral disorder defined by the St. Louis group as including a history of police trouble in addition to other variable features (e.g., a history of excessive fighting, school deliquency, poor job record, wanderlust). Guze's survey revealed that 43 percent of the sample manifested definite alcoholic problems, and 11 percent of the felons had questionable alcoholic problems; 85 percent of those interviewed were diagnosed as either sociopathic, alcoholic, or drug-dependent. Other estimates of the proportion of prison inmates manifesting "personality disorders" have arrived at a far smaller proportion of diagnosable disorders.[107] Bach-y-Rita has reviewed the problems of trying to establish such diagnoses in prisons. The physician may fail to appreciate both the cultural and the institutional determinants of the inmate's prison behavior and psychology.[107] The diagnosis of personality disorder is also variably made by attending to behavioral criteria, psychological criteria, or to a combination of these. Guze's work illustrates the conceptual and definitional problems for correctional psychiatry. Though antisocial personality is both a social and personal tragedy, equating correctional psychiatry with the treatment and management of personality disorders overwhelms and bankrupts meager psychiatric resources.

Some brief observations should be offered concerning the management of personality disorders in prison since these are the "disorders" most likely to be encountered. Traditionally, individuals with personality disorders manifest rather fixed or long-standing character traits or behaviors which may trouble others as much as, or more than, these traits or behaviors trouble the person himself. A number of personality disorders may be found among prison inmates, including passive-aggressive personality disorders, antisocial personality disorders (sociopathy—psychopathy), and explosive personality disorders.[107] A central problem in prison for these men is one of behavioral inhibition, the prevention or modification by the closed prison environment of the inmate's traditional methods of coping (e.g., taking immediate physical action, self-medication, or flight). Vaillant has nicely summarized this issue.[108] In the closed prison setting where flight is impossible and where behavior is under stricter control, anxiety and depression may be both feared and experienced, even by those inmates who are seemingly "sociopathic."[108] Such is not always counterproductive. During crises the task for the correctional psychiatrist is to communicate to the inmate, "I am sorry that you are feeling bad, but I think that you can manage the feeling."[108] The inmate's request for medication, for some "time-out" in the prison hospital, or for a facilitated change from his present living quarters to other quarters in order to avoid either perpetrating or being the victim of violence should be neither immediately acceded to, nor rejected out of hand as "manipulative." Rather more information should be gathered by the psychiatrist while he makes simultaneous efforts to reassure the inmate concerning the inmate's own competence and potential to manage both his feelings and his behavior. While occasionally one of the above interventions may be appropriate, the overriding goal is to help the inmate to directly confront, to understand, and to handle the frustrations of the prison experience without necessarily having to act upon them.[109] For example, aiding the impulsive inmate to experience, but also to tolerate, "depression" or anxiety may prevent rather than encourage other potential outcomes of prison frustrations for inmates with personality problems (e.g., violence, time spent in isolation-segregation, self-mutilation, drug abuse, reactive psychoses).[109,110]

In-prison management or treatment of inmates with personality disorders should be distinguished from attempts at "rehabilitation." With regard to rehabilitation there is some consensus, namely, that individual psychotherapy, at least insofar as it might be hoped to substantially increase future law-abiding behavior, is not likely to do so. This is particularly true when the inmate is both young and has an extensive criminal record.[111] Group therapy, peer pressure (milieu) approaches,[67,108] or behavioral approaches seem more promising here.[112] However, whatever the modality of treatment used for this type of inmate, scrupulous honesty, consistency of approach, limit-setting when necessary, and a "here and now" orientation are required.[113] It is important for the correctional psychiatrist not to maintain a pejorative attitude toward these men and their treatment; neither, however, is excessive sympathy or "excuse-making" valued or useful for the inmate. If genuine respect for the inmate is communicated there may be an opportunity for the individual inmate and the psychiatrist to form a working alliance.[22] This is particularly feasible when, as a matter of previous years of frustration and failure, the inmate himself comes to realize that his behaviors, past and present, are dysfunctional, that he welcomes some help in changing these behaviors, and when the psychiatrist may have already demonstrated his "wares" through aiding in the resolution of some in-prison minimum crisis.

Other Psychiatric and Psychological Profiles

Inadequacy, rather than stereotypic "meanness" or "badness," is a clinically more impressive finding in many prison or jail inmates. The statistical unlikelihood that incarceration will follow most offending behavior ensures that offenders either less adept at crime commission or otherwise socially least able to defend themselves against the law are the ones who will be incarcerated. For example, since serving time is in some respects more statistically normative for blacks than for whites, black prisoners often impress the psychiatrist as more "normal," more "put together" than white prisoners. Women prisoners, less than 5 percent of all inmates, may appear even more deviant, when compared to the stereotype or ideals of womanhood, than do male prisoners compared to other men.

Whether one considers male or female inmates, however, the vast majority of them are minimally educated, originate from lower socioeconomic strata, and have experienced frequent parental and otherwise severe social deprivation.[25,114,115] For men (in addition to the aforementioned diagnoses of antisocial personality, alcoholism, and drug dependency), schizophrenia, mental retardation, and perhaps epilepsy may be overrepresented in prison and jail populations.[23,25,48,116,117] From the epidemiologic perspective these last three diagnoses are probably not significantly related to crime causation but may represent the effect of differential handling of offenders (i.e., less competent offenders may more likely be sent to, and spend longer times in, institutions). For women offenders the remaining psychiatric diagnosis likely to be encountered is hysteria.[25] Some discussion is appropriate concerning prison and jail treatment for the most difficult of these psychiatric and psychological problems—the psychoses (frequently of schizophrenic type) and mental retardation.

Jail Psychoses

Psychotic jail inmates frequently fail to obtain needed medical help. One problem is the aforementioned lack of medical personnel available to adequately evaluate, diagnose, and treat these conditions.[11] In jails, in addition to the functional psychoses, attention must be given to an adequate differential diagnosis including both substance abuse and substance withdrawal (typically amphetamines, sedative-hypnotics, opiates, or alcohol), other metabolic and organic conditions, head trauma, post-convulsive states, and reactive psychoses secondary to incarceration. In theory the treatment of these conditions should be similar to treatment in other locales, but numerous bureaucratic, political, and administrative considerations seemingly overwhelm a decent medical approach.

The jail which contains an adequate medical component is the rare exception.[80] Formulation of comprehensive national, state, or local standards for jail and prison medicine,[13,118,119] or even certification for jail medical units, is on the horizon but is presently more a matter of rhetoric than reality. The psychotic inmate must be detected and then treated in some continuing fashion. All too frequently known psychotic inmates are transferred from jails to hospital settings for a brief stay, inadequately or too briefly treated, returned to the jails, frequently not on medication or without instructions as to the manner of continuing necessary care, and thus, again untreated in jail, the cycle is repeated.[120] If transfer to a hospital is possible, it cannot be quickly expedited because of legal considerations. The psychotic inmate may never be detected or evaluated because of the absence of trained jail personnel, the attitudes of jail personnel toward inmates, or the nonavailability of physicians. Though there is no magic solution to these problems, they should be confronted, and certain recommendations can be made.

Jail personnel need to be trained in the recognition of psychotic conditions and given the best current explanations for their emergence. This is best accomplished through the traditional "case approach" rather than didactically. Daily or twice daily physician contact with newly admitted, disturbed inmates is recommended. "Voluntary" transfer to a hospital setting may be advisable and possible for some inmates, and is required in cases of alcohol or sedative-hypnotic withdrawal. Though mental hospital treatment may need to be mandated for some inmates, a surprisingly large number of psychoses may be successfully managed in the jail itself, if adequate facilities and manpower are provided. Ideally, the jail should include a separate section or infirmary, adequately staffed on a 24-hour basis, for the care and management of such clearly ill inmates. Isolation and "strip cells" are not necessary and only confound the treatment.

Ensuring adequate detection, treatment, and continuing follow-up of jail inmates within the jail, as opposed to transfer, although not desirable in all cases, is practically the only way that institutional "ping-pong" can be avoided with no one taking genuine medical responsibility for the inmate. Providing for this type of jail health care should be the responsibility of a civilian health care organization or community department of health, rather than the jail per se, though the care is provided in the jail. "Contracting out" to local hospitals, clinics, or medical partnerships to provide treatment is one mechanism to ensure that the inmate is afforded treatment equal to that which he might receive if he were not in jail.[119]

Prison Psychoses

The psychotic inmate in the general prison population may be feared and victimized, and there is tremendous pressure on the prison psychiatrist to "dispose" of this inmate in some manner. In one study of Federal prisoners, it was found through record review that 4 percent of inmates had apparently suffered a first psychosis while incarcerated.[23] Again a differential diagnosis should be pursued, and the automatic response should be neither "schizophrenia" nor "transfer."

The successful management of prison psychoses may often be accomplished by voluntary transfer within the prison to a hospital section, to an infirmary, or even to "outpatient" care within the prison, though prison officials often resist or sabotage such handling.[121] Providing medication in prison poses certain problems. Its administration must be supervised. Abuse of the major tranquilizers by inmates is generally not a problem. Antipsychotic drugs simply do not make the nonpsychotic inmate "feel good." Unlike the antianxiety agents (e.g., Valium) or the sedative-hypnotic drugs (e.g., barbiturates or Doriden), antipsychotic drugs are not useful prison currency. More problematic here is inmate refusal of treatment, a right increasingly recognized and one that should be accorded, at least in the absence of clear-cut, severe, and imminent danger to self or others.[122] Psychotic inmates are not the main perpetrators of prison violence. In the absence of previous history of physical aggression, many so-called "paranoid" and even frankly delusional inmates may nevertheless avoid overt difficulties, even though they are at risk of being "gotten" first by other inmates who misinterpret their behavior or who are afraid of them. If involuntary treatment is necessary, the increasing trend is to follow procedures providing the equivalent civil protections prior to, and accompanying, such involuntary treatment.[100,101,123] Various recent court cases[101,124] have raised the specter that treatment of institutionalized offenders with antipsychotic drugs (or the use of certain behavioral techniques) may constitute more of a management or "control" device than a medical one per se. The individual practitioner must look to his heart and his training, ensuring that his approach is in fact a professional one, that appropriate medical orders and examinations have been provided, and that an individual treatment plan has been formulated. He or she is also advised to consult the most recent case of statutory law in his jurisdiction regarding in-prison treatment. Psychopharmacology, although generally required and helpful in the management of psychotic conditions, should not be automatic or administered without simultaneous attempts at supportive counseling and efforts to understand and modify any intercurrent stresses contributing to the inmate's presenting picture.

Mention should be made here of segregation and the impact of isolation (sensory deprivation) upon all inmates, including "normal" individuals and those suffering personality problems or the more severe varieties of mental illness. Surprisingly, there is poor documentation of a systematic sort concerning the impact of segregation, though numerous case reports and clinical accounts do testify to the negative impact of the segregation experience on some inmates.[1,107] A visit to any set of segregation cells reveals great commotion, banging on pipes, and mirrors extended through bars, permitting one man to communicate with another. In the absence of communication and sometimes even despite it, deterioration may occur. Agitation, lethargy or withdrawal, and self-mutilation in order to "experience" something or for purposes of attention-getting may occur.[107,125] Hallucinatory or delusive experiences emerge or are exacerbated. For example, a recent study of the seclusion experience at a psychiatric hospital showed a possible increase in patient hallucinatory experiences consequent to seclusion as well as patient delusional and affective responses of fear, terror, anger, and resentment.[126]

The correctional psychiatrist should institute a daily "rounding" to check on the conditions of those inmates who may have been placed in segregation. Though ethical and professional conflicts emerge, especially when the psychiatrist contemplates transfer of the disturbed inmate to a setting other than segregation, these uncertainties must be faced. The psychiatrist should ask himself, "How would I treat this inmate in a conventional hospital setting?" and then attempt to come as near this ideal as is possible. The problem is that the psychiatrist may be seen as attempting to lessen the punishment without his having the final authority to modify a system of management or control which he may deplore. Isolation-segregation cells are "prisons within prisons" and raise a similar debate concerning the functions of correctional psychiatry as does the prison itself. In the face of clear-cut psychoses, psychiatrists cannot fail to treat or, at a minimum, offer the opportunity for treatment to the disturbed inmate. As a quid pro quo for his willingness to treat and to examine inmates in segregation, the psychiatrist should simultaneously attempt to alter the basic prison handling of these men.

Mental Retardation

Mentally retarded inmates, numbering perhaps 10 percent of all inmates (with some variation in this overall percentage from one jurisdiction to another), are seldom served by meaningful prison programs or by prison personnel devoted to their special needs.[127,128] Recent court cases are emphasizing that more must be offered these men. For example, in the previously mentioned litigation from Alabama, the court noted:

> The evidence further reflects that there are also a number of mentally retarded inmates who need to be, according to any humanitarian concept, identified and placed in an appropriate environment.[129]

Mentally retarded inmates are more easily and more frequently victimized by other inmates. They are impaired in social intelligence as well as intellectual functioning. They have more difficulty understanding institutional rules and regulations and more frequently violate them with subsequent punishment.[127] Prisons lack the special programs necessary for habilitation of the retarded. These problems have underscored the continuing question. Should not these mentally retarded offenders be handled differently, preferably from the onset of their legal involvement? For example, the illegal behavior of the retarded could be reviewed by an Exceptional Offender's Court,[130] and more attention could be devoted to determining whether or not retarded offenders are competent to stand trial.[131] The retarded offender's disposition could more frequently be that of community supervision, or supervision in a special institutional setting, rather than that of a prison.[127] These remedies are attractive, but until now such suggestions have come against hard reality, namely, the nonavailability of adequate alternative programs to implement these ideas. This is particularly true with regard to special institutions. There is little benefit for the mentally retarded offender, especially for the nondangerous offender, in being lumped together with sexual psychopaths,[37] with severely mentally ill offenders, or, some would argue, even with "defective delinquents," as is the case at the Patuxent Institution.[127] The needs of the retarded are different, and it is pointless for such persons to spend years languishing in "special institutions" awaiting nonexistent treatment. For now the best that can be said is that the correctional psychiatrist needs to be aware of the existence and the special vulnerabilities of this group of offenders and to know that the stresses of incarceration may fall particularly hard upon them. On the more positive side it will also be noted that much of the pessimism of the past concerning the habilitation of the retarded is lessening. For some, though not all, retarded offenders, and in accord with the principle of "normalization,"[132] the routines and reinforcements of the normal prison setting may be even more therapeutic than other poorly conceived special treatment programs. For other offenders, more structured programs of a behavioral or operant sort might be warranted.[116] As noted by Rowan, what is truly needed for the retarded offender, and what is now missing, is a "wide range of alternative" approaches to meet the varying needs of all such inmates.[127]

Prison Violence

To recall the words of Rap Brown, violence within prisons and jails is now as "American as cherry pie."[84,133,134] Though inmates seldom injure prison or jail staff, they are, with increasing frequency, hurting and even killing one another. In 1970, an inmate in California ran one chance in a hundred of suffering serious injury during the year; by 1974, his chances of injury had increased fourfold.[134] From mid-1974 to mid-1976, a period of a little more than two years, there were eight homicides at the Federal penitentiary at Lewisburg, Pennsylvania.[84]

The great majority of episodes of inter-inmate violence are neither random nor inexplicable. The Federal Board of Inquiry, studying the homicides at Lewisburg, noted that "in most of the homicides the victims were assaulted for some specific reason. They apparently were not killed indiscriminantly but in retaliation for something they had done."[84] This "something" frequently related to homosexual entanglements. Both assailants and victims had long prior records. Other studies or reviews have come to similar conclusions. Inter-inmate violence is associated with homosexuality, racial and political tensions, hustling (i.e., inmate squabbles concerning cigarettes, drugs, or contraband),[135] enforcement of debts, paybacks to informers, and paybacks or exchanges between members of rival prison gangs or cliques.[134] These situational precipitants to violence need not, of course, always culminate in violence. Rather such precipitants interact with inmate behavioral predispositions, inmate psychology and psychopathology. As Toch has observed, although the relationship is not one-to-one, there is some association between the likelihood of an inmate committing a violent act in prison and his having a previous history of violence while on the street.[134] In California, for example, Mexican-American inmates are proportionately overrepresented among prison aggressors, perhaps a reflection of the special concern of this group with demonstrating *machismo*, or "manliness." Similar to street violence, prison violence is generally committed by the younger inmates.[136] These facts highlight the irony of the debates of the 1970s concerning corrections and rehabilitation. Limiting the prison to "dangerous" offenders, or decreasing discretionary handling of dangerous offenders so as to result in their automatic incarceration, makes the prison all the more volatile and destructive to its residents.

Studies of prison violence point to other factors now likely contributing to increases in interinmate violence, namely, the progressive overcrowding of prisons and jails.[73,135] Violent prisoners have been shown to be hypersensitive to physical encroachment,[137] while other researchers have demonstrated a positive correlation between disruptive behavior of inmates and the average number of square feet of living space available to the inmate.[138] Separation of aggressive or rapist inmates one from another appears to promote a reduction of group violence.[139] These studies suggest that despite the concerns of the critics, if prison violence is to be reduced, either additional, smaller and more personalized prisons must be built, or alternatively, inmate sentences must be reduced in duration so as to decrease present overcrowding.

The relationship between prison violence and inmate psychopathology or mental illness has not, however, been as adequately studied. Probably no more than 10 to 15 percent of inmates who are seriously violent or disruptive in prisons suffer from the psychoses, and even these figures are high estimates.[91,140] Bach-y-Rita and Veno have described a group of 62 men, habitually violent both within and without prisons. One group of men was notable for the extent of their associated self-mutilation and scarring; this group warranted a diagnosis of explosive personality or impulsive character disorder. These men described episodes of intolerable anxiety, restlessness, and depression. Another subgroup (13 of 62 men) were quiet and withdrawn and had subtle delusional systems not apparent to an unskilled examiner.[141] In another recent survey, Uhlig reviewed the records of 365 mentally disturbed and disruptive New England offenders, most of whom were apparently violent or aggressive in prison.[140] Of these 41.9 percent were diagnosed as severe character or personality disorders, 11.5 percent were identified as having a functional psychosis, and the remainder were apparently undiagnosed. It was found that 41.6 percent of the men had spent previous periods in state mental hospitals (beyond time for evaluation), though at the time of the survey almost all of them were back in the prisons. Uhlig's study demonstrated that an adequate approach to these men remains to be developed; neither the traditional mental hospital nor the prison has been able to offer very much.

Achieving significant reductions in inter-inmate violence will require changes in the prison milieu and penological practices over which the correctional psychiatrist may have little control. Furthermore, some violence in the prison is adaptive and necessary and should be extinguished only with caution (e.g., the inmate in danger of being raped must learn either to fight back, or, alternatively, he may need to spend a great deal of time in self-sought segregation). Nevertheless, the psychiatrist has a role to play in violence prevention in the prison.

The mentally ill violent inmate deserves psychiatric evaluation in addition to, if not instead of, repetitive handling in the prison segregation unit. Correctional officers may fail to detect psychosis which may be treatable via conventional means.[141] With the cooperation of the inmate, a complete medical workup should be performed, including attention to situational precipitants of violence, to inmate psychology, and to psychobiological and neurological factors which may be associated with violence.[38] Crisis intervention may prove useful for inmates who, with support, will communicate a wish to be less violent, and who view their violent outbursts as distasteful or upsetting rather than as absolutely necessary for survival in the prison. Psychological interventions addressed to issues of dependency or passivity, hurt masculine pride or helplessness, or the need for retaliation will usually hit home.[142,143] Finally, though no medication is as yet specific for "violence," the pharmacopoeia for aggression is expanding.[144] Assuming the request of the inmate, medication trials directed at decreasing violent outbursts may be considered for selected inmates whose response to prison provocation seems excessive, even given the nature of the prison milieu. Lithium carbonate treatment seems particularly promising.[145,146]

Suicides in Prisons and Jails

Preventing all suicides or attempted suicides in prisons and jails is a task lying beyond the capabilities of the correctional psychiatrist. Nevertheless, more studies are being performed in this area,[78,87,90,147,148] and some guidelines may be given. The risk of completed suicide is far greater in jails or in holding areas, at the time of initial confinement or pretrial, than later on during a prison term.[149] In fact, considering the deprivations associated with the typical prison experience, the psychiatrist may wonder why even more men do not take their lives in prison.[87] Those who successfully commit suicide within jails are generally older than those who merely attempt self-injury, but this rule is not absolute.[149] Youths may kill themselves in jail as well. A number of profiles have been given for jail inmates who are at risk for completed suicide, including (1) the young, impulsive inmate charged with a violent crime who is hypersensitive to confinement and makes a lethal attempt within the first day or week of incarceration; (2) the slightly older inmate who is hopeless and clinically depressed, who may have a past psychiatric history, and who threatens suicide and is reacting to a loss of supports from outside the jail;[150] (3) the good-citizen type charged with a first offense who is shamed by arrest; and finally (4) the more chronic offender who has lost his moorings to the world and cannot face doing any more time.[151] Successful suicides in jail are frequently drug or alcohol users or those charged with these offenses.[150,152] Whether within jails or prisons, hanging is the most frequent method of successful self-destruction, though other methods may be attempted, including cutting, overdosage, and ingestion of poisons or cleaning materials. To be distinguished from the above profiles are more manipulative suicide attempts, such as cuttings or nonlethal swallowings (as of glass or razor blades), which are generally accomplished by younger inmates with previous histories of violence and/or self-mutilation. In addition to manipulation, some cutters do so for purposes of tension reduction, to serve as a defense against depersonalization. These latter profiles, though in some sense more benign, do not ensure that the inmate will not go on to completed suicide.

Suicides within prisons have not been well studied. Toch presents some useful psychological autopsies of men who took their lives in prison;[78] for example, the seemingly gentle inmate, nine years in prison, who becomes progressively fearful of other inmates, who is drawn into fights, who eventually clashes with correctional staff for the first time, and who then, within a few months, electrocutes himself in a segregation unit.[78] As noted by Sloane, "anomic [suicide] attempts develop after a period of months or years of imprisonment as gradual feelings of helplessness and hopelessness envelope the individual who finds himself powerless to change his situation."[148] While severe depressions are unusual in prison settings, loss of loved ones and abandonment by formerly involved friends, lovers, or spouses may provoke clinical depressions with some potential for completed suicide in prison.

Toch has summarized in great detail the social psychology of nonlethal inmate suicide attempts in jails and prisons, a valuable work which should be consulted. It is instructive to note that the demography of attempts differs between jails and prisons.[78] In jails the men at greatest risk for suicide attempts are the older, the married, the drug user, the violent, and the white or Latin. In prison the men at greatest risk for suicide attempts are the young, the single, the non-drug user, the violent, and the white or Latin. For women inmates the risk factors include youth, drug use, violence, and Latin background. Demographic differences parallel psychological ones. For example, Latin inmates are particularly vulnerable to abandonment by relatives, and women inmates tend to have their greatest problem with loneliness.

Management of the suicidal inmate and prevention of jail or prison suicides pose similar problems to those noted in the area of prison violence. Truly ameliorative efforts require improvement of the jail or prison milieu; [148] for example, in the jail, increasing the frequency and improving the quality of exchanges between prisoners and their families so as to decrease the shock of incarceration. As another example, suicide may seem an attractive possibility to a not so powerful inmate, both shamed and angered by a homosexual rape.[153] Preventing the suicide would require preventing the rape, which might require providing all inmates with their own cells, providing increased opportunities for family visits or furloughs,[154] and altering the prison or jail environment to a less challenging one to the "manhood" of inmates likely to commit rape. On the more modest individual level, certain actions can be recommended. Correctional psychiatrists and other correctional workers, particularly jail personnel, should be acquainted with the high-risk profiles mentioned above. The risks are, of course, only comparative and not absolute. Firm predictions cannot be made. On the other hand, correctional officers can be trained to pick up danger signals in certain men in order that they be placed under surveillance. An adequate history must, of course, be obtained when the inmate is admitted to jail, and correctional staff must be acquainted with clinical profiles of depression. The use of isolation cells or the typical padded cell is not recommended for the suicidal inmate. Such sensory deprivation merely compounds the problem. Inmates at risk of suicide or threatening suicide should instead be transferred to a specially staffed portion of the jail or prison unit where around the clock surveillance is possible. In jails, most successful suicides occur at night or early in the morning, and coverage throughout these hours is necessary. In addition to this general approach, attention should also be given to the general medical problems of the inmate, particularly that adequate facilities and techniques for drug detoxification (Methadone treatments) are available. A decrease in both violence and suicide in jails consequent to an adequate program of detoxification has been reported.[155] Some depressed inmates will respond to conventional treatments for depression. Severe cases will probably require transfer to a mental hospital.

A difficult problem is the inmate with a history of self-cuttings who again threatens to kill himself or who has made a minor gesture, either in the jail or in the prison. A psychological or "investigative" approach should be pursued. It is well to begin by asking the inmate what it is he is trying to achieve or to communicate. With adequate exploration, some purposes may be judged to be manipulative and may need to be refused.[90]

Difficult Characters

The correctional psychiatrist may be asked to evaluate or treat prison or jail inmates whose behavior is both puzzling and annoying to the prison workers, such as the inmate manifesting brief, confusional episodes, who is hyperactive or who has "down" periods; the inmate whose talk makes no sense; and the inmate who feels perpetually abused and who is in continuous conflict with prison workers concerning his handling and his rights. Differential diagnosis should be pursued in these instances, giving careful attention in puzzling cases to the possibility of institutional drug or alcohol abuse, glue or solvent sniffing, or other uses of prison contraband.[156] A high proportion of prison inmates have been drug or alcohol abusers.[117,157] In selected institutions the proportions run as high as 40 to 60 percent. "Turning on" with drugs or alcohol is one of the few prison diversions; drugs and alcohol are nearly always available in prisons, and overdoses may culminate in death. Treatment of these substance-abusing inmates may be quite difficult as inmate denial of abuse is the norm, and the "pleasures" of abuse are great. Urine drug screens may need to be run as well as other routine laboratory work (e.g., testing of hepatic enzymes for liver damage). The thrust of the psychological treatment should be to achieve some consensus with the inmate that substance abuse is dysfunctional for him or her[158] and that more meaningful activities for the inmate may yet be found or created in the prison or jail.

The Ganser syndrome requires brief mention as an entity especially associated with forensic psychiatry and prisons. This is a disorder occupying an intermediate position between disease and malingering, psychosis and neurosis.[159] In this rare condition, the patient, frequently an inmate, gives clearly wrong or nonsensical answers to questions. The nature of the answers given, however, suggests that the patient understands the questions. An hysterical mechanism is presumably involved, but "organic" etiology should be excluded. Benefits may accrue to the inmate by virtue of his being believed to be mentally ill or "insane." The Ganser syndrome is short-lived. The treatment should be watchful waiting, monitoring of the realistic pressures which are upon the inmate, and confronting him with the consequences of his behavior, at least until it is possible to determine whether this is an instance of malingering or genuine psychosis.[160]

Regarding inmates who are in continuous conflict with prison staff (or with the prison medical department) concerning their rights or handling, the watchword is "be wary." This type of inmate is a repetitive visitor to the prison sick call and the correctional psychiatrist's station, and will complain to anyone who will listen, including the chaplain, the caseworker, and the warden. Many of these men have every reason to complain, and their complaints should be remedied. For others, such complaints may be more defensive. One set of complaints is replaced by another in a never-ending psychological rejection of the prison experience. Paradoxically, "curing" these men, ridding them of their complaints, may make them worse, even precipitating a prison psychosis. The main way these inmates relate to others within the prison is through complaints.

Mentally Abnormal Offenders

Achieving the goals of fair, just, and effective handling for the mentally abnormal offender seems utopian.[95-98,101,162-164] An entire monograph or two, not a portion of a chapter, would be required to discuss the problems posed, including the historically confused response to these offenders characteristic of both legal and mental health professionals. The lumping appellations "mentally abnormal offender" or "mentally disordered offender" have not helped; these terms are hardly an improvement over the terms "criminally insane" or "insane criminals."

For the present purposes, the following prisoners may be defined as "mentally abnormal offenders": offenders undergoing observation for their competency to stand trial or for criminal responsibility;[165-167] offenders deemed incompetent to stand trial; offenders found not guilty by reason of insanity (a very small proportion of all mentally abnormal offenders);[97] certain sexual offenders;[37] sentenced offenders who are or who become mentally ill;[168] "defective delinquents"[30,42,101,127] and other repetitive or dangerous criminals judged in need of special psychological handling.[162] These disparate offenders are, because of putative mental illness and putative dangerousness, frequently evaluated or treated in maximum security or other inpatient settings. These may be penal or medical in name.[98] Whatever they are called, in most cases such settings usually resemble prisons more than hospitals, as the following quotations graphically reveal:

> The story is the same everywhere. The mentally ill offender is confined in a grim storehouse. Treatment is grossly inadequate. There is virtually no therapy.[163]

> These hospitals . . . suffer . . . the traditional ailment of hospitals for criminally insane and dangerous mentally retarded patients. Geographic and professional isolation, staff difficulties, preoccupation with security measures and uncertain but probably overcautious release policies are among those usually mentioned in this context.[169]

In the last decade leading mental-health law cases[171-175,104] have addressed the rights of these offenders. Litigation has involved both the right to treatment and the right to refuse treatment.[101,122] Variable progress has recently been reported in some jurisdictions concerning the care of these persons.[170] The correctional psychiatrist's relationship to these offender-patients is complicated as compared to the prison or jail setting. By virtue of written reports or testimony given to the court about the offender's mental state or dangerousness, the correctional psychiatrist may hold the key to the offender's release or commitment. The treater (de facto if not de jure) may also be the keeper. Although this dilemma may be partly avoided (and should be avoided) by the provision of independent forensic examination related to release and recovery, such is not always possible.[176] Moreover, and unfortunately, the psychiatrist and the court may not be acquainted with the legal criteria upon which judgments are to be made concerning these offenders and by which the relevance of psychiatric evidence is established.[163,170] Finally, both the legal criteria and the medical data may be distorted or ignored by all parties in order to accomplish a hoped-for disposition for the offender. The mentally ill jail inmate, a "minor offender," may be ostensibly transferred to the maximum security hospital under the suspicion of incompetency to stand trial, but actually to obtain treatment not otherwise available. The violent offender may be temporarily diverted from his probable fate into a status of incompetency to stand trial that suits the strategic needs of either the prosecution or the defense.[177] The violent but non-mentally ill inmate may be defined as mentally ill in order to rid the prison of him. The patient declared not guilty by reason of insanity, who is not mentally ill but nevertheless judged "dangerous," may be retained for further treatment as mentally ill. Balancing the needs of society with the needs of the offender-patient, though a valid societal goal, encourages psychiatric and judicial hypocrisy, both knowingly and unknowingly.

Correctional psychiatrists working with mentally abnormal offenders must therefore always be pro-active. This includes their acquiring an understanding of the laws and the legal concepts involved, in addition to evidencing a willingness to challenge these laws and their operation when such jeopardize the treatment of offender-patients.[178] Without a pro-active stance the psychiatrist working with mentally abnormal offenders becomes mainly "dispositional grease," allowing a nonrational system to escape scrutiny.

A thorough review of the status and the treatment of the varying classes of mentally abnormal offenders is beyond the scope of this chapter but some major points are discussed below.

Incompetency to Stand Trial

Offenders held pending determination of competency to stand trial constitute the greatest proportion of mentally abnormal offenders.[97,166] The need for inpatient handling for many of these offender-patients has been greatly overestimated. Brief screening examinations performed in jail or upon an outpatient basis, if addressed to relevant legal criteria,[179,180] will avert the need for inpatient handling for many of these offenders.[165,166] Tasks that might (and usually do) take about 15 minutes to 1 hour of examination time may instead take 30 to 60 days.[181] This is either "bootleg" mental health care or misuse of an insufficient pool of mental health professionals in order to accomplish tactical legal maneuvers.[181]

Offenders found incompetent to stand trial are in danger that they will neither go to trial nor be released from the criminal hospital for many years.[182] Such continuing hospitalization can only be justified if there is the likelihood that competency will shortly be achieved. By the end of 6 months of treatment this should be apparent.[166] Because of misuse of the competency issue, some commentators favor abolition of the plea.[104] Alternatives to retention in criminal hospital status for incompetent offenders include release with dropping of criminal charges, civil commitment as mentally ill, and undergoing trial with added protection furnished.

The issue of incompetency to stand trial is illustrative for the purpose of the present discussion. These offenders should not merely be lumped or defined as "mentally abnormal offenders" and their problems considered along with other mentally abnormal offenders. Solutions to the problems of incompetency (better outpatient screening of offenders, adherence to legal criteria in decision-making, developing alternatives to criminal hospitalization) separate rather than lump the care of these offenders with other mentally abnormal offenders.[101]

Not Guilty by Reason of Insanity

The excessive attention given to the semantics of the insanity defense is philosophically interesting, understandable, and no doubt important. However, as noted by Dershowitz, perhaps less than 0.2 percent of cases (in the Federal system) culminate in this verdict.[183] In reaching its verdict, the jury attends to other data in addition to the legal instructions. What happens then to these offenders? Very few, if any, of them go free immediately.[184] Subsequent estimates of the offender's future dangerousness and his length of time in hospitalization are based primarily on the crime he has committed and not on the degree of his mental disorder.[185] Social factors such as whether or not the offender-patient is married, better educated, or possesses a skill, also affect the length of hospitalization.[185] Post-hospital follow-up studies demonstrate that failure (recidivism and rehospitalization) in such patients is predicted by two variables: the offender's age at release (the younger the offender, the greater the danger) and the extensiveness of his previous criminal history.[186,187] These studies illustrate the continuing conceptual problem concerning patients who are not guilty by reason of insanity. These offenders more nearly resemble other offenders than they do typical psychiatric patients. Curing the "mad" may not necessarily remove the "bad" or alter the social prognosis. Reconciling this side of the coin with a need for fair and proper commitment and release standards, as well as ensuring such offenders a "right to treatment," is a task for the future.[188,189] Under an equal protection rationale, some courts are ruling that such offenders must be committed and released according to procedures similar to those utilized for all other mental patients.[188]

Sex Offenders

This subject has been comprehensively reviewed by the Committee of Psychiatry and Law of the Group for the Advancement of Psychiatry.[37] For approximately 35 years, in various jurisdictions, dangerous sexual offenders have been subject to indeterminate civil commitment as "sexual psychopaths." GAP describes the statutes as "approaches that have failed," noting also that the concept of "sexual psychopathy" lacks clinical validity, that there are inherent dangers to both society and to sexual offenders in the concept of coercive cure, and that the sex psychopathic statutes should be repealed.[37] Psychological pitfalls for treatment staff involved with these offenders include problems in predicting dangerousness and in distinguishing genuine from sham cures.[101,190] One of the worst errors that can be made is to regard the management of sexual offenders as solely a matter of clinical psychiatric judgment,[191,192] thereby neglecting the obvious, namely, that these offenders, similar to many offenders not guilty by reason of insanity, also show many similarities to "normal" offenders.[190] Logically, sex offenders should be handled or treated similarly to other offenders. This is *not* to gainsay that such offenders should be provided opportunities and access to self-sought treatment, if that is their choice, within the conventional structure of a probation or prison experience. The recent debate concerning the propriety of castration for sex offenders highlights the problem of coercive treatment. Some offenders have been asked to make a "forced choice" between an indeterminate life sentence and the possibility of an irreversible alteration in their biology.[40] The issue is hardly that of informed consent, but rather a dramatic illustration of the problem of indeterminate confinement dependent upon "cure." For those offenders who genuinely seek them, behavioral treatments, especially the less risky ones such as systematic desensitization and assertive training,[37] do offer some hope for change.

Mentally Ill Prisoners

The care and treatment of mentally ill offenders has to some extent been discussed previously. It has been noted that such prisoners should not be treated involuntarily without their having been afforded the civil protections of due process hearings similar to those available to the nonincarcerated.[101] Another trend relates to the regionalization of forensic facilities, to the disbanding of conglomerate statewide maximum security prison-hospitals or hospital-prisons, and to their replacement, as much as is possible, with smaller hospitals or satellite clinics located within wings of conventional state hospitals or prisons.[101,102,161,162,170,193] The dangerousness of these mentally ill offenders has been overestimated in the past. This is another illustration of the fallacy of lumping together mentally abnormal offenders in maximum security hospitals on the basis of alleged, though unproven, common characteristics. The care of mentally ill offenders in the future will occur to a greater extent in traditional institutions (conventional prisons or hospitals) rather than in "hybrids" (in between special security institutions). These "third alternatives" pose nearly insurmountable administrative problems and have manifested a very poor track record.

In the past, prisoners who have become mentally ill in prison or jails have not been permitted to seek care voluntarily in hospitals. Such care had to be mandated. Furthermore, the prisoner typically lost certain benefits while in hospital (i.e., loss of good time or denial of parole eligibility). These practices are being criticized as unfair to prisoners and a denial of their right to medical care.[101,170] With the development of smaller, less onerous treatment alternatives for the mentally ill inmate, such practices ought to be modified.

Finally, the question arises concerning responsibility for the delivery of mental health care to mentally ill offenders. Who should be responsible, the prison or jail which hires its own personnel or a Department of Mental Health or other equivalent medical organization?[119] The latter is practically the only way to ensure that the medical needs of the offenders are not completely subsumed to those of custody. Yet prison hospitals run by doctors are nonetheless prisons. A compromise (one that cannot always be achieved and is not perfect for every inmate) is that the inmate be treated within a hospital that is within a prison.[161,193] The prison hospital should have some autonomy operating under the aegis of medical rather than penal administration. This is the least hypocritical solution to a difficult problem. Mentally ill offenders are, nevertheless, offenders. Their handling thus involves consideration of social factors which go considerably beyond the medical. As with prisoners with other types of health problems, the offender's access to high-quality mental health care should be similar to that of patients who are not incarcerated.[176] Developing quality medical facilities within jails and prisons, adequately staffed and medically administered, is one way out of this dilemma and is far preferable to the proliferation of special security hospitals.

Defective Delinquents

This concept,[30,42,101,127] similar to the concept of sexual psychopathy, is itself probably "defective." The defective delinquent is defined "as an individual who, by the demonstration of persistent, aggravated, antisocial or criminal behavior, evidences a propensity toward criminal activity, and who is found to have either such intellectual deficiency or emotional unbalance, or both, as to clearly demonstrate an actual danger to society so as to require such confinement and treatment, when appropriate, as may make it reasonably safe for society to terminate the confinement and treatment."[30] Though the definition of "defective delinquents" has been interpreted to involve psychiatric and medical concepts,[194] in practice this concept is a legally mandated approach permitting quasibehavioral and quasipenal management of recurrent criminality. The care and treatment of offenders at Patuxent Institution have generated considerable national controversy concerning behavior control.[45,195] Though no clear-cut "abuses" have occurred (treatment at Patuxent involves primarily vocational, group, and milieu therapy with progression through tiers), neither have the Patuxent results justified this type of involuntary handling.[104] The "cure" is the indeterminate sentence designed to motivate within the institution but also, as Patuxent's own figures suggest, to function as a "backup" or threat once the offender is released.[196] Patuxent claims dramatic reductions in recidivism (a 7 percent rate in fully treated men), but such results are achieved only for men for whom Patuxent itself has recommended termination of parole supervision. For offenders discharged from Patuxent under parole supervision by the courts, the recidivism rate is 39 percent. These figures are a dramatic refutation of the Patuxent approach, namely, that genuine personality changes in offenders may be achieved consequent to forced institutional "treatment." The type of parole supervision afforded, rather than the institutional treatment provided, appears more significant in reducing recidivism. There have been other telling criticisms of Patuxent's data.[101,195] Furthermore, even if the type of treatment at Patuxent were successful, considerable challenge may be raised to the indeterminate sentence on the basis of equity alone.[101,197] Because of objections to the principle of indeterminacy (even in Denmark, the home country of the famous Herstedvester Treatment Centre), use of this type of sentence has been cut back considerably. Similar to Patuxent, the results of treatment in Denmark simply have not justified the rhetoric.[162]

None of the above criticisms need prevent an inmate having a fixed release date from being handled as "a defective delinquent" if he so wishes. Providing prisoners with the opportunity for rehabilitation must not be confounded with forcing them to be rehabilitated.

Dangerous Psychopaths

Psychopathic offenders are the most controversial of inmates. This chapter cannot resolve the issue of whether psychopathy is a mental disorder.[63,64,162] The British, in particular, have been plagued by uncertainties as to how to manage and to conceptualize the handling of these offenders. As a practical matter, in the United States, psychopathy is most often not treated as a mental disorder. At any rate, neither British nor American psychopathy is with any degree of reliability "medically treatable."[162] The term itself is objectionable and pejorative. Psychiatrists more optimistic about the possibility of psychiatric intervention point out that:

> Psychopathy is an administrative term comprising patients whose only common feature is their persistently difficult behaviour and in whom three causative areas can be found, often in complex combination: (1) extremes of personality types . . .; (2) extreme mishandling in childhood . . .; and (3) *formes frustes* of organic brain damage . . . and psychosis . . . To make generalizations for psychopaths any more than one does for schizophrenia, alcoholism or nephritis, may be proved wrong in the long run.[198]

The above citation is relevant to whether any of these men (who may be extremely difficult to manage in prison) should be placed in special prisons or special prison units having medical input, or whether such offenders should be handled in regular prisons. This issue most clearly confronts the "behavior control" issue since the great majority of these men are not classically mentally ill, and they may also resist such special handling. In Britain it has been recently recommended that psychopathic offenders be treated in prisons rather than in hospitals, not in prison-hospitals or in "special" hospitals, but in "training units" established in prisons and featuring regimes of intensive work and social activities.[162] Psychiatrists, though, are to head the unit "because of the long association of the medical profession with the treatment of personality disorders."[162] It is important that admission to the units be voluntary.

In the United States, this debate has been manifested in several contexts. In order to maximize resources and to defuse the regular prisons, consideration has been given to whether regional penal facilities should be established which would receive and treat "special offenders" (e.g., "special offenders" resident in New England prisons).[140] These "special offenders" are not too precisely defined. As a common feature they seem to be not only violent and/or mentally ill, but also troublesome to the prison authorities. Although the problem addressed is no doubt real, this proposal and other recommendations for special prisoners have been viewed by some with skepticism.[140,199]

Better known nationally have been other controversies concerning programs of behavior modification for "troublesome" or violent prisoners. For example, the START program of the Federal Bureau of Prisons consisted of the involuntary transfer of inmates to living conditions involving considerable deprivation (isolation cells) with subsequent progressive amenities provided the offender commensurate with progress.[101,200] START was "stopped" by the Federal Bureau of Prisons consequent to litigation and to the controversy engendered. A Federal district court ruled that transfer to the START program involved "a major change in the conditions of confinement" and that the inmate "is entitled, at a minimum, to the type of hearing required by the Supreme Court in *Wolff v. McDonnell.*"[201] A similar, even more bitter, controversy erupted over the function of "Adjustment Centers" in the California prison system, especially the MPDU (Maximum Psychiatric Diagnostic Unit), the statewide "Adjustment Center" for all other adjustment centers.[17]

What is the correctional psychiatrist to make of this? A previous section of this chapter has suggested that psychiatric management and treatment of some violent prisoners might be helpful to the prisoners and indirectly to potential victims; such help, if voluntarily requested by inmates, should be encouraged. Morris has provided a useful description of a voluntary prison treatment program for violent offenders, noting also that such a program cannot be directed solely or even primarily toward institutional troublemakers.[20] On the other hand, coercion and isolation must not be euphemistically labeled treatment. What is treatment from the perspective of society may constitute yet another form of punishment to the offender. Given the past failures of psychiatric approaches in this area,[162] and considering the ethical dilemmas, correctional psychiatric participation in the treatment of "dangerous psychopaths" is not recommended unless (1) such treatment is self-sought by the inmate, and (2) the inmate's decision either to enter into or to continue in the treatment bears no direct relationship to subsequent release from the prison. Assuming that these conditions are met, such treatment would then in no way resemble the alleged characteristics of the aforementioned "Adjustment Centers" in California.

THE ROLE OF THE CORRECTIONAL PSYCHIATRIST

This chapter has articulated a point of view not always highlighted in discussions of prison and jail work, namely, that the primary purpose of correctional psychiatry is to make available to inmates on a voluntary basis those medical and psychological opportunities that would or should be available to them in the outside community. Treatment should be addressed to the mental disorder per se, to the prison-induced mental instability, or to the behavioral disorder as this is defined by the inmate. Furthermore, it is advocated that release generally not be dependent upon the psychiatrist's estimate of "cure," either of mental disorder or of criminality. This position is the middle ground between the unacceptable opposites of the "crime of treatment" and the "crime of no treatment."[8] Society defines the punishment; the inmate defines the subsequent treatment and requests it.

Experts in correctional psychiatry, however, conceptualize the role of the correctional psychiatrist differently.[67,202-206] A brief review illustrates both strengths and problems of other correctional roles, in addition to the clinical, which the correctional psychiatrist may play.

The Psychiatrist as Agent of Change

Some believe that the psychiatric interventions with inmates discussed above are relatively fruitless and that the correctional psychiatrist can function more broadly as a consultant to, and a shaper of, the institutional milieu (e.g., by promoting decarceration; the abolition of large, inhumane prisons; training or sensitizing correctional officers to be less punitive or more psychologically minded; advocating reforms to decrease the deprivations of incarceration; and advocating use of prison furloughs, conjugal visits, etc.). As Suarez put it, "Psychiatry would do better to spend its time treating the institution itself rather than the individual inmates within it."[205] Considering the small number of correctional psychiatrists available, it is only through directing attention to the overall milieu that the psychiatrist can influence the treatment of more than a few inmates.[203] This consultative approach, which may involve "taking the warden home to dinner," properly aims at making the prison environment more humane and constructive.

Often, however, this consultative approach does not stop at this point. It may be traditionally argued that "the wall that exists between custody and treatment must go,"[203] or that psychiatry should help "the staff members change their focus toward rehabilitation and away from infantalizing custody."[205] This is the point of departure between the present author and other commentators. Though prisons must become more humane (and making a full range of services and opportunities, including psychiatric services, available to inmates is a step in this direction), American penology has repetitively confirmed that prisons and jails will never be primarily treatment- rather than punishment-oriented institutions. Correctional officers confronted by problems of inmate violence and recidivism; correctional administrators confronted with a poverty of resources; treatment staff confronted by the limitations of closed or semiclosed institutions; and all others, including inmates, know that these institutions do not and cannot exist primarily for purposes of treatment. To assert that this is possible is to defy the logic of the word prison. Furthermore, the psychological reality of the inmate is that:

> Deprivation of freedom is punishment and no amount of semantics will make it otherwise. Inmates know and feel this and staff should admit it. There are no more bitter inmates than those who are sentenced for 'rehabilitation' and who find only a long period of isolation and sometimes repression behind the walls.[22]

Paradoxically, the ability of psychiatrists to influence the milieu and to communicate with inmate-patients is notable only when they are willing to admit that treatment is not the sole or even the major purpose of incarceration.[22] Above all, the correctional psychiatrist must always play it straight: "The lesson perhaps is that in prison one may be a more effective therapist if he does not claim to be one."[206]

Thus, while consultation to the milieu can be very much encouraged as a role complementary to that of individual inmate treatment, the correctional psychiatrist should not believe that even with changes in the milieu, prisons or jails will become genuine treatment-type institutions. Furthermore, because of external constraints, more often the milieu does not change, or milieu changes which are instituted are not maintained. The psychiatric consultant, despairing of providing any type of treatment in such a milieu, leaves the prison or jail, and once more mentally ill inmates are left with no access to traditional services. This is the danger of preoccupation with consultation to the milieu as the sole or major role for the correctional psychiatrist.

Rehabilitation

This chapter has not presented a very optimistic view concerning rehabilitation of inmates. This is the payoff which law and society hope for from correctional psychiatry, a payoff which traditionally has been associated with psychiatric participation in sentencing, in institutional classification procedures, in preparole assessment, and in other diagnostic activities.[44,48,49] Again, it is beyond the scope of this chapter to explore these areas in any depth or to review the voluminous and discouraging literature on rehabilitation. From the perspective of the present author, it is quite unwise to condition the provision of psychiatric services to inmates on the premise that such will be rehabilitative or will decrease recidivism. First, with few exceptions,[111] there is no evidence for such a claim. One would not want to take the position that the value of fixing a fractured leg in prison is dependent upon whether or not the inmate steals again. Furthermore, forcing characterologic change (necessary in some inmates for purposes of "rehabilitation") in the absence of clear-cut mental illness, dangerousness, mental incompetence, and treatability would constitute very questionable behavior for psychiatrists.[207] The paradox is that behavioral interventions which truly "work" in correcting offenders (assuming such interventions are not genuinely accepted by inmates) may be either unethical, illegal, or both. Finally, orienting the provision of psychiatric services in prison to reducing recidivism, given the present state of knowledge, exposes the correctional psychiatrist and inmates to a series of embittering encounters, encounters which jeopardize legitimate institutional treatment endeavors. The correctional officers jibe the psychiatrist—"He's back again, Doc; I thought you treated him already"—while the correctional psychiatrist knows, or should know, that psychological, social, and situational factors which contribute to inmate recidivism easily overpower psychological changes seemingly accomplished during incarceration. Despite the data, there are always new enthusiasts for rehabilitation, new nostrums proposed for old problems.[208]

Some brief comments are relevant concerning sentencing, classification, and psychiatric activities relevant to parole. These activities, which may bear some utility for the inmate but which even more frequently are of utility to the institution, must immediately be distinguished from activities falling under the mantle of the doctor-patient relationship. Confidentiality is absent, the information is shared with others, and it cannot be predicted whether the information gathered will help or hurt the inmate, at least from the inmate's perspective. All this must be explained to the inmate from the outset. Maintaining the confidentiality of even conventional treatment efforts may be very difficult in prison. The inmate must be apprised of the extent of confidentiality of communications. When inmates threaten violence or discuss escape, the psychiatrist is placed in a tenuous position. The correctional bureaucracy presses for information which the psychiatrist possesses and which constitutes a threat to the institution. The resolution of this dilemma relates to informed consent. Coincident with treatment—individual treatment, group treatment, crisis intervention—the psychiatrist should be forthright regarding information which, if it were known to him, he would feel necessary to act upon.[209] The psychiatrist must also know that no records, kept anywhere in the prison, are immune from scrutiny. If it is to be "confidential," it must be kept in the head. Moreover, the correctional psychiatrist who participates in institutional decision-making concerning an inmate should generally not be doing the treatment.

Mental health professionals who participate in administrative decision-making processes, such as, but not limited to parole and furlough relating to a prisoner, should be other than those mental health professionals providing direct therapeutic services to that prisoner (*Standards of the American Public Health Association*).[176]

Sentencing and classification issues may be considered jointly. Regarding sentencing evaluations, it is noted:

> We devote our evaluation to understanding what is happening with the individual, how the offense fits in this context, and what the individual needs in terms of therapy and rehabilitation, including some specific discussion of these needs and the agencies that might meet them.[205]

Psychiatric evaluations for purposes of sentencing may help avert prison sentences for some offenders. In the federal prison system, offenders may be sent to institutions for brief periods of observation prior to final sentencing. The assumptions concerning the utility of psychiatric participation in sentencing are as follows: first, that differential programming or treatment is available and that its pursuit will make a difference;[55] and second, that the court will be influenced by the psychiatrist's recommendation. One of the few empirical studies of this latter issue discovered this not to be the case. Psychiatric reports did not generally affect the type of sentence given.[210] If this is to be a useful activity for the correctional psychiatrist, psychiatrists must request, and should receive, feedback concerning the utility of reports, whether they are followed, and whether they make a difference. As in the area of classification, the most worthwhile psychiatric contributions involve identifying clear-cut mental illness and maintaining sensitivity to mental retardation and other factors which might contribute to institutional victimization in the event that the offender is incarcerated. The dynamics of the offender's behavior, and not merely conclusions, should be given. It is highly doubtful whether a psychiatrist's diagnosis of "personality disorder with a need for a structured setting" is very enlightening to a court.

The classification controversy may be briefly summarized. Classification is a type of diagnostic workup or evaluation from multiple perspectives, which occurs prior to or shortly after incarceration. There are no psychiatric classification systems in widespread use today. A few such psychiatric systems have been described.[55,89] A recent effort by Yarvis, dividing 25 incarcerated offenders into three groups, is illustrative. One group is essentially psychiatric in nature, neurotic offenders with minor histories of criminality. The second is a social deviance group, offenders with lengthy criminal histories. The last group of offenders manifested a clear-cut psychiatric illness as well as recurrent criminality.[211]

The critical question regarding classification is why do it? Ideally the goal is classification in some form of "treatment" (i.e., matching offender types and needs with individual programs designed to meet these needs). In practice, most classification systems are utilized for purposes of institutional "management," such as evaluating risk (Can the offender be in the community rather than the institution?) or the inmate's need for a security level within an institution, or deciding what part of the institution's resources it is worthwhile or efficient to devote to the inmate.[89,74] Compromising most classification efforts is the lack of adequate backup programs and resources which might accomplish the goals of classification. The correctional psychiatrist involved in the classification effort often experiences this effort, like other institutional "diagnosis," as a haphazard, nontheoretical attempt.[212] In practice, the choices involve such matters as assignment to one cellblock or another, whether or not the inmate will be recommended to obtain a GED, and what type of security is required for visits. Similar to other types of consultative work, the psychiatrists' dilemma is whether to recommend what they believe is necessary but which may not be available, or simply to choose on the basis of what the prison has to offer. Psychiatrists make their chief contribution, however, in adequately diagnosing mental illness, mental retardation, and neurological illness, and in clinically identifying other conventional medical entities which may require attention. Additionally, the inmate may discuss fears of victimization in the prison environment or sexual anxieties which, with the inmate's consent, may be communicated to other correctional workers for purposes of prevention.

Chapter 32 reviews the prediction of dangerousness, which is the variable of greatest interest to the parole authority. The trend in corrections is toward decreased discretionary handling with regard to parole. Some states have ended indeterminate sentencing. The critical questions concerning psychiatric participation in parole relate to the uncertain status of the psychiatrist's expertise in these matters[213] and to the propriety of psychiatric participation in this phase of corrections. To know that youth and a previous history of violent episodes, or a history of alcohol abuse, bespeak a poor prognosis is useful, but a psychiatrist is not needed to point this out, as such information is contained in the record. A psychiatrist can profitably comment on whether the inmate is presently mentally ill if the inmate is known to have been so previously and if this remains a question. The psychiatrist can review the stresses previously or presently operative on the inmate and can explain their relationship to the inmate's behavior and give some pointers concerning danger signals or situational variables that should be considered following release. Transitional mental health care can be recommended.

The assumption here is that such reports will not be presented or written by correctional psychiatrists whose roles in the prison have been in the treatment area. This is a difficult point. As the treating psychiatrist grows to know an inmate, he may clearly be of the opinion that the inmate has shown psychological growth and that further incarceration would not be helpful, or that the inmate is no longer dangerous. The temptation is to want to present this material to the parole board, especially if the inmate requests or allows it.[27,176,206] Unfortunately, such psychiatric behavior eventually confounds the prison treatment efforts. A further problem is that the inmate's release, as a realistic matter, may not depend to a great extent on the psychiatric report. Like other inmate reports from educational or vocational counselors, or Alcoholics Anonymous supervisors, these reports become excuses not to release the inmate, but instead to recommend more treatment or improvement. The punishment and the treatment are again confounded. Because of these complexities, it is again stressed that it is best for the treating psychiatrist to separate his work from that of the evaluating psychiatrist. Agreement on this matter should be reached by negotiation and discussion between the treating psychiatrist and the inmate at the outset of any treatment effort. Moreover, it is important for the evaluating psychiatrist to explain to the inmate that the purpose of a diagnostic or preparole interview is to help the parole board in reaching its decision. What inmates most want from prison is to get out. This is completely understandable but must be taken into account as the psychiatrist assesses the value of his own participation in release decision-making.

The Preservation of Therapeutic Identity

Numerous factors in the prison and jail conspire to degrade the correctional psychiatrist's identity. Some readers might argue that the skepticism evinced in this chapter concerning prison "treatment" (rehabilitation as the rationale for correctional psychiatric services) does exactly this. Such a conclusion would be a misreading of the chapter. The point has been to argue for the provision of standard medical services for inmates, whether or not these are rehabilitative. Prisoners require access to psychiatric services, not because they are prisoners, nor because such services will necessarily reduce crime, but because prisoners are people. For that matter, a similar point of view could be expressed concerning other human service programs in prisons and jails (e.g., providing adequate programs of educational or vocational training for inmates). Given the fact of imprisonment, utilizing prison opportunities should be a matter of choice for the inmate, a choice, however, that he or she must be able to make. It is in this sense that psychiatry as well as other human services can contribute to a humanizing of the prison environment, a lessening, though not an abrogation, of punishment.

Whatever the role of the correctional psychiatrist may be, there are many strains placed upon it.[6,206] For example, doing crisis intervention (e.g., dealing with problems of prison violence, suicide, drug-taking, or other disequilibriums), as well as treating the acutely mentally ill, exposes the correctional psychiatrist to the charge that he or she is mainly an institutional "pacifier" or "tranquilizer"—not a very appealing role. It has been said by experienced therapists that "to be limited to such a role, however useful it might be, is in fact a prostitution of . . . basic orientation as a therapist."[203] The role of "troubleshooter," if accomplished with empathy, may profit inmates as well as the institution. Such a role, however, if delivered with cynicism or disregard for longer-term gains that the offender might make by coping with his crisis, makes the correctional psychiatrist nothing but a "cop doctor," a doctor interested mainly in the control of inmates for the purposes of others. This custodial role must be strongly condemned.[6] The psychiatrist must therefore continually reassess and re-evaluate his approach to in-prison problems, reviewing both the frustrations and the satisfactions that such problem-solving has engendered, the psychiatrist asking himself whose agent he is, or whose agent he has become.

Other sources of ambiguity concerning the correctional psychiatrist's role are the attitudes of the inmates and the correctional officers. The prisoners, mentally ill and non-mentally ill alike, "may hold no special reverence for psychiatrists or physicians, who are considered just some more authority figures with whom to contend." Although the physician may consider himself "a helping person in the medical and mental health tradition, inmates [are] naturally disbelieving."[206] Inmate skepticism concerning the value of psychiatry is sometimes reinforced by the correctional officers, even when psychiatric intervention may be appropriate: "Why do you want to mess around with those shrinks? If you don't watch what you say, you'll end up on the funny farm for good . . . You're not crazy, what do you need those shrinks for?"[214] The majority of inmates are not mentally ill, nor do they wish to be so labeled or so handled.[206]

Halleck was one of the first to write of "the criminal's problem with psychiatry."[68] The inmate is loath to give up a "bad" role which has adaptive as well as destructive components, and instead to adopt a "sick" role.

The resolution of these problems is not simple. The correctional psychiatrist must maintain a straightforward approach in dealing with both inmates and correctional officers. The "sick" metaphor, though only a metaphor, is too powerful and has too many connotations to be usefully applied to most inmates. Even when treating those inmates who are mentally ill, the correctional psychiatrist does better to focus on inmate behaviors or feelings that are presently dysfunctional or painful, and where some agreement can be reached with the inmate that the treatment is for his or her sake rather than for others. Word spreads quickly in prison or jail about "who is on whose side." If the correctional psychiatrist is honest and consistent in his dealings with inmates, help will be sought, even if the inmate does not view his own behavior as sick or crazy.

Correctional officers sometimes ridicule psychiatric treatment because they view it as often ineffective and because they view the psychiatrist as hopelessly naive, as someone, for example, who does not realize how dangerous the inmates really are and who fails to grasp that inmates can "never be trusted." Correctional workers "often look upon the clinician as a menacing figure who wishes to unleash recklessly all the uncontrolled impulses of the criminal. . . ."[203] Correctional officers may resent the opportunities for treatment or for other types of training that may be afforded to inmates "who have done bad things," the kinds of treatments or opportunities that many correctional officers themselves have never had. These attitudes will not disappear entirely, nor is remedying them entirely within the correctional psychiatrist's purview. If, however, the correctional psychiatrist maintains his "cool" and attempts to understand the problems that beset the officers as well as the inmates, then communication is facilitated.[215] Correctional officers are generally neither cruel nor inhuman. In the main they are persons with limited future options, persons struggling hard to do a difficult and sometimes dangerous job. The continuing confrontation of the correctional officers with the failures, yet never with the successes, of the prison or jail system culminates too frequently in anger or apathy. As the correctional psychiatrist comes to experience the prison or jail environment, he begins to appreciate the problems of the correctional officers. Informal exchanges between psychiatrists and correctional officers may then obviate some of the difficulties. As is true of the psychiatrist, what the correctional officer (and admittedly also the inmate) really needs is time away from the prison.

One solution to these problems is clear-cut. Few psychiatrists should work full time in a prison or a jail for very long. Psychiatrists who maintain affiliations outside the prison or jail or who themselves are known to be "short-timers" may be better trusted by inmates than the career correctional psychiatrist.[206] Working elsewhere while doing prison or jail work permits the correctional psychiatrist to maintain professional standards and other professional associations while providing time for reflection about what he or she is doing in the prison. Similarity of psychiatric practice is thereby encouraged, whatever the setting. The cross-fertilization between the community and the prison improves the quality of mental health work that may be performed by correctional psychiatrists and by other professionals under their supervision.[170] The unwelcome outcome of full-time work in correctional psychiatry, similar to that experienced by the correctional officers (e.g., anger, apathy, or a custodial mentality), is thus avoided. As Halleck points out, many correctional psychiatrists do very little work,[1] a problem that is essentially similar to "institutionalization" of the inmates and the guards.

Related to the point that professionals can function best on a part-time basis in prisons and jails is the recommendation that medical units in prisons and jails be staffed and run autonomously from the prison administration. Ideally, university-based personnel, residents in psychiatry (with supervision), and public health and private psychiatrists who are members of a group or a hospital should provide part-time psychiatric coverage for prisons or jails. This concept, however, is often resisted by the prison administration which has a vested interest in maintaining control over its personnel. To some degree, of course, the prison officials are correct—a naive psychiatrist can wreak havoc in an institution—but the point here is one of achieving the proper balance. The proper mix for a prison psychiatric unit might include both full-time and part-time professionals, the full-time professionals serving as a liaison to the institution and the milieu, and helping to teach the part-time personnel the institutional mores, while the part-time personnel maintain community contacts and stimulate an up-to-date professional attitude for the unit.

Why Work in a Prison?

If what has been presented so far seems dismal, there is another side. Why would a psychiatrist want to work in a prison or jail? This is an interesting question. At least judged by their behavior, most psychiatrists have answered this question in the negative, namely, they wouldn't. Nevertheless, many psychiatrists exposed initially through the military service, the public health service, or even through psychiatric residency experience, get "bitten" by prisons and jails and eventually do at least some part-time work. The psychiatrist who takes the time, who can be persuaded even to visit a prison or jail, requires no convincing that (1) the need for his or her service is great, (2) the milieu is simultaneously deplorable and yet of considerable intellectual interest, and (3) with a clever approach it simply must be the case that something better could be happening there. Grandiosity and messianic zeal are, of course, no long-term friends for correctional psychiatry, yet given the indicting picture that prisons and jails present, it is not that difficult for the psychiatrist to be inspired to make some contribution. There are, of course, other motivations. Every correctional psychiatrist recalls many positive relationships established with inmates (and some with correctional officers, too), even if the inmate has continued to be in difficulty or the outcome was not known. A great deal can be learned in prisons and jails concerning social organization, individual and group adaptation to stress, problems of violent and antisocial behavior, and problems of health delivery and health planning for underserved groups. Prisons and jails are logical catchment areas and in this sense can serve as testing grounds for concepts in social and community psychiatry. Curiosity and a willingness to provide service for an underserved population are well rewarded. For at least some psychiatrists it can honestly be said, "Try it, you'll like it, at least a little bit." Providing better service for patients, rather than preventing crime, is, however, the orientation most consistent with the psychiatrist's experience and expertise.

REFERENCES

1. Halleck, S. L.: *Psychiatry and the Dilemmas of Crime, A Study of Causes, Punishment and Treatment.* Harper & Row, New York, 1967.
2. Halleck, S. L.: American Psychiatry and the Criminal: A Historical Review. *Int. J. Psychiatry* 6:185–208, 1968.
3. *A Handbook of Correctional Psychiatry* (Vol. 1, U.S. Bureau of Prisons, Department of Justice), Washington, D.C., 1968.
4. Cormier, B. M.: The Practice of Psychiatry in the Prison Society. *Bull. Am. Acad. Psychiatry Law* 1:156–183, 1973.
5. Cormier, B. M.: *The Watcher and Watched.* Scribner Tundra Books, New York, 1976.
6. Powelson, H., and Bendix, R.: Psychiatry in Prison. *Psychiatry* 14:73–86, 1951.
7. Cumming, R. G., and Soloway, H. J.: The Incarcerated Psychiatrists. *Hosp. Community Psychiatry* 24:631–632, 1973.
8. Psychiatry in Prisons: Treatment or Punishment? (Symposium). *Psychiatric Opinion* 11(3), 1974.
9. Thorne, F. C., and Forgays, D. G.: A Study of the Mental Health Services of a Correctional Mental Hospital. *J. Community Psychol.* 1:243–249, 1973.
10. Lack of Prison Psychiatrists Puts Strain on Psychologists. *Behavior Today* 7(30), July 26, 1976, pp. 2,3.
11. *Medical Care in U.S. Jails.* American Medical Association, Chicago, 1973.
12. Massachusetts Department of Public Health: Prison Health Services. *N. Engl. J. Med.* 290:856–857, 1974.
13. Ciba Foundation: Medical Care of Prisoners and Detainees. Symposium 16. Associated Scientific Publishers, Amsterdam, 1973.
14. Menninger, K.: *The Crime of Punishment.* Viking Press, New York, 1968.
15. Bailey, W. C.: Correctional Outcome: An Evaluation of 100 Reports. *J. Criminal Law Criminol. Police Sci.* 57:153–160, 1966.
16. Martinson, R.: What Works? Questions and Answers About Prison Reform. *The Public Interest,* Spring 1974, pp. 22–54.
17. Coleman, L.: Prisons: The Crime of Treatment. *Psychiatric Opinion* 11(3):5–16, 1974.
18. Klerman, G. L.: Behavior Control and the Limits of Reform. *The Hastings Center Report* 5(4):40–45, 1975.
19. American Friends Service Committee: *Struggle for Justice. A Report on Crime and Punishment in America.* Hill & Wang, New York, 1971.
20. Morris, N.: *The Future of Imprisonment.* University of Chicago Press, Chicago, 1974.
21. von Hirsch, A.: *Doing Justice: The Choice of Punishments. Report of the Committee for the Study of Incarceration.* Hill & Wang, New York, 1976.
22. Roth, L. H.: Treating the Incarcerated Offender. *Corrective Psychiatry J. Social Therapy* 15(1):4–14, 1969.
23. Roth, L. H. and Ervin, F.: Psychiatric Care of Federal Prisoners. *Am. J. Psychiatry* 128:424–430, 1971.
24. Mesnikoff, A. M. and Lauterbach, C. G.: The Association of Violent Dangerous Behavior with Psychiatric Disorders: A Review of the Research Literature. *J. Psychiatry Law* 3:415–445, 1975.
25. Guze, S. B.: *Criminality and Psychiatric Disorders.* Oxford University Press, New York, 1976.
26. Patients or criminals? (Editorial). *Br. Med. J.* 11 October 1975, p. 70.
27. Shestack, J. J.: Psychiatry and the Dilemmas of Dual Loyalties. *Am. Bar Assoc. J.* 60:1521–1524, 1974.
28. Goldfarb, R. L., and Singer, L. R.: After Conviction. A Review of the American Correction System. Simon & Schuster, New York, 1973.
29. Goldfarb, R.: *Jails: The Ultimate Ghetto.* Anchor Books, New York, 1976.
30. Rappeport, J. R.: Enforced Treatment—Is it Treatment? *Bull. Am. Acad. Psychiatry Law* 2:148–158, 1974.

31. Allen, H. E., and Simonsen, C. E.: *Corrections in America: An Introduction.* Glencoe Press, Beverly Hills, 1975, pp. 18–66.
32. Ibid., pp. 42, 43.
33. MacMahon, B., and Pugh, T. F.: *Epidemiology Principles and Methods.* Little, Brown, Boston, 1970, p. 7.
34. Fitzpatrick, J. J.: Psychoanalysis and Crime: A Critical Survey of Salient Trends in the Literature. *Ann. Am. Acad. Political Social Sci.* 423:67–74, 1976.
35. Rubin, S.: Psychiatry and the Prison: A Negative Report. *Int. J. Psychiatry* 6:214–218, 1968.
36. Russell, D. H.: Dimensions of Forensic Psychiatry. *Int. J. Psychiatry* 6:219–221, 1968.
37. Group for the Advancement of Psychiatry: Psychiatry and Sex Psychopath Legislation, the 30's to the 80's. 9(98):831–956, 1977.
38. Shah, S. A., and Roth, L. H.: Biological and Psychophysiological Factors in Criminality, in Glaser, D. (ed.): *Handbook of Criminology.* Rand McNally, Chicago, 1974, pp. 101–173.
39. Witkin, H. A., et al.: Criminality in XYY and XXY Men. *Science* 193:547–555, 1976.
40. Roth, L. H.: "Voluntary" Castration. *The Hastings Center Report* 6(5):4,30, 1976.
41. *Newman v. State of Alabama,* 503 F2d 1320, 1322–24, (5th Cir 1974), cert. den. 421 US 948 (1975).
42. Sidley, N. T.: The Evaluation of Prison Treatment and Preventive Detention Programs: Some Problems Faced by the Patuxent Institution. *Bull. Am. Acad. Psychiatry Law* 2:73–95, 1974.
43. Levinson, R. B.: Treatment in Correctional Facilities, in Carnahan, W. A. (ed.): *Legal Problems of Correctional, Mental Health and Juvenile Detention Facilities.* Practicing Law Institute, New York, 1975, pp. 551–557.
44. Smith, C. E.: Recognizing and Sentencing the Exceptional and Dangerous Offender. *Fed. Probation* 35(4):3–12, 1971.
45. Stanford, P.: A Model, Clockwork-Orange Prison. *New York Times Magazine,* September 17, 1972, pp. 71–84.
46. Stürup, G. K.: *Treating the "Untreatable"—Chronic Criminals at Hertstedvester.* The Johns Hopkins University Press, Baltimore, 1968.
47. Groder, M.: An Angry Resignation. *Corrections* 1(6):27–36, 1975.
48. Kim, L. I. C., and Clanon, T. L.: Psychiatric Services Integrated into the California Correction System. *Int. J. Offender Therapy* 15:169–179, 1971.
49. Karpman, B., cited by Robitscher, J.: Definition, Description and Dynamics of the Mentally Ill Offender as Seen from the Law and Psychiatry. Address at Institute of "The Mentally Ill Offender." Thomas Jefferson University, Philadelphia, 1970.
50. Glueck, S., cited in Russell, D. H.: Dimensions of Forensic Psychiatry, *Int. J. Psychiatry* 6:219–221, 1968.
51. Zitrin, A.: Comments in N.Y.U. Colloquium: President Nixon's Proposal on the Insanity Defense. *J. Psychiatry Law* 1:297–334, 1973.
52. Wooton, B.: The Place of Psychiatry and Medical Concepts in the Treatment of Offenders: A Layman's View. *Canadian Psychiatric. Assoc. J.* 17:365–375, 1972.
53. Quay, H. C.: What Corrections Can Correct and How. *Fed. Probation* 37(2):3–5, 1973.
54. MacDougall, E. C.: Corrections Has Not Been Tried. *Criminal Justice Rev.* 1:63–76, 1976.
55. Warren, M. Q.: Classification of Offenders as an Aid to Efficient Management and Effective Treatment. *J. Criminal Law Criminol. Police Sci.* 62:239–258, 1971.
56. The Non-Dangerous Offender Should Not Be Imprisoned. *Crime Delinquency* 21:315–322, 1975.
57. National Advisory Commission on Criminal Justice Standards and Goals: *Corrections.* Washington, D.C., 1973, pp. 595–606.

58. Serrill, M. S.: Critics of Corrections Speak Out. *Corrections* 2:3–8, 21–26, 1976.
59. Bronstein, A. J. Rules for Playing God. *Civil Liberties Rev.*, Summer 1974, pp. 116–121.
60. Dershowitz, A.: Let the Punishment Fit the Crime. *New York Times Magazine*, December 28, 1975, p. 7.
61. Levinson, R. B., and Deppe, D. A.: Optional Programming: A Model Structure for the Federal Correctional Institution at Butner. *Fed. Probation* 40(2):37–44, 1976.
62. Flynn, E. E., Turning Judges into Robots. *Trial*, March 1976, pp. 17–23.
63. Gunn, J., and Robertson, G.: Psychopathic Personality: A Conceptual Problem. *Psychological Med.* 6:631–634, 1976.
64. Lewis, A.: Psychopathic Personality: A Most Elusive Category. *Psychological Med.* 4:133–140, 1974.
65. *Clinical Aspects of the Violent Individual.* Task Force Report 8. American Psychiatric Association, Washington, D.C., 1974.
66. van der Kvast, S.: Can the Psychiatrist Foretell Criminal Behavior? *Int. J. Offender Therapy Comparative Criminol.* 20(2):148 152, 1976.
67. Halleck, S. L.: Rehabilitation of Criminal Offenders—A Reassessment of the Concept. *Psychiatric Annals* 4(3):61–85, 1974.
68. Halleck, S. L.: The Criminal's Problem with Psychiatry. *Psychiatry* 23:409–412, 1960.
69. Gettinger, S.: U.S. Prison Population Hits All-time High. *Corrections* 2(3):9–20, 1976.
70. Mattick, H. W.: The Contemporary Jails of the United States: An Unknown and Neglected Area of Justice, in Glaser, D. (ed.): *Handbook of Criminology*. Rand McNally, Chicago, 1974, pp. 777–848.
71. Vinter, R. D., Downs, G., and Hall, J.: *Juvenile Corrections in the States: Residential Programs and Deinstitutionalization.* Preliminary Report. National Assessment of Juvenile Corrections. University of Michigan, Ann Arbor, 1976, p. 13.
72. *Holt v. Sarver,* 309 F Supp 362 (ED Ark 1970) aff'd 442 F 2d 304 (8th Cir 1971).
73. *Costello v. Wainwright,* 397 F Supp 20 (MD Fla 1975), mod, 525 F2d 1239 (5th Cir 1976), 539 F 2d 547 (Sept. 27, 1976).
74. *Pugh v. Locke; James v. Wallace,* 406 F Supp 318, (MD Ala 1976).
75. Prigmore, C. S., and Crow, R. T.: Is the Court Remaking the American Prison System? A Brief Overview of Significant Court Decisions. *Fed. Probation* 40(2):3–10, 1976.
76. *Pugh v. Locke; James v. Wallace,* 406 F Supp 318, 329–330 (MD Ala 1976).
77. Irwin, J.: *The Felon.* Prentice-Hall, Englewood Cliffs, N.J., 1970.
78. Toch, H.: *Men in Crisis, Human Breakdowns in Prison.* Aldine, Chicago, 1975.
79. Swank, G. E., and Winer, D.: Occurrence of Psychiatric Disorder in a County Jail Population. *Am. J. Psychiatry* 133:1331–1333, 1976.
80. Petrich, J.: Psychiatric Treatment in Jail: An Experiment in Health-Care Delivery. *Hosp. Community Psychiatry* 27:413–415, 1976.
81. Cleaver, E.: *Soul on Ice.* Dell, New York, 1968.
82. Jackson, G.: *Soledad Brother, The Prison Letters of George Jackson.* Bantam Books, New York, 1970.
83. Inmate 66 Years Finds Life in Prison is What He Prefers. *New York Times*, August 19, 1976, p. 30, col. 3.
84. Board of Inquiry, United States Penitentiary, Lewisburg, Pa., June 8–June 15, 1976. U.S. Bureau of Prisons, Washington, D.C., 1976.
85. Banister, P. A., et al.: Psychological Correlates of Long-term Imprisonment. I. Cognitive Variables. *Br. J. Criminol.* 13:312–323, 1973.
86. Heskin, K. J., et al.: Psychological Correlates of Long-term Imprisonment. II. Personality Variables. *Br. J. Criminol.* 13:323–330, 1973.
87. Payson, H. E.: Suicide Among Males in Prison—Why Not? *Bull. Am. Acad. Psychiatry Law* 3:152–161, 1975.
88. Roth, L. H. The Bugaboo of Control—The Universal Prison Dynamic. *Newsletter Am. Acad. Psychiatry Law* 3(3):20–22, 1972.

89. Classification of Offenders, in *Corrections*. National Advisory Commission on Criminal Justice Standards and Goals, Washington, D.C., 1973.
90. Rieger, W.: Suicide Attempts in a Federal Prison. *Arch. Gen. Psychiatry* 24:532–535, 1971.
91. Roth, L. H., Rollins, A. M., and Ervin, F. R.: Violent and Non-Violent Prisoners: A Comparison. Paper given at session on institutional violence. Annual meeting, American Psychiatric Association: Dallas, 1972.
92. Twaddle, A. C.: Utilization of Medical Services by a Captive Population: An Analysis of Sick Call in a State Prison. *J. Health Social Behavior* 17:236–248, 1976.
93. Parole, Release, Supervision and Recommitment of Prisoners, Youth Offenders, and Juvenile Delinquents. Paroling, Recommitting and Supervising Federal Prisoners. *Fed. Register* 41(173):37316–37331, 1976.
94. Sigler, M. H.: Abolish Parole? *Fed. Probation* 39(2):42–48, 1975.
95. Eynon, T. G.: The Mentally Disordered Offender, in Irvine, L. M., and Brelje (eds.): *Law, Psychiatry and the Mentally Disordered Offender*. Vol. II. Charles C Thomas, Springfield, Ill., 1973, pp. 3–17.
96. de Reuck, A. V. S., and Porter, R.: *The Mentally Abnormal Offender. A Ciba Foundation Symposium*. Little, Brown, Boston, 1968.
97. Scheidemandel, P. L., and Kanno, C. K.: *The Mentally Ill Offender. A Survey of Treatment Programs*. The Joint Information Service of the American Psychiatric Association and the National Association for Mental Health, Washington, D.C., 1969.
98. Eckerman, W. C.: *A Nationwide Survey of Mental Health and Correctional Institutions for Adult Mentally Disordered Offenders*. National Institute of Mental Health, Center for Studies of Crime and Delinquency, DHEW No. (HSM) 73-9018, Washington, D.C., 1972.
99. Matthews, A. R.: *Mental Disability and the Criminal Law: A Field Study*. American Bar Foundation, Chicago, 1970.
100. Hearing Must Precede Inmate's Transfer to Mental Hospital. 20 Cr.L. 1045, 1976.
101. Wexler, D. B.: *Criminal Commitments and Dangerous Mental Patients: Legal Issues of Confinement, Treatment, and Release, Crime and Delinquency Issues*. National Institute of Mental Health. DHEW No. (ADM) 76-331, Washington, D.C., 1976.
102. Matteawan State Hospital to Shut Down by April 1. *New York Times*, August 2, 1976, p. 51, col. 7.
103. *Negron v. Ward*, I MDLR 191 (SD NY, July 13, 1976.)
104. *Davis v. Watkins*, 384 F Supp 1196 (ND Ohio 1974).
105. Alabama is Resuming Accepting Prisoners. *New York Times*, December 5, 1976, p. 43, col. 1.
106. Kaufman, E.: Can Comprehensive Mental Health Care be Provided in an Overcrowded Prison System? *J. Psychiatry Law* 1:243–261, 1973.
107. Bach-y-Rita, G.: Personality Disorders in Prison, in Lion, J. R. (ed.): *Personality Disorders, Diagnosis and Management*. Williams & Wilkins, Baltimore, 1974.
108. Vaillant, G. E.: Sociopathy As a Human Process, A Viewpoint. *Arch. Gen. Psychiatry* 32:178–183, 1975.
109. Lion, J. R.: The Role of Depression in the Treatment of Aggressive Personality Disorders. *Am. J. Psychiatry* 129:347–349, 1972.
110. Bach-y-Rita, G. E.: Habitual Violence and Self-Mutilation. *Am. J. Psychiatry* 131:1018–1020, 1974.
111. Carney, F. J.: Evaluation of Psychotherapy in a Maximum Security Prison. *Semin. Psychiatry* 3:363–375, 1971.
112. Braukmann, C. J., et al.: Behavioral Approaches to Treatment in the Crime and Delinquency Field. *Criminology* 13:299–331, 1975.
113. Donnelly, J.: Aspects of the Treatment of Character Disorders. *Arch. Gen. Psychiatry* 15:22–28, 1966.
114. Sutker, P. B., and Moan, C. E.: A Psychosocial Description of Penitentiary Inmates. *Arch. Gen. Psychiatry* 29:663–667, 1973.

115. Koller, K. M., and Castanos, J. N.: Family Background in Prison Groups: A Comparative Study of Parental Deprivation. *Br. J. Psychiatry* 117:371–380, 1970.
116. Giagiari, S.: The Mentally Retarded Offender. *Crime Delinquency Lit.* 3:559–577, 1971.
117. Roffman, R. A., and Froland, C.: Drug and Alcohol Dependencies in Prison, A Review of the Response. *Crime Delinquency* 22:359–366, 1976.
118. *Medical and Health Care in Jails, Prisons, and Other Correctional Facilities, A Compilation of Standards and Materials.* Report to the American Bar Association, Commission on Correctional Facilities and Services, Resource Center on Correctional Law and Legal Services, in conjunction with American Medical Association, Division of Medical Practice, Washington, D.C., 1974.
119. Brecher, E., and Della Penna, R. D.: *Health Care in Correctional Institutions.* Law Enforcement Assistance Administration, U.S. Dept. of Justice, Washington, D.C., 1975.
120. Psychotic Inmates Aided Little by the Cell-to-Hospital Shuttle. *New York Times,* August 7, 1974, p. 1, col. 5.
121. Peck, A. H.: A Psychiatric Ward Run by Inmates in a Prison Setting. *Bull. Am. Acad. Psychiatry Law* 2:220–222, 1974.
122. *Scott v. Plante,* 532 F 2d 939 (3rd Cir., 1976) 1 MDLR 121, 1976.
123. New York Enacts Legislation for Mentally Ill Inmates of Correctional Facilities. 1 MDLR 207, 1976.
124. *Nelson v. Heyne,* 491 F 2d 352 (7th Cir., 1974) cert den 417 US 976 (1974).
125. Virkkunen, M.: Self-Mutilation in Antisocial Personality (Disorder). *Acta Psychiat. Scand.* 54:347–352, 1976.
126. Wadeson, H., and Carpenter, W. T.: Impact of the Seclusion Room Experience. *J. Nerv. Ment. Dis.* 163:318–328, 1976.
127. Rowan, B. A.: Corrections, in Kindred, M., et al. (eds.): *The Mentally Retarded Citizen and the Law.* The Free Press, New York, 1976, pp. 650–675.
128. Brown, B. S., and Courtless, T. F.: The Mentally Retarded in Penal and Correctional Institutions. *Am. J. Psychiatry* 124:1164–1169, 1968.
129. *Pugh v. Locke; James v. Wallace,* 406 F Supp 318, 324 (MD Ala 1976).
130. Fox, S. J.: *The Reform Movement and Tactical Problems,* in Kindred, M., et al. (eds.): *The Mentally Retarded Citizen and the Law.* The Free Press, New York, 1976, pp. 627–638.
131. *U.S. v. Masthers,* 539 F 2d 721, 1 MDLR 187, 1976.
132. Wolfensberger, W.: *The Principle of Normalization in Human Services.* National Institute on Mental Retardation. Leonard Crainford, Toronto, 1972.
133. Cohen, A. K., Cole, G. F., and Bailey, R. G. (eds.): *Prison Violence.* D. C. Heath, Lexington, Mass., 1976.
134. Toch, H.: *Police, Prisons, and the Problem of Violence.* Crime and Delinquency Issues. NIMH, Center for Studies of Crime and Delinquency. DHEW Publication No. (ADM) 76-364, 1977.
135. Flynn, E. E.: The Ecology of Prison Violence, in Cohen, A. K., Cole, G. F., and Bailey, R. G. (eds.): *Prison Violence.* D. C. Heath, Lexington, Mass., 1976, pp. 115–133.
136. Bennett, L. A.: The Study of Violence in California Prisons: A Review with Policy Implications, in Cohen, A. K., Cole, G. F., and Bailey, R. G. (eds.): *Prison Violence.* D. C. Heath, Lexington, Mass., 1977, pp. 149–168.
137. Kinzel, A. F.: Body-Buffer Zone in Violent Prisoners. *Am. J. Psychiatry* 127:99–104, 1970.
138. Megargee, E. I.: Population Density and Disruptive Behavior in a Prison Setting, in Cohen, A. K., Cole, G. F., and Bailey, R. G. (eds.): *Prison Violence.* D. C. Heath, Lexington, Mass., 1976, pp. 135–144.
139. Roth, L. H.: Territoriality and Homosexuality in a Male Prison Population. *Am. J. Orthopsychiatry* 41:510–513, 1970.
140. Uhlig, R. H.: Hospitalization Experience of Mentally Disturbed and Disruptive, Incarcerated Offenders. *J. Psychiatry Law* 4:49–59, 1976.
141. Bach-y-Rita, G., and Veno, A.: Habitual Violence: A Profile of 62 Men. *Am. J. Psychiatry* 131:1015–1017, 1974.

142. Woods, S. M.: Violence: Psychotherapy of Pseudohomosexual Panic. *Arch. Gen. Psychiatry* 27:255–258, 1972.
143. Lion, J. R.; *Evaluation and Management of the Violent Patient.* Charles C Thomas, Springfield, Ill., 1972.
144. Drugs in the Treatment of Human Aggression. *J. Nerv. Ment. Dis.* 160:75–145, 1975.
145. Sheard, M. H., et al.: The Effect of Lithium on Impulsive Aggressive Behavior in Man. *Am. J. Psychiatry* 133:1409–1413, 1976.
146. Tupin, J. P., et al.: The Long-term Use of Lithium in Aggressive Prisoners. *Comprehensive Psychiatry* 14:311–317, 1973.
147. Danto, B. L. (ed.): *Jail House Blues, Studies of Suicidal Behavior in Jail and Prison.* Epic Publications, Orchard Lake, Michigan, 1973.
148. Sloane, B. C.: Suicide Attempts in the District of Columbia Prison System. *Omega* 4:37–50, 1973.
149. Esparza, R.: Attempted and Committed Suicide in County Jails, in Danto, B. L. (ed.): *Jail House Blues, Studies of Suicidal Behaviors in Jail and Prison.* Epic Publications, Orchard Lake, Michigan, 1973.
150. Fawcett, J., and Marrs, B.: Suicide at the County Jail, in Danto, B. L. (ed.): *Jail House Blues.* Epic Publications, Orchard Lake, Michigan, 1973, pp. 83–106.
151. Danto, B. L.: The Suicidal Inmate, in Danto, B. L. (ed.): *Jail House Blues.* Epic Publications, Orchard Lake, Michigan, 1973, pp. 17–26.
152. Heilig, S. M.: Suicide in Jails—A Preliminary Study in Los Angeles County, in Danto, B. L. (ed.): *Jail House Blues.* Epic Publications, Orchard Lake, Michigan, 1973, pp. 47–55.
153. Sagarin, E.: Prison Homosexuality and Its Effect on Post-prison Sexual Behavior. *Psychiatry* 39:245–257, 1976.
154. Serrill, M. S.: Prison Furloughs in America. *Corrections* 1(6):3–12, 53–56, 1975.
155. Dole, V. P.: Detoxification of Sick Addicts in Prison. *J.A.M.A.* 220:366–369, 1972.
156. Guenther, A. L.: Compensations in a Total Institution: The Forms and Functions of Contraband. *Crime and Delinquency* 21:243–254, 1975.
157. Roth, L. H., Rosenberg, N., and Levinson, R. B.: Prison Adjustment of Alcoholic Felons. *Q. J. Studies Alcohol* 32:382–392, 1971.
158. Ziegler, R., Costello, R., and Horvat, G.: Innovative Programming in a Penitentiary Setting: Report from a Functional Unit. *Fed. Publication* 40(2):44–49, 1976.
159. Lehmann, H. E.: Unusual Psychiatric Disorders and Atypical Psychoses, in Freedman, A. M., Kaplan, H. I., and Sadock, B. J. (eds.): *Comprehensive Textbook of Psychiatry.* Vol. 2. Williams & Wilkins, Baltimore, 1975, pp. 1724–1725.
160. Bellino, T. T.: The Ganser Syndrome: A Contemporary Forensic Problem. *Int. J. Offender Ther. Comparative Criminol.* 17:136–137, 1973.
161. Liss, R., and Frances, A.: Court-mandated Treatment: Dilemmas for Hospital Psychiatry. *Am. J. Psychiatry* 132:924–927, 1975.
162. Report of the Committee on Mentally Abnormal Offenders (Butler Report). Her Majesty's Stationery Office, London, 1975.
163. Brooks, A. D.: The Mentally Disabled Offender, in Brooks, A. D. (ed.): *Law, Psychiatry and the Mental Health System.* Little, Brown, Boston, 1974.
164. Shah, S. A.: The Mentally Disordered Offender, in Allen, R. C., Ferster, E. Z., and Rubin, J. G. (eds.): *Readings in Law and Psychiatry.* The Johns Hopkins University Press, Baltimore, 1975, pp. 571–586.
165. McGarry, A. L., et al.: Competency to Stand Trial and Mental Illness. Crime and Delinquency Issues, NIMH, Center for Studies of Crime and Delinquency. DHEW Publication No. (HSM) 73:9105, Washington, D.C., 1973.
166. Group for the Advancement of Psychiatry: *Misuse of Psychiatry in the Criminal Courts: Competency to Stand Trial.* Vol. 8, Report No. 89, February 1974.
167. Malmquist, C. P.: Empirical Problems in the Selection of the Insanity Defense. *Psychiatric Annals* 4(8):48–66, 1974.

168. Steadman, H. J., and Cocozza, J. J.: *Careers of the Criminally Insane: Excessive Social Control of Deviance.* D.C. Heath, Lexington, Mass., 1974.
169. Psychiatry and the Dangerous Offender. *Med. J. Australia* 1:1–3, 1972.
170. Laben, J. K., and Spencer, L. D.: Decentralization of Forensic Services. *Community Mental Health J.* 12:405–414, 1976.
171. *Baxstrom v. Herold,* 383 US 107 (1966).
172. *Bolton v. Harris,* 395 F 2d 642 (DC Cir 1968).
173. *Nason v. Superintendent of Bridgewater State Hospital,* 233 NE2d 908 (Mass 1968).
174. *United States ex rel. Schuster v. Herold,* 410 F 2d 1071 (2nd Cir 1969) cert den 396 US 847 (1969).
175. *Jackson v. Indiana,* 406 US 715 (1972).
176. Jails and Prisons Task Force: *Standards for Health Services in Correctional Institutions.* American Public Health Association, Washington, D.C., 1976.
177. Steadman, H. J., and Braff, J.: Crimes of Violence and Incompetency Diversion. *J. Crim. Law Criminol.* 66:73–78, 1975.
178. McGarry, A. L., and Bendt, R. H.: Criminal vs. Civil Commitment of Psychotic Offenders: A Seven-year Follow-up. *Am. J. Psychiatry* 125:1387–1394, 1969.
179. *Dusky v. United States,* 362 US 402 (1960) (per Curiam).
180. *Wieter v. Settle,* 193 F Supp 318 (1961).
181. *Assessment of Pretrial Competency Examinations in the District of Columbia Superior Court.* The American University Criminal Courts Technical Assistance Project. Institute for Advanced Studies in Justice, The American University Law School, Washington, D.C., 1975.
182. McGarry, A. L.: The Fate of Psychotic Offenders Returned for Trial. *Am. J. Psychiatry* 127:1181–1184, 1971.
183. Dershowitz, A. M.: Abolishing the Insanity Defense: The Most Significant Feature of the Administration's Proposed Criminal Case—An Essay. *Crim. Law Bull.* 9:434–439, 1973.
184. Leavy, M. R.: The Mentally Ill Criminal Defendant. *Crim. Law Bull.* 9:197–252, 1973.
185. Cooke, G., and Sikorski, C. R.: Factors Affecting Length of Hospitalization in Persons Adjudicated Not Guilty by Reason of Insanity. *Bull. Am. Acad. Psychiatry Law* 2:251–261, 1974.
186. Morrow, W. R., and Peterson, D. B.: Follow-up of Discharged Psychiatric Offenders—"Not Guilty by Reason of Insanity" and "Criminal Sexual Psychopaths." *J. Crim. Law Criminol. Police Sci.* 57:31–34, 1966.
187. Quinsey, V. L., Pruesse, M., and Fernley, R.: Oak Ridge Patients: Pre-release Characteristics and Post-release Adjustment. *J. Psychiatry Law* 3:63–77, 1975.
188. Tougher Release Standards Approved for Patients Held after Insanity Acquittal. *U.S. v. Ecker,* No 75-1074 (DC Cir Apr. 2, 1976) 1 MDLR 116–117, 1976.
189. Right to Treatment Affirmed for Insanity-Acquitted Defendant and One-to-One Therapy Ordered. Interest of R. G. W., No. J 1472–73 (Passaic City Juvenile and Domestic Relations Court, October 20, 1976) 1 MDLR 186, 1976.
190. Dix, G. E.: Determining the Continued Dangerousness of Psychologically Abnormal Sex Offenders. *J. Psychiatry Law* 3:327–344, 1975.
191. *Semler v. Psychiatric Institute of Washington,* 538 F2d 121 (4th Cir, 1976) cert den 97 SCt 83 (October 4, 1976).
192. Robitscher, J.: The Prediction of Dangerousness and the Protection of the Public (editorial). *Bull. Am. Acad. Psychiatry Law* 3:5–7, 1975.
193. Jablon, N. C., Sadoff, R. L., and Heller, M. S.: A Unique Forensic Diagnostic Hospital. *Am. J. Psychiatry* 126:1663–1667, 1970.
194. *State v. Williams,* 361 A2d 122 (Md CT App, 1976).
195. Behavior Control in Prisons. *The Hastings Center Report* 5(1), February 1975.
196. Carney, F. L.: The Indeterminate Sentence at Patuxent. *Crime and Delinquency* 20:135–143, 1974.
197. Schreiber, A. M.: Indeterminate Therapeutic Incarceration of Dangerous Criminals: Perspectives and Problems. *Va. Law Rev.* 56:602–634, 1970.

198. Scott, P. D.: The Butler Committee's Report. II. Psychiatric Aspects. *Br. J. Criminol.* 16:177–178, 1976.
199. Desroches, F.: Regional Psychiatric Centers, A Myopic View? *Can. J. Criminol. Corrections* 15:200–218, 1973.
200. Holland, J. G.: Behavior Modification for Prisoners, Patients and Other People as a Prescription for the Planned Society. *Prison J.* 54(1):23–37, 1974.
201. *Clonce v. Richardson*, 379 F Supp 338, 348 (WD Mo, 1974).
202. Smith, C. E.: Psychiatry in Corrections: A Viewpoint. *Miss. Law J.* 45:675–683, 1974.
203. Pacht, A. R., and Halleck, S. L.: Development of Mental Health Programs in Correction. *Crime and Delinquency* 12:1–8, 1966.
204. Heller, M.S.: The Private Reflections of a Prison Psychiatrist. *Prison J.* 54(2):15–33, 1974.
205. Suarez, J. M.: Psychiatry and the Criminal Law System. *Am J. Psychiatry* 129:293–297, 1972.
206. Ketai, R.: Role Conflicts of the Prison Psychiatrist. *Bull. Am. Acad. Psychiatry Law* 2:246–250, 1974.
207. Halleck, S. L.: Legal and Ethical Aspects of Behavior Control. *Am. J. Psychiatry* 131:381–385, 1975.
208. Yochelson, S., and Samenow, S. E.: *The Criminal Personality.* (2 vols.) Jason Aronson, New York, 1976, 1977.
209. Roth, L., and Meisel, A.: Dangerousness, Confidentiality and the Duty to Warn. *Am. J. Psychiatry* 134:508–511, 1977.
210. Bohmer, C. E. R.: Bad or Mad: The Psychiatrist in the Sentencing Process. *J. Psychiatry Law* 4:23–48, 1976.
211. Yarvis, R. M.: Psychiatric Pathology and Social Deviance in 25 Incarcerated Offenders: An Assessment. *Arch. Gen. Psychiatry* 26:79–84, 1972.
212. Shover, N.: "Experts" and Diagnosis in Correctional Agencies. *Crime and Delinquency* 20:347–358, 1974.
213. Ennis, B. J., and Litwack, T. R.: Psychiatry and the Presumption of Expertise: Flipping Coins in the Courtroom. *Cal. Law Rev.* 62:693–752, 1974.
214. Edelman, S. E., and Felthous, A. R.: Some Methodological Problems in Studying Violent Offenders. *Bull. Am. Acad. Psychiatry Law* 4:67–72, 1976.
215. A Day on the Job—in Prison. *Corrections* 2(6):6–12, 36–40, 44–48, 1976.

CHAPTER 29

Herbert C. Modlin is Professor of Community and Forensic Psychiatry at the Menninger Foundation, Associate Clinical Professor of Psychiatry at the University of Kansas Medical School, and Vice-President of the American Board of Forensic Psychiatry. Dr. Modlin was educated at the University of Nebraska and is a graduate of the Topeka Psychoanalytic Institute. He is a Life Fellow of the American Psychiatric Association, a former President of the Group for the Advancement of Psychiatry, and a Founding Fellow of the American College of Psychoanalysts.

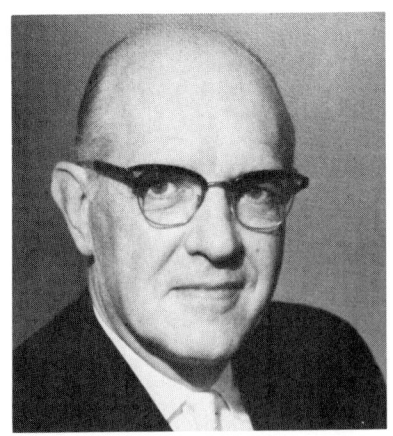

PSYCHIATRY AND THE CIVIL LAW

Herbert C. Modlin, M.D.

Forensic psychiatry has traditionally been associated with criminal law—in the courtroom with the determination of litigants' sanity and in prisons with rehabilitation. However, only a small part of modern legal practice concerns criminal law. In the average three-year law school curriculum, instruction in criminal law is given in a three-hour course for one semester. Most attorneys practice civil law; correspondingly, the collaboration of most practicing psychiatrists with lawyers occurs in connection with legal problems focused on matters of civil law. Moreover, among psychiatric patients whose problems include involvement with the law, those problems are more likely to be civil than criminal: personal injury suits, worker's compensation claims, divorce actions, child custody disputes, altercations with the Internal Revenue Service, efforts to break or preserve wills, deeds and contracts, and malpractice claims.

PERSONAL INJURY SUITS

In personal injury suits and malpractice claims that most commonly occupy potential, current, or former psychiatric patients, the law of torts applies. The field of torts is complicated; "a really satisfactory definition of a tort has yet to be found."[1] A tort is a civil wrong (as opposed to a criminal wrong) perpetrated against one citizen by another. Tort refers to a transgression of legitimate rights as in invasion of privacy, defamation, misrepresentation, nuisance, negligence, trespass on real property, false imprisonment, assault and battery, and product liability.

In essence the law imposes upon each of us a civil duty to respect the person, name, reputation, property, privacy, and liberty of others. If we violate the rights of, or injure, another regarding any of these, we may be liable to a tort claim for money damages. For a successful tort action to be pressed, X must prove that Y owed him a civic duty, that Y breached that duty, and that X suffered injury as a result.[2]

It has been estimated that about 70 percent of all the cases (not including divorce actions) on all the dockets of all the courts in the land are personal injury suits. In nearly all such claims, medical testimony is crucial; several physicians are ordinarily drawn into each case. Even when an attorney can prove liability, that a tort was committed, unless he can also establish through his medical witnesses that the tort effected injury to his client, there is no suit.

Statistics compiled by the National Safety Council over the past several years consistently reveal that about 2 million persons annually are injured in highway accidents, 1.8 million in industrial accidents, and 2 million or more in home accidents. A small number of these, perhaps no more than 2 or 3 percent, suffer an incapacitating psychiatric reaction.

The functioning of psychiatrists in personal injury suits is usually in connection with the concept of traumatic neurosis. Although "traumatic neurosis" appears repeatedly in medical and legal literature, it is not an officially accepted diagnosis; it is not listed in the *Diagnosis and Statistical Manual II* (DSM-II), published by the American Psychiatric Association. The phrase has been applied in so many contexts and varying senses that its meaning is blurred and nearly useless.

In psychoanalytic literature, traumatic neurosis generally refers to a neurosis stemming from childhood experiences in which the immature ego is called upon to cope with untoward excitations or stresses.[3] The traumatic neuroses of war refer to a hodgepodge of reactions to a wide variety of precipitating agents.[4,5] World War II spawned the tragic long-term "traumatic neuroses" engendered by concentration camp ordeals and the aftermath of atomic bombing.[6] In recent years the psychotraumatic effects of fires, tornadoes,[7] floods,[8] earthquakes,[9] sinking ships,[10] and other massive disasters have been studied and the term "traumatic neurosis" applied broadly. A companion phrase, "survivor syndrome," is becoming popular.

Since most of the clinical conditions referred to as traumatic neuroses can be classified under the standard nomenclature of DSM-II, the phrase is vocabulary of the law and, in speaking with lawyers, judges, and worker's compensation commissioners, it is tolerable, sometimes necessary jargon.

The clinical syndromes commonly seen postaccident are (1) anxiety neurosis in which free-floating anxiety may be experienced for months and sometimes for years; (2) conversion reactions, including anesthesias, paralyses, and torticollis; (3) psychophysiologic reactions, including chronic back pain, prolonged concussion syndrome, and cardiac neurosis; and (4) dependency reaction, an exacerbation of a characterologic passive-dependent reaction to stress. Depression, hypochondriasis, or dissociative reactions are rare.

ANXIETY NEUROSIS

One variety of anxiety neurosis occurs only after sudden, frightening accidents and deserves the appellation "traumatic neurosis" if anything does.[11] All the components of the syndrome are subjective complaints voiced by the victim or his family. Objective findings are minimal; thus diagnosis rests on accurate history-taking. It is exceedingly important for the physician to interview the patient's spouse and close family members since, characteristically, he is, himself, concrete, unimaginative, verbally unproductive, and an inept observer of his own feelings and behavior. The symptoms of the syndrome are as follows:

1. *Anxiety.* Patients describe chronic, free-floating anxiety: "something is about to happen." The accident to which they are reacting is long past, but the persistent protective psychophysiologic set is anticipation of an imminent recurrence. His anxiety often becomes acute if the patient finds himself again at the scene of the accident or in circumstances reminiscent of it. A phobic-avoidance reaction may be the patient's most serious occupational disability. I have seen as patients three structural steel workers following falls which were not physically damaging; none of them went "back up" again. Following a frightening accident, a heavy construction equipment operator could not tolerate visiting construction sites, much less climbing into the cab of a vehicle. He is now working as a plant night watchman, earning a third his former wages.

2. *Muscular tension.* Symptomatic complaints are restlessness, fatigability, insomnia, and a reiterated "I just can't seem to relax." The patient's spouse, often with some impatience, can vividly describe his inability to sit still for long.

3. *Irritability.* When questioned, the patient will frequently acknowledge being a bit more difficult to live with, but here again his wife waxes eloquent about his touchiness, flare-ups of anger, impatience, and loss of his former sense of humor. In over half the cases, the well-known "startle reaction" to sudden noises is an accompaniment. Radio, television, or conversation of well-meaning friends may occasion an irritable lashing out or withdrawal. His offspring, with some bewilderment and resentment, learn to avoid their explosive parent.

4. *Impaired concentration and memory.* Although these are common complaints, repeated psychological testing demonstrates no real memory loss at all. The patient's subjective sense of poor memory reflects his self-preoccupied inattention to reality in his environment.

5. *Repetitive nightmares.* Frightening dreams directly or symbolically reproducing the experienced accident occur in about 75 percent of the cases and are pathognomonic of the syndrome. A spouse may report waking during the night to find the patient violently trembling and sitting bolt upright in bed.

6. *Sexual inhibition.* A notable lowering of sexual capacity is characteristic, sometimes to the point of complete impotence or frigidity. In working-class men this may be the most disturbing symptom of the syndrome, yet one that they can rarely talk about spontaneously.

7. *Social withdrawal.* Interpersonal involvement with relatives, friends, and neighbors is avoided. The patient discontinues regular church attendance, participation in recreational activities, movie-going, and drops his club memberships. As evidenced by his behavior, he is seeking "peace at any price."

The automobile of a 52-year-old salesman, traveling in a midwestern town at dusk, stalled on some railroad tracks. In attempting to restart the car, he flooded the engine. As he waited a moment for the carburetor to drain, a slowly moving switch engine appeared, turned on its headlight, and for 8 or 10 terrorized seconds the motorist helplessly gripped the steering wheel while the fiery-eyed monstor bore down upon him. He received no physical injury from the impact, which nudged his car off the tracks, but he was so shaken that his legs buckled when he stepped from the car. When seen for psychiatric evaluation 8 months later, he complained of fearfulness, tension, restlessness, tearfulness, insomnia, repetitive nightmares, impaired concentration, irritability, and total sexual impotence. He had lost 20 pounds in weight and had been dismissed from his job. Almost anyone would be considerably shaken psychologically by such an experience but would recover in a few days or a week. For this particular man, the accident was disastrous.

Any of these symptoms may be part of other psychic illnesses, but together they constitute a specific handicapping reaction to the stress of an accident. Whenever three key symptoms—anxiety, startle reaction, and repetitive nightmares—are coexistent, a psychologically traumatic accident manifestly has occurred. In a few patients the syndrome may be complicated by a "spillover" of anxiety into the autonomic nervous system, resulting in familiar functional complaints such as palpitation, dyspnea, headache, dizziness, gastric distress, urinary frequency, and menstrual irregularity.

HYSTERICAL NEUROSIS (CONVERSION TYPE)

The postaccident conversion reaction usually consists of symptoms referable to the body site of a physical impact. Suggestibility is a prominent feature.

> On a construction job a 10-pound sandbag fell from the third floor and struck a workman on the shoulder, knocking him to the ground. An hour later the victim, unable to work because of pain, was examined by the company physician who found no evidence of serious injury. After a week of physiotherapy he was deemed ready to return to the job, but he reported for work with a torticollis, his chin fixed over his left clavicle. Further examination revealed no physical basis for the distorted position, and psychiatric referral was accomplished. Hypnotic treatment relieved the disability, and the patient returned to work, although with some conscious anxiety.

> A 55-year-old carpenter, stepping back to admire a piece of work, fell into a hole 12 feet deep. Momentarily out of breath, he lay limply while fellow workers gathered around and warned him not to move "because something might be broken." He was raised by an improvised stretcher and transported to the nearest physician whose cursory examination revealed considerable back pain and absent patellar reflexes. The physician unwisely mumbled something about "broken back," and the patient was sent by ambulance to a hospital nearby. Unfortunately, he shared a room with a multiple sclerosis patient. When examined an hour after admission he was hysterically paralyzed from the waist down.

The serious disability of such a patient is often traceable to therapeutic mismanagement. If time passes and the symptoms remain unalleviated, and if secondary gain of illness sets in—a limp, blindness, loss of voice, or torticollis becomes part of a chronic invalidism—remedial help is hard to apply.

PSYCHOPHYSIOLOGIC REACTION

The well-known but poorly understood interweaving of psyche and soma is the postaccident condition least amenable to successful management. The persistent low back pain, the prolonged concussion syndrome, the cardiac neurosis—these are the most refractory problems.

A laborer lifts a heavy load, "something snaps," and pain develops quickly. Soft tissue injury is diagnosed and orthopedic treatment instituted. After 6 months the orthopedist, stating that the tissues should be well healed, can no longer attribute the persistent pain and disability to organic trauma. Eventually the patient may be persuaded to seek psychiatric evaluation, and the psychiatrist may be hard put to explain the disability convincingly on purely psychiatric grounds. The probable factor of secondary gain may loom large, but the primary mechanisms remain obscure.

DEPENDENCY REACTION

The exacerbation of a latent, passive-dependent solution to stress may appear in relatively pure culture or may complicate numerous other clinical syndromes. One common personality characteristic of these accident casualties might be labeled "inadequate." They often seem psychologically underdeveloped.

> A middle-aged plasterer working on a ceiling fell 8 feet to a terrazzo floor when his scaffold collapsed. He was badly frightened and suffered leg pain, but medical findings were essentially negative except for a linear hairline fracture of the right os calcis requiring no specific treatment. He sought psychiatric evaluation 2 years later because of persistent inability to work and chronic diffuse pain in both legs and hips, unconfirmed by physical findings. He lived with his widowed mother who devoted much attention to his welfare. While on maneuvers during World War II, he twisted a knee and spent a year in Army hospitals. He was unable to work for an additional year after discharge from the service. In 1955, gastric symptoms were diagnosed as a pre-ulcer state and diet and medication prescribed. A subsequent acute perforation of the stomach required only simple closure, but he could not work for 18 months.

This seemingly uncomplicated man struggled through life at a marginal level of adjustment. At a casual, uncritical glance, one might view him as an undistinguished but solid member of society—good to his mother, friendly to his peers, adequately performing his work. Closer inquiry revealed that he had a sixth-grade education, was pathetically awkward and fruitless in his approaches to women, and maintained continued psychological dependence on his mother and a steadily employed brother. Physicians, insurance companies, and the general public tend to find such a person irritating or contemptible. He may be called lazy, dishonest, or mercenary. To psychiatrists these are not sufficient explanations of his behavior, nor should they be. Human psychology is not that simple.

Any kind of accident, life-threatening or inconsequential, may trigger one of the psychopathologic reactions I have discussed. The unexpected, potentially dangerous near miss, in the absence of physical damage to the victim, usually triggers the anxiety reaction. The scaffold collapses, the steam pipe bursts, the crane tips over, the gasoline fumes flare into a flash fire. Such experiences undoubtedly would produce at least a degree of psychic disequilibrium in even "normal" persons.

Minor accidents—mild concussions, wrenched back, pratfall—usually produce a psychophysiologic reaction manifested by backache, recurrent headache, palpitation and dyspnea, leg weakness, and dizzy spells.

> A young woman slipped and fell in a sitting position on a ramp in a department store. When examined by a psychiatrist a year later she was tense, hypersensitive, tearful, and unable to work because of diffuse low-back pain unexplained by findings of repeated orthopedic examinations.

This type of valid postaccident disability is difficult for the average person to understand and credit; he is prone to suspect malingering.

As a generality, there is a compensatory relationship between physical and psychic damage. The more extensive the tissue damage—fractures, lacerations, contusions, hemorrhage—the less likely a postaccident psychiatric disorder. Significant physical damage seems to bind or neutralize the reactive anxiety or depression that the patient might reasonably be expected to exhibit; he has something "real" to cope with instead of something intangible. The medical and nursing ministrations; bed rest; traction harness and plaster cast; visible evidence of "battle" injury to display; sedatives, analgesics, and narcotics; an acceptable, even required, temporary state of regressed invalidism; a legitimate, socially condoned period of convalescent inactivity—all these factors tend to inhibit the development of a complex of neurotic symptoms.

Conversely, a sudden, frightening accident causing little or no physical damage is more likely precipitant of psychiatric disorders. After the fact, the traumatized psyche is not put at rest between cool white sheets; the hyperirritable nervous system is not soothingly bandaged, poulticed, and fed intravenously; the invisible ego laceration is not legal tender for special considerations; and the victim's desire to retreat temporarily from everyday stresses is not socially approved. Incidentally, all these psychophysiologic treatments—immediate rest, sedation, isolation, enforced quiet, special attention under empathic medical authority—were encountered routinely by disturbed soldiers in Viet Nam with a resultant, remarkable low incidence of psychiatric casualties. It is unfortunate that those hard-taught lessons of military psychiatry have not been more tellingly applied to counterpart civilian problems.

The course of the accident syndrome can be influenced by a variety of factors. Keiser devotes separate chapters to the roles of physician, attorney, employer, insurance company, psychiatrist, family, and society.[12]

The havoc consequent to a severe stress depends upon the intrinsic strength of the target personality. The weaker the adaptive capacity of the psyche, the less insult is necessary to unbalance it. The more sudden and potentially dangerous the accident, the more likely it is to be psychologically unsettling, especially to an already teetering balance.

> A young man involved in a head-on highway collision miraculously escaped physical injury. The girl riding with him was killed and a passenger in the other car seriously injured. His postaccident anxiety and depression are easy to understand; so severe a stress would be difficult for the most stable person to handle with unruffled poise.

It follows that observers using a common sense frame of reference are puzzled by, if not suspicious of, the considerable disability some persons manifest after seemingly minor or even trivial accidents. Their skepticism is based on the conviction that life consists only of what can be seen, that all people are approximately alike ("like me" is the usual point of comparison), and that *a* cause produces *an* event. Psychological science considers such thinking erroneous. Individuals vary greatly in their personality strengths and weaknesses, and the capacity for flexible tolerance a victim brings with him to an accident must be duly weighed as one determinant of his postaccident recovery from its psychological impact. "One man's meat is another man's poison." What to an observer appears a minor stress may constitute a major psychic assault to a given victim's uniquely vulnerable arrangement of internal resources and the particular set of external circumstances that happen at that time to be impinging upon him. Outsiders may well be unaware that he is already near the breaking point from antecedent stresses of which the victim himself may not consciously be fully aware. The accident, then, can be a "last straw" phenomenon.

WORKER'S COMPENSATION CLAIMS

The broad intent of state worker's compensation law is to provide subsistence in lieu of salary for employees unable to work because of medical disability due to job-related incidents. Additionally, the employee's medical expenses are paid. In cases of permanent disability, the weekly payments can be extended for a definite time period, usually 5 to 10 years.

Unlike tort law, worker's compensation law is not primarily concerned with proving fault or assessing penalty against a negligent other. If the employee is involved in a damaging accident or becomes ill because of his work environment, he is automatically compensated. All employers carry worker's compensation insurance; if there is a dispute, the contesting parties are usually the employee and the insurance carrier.

In a representative case, a worker is injured. He is examined and treated by an orthopedist and in due course is declared able to return to work. The man objects because he is still tense, nervous, depressed and suffering back pain. The insurance carrier, acting on the doctor's report, promptly stops weekly payments and refuses to honor further medical bills. The worker engages an attorney, usually through the union office, and the battle is joined: enter the psychiatrist.

Persons suffering psychological decompensation from industrial accidents differ little clinically from psychologically injured victims of highway accidents. However, the incidence of psychophysiologic reactions in industrial cases is greater and the factor of secondary gain more frequently complicates recovery. Industrial environments hold possibilities for a multitude of frightening accidents, some of them bizarre: a crane tips over; dynamite goes off prematurely; an operator's hair is caught in a whirring machine.

Worker's compensation laws cover most illnesses (called "industrial illnesses") identifiable with the employment situation, not just traumatic accidents. The proof of a causal link between the development of the illness or its exacerbation is often difficult. The issue of job stress that triggers psychiatric illness presents challenging evaluative problems to the psychiatrist; for example, the inherent chronic stress in the air traffic control officer's job, or the unrelieved pressure of a ceaselessly moving assembly line belt.

The dean of a graduate school resigned and a senior professor was appointed acting dean. He assumed the new responsibilities and maintained his full teaching load. His double duty required much overtime work. One Sunday he suffered a severe coronary thrombosis in his office and, following complicated litigation, was held to have been a victim of job stress, entitled to full worker's compensation, including that for loss of future earnings. The psychiatrist's explanation of the compulsive, overconscientious professor's psychophysiologic mechanisms was helpful in winning his claim.

Evaluation of psychiatric disability in worker's compensation claims is frequently complicated by variables of the "system" encapsulating the employee—variables imposed by employer, insurance company, worker's compensation laws, doctors, the claimant's family, and patterns of his culture.

A welder, at the beginning of the day's work, stooped to get a welding rod and, on straightening up, cracked his head sharply against a steel beam. Briefly dazed, he fell to his knees. Half an hour later, complaining of severe headache and blurred vision, he told his foreman he needed to go to the emergency room of a hospital nearby. The foreman said, "Get out your toolbox or quit"—hardly an enlightened personnel policy. After another half hour he went to the hospital, was examined and sent home with medication and instructions to see his family doctor if he did not improve. The following morning his headache and neck pain were so severe that he could not lift his head from his pillow. The welder returned to the hospital and was admitted because of the neck problem, poor eye convergence, and a fleeting nystagmus. He was treated for brain concussion and cervical sprain, and discharged 10 days later to continue in treatment as an outpatient. At the end of 2 months he was pronounced sufficiently recovered for light work. In that postaccident period he experienced tension, restlessness, insomnia, sensitivity to noise, moodiness, and irritability. He snapped at his wife and railed at their children. His behavior proved a last straw for an already tottering marriage; his wife left with their children and sued for divorce. Through his union's assistance, he applied for worker's compensation and did receive two monthly checks. When the doctor reported him able to work, the checks were stopped without explanation. Thus within 3 months the patient had lost his job, his income, and his employability (because of incapacitating symptoms), as well as his wife, his offspring and the ownership of his house. He was bewildered, demoralized, depressed, and nervous. He took his troubles to an attorney whose investigative procedure included sending him to be examined by an orthopedist, a neurologist, and a psychiatrist. Armed with appropriate medical information, the attorney got the compensation checks restarted and instituted suit against the former employer whose insurance carrier then arranged for the man to be examined by its company's orthopedist, neurosurgeon, and psychiatrist. So the months dragged on while his bewilderment and self-preoccupation were intensified by diagnoses in the medical reports that ranged from malingering to brain damage to neurosis.

Although the liberal worker's compensation laws tend to encourage a dependency reaction, the possible monetary gain is of negligible psychological importance in most cases. Nearly all workmen receiving compensation lose financially since the payments are less than they earn on the job.

SECONDARY GAIN

The primary gain of psychiatric illness is inwardly directed. The patient's symptoms serve to maintain a degree of personality integration and balance, although at a level below health. Secondary gain may be thought of as outwardly directed and is an attempt to achieve interpersonal balance or gratification.[13] As a consequence of his legitimate illness, the patient may realize relief from stress, pressure, and responsibility. He may have his dependency needs met by a concerned and devoted spouse; he may acquire a morally condoned outlet for counter-aggression toward his employer; or he may discover the seeming solution to concomitant life problems.

The 55-year-old construction worker may be able to avoid consciously acknowledging his slowly fading physical strength, his diminishing muscular agility, his increasing weariness at the end of the day, and his mildly waning sexual virility. He needs to believe "I am as good a man as I ever was" and "experience is what counts on my job." He needs to maintain self-esteem, to deny how he is struggling to keep pace with the vigorous young apprentice working beside him. When this man suffers a sprained back, a bruised shoulder, a period of heat exhaustion in mid-summer, or a brief coma from a minor blow to the head, his unconscious coping efforts are facilitated by a legitimate, face-saving way out of a troubling situation. Thus a protective, problem-solving invalidism may set in—it is a common psychological maneuver. In medicine it may complicate any illness—medical, surgical, obstetrical, or psychiatric—and it is not peculiar to postaccident reactions. In fact the psychological mechanism of solving Problem A by succumbing to Problem B is a universal phenomenon of human behavior and is not peculiar to beneficiaries of medical or legal expertise.

> An oil well troubleshooter earned a comfortable living for his wife and three children through his skill in returning faltering wells to production; he frequently collected overtime pay since he and his small crew were on call day and night. The work was often hazardous, and several of his workmen were commonly out of work with injuries, but he accepted all job assignments and accomplished them with conscientious thoroughness, secure in the belief that he was immune to injury. At one difficult job on a freezing, snowy night, he slipped and fell twice from a truck, landing in a sitting position each time. He gave up and pulled his crew off the job for the first time in years. Although not seriously injured, incapacitating low back pain set in, became chronic, and he was "forced" to leave the oil wells for much less remunerative work as a salesman.

Many authors point to the inappropriateness of "gain" in secondary gain.[13-16] For such paradoxical gains the patient pays a high price and in the long run is always the loser. The "gain" is illusory and irrational and becomes part of the neurotic matrix of the disability. According to Slawson, "because it affords dependent gratification, it can complicate recovery by triggering neurotic decompensation. Marked psychophysiologic regression may follow."[15]

Monetary reward for illness may be an additional complication. "Compensation neurosis" is another piece of jargon in our working vocabulary. Its meaning is even more vague than "traumatic neurosis" because of the bias and emotion usually associated. It often takes on the character of an epithet. Here again, the reality of monetary gain is often an illusion, but the symbolism of money is part of our contemporary mythology. The dollar may represent emotional security, just compensation for suffering, a symbolic taking away of that which is precious from the aggressor, in short a righteous retribution.[17]

MALINGERING

Malingering is the conscious, planned simulation of illness for the sake of gain. Individuals who simulate mental illness are uncommon, and those who do it successfully are rare. In contrast, patients who simulate health are a common clinical experience. In the personal injury problems in which we have been involved, time is on the clinician's side diagnostically. The symptoms have been present for months or years and have produced a consistent pattern of impaired functioning in most aspects of the patient's life.

The vast majority of patients who fail to improve from the effects of an industrial injury after a reasonable treatment effort are not malingering. Enelow[14] has classified these long-term nonrecoverers as (1) depressed patients; (2) hysterical personalities; (3) dependent, immature persons; (4) pseudo-self-sufficient persons; and (5) aging workers. A sixth category, sociopathic exploiters, will contain most of the would-be malingerers.

Insurance company investigative and legal personnel must see some claimants who seem at least partly motivated by cupidity and who are prone to exaggerate complaints. Some claimants must perceive the insurance company as skeptical, resistive, withholding, and even insulting, particularly where psychological disability is concerned. Commonly both tort and worker's compensation cases drag on for months or years, and the patient is caught up in the legal system which has only one method, the dollar, for compensating him for pain, suffering, disability, insecurity, fear, and economic loss. He is, in effect, required to maintain his illness in order to live in peace with his own conscience. If he is no longer ill, then his claim is dishonest. Thus he continues to wear the neck collar, carry the cane, turn on the heat lamp, take the medication, and settle into a state of chronic invalidism. The clinical problem is to define which aspects of his symptom picture should be placed where on the continuum: primary illness, secondary gain, compensation, exaggeration, cupidity, or malingering.

SPECIAL PSYCHIATRIC-LEGAL PROBLEMS

It is beyond the scope of this chapter to review the extensive literature and present illustrative cases on a number of special clinical-legal problems that complicate the lives of patients and the attorneys on both sides of a dispute. A brief discussion of those special concerns, together with references to leading books and articles about them, is offered below.

BURNS. The severely burned patient, once the fright stemming from the fire and the acute pain of the burn have subsided, faces a prolonged ordeal. A "traumatic neurosis" may ensue with the typical nightmares prominent. Usually this phase is short and the patient's attention focuses on his unfamiliar body surface as he goes throught debridement, baths, dressings, removal of dressings, aseptic isolation, skin grafting, infection, regrafting, and painful exercises for contractures. Regression is the rule, particulary in children.[18] Usually it is a reversible retreat, but often not entirely. Particularly if the reparative plastic surgery goes on, as it commonly does, for a matter of years, the process of return to "normalcy" is impeded. One patient has had 12 operations in 3 years, another 15 surgical procedures over a period of 4 years. Children are often less psychologically scarred than adults, who may have fluctuating depression and social withdrawal. After healing comes the adaptation to residual scarring, the stares of strangers, the partly disguised discomfort of relatives, refusal to eat in public, and a gnawing concern about the future of interpersonal relationships, particularly about sexual intimacy.[19]

AMPUTATIONS. The phantom limb phenomenon has been well documented, but significant psychiatric sequelae are uncommon since the limb in most cases disappears by telescoping into the amputation stump. A period of mourning for the lost member is common, occasionally intense enough to be called depression, but on the whole amputees are not particularly susceptible to disabling psychiatric illnesses.[20]

SCARS. Cosmetic scarring is a problem with special implications for girls and young women on the basis of conventional social-sexual values. The scar victim, complaining less than her concerned mother and lawyer, is often protected by her own intact body image. She may experience the stares and questions of friends and strangers as odd, intrusive, and crude, since she rapidly learns not to see the scar in her mirror. The psychiatric consultant may have seen little definable psychological impairment, but the lawyer still presses him for an opinion about the possible effects of the scar on his client's marital and occupational prospects.

PROLONGED PAIN. Much of the postaccident pain that psychiatrists hear described by patients is psychogenic, although an organic insult may have initiated it.[21] Occasionally there is a patient who has endured organic pain over a long period: persistent phantom limb pain, only partially relieved tic doloreux, or inoperable spinal root irritation. A common result is a chronic, partially incapacitating personality change with tension, irritability, explosions of temper, loss of humor, impatience, fatigue, and self-preoccupation.

CHILDREN. The extent of postaccident disability in a child is primarily dependent upon his family's attitudes.[22,23] If his mother repeatedly wails, "My baby is ruined," a child may well come to believe it. If he receives special attention and privileges and is excused from domestic chores and responsibility for erratic behavior, he may adapt with alacrity, and his development will be impeded. Given a wholesome home environment, the power of the natural growth process, the merciful capacity to forget, and the need for peer companionship, it is unlikely that untoward psychic sequelae will permanently affect the child.

SEXUAL MOLESTATION INCLUDING RAPE. Recent cases of note have included a young woman who was abducted from a dark and deserted plant parking lot, a woman of 62 who was attacked by a soldier on a military reservation, a girl of 6 who was molested by a utility meter reader, and the 15-year-old daughter of a hospitalized patient, who was seduced by a male social worker. Civil suit was entered in all of these cases against the company, the government, or the hospital, claiming negligence, breach of civil duty, and damage. The current literature regarding such offenses is voluminous, and a "rape syndrome" has been described. Long-term effects of rape are measurably influenced by the quality of supportive understanding from intimates of the victim. Often her most important "therapeutic" aid is afforded by her husband. For further extensive discussion, see Chapter 18, "The Rape Experience."

Problems of Causality

The law seeks certainty. Did the accident cause the plaintiff's present disability? If there were several "causes," what percentage of the disability was due to the accident? The Worker's Compensation Commissioner and trial judge must resolve the dispute—"the buck stops there." The psychiatric witness will be pressed by both attorneys to be definite as possible, and may well feel pressured and beleaguered. If he can only ethically say "maybe," "in part," or "yes and no," he should resist dissuasion. The legalists have to do the best they can with his imprecise testimony.

The law is of some help, if the psychiatrist can accept it. The law states that if the accident caused the disability, activated a latent condition, or aggravated a pre-existing condition, the person at fault is liable. The tort offender takes his victim as he finds him. The employer takes his employee as he finds him. In other words, factors of predisposition are legally irrelevant. In practice, the opposing attorney tries to present all possible predisposing factors to influence the jury, in spite of the letter of the law.

The law also recognizes the "chain of events theory" with the accident forming the first "link." The case of the welder is illustrative: the original blow on the head, with legitimate organic and psychiatric disability, became compounded by the losses attendant to the accident (his wife, his home, etc.). The law finds it impossible to sort out and assign percentages of blame in so complex a series of misfortunes besetting a life, and so do I. In this case the State Compensation Commission assigned full responsibility to the welder's employer.

A typical "chain of events" begins with a back injury from lifting a heavy load and continues with pain, disability, loss of income, medical examination, differing medical opinions, myelogram, surgical disc removal, continued pain, nervousness, tension, insomnia, discouragement, silent concern over impotence, spinal fusion, continued disability, depression, lawsuit—and permanent invalidism.

Percentage of Disability

Particularly in worker's compensation cases, the doctor is expected to grade the client-patient's disability according to a table of percentages. The orthopedic surgeon is comfortable in estimating 50 percent impairment of a hand, 25 percent impairment of the body as a whole; the psychiatrist is expected to offer similar estimates. A useful guide is the rating system devised by an expert committee of the American Medical Association.[24] It is a guide, and the psychiatrist may deviate from it, but adherence to it does enable the clinician to maintain a consistency in communicating his findings and conclusions.

In worker's compensation cases only occupational disability is relevant. In tort cases everything may be thrown in, including pain and suffering, loss of consortium, social incapacity, and reduction in the enjoyment of life.

Prediction

Lawyers frequently remind me of a reality: the client has his day in court, and that is it. He cannot sue again, 5 to 10 years later, for lingering impairment from the original injury. Thus the attorney presses for a statement about the long-term effects of the accident: the persistent pain, the scar, the burn disfigurement, the sexual insult, and the occupational limitation. His questions are appropriate; so are vague answers. Psychiatrists are handicapped by a dearth of adequate follow-up studies and usually must reply according to their individual clinical impressions.

Legal Competency

Competency, in the law, is judged and defined variously: competency to stand trial, the related issue of mental competency or responsibility at the time of commission of an offense; competency to manage one's affairs; and competency to make a will or enter into a contract. We will deal briefly with each of these in the following pages.

WILLS

Elderly persons occasionally alter their wills in a seemingly capricious fashion, and suits to "break" a will are not uncommon. In a recent case, a woman of 84 bequeathed her sizable estate equally to two nephews. One of them visited her regularly; the other ignored her. In a codicil she left the negligent nephew $1,000 and the attentive one the rest of her property.

In will contests there is no patient for the psychiatrist to examine. His professional opinion must be based on material the attorney presents as well as on information garnered from his own interviews of persons with knowledge about the testator on the day of the signing of the will or codicil. In court, the attorney will ordinarily propound a hypothetical question: "Doctor, assume that an 84-year-old woman with two nephews . . . " It is appropriate for the psychiatrist to assist in preparing the hypothetical question to include the data that substantiate his opinion; for example, the old woman's developing cataracts; her reduced social contacts; her periods of confusion and disorientation at night; and her bitter, sometimes irrational views and remarks about the nephew in disfavor.

The law offers a guiding definition of competency to make a will. Did the testator, at the time he executed his will (1) understand the objects of his natural bounty and (2) the nature and extent of his property? Those are the issues to be settled in court. As indicated by the preponderance of evidence he has gained, the psychiatrist says yes or not to the questions. If he says "no," he should add "by reason of mental illness." He will then be asked to expand and explain. For an example of a psychiatric report in a will-contest case, see the illustrative report at the conclusion of Chapter 30.

CONTRACTS

The ruling legal questions here are: (1) did the party to the contract understand the legal instrument he signed, and (2) did he understand the probable consequences of his act? A recently widowed man, hoping to regain social contacts, signed a contract for $1,700 worth of lessons at a dance studio. After two lessons he realized the error of his decision and sued for contract release on the plea of his disabling depression and faulty judgment. A discouraged, aging farmer sold his property, then became more depressed when he found himself homeless and unemployed. He sued for return of his property on the basis of incapacitating depression and mental inability to anticipate the consequences of his action.

COMPETENCY TO MANAGE ONE'S AFFAIRS

The usual outcome of a personal competency issue in court is appointment of a guardian, conservator, or power of attorney for the impaired subject. The plea for a guardian is regularly entered by someone other than the subject, and legal dispute may arise.

An elderly woman, living with one of three nieces, began showering her and her family with gifts. The other two nieces became concerned and moved to have a guardian appointed. A man disturbed by his 65-year-old mother's liaison with a traveling salesman and her generous gifts of money to him, petitioned the court to have a guardian appointed for his mother. Both women contested guardianship and jury trials resulted.

The primary clinical problem in such cases is estimation of judgment. There may be evidence of minor defects in recent memory and occasional behavioral errors, such as writing a check on the wrong bank or forgetting to pay a bill, but lack of evidence of personality deterioration or significant defects in business and social judgment. A full psychological test battery yields reliable evidence of the defendant's competency (see the description of such psychological tests in Chapter 31). My inclination, and that of the law, is to support the subject's freedom.

Medical Malpractice Cases

In the light of the current malpractice involvements, it seems incumbent on the medical profession to better its past performance in the art of self-policing, to break its traditional "conspiracy of silence," and to expose the incompetent practice of colleagues. Many malpractice suits are petty, ill-advised, or opportunistic; some are legitimate. We are currently involved in seven such suits, three against surgeons and four against psychiatrists and psychiatric hospitals. In two cases we are appearing for the doctor, and in two others we have advised the attorneys concerned that we consider their client's case against the physician to be very weak. The crucial question in all such cases is, did the doctor or the hospital deviate significantly from a generally accepted standard of care?

The four psychiatric cases involved patients' suicides and, again, there is no patient to question. The procedure is the "psychological autopsy," including interviewing those with pertinent evidence to give, perusal of records, and preparation of a hypothetical question. The particular burden in such cases is how one substantiates and documents "a standard of care," and demonstrates that if the proper standard had been adhered to, suicide might have been prevented.

As an expert witness in medical malpractice suits, a psychiatrist is primarily a consultant to the legal firm, evaluating the evidence, pointing to the strengths and weaknesses regarding medical facts and ethics in the lawyer's brief, and suggesting further inquiry. The psychiatrist is not a legal investigator; it is the attorney's task to find and present the evidence.

CONCLUSION

A survey of 100 consecutive civil law litigant-patients referred to the Menninger Clinic in 1976 and 1977, reveals that all were referred by attorneys who possibly were alerted to their clients' need of psychiatric attention by the tenor of reports submitted to them from orthopedists, neurosurgeons, and other physicians: "the patient is very nervous," or, "there is a psychosomatic complication," or, "there is a functional overlay," or a similar avoidance of the term "psychiatric."

In such referrals the psychiatrist may feel a dual responsibility—to the attorney and to the patient. The psychiatrist works as an agent of the lawyer in that his clinical report becomes part of the lawyer's legal evidence. This consulting role is in a sense concretized by fee arrangements. Lawyers are aware that doctors do not accept a contingency fee and, if the client is unable to pay, it is desirable that the lawyer understand that he is responsible for the doctor's charges.

The written report to the attorney should be complete; it should inform the attorney as to what the psychiatrist can and cannot disclose if he is called into court to testify. A further advantage of a complete report is that it frequently negates the need for a court appearance. Armed with an authoritative report, the attorney may negotiate a settlement and avoid a trial. In 1975, we evaluated 15 "traumatic neurosis" cases and went to court only four times.

The report to the attorney will be shared with the opposing lawyer, the Worker's Compensation Commissioner, the judge, and even with his client. Therefore it is necessary to have the patient understand that material he wishes not divulged will be kept confidential. Such facts as that the patient was of illegitimate birth, has had an abortion, or smokes marijuana may have no bearing on matters relevant in his civil suit. Moreover, certain of the psychiatrist's speculations or educated hunches about the patient are better conveyed to the attorney orally, if at all, rather than in writing. Such imprudently dropped phrases as "latent homosexuality," "seductive hysterical character," or "sadistic fantasies" can be pursued in court by an astute cross-examining attorney to the point that their author regrets his conjectural excursion from clinical exactness.

REFERENCES

1. Prosser, W. H.: *Handbook of the Law of Torts*. ed. 3. West, St. Paul, 1964.
2. Black, H. C.: *Black's Law Dictionary*. West, St. Paul, 1951.
3. Furst, S. (ed.): *Psychic Trauma*. Basic Books, New York, 1967.
4. Kardiner, A.: *The Traumatic Neuroses of War*. National Research Council, Washington, D.C., 1941.
5. Grinker, R., and Spiegel, J.: *Men Under Stress*. Blakiston, Philadelphia, 1945.

6. Krystal, H. (ed.): *Massive Psychic Trauma.* International Universities Press, New York, 1969.
7. Taylor, J., Zercher, L., and Key, W.: *Tornado.* University of Washington Press, Seattle, 1970.
8. Special Section: Disaster at Buffalo Creek. *Am. J. Psychiatry* 133:295–316, 1976.
9. Wolfenstein, M.: *Disaster.* The Free Press, Glencoe, Ill., 1957.
10. Leopold, R. L., and Dillon, H.: Psychoanatomy of a Disaster. *Am. J. Psychiatry* 119:913–921, 1963.
11. Modlin, H.C.: The Postaccident Anxiety Syndrome: Psychosocial Aspects. *Am. J. Psychiatry* 123:1008–1012, 1967.
12. Keiser, L.: *The Traumatic Neurosis.* J. B. Lippincott, Philadelphia, 1968.
13. Laughlin, H.: *The Neuroses.* Butterworth, Washington, D.C., 1967.
14. Enelow, A.: Malingering and Delayed Recovery from Injury, in Leedy, J. (ed.): *Compensation in Psychiatric Disability and Rehabilitation.* Charles C Thomas, Springfield, Ill., 1971.
15. Slawson, P.: Compensable Psychiatric Disability and the Problem of Secondary Gain, in Leedy, J. (ed.): *Compensation in Psychiatric Disability and Rehabilitation.* Charles C Thomas, Springfield, Ill., 1971.
16. Modlin, H. C.: Accidents and Traumatic Neurosis. *Lawyers Medical Cyclopedia.* Allen Smith, Indianapolis, 1973.
17. Knight, J.: Money Attitudes in Rehabilitation, in Leedy, J. (ed.): *Compensation in Psychiatric Disability and Rehabilitation.* Charles C Thomas, Springfield, Ill., 1971.
18. Goldston, R.: The Burning and the Healing of Children. *Psychiatry* 35:57-n66, 1972.
19. Jorgensen, J., and Brophy, J.: *Psychiatric Treatment Modalities in Burn Patients.* Grune & Stratton, New York, 1975.
20. Parks, C.: Psycho-social Transitions: Comparison Between Reactions to Loss of a Limb and Loss of a Spouse. *Br. J. Psychiatry* 127:204–210, 1975.
21. Shanfield, S., and Killingsworth, R.: The Psychiatric Aspects of Pain. *Psychiat. Ann.* 7:24–35, 1977.
22. Macgregor, F., et al.: *Facial Deformity and Plastic Surgery: A Psychosocial Study.* Charles C Thomas, Springfield, Ill., 1953.
23. Watson, E. J., and Johnson, A.: The Emotional Significance of Acquired Physical Disfigurement in Children. *Am. J. Orthopsychiatry* 28:85–97, 1958.
24. Committee on Rating of Mental and Physical Impairment: Mental Illness. *J.A.M.A.* 198:1284–1293, 1966.

CHAPTER 30

A. Louis McGarry is Professor of Clinical Psychiatry at the State University of New York at Stony Brook and Director of the Division of Forensic Services at the Nassau County Medical Center in East Meadow, New York. A graduate of Harvard College and Boston University Medical School, he is a Fellow of the American Psychiatric Association and a member of the Committee on Psychiatry and Law of the Group for the Advancement of Psychiatry. Dr. McGarry is a former Associate Clinical Professor of Psychiatry at Harvard Medical School. He has also served as Assistant Commissioner of Mental Health for Legal Medicine in the Massachusetts Department of Mental Health and as Associate Professor of Legal Psychiatry in the Law-Medicine Institute at Boston University. The author of numerous professional papers and monographs, Dr. McGarry is former Chairman of the Editorial Board of the *Massachusetts Journal of Mental Health* and is currently a member of the Editorial Board of *Psychiatric Opinion*.

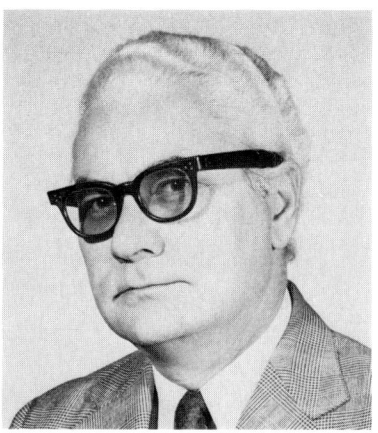

PSYCHOLEGAL EXAMINATIONS AND REPORTS*

A. Louis McGarry, M.D.

The involvement of behavioral science clinicians in legal proceedings usually begins and ends with the submission of a report either to one of the adversaries or, perhaps most frequently, to the court in the early stages of the proceedings. Psycholegal reports are of great importance and can substantially affect the outcome of legal actions.[1] This is particularly true in such proceedings as guardianship and child custody matters. The person proposed for a guardianship or conservatorship is rarely in a position to challenge the report of a psychiatrist.

This chapter is devoted to a delineation of the elements which should be covered in the preparation of such reports. I have touched on some of these elements in Chapter 26, but they bear repeating and further expansion. Briefly, what is required is as follows:

1. A clear understanding on the part of the examiner of what legal questions are being asked.
2. An understanding of the circumstances relating to the legal action, including the party for whom the examiner acts when conducting the evaluation.
3. The collection and review of relevant legal and medical documents, particularly if there have been prior hospitalizations (nurses' notes as well as physicians' notes are often of great value).
4. An adequate past history.
5. The conducting of an adequate mental status examination with particular attention to those areas of ability or disability which have relevance to the legal questions asked.

---

*This chapter was supported in part by Grant No. RO1 MH25955 from the Center for Studies of Crime and Delinquency of the National Institute of Mental Health.

6. A description of the degree to which psychic disability, if any, can be related to the legal questions asked, together with the degree of medicolegal certainty with which the examiner offers his opinion.

Psycholegal examinations may be very broad in their scope or relatively narrow (i.e., the complexity of a child custody proceeding as compared to an examination for competency to stand trial). Nevertheless, in my opinion, the elements outlined above should be adhered to. Of particular importance is the last element, relating to the degree of medicolegal certainty with which an opinion is offered. The competent expert will offer an opinion with that degree of certainty which his data will support. This can range from "no opinion," to "more likely than not," to "probably," to "within reasonable medical certainty."

A corollary to the above is that there must be adequate time for the clinician to develop the data required to form an opinion. It is recognized that clinicians involved in psycholegal examinations may indeed be overburdened, particularly those in public service. It is this fact that has been responsible for much of the justified criticism of the involvement of the behavioral-science disciplines designed to assess competency to stand trial (Fig. 30-1). In our hands, the conducting of a structured interview and completion of a one-page scoring instrument rarely took more than 1 hour.

In the interest of further understanding of these elements, four psychiatric reports are presented which exemplify them. The reader will note the use of quotations from the examinee and from other professionals, as well as written behavioral observations by hospital nurses and a focus on phenomenologic, direct behavioral description by the examiner. All of these devices, in my experience, have added to the probative value of such psycholegal reports. The following examples are of actual reports on a variety of psycholegal evaluations. Names and places have been changed to protect the privacy of the examinees and others.

TESTAMENTARY CAPACITY

The first of these reports relates to a question of testamentary capacity in an elderly widow. The facts and circumstances are delineated in the report.

Psychiatric Report

QUALIFICATIONS OF THE EXAMINER

My professional qualifications are attested to in my attached curriculum vitae. I am certified in psychiatry by the American Board of Psychiatry and Neurology.

CIRCUMSTANCES OF THE EXAMINATION

In this matter, I was retained by Attorney Schofield, who represented several of Mrs. Farfield's children other than Mrs. Hester Johnson. The examination took place at Mrs. Johnson's home, where Mrs. Farfield resides, between the hour of 10:30 a.m. to 11:30 a.m., Saturday, January 8, 1972. Present were Mrs. Farfield, myself, and Mr. Andrew Campbell, Jr., of the law firm of Brewster and Standish, who appeared to represent the

	Total	Severe	Degree of Incapacity Moderate	Mild	None	Unratable
1. Appraisal of available legal defenses	1	2	3	4	5	6
2. Unmanageable behavior	1	2	3	4	5	6
3. Quality of relating to attorney	1	2	3	4	5	6
4. Planning of legal strategy, including guilty plea to lesser charges where pertinent	1	2	3	4	5	6
5. Appraisal of role of:						
a. defense counsel	1	2	3	4	5	6
b. prosecuting attorney	1	2	3	4	5	6
c. judge	1	2	3	4	5	6
d. jury	1	2	3	4	5	6
e. defendant	1	2	3	4	5	6
f. witnesses	1	2	3	4	5	6
6. Understanding of court procedure	1	2	3	4	5	6
7. Appreciation of charges	1	2	3	4	5	6
8. Appreciation of range and nature of possible penalties	1	2	3	4	5	6
9. Appraisal of likely outcome	1	2	3	4	5	6
10. Capacity to disclose to attorney available pertinent facts surrounding the offense including the defendant's movements, timing, mental state, actions at the time of the offense	1	2	3	4	5	6
11. Capacity to realistically challenge prosecution witnesses	1	2	3	4	5	6
12. Capacity to testify relevantly	1	2	3	4	5	6
13. Self-defeating versus self-serving motivation (legal sense)	1	2	3	4	5	6

Examinee _____ Examiner _____

Date _____

FIGURE 30-1. Competency to stand trial assessment instrument.

interests of Mrs. Farfield and, possibly, those of Mrs. Johnson as well. It later appeared that although Mrs. Johnson did not remain in the examination room, she remained within hearing of the examination. This assumption rests on the fact that at the conclusion of my examination, which was not interfered with in any fashion by either Mr. Campbell or Mrs. Johnson, Mrs. Johnson abruptly appeared at a point at which Mrs. Farfield began to cry in the context of remembering her deceased husband. Mrs. Johnson proceeded to embrace and comfort her mother, and in responding to my remark that "I hoped the examination had not been too stressful," Mrs. Johnson answered, "Yes, it had been." Mrs. Johnson was gracious and courteous to this examiner throughout my stay in her home.

PURPOSES OF THE EXAMINATION

On January 30, 1970, Mrs. Farfield signed a legal instrument which was notarized by Attorney Arthur James and which is effect, as I understand it, appointed Mrs. Johnson as trustee of Mrs. Farfield's estate and awarded the entire estate to Mrs. Johnson and her two sons, John and Able Johnson, on Mrs. Farfield's death. Mrs. Johnson accepted responsibility as trustee by her signature on the instrument dated February 24, 1970. The instrument, as I understand it, comprises both a trust during Mrs. Farfield's lifetime and, in effect, a will when she dies.

With regard to the other living children of Mrs. Farfield, the trustee, Mrs. Johnson, is directed in the instrument as follows:

> "She shall not make any distribution to my children, James S. Farfield, Sr., Andrew Farfield, Jane Farnsworth, and Estelle Cermesoni. They have either been provided for or are in excellent circumstances and have no need."

In view of what they have observed and regarded as abnormal behavior and defective memory on the part of Mrs. Farfield, several of Mrs. Farfield's children retained Attorney Schofield in order to challenge Mrs. Farfield's testamentary capacity and the legal validity of the instrument of January 30, 1970.

The purpose of this examination and my review of available medical records, therefore, was to arrive at a psychiatric assessment, if possible, of Mrs. Farfield's testamentary capacity on January 30, 1970.

PREPARATION FOR THE EXAMINATION AND THE QUESTIONS TO BE ANSWERED

In preparing for the examination, I studied for 2 hours the medical records of the Mercy Hospital relating to a hospitalization there of Mrs. Farfield between December 14, 1968 and January 5, 1969, in order to assess whether there was evidence of a psychiatric disorder in Mrs. Farfield at that time, it degree, and its relevance to the legal instrument executed by her approximately 1 year later.

I also briefly studied the legal instrument signed on January 30, 1970. As I see it, the relevant questions to be answered were as follows:

1. Is Mrs. Farfield mentally incapacitated at this time and if so, to what degree is she likely to have been mentally incapacitated on January

30, 1970, and, if so, to what degree did her likely mental state on that date impair her ability to:
   a. know the natural heirs to her bounty?
   b. know that she was signing, in effect, a will?
   c. know the value and extent of her estate?
   d. know the beneficiaries of her will?
2. Since representations had been made to me by Attorney Schofield to the effect that Mrs. Farfield's trust and will was at variance with her deceased husband's will, which provided for the estate to be equally divided among his children, I elected to inquire into Mrs. Farfield's attitude toward her husband's testamentary intentions.

RELEVANT PAST PSYCHIATRIC HISTORY

The available medical history relevant to her previous psychiatric status consists of the Mercy Hospital record of Mrs. Farfield's admission there between December 14, 1968 and January 5, 1969. Based upon frequent nurses' observations of Mrs. Farfield's "confusion," the necessity to restrain her in bed on two occasions, an abnormal electroencephalogram "consistent with cerebral atrophy," and a presumptive diagnosis of "arteriosclerosis, cerebral, generalized and cortical atrophy," it is clear that a substantial organic brain syndrome was manifest in Mrs. Farfield 1 year before the disputed instrument was signed.

MENTAL STATUS

General Appearance

Mrs. Farfield, an 85-year-old widow, sat comfortably on a couch throughout the interview. She was attractively dressed in a suit and was neatly and appropriately groomed. On occasion during the interview she picked at what appeared to be a too tight garter. Her attitude was friendly and courteous. She appeared to be in good physical health except for the presence of a cane and obvious osteoarthritic changes in her hands.

Perceptions

No hallucinations were noted. Mrs. Farfield appeared to have the illusion that her two Johnson grandsons were her own sons.

Affect

Labile, shallow and, at times, inappropriate affect was noted. There was frequent chuckling, often appearing when Mrs. Farfield did not understand a question or could not come up with an answer. Affect ranged to open weeping associated with the memory of her husband.

Thought Processes

There was a good deal of circumstantiality and some loose associations, usually in the relating of family events and memories.

Thought Content

Two themes kept re-emerging, particularly when Mrs. Farfield's associations would wander. One had to do with the virtues of those family members that she could remember (specifically, her husband, her daughter, Mrs. Johnson, and Mrs. Johnson's two sons); the second concerned her comfort and satisfaction with her living arrangements with her daughter: "I couldn't live without Hessie. This is my home." And, "I have a beautiful thing here."

Memory

This was strikingly defective. Mrs. Farfield could not give me the names of her living children other than Mrs. Johnson (Hessie), and when their names were read to her, she did not remember who they were (although she did correct my pronunciation of Mrs. Cermesoni's name). Her other children's names were misidentified by her as "cousin" or "not related," or, "He'd come home nightly and help my father." Further reference was made to the "others" (not otherwise identified) who were described as "rich" and not in need of money. The names Mrs. Farfield finally produced as the names of her "eight or ten" children were "Harry, Wilber, Billy, and Alice." These do not correspond to the names listed as those of her actual children, and unless they are nicknames, I am assuming that they are either misidentified persons or bad guesses. Finally, when asked if John and Henry (also apparently identified as "Harry"), the two Johnson children, were her sons or her grandsons, she replied that they were her "sons" and the "sons of my husband."

Orientation

Mrs. Farfield knew that I was a doctor and that she was living with her daughter "Hessie," whom she clearly knew. Beyond this, as documented above, there was gross disorientation as to persons, notably for her children other than Mrs. Johnson.

Judgment

Based largely on the severe defects in her memory, Mrs. Farfield must be regarded as obviously defective in her judgment. For example, when she was asked if she would keep her will consistent with her husband's intentions, she answered, "I'd go right by his," whereas it appears that she has substantially changed what are represented to be her husband's testamentary intentions. When asked, "Did you change his will?" she answered, "Of course I wouldn't."

Intelligence

Mrs. Farfield clearly manifested a severe degree of intellectual deterioration. Simple repetitive questions were often not understood, and when asked for expansion on statements she did make, she was unable to understand or expand, even when her own words were repeated for her.

Summary and Diagnosis

At the time of examination, Mrs. Farfield manifested severe defects in memory, intelligence, orientation, affect, and judgment which are characteristic of a moderately severe organic brain syndrome.

My diagnosis is psychosis with cerebral arteriosclerosis.

Answers to the Formulated Questions

Mrs. Farfield is severely mentally incapacitated at this time. Based on the antecedent history of symptoms and medical findings which antedated her signing of the instrument of January 30, 1970, it is within reasonable medical certainty that she was mentally incapacitated on that date to a severe degree.

1. Mrs. Farfield does not know the natural heirs to her bounty at this time, and it is likely that there was a severe degree of impairment of this knowledge on January 30, 1970.
2. Mrs. Farfield knows that she signed, in effect, a will and remembers that Attorney Arthur James "made the will." She estimates that this will was "five years ago."
3. Mrs. Farfield appears to know roughly the value of her property, "eighty thousand dollars." According to Attorney Schofield, the value is $100,000.
4. Mrs. Farfield knows that her will provides that her daughter Hessie (Hester Johnson) and her "sons" "John and Harry" (also called "Henry" by Mrs. Farfield) are the beneficiaries of her will.

Clearly, assuming that her husband's will provided otherwise, Mrs. Farfield is not aware and does not intend that her will should be different from that which her husband had intended. This unawareness of her husband's intentions is very likely to have been present on January 30, 1970.

Summary

In my opinion, within reasonable medical certainty, Mrs. Farfield does not have the testamentary capacity at this time to make a valid will. In my opinion, there is very serious doubt that she had the testamentary capacity to make a valid will on January 30, 1970.

GUARDIANSHIP

The second case relates to a question of guardianship of an 80-year-old retired businessman with a substantial estate. The facts and circumstances are recorded in the report.

Psychiatric Report

QUALIFICATIONS OF THE EXAMINER

My curriculum vitae is attached. I am certified in psychiatry by the American Board of Psychiatry and Neurology. I am licensed to practice medicine in this state.

CIRCUMSTANCES OF THE EXAMINATION

Mr. Goldman was examined for 1 hour at his apartment on Saturday, February 24, 1973. The purpose of the examination was to inquire whether Mr. Goldman is mentally ill, and whether by reason of such mental illness a permanent guardianship is required for his protection. The examiner was retained by Miss Ella Goldman, Mr. Goldman's daughter (and temporary guardian), and by her attorneys, Mrs. James Levine and Mr. Peter Platt. In preparation for the examination, the medical and psychiatric records of Mr. Goldman's hospitalizations at the Memorial General Hospital (covering 1969 through January 1973) and the Johnson Hospital (January and February 1973) were reviewed by this examiner for 2 hours.

RELEVANT PAST HISTORY

In July 1969, Mr. Goldman had a carcinoma of the rectum resected, and he has lived since with a colostomy. Three days postoperative of this resection, Mr. Goldman had an episode of mental illness, documented in the hospital record, characterized by confusion, suicidal ideation, and paranoid thinking regarding his wife. This apparently cleared up after discharge from the hospital.

In January 1971, he had an episode of left hemiparesis from which he made a good functioning recovery. However, by the fall of 1972, Mr. Goldman suffered from increasing weakness in his legs, such that he had to be confined to a wheel chair. There were a number of admissions to the Memorial General Hospital for the purpose of diagnosing and correcting a recurrent fever of unknown origin. Ultimately, by radioactive liver scan, the diagnosis of metastatic carcinoma to the right lobe of the liver was confirmed on November 16, 1972. Subsequently, both Mr. Goldman and his daughter were informed as to the nature of Mr. Goldman's illness by the attending physician, Dr. Palmer, to the effect that (1) "His illness is very serious;" (2) "It may be related to the operation;" and (3) "I emphasized that it would not get better." At the time, Mr. Goldman indicated that he understood Dr. Palmer by nodding his head affirmatively.

In terms of recent psychiatric history during his hospitalizations in November 1972 and January 1973 at the Memorial General Hospital, there were two well-documented episodes of acute psychosis. On these occasions, two psychiatrists (Doctors Litner and Bragg) and Mr. Goldman's attending physician, Dr. Palmer, described these episodes in the record. The symptoms included allegations of infidelity by his wife, illusions, disorientation, and defective reality testing. Dr. Bragg, a psychiatrist who has examined Mr. Goldman on several occasions in the recent past, wrote on January 13, 1973, that "He has deteriorated physically and mentally since my last contact with him four months ago. He is quite suspicious (paranoid), at times disoriented with reality testing impaired." Dr. Litner, on November 11, 1972, and Dr. Palmer, on January 12, 1973, recorded their opinions in the record to the effect that Mr. Goldman was incompetent to manage his affairs.

In later January and early February 1973, Mr. Goldman had a brief voluntary admission at the Johnson Mental Hospital, which was subsequently terminated by Mr. Goldman. Johnson petitioned for the involuntary commitment of Mr. Goldman, but voided this petition by discharging Mr. Goldman prior to the scheduled judicial hearing. By this time, Miss Goldman, through her attorney, Mr. Levine, had succeeded in obtaining a temporary guardianship over her father. According to an extract of the Johnson Hospital records on Mr. Goldman, prepared by Attorney Platt, a Dr. Henderson of the Johnson staff wrote in a memo dated January 26, 1973, that "Family is prepared to file for guardianship which seems appropriate for this depressed, panicky man with inadequate judgment and periods of confusion and disorientation with some [paranoia]."

Mr. Goldman is currently married for the second time, although he and his current wife are separately domiciled. His first wife died in 1965 after a prolonged illness (Parkinson's disease). Two children were born of the first marriage: Alan, who died in World War II, and Ella, who has lived abroad for most of the last 19 years, but who returned to be with her father in mid-January 1973. Mr. Goldman has one living sibling, a brother, Jonathan, who lives in Florida. At the time of the examination, Mr. Goldman was living alone in his apartment with round-the-clock nursing coverage.

PRELIMINARY CONSULTATION WITH MISS ELLA GOLDMAN

This examiner was met in the apartment house lobby on the day of the examination of Mr. Goldman by his daughter, Ella, and her companion, Edwardo. According to Miss Goldman, her father had become extremely angry at her and suspicious of both her and Mr. Levine, formerly Mr. Goldman's attorney and now representing Miss Goldman. This anger and suspicion centered around both the hospitalization at Johnson and the temporary guardianship proceedings.

During the first two of the previous five days, Miss Goldman reported that her father had been extremely agitated and confused. Three days before my visit, however, Mr. Goldman had been placed on heavy dosage of the tranquilizer Valium, and associated with this, he had been relatively calm.

Miss Goldman further expressed her concern about the possible impending visit to Mr. Goldman by his brother, Jonathan. According to Miss Goldman, Jonathan's recent contacts with her father had been very disturbing to him. Jonathan's visits to Mr. Goldman at Johnson had been characterized in the Johnson record as "intrusive" and a "disquieting influence on the patient." According to Attorney Platt, this led to the hospital's limiting the length of Jonathan's visits to Mr. Goldman.

THE EXAMINATION AND MENTAL STATUS

Mr. Goldman was asleep when I arrived at the apartment. He was awakened by the attending nurse. I introduced myself as a psychiatrist and identified myself as having been sent by his daughter and her attorneys, Mr. Levine and Mr. Platt. I further explained that my visit related to the "guardianship business."

General Appearance

Mr. Goldman is 80 and appears physically to be a very ill man. A moderate ptosis on the left eyelid was noted. He remained on his back in bed under a blanket throughout the interview, dressed in a stained blue formal shirt. There was extreme psychomotor retardation. Movements and speech were sluggish and halting. At times his speech was inaudible. His full moustache was neatly groomed, but there appeared to be about a day's growth of unshaven facial hair. During the interview, the nurse retired to the next room.

Despite the psychomotor retardation, he was in good contact. One sensed, however, a certain guardedness, or at least reluctance or inability to pursue any subject in any depth. For example, in answer to the question, "Do you understand about this guardianship business?" he said, "No I don't care to." In response to a comment from me that Mr. Levine was vacationing in the Virgin Islands, he said, "Let him stay there." Later, on my returning to the guardianship issue, he called it a "put-up job" but would not elaborate. With respect to an inquiry on my part regarding his financial affairs, he told me to "ask Mr. Adams at the First National Bank." In short, his responses had the effect of closing off inquiry in any depth on virtually any subject that was broached. The single exception to this was some expansion on his 18-month service in the Navy as a Chief Petty Officer (Commissary) during World War I.

Thought Content and Processes

As reflected by Mr. Goldman's responses, thought content at the time of the examination tended to be concrete and superficial with little in the way of elaboration or association. No delusions were elicited. There are paranoid ideation and delusions by history.

Perception

Mr. Goldman misread the time on his watch, although he had his glasses on, reading 3 o'clock instead of the actual 12:15. No illusions or hallucinations were noted or elicited. However, there are illusions by history in which Mr. Goldman interpreted sounds outside his hospital room as sexual activity between doctors and nurses.

Affect

As noted above, there was extreme psychomotor retardation reflective of a sad and depressed mood. Affect remained constricted with a single exception on the mention of Mr. Goldman's dead son, Alan, at which point his face abruptly contorted and he cried for several minutes.

Memory

Distant memory did not appear to be impaired, at least with respect to Mr. Goldman's Navy days. Neither did recent memory appear impaired. He recalled accurately what he had had for breakfast and remembered that his brother Jonathan was about to visit from Florida. This proved to be the case. The brother arrived as I left.

Orientation

Mr. Goldman thought it was Sunday (it was Saturday), but otherwise there appeared to be no defect in orientation as to time, place, or person during the examination.

Intelligence

Due to Mr. Goldman's underresponsiveness and concreteness, it was difficult to assess his intelligence. My impression is that he is of at least average and probably above-average intelligence.

Insight and Judgment

During the interview I did not elicit any significant defects in judgment. However, Mr. Goldman's recorded medical and psychiatric history of the last few months indicates that his judgment at times is very poor. His daughter reports that he recently sold some valuable books for $13,000 which were easily worth $25,000. He has spoken of unrealistic, indeed in view of his weakened physical state, dangerous plans to go to Spain to do business in art.

His recorded delusions regarding his wife's infidelity, his dismissal of his formerly trusted attorney and friend of 50 years and what appears to be the unwarranted castigation and suspicion of his daughter, all raise very serious doubts as to his judgment.

There is little evidence that Mr. Goldman has any significant insight into his pathological behavior. Rather, he is reacting to his tragic situation with denial, projection, avoidance, and episodic dementia.

Diagnosis

My diagnosis is depressive reaction, with paranoid features and episodic acute organic brain syndrome.

Formulation

Although this examination, in and of itself, elicited relatively mild pathology, the recent history is replete with episodes of serious psychological pathology in Mr. Goldman. I see him at best maintaining an extremely fragile balance which is highly vulnerable to intercurrent physiological and psychological stress with recurrent episodes of psychotic thinking and behavior resulting. With the inevitable physical deterioration which he faces, it is very probable that his psychological functioning will continue to deteriorate as well. In my opinion, it is necessary for his own welfare that he be protected in body and estate from making ill-advised testamentary and personal decisions which may be based on episodic psychotic thinking.

EXAMINER AS AGENT OR IMPARTIAL EXPERT

Of great importance in the preparation of psycholegal examinations and reports is the question of which party the examiner represents and what use is then made of the report. Subtle and not so subtle issues emerge in this context. If the examiner is hired by an adversary, then the adversary will obviously have his own purposes in mind and will want the examiner to support these purposes. The adversary or his attorney may wish the report to be modified and certain findings stressed. If the examiner can technically accept such modifications, this is acceptable, but there is a point beyond which so much violence can be done to the original findings that it becomes unethical. The adversary who has hired the expert may choose not to use the report if it does not adequately serve his purposes, and that is his right. Those examiners in a particular community who are excessively accommodating to those who hire them do not go unnoticed in the medical and legal professions, and their credibility obviously suffers, as it should. (These issues are further discussed in Chapter 17 concerning courtroom presentation.)

A more desirable model, in my experience, is the appointment of an examiner acceptable to both sides in an adversary proceeding. Appropriate stipulations as to the payment of the fee and to the effect that both sides will receive the report and may use or not use it as they choose can also be worked out. This avoids the ethical issues raised above.

In the public service area where the examiner is paid by governmental sources, the impartial expert model suggested above is generally the case. The examiner is the agent of the judge or the court and need not deal with the problem of accommodation to the purposes of either adversary. This model has been criticized in view of the observation that no one is completely impartial. Psychiatrists, for example, are usually defense-minded in criminal proceedings. In my opinion, the competent, ethical, mental health professional should not have difficulty with either model. What matters is that the quality of the examination be high and that it be based upon adequate, accurate data.

COMPETENCY TO STAND CRIMINAL TRIAL

The following two reports relate to psychiatric examinations on the issue of competency to stand criminal trial. In terms of the impact on the lives and freedom of people, this issue is most important. Many thousands of defendants are affected each year. Accurate aggregate data are not currently available, but in Massachusetts alone, with a population of about 6 million, about 1000 people a year are hospitalized for competency determinations.

Psychiatric Report No. 1

QUALIFICATIONS OF THE EXAMINER

My curriculum vitae is attached. Briefly, I am fully licensed to practice medicine in this state. I am certified in psychiatry by the American Board of Psychiatry and Neurology, and I have been designated a qualified physician for forensic matters in this state.

CIRCUMSTANCES AND PURPOSES OF THE EXAMINATION

James C. Colburn is accused of first-degree murder. By reason of recent bizarre behavior on his part, a question of his competency to stand trial has again been raised as it has on a number of occasions in the past. On or about April 12, 1974, I was contacted by Assistant District Attorney Cameron who requested that I examine Mr. Colburn on the question of his competency to stand trial. After a brief telephone discussion about the facts of the case, I agreed to participate. Mr. Cameron had certain written materials (which will be described below) delivered to me late on the same day. During the following weekend I studied these materials. On Tuesday, April 16, 1974, I talked to Assistant District Attorney Cameron. At that time I indicated that I preferred not to be called by either of the adversaries in the case, but rather to be appointed by the Court as an expert under the provisions of Massachusetts General Law, Chapter 123, Section 19. Mr. Cameron agreed to this and indicated that he would arrange for such an order of appointment by the Court.

After confirming through Mr. Colburn's social worker at the state hospital at Bridgewater, where Mr. Colburn was and is currently hospitalized, that Mr. Colburn would be willing to be examined by me, I proceeded to Bridgewater on Thursday, April 18, 1974.

Finally, it should be noted that the two most recent psychiatric examinations of Mr. Colburn (by Dr. Arthur Consuelo of Bridgewater, on April 2, 1974, and by Dr. Michael Galvin, on or about March 15, 1974) indicated that Mr. Colburn was now incompetent to stand trial by reason of mental illness.

DOCUMENTS REVIEWED

In preparation for my examination of Mr. Colburn, I studied various clinical and legal records. These included the extensive clinical file at Bridgewater pertaining to Mr. Colburn (his current admission is his fourth there), a summary of the State's case against Mr. Colburn, a previous psychiatric report on Mr. Colburn, dated May 10, 1973, by Dr. Eugene Barnes, and certain other legal documents pertaining to Mr. Colburn's current hospitalization. I spent 5 to 6 hours reviewing these documents prior to my examination of Mr. Colburn at Bridgewater.

RELEVANT PAST PSYCHIATRIC HISTORY

Prior to the current admission at Bridgewater, Mr. Colburn had been admitted there on three previous occasions in connection with criminal proceedings against him (1966, 1971, and 1973). He has also been a patient at the Metropolitan State Hospital in the past (1953, 1956, and briefly on a voluntary in 1965). Two of the three Metropolitan State Hospital admissions were in connection with alleged delinquent or criminal acts. On all of these prior hospitalizations, Mr. Colburn was found to be competent to stand trial and on all of these occasions he was diagnosed as a personality disorder of varying types, predominantly that of a passive-aggressive or antisocial type. On no occasion was he found to by psychotic. Mr. Colburn has a fairly extensive criminal history largely consisting of alleged and convicted assaults on women.

RECENT RELEVANT PSYCHIATRIC HISTORY

I think it most useful to give a chronology or description of Mr. Colburn's recent behavior which gave rise to the renewed question of his competency to stand trial. It begins on March 6, 1974, at the end of a visit from the mother of his infant son, Ms. Johnson, in the Billerica House of Correction visiting room. After what was described as a "cheerful and light" conversation, Mr. Colburn reportedly seized Ms. Johnson, announced that he "wanted to kill himself" and "that he was going to take her down with him." Using "a homemade ice pick," he allegedly inflicted what apparently were superficial lacerations on her before he was restrained. Shortly afterward he allegedly assaulted a correctional officer. Later that day, on examination by a physician whose name is illegible, Mr. Colburn was described as "polite, coherent, and well-oriented. He shows no clear evidence of delusions and hallucinations or psychosis . . . He appears very much in control of himself and was appropriately guarded, but laughed most inappropriately and complained of chest and abdominal pains. . . ."

Subsequently, on March 16, 1974, the defendant was readmitted to Bridgewater for the fourth time. On March 18, 1974, in a note dictated over the telephone, Dr. Michael Galvin reported that in his opinion Mr. Colburn was "paranoid" and "vain and narcissistic and that he feels his lawyer is part of the system" and is "not competent."

In a long staff note describing a conference attended by Bridgewater clinical staff, dated April 2, 1974, Dr. Arthur Consuelo described an emotional outburst at the staff by Mr. Colburn when he was "in tears, anxious and depressed. . . ." Dr. Consuelo, concluding that the defendant was a "passive-aggressive personality, aggressive type, decompensating into schizophrenic reaction, paranoid type," found him to be incompetent to stand trial. It is noted that Mr. Colburn was placed on tranquilizer medication at that time—Thorazine, 200 mg daily, and Stelazine, 10 mg twice daily.

On or about April 16, 1974, in the visiting room, Mr. Colburn abruptly manifested a "crick" or spastic neck. This was attributed to the side effects of medication and so treated. At this time, Dr. Ronald James, at the request of the district attorney's office, was examining Mr. Colburn.

PSYCHIATRIC EXAMINATION

Mr. Colburn abruptly terminated my examination of him after, at most, 5 minutes of interview time. Despite its brevity, in my opinion, the examination has significant clinical and probative value.

As I approached Mr. Colburn in the visiting area of the Bridgewater State Hospital, accompanied by a correction officer, the defendant was sitting on a bench in a rigid position, looking straight ahead with a fixed stare. When I introduced myself to him, he was initially unresponsive, then turned his head toward me and slowly said in a rather vague tone of voice, "Dr. Barnes . . . Dr. James. . . ." I reminded him that his social worker had gotten consent from him the day before for me to examine him. At this point his demeaner abruptly changed and he stood up with alacrity, moving toward an interviewing room. The officer who noted the odd behavior of the defendant suggested that the interview take place in the large visiting room in sight of several correctional officers, rather than in the relatively secluded interview room.

As the interview opened, I again identified myself, and I reiterated that he did not have to speak to me if he chose not to. I further explained that I had been asked by the Court to examine him on the question of whether he could adequately assist in his defense and protect himself. Abruptly at this point, he took over the questioning. His manner, speech, and facial expression were quite hostile. He asked me what Dr. Consuelo had decided about his competency. I answered. Then he asked about Dr. Galvin's opinion. I answered. He then asked me about Dr. James' opinion. I told him I did not know. He said, "Yes you do, you're both from the Court, you talked to each other." Then he said, "I don't want to talk with you. I'm afraid of you. Someone is trying to poison me. You may be the one who wants to poison me." At this point I asked him if he wanted to go back for trial. He answered, "Yes, I do," and then I tried to inquire into his relationship with his lawyer. He said, "I'm not interested in that," and then a second time, "Somebody wants to poison me." I said, "Well, I repeat, you don't have to talk to me, but it does make a rather wasted trip for me." He retorted rather sharply, "You get paid. It's a nice, beautiful day for a drive in the country." He then stood up abruptly with a questioning gesture, opened his hands, and said, "I'm all set. No more questions. I've seen too many doctors," and returned to the seat on the bench where I initially encountered him. I went to the other end of the long visiting room, but I was able to note that Mr. Colburn had returned to his rigid, staring posture. This attitude was totally at variance with Mr. Colburn's behavior during the interview, at which time his movements and gestures were quite natural and normal. At this point, one of the officers noted that "He has the zombie look." Another officer added, "He was all right when we brought him up here."

Because of the brevity of the interview and my not being able to do a full mental status examination or to explore the substantive issues of competency, I elected, at this point, to interview one of the correctional officers on the defendant's ward so that I could get a more longitudinal picture of the defendant's behavior. Officer James Ward of H Ward met me in the visiting room. Mr. Ward told me that Mr. Colburn, during the many hours that he had observed him on H Ward, was "a good worker, very cooperative, very polite, does odd jobs on the ward, very diligent, in a good mood most of the time, has friends, gets along good with the other patients." To my question as to whether he had ever noticed anything "odd" about Mr. Colburn, he answered, "No, he's just the same as the last time he was here."

SUMMARY AND OPINIONS

Given the brevity of the direct examination of the defendant, Mr. Colburn, I have been forced to rely on the fortunately extensive historical and descriptive data available from others in order to reach an opinion which is within reasonable medical certainty.

Based upon the multivariant, bizarre behavior of this man from March 6, 1974 until April 18, 1974, I am unable to integrate a reasonable psychiatric hypothesis, which I could defend, which would lead to a diagnosis of one or more mental illnesses in the defendant. There are a plethora of symptoms, but they do not hang together clinically; they are inconsistent, unsustained, contradictory, and most unlikely to exist in the same mentally ill person over the time period which I have described in some detail in the report. The only clinical conclusion that I can reach is that this is a desperate man seeking desperately, but in an unsophisticated fashion, to demonstrate that he is mentally ill. In my opinion he is not mentally ill, and the symptomatology and behavior I have described yield the only viable clinical conclusion—that Mr. Colburn is feigning mental illness.

Observations of this man move from suicidal behavior to homicidal behavior, to inappropriate laughter, to chest and abdominal pain, to paranoid statements regarding the system of criminal justice, to paranoid thinking about defense counsel, to tears and anxiety in an emotional outburst, to neck spasm (possibly valid), to the total opposite of all this discharge of emotion—that of an emotionless, dazed, staring, rigid, catatonic performance—and finally, to his at least twice repeated paranoid delusions regarding poison.

I use the word "performance" above because my few minutes with Mr. Colburn were instructive. He began as a mute, distant, physically rigid person and abruptly became a sharply retorting, naturally moving, poison-fearing, hostile interviewee, only then to return to a catatonic-like appearance. This episode is completely inconsistent with clinical reality. Neither the catatonic schizophrenic nor the psychotically depressed person nor certain organic or toxic states, all of which could be the basis of such bizarre withdrawn behavior, are consistent with popping out of such a state for 5 minutes and then popping back in. It just doesn't happen with the truly mentally ill.

It is noteworthy that Mr. Colburn's most bizarre behavior is reserved for the most public places, such as visiting rooms and staff conferences, and is reserved, for the most part, for examining clinicians. On his ward with only custodial staff observing his behavior, he is ostensibly normal. He may well carry his performance into the courtroom.

My opinion is that his man is malingering. It is highly likely that he is just as competent to stand trial now as he has been repeatedly in the past. I see no valid grounds at this time to support a finding of incompetency to stand trial.

Diagnosis

My diagnosis is personality disorder, antisocial personality. In my opinion the defendant, James C. Colburn, has a rational as well as factual understanding of the nature of the criminal proceedings against him, is aware of his position and his peril with relation to these proceedings, and is able to adequately assist counsel in his defense if he chooses to exercise such ability.

Psychiatric Report No. 2

QUALIFICATIONS OF THE EXAMINER

The curriculum vitae of the examiner is attached. Briefly, I am board certified to practice psychiatry. I am licensed to practice medicine in this state. I am an Associate Clinical Professor of Psychiatry at the University Medical School.

PURPOSE OF THE EXAMINATION

I examined Mr. Clifton at the request of Judge Gordon of the Municipal Court and with the concurrence of both prosecution and defense counsel in a criminal case currently being litigated against Mr. Clifton. According to Assistant District Attorney Hier, Judge Gordon is specifically concerned about (1) the degree, if any, of Mr. Clifton's short-term memory loss and (2) the effect such short-term loss, if any, will have on his competency to stand trial. The purpose of the examination, therefore, was a psychiatric assessment of Mr. Clifton's competency to stand trial at the present time with particular reference to the memory deficit mentioned above.

MATERIALS REVIEWED

In preparation for this examination, I reviewed a letter, dated November 29, 1976, from Andrew P. Hier, Assistant District Attorney, which briefly outlined the alleged facts of the criminal action which has been taken against Mr. Clifton. I also reviewed a letter from Andrew Foley, defense counsel for Mr. Clifton, in which he added certain facts not mentioned in the communication from Mr. Hier. Finally, through the good offices of Mr. Foley, I reviewed the most recent case law on the subject of competency to stand trial and not guilty by reason of insanity, as reflected in *Commonwealth v. Paul H. Kostka*.

MENTAL STATUS EXAMINATION

General Appearance

Mr. Clifton was accompanied to the interview by his wife, and she sat with the examiner. Mr. Clifton, an attorney, was a neatly and appropriately groomed, 87-year-old man carrying a cane, but with a fairly firm, assured gait. He was wearing glasses and had a bandage over his nose due to some recent minor surgery. As he greeted me, he asked whether I was related to Bernie Jameson, a well-known Boston figure. Mr. Clifton's bearing was for the most part dignified and appropriate. He related to the examiner in a direct though somewhat guarded manner. Frequently, he looked to his wife for assistance in responding to questions. At my request, however, his wife desisted from answering for him most of the time.

Perceptions

No abnormalities were noted; neither were illusions or hallucinations.

Affect

Although for the most part composed, there were several occasions where Mr. Clifton broke into shallow, tearful emotionality. These episodes were of short duration.

Thought Processes

Mr. Clifton was quite concrete in his thinking. For example, when asked what habeas corpus meant, his answer was "body or person." I found no evidence of delusions or looseness of association. There was a tendency for him to be somewhat garrulous with respect to old acquaintances and colleagues.

Thought Content

A persistent theme was Mr. Clifton's total denial of any wrongdoing in connection with his case. He was quite resistant to discussing the case or any of the alleged facts of the case. He even denied initially that there was such a case against him. Later, however, he went into some detail with respect to his version of the history of the trust arrangement, its origins, and the motivation of the complainant. A second theme that was noted could be described as name-dropping of various judicial and other well-known Boston citizens.

Orientation

Mr. Clifton knew my name and addressed me by name a number of times during the interview. He knew that I was a physician, and he knew the Court had authorized the examination and expressed a willingness to cooperate. He could tell me that it was afternoon, but could not give the hour. He knew the month, but not the date. He could give me his address and was able to describe accurately various locations in the town of Dover where he lived for many years. It is clear, however, that he required the assistance of his wife in finding my office.

Memory

Mr. Clifton's recent memory appears to be substantially impaired. However, the defects in memory are somewhat selective, and it is difficult to determine whether one is dealing with resistance or evasiveness with particular respect to the criminal proceedings in which he is engaged. On the one hand, he denied being involved in a criminal matter altogether, but then later when I asked about the last time he had seen Judge Gordon, he reported "about a month ago when they were trying me." However, he quickly disclaimed any knowledge of the trial, stating, "I haven't got anything to say on that," despite his reference to a trial proceeding in his prior response. Again inconsistently, at one point he denied knowing anything about the alleged facts of the case and then subsequently made the following statement: "She claims I have her money and I haven't got her money." When asked about the fact that John (Mr. Clifton's son) had offered money, his answer was, "He wanted to dispose of the matter, that's all." I have gone on at length here to try to demonstrate the inconsistency and selectivity of Mr. Clifton's memory loss. Nevertheless, I have no question in my mind that there is memory loss of a substantial degree. For example, although he could remember my name consistently throughout the interview, he was unable to remember the name of his attorney, even though his attorney's name was mentioned several times.

His distant memory, however, was much less affected than his recent memory. He was able to describe events in his early life, high school graduation, time spent in the Army during World War I, and the two offices that he used during his 60 years as a practicing attorney. He also remembered the telephone number of his former law office.

Intelligence

Although as indicated, Mr. Clifton tends to be concrete and simplistic in his answers, he continues to show evidence of a man who obviously had been active in professional life. When I attempted to question him about his case using a hypothetical model, he responded, "Of course we used hypotheticals, but it is not appropriate in this situation." In my opinion there is some deterioration in intelligence of this man, but it is not of a profound degree.

Insight

Mr. Clifton is very aware of his failing faculties. He said, "My brain has deteriorated" and added, "What do you do for a bullfighter when he can no longer be in the ring?"

Diagnosis

My diagnosis is nonpsychotic organic brain syndrome with senile brain disease.

OPINION REGARDING COMPETENCY TO STAND TRIAL

The principal question here is whether Mr. Clifton's defect in recent memory so compromises his capacity to assist counsel in his defense that he would be unable to bring before the Court a defense which might be available if his memory were not so compromised. This defect would assume greater or lesser importance, depending on whether the facts in this case, established through records, can be developed independently of Mr. Clifton's participation. As I have indicated in the mental status examination above, Mr. Clifton's defect in recent memory appears to be rather selective and has the effect of avoiding participation in the legal proceedings against him. I am of the opinion that if Mr. Clifton chose to, he could more actively participate. He appears to have taken the stance that if he ignores these matters, they will somehow be resolved without his acting or accepting any possibility of wrongdoing on his part. Of course, the ultimate decision about whether Mr. Clifton is competent or not rests with the Court. It is my opinion that Mr. Clifton is more likely than not to be competent to stand trial at this point in time, based upon examination of him, and considering the alleged facts of the case. The latter consideration, it seems to me, is relevant in the sense that the alleged facts of this case are of a relatively simple matter to litigate as compared, for example, to the complexity of a tax fraud case.

Usually requests or orders for psychiatric evaluations of competency to stand trial are broadly put. The examining psychiatrist is in the position of conducting a comprehensive evaluation with a complete mental status examination and then articulating the way or ways discerned ego deficits impinge on the ability of the defendant to understand the nature of the proceedings and rationally to assist counsel in his defense. What is required is the translating of psychiatric data into a legally useful report. My early experience in observing competency for trial examinations made it abruptly clear that a global, simplistic, medical standard was being applied, and this standard was the presence or absence of psychosis.[2] It uniformly followed that the psychotic was incompetent according to the examining psychiatrist, and the nonpsychotic, including the moderately retarded, was declared competent. American case law has rejected the equating of psychosis and trial competency.[3]

What was even more important was that neither the legal profession nor the psychiatrists involved made any attempt to translate the psychiatric findings into concepts which would permit meaningful communication between the two professions. Accordingly, this author and colleagues, as a part of a research study[4] on competency to stand trial, set about to design an instrument which would facilitate such communication. The approach to this task was interdisciplinary, involving psychiatrists, lawyers, and psychologists. The competency-assessment instrument we developed, along with a handbook,[5] has been published in various sources (see Fig. 30-1).[6]

We surveyed all of the legal grounds for a finding of incompetency. Ultimately 13 areas of functioning and understanding on the part of the defendant were delineated. On the assessment sheet, each area is quantitatively scored, ranging in degrees of incapacity from total, to severe, to moderate, to mild, to none. A rating of 6 is provided when the data do not permit a rating which can be adequately supported. By a process of multiple-observer, simultaneous ratings with subsequent consensus seeking, high interrater reliability (consistency) was established, even with relatively inexperienced evaluators.[7] The handbook includes three structured interview questions for each of the 13 areas of assessment with definitions of each and brief clinical examples of patients functioning at the various levels of incapacity.

The instrument provides the means of translating psychiatric data into legally relevant language and concepts and has improved communication in this legal area between mental health professionals and the courts and lawyers.

CRIMINAL RESPONSIBILITY

Forensic psychiatric reports and testimony have frequently been criticized when they have dealt with the issue of criminal responsibility. There has been a preoccupation with the language of the various legal tests* designed to guide and instruct the trier of fact in determining criminal responsibility.[8] There are difficulties here, arising, in part, because psychiatric evaluations on the issue are *ex post facto,* often weeks and even years after the alleged criminal act. First, there must be retrospectively credible corroboration in order that a valid and defensible opinion can be reached. Second, it is necessary to establish a causal relationship between any mental illness at the time of the crime and the crime itself. The third consideration which, in my view, is the most confounding of all, is that the determination of criminal responsibility is in large measure a question of morality and social policy. Such questions do not lend themselves easily to a high degree of scientific accuracy.

Despite the difficulties, I do not join with those who would eschew any role for the psychiatrist or psychologist in determining criminal responsibility. (Dr. Pollack, in Chapter 27, also provides a useful ethical discussion of the role of the psychiatrist in assessing criminal responsibility.) It is possible in retrospect to establish the existence of severe mental illness at the time of a criminal act with adequate credible and corroborative data.

There is probably greater difficulty, however, in developing a defensible opinion with respect to a causal relationship between a retrospectively established mental illness and a particular criminal act. Case law in the District of Columbia Court of Appeals[9] had been helpful in this regard where the causal connection can be established (to the jury's satisfaction) that "without which" or "but for" the existence of mental illness, the criminal act would not have taken place. More recent law[10] in the same

---

*Counsel should provide the language of which test is applicable in a given jurisdiction, together with locally relevant case law. The tests vary among jurisdictions, but, increasingly, the language developed by the American Law Institute has been adopted in the United States. It reads as follows:

A person is not responsible for criminal conduct if, at the time of such conduct, as a result of mental disease or defect he lacks substantial capacity either to appreciate the criminality of his conduct or to conform his conduct to the requirements of the law.

court, however, may have weakened the precedential weight of this yardstick of causality.

Fortunately, the question of the criminal responsibility of the mentally ill is rarely litigated. If the principles proposed in this text are adhered to, then the poor quality of psychiatric testimony on this issue can be decreased. I am quite aware that our overtaxed courts will not be pleased with the psychiatrist who will not give an opinion relating to criminal responsibility unless he is satisfied that he has adequate grounds, especially if that psychiatrist is a public servant. Yet, the criminal justice system cannot have it both ways—it cannot have credibility in psychiatrists and also have psychiatrists who always have an opinion, defensible or not.

AMNESIA

American courts have generally rejected amnesia as a basis for a finding of incompetency to stand trial or of criminal irresponsibility, largely because the condition is thought to be feigned.[11] An exception to this generalization is amnesia arising from severe head injury.[12] On those few occasions when I have been willing to offer an affirmative opinion on amnesia of psychogenic origin, as in a fugue or dissociative state, it has been noteworthy that the amnesia was not total. Scraps and flashes of the otherwise amnestic state were remembered. In contrast, the claimed amnesia of the malingerer, as well as amnesias of genuine physical origin, is total.

MALINGERING

When the suspicion of malingering is aroused, one first looks for possible secondary gain. In some jurisdictions where release procedures are onerous, a defendant is worse off after a finding of not guilty by reason of insanity, and malingering with such a plea gains little. In others, notably New York State, much more can be gained by malingering, and it is therefore a greater problem. As indicated in the sample report on James C. Colburn, naivete about clinical psychiatric syndromes, as manifested by a multiplicity of inconsistent signs and symptoms, should raise one's suspicions. Again, as in the Colburn case, it is difficult for the malingerer to sustain his feigned symptoms over prolonged periods. Often when out of sight and hearing of the mental health professionals there is a reversion to normal behavior. One should, therefore, inquire regarding behavior as observed by correction officers, attendants, other nonprofessionals, and even other patients. The bottom line, however, is that it is most often not possible to detect, within reasonable certainty, when a mental disorder is being feigned.[13]

REFERENCES

1. Balcanoff, E. J., and McGarry, A. L.: Amicus Curiae: The Role of the Psychiatrist in Pre-trial Examinations. *Am. J. Psychiatry* 126:342–347, 1969.
2. McGarry, A. L.: A Survey of Court Observation Cases at Boston State Hospital in 1960. *Boston Med. Q.* 16:59–63, 1965.
3. *State v. Severns*, 184 Kan. 213, 336, p. 2 d. 447, 452 (1959).
4. McGarry, A. L., et al.: Competency to Stand Trial and Mental Illness. Crime and Delinquency Issues: monograph Series. DHEW Publication No. (HSM) 73-9105, Washington, D.C.

5. Brooks, A. H.: *Law, Psychiatry and the Mental Health System.* Little, Brown, Boston, 1974, pp. 349–361.
6. Allen, R. C., Ferster, E. F., and Rubin, J. G. (eds.): *Readings in Law and Psychiatry.* rev. ed. The Johns Hopkins University Press, Baltimore, 1975.
7. McGarry, et al., op. cit., p. 115.
8. McGarry, A. L.: Law-Medicine Notes: Criminal Responsibility—A New Test for Massachusetts. *N. Engl. J. Med.* 278:1003–1004, 1968.
9. *Carter v. United States,* 252 F. 2d, 614; *Douglas v. United States,* 239 F, 2d, 52.
10. *United States v. Brawner,* 471 F. 2d, 969, D.C. Cir. (1972).
11. Amnesia: A Case Study in the Limits of Particular Justice. *Yale Law J.* 71:109–120, 1961.
12. *Wilson v. United States,* 391 F. 2d, 460 (D.C. Cir. 1968).
13. Rosenhan, D. L.: On Being Sane in Insane Places. *Science* 179:250–258, 1973.

CHAPTER 31

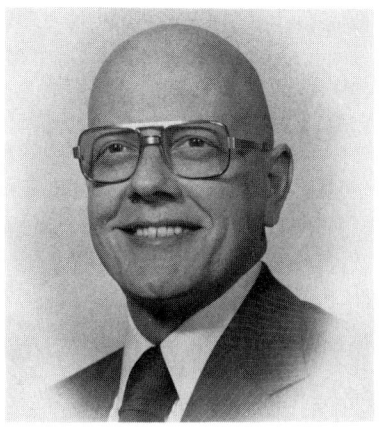

George V. C. Parker is a clinical psychologist currently in private practice in Austin, Texas. He is a former faculty member of the Department of Psychology of the University of Texas at Austin. In 1963, Dr. Parker received his doctorate at the State University of Iowa, where he was also on the faculty. He is a member of the American Psychological Association.

PSYCHOLOGICAL TESTING IN LEGAL SETTINGS*

George V. C. Parker, Ph.D.

The value of psychological testing for improving accuracy of prediction and understanding of human behavior has been widely recognized for some time. Karl Menninger has written, "The practice of psychiatry without the assistance of modern psychological testing is as old-fashioned and out-of-date as would be the practice of orthopedics without the x-ray."[1] Menninger's statement underscores the growing recognition of the degree to which psychological testing can provide significant and relevant data for professional people who are called upon to make responsible decisions having long-range effects upon the lives of other human beings.

BASIC CONCEPTS AND GUIDELINES

The function of psychological testing is the measurement of individual psychological differences in humans (i.e., the extent to which one person being tested differs from a reference group of other individuals). One of the first problems which stimulated the development of psychological tests was the identification of the mentally retarded, and even today the diagnosis of intelligence deficiency remains a major application of certain psychological tests. While there are many such tests, and numerous ways to group them, the most useful psychodiagnostic tests can be grouped into three major categories:

---

*This chapter is adapted and updated from an earlier mimeographed manuscript by Dr. Parker, entitled "A Handbook of Psychological Testing for Juvenile Court Judges" (1967), used in training programs for the judiciary. The illustrative figures have been added for this publication. Additional support was provided through Grant No. R01 MH25955 from the Center for Studies of Crime and Delinquency of the National Institute of Mental Health.

1. Tests used to measure intelligence, or general ability and its deficiencies;
2. Tests to detect brain damage;
3. Tests to assess personality, either in terms of specific traits or in overall dimensions.

PSYCHOLOGICAL TESTS DEFINED

A psychological test is essentially an objective and standardized measure of a sample of behavior. Like tests in any other science, psychological tests are observations made of a small, carefully chosen segment of an individual's behavior. The process is similar, in many ways, to that followed by a chemist who analyzes a water source on the basis of samples from it.

TEST SCORES

It is important to keep in mind that a test score obtained on the basis of standardized psychological procedures is not absolute or without some degree of error. Consequently, it is often useful to think of an individual's true score on a particular scale as being very close to (within a band on either side of) the obtained test score. For example, if an individual's obtained IQ score on the full scale of the *Wechsler Adult Intelligence Scale* is 100, it is more accurate to think of this as being the centerpoint of a range, and the individual's true score, in all likelihood, as being within a few IQ points on either side of this (i.e., a true score between 95 and 105). The reason for this, of course, is that a psychological test, like any other scaling technique, contains some small degree of error of measurement.

When psychologists refer to the question of how stable an individual's test score is, they will call it the test's reliability (i.e., how likely it is that A will obtain the same score on test X if he is retested several times over a period of time, or if he is tested by different examiners). Psychological tests vary, of course, in the extent to which they are reliable. However, the psychological tests most frequently used by qualified examiners, those of an objective, structured character, have empirically demonstrated high reliability. The more subjective, projective tests (see below) are more vulnerable to differing interpretations.

PSYCHODIAGNOSIS

When a test is used to draw conclusions about other, nontest, broader characteristics of the individual, we are interested in its diagnostic or predictive value. To the extent that a sample of behavior (test) is empirically useful in drawing accurate inferences about past, present, or future personality traits of an individual (i.e., external characteristics, or nontest criteria), the test is said to be valid for the purpose. The psychodiagnostic utility of a test is unquestionably the single most important consideration bearing on its purpose. Consequently, several points related to validity should be stressed here.

First, it should be clear that an individual's obtained score on a psychological test, in and of itself, is meaningless. If you knew only that A had a score of 25 on test X, this would not provide you with very useful information about A. If, however, you knew that A's score of 25 on this test is usually exceeded by 95 percent of other men of his age and education, and if you knew that test X is a test of general intelligence, then you would have considerably more information about *A*. Such information could then be used to make other inferences about *A* in terms of the kind of work that he would be able to do and how easily he could be trained to perform in a specified array of vocational activities. This means, of course, that it is necessary that there be an appropriate normative group with which to compare any obtained test score. For example, it would be inappropriate and unjustifiable to compare the performance of a non-English-speaking 10 year old on the *Wechsler Intelligence Scale for Children* with the performance of English-speaking students from different socioeconomic backgrounds and different cultural and educational experiences.

Finally, it must be noted that the results of no test can be useful, meaningful, or valid unless the results have been obtained by a properly trained, skilled psychological examiner. The results of such testing can be only as good as the professional competence and integrity of the psychologist making the evaluation. Inferential interpretations of such test results by a poorly trained examiner, aside from being inaccurate and useless, may indeed be misguided and harmful. A cautionary note must thus be interjected here, emphasizing that the professional qualifications of any psychological examiner employed professionally or otherwise must be unquestionable. Generally, the safest and most expeditious manner in which to assure that this is accomplished is to have such testing done directly by, or closely supervised by, a qualified clinical psychologist who has graduated from a recognized, accredited doctoral program.

MAJOR AREAS OF PSYCHOLOGICAL TESTING

The Evaluation of Intelligence

At the very foundation of psychodiagnostic testing is the evaluation of intelligence. Of great value to the clinical psychologist for diagnostic purposes is a good indication of the level of an individual's intellectual functioning. Even though not all experts agree about the definition of intelligence, it is widely held that intelligence involves the ability of the individual to integrate his present patterns of behavior, as well as his ability to modify these patterns, as a result of a new experience. In other words, the individual's intelligence is held to be related directly to his ability to profit from learning experiences. It may seem initially that intelligence is relevant only to the question of whether or not an individual is mentally retarded. In such cases the determination of intellectual level is certainly of critical importance and may very well mean the difference between whether the individual is institutionalized or permitted to attempt to make himself a member of a society which is intellectually superior to him. However, the measurement of intelligence for these purposes is but one aspect of the overall usefulness of the evaluation of intelligence in psychodiagnosis.

Through the measurement of intellectual functioning, the psychologist can study the ways in which the individual's intellectual ability is threatened by personality problems. Because different forms of pathology affect intelligence in different ways, it is diagnostically useful to have a clear picture of the present level of general ability, even though the present level of ability is not a completely accurate reflection of the true potential or ability of the individual. A variety of personality factors, such as hostility, poor motivation, lack of interest, impairment of memory, inattention, apathy, and organic deficiency, may operate to obscure the individual's real ability.

The psychologist's task is not only to measure present ability, but also to estimate potential ability and to judge accurately the reasons for any discrepancy between effective intellectual functioning and potential level of functioning. Actually there is still another way in which the measurement of intelligence is important in psychodiagnosis. It permits the psychologist to observe the individual under relatively standard conditions. By noting the individual's reactions to the various questions and tasks required by the clinical tests of intelligence, the examiner is able to see such characteristics as tolerance for frustration, perseverance, ability to maintain attention, determination, reaction to stress, emotional stability, and similar personality dimensions which may be of real significance prognostically for the court officer.

Regardless of the purpose for which the evaluation of intelligence is intended—diagnosing mental retardation, studying the effects of personality problems on intelligence, or using the test situation as a means of understanding personality dimensions—the psychologist has at hand a variety of techniques for accomplishing his purpose.

Tests of Intelligence

Tests of intelligence can be divided into two major categories: group tests and individual tests. While the group intelligence tests serve a wide variety of purposes in such settings as schools and the military, in the clinical situation the most widely used test is the individual test. The latter tests are generally much more satisfactory for the kinds of questions and diagnostic issues of relevance to courts of law.

Individual tests of intelligence which do not require the use of language (verbal behavior) are called performance tests. Those tests which depend essentially upon words and numbers are referred to as verbal tests. The most valuable and widely used clinical tests of intelligence consist of combinations of both verbal and performance subtests. Among the more widely used performance (nonverbal) tests in intellectual assessment today are the *Goodenough Draw-A-Person Test* and the *Raven Progressive Matrices Test*. The Goodenough method consists of estimating general nonverbal ability from the individual's drawing of a person. Credit points are given for various details of the body and clothing. For example, one point is given for each of the following: head, legs, arms, length of trunk greater than breadth of trunk, eyes, nose, at least two articles of clothing, fingers, leg joint, and similar details. The total number of points is then converted into a quantitative measure of intelligence. This test has a natural appeal to youngsters and is a useful way of "breaking the ground" in a diagnostic testing session. The test can provide evidence for personality functioning and conflicts as well as an intelligence estimate.

The Progressive Matrices test consists of a series of designs in each of which a part is removed, and the individual is presented with six alternative parts from which to choose the part which is missing in the original design. The instrument can be useful in measuring the person's ability to reason by analogy, to form comparisons, and to indicate his logical method of thinking. The major appeal of a strictly nonverbal test such as this is that it has considerable utility with individuals who are unable to talk. For example, where a brain trauma has led to expressive aphasia, the individual may select his correct response simply by pointing. Consequently an indication of his intelligence may be obtained without his having to talk during the examination period.

Some time ago, most clinical psychologists came to the conclusion that a more valid measure of intelligence may be obtained when both verbal and performance tasks are combined. Replacing earlier tests for the most part are the Binet tests and the Wechsler tests of intelligence. Both of these are relatively comprehensive and combine both verbal and nonverbal subtests.

THE BINET TESTS

The first of the modern intelligence tests, devised by Alfred Binet in 1905, are actually age scales in that subjects are given credits in months for tasks completed successfully. The individual's total score is the sum of the months of credit received for items passed. This total credit in months is known as the *mental age* (MA) which is, in conjunction with the individual's chronological age, converted into an intelligence quotient (IQ). Even though the Binet Scales are widely used, their diagnostic value has been limited in several ways. The most important limitation concerns the fact that the Binet tests were originally designed for working with children. As a result, the test continues to be more useful with children than with adults. Even though the scales have limited clinical usefulness beyond the determination of the intelligence quotient, they continue to be a valuable test for children under 10 years of age.

The most important diagnostic index which may be derived from the Binet Scales is scatter. Of concern is the irregularity of test performance, or the extent to which difficult items are passed while easier items are failed. The amount of scatter is generally thought to be an indication of the severity of psychopathology.

THE WECHSLER TESTS

Largely because of the shortcomings of the Binet Scales, and because of problems with the age ceiling, a new type of intelligence measure permitting better assessment of upper age levels, including adults, was devised in 1939 by David Wechsler of Bellevue Hospital in New York City. The most recent revisions of the Wechsler tests are the *Wechsler Intelligence Scale for Children–Revised* (WISC-R), which was introduced in 1974, and the *Wechsler Adult Intelligence Scale* (WAIS), introduced in 1955.

The WISC-R, which is applicable for the age of 5 years to 15 years 11 months, consists of 12 subtests, six verbal and six nonverbal. Examples of verbal subtests include: Information (Who discovered America? What is a hieroglyphic?); General Comprehension (What should you do if you see a train approaching a broken track? Why should a promise be kept?); Arithmetic (At 7¢ each, what will three cigars cost? 36 is ⅔ of what number?); Similarities (In what ways are a piano and a violin alike? In what way are liberty and justice alike?); and Vocabulary (What is the meaning of these words: letter . . . microscope . . . aseptic . . . traduce?). The Performance subtests of the WISC-R consist of a variety of scales, including the Picture Completion, in which the individual indicates what essential part is missing from a drawing; Picture Arrangement, in which the individual arranges a series of pictures to tell a logical, meaningful story; and Block Design, involving the arranging of blocks to conform with a picture model. Even though the WISC-R is available in clinical testing, it has not replaced the Binet Scales in evaluation of intelligence with children under age 10.

The WAIS is designed to be used with individuals who are older, (i.e., ages 16 and above). The subscales of the WAIS are similar in format to the WISC-R, although, of course, the demands of the tasks are greater because of the higher age of the individuals for whom it is intended. While the Binet test consists of age scales, the WISC-R and WAIS are point scales. The raw score for each subtest is converted to an equivalent weighted score, permitting direct comparison with other subtests. The individual's obtained scores may then be put upon a profile, allowing easy identification of gross subtest discrepancies and scatter. When the weighted scores are added together, the clinician can obtain three different intelligence quotients: verbal, performance, and full-scale.

The significant advantages of the Wechsler tests are: (1) the scales for teenagers and adults contain materials for, and have been standardized on, teenagers and adults; (2) an individual's performance is compared with the average for his own age group; (3) verbal and nonverbal items receive appropriate weight which permits direct comparisons between subtests; and (4) the three separate intelligence quotients permit increased flexibility in interpretation. Finally, although special training is needed to administer, score, and interpret the Wechsler tests, they are not unusually difficult or time-consuming procedures with which to obtain IQ estimates.

Educational Achievement Tests

Even though tests of educational achievement are not, strictly speaking, intelligence tests, the two do have much in common. Basically, the former focus largely upon the quality and quantity of learning reached in a specific area of study or skill (e.g., arithmetic or language comprehension). The content of both kinds of tests is similar, although intelligence tests are much broader in scope. In any event, because achievement tests can be of importance in the court psychologist's assessments, particularly of learning problems, there are several which will concern us here.

A serious problem facing a youth in the latency or adolescence period is the development of his basic academic skills. Regardless of what other problems may bring a youth to the attention of law enforcement agencies, learning problems may often play an important role in his pattern of difficulties. Indeed, authorities generally agree that learning problems may be the precursor for the emergence of serious behavioral and psychological problems.

Educational achievement tests are wide in range, and the instrument chosen in a particular case would depend largely upon the specific problem areas of concern. The sounder, more widely used batteries include the following:

> *California Achievement Tests:* Appropriate for grades 1 through 14. Tests for reading vocabulary, reading comprehension, arithmetic fundamentals, arithmetic reasoning, mechanics of English, and spelling.
> *Iowa Tests of Basic Skills:* Grades 3 to 9. Tests in vocabulary, reading comprehension, arithmetic skills, and work-study skills.
> *Metropolitan Achievement Tests:* Grades K through 9. Tests in vocabulary, reading, arithmetic, science, social studies, and study skills.
> *equential Tests of Educational Progress:* Grades 4 through college. Tests

for reading, writing, mathematics, science, social studies, listening comprehension, and essay writing.

SRA Achievement Series: Grades K through 12. Tests for reading, language perception, language arts, arithmetic, and work-study skills.

Stanford Achievement Test: Grades 1 through 13. Tests for arithmetic, reading, science, social studies, and study skills.

These batteries of tests are designed to assist in the evaluation of educational achievement in several ways. For example, they indicate intraindividual discrepancies within the subtests, suggesting areas where the individual may need intensive remedial training. They may reflect a serious discrepancy between an individual's IQ score (and, hence, his expected or potential level of performance) and his actual achievement level, indicating difficulties in maximizing one's potential. A superior IQ coupled with deficient achievement scores is not uncommon with an individual who has internal conflicts leading to external adjustment problems. The nature and extent of such discrepancies may provide the psychologist with both diagnostic information and clues for recommendation of remedial steps.

A specific kind of achievement test for the assessment of reading problems (dyslexia) is available. Reading skills are so basic to success in the educational process—and much of the rest of adjustment in our highly verbal society—that difficulties in this area can have far-reaching, detrimental ramifications for many aspects of an individual's life. When dyslexia problems are suspected, the examiner may choose any of several useful, reliable instruments with which to assess the magnitude and scope of the reading deficiency:

Stanford Diagnostic Reading Tests: Grades 1–13
  a. Vocabulary: in English, mathematics, science, social studies
  b. Comprehension: silent, auditory
  c. Rate of reading: general, science, social studies
  d. Word attack: oral and silent

Gates-McKillop Reading Diagnostic Tests: Grades 1–12
  a. Oral reading errors: omissions, reversals, mispronunciations, etc.
  b. Vocabulary
  c. Phrase perception
  d. Visual perception: syllabication, blending, etc.
  e. Auditory perception
  f. Spelling

Gilmore Oral Reading Test: Grades 1–8
  a. Substitutions
  b. Mispronunciations
  c. Assistance in pronunciation
  d. Disregard of punctuation
  e. Insertions
  f. Hesitations
  g. Repetitions
  h. Omissions

These tests are intended to identify specifically and accurately the elements causing the individual's difficulties in reading. Their usefulness is probably enhanced when two points are kept in mind. First, with regard to the assessment of the speech components of oral reading difficulties, consultation with a trained speech correctionist is highly advisable. Second, use of current diagnostic reading tests should be coupled with examination for visual anomalies and auditory deficiencies that may interfere with learning and reading efficiency.

Interview Data

It should be stressed in this section that even though the examiner is formally obtaining information with regard to intelligence while administering such tests, there is a great deal of other information which the examiner is obtaining simultaneously. Actually, the skilled clinician will obtain this information regardless of the specific nature of the test being administered, and this information will often have considerable value for making nontest interpretations about the individual being examined. For example, clinicians commonly attend very closely to what the individual says during the interview; his choice of words (vocabulary), the clarity and organization of his thinking, and the appropriateness of what he says are all data which can be valuable in trying to understand the person being examined. Moreover, the way that the individual responds emotionally provides useful information to the clinician. The affect which is expressed, its appropriateness, and the correspondence between what the individual is saying and the affect associated with it can suggest both strengths and weaknesses in the individual's adjustment to his environment. The examinee's overt behavior, such as the way that he walks, dresses, and seats himself during the psychological examination, can provide useful clues as to the way in which he relates to authority figures in his environment. Finally, during an interview, an examinee may express a wide variety of attitudes, such as subtle or overt hostility toward the examination, indifference or resentment, or friendly cooperation and openness, all of which may be employed by the clinician in drawing his conclusions and making his recommendations to the court. In sum, the obtained IQ score for an examinee is but one part of the result of the examination. Although indeed valuable, there is a great deal more information of equal importance which must be considered in assessing the overall results of the examinations. An IQ score by itself, with no other background or personality information about the examinee, is of limited value. This, of course, is one of the many reasons why it is imperative that the clinician be highly trained and have demonstrated professional competence.

The Evaluation of Organic Deficiency

Behavioral problems can arise naturally from a variety of sources and can bring an individual into conflict with his environment. In every case referred to the clinical psychologist for diagnosis, the possibility exists of an underlying destructive process in the nervous system. In many cases this can be eliminated rather easily as a possibility, although in some cases it is a question which must be seriously explored. The point may be illustrated by noting the well-recognized fact that people tend to do more and more of the things which they do best. A youngster may have an organic problem leading to reading difficulties, for example, which for a variety of reasons may cause him difficulties with school authorities. Recoiling from the pressure to do better and the embarrassment associated with looking bad in the eyes of his peers, a youngster with a reading problem may handle his frustrations by becoming a school delinquent and devote his time to socially unacceptable activities which bring him into conflict with the law. Such difficulties can have an organic etiology, and where organic changes are pronounced, various neurologic techniques can be useful in identifying the source of the problem. These physical methods, however, are often insensitive to early and subtle changes in the nervous system, with the result that there is growing attention to various psychological tests of organicity.

During the past 10 years there has been considerable development of psychologic tests that measure brain function. The major psychological approaches to the evaluation of organic brain damage are through the use of tests that assess (1) intellectual-cognitive, (2) sensory-perceptual, (3) visual-motor, (4) verbal-language, and (5) spatial-perceptual functioning.

NEUROPSYCHOLOGICAL TESTS

Traditionally the Bender-Gestalt (B-G) has been used as a screening test for organicity. Administration of the B-G (Fig. 31-1) is straightforward. The examinee, using pencil and paper, is asked to reproduce nine designs which are shown to him one at a time. The first design is shown, and after the examinee has copied it, he is shown a second drawing, and so on until the series of nine drawings has been copied. As with other visual-motor tests of organicity, the more important, general deviations of the B-G designs are oversimplification, fragmentation, displacement, distortion, elaboration, rotation, and in very serious cases, complete destruction of the pattern of the design (Fig. 31-2). However, by itself the B-G is no longer considered sufficient. Screening examinations for organic dysfunction should include a combination of task-specific tests.[2] By combining the B-G with a sensory-perceptual test (e.g., Reitan-Klove Sensory Perceptual Examination) and a verbal-language test (e.g., Reitan-Indiana Aphasia Screening Test), along with a measure of intelligence, an adequate screening examination can be made.

Probably the best standardized and comprehensive test for assessing organic brain dysfunction is the Halstead-Reitan Neuropsychological Test Battery.[3] This battery of tests, which requires 3 to 5 hours of administration time, is comprehensive and evaluates in detail all of the above-mentioned areas. Results of such examination are definitive for the presence of organic dysfunction as well as delimiting specific neurologic areas of systems that are damaged or dysfunctional. There are several excellent reviews of neuropsychologic testing in individuals with suspected neurologic damage/dysfunction using the Halstead-Reitan and other test procedures.[2,4,5] Any individual with a known history of brain damage/dysfunction should be evaluated with a more comprehensive test battery, and the results must be evaluated only by a qualified examiner.

Evaluation of Personality Functioning

Most psychologists probably find the area of personality evaluation the most interesting of their activities. By its very nature it is the most complicated and involves the least routine procedures. Like other tests, they are a means of obtaining answers to many, but not all, questions which may be asked of the clinician. As a case in point, the author recalls a time when he was asked to ascertain whether two girls, aged 8 and 10, were telling the truth when they asserted that their father had been having

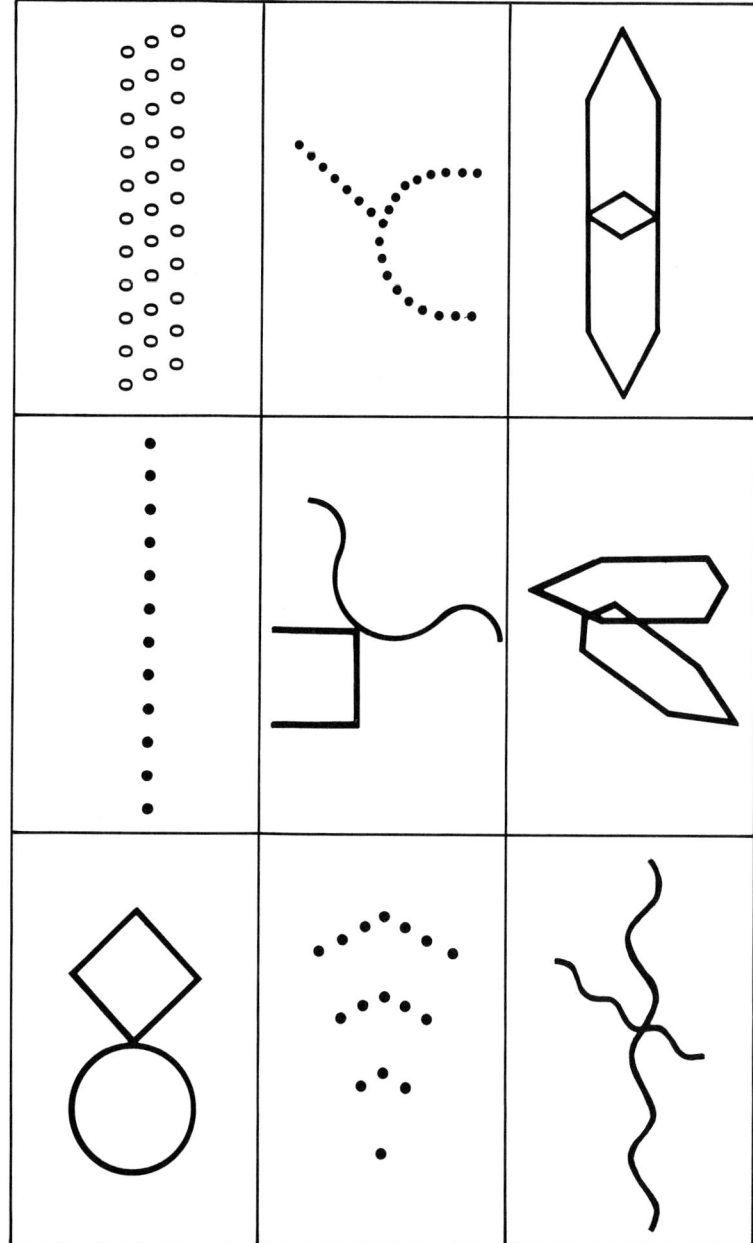

FIGURE 31-1. A reproduction of the original Bender-Gestalt stimulus figures that the examinee is asked to copy one at a time.

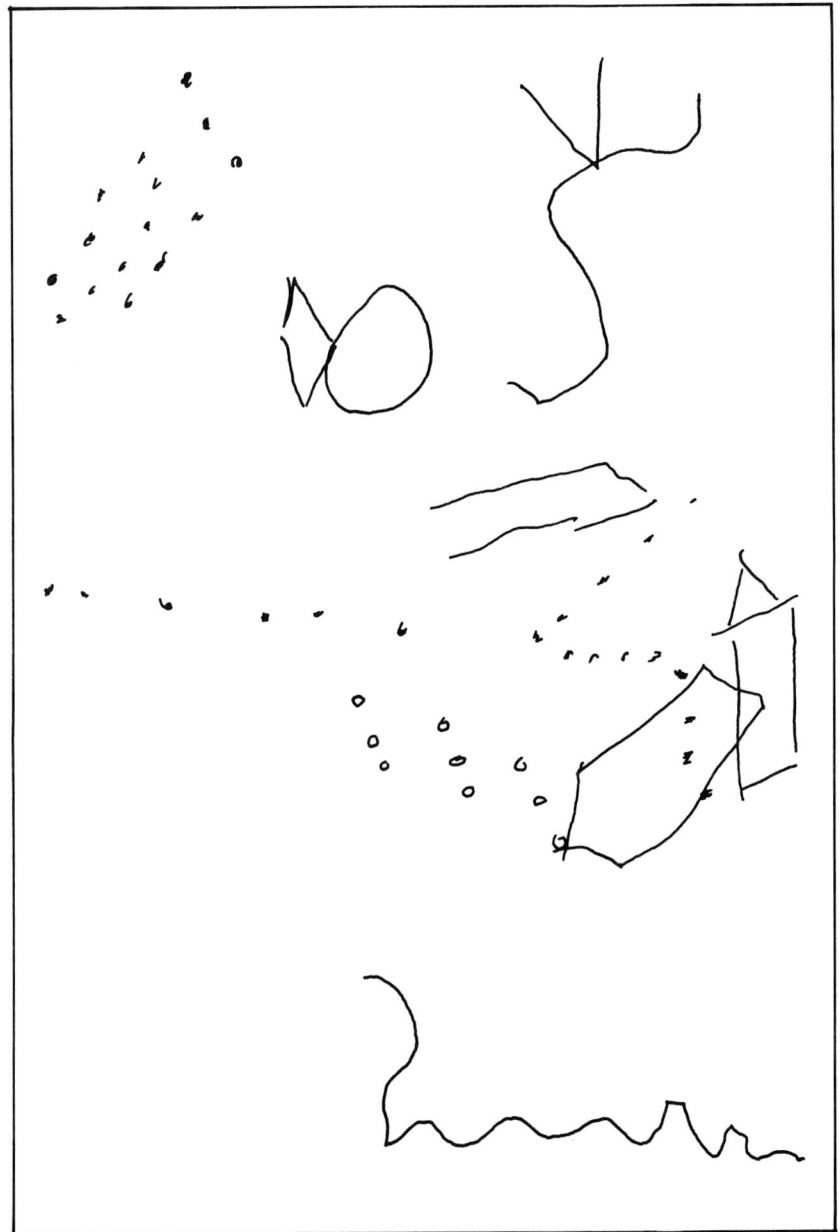

FIGURE 31-2. This Bender-Gestalt test reproduction is by a 22-year-old black male before the court for threatening his neighbors and resisting arrest. Analysis of the test reproductions suggests a marked perceptual-motor deficit commonly found in brain-damaged individuals. A subsequent neurologic examination revealed a tumor in the left temporal and occipital areas of the brain. The screening of this case by the court clinic resulted in a diversion from the criminal justice system to a medical hospital where surgery was performed to prevent further organic deterioration.

incestuous relations with them. Because of the gravity of the consequences, it was of obvious importance to be very sure that the girls were not lying about their father, perhaps because of instructions from their mother. The court authorities had hoped that the examiner could "give some personality test to make sure that the girls were not lying." The point is that there is no such test and that the psychologist had to rely on his best judgment in assessing evidence similar to that available to other court officers. He could talk with the girls, attempt to gain their confidence and encourage their honesty, but there is nothing infallible in the psychologist's arsenal.

The psychologist has many tests and techniques available for the study of personality. These serve many purposes, although not all of them are of equal value for a single purpose. Some methods are designed for examining the structural characteristics of an individual's personality, while others are more suited for assessing unconscious personality dynamics. Basically, there are two broad classes of tests for the assessment of personality which will concern us here: the *objective* approach and the *projective* approach.

OBJECTIVE APPROACHES

The psychologist has available a variety of instruments which fall into the category of objective testing. Some of the more commonly employed instruments are the *California Psychological Inventory*, the *Guilford-Zimmerman Temperament Survey*, the *Edwards Personal Preference Schedule*, the *Adjective Check List*, and the *Minnesota Multiphasic Personality Inventory*. Most of these objective instruments, while providing a multidimensional survey of personality functioning and structure, are intended for use with adult populations including, in most instances, late high school and college years. Probably the best known and most widely used of these instruments is the *Minnesota Multiphasic Personality Inventory* (MMPI), which we will explain herein.

The MMPI, which may be scored manually or by computer, is appropriate for use with individuals who are no less than 13 years of age and who have at least an eighth grade reading ability. Of interest particularly to the psychologist concerned with psychodiagnosis, the MMPI consists of more than 500 statements which the examinee designates as being "true" or "false," insofar as the statement applies to the examinee himself. The responses are scored and the results are recorded for ten major diagnostic classes such as hysteria, hypochondriasis, schizophrenia, psychasthenia, hypomania, and psychopathy. Specific items in the test are in the following format: "I am often frightened by strangers," and "I don't worry more than most other people." The skilled clinician, trained in the use of this test, can evaluate an MMPI profile and draw a number of psychodiagnostically useful conclusions from it. For example, some profile patterns indicate deep-seated conflicts with parental figures and strong hostility toward authority. Other patterns can indicate bizarre and distorted thinking patterns which may lead the individual to behave in openly aggressive and hostile ways. The MMPI is a very useful instrument, but because of the deceptive simplicity of the test, the results must be interpreted by an expert in the field.

The *Jesness Inventory* is another instrument that has been used successfully with disturbed children and adolescents, particulary juvenile delinquents, to obtain a profile of personality characteristics. The Inventory consists of 155 true-false items which measure the reaction of youngsters to a wide range of content. There are 11 scales in the instrument that are a reflection of various clusters of responses to the items. Scales reflect such dimensions as social adjustment, values, maturity, manifest aggression, and anxiety. The range of items provides an opportunity to view various facets of the youngster's personal life. For example, items such as "My life at home is always happy" reflect the reaction to family life. Within the context of other items, a "yes" response may indicate a denial of problems that may exist. On the other hand, how a youngster responds to "If I could, I'd just as soon quit school now" may reflect attitudes toward school, but also is correlated with the manifest aggression side, reflecting an awareness of feelings, especially anger and frustration.

This instrument can be scored manually or by computer. Normative sample delinquents and nondelinquents have indicated differences, even when socioeconomic class is taken into consideration. An added characteristic of the Jesness Inventory is that a computer-scoring service can extrapolate from the information into a classification system based on the work of Marguerite Warner and her colleagues, who have developed a concept of interpersonal maturity based on levels of integration of personality. Working with the California Youth Authority as well as in other settings, Warner and her assoicates found that most youngsters fall into integration levels 2, 3, and 4.* These levels of integration measure the individual's perception of himself and others. Within these maturity levels, subtypes are distinguished according to the manner in which the individual responds to events in his environment, particularly in relationship to others.

Below are listed the integration levels (I levels) most commonly attained by youngsters when appearing before juvenile courts, including subtypes and code names:

Code Name		Delinquent Subtype
I_2	Aa	Unsocialized aggressive
I_2	Ap	Unsocialized, passive
I_3	Crm	Conformist, immature
I_3	Cfc	Conformist, cultural
I_3	Mp	Manipulator
I_4	Na	Neurotic, acting out
I_4	Nx	Neurotic, anxious
I_4	Ci	Cultural identifier
I_4	Se	Situational, emotional reaction

The age limits and educational-level requirements of most objective tests seriously curtail their breadth of application with very young individuals. Consequently, for personality evaluation of juveniles, the examining psychologist will probably depend more explicitly upon projective instruments.

PROJECTIVE APPROACHES

Personality diagnosis through the projective approach involves assessment of the individual's responses to relatively unstructured test materi-

---

*Integration level 1 theoretically exists but would be of such severe primitiveness that children at this level are likely to be institutionalized at an early age. As a practical matter, therefore, such children do not come before the courts and in establishing norms for the various integration levels were not available.

als. The examinee expresses his characteristics in response to ambiguous situations in such a way that he unconsciously reveals the basic structure and dynamics of his personality. The basic nature of projective assessment can be seen in many clinical questions used in personality evaluations. When a youngster is asked what kind of animal he would like to be, he may reply that he would like to be an elephant because he could then step on people and hurt or squash them; another youngster may reply that he would like to be a puppy dog because then people would cuddle him and love him. The implications of these different responses for personality differences are obvious and can easily be seen by someone with less psychological training than a psychiatrist or a psychologist.

Some of the most useful projective techniques, such as the *Rorschach test*, the *Thematic Apperception Test*, the *Children's Apperception Test*, the *Draw-A-Person test*, the *Make-A-Picture Story test*, the *Michigan Picture Story Test*, and the *Sentence Completion Test*, are familiar to the lay public because of the widespread attention they have received. They are intrinsically interesting and are usually the kind of test the public associates with the role of the psychologist. Several of these will be examined below.

Thematic Apperception Test

The Thematic Apperception Test (TAT) requires the examinee to make up a story about a series of pictures that are presented to him one at a time. He may either write his own stories or the examiner may write the stories as dictated by the examinee. He is asked to explain what is going on at the present time in the picture, what led up to the situation, what the characters in the picture are thinking and feeling, and what the most likely outcome would be.

The stories produced from the TAT are regarded as having implications for relatively conscious current conflicts and problems which the examinee may be experiencing. The clinical interpretation involves focusing upon such dimensions as the way in which the characters interact, the degree of warmth or conflict in their relationships, the kinds of goals they hold for themselves, the kinds of expectations they have for themselves and others from the environment, and the general level of maturity indicated by the patterns of the stories. Since the pictures depict both children and adults, as well as scenes of pure fantasy, the results of TAT stories can cover a rather broad spectrum of personality functioning. TAT themes can be very useful in identifying the major sources of conflict and can suggest what sorts of remedial or therapeutic intervention would be most appropriate in a particular case. TAT stories basically suggest what kind of environment a person sees around himself, and what kind of people he feels live in the world with him.

There have been a number of modifications of the TAT. One has been that of changing the faces and figures of the characters in the pictures to make it easy for various racial groups to identify with the situations portrayed. Another modification has resulted in a series of ten cards for use with children. This modification, known as the *Children's Apperception Test* (CAT), provides pictures which center around feeding conflicts, parental relationships, sibling rivalry, toilet training, and other situations common to children (Fig. 31-3).

Similar to the TAT and CAT is the *Michigan Picture Story Test* (MPST), which consists of test materials depicting the youngsters in relationship

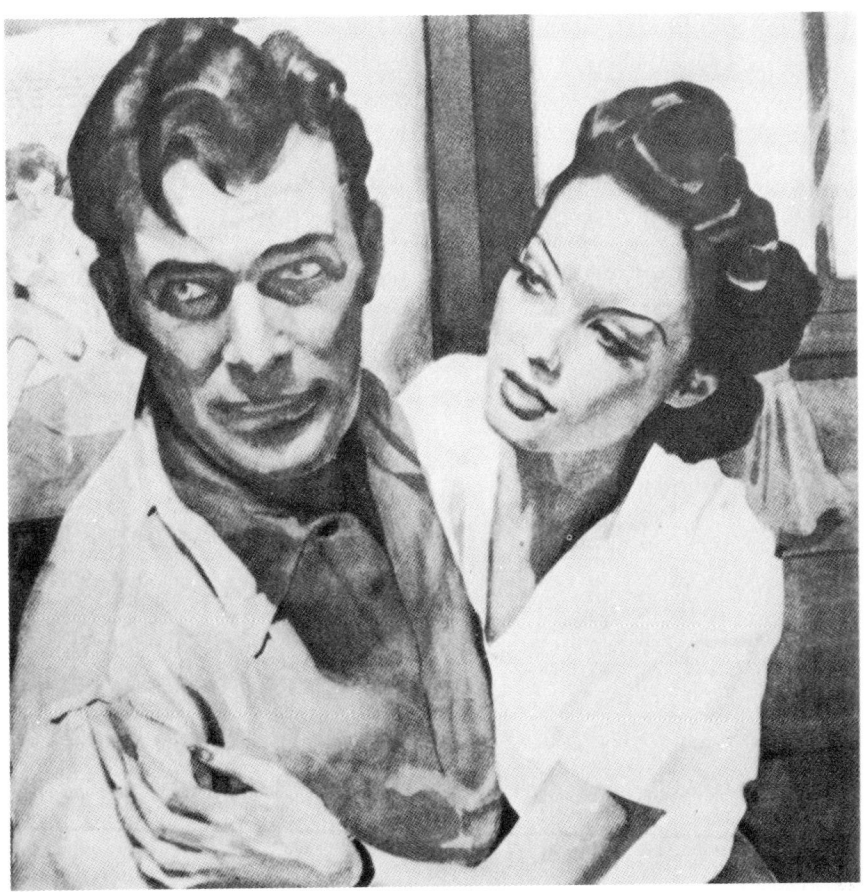

FIGURE 31-3. Thematic Apperception Test. The defendant is before the court on a charge of aggravated assault on his girlfriend, assault on the arresting police officer, and drunkenness. The defendant is white, 32 years old, a divorced male who is employed as a shipper in a shoe factory. He has two prior charges of physical assault on family members and one charge of armed robbery. The defendant was referred to the court clinic by the judge to determine his capacity and willingness to profit from psychiatric treatment. He was given a full battery of psychological tests. The following is his response to TAT card No. 4 (the tester's questioning and elicitation of fuller responses have been deleted): "This guy here looks like he just had a beef with someone. Somebody made a pass at his girlfriend and called her a name. She's just told this guy here that this happened last night. He looks mad as hell. He's going out to get the guy. She's trying to stop him and cool him off. But he won't listen to her. He shoves her off and goes out looking for the guy. He finds him in a pool room and beats the hell out of him. He don't like people making passes at his girl."

to parents, policemen, and other authority figures, as well as peers. This test can be very useful in assessing the structure of a youngster's attitudes toward adults and peer figures as well as evaluating the extent of problems in this regard.

Included in this category is the *Make-A-Picture Story test* (MAPS), which is similar to the MPST in terms of purpose and interpretive potential. The distinction of the MAPS from the other tests is that it affords more flexibility in allowing the examinee to select his own characters to be put on a small stage background, and to base a story upon this situation.

Figure Drawing

Several approaches to the evaluation of personality by means of drawings made by the examinee have been developed. By and large, the drawing skill of the examinee is not a major factor. With the *Draw-A-Person test* (DAP), the examinee is simply asked to draw a picture of a male and female figure, using pencil and paper. Figure drawings can give immediate first impressions, as with clearly hostile or aggressive figures or with passive and submissive figures. Interpretations are also based upon the size of the figures, their positions, their postures, whether they appear to be confident, outgoing, and so forth. The particular area of the body or clothing which is emphasized is regarded as having significance for personality assessment.

Interpretations based upon figure drawing tests are highly inferential and should be based upon findings from other tests as well (Fig. 31-4).

Incomplete Sentences Test

Several sentence completion and incomplete sentence tests exist, any of which may be of value to the psychologist called to court. These are pro-

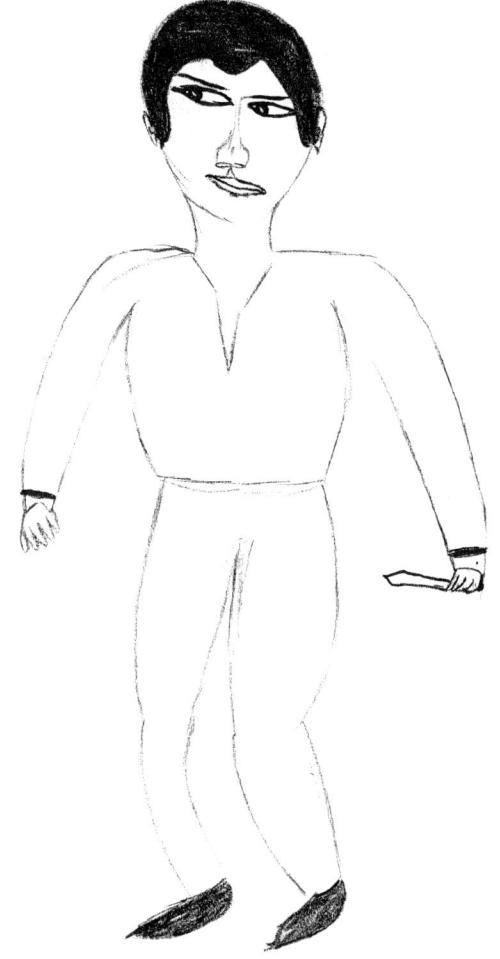

FIGURE 31-4. The following Draw-A-Person test (DAP) is of a 35-year-old white male before the court on a charge of murdering his wife. He has an extensive prior record for armed robbery and extortion. The client has a seventh grade education and has worked as a truck driver, but he is presently unemployed. The DAP often succeeds in uncovering a person's major problem area, of which he may or may not be conscious. This subject's DAP graphically depicts his preoccupation with aggressive impulses.

jective methods in which the examinee is presented with a series of partial sentences and required to complete the meaning of the sentence. Examples of such sentences are: "I think that most women are . . ."; "I have always wished I could . . ."; "If given the chance, most people would like to . . . ." The stems of the sentences tend to focus on sexual preoccupations, religious feelings, autistic tendencies, relationships with parents and peers, fears, anxiety, guilt feelings, and hostile and aggressive impulses. The pattern of the examinee's responses can often give the clinical psychologist considerable insight into areas of conflict, as well as strengths and weaknesses of the examinee's personality.

Competency Screening Test

Psychologists are frequently called upon by the court to evaluate an individual's mental status or intelligence, not for its own sake, but to aid in the resolution of a legal issue. Competency to stand trial is based on a legal definition rather than a psychiatric diagnosis. In order to aid the court in determining an individual's fitness to stand trial, the Competency Screening Test was developed.[6] This instrument is a sentence completion test consisting of 22 sentence stems, each of which relates to an aspect of playing the role of a defendant in a criminal court (Fig. 31-5). Thus the response to a stem which states "When I go to court the lawyer will . . ." should help to evaluate the defendant's ability to cooperate with his attorney in his own trial. Other items elicit responses that aid in determining one's awareness and understanding of the nature and object of the proceedings. Each items is scored as 0, 1, or 2, with the aid of a scoring manual. Defendants with scores of 21 and above have been found to be competent for trial with a high level of confidence. Those with lower scores may require more intensive evaluation before making a determination as to their competency. The first-order production by the defendant has the advantage of providing direct data to the court in arriving at a judicial determination of competency to stand trial. This test takes 15 or 20 minutes to administer and about the same time to score. Feminine and vernacular Spanish versions of the test have also been developed.

Rorschach Test

Probably the most well-known and widely used of the projective methods for personality assessment is the Rorschach test. This test requires that the examinee interpret a series of ten inkblots, all of which are on cards. Five of the inkblots are in black, white, and shades of gray; the remaining five involve some degree of color. Most experts agree that the Rorschach is a psychodiagnostic technique of significant sensitivity. It evaluates the emotional life of the examinee, provides an estimate of his intellectual level, and helps illuminate many components of his personality.

There are three essential categories in the scoring of the Rorschach test. The first is location, or where the response is seen on the card; the second is the determinants, or how and why it is seen; and the third is the content, or the specific nature of what is seen.

Clinical experience with the Rorschach test, both with responses of children and adults, has indicated that some types of personality problems have relatively characteristic test patterns. Test records of individuals who are severely disturbed, such as psychotics and other schizophrenics, are characterized by peculiar and often bizarre responses. The form qual-

Score		
1	1. The lawyer told Bill that	not to worry.
2	2. When I go to court the lawyer will	do his best for me.
0	3. Jack felt that the judge	was too old.
2	4. When Phil was accused of the crime, he	panicked.
2	5. When I prepare to go to court with my lawyer,	I will help him all I can in my defense.
1	6. If the jury finds me guilty, I	will abide with their decision.
2	7. The way a court trial is decided	is by the presentation of the facts.
1	8. When the evidence in George's case was presented to the jury,	he felt much relieved.
2	9. When the lawyer questioned his client in court, the client said	the truth.
2	10. If Jack had to try his own case, he	probably would get all fouled up.
2	11. Each time the D.A. asked me a question, I	answered.
2	12. While listening to the witnesses testify against me, I	paid strict attention.
2	13. When the witness testifying against Harry gave incorrect evidence, he	was told about it to his attorney.
2	14. When Bob disagreed with his lawyer on his defense, he	told him.
2	15. When I was formally accused of the crime, I thought to myself	was I really responsible?
1	16. If Ed's lawyer suggests that he plead guilty, he	would hesitate.
2	17. What concerns Fred most about his lawyer	is his unquestionable competence.
1	18. When they say a man is innocent until proven guilty,	he has a good chance to be freed.
2	19. When I think of being sent to prison, I	am scared.
1	20. When Phil thinks of what he is accused of, he	regrets the crime.
2	21. When the jury hears my case, they will	judge me fairly.
2	22. If I had a chance to speak to the judge, I	would explain my condition at the time of the incident.

FIGURE 31-5. Competency Screening Test. The defendant was before the court for murdering his brother-in-law during a drinking party when an argument resulted in a physical confrontation. He is 27 years old, married with two children, and employed as a truck driver. On this sentence completion test he earned a score of 35, placing him in the range of scores for persons who have been considered competent to stand trial. The test protocol indicates that he has sufficient awareness of the court proceedings, an appreciation of the consequences of his act, and the ability to communicate with his attorney in developing a defense. The hospital maintained that the defendant was physically able to return to trial, and subsequently the defendant was found to be competent to stand trial.

ity is usually poor; schizophrenic examinees see things in the blots which are quite discrepant from the actual stimulus properties of the inkblot. They may focus all their attention on very minute details of the blots while ignoring major components, or they may become quite emotionally involved with the blots and personalize their percepts in such a way that they are unable to differentiate between themselves and the Rorschach card.

In any diagnostic case where there is a serious question of psychological problems such as a significant thought disorder, it is probably advisable that a Rorschach be used. While the Rorschach technique is relatively straightforward in administration and test scoring, interpretation of the data is quite a different matter. The test can be extremely revealing in the hands of a skilled clinician.

REFERENCES

1. Menninger, K., et al.: *Am. J. Psychiatry* 103:473, 1947.
2. Strub, R.L., and Black, F.W.: *The Mental Status Examination in Neurology.* F.A. Davis, Philadelphia, 1977.
3. Reitan, R.M., and Davison, L.A.: *Clinical Neuropsychology: Current Status and Applications.* V.H. Winston, Washington, D.C., 1974.
4. Lezak, M.D.: *Neuropsychological Assessment.* Oxford University Press, New York, 1976.
5. Smith, A.: Neuropsychological Testing in Neurological Disorders, in Friedlances, W.J. (ed.): *Advances in Neurology.* Raven Press, New York, 1975.
6. Lipsitt, P.D., Lelos, D., and McGarry, A.L.: Competency for Trial, A Screening Instrument. *Am. J. Psychiatry* 128:105-109, 1971.

ADDITIONAL READING

Anastasi, A.: *Psychological Testing.* ed. 4. Macmillan, New York, 1976.
Houts, M.: The Psychological Tests, in Houts, M. (ed.): *Lawyers' Guide to Medical Proof.* Matthew Bender, New York, 1966.
Hutt, M. L., and Briskin, J. J.: *The Clinical Use of the Revised Bender-Gestalt Test.* Grune & Stratton, New York, 1960.
Klopfer, B., and Davidson, H. H., *The Rorschach Technique: An Inventory Manual.* Harcourt, Brace, New York, 1962.
Marshall, K.: Evidence, Psychology, and the Trial: Some Challenges to the Law. *Columbia Law Rev.* 63:197–220, 1963.
Nunnally, J. C.: *Educational Measurement and Evaluation.* ed. 2. McGraw-Hill, New York, 1972.
Silber, D. E.: Clinical Psychology—Its Role and Methods, in Allen, R. C., Ferster, E. Z., and Ruben, J. G., (eds.): *Readings in Law and Psychiatry.* rev. ed. Johns Hopkins University Press, Baltimore, 1975.
Sunderberg, N. D.: The Practice of Psychological Testing in Clinical Services in the United States. *Am. Psychologist* 16:79–83, 1961.
Sunderberg, N. D., and Tyler, L. E.: *Clinical Psychology: An Introduction to Research and Practice.* Appleton-Century-Crofts, New York, 1962.
Thorndike, R. L., and Hagen, E. P.: *Measurement and Evaluation in Psychology and Education.* ed. 3. Wiley, New York, 1969.

CHAPTER 32

R. Kirkland Schwitzgebel is Associate Professor of Psychology at California Lutheran College. After completing undergraduate studies at the Ohio State University, Dr. Schwitzgebel entered the Graduate School of Education at Harvard, where he received his doctorate in 1962. He subsequently earned a law degree from Harvard Law School. Dr. Schwitzgebel is Chairperson of the Committee on Scientific and Professional Ethics and Conduct of the American Psychological Association. He is also a member of the Editorial and Advisory Board of the *Journal of Law and Human Behavior*. Dr. Schwitzgebel has authored numerous articles and several books and monographs dealing with the adolescent offender and behavior modification techniques.

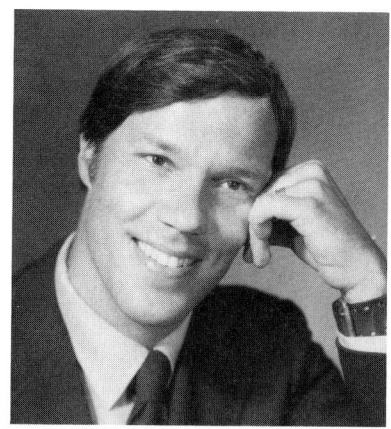

PREDICTION OF DANGEROUSNESS AND ITS IMPLICATIONS FOR TREATMENT*

R. Kirkland Schwitzgebel, Ed.D., J.D.

The following discussion briefly examines some of the major issues and current trends in the prediction and treatment of mentally ill persons considered dangerous. The discussion does not include a consideration of persons who are dangerous only to themselves, such as suicidal or gravely disabled persons. The focus is upon mentally ill persons who present a substantial risk of physical harm to others. The concluding suggestions for improving predictive accuracy and treatment efficacy are frankly speculative and are offered to stimulate further clinical investigation and research.

Persons attempting to predict and treat dangerous patients currently find themselves in a difficult social and legal situation. On one hand, there is legislative and judicial pressure upon treatment personnel to find the "least restrictive alternative" for handling the dangerous mental patient consonant with the patient's or public's safety.[1,2] On the other hand, treatment personnel may be legally responsible if they prematurely release a dangerous person or fail to notify potential victims of the patient's dangerousness.[3] This situation is further complicated by the varying legal definitions of dangerousness found in different states and the clinical difficulty of predicting future behavior likely to be considered dangerous.

PREDICTIVE ACCURACY

Perhaps one of the best known studies of the prediction of dangerousness is that of the "Baxstrom patients" made by Steadman and his associates.[5,6] As a result of a legal decision by the United States Supreme Court,[4] 967

---

*This chapter was supported in part by Grant No. R01 MH25955 from the Center for Studies of Crime and Delinquency of the National Institute of Mental Health.

patients who were involuntarily committed to Dannemora and Matteawan State Hospitals as dangerous persons were released to 18 civil facilities in their respective communities in New York State. Four years later, only 2.7 percent of these patients were returned to the hospitals to which they had originally been committed. A more intensive follow-up study of a subsample of these patients found that 17 percent had been arrested and 7 percent were convicted. Not all of the convictions resulted in confinement. In summary, the vast majority of these supposedly dangerous patients were not in fact dangerous when released into the community within the 4 years of the follow-up study.[5,6,7]

Other studies of patients released by court or administrative order, contrary to psychiatric diagnoses of dangerousness, have generally produced similar results. For example, in Illinois, Rubin[8] has studied "the Menard 18." Because of an "administrative error," 17 of these 18 patients spent a total of 425 years in confinement after they legally should have been placed in less restrictive treatment or community settings. Rubin's follow-up study also indicated that these illegally confined men were probably not very dangerous, even at the time of their initial commitment. (One of "the Menard 18" has been so administratively misplaced that he cannot be located.)

In 1967, a new statute in Massachusetts required the judicial review of involuntarily committed mental patients at the Massachusetts Correctional Institution at Bridgewater. The patients there at that time were reviewed in light of the Baxstrom decision which required new, legal safeguards prior to commitment. Out of a sample of 234 patients transferred to other civil hospitals, a 33-month follow-up study found that 93 (39.7 percent) were released or escaped into the community. After an average of 13 months in the community, 15 of the patients (16.1 percent) appeared in court. There was only one conviction for a felony. All the other charges were misdemeanors, usually drunkenness.[9] It could be reasonably concluded that at least one-third of the men being detained in Bridgewater were not dangerous. A higher rate of release into the community might have revealed an even higher percentage of nondangerous patients.

The professional literature almost uniformly affirms low predictive accuracy with regard to the dangerousness of mental patients. One study, however, by Kozol, Boucher, and Garofalo[10] claims that dangerousness can be "reliably diagnosed and effectively treated." The senior author, a psychiatrist, and his associates examined 592 male convicted sex offenders who had been sent to the Bridgewater Institution for diagnosis as potentially sexually dangerous persons. On the basis of initial diagnostic studies, the authors concluded that 304 of these persons were not dangerous, while 257 were diagnosed as dangerous. The remaining 31 patients were returned to prison for legal reasons and were not included in the reported diagnostic studies. After receiving treatment for an average period of 43 months, 82 patients were released. Of these, five subsequently committed serious assaultive crimes, thereby producing a recidivism rate of 6.1 percent, according to the authors.

This appears to be an excellent record of diagnosis and treatment. Fortunately, the authors also provide data on 49 patients, diagnosed and treated by them as dangerous, whom the court released from Bridgewater contrary to the medical staff's recommendation. Of these patients, 34.7 percent subsequently committed serious assaultive crimes. Conversely, 65.3 percent did not commit such crimes after approximately 5 years in the community. Thus nearly two-thirds of those patients released contrary to predictions of dangerousness by Kozol's group were not subsequently dangerous.[11] This represents a serious overprediction of dangerousness.

There has been even further criticism of the Kozol study. A reanalysis of the data in this study by Evenson and Altman[12] found an expected base rate of recidivism of 11 percent for the total group of 435 released patients. (There were 304 patients released as not dangerous at the initial diagnosis; 82 were released as not dangerous after treatment; and 49 were released by the court contrary to a diagnosis of dangerousness.) It would have been possible to obtain 89 percent accuracy with this group of patients merely by predicting that all of the patients were not dangerous. Most of the project staff's predictive accuracy came from correctly identifying the large number of patients who were not dangerous. If one statistically compensates for correct prediction occurring merely by chance, one finds that the staff's predictive accuracy was about 27 percent.

A study by Carney at the Patuxent Institution of Maryland also seems to support the ability of psychiatrists to predict dangerousness or the absence of it. However, the medically released group had community placements while on parole and the court-released group did not. Moreover, the data utilized in the study are incomplete.

Ennis and Litwack[14] have sharply questioned the legal qualification of psychiatrists to testify as experts on the issue of dangerousness. They comment:

> An exception to the ordinary rules of evidence has been created to permit experts to testify in court as to their opinions, conclusions, and judgment. With the exception of psychiatrists, witnesses are required to prove their expertise before courts will permit them to testify as experts. If that same proof were required of psychiatrists, they could not qualify as expert witnesses. Support for this proposition may be provided by analogy to the judicial treatment of polygraph results.
>
> There is no question that psychiatric judgments are far less reliable and valid than polygraph judgments. Although the evidence is still accumulating, a conservative estimate is that an experienced polygraph examiner can correctly detect truth or deception about 80 to 90 percent of the time.
>
> Significantly, one study has indicated 'that an examiner is more inclined to report a guilty subject innocent than he is to report an innocent subject guilty.' The converse is true of psychiatrists; if doubt exists, it almost always is resolved to the patient's disadvantage; predictions of dangerousness afford the prime example.
>
> Despite this proven reliability and validity of polygraph tests, only a handful of state and federal trial courts have received polygraph reports in evidence, and then usually for only limited purposes. Moreover, no appellate court has approved the admission of polygraph reports over the objection of a party.
>
> Whatever may be said for the reliability and validity of psychiatric judgments in general, there is literally no evidence that psychiatrists reliably and accurately can predict dangerous behavior. To the contrary, such predictions are wrong more often than they are right. It is inconceivable that a judgment could be considered an 'expert' judgment when it is less accurate than the flip of a coin.
>
> Accordingly, psychiatrists should not be permitted to testify as ex-

pert witnesses until they can prove through empirical studies that their judgments are reliable and valid.

In an experimental study by Sweetland,[15] college students and psychiatrists agreed extensively on the degree of "dangerousness" and "nondangerousness" as indicated by various personality characteristics. This suggests the possiblity that psychiatric judgment is not based upon any special knowledge or expertise beyond that of educated laymen. There are also several studies indicating that the diagnostic classifications made by psychologists are not more reliable or valid than those made by laymen.[16]

More recently, Steadman and Cocozza[17] have studied the predictive accuracy of psychiatrists evaluating the dangerousness of 257 felony defendants found incompetent to stand trial. The study groups had an average (mean) age of 31 and were predominately nonwhite; approximately two-thirds came from the New York City area, and the alleged offenses more often involved violent acts against persons rather than property or drugs. Data collected over a 3-year follow-up period indicated that the group of defendants diagnosed as dangerous was not statistically more dangerous than the group of defendants diagnosed as nondangerous. The researchers concluded: "The level of accuracy by the psychiatrists was no greater than that obtainable by chance. These findings suggest that psychiatric testimony to the court in regard to applying the dangerousness standard currently should not be considered expert."

Stone[18] has commented: "The law, influenced by the reforms I have described, asks the psychiatrist to prognosticate dangerous behavior. That is absurd because it is a rare event, and the capacity for such prognostication is absent. What the mental health profession can prognosticate is the mental state and the likely course of the illness of the patient." Legal attacks upon the assumption of psychiatric expertise in the prediction of dangerousness will probably increase in the near future unless better predictive accuracy can be scientifically demonstrated.

APPROACHES TOWARD INCREASING PREDICTIVE ACCURACY

Some Immediate Steps

Long-term prediction of behavior is more difficult than short-term prediction. Accurate prediction is more likely for one day in the future than for one year in the future or for an indefinite period of time. Therefore, clinicians might consider shortening, or at least specifying, the time frame of their predictions. This may require the more frequent examination of patients because the time frame is shortened.

If the psychological and social conditions surrounding a patient change, prediction becomes more difficult. Therefore, prediction might be made with reference to particularly critical conditions for each patient (e.g., continued employment, a stable marriage, or abstinence from alcohol). As circumstances change, the clinician should be notified and the patient reassessed. Courts do not always require an evaluation of dangerousness projected indefinitely into the future. In fact, the trend is to require more time-limited predictions. For example, the predicted dangerous act necessitating confinement must, in some states, be expected to occur within the "reasonably foreseeable future."[19] It is reasonable to require no greater prediction into the future for the release of patients.

The definition of dangerousness should be clarified prior to prediction. Does the dangerousness include harm to self? Does it include financial harm to others? Does it include public drunkenness? Does it include verbal threats or abuse? Does it include preparation or plans that might lead to violence such as the purchase of a firearm? Without prior agreement about what behavior constitutes a dangerous act, it is likely that there will be considerable disagreement, and predictive accuracy will be poor. Increasingly, civil commitment statutes are requiring evidence of specific acts, attempts, or threats of physical harm prior to commitment. An Arizona statute defines "danger to others" as "behavior which constitutes a danger of inflicting substantial bodily harm upon another person based upon a history of having inflicted or having attempted to inflict substantial bodily harm upon another person within 12 months preceding the hearing on court ordered treatment. . . ."[20]

Another strategy for improving predictive accuracy involves the use of two or more professionals rating or assessing the patient independently, then comparing the results.[21] In this way, factors overlooked or overrated by one person may be detected by the other. It is important that the initial assessment by the two persons be conducted independently, rather than having the initial assessment passed on to the second person for confirmation. When there is poor agreement (low interrater reliability) between two persons making an assessment, it is fairly certain that at least one of them is incorrect. Low interrater reliability usually establishes the upper limit of valid (truthful) assessment. Thus, if one physician detects mammary cancer by clinical examination and another physician using the same procedure does not, one of them is in error, and the validity of the result is in question. Sometimes independent assessment and comparison using different procedures or approaches is necessary to obtain sufficient validity.*

Clinical experience alone may not be sufficient to guarantee validity or even agreement among the "experts." As a part of a study of the competency of patients to stand trial, the agreement (interrater reliability) among eight psychiatrists with an average (mean) of 287 competency examinations was examined. These expert psychiatrists were generally mental hospital superintendents or chief psychiatrists. They had no greater agreement among themselves on patient's competency (R of .67) than psychiatrists with no previous experience in competency examination (R of .68).[23] In general, even among experts, agreement about assessment criteria, discussion of areas of disagreement, and the feedback of results over a series of patients can be expected to increase substantially both assessment reliability and potential validity.

Consideration of Social-Environmental Factors

There are many theories about the etiology of dangerous behavior. A part of the reason for so many theories is that the concept of "dangerousness" subsumes many different behaviors ranging from the carefully planned execution of a political enemy to rage reactions inadvertently harming

---

*For example, in a study involving the screening and follow-up of 20,211 women for mammary cancer,[22] almost two out of five of the prevalent cancers in the initial screening would have been missed by clinical examination. Conversely, mamography alone would have missed more than two out of five cancers subsequently detected. Both clinical examination and mamography were necessary.

innocent bystanders.† Presumed causes may range from social discontent to neurologic disorders such as temporal lobe seizures.[24,25] Traditionally, legal and psychiatric conceptualizations of dangerousness have focused upon the individual as the source of these behaviors. More recently, a view has been emerging which focuses upon the interaction of a person with his physical and social environment in the production of behavior considered dangerous. In this view, there must be a behavior, a social context for that behavior, and an observer who labels the behavior as dangerous.[26]

The conceptualization of dangerous behavior as a product of person-environment interactions can have important legal and clinical consequences. For example, consider the proverbial "little old lady" who accidentally leaves the gas jets turned on in her apartment after using her stove. She may not only kill herself, but also some of her neighbors and is, therefore, committable under many states statutes as a dangerous person. But does the "dangerousness" lie within her, within her environment, or both? The dangerousness in this case is correctable not only by committing this woman to an institution for treatment, but also by replacing her gas stove with an electric one.

Some people may be dangerous only in particular situations (e.g., in barrooms), under particular conditions (e.g., when intoxicated), and in particular interpersonal context (e.g., threats to self-esteem). Too often, clinicians may infer enduring personality traits from behaviors which are, in fact, responses to specific environmental conditions. A child may hit another child primarily when he is struck first or is insulted. This aggressive behavior may persist if it is reinforced by praise for being "tough" or by the other child's surrender of territory. The importance of antecedent and consequent environmental events has been frequently observed and demonstrated in experimental studies with children.[27] From a community viewpoint, O'Neal and McDonald[28] have extensively reviewed various environmental factors that might be related to increased aggression. Among these factors are noise, heat, territoriality, crowding, anonymity, diffusion of responsibility, and audience approval. In a survey of studies of animal aggression, Moyer[29] has suggested several general categories of aggression that are responsive to the environmental context. Some of these categories are fear-induced aggression, sex-related aggression, and instrumental (rewarded) aggression. The specification of the environmental factors associated with aggression would seem to be a more promising approach to predicting physically harmful acts than a general and diffuse concept of dangerousness. As will be discussed later, the consideration of environmental factors may significantly influence treatment and release decisions.

Base-Rate Information in Case-Specific Decisions

Mental health personnel rather consistently overpredict dangerousness,[30] which leads to extensive confinement of patients who are allegedly dangerous but who are, in fact, not so. The reason for this overprediction is probably, in part, the strong negative reaction of the public to errors

---

†The issue has sometimes been raised as to whether a "hired killer" may be involuntarily committed under civil statutes because, although he is dangerous, he may not also be mentally ill. Use of habitual offender statutes may be a more appropriate approach.

associated with the release of dangerous persons, whereas there is relatively little concern about unnecessary confinement.[31,32] Those persons clinically predicted to be dangerous, but who are in fact not dangerous, represent false-positive errors in prediction. In contrast, those persons clinically predicted to be not dangerous, but who are in fact dangerous, represent false-negative errors in prediction. It is likely that both false-positive and false-negative errors might be reduced by incorporating statistical prediction techniques into clinical decision-making.[33]

For over two decades, research has been conducted comparing clinical with statistical prediction techniques.[34] A review of 45 studies by Sawyer,[35] comparing statistical and clinical evaluations, revealed that statistical methods were at least equal to, and generally superior to, clinical methods. It would seem desirable, therefore, to use statistical methods at least in combination with clinical methods. Shah[33] has described one possible method of combining clinical and statistical methods:

> A fundamental rule of statistical prediction is that expected accuracy must control the relative weights assigned to the specific evidence being used for predictions (e.g., various clinical indices and 'signs') and to the prior information (viz., the base rates). As the expected accuracy of the [clinical] predictions decreases (viz., in situations where the base rates are very low and the available evidence not very reliable), the prediction should become regressive and should shift closer to the base rates or the prior probabilities. For example, if only 10 percent of a particular group are expected to engage in future violent behavior on the basis of prior probability (base rates), and if the specific evidence concerning predictions is of poor reliability (e.g., clinical assessments and certain psychological test indices), then the predictions should remain close to the base rates. The greater the move away from the base rates under the above conditions, the greater will be the probability of error.
>
> Experiments conducted by Kahneman and Tversky[36] demonstrated, nevertheless, that individuals engaged in a predictive task very commonly disregard information concerning prior probability when some specific current information is provided. There is a tendency instead to resort to the representativeness heuristic, even to the extent that involves gross departures from the prior probabilities.

It appears that specific case history information often strongly influences clinical prediction, whereas relevant statistical information does not have great influence. In fact, valuable statistical information may be ignored when completely worthless case history information is given to persons making predictions. Carroll[37] found that brief, case history descriptions were subjectively compelling enough to negate the use of important statistical information.

Parole Board Prediction System

One potentially useful approach involving both clinical and statistical information is the two-dimensional system used by the United States Board of Parole.[38] In actual practice, the parole board member rates the prospective parolee on the severity of his prior offense and his parole prognosis (risk of recidivism). The severity is rated from low severity (e.g., minor theft) to highest severity (e.g., willful homicide). Parole prognosis is determined by considering eleven factors generally found to be related to recidivism, such as age, prior incarcerations, and employment. These eleven factors are scored to produce a parole prognosis ranging from a very high probability of success to a very low probability of success. After rating the prospective parolee on offense severity and parole prognosis, the parole board member examines a statistical table that suggests a range of time to be served before release (e.g., 20 to 24 months). This table is based upon the statistical analysis of the parole success and failure of similar parolees. If the parole board member wants to make a recommendation outside the suggested range, he must justify his decision by providing information that makes this particular case unique. The decision-maker is therefore not obligated to follow a statistical formula, but an additional burden of proof is placed upon him if he wishes to exceed the statistically generated guidelines for discretion.[39] Under these conditions, decisions appear to be more uniform and in line with statistical prediction. But there still remains much room for subjective evaluation and input which may be of critical importance in certain cases.

It is not likely that such a system will soon be used in predicting dangerousness in the civil commitment area because of an inadequate data base and because of the reluctance of mental health personnel to subject their decisions to empirical and administrative review. The individual clinician can, however, begin to decrease his reliance upon clinical case material when such reliance results in the exclusion of factors generally shown to be related to subsequent dangerous acts. In summarizing several studies, Burnham[40] has concluded that "the maximum number of data items along different dimensions which can be processed profitably at the same time, without any formal decomposition and restructuring of the decision process, is about eight. Above that number, confusion does set in resulting from a decline in decision quality . . . We must be aware that information overload is real, likely, important, and damaging."

The above example of parole decision-making required only the simultaneous consideration of two data items. Among the eight or fewer items to be considered would be those items statistically shown to be related to subsequent dangerousness for the particular population being evaluated. At least this information, even if not used, would not be as damaging to the decision-making process as irrelevant case history material. Perhaps with training and exposure to statistical data, clinicians could begin to feel more comfortable about integrating clinical and statistical information.

TREATMENT IMPLICATIONS

Although some individual patients may be greatly helped by traditional psychotherapeutic methods, the overall effectiveness of these methods is subject to serious question. There are many studies reporting negative results.[41-45] Generally it appears that the more carefully studies are designed to control for factors such as improvement without treatment (spontaneous remission), placebo effects, self-report bias, and attrition rates, the more likely they are to find negative treatment outcome. Traditional treatment methods are not necessarily to be abandoned but may be augmented by some newer forms of treatment or behavioral intervention. Although there is a great need for more research on treatment methods, relatively little research is presently being done on this important problem. The present situation with regard to public policy is somewhat like building tuberculosis sanitariums rather than treating or preventing tuberculosis. The following discussion briefly presents some speculations about new directions for psychotherapeutic intervention.*

Desensitization Techniques

One possible approach involves the desensitization of patients to stimuli that usually elicit anger or aggressive responses. In one study,[48] research subjects who became angry while driving and also exhibited behaviors such as swearing, tailgating, or driving at excessive speeds were gradually exposed to descriptions of driving situations that made them angry. Prior to and during this exposure, the subjects engaged in deep muscle relaxation. (Most people find it difficult to be deeply relaxed and impulsively angry at the same time.) Following this treatment, the subjects reported less anger in response to driving scenes. These reports tended to be confirmed by galvanic skin response measures, but not by the heart rate measures. Further study of this treatment approach is needed. To the extent that stress or fear precedes the feeling of anger, as in situations of threat, a desensitization procedure might be a reasonable approach. Systematic desensitization has rather consistently been shown to be clinically useful in reducing fear responses.[49,50]

A related approach is called "stress inoculation."[51] It assumes that anger and aggression may be produced, at least in part, by a person's perception, thoughts, and self-statements in a situation. This approach attempts to strengthen self-control primarily through cognitive means, although some relaxation procedures may also be used.[52] The person may be taught to make statements to himself such as, "Stay calm," "Stay cool, this will soon be over." The person may also be taught to observe himself in the situation to provide emotional distance and thus reduce the impact of the situation. The person might also attempt to think about other matters or to recall a previously practiced relaxing scene.[53] Rehearsing and role playing these procedures with a therapist may be useful or even essential.[54,55,56]

A different approach has been used with extremely aggressive, chronic schizophrenic patients. These patients had to be restrained because their aggression presented a danger to themselves and others. Some of these patients frequently attempted to smash windows or other glass. During counter-conditioning sessions, the patients received electric shocks while visualizing breaking glass. Follow-up studies indicated marked reduction of their glass-breaking behavior.[57]

More recently, covert sensitization has sometimes been used in the place of electric shock or other aversive stimuli. In covert sensitization, the patient imagines an aversive stimulus or situation, such as getting nauseous and vomiting, immediately after imagining the performance of the prohibited behavior.[58] This method has been used with a patient having sadistic fantasies[59] and with exhibitionists.[60] This last study involved ten exhibitionists and included the use of valeric acid which the patient inhaled while imagining a nausea-inducing scene. Later the subjects were given small bottles of valeric acid from which they were to inhale in those circumstances which would ordinarily have elicited exhibitionist behavior. The subjects returned for "booster" treatment at 3, 6,

---

*An extensive survey of contemporary treatment methods using learning theory approaches can be found in *Analysis of Delinquency and Aggression* by Ribes-Inesta and Bandura,[46] and in Chapter 5 of *Aggression in Man and Animals* by Johnson.[47]

and 12 months. The results indicated a very substantial reduction of exhibitionist behavior and fantasies during the 12 months.

This last study illustrates an increasing concern about the limitations of treatment confined entirely to hospital, clinic, or office settings. Patients may have difficultly in generalizing experiences in an office to their daily life situations. Furthermore, the therapist may not be able to observe directly the behavior to be changed or even get a clear description of it. In the treatment of phobias, therapists have sometimes accompanied patients on elevators, across streets, or on airplanes while using relaxation procedures. These in vivo treatment procedures have been particulary effective with some patients.[50] A mid-range procedure is to bring objects into the treatment session which elicit the problem behavior or alternatively to film or videotape scenes in the natural setting in which the behavior occurs. These scenes may then be played during the treatment session. Of course, it is difficult to duplicate exactly the natural world of the patient in a hospital or clinic because he will usually be aware that he is in an alternative setting. In some cases, there may be no adequate substitute for real-world experiences.

Conditional Release

On a limited scale, it might be desirable to release certain patients from a hospital under close supervision and conditions that are likely to protect both the patient and public. A conditional release procedure might be used. For example, in *People v. Thingvold*,[61] a patient asserted that he was no longer a sexually dangerous person and should be released from the hospital. Four psychiatrists were uncertain. The Court permitted a conditional release of the patient, citing an Illinois statute that read in part:

> If the court finds that the patient appears no longer to be sexually dangerous but that it is impossible to determine with certainty under conditions of institutional care that such person has fully recovered, the court shall enter an order permitting such person to go at large subject to such conditions and such supervision by the Director as in the opinion of the court will adequately protect the public. In the event the person violates any of the conditions of such order, the court shall revoke such conditional release and recommit the person under the terms of the original commitment.

The Court requested a lower court to consider the placement of the patient in a half-way house under whatever provisions the trial court would consider appropriate to protect the public.

Conditional releases for short periods of time with close supervision would seem preferable to the long-term confinement of patients on the basis of uncertain probabilities of future dangerous conduct. Treatment such as in vivo desensitization could then be conducted in these settings.

Because adequate predictive accuracy about future dangerousness is difficult to obtain, it might be desirable in some situations to release the patient conditionally under very precise conditions to observe his behavior in natural settings. These releases might be considered a part of controlled clinical studies or tests of the effects of various environments upon the patient. The patient might, for example, be interviewed and tested immediately prior to and following his conditional release. If the patient were visited in his natural environment, he might be tested there as well.

Released patients have sometimes been requested to mail a postcard to the therapist each day. The postcard may contain a schedule of the previous day's activities and the medication taken. Unusual patterns of activity, sleep, medication, or even the failure to send in a card may provide useful information about the patient. Verification of some of the information reported can be made by phone calls or visits.

Alcohol in Treatment Program

The use of alcohol in natural settings might be an important factor related to aggression in some patients, but it is seldom tested in institutions. Alcohol has also been found to increase the intensity of electric shock that subjects are willing to administer to others.[62,63] In a different experiment conducted in an informal group setting, male volunteers from the general public showed statistically significant increases in aggressive behavior after drinking.[64]

Studies have frequently reported the involvement of alcohol with aggressive crimes. In a study of persons arrested during or shortly following the commission of a felony, it was found that 47 out of 60 persons committing physical assaults had blood alcohol levels greater than 0.10 percent at the time of their arrest.[65] In a study of 588 homicides over a 5-year period in Philadelphia, alcohol was found to be present in either the offender or the victim in 64 percent of the cases.[66] A study of 77 committed rapists in California indicated that 43 percent were drinking alcohol heavily, and 6 percent were drinking moderately or lightly, at the time the offense was committed.

There are several theories that might account for the relationship between alcohol consumption and aggression in certain patients. One theory postulates that aggression is inhibited by feelings of anxiety, fear, or guilt. If alcohol reduces these emotions, aggression may be disinhibited or released. Another, but not incompatible, theory is related to state-dependent learning (sometimes called dissociated learning). State-dependent learning refers to a phenomenon in which information learned under a drug condition is not transferred or remembered in a nondrug state. For example, normal persons who learn material such as nonsense syllables following the ingestion of alcohol may subsequently experience greater recall of the learned material after ingesting alcohol than without it.[68,69] In a study involving marijuana, Stillman and coworkers[70] concluded: "As predicted by a state-dependent model, subjects reproduced material best when they were in the same drug state as they had been when they first encountered the material to be recalled. In particular, marijuana-marijuana reproduction surpassed marijuana-placebo or placebo-marijuana reproduction; that is, material first encountered in a drug state was better reproduced when the subject was again in the drug state than when he was sober." State-dependent effects have also been suggested for amphetamine and amobarbital.[71] The extent to which learning is affected by state-dependency is a matter of speculation with a low estimate of about 15 percent of the learned material influenced by the alcohol.[72] That 15 percent may be socially significant or important in daily life situations. Demonstrations of state-dependent learning with socially significant material related to aggression need to be conducted.

If it is assumed that the state-dependent learning phenomenon applies to the learning and display of aggressive behavior, it is possible to hypothesize why alcohol may be related to aggression in some individuals but not in others. For certain individuals, alcohol may facilitate the recall of previously successful aggressive behaviors emitted while intoxicated, such as fights in a barroom. The recall of these behaviors and the events surrounding them may alter both the perception of the present environment and the anticipated consequences of aggression. The altered perception, combined with the anxiety-reduction effects of alcohol, may encourage learned patterns of aggression.

If certain behaviors learned during one internal state (e.g., sobriety) do not generalize well to other internal states (e.g., alcohol intoxication), then we could expect little therapeutic benefit from treating a sober person in a clinic setting for those aggressive behaviors which usually occur while he is intoxicated in a different setting. Therapeutic failure would be likely, and that is what is generally found. If the consumption of alcohol cannot be readily reduced or controlled, it might be useful to consider the possibility of treating aggression under state-dependent conditions. Shealy and Shen[73] treated a patient, in a hospital setting, who presented himself to the hospital for treatment of homicidal impulses which were manifested when he was extremely intoxicated with alcohol. The treatment involved two aspects. One aspect was a cognitive technique aimed at the patient's ideas concerning his masculinity. The second aspect used a behavior rehearsal technique which included alcohol. Following intoxication, the patient was taught to walk away from taunts from two of his brothers. This was a situation that usually evoked aggression.

In a study of "state-dependent therapy" currently being conducted by the author, the feasibility of treating patients while they are moderately intoxicated for behaviors occurring during intoxication is being explored. In one case involving aggressive behavior, the patient was systematically desensitized to insults while intoxicated. The initial treatment sessions were conducted in a laboratory setting. After the procedures appeared to be effective and efficient in preventing aggression in the laboratory setting, treatment was conducted in barroom settings where the aggression usually occurred to further increase generalization and the relevance of the treatment. Preliminary results during the past several months appear very positive.

CONCLUSION

Much more research is necessary to develop effective treatment interventions with dangerous behavior. If treatment could become brief and effective with minimal side effects, the issue of the accurate prediction of dangerousness would not be as critical as it is today because false-positive errors would not result in extensive deprivations of liberty. Until that time, mental health professionals may have to tolerate considerable ambiguity and legal risk while moving toward more empirical modes of prediction and more innovative forms of treatment.

REFERENCES

1. *Covington v. Harris*, 410 F.2d 617, 1969.
2. *Delaware Code Ann.* tit. 16 S 5125, 3, Supp. 1974.
3. *Tarasoff v. Regents of University of California*, 551 P.2d 334, 1976.
4. *Baxstrom v. Herald*, 383 U.S. 107, 1966.
5. Steadman, H. J., and Halfon, A.: The Baxstrom Patients: Background and Outcomes. *Semin. Psychiatry* 3:376–385, 1971.
6. Steadman, H. J., and Keveles, G.: The Community Adjustment and Criminal

Activity of the Baxstrom Patients: 1966–1970. *Am. J. Psychiatry* 129:304–310, 1972.
7. Steadman, H. J.: Implications from the Baxstrom Experience. Paper presented at the American Academy of Psychiatry and the Law Convention, Atlanta, March 16, 1973 (Mental Health Research Unit, New York State Department of Mental Hygiene, Albany, New York).
8. Rubin, B.: Prediction of Dangerousness in Mentally Ill Criminals. *Arch. Gen. Psychiatry* 27:397–407, 1972.
9. McGarry, A. L., and Parker, L. L.: Massachusetts' Operation Baxstrom: A Follow-up. *Mass. J. Mental Health* 4:27–41, 1974.
10. Kozol, H. L., Boucher, R. J., and Garofalo, R. F.: The Diagnosis and Treatment of Dangerousness. *Crime and Delinquency* 18:371–392, 1972.
11. Monahan, J.: Dangerous Offenders: A Critique of Kozol et al. *Crime and Delinquency* 19:418–420, 1973.
12. Evenson, R. C., and Altman, H.: A Re-Evaluation of "The Diagnosis and Treatment of Dangerousness." Unpublished paper, Missouri Institute of Psychiatry, University of Missouri School of Medicine, St. Louis, 1975.
13. Carney, F. L.: The Indeterminate Sentence at Patuxent. *Crime and Delinquency* 20:135–143, 1974.
14. Ennis B. J., and Litwack, T. R.: Psychiatry and the Presumption of Expertise: Flipping Coins in the Courtroom. *Cal. Law Rev.* 62:693–752, 1974.
15. Sweetland, J. P.: "Illusory Correlation" and the Estimation of "Dangerous" Behavior. Ph.D. dissertation, Department of Psychology, Indiana University, 1972. (Cited in Shah, S. A.: Dangerousness: A Paradigm for Exploring Some Issues in Law and Psychology. Paper presented at the American Psychological Association Convention, September 5, 1976.)
16. Ziskin, J.: *Coping with Psychiatric and Psychological Testimony*. Law and Psychology Press, Beverly Hills, 1970, pp. 147–158.
17. Steadman, H. J., and Cocozza, J. J.: A Natural Experiment in the Psychiatric Prediction of Dangerousness. Unpublished paper, Mental Health Research Unit, New York State Department of Mental Hygiene, Albany, New York, 1976, p. 11.
18. Stone, A. A.: *Mental Health and Law: A System in Transition*. Center for Studies of Crime and Delinquency, NIMH, Washington, D.C., 1975, p. 67.
19. *Rosenfield v. Overholser*, 262 F.2d 34, 1958.
20. *Arizona, Rev. Stat. Ann.* ch. 36–501, 3, 1974.
21. Tversky, A., and Kahneman, D.: Judgment under Uncertainty: Heuristics and Biases. *Science* 185:1124–1131, 1974.
22. Stran, P., Venet, L., and Shapiro, S.: Man Screening in Mammary Cancer. *Cancer Res.* 23:875–878, 1969.
23. McGarry, A. L., et al.: Competency to Stand Trial and Mental Illness. Center for Studies of Crime and Delinquency, NIMH, Washington, D.C., 1973, reprinted 1974.
24. Clemente, D. C., and Chase, M. H.: Neurological Substrates of Aggresssive Behavior. *Ann. Rev. Physiol.* 35:329–356, 1973.
25. Bach y Rita, G., and Veno, A.: Habitual Violence: A Profile of 62 Men. *Am. J. Psychiatry* 131:1015–1017, 1974.
26. Shah, S. A.: Dangerousness: Some Definitional, Conceptual, and Public Policy Issues, in Sales, B. D. (ed.): *Perspectives in Law and Psychology*. Vol. 1. Plenum, New York, 1977, pp. 91–119.
27. Patterson, G. R., and Cobb, J. A.: Stimulus Control for Classes of Noxious Behaviors, in Knutson, J. F. (ed.): *The Control of Aggression*. Aldine, Chicago, 1973, pp. 145–199.
28. O'Neal, E. C., and McDonald, P. J.: The Environmental Psychology of Aggression, in Geen, R. G., and O'Neal, E. C. (eds.): *Perspectives on Aggression*. Academic Press, New York, 1976, pp. 169–192.
29. Moyer, K. E.: The Physiological Inhibition of Hostile Behavior, in Knutson, J. F. (ed.): *The Control of Aggression*. Aldine, Chicago, 1973, pp. 9–38.
30. Wenk, E. A., Robinson, J. O., and Smith, G. W.: Can Violence Be Predicted? *Crime and Delinquency* 18:393–402, 1972.

31. Shah, S. A.: Some Interactions of Law and Mental Health in the Handling of Social Deviance. *Catholic U. Law Rev.* 23:674–719, 1974.
32. Shah, S. A.: Dangerousness and Civil Commitment of the Mentally Ill: Some Public Policy Considerations. *Am. J. Psychiatry* 132:501–505, 1975.
33. Shah, S. A.: Dangerousness: A Paradigm for Exploring Some Issues in Law and Psychology. Paper presented at the American Psychological Association Convention, Washington, D.C., September 5, 1976.
34. Meehl, P. E.: *Clinical Versus Statistical Prediction.* University of Minnesota Press, Minneapolis, 1954.
35. Sawyer, J.: Measurement and Prediction, Clinical and Statistical. *Psychol. Bull.* 66:178–200, 1966.
36. Kahneman, D., and Tversky, A.: On the Psychology of Prediction. *Psychol. Rev.* 80:237–251, 1973.
37. Carroll, J. S.: Prediction of Recidivism: Conflicts Between Clinical Strategies and Base-Rate Information. Unpublished paper, Carnegie-Mellon University, Pittsburgh, 1977.
38. Gottfredson, D. M., Hoffman, P. B., Siegler, M. H., and Wilkins, L. T.: Making Paroling Policy Explicit. *Crime and Delinquency* 21:33–44, 1975.
39. Genego, W. J., Goldberger, P. D., and Jackson, V. C.: Parole Release Decision-Making and the Sentencing Process. *Yale Law J.* 84:810–902, 1975.
40. Burnham, R. W.: Modern Decision Theory and Corrections, in Gottfredson, D. M. (ed.): *Decision-Making in the Criminal Justice System: Reviews and Essays.* Center for Studies of Crime and Delinquency, NIMH, Washington, D.C., 1975, pp. 92–123.
41. Miller, R. B., and Kenny, E.: Adolescent Delinquency and the Myth of Hospital Treatment. *Crime and Delinquency* 12:38–48, 1966.
42. Morris, H. H., Escoll, P. J., and Wexler, R.: Aggressive Behavior Disorders of Childhood: A Follow-Up Study. *Am. J. Psychiatry* 112:991–997, 1956.
43. Schorer, C. E., Lowinger, P., Sullivan, T., and Hartaub, G. H.: Improvement without Treatment. *Dis. Nerv. Syst.* 29:100–104, 1968.
44. Singer, J. E., and Grob, M. C.: Patients Discharged Against Medical Advise: A Follow-Up Study. *Mass. J. Mental Health* 5:57–66, 1974.
45. Wolkon, G. H., Karmen, M., and Tanaka, H. T.: Evaluation of a Social Program for Recently Released Psychiatric Patients. *Community Mental Health J.* 7:312–322, 1971.
46. Ribes-Inesta, E., and Bandura, A.: *Analysis of Delinquency and Aggression.* Wiley, New York, 1976.
47. Johnson, R. N.: *Aggression in Man and Animals.* W. B. Saunders, Philadelphia, 1972.
48. Rimm, D. C., et al.: Systematic Densenitization of an Anger Response. *Behav. Res. Ther.* 9:273–280, 1971.
49. Paul, G. L.: Outcome of Systematic Desensitization. II. Controlled Investigation of Individual Treatment, Technique Variations, and Current Status, in Franks, C. M. (ed.): *Behavior Therapy: Appraisal and Status.* McGraw-Hill, New York, 1969, pp. 105–159.
50. Schwitzgebel, R. K., and Kolb, D. A.: *Changing Human Behavior: Principles of Planned Intervention.* McGraw-Hill, New York, 1974, pp. 14–31.
51. Meichenbaum, D., and Cameron, R.: Stress Inoculation: A Skills Training Approach to Anxiety Management. Unpublished manuscript, University of Waterloo, 1973.
52. Novaco, R. W.: *Anger Control: The Development and Evaluation of an Experimental Treatment.* D. C. Heath, Lexington, Mass., 1975.
53. Bower, S. A., and Bower, G. H.: *Asserting Yourself: A Practical Guide for Positive Change.* Addison-Wesley, Reading, Mass., 1976, pp. 56–63.
54. Kanfer, F. H.: Self-Management Methods, in Kanfer, F. H., and Goldstein, A. P. (eds.): *Helping People Change: A Textbook of Methods.* Pergamon Press, Elmsford, N.Y., 1975, pp. 309–355.
55. Nolan, J. D.: Self-Control Procedures in the Modification of Smoking Behavior. *J. Consult. Clin. Psychol.* 32:92–93, 1968.

56. Roberts, A. H.: Self-Control Procedures in Modification of Smoking: Replication. *Psychol. Rep.* 24:675–676, 1969.
57. Agras, W. S.: Behavior Therapy in the Management of Chronic Schizophrenia. *Am. J. Psychiatry* 124:240–243, 1967.
58. Cautela, J. R.: Covert Sensitization. *Psychol. Rec.* 20:459–468, 1967.
59. Davison, G. C.: Elimination of a Sadistic Fantasy by a Client: A Controlled Counterconditioning Technique. *J. Abnorm. Psychol.* 73:84–90, 1968.
60. Maletzky, B.: Assisted: Covert Sensitization in the Treatment of Exhibitionism. *J. Consult. Clin. Psychol.* 42:34–40, 1974.
61. *People v. Thingvold,* 251 N.E. 2d 553, Ill. App. 1969.
62. Shuntick, R. J., and Taylor, S. P.: The Effects of Alcohol on Human Physical Aggression. *J. Exp. Res. Personality* 6:34–38, 1972.
63. Taylor, S. P., and Gammon, C. B.: The Effects of Type and Dose of Alcohol on Human Physical Aggression. *J. Personality Social Psychol.* 32:169–175, 1975.
64. Boyatzis, R. E.: The Effect of Alcohol Consumption on the Aggressive Behavior of Men. *Q. J. Studies Alcohol* 35:959–972, 1974.
65. Shupe, L. M.: Alcohol and Crime: A Study of the Urine Alcohol Concentration Found in 882 Persons Arrested During or Immediately After the Commission of a Felony. *J. Crim. Law, Criminol. Police Sci.* 44:661, 664, 1954.
66. Wolfgang, M. E., and Strohm, R. B.: The Relationship Between Alcohol and Criminal Homicide. *Q. J. Studies Alcohol* 17:411–425, 1956.
67. Rada, R. T.: Alcoholism and Forcible Rape. *Am. J. Psychiatry* 132:444–446, 1975.
68. Goodwin, D. W., et al.: Alcohol and Recall: State-Dependent Effects in Man. *Science* 163:1358–1360, 1969.
69. Overton, D. A.: State-Dependent Learning Produced by Alcohol and Its Relevance to Alcoholism, in Kissin, B., and Begleiter, H. (eds.): *The Biology of Alcoholism. Vol. 2, Physiology and Behavior.* Plenum, New York, 1972, pp. 193–217.
70. Stillman, R. C., et al.: State-Dependent (Dissociative) Effects of Marihuana on Human Memory. *Arch. Gen. Psychiatry* 31:81–85, 1974.
71. Bustamante, J. A., et al.: State-Dependent Learning in Humans. *Physiol. Behavior* 5:793–796, 1970.
72. Weingartner, J., and Faillace, L.: Alcohol State-Dependent Learning in Man. *J. Nerv. Ment. Dis.* 153:395–405, 1971.
73. Shealy, A. E., and Shen, J.: The Use of State-Dependent Learning Principles in Treatment: A Case Report. *J. Community Psychol.* 1:232–234, 1973.

CHAPTER 33

Simon Dinitz is Professor of Sociology at Ohio State University. He is a Past President of the American Society of Criminology and Editor of *Criminology,* the official journal of the Society. He was also Associate Editor of the *American Sociological Review.* Dr. Dinitz was a member of the Ohio Governor's Task Force on Corrections in 1971. He was an advisor to the United Nations Social Defense Research Institute from 1969 to 1974, and is currently a member of the international advisory board of the University of Tel Aviv. In 1967, he received the Hofheimer Prize for Research of the American Psychiatric Association. Dr. Dinitz is the author of several books, research papers, and articles on various aspects of criminology, delinquency, victimology, and the treatment and prevention of schizophrenia.

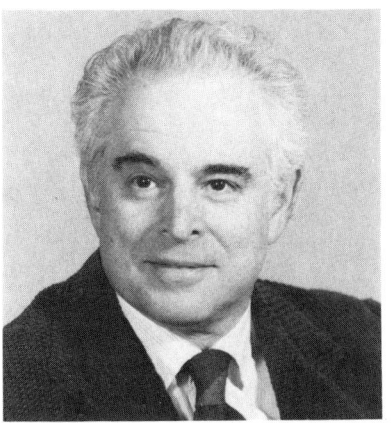

THE ANTISOCIAL PERSONALITY

Simon Dinitz, Ph.D.

Antisocial personality is a clinical disorder whose course, mechanism, and etiology remain unknown.[1] Genetic, physiologic, interactional, and sociocultural etiologies have been advanced to explain this intractable behavioral disorder which is not recognized as a form of mental illness by present legal standards. From M'Naghten to the American Law Institute Model Penal Code, the sociopath has been considered to be fully responsible for his conduct. In this, as in other spheres, the law and psychiatry are at odds. Thus the 1952 *Diagnostic and Statistical Manual of Mental Disorders* of the American Psychiatric Association described antisocial sociopaths as:

> ... chronically anti-social individuals who are always in trouble, profiting neither from experience nor punishment and maintaining no real loyalty to any person, group, or code. They are frequently callous and hedonistic, showing marked emotional immaturity with lack of sense of responsibility, lack of judgment, and an ability to rationalize their behavior so that it appears warranted, reasonable and justified.

The second (1968) edition of the *Manual* and the 1969 APA glossary contain no mention at all of such traditional and now obsolete terms as sociopathy and psychopathy. This most recent change in classification replaces sociopathy with antisocial personality, the latter described as follows:

> This term is reserved for individuals who are basically unsocialized and whose behavior pattern brings them repeatedly into conflict with society. They are incapable of significant loyalty to individuals, groups, or social values. They are grossly selfish, calloused, irresponsible, im-

pulsive, and unable to feel guilt or to learn from experience. Frustration tolerance is low. They tend to blame others or offer plausible rationalizations for their behavior . . . .

Previously and less specifically referred to as psychopathy,* constitutional psychopathic state, and psychopathic personality, sociopathy has been attributed to genetic, biologic, interpersonal, and cultural causes.[2]

Clinical evidence indicates that the antisocial personality constitutes from 1 to 3 percent of all adults of both sexes.[3] Even if this estimate is somewhat overdrawn numerically, sociopathy is an economically and socially expensive mental disorder. Furthermore, this chronic and disabling disease, which is probably characterized by a shortened life span,[4] is estimated to affect approximately 20 percent of the adult correctional population in the United States.† These institutionalized offenders are at best difficult to rehabilitate[5] and are often disruptive to the point of negating rehabilitative efforts for the remaining 80 percent of the inmates.

In contrast to the relative ease of management of the antisocial person in the smaller, more homogeneous community, the sociopath today represents an increasingly serious problem in the complex urban setting.

Whatever the precise etiology—the extraordinary disruption of the modern family, the increased geographic mobility, the "eclipse" of community, the elaboration of the female-headed household as a major type—the increased social disorganization occasioned by urbanization seems to have exacerbated the problem. The sociopath creates problems for the urban community; the urban community negatively influences the sociopath. The spiral effect is to be seen in *Children Who Hate*,[6] the "core" members of gangs,[7] and the changing composition of inmate populations. Experienced corrections people are more than ever disturbed by this trend and freely confess that they are unable to deal successfully with these highly disruptive inmates.

Despite the size of the sociopathic population and the belief of many clinicians that sociopathy is probably an irreversible personality disorder, little headway has been made in effective treatment techniques. In general, most correctional officers feel that no effective therapy exists and, even worse, that antisocial sociopaths are not amenable to treatment.[8] If sociopathy could be studied, its epidemiology delineated, and its social and biomedical characteristics elucidated, some of the defeatism which now characterizes the corrections system might be alleviated.

EARLY FORMULATIONS

The contemporary conception of the antisocial personality which forms the theoretical basis of present conceptions of the nature of sociopathy

---

*Psychopathic personality was the generic term used to refer to a large group of disorders which were regarded by many physicians and clinicians as diverse in nature and as having too little in common to justify subsuming them under the general term. Furthermore, practitioners seldom used the term except to refer, not to the more heterogeneous group, but to one and only one of the disorders—psychopathy.

†Cleckley, H., *The Mask of Sanity* (C. V. Mosby, St. Louis, 1950), Appendix A. Bernard Glueck investigated 608 Sing Sing inmates, 18.9 percent of whom were found to be sociopaths (quoted in S. Maughs, A Concept of Psychopathy and Psychopathic Personality: Its Evolution and Historical Development, *J. Crim. Psychopathol.* 2:480, 1941).

has evolved from formulations that have been advanced by numerous investigators, most of whom have derived their theories and insights from clinical experience.

Pinel is credited with first describing this phenomenon in modern terms.[9] His classification and description of *manie sans delire* (mania without delusions), while mixing a variety of disorders, dealt with this previously unexplained phenomenon. His tripartite classification (impulsive insanity and moral idiocy, hypomania, and melancholia activa), broadened the conception of mental illness and led others to question the prevailing notion of the time that the intellect is always involved in mental illness.

The American psychiatrist Benjamin Rush expressed similar ideas as early as 1812, speaking of moral alienation, defective organization of moral faculties, and deranged will. While postulating a special moral sense, in accordance with faculty psychology, Rush, like Pinel, recognized that mental illness may involve other than intellectual faculties.

These formulations influenced the English physician, J. C. Prichard. His comprehensive descriptions of sociopathy (under the titles of moral insanity and moral imbecility) drew attention to states characterized by an affective and feeling disorder, rather than by understanding and intellect. While his description of nonintellectual "insanity" was a bold step in the classification of mental diseases, he grouped all disorders on the basis of symptomatology and consequently included disorders other than sociopathy.

Garofalo,[10] one of the major founders of positive criminology, attempted to evade the issue of moral insanity by suggesting that biological factors might be present:

> Should [such moral anomalies as the sociopath] be regarded as a new nosologic form—the moral insanity of the English writers? The existence of this form of alienation is questionable, to say the least. In spite of utmost efforts to discover traces of insanity, one is often obliged to admit that the individual under examination possesses an intelligence which leaves nothing to be desired, that he exhibits no nosologic symptom, unless it be the absence of a moral sense, and that, to quote a French physician, whatever be the subject's unity of mind, 'the psychic keyboard has only one false note and only one.'

Garofalo further noted that these children are born with "ferocious instincts." For these criminals with imprudence, lack of insight, and moral insensibility, who exhibit complete indifference to shame, he substituted the term "constitutional inferiority" for "moral insanity."

Lombroso,[11] the father of modern criminology and a forensic psychiatrist, embraced the conception of the chronically antisocial individual as a moral imbecile, noting that he was guiltless, highly aggressive, impulsive, boastful, and particularly insensitive to social criticism and physical pain. Lombroso wanted such persons placed in asylums:

> At first sight this proposition seems absurd . . . But proper attention has not been paid to the fact that it is just such . . . cases, intermediate between reason and insanity, in which, therefore, the criminal asylums are most useful and of most service in guaranteeing the public safety.[12]

Partridge is credited with the introduction of the term sociopath, suggesting that persons with this disorder should be considered defective as a consequence of improper socialization.[13] Utilizing psychoanalytic theory, Partridge located the sociopath's maladjustment in the developmental process. A study of 50 sociopaths revealed, Partridge contended, that the sociopath fails to progress through the stages of normal child development and retains adjustment techniques common to early childhood. He described this disorder as a permanently fixed concentration on oral needs. His studies led him to conclude that:

> [The sociopathic] personality is a persistent behavior pattern or tendency in which there is usually excessive demand . . . which when there is a failure of direct or immediate satisfaction, is reacted to by a tendency to develop characteristic ways of dominating situations; by emotional displays we call tantrums, by sulks; by running away . . . .[14]

Thompson[15] offers a somewhat similar conception. To him, sociopathy is a personality deviation characterized by an inability to adjust adequately and consistently to social standards. Thompson maintained that this deviation stems from a basic mental defect which renders the sufferer incapable of developing an adequate sense of time, particularly with regard to self. Lack of guilt, insufficient judgment, impulsiveness, and inability to profit from experience are secondary symptoms which result from this basic defect.

Henderson[16] used the term psychopathic state to refer to the antisocial sociopath and included three groups under this rubric: the predominantly aggressive, the predominantly passive or inadequate, and the predominantly creative. The latter state suggests the genius as a variant of the sociopath.* In essence, Henderson described the sociopath as unstable, explosive, and egocentric. Psychic immaturity is the prime feature of his condition:

> He cannot accept things as they are; he is unable to fit into the life of the herd, but tends to lead an independent, individualistic type of existence with no thought or feeling for his family, his friends, or his country. He is blunted emotionally . . . for a time he may prove charming . . . For some inscrutable reason he fails to grow up, he remains at the level of a primitive savage with a distaste for reasoning and an 'impermeability to experience' . . . . The judicial, deciding, selecting process described as intelligence, and the energizing, emotivating, driving powers called character, are not working in harmony.[17]

Cleckley[18] has provided the most inclusive and thorough conceptualization of the antisocial sociopath, maintaining that the latter is a distinguishable, deeply rooted clinical entity. The disorder adversely affects

---

*Kozol, a more recent contributor, also related genius and sociopathy, and stated that the same dynamics operate in both. The level of assault differs—the genius creates, whereas the sociopath makes his attacks for "kicks;" yet both are characterized by identical factors, Kozol maintained. There is dissociation between basic impulse patterns and the development of social pseudo-conformity. Sociopaths learn to conform for their own benefit; however, this educative process appears unrelated to the primitive impulse structure. This separation accounts for the lack of internal control and the primitiveness of goals which characterizes them (Maughs, op. cit., p. 484).

interpersonal relations and is demonstrated best when the sociopath confronts problems of living.

The antisocial sociopath, according to Cleckley,[19] is characterized by:

1. Superficial charm and good intelligence.
2. Absence of delusions and other signs of irrational thinking.
3. Absence of nervousness and other psychoneurotic manifestations.
4. Unreliability.
5. Untruthfulness and insincerity.
6. Lack of remorse or shame.
7. Inadequately motivated antisocial behavior.
8. Poor judgment and failure to learn by experience.
9. Pathologic egocentricity and incapacity for love.
10. General poverty of major affective relations.
11. Specific loss of insight.
12. Unresponsiveness in interpersonal behavior.
13. Fantastic and uninviting behavior, with drink and sometimes without.
14. Suicide rarely carried out.
15. Sex life impersonal, trivial, and poorly integrated.
16. Failure to follow any life plan.

More precisely, Cleckley described the sociopath who is likely to end up in prison as easy to talk with, friendly, and frequently of superior intelligence. Outer perceptual reality is not distorted; social values may be accepted verbally, and excellent logical reasoning prevails. The sociopath with great verbal facility foresees consequences of action and criticizes former mistakes. These excellent rational powers, so apparent verbally as well as in hypothetical situations, do not carry over into behavior. Despite his rationality, the sociopath shows poor judgment in behavior and has a perplexing ability for creating situations in which no rational person would participate. Furthermore, he suffers from specific loss of insight. He neither knows how others feel in relation to him nor appreciates subjectively the values and major emotional concerns others have for him. There is a total absence of appraisal of self as a real and moving experience. The sociopath has all the qualities by which insight is gained, and awareness of major facts, all the words of understanding; yet these facts neither enter into his evaluations nor prompt him to change his behavior. The discrepancy between his favorable orientation and ability to reason and his behavior is enigmatic.

This baffling paradox is clearly revealed in the sociopath's inadequately motivated antisocial behavior, his failure to develop a life plan, and his untruthfulness. As part of his antisocial conduct, he often commits crimes for small stakes and under great risks. Yet there is no evidence of a compulsive or neurotic component. He does not formulate long-term goals, but seems to be motivated to fail in life. He cannot be trusted in his accounts of the past, statement of present intentions, or promises for the future. He lies, seemingly without purpose, and, with ready sincerity, manipulates truth to gain his immediate ends.

The sociopath's untruthfulness is coupled with personal unreliability and irresponsibility. He is irresponsible, no matter how binding the obligation, in trivial as well as in serious matters. While the antisocial sociopath intermittently reveals convincing and conforming loyalty,[20] predicting when he will or will not be responsible appears to be impossible. It does not seem to be related to mood, objective stress, or amount at stake for himself or for others. Furthermore, he feels no shame or remorse; the antisocial sociopath usually projects blame on others, and his blaming of himself is hollow, casual, and instrumental. He is seemingly incapable of object love and is generally unresponsive in interpersonal behavior. While he may be attentive to small courtesies, perhaps even obliging and generous, he cannot show consistent, ordinary responsiveness to kindness and trust. He is not usually motivated by altruistic concern, although he may superficially claim to be; nor can he express genuine human emotions. In brief, the sociopath is impoverished in affective reactions.

Cleckley suggests that the sociopath has no deep commitment either to persons or ideas. He often overindulges in sexual behavior, alcohol, drugs, and other "thrill-producing" substances. Sexual behavior is random, provoked frequently by whimlike impulses of little intensity, and is free of emotional involvement.

Cleckley adopted the term "semantic disorder" or "semantic psychosis" to refer to the clinical entity characterized above. The sociopath mimics the human personality and wears a "mask of sanity." He is unaware of and lacks the ability to become cognizant of what the most important life experiences mean to others. Major emotional accompaniments or affective competencies are missing. His response to life is dissociated, and components of normal experience are not integrated into a wholly human reaction.

Gough,[21] in a social psychological treatment of sociopathy, contends that the sociological theory of role-playing as described in the work of the symbolic interactionists, such as Harry Stack Sullivan in psychiatry, provides a synthesis of known facts of sociopathy and formulated deductive hypotheses for empirical testing. The antisocial personality, according to Gough, is pathologically deficient in role-taking ability. This deficiency is characterized by an inability to view the self as an object and to identify with another's point of view. Since other aspects of sociopathy are associated with this deficiency, Gough concluded that the causes of sociopathy must be sought in the causes of inadequacy in role-playing ability.

ETIOLOGIC PERSPECTIVES

Defective Role-Taking

Apart from clinical studies, the antisocial sociopath has been relatively neglected as a subject of research. There have been very few social psychological studies.

Following Gough, Baker[22] investigated skill in taking the role of the other and hypothesized that in a group of male prisoners, antisocial sociopaths would be less able than nonsociopaths* to empathize with their cellmates, all of whom had shared a cell with these cellmates for at least 4 weeks. Each subject and his cellmate filled out four adjective checklists: for self *(A)*; for cellmate *(B)*; prediction of self-checks for cellmate *(C)*; and subject's guesses as to how he appears to his cellmate *(D)*. Predictions made by each subject on checklists *C* and *D* were compared with the cellmate's actual choices on checklists *A* and *B*, thus providing two measures of empathy, including the percentage of correct predictions on check-

---

*Subjects were assigned to categories on the basis of MMPI profiles.

list C and the percentage of correct predictions on checklist D. The first indicates ability to perceive qualities or traits others use in assessing one's self. While the samples are small (21 sociopaths and 13 nonsociopaths), the differences in C and D percentages are statistically significant; sociopaths are less able to empathize with others.

Albrecht and Sarbin,[23] arguing that antisocial sociopaths cannot take the time to put themselves in the role of the other before they act,† and therefore are poor tension binders, hypothesized that such persons would be most responsive to annoying stimuli. Administering a 172-item annoyance questionnaire to 60 male subjects (20 diagnosed as sociopaths, 27 diagnosed as neurotics, and 13 without psychiatric diagnosis), they found significant differences between groups on total mean scores, with sociopaths having the highest, normals intermediate, and neurotics lowest mean annoyance scale scores.

McCord and McCord offer one of the more recent formulations of the sociopath and specify guiltlessness and lovelessness as the core characteristic of the antisocial sociopath:

> The [antisocial personality] is an asocial, aggressive, highly impulsive person, who feels little or no guilt and is unable to form lasting bonds of affection with other human beings.[24]

These characteristics, it would appear, are considered basic to the antisocial sociopath syndrome; they are consistently employed in almost all contemporary uses of the concept.

The McCords attempted to evaluate the contributions of milieu therapy on young, aggressive, sociopathic boys at the Wiltwyck school in New York, wherein both individual and group therapy were combined in a warm, permissive environment. After painstaking study, the authors concluded that milieu therapy causes radical alterations in personality of the subjects. However, such an environment is easily manipulated by sociopaths; if the subjects had been followed after release, much of the optimism concerning successful treatment might have been dispelled by observing the behavior of sociopathic boys in a nonaccepting environment.

Sociological and Psychiatric Variables

Robins,[25] in the most thorough sociological and psychiatric study of the antisocial personality to date, directed a 10-year research project representing a 30-year longitudinal study of the adult status of 524 child-guidance clinic patients at the St. Louis Municipal Psychiatric Clinic. This patient group was made up predominantly of male offspring of American-born Protestant parents of low socioeconomic status; blacks were excluded from the investigation. Ninety percent of the subjects were located, 82 percent were interviewed, and 98 percent were successfully traced through adult records. On the basis of interview and record information, and for each of the 19 areas of the subject's life in which he might have failed to conform to societal norms,[26] specific criteria for sociopathic

---

†This point is basic to Gough's role-taking theory of sociopathy, following Mead (G. H. Mead, *Mind, Self and Society*, University of Chicago Press, 1934).

behavior were established.* These criteria allowed two psychiatrists to agree as to whether 80 percent of the subjects were well or ill,† and to make reasonably specific diagnoses for 71 percent of the subjects. Robins does not indicate the degree to which the remaining 29 percent, who could not be specifically diagnosed, differed from those who were successfully diagnosed. (This latter point introduces possible unkown biases.)

The 94 sociopathic personality subjects from St. Louis were compared with four other specific diagnostic groups that occurred frequently enough to permit statistical comparisons (anxiety neurosis, hysteria, schizophrenia, and alcoholism), and with a group of 100 control subjects from the same city, matched on race, area of residence, sex, age, and IQ.

This important research was concerned basically with three areas of delineation: distinctive symptoms of the sociopathic personality; a portrait of adult sociopathic personality; and childhood behavior predictive of later diagnosis. The findings in these three areas are complex, subject to differences in interpretation, and were not analyzed or presented in a wholly satisfactory fashion.

As for symptoms, persons diagnosed as sociopathic personalities in the St. Louis study had more symptoms than any other diagnostic group, the three most common symptoms being financial dependency, poor work history, and multiple arrests. Four symptoms distinguished the sociopathic personality group at a statistically significant level from the other four groups: poor marital history, impulsiveness, vagrancy, and the use of aliases. The presence of one or more of the latter symptoms turned out to be among the best indicators of later sociopathic personality diagnosis.

The portrait of the St. Louis patient diagnosed as a sociopathic personality as an adult is contaminated by the use of the 19 symptom areas to diagnose subjects; the very criteria used for diagnosis were later treated as characteristics of the sociopath. However, four noncircular aspects of sociopathy are also presented: social adjustment, health, psychiatric symptoms, and treatment.

In general, persons diagnosed as sociopathic personalities in the St. Louis study had a disproportionately high death rate, more than twice the national rate; felt themselves to be sicker than other groups; were extremely mobile; more often lived in the core city; were currently more often unemployed; had experienced long periods of unemployment; usually held a low-ranking blue-collar job; rarely held a job for long; functioned longer in jobs in which they had little supervision; earned less when employed; were downwardly mobile in occupation; had low educational attainment; experienced little upward mobility from their fathers; were more frequently recipients of aid from public agencies; had the lowest percentage with established credit ratings; were more often divorced than any other group, and less often currently living with spouse;

---

*The median number of areas in which subjects given the diagnosis of antisocial sociopathic personality met the various criteria for failure to conform to societal norms was first reported to be 11. In the next paragraph it was reported that 13 of the 19 symptoms occurred in at least half the subjects diagnosed as antisocial sociopathic personalities. Five pages later it was noted that 69 percent of the sociopathic group had at least nine of these 19 symptoms.

†The psychiatrists were aware that the topic of interest was antisocial sociopathic personality; a relatively high proportion (15.6 percent) were diagnosed sociopathic. It may well have been that "blind" evaluators would not have found such a high proportion to be sociopathic.

tended to marry spouses with serious behavior problems; married somewhat younger than either patient or control groups; were slightly more often childless; were parents to children who were already showing marked emotional problems, few of whom graduated from high school; had the lowest rates of induction into the armed forces; were extreme medical and disciplinary problems in the service; and had aborted terms of military service.

The St. Louis patients also had unusually high proportions of nontraffic arrests, being arrested at least once for a major crime; had more convictions when arrested than all other subjects; were less likely to "burn out" in criminal behavior over time; evinced high rates of problem drinking; and were either currently experimenting with drugs (5 percent) or were or had been addicted to drugs (10 percent).

The sociopaths in the St. Louis study were also more often isolated from relatives and neighbors; belonged to very few formal organizations; had many neurotic and somatic symptoms; had rarely sought psychiatric care; had been frequently hospitalized in mental hospitals (21 percent); and had been more often previously diagnosed as sociopathic when hospitalized.

The above characteristics have been closely linked with lower social class status by sociologists, especially Matza,[27] Kahl,[28] and Komarovsky.[29] Social class may well be intervening to produce these marked differences and traits, although Robins made a concerted but somewhat ineffectual and unconvincing effort to contraindicate social class as an explanatory variable.

Robins' treatment of social class as a variable is at best less than ideal. Her study group is somewhat vaguely broken into "blue collar" and "white collar" on the basis of father's occupation; 24 percent of the former and 13 percent of the latter were found to be sociopathic. This represents a ratio of almost 2:1. It may be that sociopathy is concentrated in the lower class, owing to the relative breakdown in socialization or to the sociopaths' having drifted downward. Another possible alternative is that psychiatrists see such antisocial behavior of the lower class as sociopathy, exhibiting middle-class perspective as professional judgment. Perhaps all three may be operating, although Robins argues against the latter. However, the argument would have been stronger if she had presented the average number of symptoms necessary for diagnosis as sociopath for the lower and middle class, separately.

Finally, as for childhood behavior predicting sociopathy, Robins suggested that these symptoms would include aggression or theft for a boy; many episodes of diverse antisocial behavior, at least one of which could bring the child before a juvenile court; antisocial involvement with strangers and organizations as well as with parents and teachers; gratuitous lying; a history of truancy, staying out late, and refusing to obey parents; little guilt over behavior; irresponsibility concerning both being where one was supposed to be and taking care of money; interest in sexual behavior and experimenting with homosexual behavior; bed-wetting; and poor grooming. Only self-exposure and vandalism, among the antisocial symptoms, were innocuous. Girls resembled boys in the antisocial symptoms, except that they exhibited sexual misbehavior more frequently and prominently and experienced the onset of difficulties more visible at a later age.

Robins noted that antisocial behavior by the fathers of the patients is predictive of antisocial behavior for patients, particularly paternal desertion, arrest, excessive drinking, failure to support the family, and chronic unemployment. However, as for the effects of the family setting on sociopathic personality per se, Robins noted only that parental rejection does not appear to lead to sociopathy, and early separation from an antisocial father does not appear to prevent the development of sociopathy in the child. In the latter case, this may be due to the lessened ability of the mother alone to exercise control over the child.

In conclusion, Robins suggested that a more precise study of the sociopathic personality could be made from a longitudinal study of consecutive births, thus minimizing the selectivity inherent in subjects volunteering or being forced to seek attention at mental health or child guidance clinics. Such would be a difficult but potentially rewarding enterprise.

BIOLOGICAL SUBSTRATES OF SOCIOPATHY

Despite the long-standing interest, particularly on the part of European criminologists, in the biologic substrates of chronically antisocial behavior, few modern American criminologists have considered it relevant to examine these aspects of criminal conduct. There are, of course, a variety of justifications for this neglect. For one thing, academic criminology in the United States is located in departments of sociology rather than in schools of law or medicine, as has been traditional in Europe and Latin America. Given their training and orientation, few sociologists are versed in, or sympathetic to, a biologic perspective. Instead, American criminology has been distinguished by its strong sociocultural emphasis and its view of criminal behavior as essentially learned and adaptive conduct. Another and perhaps even more important reason for this neglect of biologic investigation has been the sorry history of the biological perspective in the last hundred years. The extravagant claims, meager empirical evidence, naivete, gross inadequacy, and stated or implied concepts of racial and ethnic inferiority in the work of the constitutionalists, the morphologists, the European traditionalists, and the early endocrinologists deservedly discredited the biological framework in the study of crime. Finally, American psychiatrists, at least those interested in criminology, have long been wedded to a psychodynamic orientation in which the focus is on the psychogenic and familial bases of intrapsychic and interpersonal pathologies rather than the psychophysiologic. Given this intellectual climate and disreputable history of biological theorizing, it is little wonder that even the very few important empirical observations of a biologic nature have been generally overlooked by criminologists.

Nevertheless, recent, though limited, studies of the antisocial sociopath have been conducted by physiological psychologists, biologists, and physicians, most of whom have focused on the physiologic responses of the sociopath as distinguished from other inmates. It was in 1949 that Funkenstein and associates[30] parenthetically mentioned the cardiovascular lability of chronically antisocial individuals. Funkenstein, a psychiatrist, and his colleagues reported on 15 sociopaths (13 men and 2 women) selected from a group of court referrals to the Boston Psychopathic Hospital. They characterized these subjects, ranging in age from 21 to 39 (mean = 25), as hostile recidivists. All had committed crimes of violence and exhibited no clinical signs of anxiety, although they often claimed to be "nervous." Even though none of these subjects volunteered any complaint of subjective discomfort, after an injection of 50 mg of epinephrine, 13 of the 15 sustained a systolic blood pressure rise of 75 mm Hg as compared to only 19 of the 85 psychotic and neurotic patients and five of the 15 controls.

In 1955, a psychologist, Lykken,[31] reported on the performance of 19 "primary" sociopathic felons (12 of whom were men) on eight assorted psychological tests. On the two tests measuring autonomic function, the "primary" sociopaths produced a diminished galvanic skin response (GSR) to lying and a diminished conditionability of the GSR as compared to the noninstitutionalized controls. The first difference, the GSR to lying, approached the 0.05 level of significance. These differences were statistically different when the "primary" sociopaths were compared with a group of 19 incarcerated "neurotic" sociopaths (i.e., the inmates who were labeled sociopath by the prison staff but who did not meet Cleckley's clinical criteria).

In 1964, the social psychologists Schacter and Latane[32] reported that 15 imprisoned male sociopaths showed greater increases in pulse rate following an epinephrine injection than did 15 inmate control subjects. (Whether the controls of Schacter and Latane more closely related to Lykken's "neurotic" sociopaths or to his controls is a moot point.)

In 1965, the psychologist Lippert[33] compared 21 "sociopathic" delinquents with 21 nonsociopathic delinquents and found that their patterns of spontaneous GSR frequency were characterized by (1) lower resting levels, (2) lesser increases during experimental manipulation, (3) decreases below resting levels following experimental manipulation, and (4) increased adaption to repeated stimuli.

In 1968, Hare[34] like Lippert, found that, at rest, 21 primary psychopaths had higher skin resistance and less variability than 12 nonpsychopathic controls. Furthermore, the psychopaths' GSR, cardiovascular and orienting responses to mild stimuli, such as the solution of arithmetic problems, were less than in the controls.

Hakerem[35] observed an exaggerated pupillary response in a group of patients who were later identified as "psychopaths." This parenthetical observation was neither pursued nor published.

In the most recent and elegant assessment of the status of research in sociopathy, Hare[36] underscores the assumption, now increasingly postulated, of a physiologic basis for this disorder. Substantial emphasis has been placed on some prominent biologic correlates of sociopathy, specifically:

1. That the EEG patterns of some antisocial personalities resemble those of children. This has led some investigators to the hypothesis of delayed maturation of some cortical neuronal mechanism.[37] These abnormal EEGs, often found in their parents as well, are characterized by a predominantly slow wave pattern, a pattern found in states of hypoarousal.
2. In some antisocial personalities, Hare argues that limbic system disfunction, as evidenced in an abnormal slow wave EEG, seems to be involved.
3. From this evidence, one may conclude that psychopathy may depend on a decreased state of cortical excitability and on an attenuation of sensory input.[38]
4. Moreover, some sociopaths display not only these symptoms of hypoarousal, but those of sensory deprivation as well. For example, consistently observed is the paradoxical increase in aggressivity and other emotionality in certain sociopaths treated with drugs, such as

barbiturates, neuroleptics, and ethanol—substances which usually aggravate states of sensory deprivation and promote passivity.[39]

5. Certain antisocial personalities demonstrate a pathologic need for stimulation and appear to be at a low end of an arousal continuum.[40] One would expect from these observations that some sociopaths would avoid the use of depressants. Indeed, Robins[41] found this to be the case. On the other hand, Hill[42] found depressants to improve the behavior of aggressive sociopaths.
6. Some antisocial personalities exhibit stereotyped behavior.[43] In view of poor space-time integration and the stereotypical behavior, there is a likelihood that basal ganglia dysfunction may be involved.
7. Definite sexual differences in the median age of the onset of antisocial personality symptoms may not be entirely socioculturally determined. Whereas in boys, symptoms occur at 7 years of age, they are less severe in girls and occur later, at 13. There may be a sex-related difference in certain kinds of sociopathy together with a possible biological explanation, as indicated in the research by Robins.
8. Sociopaths or antisocial personality types improve as a function of age, supporting the concept of delayed maturation. However, only a certain type of sociopath will improve, while others will continue to demonstrate symptoms for life unless otherwise modified.
9. On the basis of the assumption that sociopathic behavior is somehow a consequence of hypoarousal, MacCulloch and Feldman[44] suggested that stimulants such as amphetamine might have utility in the treatment of sociopaths. However, Hare[45] rightly adds social processing to this chemotherapy as a potential means of rehabilitation.

HETEROGENEITY OF SOCIOPATHY

It is clear that much of the recent research in sociopathy suggests a highly probable biological etiology, yet often there has been little statistical validation of this hypothesis within and between studies from different laboratories. Possible explanations of this lack of validation may lie in the operational definitions of sociopathy and the selection of different sociopathic types for experimentation purposes.

After attempting to replicate the pioneering work of Schachter and Latane, in which a unique biologic response was described in sociopaths, it became clear to us that even the rigorous selection procedures used by them had failed to provide us with a homogeneous group; marked variability in biologic and other measures made interpretation meaningless. We soon concluded that much of this variation, also noted by others, could be explained on the basis of at least two subgroups, as described below.

Our own multidisciplinary investigation, begun in 1965 at the Ohio Penitentiary and involving 19 "primary" sociopaths (10 mixed and 14 nonsociopaths, as defined by clinical, psychometric, and criminal history criteria), revealed that the "primary" sociopaths were not homogeneous with regard to such sociocultural variables as previous antisocial history, family characteristics, psychological profiles, and attitudes. As a result, using the Lykken Scale scores as the criterion, the "primary" sociopaths were divided into two types—"hostile" and "simple." These types were clearly and significantly different from each other on nearly all of the sociocultural and psychological measures. Most importantly, only the "simple" (reasonably nonaggressive) sociopaths demonstrated the cardiac lability to epinephrine previously ascribed to sociopaths in general.[46] The exaggerated autonomic responses of simple sociopaths demonstrate that their characteristic overt behavior is paralleled by a characteristic physiologic behavior.

It is possible, based on research at various Ohio prisons, that a logical case can be made for both abnormal autonomic and abnormal social behavior in the simple sociopath, resulting from a single, simple, structural biological defect. The most parsimonious lesion consistent with the available physiologic data is simply a diminished function (partial or total) of the catecholamine-secreting nerve endings, including those involved with sensory receptors. Such a sympathetic denervation would produce a denervation sensitivity long familiar to psychologists. Such a supersensitivity—of whatever origin—is testable by current technology. This hypothesis in no way precludes extension of the defect to monoaminergic interneurons modulating both sensory input and motor output at higher levels of nervous system integration.

It is reasonable to assume that a defect already observed for three disparate effectors—heart, skin, and pupil—is general among catecholamine-secreting neurons. Since other evidence, both physiologic and anatomic,[47] indicates that the sympathetic nervous system modulates sensory input at several levels, including interoceptors and exteroceptors themselves, one result of such a general sympathetic nervous system defect would be a reduction and distortion of incoming stimuli in the simple sociopath. In point of fact, both Schoenherr[48] and Hare[49] have already demonstrated an elevated threshold for electric shock in sociopathic prisoners. Such diminution and distortion of sensory data on a chronic basis must markedly modify conditioned responses to emotion-laden stimuli, thereby distorting the attitudes and values erected during the formative years.

It is conceivable and desirable that lesions such as those mentioned could be reversed or at least compensated by medical means. Such medical treatment would probably suffice as a preventive measure when applied prior to the onset of the disease. However, in those in whom detection is delayed until the syndrome has developed, the defect will have influenced behavior already; years of faulty programming would continue to determine behavior even after any original biologic basis had been removed or compensated. Hence, even a medical solution to the sociopath's problem would be insufficient. If our assumptions are correct, therapeutic intervention, of necessity, will have to include resocialization.

The issue is far from being resolved. We are still very much in ignorance of the course, mechanisms, and etiology of the behavior pattern and mental status currently called antisocial personality. Despite increased pharmacologic treatment of those designated as sociopaths, the chronically antisocial individual is likely to tax our ingenuity and patience in the foreseeable future to perhaps an even greater extent than he has in the past. In conclusion, there is considerable room for pessimism, notwithstanding the return of the medical and biologically oriented specialists of the field.

REFERENCES

1. Kaelbling, R., and Patterson, R.: *Eclectic Psychiatry.* Charles C Thomas, Springfield, Ill., 1966, p. 371.
2. An excellent summary of these attributions may be found in Cleckley, H.: Psychopathic States, in Arieti, S. (ed.): *American Handbook of Psychiatry.* Basic

Books, New York, 1962, pp. 567–588. See also Noyes, A., and Kolb, I.: *Modern Clinical Psychiatry*. W. B. Saunders, Philadelphia, 1963, pp. 460–464; Robins, E.: Personality Disorders. II. Sociopathic Types: Antisocial Disorders and Sexual Deviations, in Freeman, A., and Kaplan, H. (eds.): *Comprehensive Textbook of Psychiatry*. Williams & Wilkins, Baltimore, 1967, pp. 955–956; and McCord, W., and McCord, J.: *Psychopathy and Delinquency*. Grune & Stratton, New York, 1956, pp. 47–81.

3. Gregory, I.: *Psychiatry*. W. B. Saunders, Philadelphia, 1961, pp. 52–67.
4. Robins, L.: *Deviant Children Grown Up*. Williams & Wilkins, Baltimore, 1966, pp. 90–92.
5. Noyes and Kolb, op. cit., p. 462.
6. Redl, F., and Wineman, D.: *Children Who Hate*. The Free Press, Glencoe, Ill., 1951.
7. Yablonsky, L.: *The Violent Gang*. Macmillan, New York, 1962.
8. Robins, op cit., p. 2; Freedman and Kaplan, op cit., p. 958; Noyes and Kolb, op cit., pp. 464–465; Cleckley, Psychopathic States, pp. 585–587; and McCarthy, D. J., and Corrin, K. M.: *Medical Treatment of Mental Diseases*. J. B. Lippincott, Philadelphia 1955, pp. 415–418.
9. Maughs, S.: A Concept of Psychopathy and Psychopathic Personality: Its Evolution and Historical Development. *J. Crim. Psychopathol.* 2:465–499, 1941.
10. Garofalo, R.: *Criminology*. Little, Brown, Boston, 1914, p. 80.
11. Lombroso, C.: *Crime: Its Causes and Remedies*. Little, Brown, Boston, 1911, pp. 365–366.
12. Ibid., p. 423.
13. Maughs, op cit., p. 487.
14. Quoted in Henderson, P. K.: *Psychopathic States*. W.W. Norton, New York, 1939, p. 27.
15. Thompson, G. N.: Psychopathy. *Arch. Crim. Psychodynamics* 4(2):736–749, 1961.
16. Henderson, op. cit.
17. Henderson, op cit., pp. 128–129.
18. Cleckley, H.: *The Mask of Sanity*. ed. 4. C. V. Mosby, St. Louis, 1964.
19. Ibid., pp. 363–400.
20. Kaelbling and Patterson, op. cit., p. 372.
21. Gough, H.: A Sociological Theory of Psychopathy. *Am. J. Sociol.* 53:359–366, 1948.
22. Baker, B.: Accuracy of Social Perceptions of Psychopathic and Non-Psychopathic Prison Inmates. Unpublished manuscript, 1954. Summarized in Sarbin, T. R.: Role Theory, in Lindzey, C. (ed.): *Handbook of Social Psychology*. Addison-Wesley, Reading, Mass., 1954, p. 246.
23. Albrecht, R., and Sarbin, T. R.: Contributions to Role-Taking Theory: Annoyability as a Function of the Self. Unpublished manuscript, 1954; Lindzey, op. cit., p. 246.
24. McCord and McCord, op. cit., p. 2.
25. Robins, op. cit., pp. 90–92.
26. Ibid., p. 80.
27. Matza, D.: Poverty and Disrepute, in Merton and Nisbet (eds.): *Contemporary Social Problems*. Harcourt, Brace & World, New York, 1966, pp. 619–669.
28. Kahl, J.: *The American Class Structure*. Rinehart & Company, New York, 1957, pp. 205–215.
29. Komarovsky, M.: *Blue-Collar Marriage*. Random House, New York, 1964.
30. Funkenstein, D. H., Greenblatt, M., and Solomon, H. C.: Psychophysiological Study of Mentally Ill Patients. *Am. J. Psychiatry* 106:359–366, 1949.
31. Lykken, D. T.: A Study of Anxiety in the Sociopathic Personality. Ph.D. dissertation, University of Minnesota; University Microfilms, Ann Arbor, 1955, No. 55-944.
32. Schacter, S., and Latane, B.: Crime, Cognition and the Autonomic Nervous System, in Levine, D. (ed.): *Nebraska Symposium of Motivation*. University of Nebraska Press, Lincoln, 1964, pp. 271–274.
33. Lippert, W. W.: The Electrodermal System of the Sociopath. Ph.D. disserta-

tion, University of Cincinnati; University Microfilms, Ann Arbor, 1965, No. 65-12921.
34. Hare, R. D.: Psychopathy, Autonomic Functioning, and the Orienting Response. *J. Abnorm. Psychol.* 73 (Suppl.):1–24, 1968.
35. Personal communication, September 1968.
36. Hare, R. D.: *Psychopathy.* Wiley, New York, 1970, p. 33.
37. Kiloh, L., and Osselton, J. W.: *Clinical Electroencephalography.* Butterworth, Washington, 1966; Lindsley, D. B.: The Ontogeny of Pleasure: Neural and Behavioral Development, in Heath, R. G. (ed.): *The Role of Pleasure in Behavior.* Harper & Row, New York, 1964, pp. 3–22; Scheibel, M. E., and Scheibel, A. B.: Some Neural Substrates of Postnatal Development, in Hoffman, M., and Hoffman, L. (eds.): *Review of Child Development Research.* Vol. 1. Russell Sage Foundation, New York, 1954, pp. 481–519.
38. Hare, op. cit., p. 36; Lindner, L. A., Goldman, H., Dinitz, S., and Allen, H. E.: Antisocial Personality Type with Cardiac Lability. *Arch. Gen. Psychiat.* 23:260–267, 1970.
39. Cleckley, H., op. cit.
40. Quay, H. C.: Psychopathic Personality and Pathological Stimulation Seeking. *Am. J. Psychiatry* 122:180–183, 1965; Petrie, A.: *Individuality in Pain and Suffering.* University of Chicago Press, Chicago, 1967; Eysenck, H. J.: *The Biological Basis of Personality.* Charles C Thomas, Springfield, Ill., 1967.
41. Robins, L. N.: *Deviant Children Grow Up.* Williams & Wilkins, Baltimore, 1966.
42. Hill, D.: Amphetamine in Psychopathic States. *Br. J. Addiction* 44:50–54, 1947.
43. Hare, op. cit., p.89.
44. MacCulloch, M. J., and Feldman, M. P.: Personality Structure and Its Relation to Success in the Treatment of Homosexuals by Anticipatory Avoidance Conditioning. Unpublished manuscript; Hare, op. cit., p. 117.
45. Hare, op. cit., p. 118.
46. Allen, H. E.: Bio-Social Correlates of Two Types of Antisocial Sociopaths. Ph.D. dissertation, Ohio State University; University Microfilms, Ann Arbor, 1969, No. 70-13971; Allen, H. E., Lindner, L. A., Holdman, H., and Dinitz, S.: The Social and Bio-Medical Correlates of Sociopathy, *Criminologica* 6:68–75, 1969; Allen, H. E., Lindner, L. A., Goldman, H., and Dinitz, S.: Hostile and Simple Sociopaths: An Empirical Typology. *Criminology* 9:27–47, 1971; Goldman, H., Lindner, L., Dinitz, S., and Allen, H.: The Simple Sociopath: Physiologic and Sociological Characteristics. *Biological Psychiatry* 3:77–83, 1971; Lindner, L. A., Goldman, H., Dinitz, S., and Allen, H.: Antisocial Personality Type with Cardiac Lability. *Arch. Gen. Psychiatry* 23:260–267, 1970; Goldman, H.: Diseases of Arousal. *Quaderni di Criminologia* (in press).
47. Bulbring, E.: Biophysical Changes Produced by Adrenaline and Noradrenaline, in Vane, J. R., Volstenholme, G. E. W., and O'Conner, M. (eds.): *Adrenergic Mechanisms.* Little, Brown, Boston, 1961, pp. 275–287; Burn, J. H.: The Relation of Adrenaline to Acetylcholine in the Nervous System. *Physiol. Rev.* 25:377–394, 1945; Chernetski, K. E.: Sympathetic Enhancement of Peripheral Sensory Input in the Frog. *J. Neurophysiol.* 27:493–515, 1964; Eldred, E., Schnitzlein, H. N., and Buchwald, J.: Response of Muscle Spindles to Stimulation of the Sympathetic Trunk. *Exp. Neurol.* 2:187–195, 1960; Lowenstein, W. R., and Altimirano-Orrego, R.: Enhancement of Activity in a Paciniam Corpuscle by Sympathomimetic Agents. *Nature* 178:1292–1293, 1956; Beidler, L. M.: Mechanisms of Gustatory and Olfactory Receptor Stimulation, in Rosenblith, W. A. (ed.): *Sensory Communication.* Wiley, and MIT Press, New York and Cambridge, Mass., 1961, pp. 294–307; Rodriguez-Perez, A. P.: On the Existence of Accessory Unmyelinated Fibers in the Meissner's Corpuscles of the Pulp of the Human Toe. *Dermatologica* 129:468–474, 1964.
48. Schoenherr, J.: Avoidance of Noxious Stimulation in Psychopathic Personality. Ph.D. dissertation, U.C.L.A.; University Microfilms, Ann Arbor, 1965, No. 64-8334.
49. Hare, R. D.: Detection Threshold for Electric Shock in Psychopaths. *J. Abnorm. Psychol.* 73:268–272, 1968.

CHAPTER 34

Donald L. Tasto is a clinical psychologist and former Director of the Center for Research on Stress and Health at SRI International (formerly the Stanford Research Institute) in Menlo Park, California. He has held faculty appointments as Assistant Professor of Psychology at the University of Arkansas and as Associate Professor of Psychology at Colorado State University. Dr. Tasto is a diplomate in clinical psychology of the American Board of Professional Psychology. He is now in private practice in the San Francisco Bay Area.

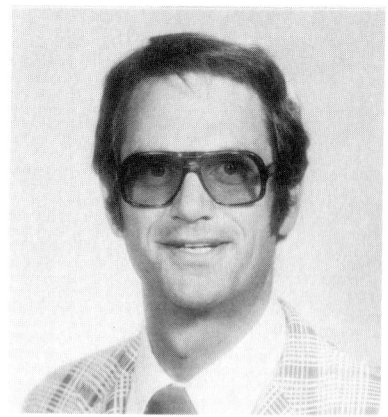

PEDOPHILIA

Donald L. Tasto, Ph.D.

THE CRIME OF PEDOPHILIA

A *pedophile* is an adult who repeatedly engages in sexual activities with prepubescent children. The prevalence of pedophilia is difficult to determine since many offenses go unreported. Statistics are difficult to interpret because child molesting is reported under many different categories, including "contributing to the delinquency of a juvenile," "indecencies with children," "indecent assault," "lewd conduct," and similar phrases. Moreover, child molesting is often included in a general category, such as "sexual offenses," in crime statistics reports. Investigators tend to define pedophilia in different ways. Some restrict the term to offenders involved with children under 12 years old, while others include those involved with person 14 to 16 years old. This is unfortunate, since several investigators have found that offenders involved with adolescent females differ greatly from those involved with prepubescent children.

It is known, nevertheless, that child molesting is a fairly common offense. Most investigators believe that offenses against children represent a large proportion of all sexual crimes. Glueck[1] estimates that one-half to two-thirds of all sexual offenses involve children. Slovenko[2] states that the largest group of sex offenders is composed of men who indulge in sexual acts with children. Mohr and associates[3] believe that sexual acts with children and exhibitionism constitute the majority of sexual offenses brought to court.

The seriousness with which pedophilia is regarded by society is reflected in the treatment of the convicted pedophile. Although first offenders may be placed on probation with provision for psychiatric treatment, recidivists are usually imprisoned or institutionalized. Special legislation in 31 jurisdictions of the United States provides for the civil commitment of the sexual offender, often for an indeterminate period. Sex-psychopath laws in a few states, such as California, Michigan, and Wisconsin, are usually aimed at sex offenders who use violence or who choose children as sexual objects. For example, at Atascadero State Hospital in California, approximately 80 percent of those committed as sexually dangerous persons and discharged between 1954 and 1960 were pedophiles.

These laws have been severely criticized on the grounds of vagueness, violation of due process, or because effective treatment was not available for the offender. If effective treatment has not been readily available for pedophiles in psychiatric hospitals, the situation has been much worse in prisons. The sex offender finds himself on the lowest rung of the prison hierarchy. Far from providing the pedophile with training in normal heterosexual behavior, the prison environment probably encourages further deviance.

CLASSIFICATION OF PEDOPHILES

Pedophiles can be classified in many ways. The broadest division of child molesters is based on the sex of their victims. A pedophile whose sexual object is a child of the opposite sex is termed a *heterosexual pedophile;* a pedophile attracted to a child of the same sex is termed a *homosexual pedophile*. Several investigators have found a subgroup of individuals whose primary problem is not sexual deviation. They are child molesters who are senile, psychotic, or mentally deficient. In these cases, sexual deviation is only part of a more general incapacity. Researchers have also identified a delinquent or psychopathic subgroup. Child molesting for offenders in this category is either only one small part of a criminal life style or is an outlet for aggressive, sadistic impulses. Pedophiles in the latter subgroups constitute only a small percentage of the total pedophile population. The remaining pedophiles, probably the majority of the child-molesting population, can be divided into three subtypes as follows:

> *Type I pedophiles* are unable to interact socially with women because of anxiety or social deficits, or both. These individuals are sexually aroused by both normal objects and children.
> *Type II pedophiles* can interact socially with adult women but are unable to become sexually aroused by them. They are sexually aroused only by children.
> *Type III pedophiles* cannot interact socially with women and are unable to become sexually aroused by them. They are sexaully aroused only by children.

PREVENTIVE FACTORS

In a society which condones some methods of sexual gratification and punishes all others by social ostracism or incarceration, deviations from the socially approved methods of sexual gratification develop because certain preventive factors prohibit individuals from obtaining sexual gratification from these methods. These factors are (1) conditioned fear of social interactions with women; (2) inadequate social skills; and (3) inability to become sexually aroused by adult females. If any of these factors is present to an extreme degree, it can prevent the individual from developing normal sexual behavior. If the anxiety, social deficit, or arousal deficit is less severe, the individual may develop an adequate or marginal sexual adjustment, which is nevertheless quite vulnerable to environmental stress. In still other cases, the individual may have made a satisfactory sexual adjustment that is interrupted by the onset of one of these preventive factors later in life.

Although the inability to form normal sexual relationships with adult women does not necessarily lead to pedophilic behavior, it does increase the likelihood that alternative sexual outlets will be sought.

Conditioned fear of social interactions with adult women may be learned through the pairing of women with unpleasant or punishing events or through modeling. If an individual is afraid of his mother, this fear may generalize to include all women. A man who repeatedly fails when attempting social or sexual initiations with women may come to fear such interactions. Regardless of the precipitating events, a conditioned fear of women will make an individual very anxious at the thought of approaching women socially, and he will therefore avoid such situations.

To establish satisfactory sexual relationships with adult women, a man must perform a variety of social skills, such as identifying potential partners, including social contacts, and participating in conversations. Inadequate social skills in any of these activities may inhibit the formation of social relationships. In some cases an individual with low-level social skills may succeed in forming a close relationship and maintaining this relationship for some time. If the relationship terminates, such an individual may be unable to seek out new partners. Sometimes a person who has had an adequate social and sexual adjustment may find himself in a situation which requires new social skills which he has not acquired. Such a person may be an older widower or divorced man who knew how to approach women in his college classes, but doesn't know how to locate prospective partners in his current social environment.

The inability to become sexually aroused by adult females is the third preventive factor. Sexual arousal as a physiologic response can be conditioned to many different environmental stimuli. In the normal course of development, male sexual arousal becomes conditioned to stimuli associated with women. In some cases, however, such an arousal pattern does not develop or is inhibited by anxiety. In other cases, if sexual relationships with adult women are punishing and unpleasant experiences, the arousal response may decrease and be extinguished.

Any one of a combination of these factors may prevent an individual from forming satisfactory sexual relationships with adult women at some point in his life. The individual may then seek alternative sexual outlets. If he happens to find himself sexually aroused by children and finds such behavior reinforcing, a pattern of pedophilic behavior may well become established.

SEXUAL AROUSAL TO CHILDREN

Human sexual arousal can be conditioned to practically any environmental stimuli. A pattern of sexual arousal to immature females may develop in a number of ways. In normal development, sex play between young children is common. A young male will come to associate young females (and males) with sexual pleasure. Ordinarily this association is quite normal and healthy; it does not interfere with, and may even facilitate, normal development. If, however, normal sexual development is inhibited by anxiety or social skills deficits, an individual may continue to turn to immature females for sexual activity. This is the adolescent pedophile described by Mohr and associates,[3] as well as Gebhard's sociosexually underdeveloped offender[4] and the pedophile-fixated type discussed by Cohen.[5]

In other cases, if sexual pleasure has been strongly associated with young girls, an individual's sexual interest may return to them if he fails with women of an appropriate age or if he becomes socially isolated. In still other instances, sexual interest in children may develop circumstantially. A person who is seeking a sexual outlet may turn to children because they are more readily available or less demanding emotionally and socially. It should also be remembered that the child, in the spontaneous enjoyment of physical pleasure, may initiate physical contact with an adult who may find himself becoming sexually aroused by the child.

Regardless of the reason for which sexual contact with a child is originally sought, pleasurable experiences of this sort will strengthen the likelihood of sexual arousal to children and sexual behavior with children occurring again. Sexual fantasies about children may also come to elicit sexual arousal; sexual satisfaction occurring in conjunction with the fantasy will further strengthen the arousal pattern.

A pattern of sexual arousal to children is most likely to develop in an individual whose various social and sexual deficits make sexual relationships with adult women impossible or unsatisfactory. While it is possible for such a pattern to develop and exist simultaneously with an adequate sexual relationship with an adult woman, this seems unlikely because of the potentially punishing consequences of the deviant behavior. However, Mees[6] notes that "sexual offenders often have a repertoire of sexual behavior which includes both 'normal' and deviant sex acts, apparently under the control of different initiating and maintaining stimuli."

Based on the work of many researchers, a composite portrait of the pedophile—his psychological and social characteristics and the nature of his offense—can be drawn.

HETEROSEXUAL PEDOPHILIA

In many respects, the heterosexual pedophile does not differ greatly from the general population, although the data are sometimes inconsistent. Mohr and his associates found no significant difference between pedophiles and the general population in terms of intelligence, occupation, and education.[3] However, McCaghy[7] found most of his sample to be of lower socioeconomic status and of low educational-occupational level. According to Gebhard's study, noted earlier, heterosexual offenders against children range in intelligence over the full spectrum, but with a higher percentage than normal controls in the subaverage groups (11 percent feeble-minded and 34 percent with an IQ between 70 and 90). He also found the group to have less education (57 percent had 8 years or less) and lower occupational status (mostly unskilled or semiskilled labor) than normal controls. Swanson[8] found that most of his sample had attended high school and that 60 percent had an adequate or better work history, while the remaining 40 percent had an inconsistent or inadequate work history. Most were of average or above average intelligence, with 33 percent low average or subnormal.

The heterosexual pedophile does not usually have a criminal background, and according to Gibbons,[9] he tends to have prosocial attitudes and a noncriminal self-concept; 60 percent of Gebhard's sample and 50 percent of Swanson's sample had not had previous nonsexual convictions.

Few heterosexual pedophiles are psychotic, although they may be psychologically disturbed to some degree. More frequently represented are the mentally retarded. Gebhard found that 10 percent of his sample were psychotic or severely neurotic at the time of the offense and that 14 to 20 percent were mentally retarded. Swanson found that 12 percent were neurotic or borderline psychotic, that 16 percent were mentally retarded, and that 68 percent had personality disorders (e.g., sociopath, schizoid, or inadequate personality).

Pedophiles range in age from adolescents to elderly men. According to Gebhard, the average age of the heterosexual pedophile is 35. Frisbie[10] found that 41 was the average age of the pedophile whose victim was under 12.

Many pedophiles are married, but their marriages are often tenuous. The majority of heterosexual pedophiles older than 20 are married, but they tend to marry later and to have more marital problems than the general population. Gebhard found that the majority of pedophiles have been married at some time but that their marriages are unstable. Only 31 percent were married at the time of the offense, and 41 percent were never married. Of the minority who were still married, 75 percent reported that their marriages were "rather happy" or "very happy." Frisbie reported a high proportion of single, divorced, and separated men, compared to the general population, among the pedophiles at Atascadero State Hospital.

Most investigators agree that some pedophiles have difficulty forming and maintaining social relationships. This difficulty is reflected in the statistics on marital status cited above. According to some investigators, pedophiles may behave in a generally unassertive and inadequate fashion.

This social and psychological maladjustment is noted in the work of many researchers. In describing the sex offenders at Atascadero State Hospital, Laws and Serber[11] note that "A significant portion of our population is virtually incapable of appropriate heterosexual social relationships." Mohr and his associates found that the pedophile tends to have an immature, inadequate personality type and is likely to be isolated from social contacts with adults. Cohen and Kozol[12] found interpersonal difficulties to be common in pedophiles. Gibbons states that the pedophile is usually a timid, retiring, unassertive person.[9] The pedophile is often regarded as inhibited, moralistic, and guilt-ridden, according to Gebhard and Gibbons. Based on their observations, Revitch and Weiss[13] believe that most heterosexual pedophiles turn to children because of personal inadequacies that prevent them from establishing satisfactory relationships with adults.

Mohr and Gebhard found that some heterosexual pedophiles suffer from sexual maladjustment, although many do have "satisfactory relationships" with adult women. Only 20 percent of Swanson's sample of pedophiles (N=25) had adequately adjusted to adult heterosexual relationships, although 75 percent had a primarily adult heterosexual orientation. Gebhard and Mohr both report that the pedophile doesn't actually prefer children, but that he doesn't discriminate against children as sexual partners. Their conclusions are based on reports by offenders themselves.

Researchers have also developed laboratory techniques to identify pedophiles. Using penile tumescence as a measure of sexual arousal, Freund[14] found that heterosexual pedophiles could be distinguished from people with normal sexual orientations by their arousal responses to pictures of naked men, women, and children, just as homosexuals could be distinguished. Compared to normal controls, heterosexual pedophiles showed higher arousal to slides of female children and lower arousal to slides of female adults. However, pictures of children did not always rank first in arousal potential. Interestingly, of the 20 pedophiles tested by Freund, 15 stated prior to examination a preference for adult females, explaining their pedophilic offenses as products of extraordinary circumstances. In half of the cases studied by Swanson, conflict or loss of the usual source of sexual gratification preceded the offense. In a study similar to Freund's, Quinsey and associates[15] found that while penile circumference responses (PCR) to slides of nude men, women, and children can differentiate pedophiles from people with normal sexual orientation, skin conductance responses (SCR) and subjects ranking the slides in order of sexual preference cannot.

Researchers differ about the offender's disposition to engage repeatedly in pedophilic behavior. This issue centers on the extent to which the offender's behavior is determined by environmental factors and the extent to which it is the result of lasting personality characteristics. For instance, Swanson sees child molesters on a continuum ranging from certain individuals to whom the child represents the sexual object of choice to those at the other end of the continuum where the choice of an immature sexual object is virtually a matter of convenience or coincidence. Revitch and Weiss[13] contrast the compulsive, repetitive offender with the impulsive, situationally determined offender.

Investigators are divided about how many pedophiles should be considered "chronic" and how many "situational." Mohr and his associates, in studies described earlier, cite recidivism figures of 5 to 8 percent for heterosexual pedophiles who are first offenders and 20 percent for those with previous offenses. Mohr believes that only 3 percent of all child molesters are chronic offenders who will persist in deviant behavior for a long time. Recidivism figures on pedophilia can, of course, be misleading since they may only indicate that the offender has become more circumspect.[16]

Pedophiles frequently mention alcohol in connection with the offense to excuse their behavior. Gebhard found that alcohol was a factor in 30 percent of the offenses studied, while Swanson put the figure at 33 percent. Gebhard, however, noted that "While many sex offenders, and especially those who offend against children, claim drunkenness in exoneration, in very few cases does intoxication seem to do more than simply release pre-existing desires."[17] Gebhard concluded that 70 percent of the pedophilic offenses studied were premeditated. Sometimes the first offense was an impulsive act, but later contacts were usually deliberately sought.

Situational factors influence pedophiles to varying degrees in different cases. For some pedophiles, sexual interest in children has persisted for many years, regardless of other circumstances in their lives. In Gebhard's sample, 30 to 40 percent of the heterosexual pedophiles had a 10-year or longer history of sexual interest in or activities with children. In other cases, pedophilic behavior does not occur unless precipitated by severe emotional stress. Once the behavior starts, however, it may become habitual and continue for some time. In still other cases, pedophilic behavior may be a single impulsive act spurred by intoxication, unusual stress, or a tempting opportunity.

HOMOSEXUAL PEDOPHILIA

A homosexual pedophile is an adult who commits sexual acts with prepubescent boys. This behavior represents two deviations in the choice of a sexual object—age and sex.

Homosexual pedophiles usually have a history of homosexual behavior. Gebhard reports that most homosexual pedophiles have had considerable homosexual experience; very few (16 percent) were married. McCaghy, believes that homosexual pedophilia may be part of a chosen life style; many such persons have previously accepted a homosexual identity. According to Gigeroff and associates,[18] homosexual pedophilia is more egosyntonic and more difficult to change than heterosexual pedophilia. The recidivism rate for homosexual pedophilia is twice that of heterosexual pedophilia.

TREATMENT

Researchers in recent years have been trying to develop treatment methods for pedophiles in prisons and hospitals. Some of the more promising techniques will be reviewed below. However, no well-researched, proven, effective treatment for pedophilia now exists. Techniques to treat pedophilia can be divided into three general groups:

1. *Physiologic techniques* are based on the fact that the sexual drive can be reduced by castration or by administering hormones. These treatment techniques, although not generally used in the United States, have been employed in the Netherlands and in some Scandinavian countries.[19] Hormonal treatment in conjunction with psychological treatment has been used to temporarily reduce the sexual drive.[20]
2. *Traditional psychotherapy* (individual and group), supplemented by recreational therapy, occupational therapy, sex education, and other activities, is used in some treatment facilities. However, reports are mixed on the effectiveness of traditional psychotherapy with pedophiles.[21] Some researchers suggest that traditional psychotherapy may be helpful when combined with behavioral techniques. McCaghy[22] wondered whether "insights" achieved by pedophiles in therapy actually change their behavior or if they merely give pedophiles different justifications for their deviant behavior.
3. *Behavioral approaches* in treating pedophiles are used to (1) increase or facilitate adequate social interaction with adult women; (2) increase sexual arousal to women; and (3) decrease sexual arousal to children, reduce sexual fantasies and thoughts involving children, and decrease urges to engage in sexual activities with children.

Systematic desensitization, assertive training, and social skill training are used to help pedophiles to increase or facilitate adequate social interaction with adult women. Treatment of various kinds of sexual deviations has often included systematic desensitization when anxiety or fear of women seemed to be an important factor. Researchers have also reported the benefits of using assertive and social skill training. Stevenson and Wolpe[23] successfully used assertive training to treat a heterosexual pedophile with a 3-year history of deviant behavior. Edwards[24] made effective use of assertive training to treat a homosexual pedophile with a 10-year history of deviance. Training in assertive behavior and appropriate social behavior (such as body posture and speech fluency) has been used to treat pedophiles at Atascadero State Hospital.

Researchers have used many techniques to increase the sexual interest of pedophiles in women. Increased sexual arousal to adult women may in itself decrease arousal to children. Beech and associates[25] treated a pedophile by conditioning his sexual arousal to pictures of mature females, using a classical conditioning model. Pictures of immature females used as unconditioned stimuli for eliciting the sexual response followed pictures of mature females used as conditioned stimuli. The patient's arousal was successfully generalized to mature women in real life.

In fading, a stimulus that produces sexual arousal is gradually modified so that arousal generalizes to an appropriate stimulus. Barlow and Agras[26] have used this procedure successfully with homosexuals. A picture of a nude male was slowly faded into a picture of a nude female so that sexual arousal could be maintained.

Shifting of fantasies involves the conditioning of masturbation fantasies. Evans[27] found that people with sexually deviant fantasies took longer to respond to treatment than those with normal fantasies. McGuire, Carlisle, and Young[28] believed that sexual aberration is strengthened by orgasmic reinforcement of deviant fantasies. They suggest that a pedophile's fantasies be shaped and that appropriate fantasies by reinforced by orgasms. In this technique, the patient may be instructed to switch to an appropriate fantasy immediately before an orgasm. In aversion relief, the cessation of an aversive stimulus is paired with an appropriate sexual stimulus, such as a slide of a mature woman.

Many efforts have been made to decrease the sexual arousal of pedophiles to children, to reduce their sexual fantasies and thoughts involving children, and to decrease their urges to engage in sexual activities with children. Cautela[29] and Barlow's group[30] have used covert sensitization to decrease sexual arousal to inappropriate stimuli. In this procedure, the subject (in this case, having a 13-year history of pedophilic behavior) imagines approaching an inappropriate object and then imagines an aversive result, such as nausea and vomiting. Imagined retreat from the object is paired with relief from the unpleasant consequence. This procedure reduced subjective and automatic arousal to young girls in the treatment sessions and in the patient's everyday life.

Callahan and Leitenberg[31] compare covert sensitization with contingent shock in treating pedophilia. In the contingent shock procedure, arousal to slides of young children was paired with a shock. Their covert sensitization procedure was similar to that described previously, except that the subject imagined not only retreating from an inappropriate object, but also approaching an appropriate object while feeling aversion relief. Physiologic measures of arousal (penile tumescence), subjective reports of sexual urges and fantasies, and masturbation and overt acts were used in the procedure. In the two cases presented, covert sensitization was the most effective, especially in decreasing deviant fantasies. In the case of one homosexual pedophile, contingent shock did not increase responses to women or change fantasies, while covert sensitization increased heterosexual fantasies.

Edwards[24] used thought-stopping in combination with assertive training to suppress the pedophilic thoughts and fantasies of a homosexual pedophile. The subject was instructed to say "Stop!" to himself and then relax whenever he became aware of an inappropriate thought or stimulus.

Shame aversion therapy used to treat a pedophile is reported by Serber.[32] (The subject had a 30-year history of heterosexual pedophilia.) The offender acts out his deviant behavior with a surrogate victim (not a child) before an audience. In a later article, Serber stresses that such procedures appear unable to suppress permanently the deviant behavior unless the individual is trained to perform alternative behavior.

CONCLUSION

Based on the case study reports of the psychological treatment of pedophiles and on the treatment programs for other deviations, researchers can now design well-controlled exploratory studies of pedophiles in the laboratory. These studies should produce empirical support for the multiple causative model of pedophilic development, a classification system for pedophiles, procedures for diagnosing the factors which maintain the deviant behavior, and a treatment program that increases adult heterosexuality and reduces or eliminates pedophilic behavior. Thus the pedophile could be offered a rehabilitative alternative to incarceration which would help him return to society free of the sexual problems which brought him to the attention of the courts.

REFERENCES

1. Glueck, B. C.: Pedophilia, in Slovenko, R. (ed.): *Sexual Behavior and the Law*. Charles C Thomas, Springfield, Ill., 1965, pp. 539–562.
2. Slovenko, R.: A Panoramic View: Sexual Behavior and the Law, in Slovenko, R. (ed.): *Sexual Behavior and the Law*. Charles C Thomas, Springfield, Ill., 1965.
3. Mohr, J. W., Turner, R. E., and Jerry, M. B.: *Pedophilia and Exhibitionism*. University of Toronto Press, Toronto, 1964.
4. Gebhard, P. H., et al.: *Sex Offenders: An Analysis of Types*. Harper & Row, Paul B. Hoeber, New York, 1965.
5. Cohen, M. L., Seghorn, T., and Calmas, W.: Sociometric Study of the Sex Offender. *J. Abnormal Psychol.* 74:249–255, 1969.
6. Mees, H. L.: Sadistic Fantasies Modified by Aversive Conditioning and Substitution: A Case Study. *Behav. Res. Ther.* 4:317–320, 1966.
7. McCaghy, C. H.: Child Molesters: A Study of Their Careers as Deviants, in Clenard, M. B., and Quinney, R.(eds.): *Criminal Behavior Systems: A Typology*. Holt, Rinehart & Winston, New York, 1967.
8. Swanson, D. W.: Adult Sexual Abuse of Children: The Man and The Circumstances. *Dis. Nerv. Syst.* 29:677–683, 1968.
9. Gibbons, D. C.: *Society, Crime and Criminal Careers*. Prentice-Hall, Englewood Cliffs, N. J., 1973.
10. Frisbie, L. V.: Treated Sex Offenders Who Reverted to Sexually Deviant Behavior. *Fed. Probation* 29:52–57, 1965.
11. Laws, D. R., and Serber, M.: *Measurement and Evaluation of Assertive Training With Sexual Offenders*. Atascadero State Hospital, Atascadero, California, 1972.
12. Cohen, M. L., and Kozol, H. L.: Evaluation for Parole at a Sex Offender Treatment Center. *Fed. Probation* 30:50–55, 1966.
13. Revitch, E., and Weiss, R. G.: The Pedophiliac Offender. *Dis. Nerv. Syst.* 23:73–83, 1962.
14. Freund, K: Diagnosing Heterosexual Pedophilia by Means of a Test for Sexual Interest. *Behav. Res. Ther.* 3:229–234, 1965; Freund, K.: Diagnosing Homo- or Hetero-sexuality and Erotic Age Preference by Means of a Psychophysiological Test. *Behav. Res. Ther.* 5:209–228, 1976; Freund, K.: Erotic Preference in Pedophilia. *Behav. Res. Ther.* 5:339–348, 1967.
15. Quinsey, V. L., Steinman, C. M., Bergersen, S. G., and Holmes, T. F.: Penile

Circumference, Skin Conductance, and Ranking Responses of Child Molesters and 'Normals' to Sexual and Nonsexual Visual Stimuli. *Behav. Ther.* 6:213–219, 1975.
16. Macindoe, I.: Therapeutic Treatments for Sex Offenders. *Reports from the Research Laboratories of the Department of Psychiatry, University of Minnesota,* No. PR-71-3, April 20, 1971.
17. Gebhard, et al., op. cit.
18. Gigeroff, A. K., Mohr, J. W., and Turner, R. E.: Sex Offenders on Probation: Homosexual Pedophiles. *Fed. Probation* 33(1):36–39, 1969.
19. Stürup, G. K.: Sex Offense: The Scandinavian Experiences. *Law and Contemporary Problems* 25(2):361–375, 1960.
20. Macindoe, op. cit.
21. Fisher, R. G.: The Legacy of Freud: A Dilemma for Handling Offenders in General and Sex Offenders in Particular. *U. Colorado Rev.* 40:242–267, 1968.
22. McCaghy, op. cit.
23. Stevenson, I., and Wolpe, J.: Recovery from Sexual Deviations Through Overcoming Nonsexual Neurotic Response. *Am. J. Psychiatry* 116:737–742, 1960.
24. Edwards, N. B.: Case Conference: Assertive Training in a Case of Homosexual Pedophilia. *J. Behav. Ther. Exp. Psychiatry* 3:55–63, 1972.
25. Beech, H. R., Watt, F., and Poole, A. D.: Classical Conditioning of a Sexual Deviation: A Preliminary Note. *Behav. Ther.* 2:400–402, 1971.
26. Barlow, D. H., and Agras, W. S.: Fading to Increase Heterosexual Responsiveness in Homosexuals. *J. Appl. Behav. Analysis* 6:355–366, 1973.
27. Evans, D. R.: Masturbation Fantasy and Sexual Deviation. *Behav. Res. Ther.* 6:17–19, 1968.
28. McGuire, R. J., Carlisle, J. M., and Young, B. G.: Sexual Deviations as Conditioned Behavior: A Hypothesis. *Behav. Res. Ther.* 2:185–190, 1965.
29. Cautela, J. R., and Wisocki, P. A.: Covert Sensitization for the Treatment of Sexual Deviation. *Psychol. Rec.* 21:37–48, 1971.
30. Barlow, D. H., Leitenberg, H., and Agras, W. S.: Experimental Control of Sexual Deviation Through Manipulation of the Noxious Scene in Covert Sensitization. *J. Abnormal Psychol.* 74:596–601, 1969.
31. Callahan, E. J., and Leitenberg, H.: Aversion Therapy for Sexual Deviation: Contingent Shock and Covert Sensitization. *J. Abnormal Psychol.* 81:60–73, 1973.
32. Serber, M.: Shame Aversion Therapy. *J. Behav. Ther. Exp. Psychiatry* 1:213–215, 1970.

CHAPTER 35

Thomas P. Hackett is Eben S. Draper Professor of Psychiatry at Harvard Medical School, and Chief of Psychiatry at Massachusetts General Hospital in Boston. Dr. Hackett has served as a Court Clinic Psychiatrist in the Division of Legal Medicine of the Massachusetts Department of Mental Health, and as an Instructor in Forensic Psychiatry at the Law-Medicine Institute of Boston University. He has frequently been a consultant to the American Heart Association and the National Heart, Lung, and Blood Institute of the U.S. Public Health Service. Dr. Hackett is a member of the Association for the Psychiatric Treatment of Offenders and the American Psychiatric Association.

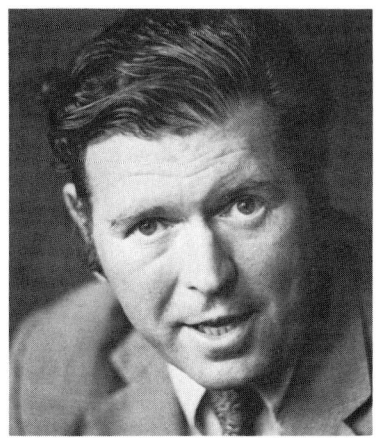

Fay A. Saber is Assistant Professor of Medicine in Society at Wright State University School of Medicine in Dayton, Ohio. A graduate of Providence College and of Boston College Law School, she is a former Teaching Assistant in Health Law at Harvard School of Public Health and Harvard Medical School.

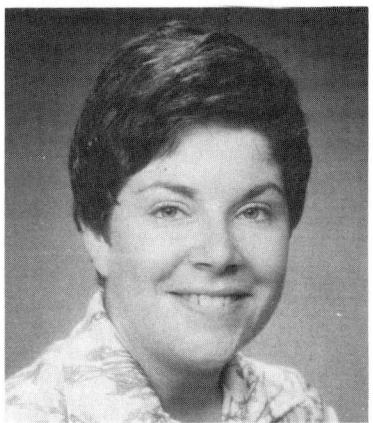

William J. Curran is Frances Glessner Lee Professor of Legal Medicine at Harvard University and Chairman of the State Medicolegal Investigation Committee of Massachusetts. Professor Curran writes regularly for the *New England Journal of Medicine* and teaches at the Medical School, Law School, and School of Public Health at Harvard. He was formerly Robert R. Utley Professor of Legal Medicine and Director of the Law-Medicine Institute of Boston University. He also served as Assistant Professor of Law and Government and Assistant Director of the Institute of Government at the University of North Carolina. Professor Curran is the author of several books in the medicolegal field including *Law, Medicine and Forensic Science* (with E. D. Shapiro); *Trauma and the Automobile; The Doctor as a Witness;* and *Medicolegal Proof in Litigation.* He is an Associate Editor of the *American Journal of Law and Medicine* and was formerly Medicolegal Editor of the *Massachusetts Law Quarterly.*

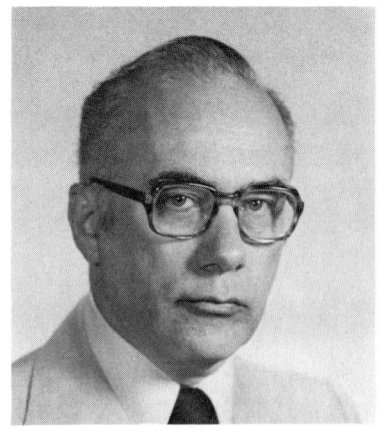

EXHIBITIONISM*

Thomas P. Hackett, M.D.,
Fay A. Saber, J.D., M.P.H., and
William J. Curran, J.D., LL.M., S.M.Hyg.

At common law it was an offense willfully and intentionally to expose the private portions of one's person in a public place while in the presence of others. Although several states still retain the common law definition of exhibitionism,[1] most jurisidictions have enacted statutes or ordinances making public display of one's genitalia a criminal offense.[2] Whether treated as a common law or statutory crime, the main elements of the offense basically remain the same: (1) intent to expose, (2) in a public place, and (3) in the presence of others. The prosecution, to obtain a conviction, has the burden of proving separately each of these aspects of the crime.

In order to establish a willful and intentional disposition to expose, many courts grant a certain amount of latitude to prosecutors by allowing proof of other similar acts to be introduced in evidence in an effort to demonstrate intent as opposed to mere inadvertence on the part of the accused. However, where a previous history of similar activity does not exist, proof of the defendant's intent will turn upon the facts adduced at trial.

The requirements of proving exposure in a public place is met by establishing that the act took place in a location open to public view where individuals other than the person who actually witnessed the indecent exposure might also have seen it had they looked. Thus convictions have been obtained where defendants exposed themselves in automobiles parked on public thoroughfares.

In establishing that the offense was committed in the presence of oth-

---

*This chapter is a revision and updating of material previously published by Dr. Hackett in *Seminars in Psychiatry,* Vol. 3, No. 3, August 1971. It is reprinted with the permission of the publisher, Grune & Stratton, New York.

ers, it is only necessary that one person actually have seen the act performed, provided that it occurred in a public place where other persons might have seen it. This follows from the element of occurrence in a public place described above.

Statutory offenses, as noted earlier, closely follow the common law definition of indecent exposure or exhibitionism. However, some statutes have modified the elements of the crime with respect to display of one's genitalia before children of a certain age. Under these statutes, as interpreted in court decisions, there is no requirement that the offense occur in a public place or where persons other than the child witnessing the act might see it. Sentences under these legislative enactments appear to be more severe, the intent being to prevent children of tender years from being subjected to physical or emotional harm.[3] Similarly, some statutes have modified the exposure in a public place requirement so that a conviction might be obtained if the offense occurs in a private place where other persons might see it or be offended by it.[4]

Recent reforms have been suggested regarding the way in which the law should treat the act of indecent exposure or exhibitionism. In many legal circles it is believed that the act is more a nuisance than a serious criminal act, and therefore it is frequently found to be classified as a petty misdemeanor.[5] However, where the offense occurs before a young child or adolescent, one often finds the crime treated as a gross misdemeanor or felony. Some statutes, moreover, treat a second and any subsequent conviction of indecent exposure as a felony.

Much of the appellate litigation following conviction for indecent exposure turns upon legal technicalities, including whether the underlying statute is overly broad or vague in its language. Many states have attempted to eliminate such appellate interpretation by redrafting their statutes to define carefully and describe terms employed in the text of the criminal code.[6]

HISTORY

In 1877, Professor Charles Lasègue published a paper entitled, "Les Exhibitionistes."[7] He apologized for using a new term because he could find no phrase in criminal argot or Parisian patois that in any way described the male exhibitionist. His observations of a century ago fit today's exhibitionist as though they had been tailored for him. Even though the number of Lasègue's cases was small, the information he extracted applies unmodified to most of today's exhibitionists. His data characterize the exhibitionist as follows: he puts a distance between himself and the victim which is never crossed; the impulse to expose is sudden and unpredictable; there are periodic occurrences of this impulse; the act itself appears meaningless in that it is devoid of sexual or logical motives; the patient's past is uneventful (he was not psychotic, a criminal, or a mental patient); the patient often appears indifferent to the consequences of his exposure, feeling little guilt about his act's effect on the victim and often seeming indifferent to the danger of being arrested. "They limit their appetite to the exhibition, which is never the point of departure for more salacious activity." This conglomerate of features, Lasègue concludes, constitutes a definite and specific syndrome sufficient to justify his new term, exhibitionism.

Wilhelm Stekel wrote of exhibitionism, underscoring its extreme impulsivity and compulsivity. He emphasized the narcissism inherent in the act and elaborated on the infantile regressive factors in exhibitionism.[8] In 1912, Krafft-Ebing described exhibitionism as "periodic insanity."[9] He believed that the act occurred during a state of clouded consciousness, and he compared it to a form of epilepsy. He divided the offenders into four groups that can easily be reduced to two: primary and secondary. The primary group included neurasthenics with periodic impulsive exhibitionism. The second group had exhibitionism as part of general cerebral disease and also had epilepsy. In his 1950 study, Rickles writes of normal exhibitionism that occurs in children, primitive people, nudists, and in precoital adult behavior.[10] He differentiates this from abnormal exhibitionism which "occurs in the depraved, psychotics (both organic and functional), the feeble-minded, epileptics and psychoneurotics."

As one can see from this review there are basically two types of exhibitionism: the primary, defined by Mohr and coworkers, and comprising all the cases in this presentation, and the secondary, in which exposure is part of another complex of illnesses such as epilepsy, dementia, or schizophrenia. Christoffel coined the phrase "male genital exhibitionism," which excludes females and is commonly used to designate the primary type.[11]

The recognition that the adult exhibitionist acts out a partial aspect of instinctual behavior normally expressed in childhood and subsequently repressed was first delineated by Freud in *The Interpretation of Dreams*[12] in 1900, and later fully described in his classic *Three Essays on Sexuality*[13] in 1905. This position was maintained with little change by Fenichel, who regarded exhibitionism simply as the "overcathexis of a partial instinct" in the service of reassurance against castration anxiety secondary to Oedipal guilt.[14] Alfred Adler viewed exhibitionism as the result of organ inferiority; that is, the individual felt that either his sexual apparatus or performance was inferior and exposed himself in order to obtain from his victim a response of awe or fear to restore his sense of adequacy.[15]

It must be added that a considerable library of data exists relating male genital exhibitionism to the ancient rituals associated with phallic worship. Both Rickles[16] and Karpman[17] regard it, in part, as an atavistic regression on a grand scale.

TREATMENT AND PATIENT MANAGEMENT

Although exhibitionism has been defined by many authors, the definition we find most satisfactory is that proposed by Mohr and associates.[18] In their opinion, exposure of the male genital apparatus is not in itself a determinant of clinical exhibitionism unless it represents the final sexual gratification without any intention of further sexual contact. This definition separates the exhibitionistic exposure from genital exposure for other reasons, such as coitus and urination, as well as from the type of exhibitionism found in mental disorders such as senile dementia and schizophrenia.

The treatment of the exhibitionist has not been dealt with nearly as extensively as have the descriptive and speculative psychodynamic aspects of the condition. Psychoanalytic treatment has not been notably successful in those reports available. More recently the use of group therapy in the treatment of these offenders has been published.[18,19,20] This is a promising method of therapy, particularly if it is required as a condition of probation. Other techniques have also been applied to a limited number of patients with some success.[21]

Although historically exhibitionism has been defined as a male phenomenon, recent literature[22] suggests that the traditional definitions of indecent exposure should be carefully reviewed. Hollender and associates[23] contend that while the psychodynamics of the female exhibitionist markedly differ from her male counterpart, the behavior patterns are quite consistent.

PSYCHOLEGAL ASPECTS

Mohr and associates[24] have written a text dealing with the more general psycholegal aspects of exhibitionism. It contains practical information on exhibitionism and pedophilia which should prove quite useful to the clinical psychotherapist.

CASE STUDIES

All of the cases to be reported were seen at the Court Clinic of the Third District Court in East Cambridge, Massachusetts. Since 1956, one of the authors has examined 214 exhibitionists and has taken 45 into psychotherapy. Data are based on 37 of the 45 individuals, because the remaining eight are still in treatment. All 37 have been terminated and have been followed for varying periods of time.

Most of the exhibitionists coming before the court are interviewed by a psychiatrist at the time of their arraignment. Those falling into the category of secondary exhibitionists (the demented and the schizophrenic) are usually hospitalized for further examination and are not included in this series. Primary exhibitionists are usually placed on probation with the stipulation that they attend the court clinic regularly for psychotherapy. Therapy is usually conducted once a week for 50 minutes. If the patient is married, a referral is made for the spouse to be followed by the social service department.

Characteristics of Patient Population

The patients ranged in age from 17 to 45 years with a mean of 26 and a median of 24. Sixteen were single, 19 were married, one was separated, and one was divorced. There were 21 Roman Catholics, 12 Protestants, one Jew, two Greek Orthodox, and one Muslim. All were high school graduates, five had bachelor's degrees, two had master's degrees, and three had doctorates. All were employed and had good work records. Salaries ranged from less than $1,000 a year, in the case of students who worked part-time, to $17,000 a year, with a mean of $5,400. Diagnostically, there was one schizophrenic who was openly psychotic and delusional for a 6-month period; four were borderline psychotics, none of whom decompensated. There were seven obvious passive-aggressive characters, one passive-dependent, and two with alcoholic problems. Both of the last were able to remain employed. Alcohol enhanced but did not generate the impulse to expose in either case. All 37 tended to use obsessive-compulsive defenses as major coping techniques. Eight had one of the following physical difficulties: diabetes, tuberculosis, facial burns, deafness, polio, seminoma, severe stuttering, or multiple abdominal surgical procedures. These physical disabilities had no discernible bearing on the patients' motives to expose.

Seventeen had previous arrests for exhibiting themselves. Fifteen of these had been convicted, five more than one time. Only one exposed to children, but 18 exhibited to early teenagers. The remainder were less selective in their choice of victims. No homosexual exhibitionists were included in the sample. The most common technique involved the use of the automobile. Either the patient would expose while asking directions from his car, or he would cruise an area to locate a victim and then leave the auto to expose. He would then return to his vehicle for a getaway. Thirty exposed with either a flaccid or semierect penis. In this group, masturbation followed the exposure, usually by minutes to hours, and took place in a setting of safety. The remaining seven all had erections. Five of them masturbated while exposing, while the other two not only masturbated, but also shouted threats or made threatening gestures during the act. One of the latter was an active frotteur and frequently pinched the victim's breast or backside as part of his technique. In no instance did the victim receive serious physical injury.

Of concomitant sexual disorders, sexual inhibition was by far the most common. With few exceptions these individuals had fewer heterosexual contacts than the average male, based on Kinsey's statistics.[25] Those married had intercourse less often per week than a comparable population polled by Kinsey. Premature ejaculation was found in seven and periodic impotence in two. Curiously, only one of the 37 was a voyeur. Frottage was practiced by one, and periodic homosexuality occurred in another.

Of the 21 who were or had been married, 10 were thought to have stable unions, a judgment based on three years of marriage without a major rift, separation, or talk of divorce. Eight were judged to have fair marriages based on one period of separation with at least the discussion of divorce, although no action was taken. Three were felt to have poor marriages because separation was or had been a part of the picture for at least one year and more than one separation had occurred.

In socioeconomic background, 28 came from middle to lower middle-class families; nine came from lower middle- to lower-class backgrounds. Fourteen had suffered parental deprivation, usually with the father away for long periods; 23 had not. Thirty-two were reared according to very strict precepts with particular emphasis on the suppression of anger. The open expression of anger in any form was seldom tolerated by either parent, but the mother tended to be the harsher enforcer. Five were reared under less suppressive circumstances, two with mothers who were quite promiscuous. Sexual matters were generally not discussed in these homes, but there was no obvious sexual suppression as was the case with anger.

On an introversion-extroversion rating scale, 23 of the patients classified themselves as introverts, five as extroverts, and nine were mixed. None was clinically depressed.

As a consequence of the above facts, a profile of the Cantabrigian exhibitionist would appear as follows: He is in his middle 20's, the product of a strict middle-class upbringing. He has had a high school education and a good work record. He is nondelinquent, inclined to introversion, had a dominant mother, and has a potential problem with expression of anger. He is also probably sexually inhibited and is apt to be shy and reticent around women. By and large, these are quiet, grass-roots people. They do little to draw attention to themselves except periodically to expose their genitalia. Possibly because of the proximity of the court to the Harvard area, their educational level, salary, and socioeconomic standing are higher than in comparable populations around the country.

Therapy

When a finding of guilty was made in these cases, the patient was placed on probation with the stipulation that he attend the court clinic. The only requirement for entering therapy was that the patient must admit that he exhibited himself. There is a small percentage of exhibitionists who initially admit guilt to avoid the threat of imprisonment but who deny it once therapy starts. They revert to the standard excuse that they had merely been urinating. When this occurred a therapeutic deadlock ensued which was impossible to work through in every case. As a consequence these patients were returned to their probation officer who saw them regularly as he would any probationer. Only those people who fully acknowledged guilt and desired to understand their problem qualified for psychotherapy.

The longest treatment period has been 14 years. Two were in treatment for 6 years, two for 4 years, one for 3 years, seven for 2 years, three for 1 to 1½ years, five for 1 year, and 16 for 6 months.

The time spent in psychotherapy diminished as the therapist's experience developed. Initially the average time of treatment was 2 to 2½ years. This steadily declined to a period of 6 months which has been held to for the last 5 years. The reason for this is that certain characteristics of the exhibitionist emerged which seemed intimately bound up with the impulse to expose. These key conflicts involved the awareness and discharge of anger. They recurred so regularly in case after case that it soon seemed advisable to focus on these issues early and to shape treatment around methods of forcing insight and teaching alternate ways of handling anger.

In general terms therapy could be divided into three phases. The first could be called enthusiastic endorsement. Most of these patients stated that they had been thinking of obtaining psychotherapy for some time, but none had done so before being apprehended by the police. Although no case could be found in which an exhibitionist has sought psychiatric help without being urged by some social agency such as the police department, each of the 37 gave every evidence of welcoming the chance of therapy once before the court. As a consequence, during this first phase, the patient freely and enthusiastically speaks of the intimate details of his past life, and one can obtain an accurate and complete account of his early development, family history, current struggles, and predominant methods of coping with stress. Attendance is regular, there is very little acting out, and the impulse to expose often vanishes during this first stage of treatment. It is as though the old pattern of behavior has been somehow magically snuffed out by treatment and probation. After a month or two the patient begins to believe that the impulse is truly gone, that simply talking about his problems—even though no insight has been gained—has done the trick. Often he can remember no comparable period of his postpubertal life when the impulse to expose has been so inactive. The patient is then told by the therapist that his tendency to expose will return and that it may do so with dramatic suddenness. He is further cautioned that he must under no circumstances yield to the impulse. This injunction has nothing to do with the court; there is no threat of reporting an offense to the probation department; rather it is explained to the patient that by thwarting the impulse, the true motive behind it may emerge and be dealt with therapeutically.

To avoid exposing, two maneuvers can be suggested. At first it was thought that masturbation might provide the best method to stave off the impulse to expose, but it turned out that many exhibitionists regarded masturbation as more heinous an act than exposing. Even when masturbation was used, it seldom provided more than a brief interim of control. Because of this a more drastic measure was suggested: inducing pain. Smokers were advised to burn themselves with lighted cigarettes or with their cigarette lighters. Others were instructed to bite their cheeks, to pinch themselves, or to bark their shins—anything to cause pain sufficient to dampen the impulse. This appeared to be remarkably effective, even though in one instance it caused a rather severe injury. One of the patients worked as a hod carrier. In the midst of being tormented by impulses to expose, he emptied the entire hod of bricks upon his foot, breaking a metatarsal. Needless to say, the resulting pain extinguished the desire to expose.

Once the impulse to expose returns, the second period of therapy begins. This usually occurs during the second month. It consists of a kind of sector analysis of the precipitating events that lead to the act of exhibitionism and to the motives these reveal. This is often implemented if, during the first phase, the doctor has paid close attention to incidents relating anger to exposing and documents these without revealing this to the patient. In general the exhibitionist regards his act as a prelude to seduction. In his fantasy, the woman often praises his penis or marvels at it. In truth the very opposite occurs. The victim rarely exclaims in joy at what is presented her, but rather screams out in fear or retreats in alarm. The fact that wish-fulfilling fantasy and fact are polar opposites when it comes to exhibitionism is used by the therapist to demonstrate that the reason for exposing must be other than a preamble to sexual intercourse. There are far better ways of approaching a women for sex than affronting her with a naked penis. Establishing this point is not difficult, although there is undoubtedly a strong sexual component to the act since masturbation invariably accompanies it, most frequently after the actual exposing has occurred.

It had originally been postulated that the essential reason for exposing had to do with the misguided expression of anger. This assumption arose from the fact that most of the patients were the products of strict upbringings in which anger was proscribed. The victims behaved as though they had been frightened, and they viewed the offense as a visual violation. Havelock Ellis referred quite correctly to exhibitionism as "psychic defloration" in terms of its effect on the prey.[26]

The initial contention was that a precipitating event would precede each act of exposure. Typically this would consist of being hurt, frustrated, insulted, or symbolically caponized by a woman. In a keen desire to find supporting evidence, a more significant source of anger was overlooked in the adult male: his employer and peers. As our experience enlarged, it was found that the precipitating event could include an immense variety of happenings all containing a common core of aggravation for the individual patient. What was annoying or frustrating for one might not be for another. Using personal responses to situations (substituting how one would feel in the circumstances the patient described) was often but not always helpful. Since most, if not all, of these patients were obsessive-compulsive to varying degrees, they had great difficulty perceiving anger as others felt it. For example, one patient had a fat boss who insisted that those in his employ light cigars and open doors for him and defer to his judgment in all matters, much the way Old World courtiers had to behave in noble company. When the patient was told that his boss sounded like a caricature out of a Dickensian sweatshop, he would not hear of it and defended the man on the basis that his position justified such arrogance. It was not the boss that had triggered his exposing, but rather a peer who was athletic, confident, and highly successful as a seducer. Whenever the patient heard stories of recent conquests, he felt inferior and angry, which in turn set off a chain of mental events leading to the desire to expose himself. He had done this in the same context since puberty; there had always been one boy or another who produced this response, and yet he was unaware of the pattern until it had been pointed out and documented with numerous examples from his past.

When the connection between anger and the impulse to expose has been established, the third phase of treatment begins. This concerns finding alternative ways of coping with anger and with the desire to expose. Originally, sublimation was considered (e.g., exposing to a wife or mistress or posing before mirrors), but this was never a success. Exhibitionists simply do not expose to wives, girl friends, or women they know, and the type of sublimation we had in mind would be unacceptable to a sexually inhibited person. The next therapeutic tack was more successful. It had to do with recognizing what specifically made the individual angry and then, to vent the anger, finding ways that were more socially acceptable than exposing. Patients were encouraged to express anger at their wives when this was called for by shouting, talking back, pounding the table, or even simulating anger that wasn't felt. The last, like method acting, sometimes worked beautifully. It was of great help when the wife of the exhibitionist was also in treatment with our social service department because she too could be taught to encourage rather than thwart nascent attempts at the expression of anger on the part of her spouse. A program of activity was also recommended, such as jogging, swimming, engaging in sports, setting up a punching bag, or hunting.

Sometimes a style of exposing could be altered to make it less conspicuous. Patients who enjoyed masturbation on the streets were told to do it in their cars with a coat or some other type of cover over the penis to hide movement.

Anticipation is a useful technique in the treatment of the exhibitionist. Once the relationship between the precipitating event and the impulse is established, the patient can learn when to anticipate the impulse. If his control is shaky, he must take pains to insure that he will not be in a position to act out his impulse. One way of doing this is to stay in the company of some family member until the desire is controllable. Wives, children, and close friends have been employed successfully in this capacity, often without realizing it. Another important treatment aspect having to do with anticipation is advising the patient to expect an exacerbation of his symptom along with a sense of lessened control over it at the time therapy is terminated. Predicting this with the patient and terminating gradually while maintaining regular contact by telephone can reduce trouble during this period.

It is of interest to note that 85 percent of the people in this series preferred to stay in psychotherapy when their probation expired and they were free to quit. It is significant that of the four who stopped therapy prematurely, all were involved in exhibitionistic acts that resulted in their return to the court within months after they stopped treatment. Following a second course of therapy, some came to the attention of the police again. These are included in the follow-up report.

Follow-Up

The longest follow-up in the series is 14 years; the shortest is 2 years. Follow-up was obtained by two methods: (1) the patient was contacted either by telephone or by letter to inquire whether the impulse to exhibit had returned and whether he had again exhibited; and (2) the chief probation officer checked both state and federal arrest records to determine whether or not the patient's name turned up on any roster of offenders. Thirty-four patients indicated no subsequent exhibition during the follow-up period after completing treatment. This was backed up by no subsequent reports of arrests in their criminal records.

There were three therapeutic failures in this series of 37 in terms of recidivism. Two of the three comprised the small subgroup described below as aggressive exhibitionists. Although these were never apprehended by the police, their exposure continued despite therapy. One of them was a schizophrenic, the only one in the series who had an overt psychotic decompensation. Mellaril was used, but the patient discontinued it because of its side effects. Another was one of the two considered dangerous by the examiner because of his sadistic frottage as well as his assaultive fantasies toward women. The third individual simply never entered into a therapeutic alliance, and therefore less rapport was possible with him than with the others. Had Depo Provera been available at the time, it or another antiandrogen preparation might have been helpful. The use of these preparations has been described by Money.[27]

Classification

The sample of 37 patients can be divided into three subcategories: (1) 30 typical male genital exhibitionists; (2) five masturbators (those who masturbate in the presence of women, sometimes openly, sometimes covertly); and (3) two aggressive exhibitionists. Most of the 37 reported that the impulse to expose had returned from time to time but that the intensity of the impulse diminished and it was not acted on.

The male genital exhibitionist simply exposes, sometimes with an erection, more often without, and never makes a menacing gesture toward his victim.

The masturbators may or may not be primary exhibitionists but enjoy masturbating in public far more than in private. Their fantasies are more active: they imagine that a woman may come over and embrace them and perhaps perform fellatio or even go on to intercourse. Their fantasies are not violent or assaultive. They could easily be categorized as male genital exhibitionists and included in the first group of 30, but they stand out because their behavior is more that of a simple masturbator than of someone who exposes to shock.

The aggressive-assaultive exhibitionists expose with an eye toward producing a maximum amount of shock and terror. They will hide in the hallways of dormitories and jump out when women come by, or they will expose to a single woman in dark places and make menacing gestures. One was a "Sunday morning" exhibitionist who would expose to solitary women taking sunbaths in lonely places in a large park. He would walk up to them with his penis out and erect, look at them menacingly, say he was going to rape them and beat them and kill them, and then ejaculate and run away. The other, the frotteur, would sometimes accompany his exposing, which usually occurred on dark streets or in back alleys, by grabbing the woman's breast and twisting it. He would sometimes look through apartment windows at women who were undressing and then knock or rattle the window, pointing to his penis, shouting that he was going to rape them, and verbalizing other obscenities to terrify the victim. Both exhibitionists, after a year or two of therapy, admitted that they had assaultive, sometimes homicidal, fantasies toward women but never carried them out. Since then two other exhibitionists with similar fantasies have appeared for therapy. This small series forms a distinct subgroup worthy of more research and attention because they may well fall into the category of dangerous sexual offenders, an appellation that is not and should not be used with the ordinary male genital exhibitionist.

Discussion

To our knowledge, this series represents the largest group of exhibitionists in individual psychotherapy for the longest period of time and with the longest follow-up that has been reported. All have been treated by the same therapist with roughly the same type of psychotherapy. Its main thrust has been to demonstrate that the basic motive behind the act is aggressive rather than sexual. Treatment is designed to demonstrate this and to teach alternative methods of handling anger. Most of the people in this sample seem to have benefited from their therapeutic encounter, although there is only presumptive evidence that the theory behind the treatment is valid. A carefully controlled study is required for that type of demonstration. Regardless of the reason, treating the exhibitionist in an outpatient setting has merit, as demonstrated by Mohr and coworkers.[28] As a group, with the exception of the aggressive exhibitionists already described, these are productive members of society who usually do not require inpatient treatment or punishment, neither of which have historically proved of any value in helping them to control their impulse. The use of group therapy, as reported by other authors, is an encouraging new avenue of therapy for the large number of sexual offenders of this type found in our courts.[29,30] The contribution of groups in which the cotherapist is female should prove especially valuable in the treatment of the adult male exhibitionist.

It is worth reemphasizing that treatment apparently must be enforced upon these individuals because so few, if any, seek help themselves for their difficulties. If information of the kind presented in this chapter were made available to state law enforcement agencies throughout the country, and a greater understanding of the exhibitionist thereby encouraged, a considerable burden could be removed from the penal facilities at these agencies. It seems likely that the more people of this type who are placed in programs of treatment, the less recidivism will occur. Perhaps the principles described in this presentation, if utilized in a group setting, would improve some of the treatment reported by others. A more vigorous approach to control along endocrinologic lines, as in the use of antiandrogens, should probably be included in the repertoire of treatment.

REFERENCES

1. *Commonwealth v. Broadland,* 315 Mass. 20, 1943.
2. *California Penal Code* S 314; *McKinney's Consolidated Laws of New York, Penal Laws* S 245.00; *Revised Code of Washington* 9A 88.010.

3. *State v. Trenary*, 79 Ariz. 351, 290 P.2d. 250, 1955.
4. *Minnesota Annotated Statutes* S 617.23; *Wisconsin Statutes* S 18.2-387.
5. *Model Penal Code* S 213.5 (Proposed Official Draft, May 4, 1962).
6. *New Mexico Statutes* 40A-9-24; *Smith-Hurd Illinois Annotated Statutes* C.38 S 11-9.
7. Leségue, C.: Les Exhibitionistes. *L'union medicale* 23:703, 1877.
8. Stekel, W.: On the Psychology of Exhibitionism. *Z. Sexualle Wissenschaft* 7:241, 1920.
9. von Krafft-Ebing, R.: *Psychopathia Sexualis.* ed. 12. Rebman, New York, 1912.
10. Rickles, N. K.: *Exhibitionism.* J. B. Lippincott, Philadelphia, 1950.
11. Christoffel, H.: Male Genital Exhibitionism, in Lorand, S. (ed.): *Perversions: Psychodynamics and Therapy.* Random House, New York, 1956.
12. Freud, S.: *Interpretation of Dreams.* Macmillan, New York, 1937.
13. Freud, S.: *Three Essays on the Theory of Sexuality.* Image, London, 1949.
14. Fenichel, O.: *The Psychoanalytic Theory of Neurosis.* Norton, New York, 1945.
15. Adler, A.: *The Neurotic Constitution.* Moffat Yard, New York, 1917.
16. Rickles, op. cit.
17. Karpman, B.: The Psychopathology of Exhibitionism. *J. Clin. Psychopathol.* 9:179, 1948.
18. Mohr, J. W., Turner, R. E., and Jerry, M. B.: *Pedophilia and Exhibitionism: A Handbook.* University of Toronto Press, Toronto, 1964.
19. Mathis, J. L., and Collins, M.: Mandatory Group Therapy for Exhibitionists. *Am. J. Psychiatry* 126:1162, 1970.
20. Witzig, J. S.: The Group Treatment of Male Exhibitionists. *Am. J. Psychiatry* 125:179, 1968.
21. Maletzky, B. M.: Assisted Covert Sensitization in the Treatment of Exhibitionism. *J. Consult. Clin. Psychol.* 42:34, 1974.
22. Zavitzianos, G.: Fetishism and Exhibitionism in the Female and Their Relationship to Psychopathy and Kleptomania. *Int. J. Psychoanal.* 52:297, 1971.
23. Hollender, M. H., Brown, C. W., and Roback, H. B.: Genital Exhibitionism in Women. *Am. J. Psychiatry* 134:436, 1977.
24. Mohr, et al., op. cit.
25. Kinsey, A. C., Pomeroy, W. B., and Martin, C. S.: *Sexual Behavior in the Human Male.* W. B. Saunders, Philadelphia, 1948.
26. Ellis, H.: *The Psychology of Sex.* Heinemann, London, 1933.
27. Money, J.: Use of an Androgen-Depleting Hormone in the Treatment of Male Sex Offenders. *J.Sex Res.* 6:165,1970.
28. Mohr, et al., op. cit.
29. Mathis and Collins, op. cit.
30. Witzig, op. cit.

ADDITIONAL READING

Bastani, J. B.: Treatment of Male Genital Exhibitionism. *Comprehensive Psychiatry* 17:769, 1976.
Brancale, R.: The New Jersey Program for Sex Offenders. *Int. Psychiat. Clin.* 8:145, 1971.
Cabanis, D.: Female Exhibitionism. *Z. Rechtsmed.* 71:126, 1972.
Exposure: Criminal Offense Predicted upon Indecent Exposure. *Am. Law Rev.* 2d. 94:1353, 1964.
Rader, C. M.: MMPI Profile of Exposers, Rapists and Assaulters in a Court Services Population. *J. Consult. Clin. Psychol.* 45:61, 1977.
Rooth, F. G.: Changes in Conviction Rates for Indecent Exposure. *Br. J. Psychiatry* 121:89, 1972.
Rooth, F. G.: Exhibitionism Outside Europe and America. *Arch. Sex. Behav.* 2:351, 1973.
Rooth, F. G.: Exhibitionism, Sexual Violence and Paedophilia. *Br. J. Psychiatry* 122:705, 1973.

Rooth, F. G.: Indecent Exposure and Exhibitionism. *Br. J. Psychiatry* (Spec. No.) 9:212, 1975.

Rooth, F. G.: Some Historical Notes on Indecent Exposure and Exhibitionism. *Medico-Legal J.* 38:135, 1970.

Rooth, F. G., and Marks, I. M.: Persistent Exhibitionism: Short Term Responses to Aversion, Self-Regulation and Relaxation Treatments. *Arch. Sex. Behav.* 3:227, 1974.

Smuckler, A. J., and Rader, C. M.: Personality Characteristics of Exhibitionists. *Dis. Nerv. Syst.* 36:600, 1975.

Student Note: Section 314(1): Nudeness or Lewdness? *Hastings Law Rev.* 24:1327, 1973.

Wagner, E. C., and Hoover, T. O.: Exhibitionistic M in Drama Majors: A Validation. *Percept. Mot. Skills* 32:125, 1971.

Zechnich, R.: Exhibitionism: Genesis, Dynamics and Treatment. *Psychiat. Q.* 45:70, 1971.

CHAPTER 36

Robert E. Litman is Co-Director and Chief Psychiatrist at the Suicide Prevention Center and the Institute for Studies of Destructive Behaviors in Los Angeles, as well as an Adjunct Professor of Psychiatry at the University of California at Los Angeles. He is a member of the Southern California Psychiatric Association and the Southern California Psychoanalytic Society and Institute, and is past President of the American Association of Suicidology.

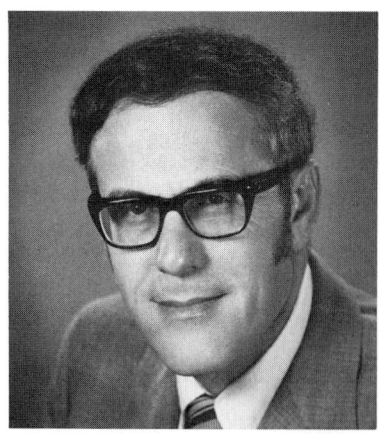

PSYCHOLEGAL ASPECTS OF SUICIDE

Robert E. Litman, M.D.

Suicide is defined as the intentional taking of one's own life. This definition, however, does scant justice either to the complexity and variability of suicidal phenomena, or to their profound ethical, philosophical, social and clinical implications. Shneidman[1] and Resnik[2] provide excellent overviews. This chapter will focus on certain important psychological and legal aspects of suicide, while at the same time emphasizing that the legal principles are rapidly changing.

THE CERTIFICATION OF SUICIDE

Traditionally, society has felt that it was necessary to assign blame for every death, either to God (natural, accidental) or to man (homicide, suicide). If God was the responsible agent, nothing more need be done, but if man was to blame, then there must be punishment for the guilty. Thus, for centuries, English law designated suicide as a special crime, punished by mutilation of the body, sanctions on the place and manner of burial, forfeiture of property, and censure of the family.

Legal requirements regarding responsibility for death have changed considerably in more recent years. The importance of God as the responsible agent has receded into the philosophical background. Both accidental and natural deaths may be investigated with great care, and responsibility is frequently assigned to some correctable circumstance. With regard to suicide, society's attitudes have become more tolerant, but are still ambivalent and contradictory. The trend is to view suicide less as a sin or crime, and more as an unfortunate consequence of mental illness and social disorganization. Judicial attitudes toward suicide have turned away from assessing guilt and enforcing punishment toward protecting suicidal persons when possible, and toward efforts to care for or compensate the surviving victims of suicide deaths. In England, the last of the penal statutes against suicide were repealed in 1961. Many people are not aware of the fact that suicide is not, and never was, a criminal act in most of the United States. Among those states which retained the common law concept of suicide as illegal, there has been an impressive move toward decriminalization. Suicide is currently a crime in only five states: Maryland, New Jersey, North Carolina, Oklahoma, and South Carolina. No penalty is provided for breaking the law against suicide, but suicide attempts are felonies or misdemeanors and could result in jail sentences, although the laws are seldom enforced. In recent years, a number of states (Alabama, Kentucky, Nevada, New York, North Dakota, South Dakota, and Washington) have repealed their anti-suicide laws. In the remaining 45 states, approximately half have no penal statutes on suicide, while the other half have no laws against suicide or suicide attempts, but they specify that it is a felony to aid, advise, or encourage another person to commit suicide.

An undercurrent of social condemnation of suicide has persisted. Frequently, the relatives and friends of persons who committed suicide feel themselves to be not only bereaved, but also stigmatized. They often attempt to persuade, coerce, or otherwise influence the authorities against the certification of suicide. For example, suicide notes may be concealed or destroyed. Evidently, certifying a death as suicide is still felt to be equivalent to a judicial verdict of "guilty." The certifying authority may be uncertain or confused because the statutory and traditional definitions of "suicide" are ambiguous, leaving a broad, borderline area between clear-cut suicide and other modes of death in which fall a number of more or less equivocal deaths. Because of the variations in standards for certifying deaths in different jurisdictions, the suicide statistics for different communities of the United States are not directly comparable. Physicians and surviving relatives have told me in confidence of many deaths which were suicides, but which had been certified as natural or accidental deaths by a physician, either through error, misinformation, or deliberate falsehood. One can only guess at the number of suicides concealed in this fashion. In the United States in recent years, approximately 25,000 suicides have been certified each year. My own estimate is that there were an additional 10,000 deaths yearly which would have been certified as suicides if there had been complete and impartial investigations.

Although it is highly desirable to define the categories of the mode of death more clearly and to insure greater uniformity in the application of the definitions, there is, I believe, no simple solution to the problem of variability in suicide death certifications. In the first place, the information available to certifying authorities varies greatly. Examination techniques and the ease and accuracy of toxicologic determinations are dissimilar. Secondly, in certifying a death as suicide, the official must make some degree of inference about the victim's intention. Intention is an ambiguous concept. It does not imply that the individual knew for certain that the act would result in death, since such a certainty is impossible. The term implies only that the person "had it in mind" that the self-destructive act might easily cause death, or that the act was likely to cause death.

A frame of reference for many certifying authorities is to view suicide as somewhat analogous to homicide, even though suicide is not illegal, and unlike murder, the intention to do wrong is not required. There might logically be various degrees of suicide, as there are various degrees of homicide, as follows:

1. First-degree suicide: deliberate, planned, premeditated, self-murder.
2. Second-degree suicide: impulsive, unplanned, under great provocation or mitigating circumstances.
3. Third-degree suicide: sometimes called "accidental" suicide. This occurs when a person puts his or her life into jeopardy by voluntary self-injury, but where we infer that the intention to die was relatively low because the method of self-injury was relatively harmless, or because provisions for rescue were made. The person was "unlucky" actually to die.
4. Suicide under circumstances which suggest a lack of capacity for intention, as when the person was psychotic or highly intoxicated from the effects of drugs, including alcohol.
5. Self-destruction due to self-negligence: for example, such self-destructive behaviors as chronic alcoholism, reckless driving, ignoring medical instructions, cigarette smoking, and similar dangerous activities. In general, such deaths are not at present classified as "suicide."
6. "Justifiable" suicide: for example, the self-destructive action of a person with a terminal illness. This last category is of considerable current interest to philosophers, theologians, and social psychologists.

We can anticipate that in the future efforts will be made to reduce the social, psychological, and quasilegal attitudes that continue to stigmatize all categories of suicide. Eventually, persons suffering from incurable disease processes may be encouraged to choose the place and time of their deaths with medical assistance.[3]

Relatively few equivocal cases are encountered under the first two categories; they are universally certified as suicides. Deaths occurring in category 5 are usually certified as natural or accidental. Equivocal cases generally arise in category 3, or third-degree suicide, where the facts may be interpreted differently by different certifying authorities. In Los Angeles a tendency has developed to recommend that equivocal cases be certified as suicides if the victim deliberately took as much as a 5 percent gamble that a given action would result in death.

Case 1

A 27-year-old male security officer, after an argument with his wife, took out his revolver and emptied out all the bullets except one. He turned the cylinder several times at random, and announcing, "This is Russian roulette," he put the barrel of the revolver to his temple and pulled the trigger. The gun discharged and killed him. Since there were six chambers in the revolver, his chance of death was 1 in 6. After some discussion, the consultants felt that this was sufficient intention to justify certification of (second-degree) suicide.

Case 2

A woman took a considerable quantity of barbiturates at 4:30 p.m. and fell asleep in front of the refrigerator on the kitchen floor. She knew that nearly every working day for the last three years her husband had come home at 5:00 p.m. and gone straight to the refrigerator for a beer. There was thus a strong possibility that she would be rescued. However, her husband was delayed and did not reach home until 7:30 p.m., when he found her unconscious. She later died in the hospital. The certification was suicide.

Case 3

A woman ingested a moderate overdose of barbiturates and fell asleep with a note pinned to her chest—"If you love me, wake me up." Her husband came home around 10:00 p.m., saw the note, threw it in the wastepaper basket, and went out to a bar for the rest of the night. When he got home early in the morning, she was dead. The certification was suicide, although the local district attorney did consider bringing charges of homicide.

Case 4

In the middle of a lovers' quarrel, a young man picked up a bottle of snail poison which contained arsenic and drank it in front of his fiancée, dramatically declaring that if she would not marry him immediately, he would kill himself. Interviewed later in the hospital, the young man said that he was not at all sure the snail poison would kill him. At the time he ingested it, he was caught up in his own drama. The arsenic, however, was eventually fatal, and the certification was suicide.

Case 5

A man wrote a suicide note and turned on the gas. However, Los Angeles gas is of low lethality. After waiting several hours, the victim became bored and lit a cigarette. There was an explosion which caused severe burns from which he died. The certification was suicide. Cases of this sort require considerable thought, but it seemed to the staff that the connection between the original suicidal intention and the eventual death was direct enough to justify the certification of suicide.

Case 6

A schizophrenic woman who had said that God wanted her to die to save the world, jumped to her death from the balcony of a psychiatric hospital. The death was certified as suicide. Unlike murder, the intention to do wrong is not necessary for a certification of suicide.

Case 7

A ship's captain became self-destructive only when he was highly intoxicated. Since he never drank alcohol at sea, he was safe there, but he had made several suicide attempts while drunk in port. He finished a night of heavy drinking in Los Angeles by shooting himself through the heart. The certification was suicide.

PSYCHOLOGICAL AUTOPSIES

A serious problem in investigating possible suicide involves the difficulties encountered in obtaining sufficient information or facts about a case to support the inference of suicide. As this author[4] and others[5] have noted, police reports are usually incomplete as sources of information. This is because the police are primarily interested in determining whether a homicide was committed, and they usually are not trained to collect extensive data on other types of cases. Nevertheless, in evaluating a possible suicide, it is highly desirable to have a description of the scene of death, including the position of the body, and to have evidence gathered at the scene, such as weapons, pills, poisons, and notes. In addition, it is important to reconstruct the habits of the victims both in connection with the method of death, such as in the use of guns or pills, and in regard to the person's general life-style. This will help to evaluate whether the person was at high risk for death by suicide or, conversely, for death by accident.

Almost 20 years ago, Norman L. Farberow, Edwin S. Shneidman, and the author, together with Theodore Curphey, who was then the Los Angeles County Medical Examiner-Coroner, began to develop a method for collecting information to assist in certifying modes of death more accurately. We obtained information by interviewing persons who knew the deceased fairly well, such as friends and family members, as well as professional persons such as teachers, physicians, and clergymen who had dealt with the deceased individual. The process came to be called a "psychological autopsy." The objective of the psychological autopsy is to reconstruct the background, personal relationships, habits, personality traits, character, and life-style of the deceased. This process can help greatly in evaluating equivocal cases. It was discovered while conducting thousands of psychological autopsies that this procedure, in addition to producing relevant investigative material, also had therapeutic value, leading to bereavement counseling, the relieving of guilt feelings, and the answers to other questions.

ACCIDENT VERSUS SUICIDE

Retrospective studies of persons who have committed suicide indicate that they could be grouped into two contrasting categories: (1) stable personality and life-style, and (2) unstable personality and life-style. People usually die in the same kind of behavior pattern as that which they followed in life. Persons who have a long history of stability in life-style and who have been conscientious and have not abused drugs seldom die accidentally under circumstances which suggest suicide. When such person die as a result of taking pills, or by gunshot wound or jumping from high places, it is usually because that was what they planned to do. By contrast, people who were unstable in their life-styles, who were erratic, irresponsible, careless, impulsive, and short-sighted, who showed poor judgment and poor planning, who often abused alcohol and other drugs, or who were mentally ill were quite capable of committing suicide. They were also capable of accidentally killing themselves in ways that might resemble suicide. It is with these latter people that equivocal cases generally occur.

It was noted earlier that cases of death due to self-negligence or self-indulgence usually are not certified as suicide, although there have been some interesting speculations that they should be. For example, deaths resulting from cirrhosis of the liver due to chronic alcoholism, or from lung cancer due to cigarette smoking are by common consensus called natural deaths. Problems are raised, however, in considering the chronic alcohol abuser who takes large amounts of sleeping pills and who also is depressed and talks about suicide. When such a person dies, how can one decide whether he or she died of the combination of alcohol and drugs used in order to feel "stoned" or whether additional drugs were ingested for a lethal purpose? In such cases, all of the evidence must be considered. If the blood-alcohol level and the amount of blood barbiturate are both insufficient to cause death, the resultant death was in all probability due to an unanticipated additive effect, and the correct certification would be accident. In those cases where there is a high level of hypnotics in addition to alcohol and where the psychological autopsy uncovers a history of recent crisis in the life of the person with consequent mood change, usually depression, then the evidence would tend toward certification as suicide.

A second subgroup of cases which most dramatically illustrates the suicide-accident problem includes persons who were physiologically drug-addicted. Such addicts may place themselves in a deep state of anesthesia almost every night or even during the day. If they have a mild respiratory infection, or twist themselves into an awkward position that obstructs the airway, they may die without suicidal intent. Investigators usually find the premises untidy and disorganized with unused pills and capsules lying about. The blood concentration of the drugs is usually in the middle-lethal range, not extremely high. On the other hand, it must be kept in mind that addicts are disturbed and depressed persons, often on the verge of deliberate suicide. Clues indicative of suicide are present if all the pills are gone (since addicts like to keep a supply on hand), if the blood concentration is extremely high, and if there is a recent history of unusually distressing disturbance of the life pattern (e.g., an arrest, the loss of a love relationship, or a physical illness). At the risk of generalizing, it appears that suicides tend to get their drugs from physicians, while accidental victims of drug abuse tend to obtain their drugs through nonmedical channels.

DRUG AUTOMATISM

The concept of drug automatism has been offered as an explanation of some drug-overdose cases. According to this hypothesis, the patient develops a state of toxic delirium after ingesting one or several doses of a prescribed drug, and in the delirious or automatism state, takes much more of the drug unintentionally. Quite a lively controversy has developed around this hypothesis, which is difficult to prove or disprove.[6] Proponents of this view argue that dangerous, even lethal, potentialities exist for drug overdose through automatism, although specific cases are difficult to demonstrate. Critics of the theory feel that it is unproven and unnecessary, and assert that it has persisted only because it serves the desires of many patients, their relatives, and physicians in order to deny the self-destructive motives and actions of the patients.

The drug-automatism syndrome was first described by Richards in a clinical note which stated: "It would appear that the knowledge of the need for another tablet persists, but the memory is so affected by the drug, that the patient does not realize that he has satisfied the need, and automatically repeats the dose at intervals."[7] However, as Long demonstrated, a gradual, one-at-a-time overdosage leads to sleep and cannot cause a blood level sufficiently high to produce death.[8] Thus, when a large concentration of barbiturates is found in the tissues, it is clear that the deceased did not take the pills one at a time over a prolonged period of time. A large concentration of drugs in the tissues of a nonaddict implies ingestion of many pills at one time.

In the period 1959–1960, my colleagues and I reviewed 100 equivocal suicides by the psychological autopsy method, and interviewed several thousand persons who had ingested drug overdoses serious enough to bring them into Los Angeles County Hospital for treatment.[9] In these studies, and in subsequent investigations, we were unable to confirm any cases of fatal drug overdose due to automatism. Furthermore, our studies of persons who had barely survived the ingestion of large amounts of hypnotic drugs failed to reveal any cases of automatism. There were a number of patients who described behavior which resembled automatism, but they had ingested low to moderate, relatively nonlethal amounts of drugs. The automatism represented a symptom of the incapacity of the patient (due to such factors as brain damage, metabolic illness, old age, infectious disease, or mental illness), rather than the specific action of any particular drug. These studies convinced me that for any individual taking a prescribed dose of barbiturates (e.g., 100 or 200 mg at night) or other hypnotic drug in an analogous prescribed dose, the possibility of a fatal automatism reaction is extremely rare. I estimate a probability of one in a million at most. On the other hand, there is a common and frequent route to fatal, accidental overdose, sometimes involving toxic delirious states resembling automatism. This road is by way of prolonged drug abuse, often combined with alcohol abuse. This type of lethal potential can be diagnosed and predicted, and there are possible avenues for prevention.

INSURANCE ASPECTS OF SUICIDE

The issue of suicide versus accident sometimes involves controversy over insurance benefits. The possibility of a contest arises from two aspects of insurance contracts. First, most life insurance policies contain a time clause covering the first one or two years, specifying that the claim for death benefits is invalidated if the insured person's death is by suicide. Legally, the company bears the burden of proving that the death was, indeed, a suicide. Second, many persons are covered by insurance contracts which specify that a certain amount of money (double indemnity) will be paid for deaths due to accident. In this situation, the burden of proof is on the beneficiary to show that the death was, indeed, an accident. Neither the insurance companies nor the beneficiaries of deceased persons are bound to accept the death certificate as a valid conclusion concerning the mode of death. A recent survey[10] demonstrated that medical examiners, given identical data, may reach opposing decisions on certification.

Either or both of the parties to any insurance contest may seek the assistance of an expert on suicide. This person may be a psychiatrist, psychologist, or other type of behavioral scientist. According to my experience, the expert can be most helpful and most believable by avoiding an overly authoritative or decision-making posture. Most court cases are not clear-cut; otherwise, they would probably not be under litigation. Furthermore, it is the task of the court, not the expert, to reach a verdict. The expert should try to clarify the facts and their relative importance, noting that some evidence may point toward suicide and other evidence may point toward accident. My best opinion, as an expert in court, is usually somewhat less than 100 percent certain. For example, I might give my opinion that, on balance, the facts indicate to me that there is a 60 percent probability that a certain death was suicide and a 40 percent probability that the death was an accident. The judge or the judge and jury together, taking all the facts and opinions into consideration, will finally draw an inference regarding the intentions of the deceased person and the relevancy of those intentions for the interpretation of suicide or accident in terms of the insurance contract.

Judges and juries are interested in motives. They feel that the victims would not have killed themselves intentionally if there were not motives to commit suicide. An expert can help to explain why people commit suicide. In my experience, the most common motive for committing suicide is severe depression. The depression is accompanied by painful feelings of worthlessness, helplessness, and hopelessness so that the person feels that he or she is doomed to suffer and be victimized and will never be able to bring about a change in the future. Therefore, suicide seems to be the only answer. An expert should be able to explain to the court that there are both psychological and physiological components in severe depression.

Most depressed people communicate how they feel to someone they trust, although some try to hide their feelings. Common-sense advice for someone who is feeling fatigued and exhausted is that they take some time off from work. One of the most distressing features of depression, however, is that the person often cannot enjoy a vacation. Going away on a trip may be perceived as a dangerous disruption of important supports such as work satisfaction. The prospect may precipitate suicide. Relatives and friends are puzzled: "How could it be suicide? We were just about to take a trip to Las Vegas."

In certain types of mental illness, there are delusions which may lead the victim to commit suicide. For example, persons may hear voices declare that they have committed unpardonable sins and God wants them dead. People may feel persecuted by the government, the communists, or other enemies so that they must commit suicide in order to save themselves and their families from a fate worse than death. In such cases, there has usually been a history of mental illness with hospitalization or prolonged, outpatient psychiatric treatment. The expert should be able to explain to the court in what ways the motivations of mentally ill persons are different in quality from those of persons who are not mentally ill.

The role of drugs, especially of alcohol, in suicide, is extremely important and should be clarified for the judge and jury. Alcohol and certain other drugs facilitate suicide by removing elements of psychological self-control and self-preservation during a crisis. Moreover, by their distressing personal and social effects, they bring about, over a period of time, a downward course in the person's life-style. Finally, many drugs, including alcohol, aggravate depression. On the other hand, drug abuse and chronic alcoholism are also important factors in causing accidents and accidental deaths.

Some people are involved in styles of living which are self-destructive

They alienate other people, move from job to job and place to place, and have very few dependable personal relationships. They may have made a number of suicide attempts in the past, and also may have had a number of accidents. Such persons are equally susceptible to suicide and to accident. Here the expert may be helpful in clarifying the relationship between circumstantial evidence and inferred motivation. Accidents tend to occur during ordinary, accustomed, or repetitive activities. For example, the great majority of serious one-car automobile accidents occur at night, to persons who frequent bars and are on their way home after heavy alcohol drinking. Suicide, on the other hand, involves an unusual set of circumstances—being at an unexpected place at an unexpected time—for which there is no good reason. An example is being hit by a railroad train at a place and time at which the person would not ordinarily be present. Sometimes the method itself is of overriding significance. For example, if there are very high amounts of hypnotic drugs in the blood of a person who was not a drug abuser, or if there is a bullet hole in the right temple of a right-handed person, suicide is a much stronger probability than accident.

WORKER'S COMPENSATION AND SUICIDE

Worker's compensation laws that provide for the medical care and support of persons injured in the course of employment have been interpreted by the courts to include the mental as well as the physical consequences of work-incurred injury. As a result, the agency which is administering these laws is required to compensate the survivors of workers who commit suicide as a result of work-related emotional trauma, and they must provide disability benefits and appropriate treatment to workers with injuries incurred in suicide attempts that are work-related. Most commonly, there is a history of a work-related physical injury, such as back strain, followed by unsuccessful treatment, with a gradually developing reaction of pain, suffering, and depression ending finally with suicide. However, there need not be physical injury. Emotional trauma related to the job such as conflict in loyalties or a promotion or demotion can produce similar anxieties and depression.

Case 1

During a robbery at a motion picture theater, a worker was tied up and threatened. For several months thereafter, he complained of tension, backache, sleeplessness, fatigue, and bad dreams. His death was by hanging. A suicide note stated that he felt that he could not continue living in a state of fear.

Case 2

A 40-year-old ex-college football star had been a successful salesman, executive, and finally president of a corporation. It was well known that he had up and down moods, mostly up, and that he had a weakness for liquor and women. Suddenly and unexpectedly, because the corporation needed a scapegoat to cover up some previous errors, he was fired from his job under humiliating circumstances. Within a week, he committed suicide.

Case 3

A middle-aged college professor was repeatedly passed by for promotion to a tenured position. Criteria for promotion were unclear, the promotion committee meetings were secret, and it was hard for the professor to know what he was doing that was wrong. Nevertheless, promotion was absolutely necessary for him to have security or success in his career. He made a suicide attempt in his car by means of carbon monoxide inhalation, but was rescued by his wife. About a month later, however, he killed himself in the same manner.

Suicide and Previous Injury

There is an increasing tendency on the part of the courts to award compensation to survivors of persons who committed suicide as a result of the injurious action of someone else. For example, a woman who had been injured in an automobile accident later committed suicide as a result of the pain, suffering, and depression. The persons who were liable for the original injury were held liable for her death. In many jurisdictions, it must be proved, not only that the suicide was the direct result of the original injury, but that the victim was unable to resist the urge to commit suicide. The testimony of an expert, usually a psychiatrist, is often sought to establish that the state of mind of the person, as a result of the injury suffered, was such that the victim could not resist the suicidal urge. It is important for the expert to discover whether the victim had become anxious, confused, severely depressed, or delusional, and to explain the significance of these mental states to the court. For example, one of the important consequences of depressive illness is the impairment of such functions as initiative, self-direction, and decision-making, so that a depressed person could not reasonably be expected to use will power to prevent suicide, especially if the person was suffering from a delusional feeling of hopelessness.

SUICIDE AND MEDICAL MALPRACTICE

The basic theme of this chapter is that the law's view of suicide faithfully mirrors society's view, which is confused, ambivalent, and contradictory. While some people think of suicide as requiring courage, independence, and self-sacrifice, the majority view continues to be that suicide represents cowardice, defeatism, selfish hostility, and social irresponsibility. The law sees suicide as a social evil, but it is quite unclear as to what extent the justice system should be involved in suicide prevention. Medical personnel and medical institutions are caught up in this conflict.

For every individual in our society who commits suicide, there are approximately 40 to 50 who suffer from depression and who seriously consider committing suicide. These suicidal people often consult physicians because of complaints such as sleeplessness, fatigue, inability to concentrate, anxiety, weight loss, muscle tension and muscle pain, indigestion, or because of recognized abuse of drugs and alcohol. If the physicians allow the patients to open up about how they feel, or if family members act as informants, physicians may discover that a patient has been thinking seriously about committing suicide. Furthermore, suicidal actions may occur in a physician's office or a general hospital, or in a psychiatrist's office or psychiatric hospital.

If a patient commits suicide, under what circumstances may physicians and hospitals be liable in lawsuits alleging negligence or malpractice? Ordinarily, the general practitioner or specialist in medicine or surgery is not expected to detect a high suicide risk in office practice, or necessarily to take preventive anti-suicide action, although ideally the physician would do both.[11] If the patient dramatically calls suicidal tendencies to the attention of a general physician, a reasonable evaluation is called for, and a consultation with a psychiatrist should be considered. One area in which physicians may be properly accused of negligently contributing to a suicide is when they prescribe large amounts of hypnotic drugs to a person who is known to have been a drug abuser or alcoholic, especially if such a person has made suicide attempts in the past. The same rule would apply to psychiatrists practicing with outpatients.

There is a growing tendency for society and its courts to expect hospitals and hospital-like institutions to prevent suicide if it can be done reasonably. In general and psychiatric hospitals, suicide is a rare event, accounting for only 1 percent of the total annual number of suicides. More than a third of hospital suicides result in lawsuits. According to experience in Los Angeles County, the average 400-bed community hospital might expect no more than one suicide every five years. If the occurrence of suicide is appreciably greater than this, it should arouse self-criticism and self-scrutiny in the administration. After any suicide in a hospital, there should be a complete investigation and a report setting forth the contributing causes and making recommendations for future prevention of a similar event. One essential for suicide prevention in medical and surgical wards is to protect patients who are temporarily depressed, agitated, or confused from falling from a dangerous height. Safety devices which limit the opening of windows and safety screens on doors and windows might prevent a majority of hospital suicides. Attention should be paid by physicians to clinical notes by nurses that a patient has been confused, demanding to go home, threatening suicide, or testing the strength of the windows. If a psychiatric consultation is requested, there should be a reasonably rapid response, and the recommendation from the consultant should include clear, direct-action recommendations.

Recently, general hospitals have encountered increasing legal difficulties in managing overdose patients in emergency care units. There has been a high incidence of malpractice suits generated by overdose patients, even those who had been successfully resuscitated. In response, we may see a growing movement toward the development of specialty units for the treatment of drug overdose cases.

The changing nature of psychiatric hospital practice has been confronted head-on by the problem of malpractice liability. In recent years, there has been a strong emphasis on the civil liberties of psychiatric patients with promotion of ambulatory crisis therapy, short-term hospitalization, open wards, and the earliest possible discharge from the hospital. There is a widespread trend in psychiatry to strip away the prisonlike features from the mental hospital, to abolish restraints, and to encourage a maximum of patient self-responsibility. Psychiatrists find themselves responsible for suicidal patients in psychiatric settings which have been deliberately designed to give the patients maximum freedom of action as part of the therapeutic milieu. Most psychiatrists regard suicide potentiality as a disturbing element complicating and sometimes restricting the therapeutic process and requiring special care and consultation. In psychiatric hospital practice, the possibility of suicide should be explicitly considered and entered into the record as part of the therapeutic program plan. The best defense against the accusation of malpractice is that the possibility of suicide was explicitly considered and a treatment decision reached.[12]

SUICIDE ASSESSMENT

I have pointed out that the assessment of suicidality can be expressed in a statement of suicide probability or risk.[13] An assessment is essential for two purposes: (1) immediate survival of the patient; and (2) long-term therapy goals for the patient who survives. The two objectives are not necessarily contradictory, but neither are they congruent. Treatment goals for most patients include achieving greater freedom, self-direction, and personal responsibility, yet short-range survival goals put the emphasis on the safety and security of the patient at the expense of independence, autonomy, and self-responsibility. Suicidal patients who are legally committed to a psychiatric institution dramatize the therapeutic dilemma. In practice we try to use common sense, knowledge, and experience to assist patients toward both survival and dignity.

If the consultant assesses the suicidal risk as high, hospitalization in a psychiatric unit is probably the best disposition, both for the patient's safety and as a place to reevaluate personal relationships and personal resources in planning for future activities. Even the best hospital units, however, are only relatively secure, and the treatment is only relatively effective. In my opinion, the most important aspect of the therapy of a truly suicidal person is the transition in the therapeutic process from preoccupation with safety, security, and survival to concern for life-style, interpersonal relationships, and self-direction. The main problem with hospitalization is that this transition can be delayed or confused. There is a serious question as to how useful legal commitment is for the purpose of preventing suicide. As legal grounds for commitment have been tightened and reduced in California, there has not been an epidemic of suicides in patients prematurely released from enforced psychiatric hospitalization. Therefore, I view psychiatric commitment as an expedient which should be used sparingly, with high selectivity and thoughtful deliberation. The argument for commitment is that the suicidal urge is time-limited and that the future of the patient should be protected against the transient turmoil of his personality. Two weeks of persuasion and discussion should be sufficient, however, to enable a patient to repair fragmented ego-controls. This should put an upper time-limit on commitment as an anti-suicide measure in all but the most exceptional cases.

From the standpoint of the patient's safety, the best precaution against suicide in or outside a hospital is the presence of other people. This may mean a continuous monitoring of a patient by family, by other patients, and by the staff of the hospital. The privacy of a single room is not an advantage for suicidal persons. Isolation is contraindicated. Common sense dictates that windows and doors be secure and that poisonous materials not be readily available. It is helpful to have regular patient meetings which include a periodic review by the patients of possible danger areas and dangerous objects in the environment. Ease of communication from patients to staff to physicians and back contributes greatly in forestalling suicidal actions in hospitals. It should be stated explicitly, however, that there is no certain way to prevent anyone from committing suicide anywhere, if the individual is wholly dedicated to self-death.

All of the problems discussed above have been and are still being presented to courts on all levels. The court decisions have been inconsistent, even contradictory. If a patient is discharged from a hospital after improving and then commits suicide, is the hospital liable? In two excellent reviews, Perr[14] describes the results of court actions. He stresses that the law demands reasonable care in foreseeable situations. The key words in the cases are "reasonable," "anticipated," "foreseeable," "preventable," and "controllable."

With regard to suicide, we are passing through a time of rapid change, both in legal attitudes and in psychiatric practice. What can reasonably be anticipated, foreseen, controlled, or prevented is limited by what is desirable and what is beneficial. We can look forward to a fairly long period of confusion, discontinuity, and contradiction as our ideas of justice and of medical and psychological practice struggle to keep pace with each other.

REFERENCES

1. Shneidman, E. S. (ed.): *Suicidology: Contemporary Developments.* Grune & Stratton, New York, 1976.
2. Resnik, H. L. P.: *Suicidal Behaviors.* Little, Brown, Boston, 1968.
3. Kastenbaum, R.: Suicide as a Preferred Way of Death, in Shneidman, E. S. (ed.): *Suicidology: Contemporary Developments.* Grune & Stratton, New York, 1976.
4. Litman, R. E.: Police Aspects of Suicide. *Police* 10:14–18, 1966.
5. Murphy, G., et al.: On the Improvement of Suicide Determination. *J. Forensic Sci.* 19:276–283, 1974.
6. Dorpat, T. L.: Drug Automatism, Barbiturate Poisoning and Suicidal Behavior. *Arch. Gen. Psychiatry* 31:216–220, 1974; Good, M. L.: The Concept of Drug Automatism. *Am. J. Psychiatry* 133:948—952, 1976; Aitken, R. C. B., and Proudfoot, A. T.: Barbiturate Automatism—Myth or Malady? *Postgrad. Med. J.* 45:612–616, 1969.
7. Richards, R.: A Symptom of Poisoning by Hypnotics of the Barbiturate Acid Group. *Br. Med. J.* 1:331, 1934.
8. Long, R. H.: Barbiturates, Automatism and Suicide. *Postgrad. Med.* 28:A56–A72, 1960.
9. Litman, R. E., et al.: Investigations of Equivocal Suicides. *J.A.M.A.* 184:924–929, 1963.
10. Curvey, C. E.: Effect of the Manner of Death in Medicolegal Cases in Insurance Settlements. *J. Forensic Sci.* 19:390–398, 1974.
11. Motto, J. A.: Toward Suicide Prevention in Medical Practice. *J.A.M.A.* 210:1229–1232, 1969.
12. Litman, R. E., et al.: Prediction Models of Suicidal Behaviors, in Beck, A. T., Resnik, H. L. P., and Lettieri, D. J. (eds.): *The Prediction of Suicide.* Charles Press, Bowie, Maryland, 1974, pp. 141–163.
13. Litman, R. E.: The Assessment of Suicidality, in Pasnau, J. (ed.): *Consultation-Liaison Psychiatry.* Grune & Stratton, New York, 1975.
14. Perr, I. N.: Liability of Hospitals and Psychiatrists in Suicide. *Am. J. Psychiatry* 122:631–638, 1965; Perr, I. N.: Suicide and Civil Litigation. *J. Forensic Sci.* 19:261–266, 1974.

CHAPTER 37

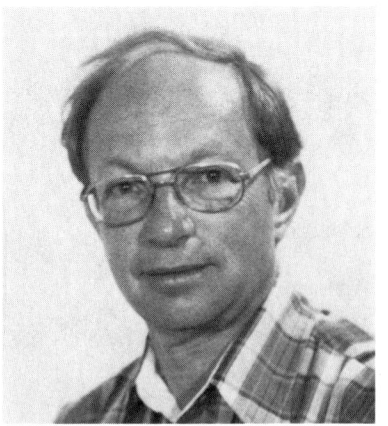

Julian Kivowitz is Senior Psychiatrist and Director of the Child Inpatient Ward of the Neuropsychiatric Institute at the University of California at Los Angeles. A graduate of Harvard College and the University of Buffalo School of Medicine, Dr. Kivowitz is a member of the American Psychiatric Association and the Southern California Psychiatric Society. He has published a number of research papers and articles in the field of mental retardation and developmental disabilities.

MENTAL RETARDATION AND THE LAW

Julian Kivowitz, M.D.

DEFINITIONAL CONCEPTS

Approximately 3 percent of the population of the United States falls into the category of the mentally retarded. Thus there are more than six million such persons in our country. They do not represent a homogeneous group, but rather have their own idiosyncrasies and differences. The American Psychiatric Association offers the following definition:

> Mental retardation refers to subnormal general intellectual functioning which originates during the development period and is associated with impairment of either learning and social adjustment or maturation, or both.[1]

For purposes of classification, four major categories are recognized. These categories are based partially on intelligence quotient (IQ) and partially on adaptive behavior. All leading authorities agree that the IQ level should not be the only determinant. The American Psychiatric Association further cautions that,

> It is recognized that the intelligence quotient should not be the only criterion used in making a diagnosis of mental retardation or in evaluating its severity. It should serve only to help in making a clinical judgment of the patient's adaptive behavioral capacity. This judgment should also be based on an evaluation of the patient's developmental history and present functioning, including academic and vocational achievement, motor skills, and social and emotional maturity.

The four major categories are (1) profound mental retardation (IQ under

20); (2) severe mental retardation (IQ 20 to 35); (3) moderate mental retardation (IQ 36 to 51); and (4) mild mental retardation (IQ 52 to 67). There is also a fifth category called borderline mental retardation (IQ 68 to 83) which is not generally recognized and will not be discussed in this chapter. At times this category is mentioned in legal proceedings in an effort to indicate a relatively low level of intellectual functioning, usually not enough to indicate legal incapacity of a general nature.

The profoundly retarded represent 0.5 percent of the retarded population. This group of individuals will be capable at most of only limited self-help. They will most likely need hospitalization or some type of environment in which constant care is available throughout their lifetime.

The severely retarded represent 3.5 percent of the retarded population. This group will be capable of habit training as children. As adults they will most likely need a controlled environment.

The moderately retarded represent 6 percent of the retarded population and can develop academic skills equal to about the second grade level. As adults they will most probably need a sheltered environment.

The mildly retarded represent by far the largest group, constituting the remainder of the retarded population, or about 5.5 million people. They can develop academic skills equivalent to about the sixth grade level. As adults they can develop social and vocational skills. Whether they are institutionalized or not depends more on their social skills and on the range of alternatives available to them than on their intellectual functioning.

LEGAL ISSUES

The legal problems of the retarded are many and varied. They have been described in the following way:

> The mentally retarded individual represents an ongoing set of legal problems throughout his life. First there is the problem of a label—how it is applied and in the criteria for its application. Second there is the problem of protecting the labeled individual as to whether he is to be institutionalized or not and at what age. Third there is a protection of his rights while institutionalized. Fourth, for the mentally retarded outside total institutions, there is need to protect and supervise the exercise of their constitutional rights and to ensure that they are provided a decent living standard and are not exploited.[2]

The remainder of this chapter will focus on these legal problems.

The diagnosis of mental retardation is applied to individuals at various ages and by different professional evaluators, depending upon the severity of the disability. The more disabled the person, the younger he is apt to be when the label is attached to him, and the more likely it is to be attached by someone in the health professions. Those with a less severe disability usually have the label applied later, most commonly during the early school years by someone associated with the educational system. A great deal of valid argument has centered on the exclusive use of psychometric tests in the labeling process. The tests are said to be culturally biased and excessively verbal, thus discriminating against the child coming from a different cultural setting. Several lawsuits have recently been brought, challenging the exclusive use of IQ tests to determine mental-intellectual functioning.

The case of *Spangler v. Board of Education*[3] is representative of these suits in which the use of traditional intelligence tests as the basis for student placement was challenged. As a result of these court cases, Article 9, Section 5 of the California State Constitution was changed. Among the new provisions are (1) that all bilingual children must be tested in both their primary and secondary languages, and (2) that test instruments which rely upon heavily loaded verbal material cannot be used in the evaluation.

Because of false labeling, not only have the retarded often been improperly placed in the school system, but they have often been excluded. This issue was considered in the case of *Mills v. Department of Education of the District of Columbia*.[4] In this case, the court found that the diagnosis-assigning process posed grave dangers of violating elemental notions of due process of law. Moreover, the *Mills* court found that there was a special obligation upon the state to provide adequate education when the state had assumed custody of the child. A Pennsylvania court prohibited state officials from denying or delaying the provisions of free public education to mentally retarded children.[5] Although these children had long been excluded from public schools as uneducable or unable to profit from formal instruction, the court declared that every child should be given the opportunity to profit from some sort of education or training.

For the less severely retarded, the labeling process is most commonly applied in relation to residential placement. Several important questions are raised in this latter situation. The major one is the problem of protecting the labeled individual from premature or unnecessary institutionalization.

INSTITUTIONALIZATION OF THE RETARDED

The question of the institutionalization of the mentally retarded is a thorny one. In the commitment procedure, the retarded have rarely been represented by legal counsel and have not received due process of law.[6]

In a survey in California,[7] only two of 40 individuals were represented by an attorney during the commitment process. Most of the parents did not think that it was necessary. Usually the decision of the professional people involved was accepted without giving those directly affected a chance to approve the decision, to participate in its formulation, or to object to it. Currently, litigation is under way which challenges these placement decisions, with parents and legal advocates for retarded persons suing the responsible professionals on the ground that due process had not been adhered to in making the decision. There is even the possibility of increased malpractice litigation against professionals for giving misleading advice in placement decisions.

RIGHT TO TREATMENT OR HABILITATION

Even more litigation is involved in ensuring that the person, once institutionalized, will receive adequate treatment, care, and habilitation. This is the so-called right to treatment for which there have been several landmark cases. Greenblatt[8] described his personal experience in the case of *Ricci v. Greenblatt*.[9] In 1970, Dr. Greenblatt was the Commissioner of Mental Health for the Commonwealth of Massachusetts. He and several other members of the state establishment were defendants in a class action suit charging them with cruel and abusive treatment of retarded individuals in Belchertown State School. The federal judge who heard the case decided, among other things, that the state schools had to draw up a plan for the adequate treatment of every resident. Greenblatt pointed out,

> Adequate care and treatment . . . required a great deal of money. No matter how modest the standards used, millions of dollars would be required. At that time, there was a taxpayers' revolt in Massachusetts. It was obvious that the state budget would have to be drastically increased, but both the legislative and executive branches were committed to levying no new taxes.[10]

Finally, an agreement was reached. Additional personnel were hired, and more treatment was given to the patients. In concluding this article, the author prophesied,

> The era of use of judicial procedures in behalf of the disenfranchised in our health system has just begun.[11]

Another landmark case on the issue of right to treatment is *Wyatt v. Stickney*.[12] The federal district court in Alabama found that with regard to the right to treatment, no viable distinction between the mentally ill and the mentally retarded could be made. It declared, therefore, that conditions in the state retardate institution (as also in the mental hospitals) violated constitutional rights of habilitation. Judge Johnson's order set forth detailed minimum standards for physical facilities, procedures, and staffing and declared that the state would have to find the funds to satisfy the order. Still another case was that of the *New York Association for Retarded Children v. Rockefeller*.[13] This case was a class action suit brought on behalf of more than 5,000 residents of New York's Willowbrook State Hospital for the mentally retarded. The institution was found to fail to conform to the minimal accreditation standards of various national and accrediting organizations.

OTHER HUMAN RIGHTS

For the mentally retarded, both within and outside of institutions, there is a need to provide, protect, and supervise the exercise of their constitutional rights and to ensure that they are provided a decent living situation and are not exploited. These constitutional rights apply both to the civil and criminal areas. In the civil area, questions of capacity to make a contract, to make a will, and to marry have been raised.

The question of whether a retarded person is legally able to make a contract is still not clear. This doubt applies especially to the committed mentally retarded patient. In a recent survey 47 judges involved in California commitment proceedings[14] were asked the question, "Can the retarded contract?" Four answered "Yes," seven answered "No," 20 answered "Don't know," and 16 did not answer. When a guardian is appointed for the committed patient, the issue becomes clearer. An order appointing a guardian of the person or the estate for an adult generally has the legal effect of rendering him incompetent to act alone. However, if the retarded person does not have a guardian, California courts have refused to merge a finding of incompetency with the commitment order, holding that an order of involuntary hospitalization, at least for the mentally ill, has the effect only of depriving the individual of his personal freedom and providing him proper care, not of rendering him incapable of contract.

In summary, then, the procedure to follow in determining whether or not a retarded person can make a contract is first to see if he is under guardianship which may render him incompetent to act alone, and if he is not, to consult legal counsel concerning the civil code of the state dealing with the power to contract. Each case would then have to be decided on its own merits within the provisions of the relevant civil code.

Problems found in contractual ability are also present in the issue of testamentary capacity. In order to have capacity to dispose of property by will, California statutory law and the laws of most states require that the person be over 18 and of sound mind. The courts generally interpret this requirement to mean that testamentary capacity exists if at the time the will is executed, the testator is possessed of sufficient mental capacity to understand and recall the nature and situation of his property and to remember and understand his relations to persons who have claims upon his bounty and whose interests are affected by the provisions of this instrument. California courts have held that an adjudication of incompetence does not prevent the incompetent from making a valid will. At most, an adjudication of incompetence raises an inference of lack of testamentary capacity upon the date of the adjudication. It follows that it is the individual's capacity at the time he executed the will that is decisive, rather than an earlier or later order of commitment.

The same questions that apply to making a contract and making a will apply to the ability to marry. The same 47 judges who were asked the question about contracting were also asked about the individual's ability to marry. Six answered "Yes," five answered "No," and 20 answered "Don't know." In California, one of the criteria used is whether or not the person is entirely without understanding at the time he marries. The trouble is that no statutory definition of persons entirely without understanding is provided. Kay[15] has commented:

> Prior adjudication of incompetence does not prevent the incompetent from subsequently entering a valid marriage, even though he has not been judicially restored to competence at the time of the ceremony. It would seem to follow that an order of commitment would not of itself render a mentally retarded person incapable of legally marrying.

Related closely to the issue of marriage are the sexual rights of the retarded, which are now being discussed with increased frequency. The issue is of concern to the law mainly in the area of sterilization. This procedure is based on at least two outmoded notions. The first is that the retarded have absolutely no judgment in the sexual sphere. Cooke quotes Dr. George Tarjan, at that time superintendent of a major hospital for the mentally retarded, as observing,

> The extramarital conception rate of our women patients would have given pride to any college president or high school principal.

The current position is that, given proper instruction, the retarded person may very well have adequate sexual judgment.

The second misconception is that intelligence is determined by a single gene or at most by a few and that the spread of mental retardation can be prevented by sterilization of all of the retarded. As recently as 1973, 26 states had sterilization laws for the mentally retarded, and in 23 states it was compulsory. The concept is now being challenged. A recent case[17] in Ohio describes the situation in which a probate judge accepted a county child welfare board's affidavit that a minor female was feeble-minded and ordered her to be sterilized. The procedure was performed. Later the parents sued both the judge and the hospital, insisting that she had not consented to the operation and furthermore that there was no statutory basis for the judge's order. The parents also contended that the participating parties were conspirators who deprived their child of her civil and constitutional rights. The federal judge ruled that the probate judge was without authority to order the sterilization. Furthermore, he stated, that because there was no Ohio law to support the judge's order of sterilization, he not only exceeded his jurisdiction, but also acted completely without authority. Consequently, he did not enjoy judicial immunity and was subject to suit by the sterilized person for the consequences of the unauthorized order. Even with statutory authority, hospitals are becoming increasingly wary of authorizing sterilization procedures. They believe that at some future time a suit might be brought by or on behalf of the female, alleging conspiracy or other wrongful act to deprive her of her procreative capabilities.

GUARDIANSHIP

In order to protect the retarded from making unwise personal and financial decisions, especially if there is no family involved, the law traditionally relied on the concept of guardianship. This concept is being revised with several assumptions about guardianship now being questioned. The initial assumption is that the interest of the family always coincides with the interest of the retarded individual. This is not always the case. Some authorities feel that a guardian should often be appointed to protect the individual from his own family. Another concept which is coming under increasing question is that of the unitary guardian. In the report of the President's Commission on Mental Retardation in 1963, it was noted that the concept of guardianship was a relic of a time when the mentally retarded individual was considered an incompetent who had to be kept away from normal social contacts. In earlier times, retarded persons were alienated from society and without rights. The President's Commission recommended that a range of guardianship plans be developed to accommodate the degree of incapacity of the retarded person and the condition of his family life. For example, there could be limited guardianship for the mentally retarded adult with the scope of the guardian's authority carefully defined by a court order. Under such a limited guardianship, the retarded person could exercise most of his rights but be controlled in the management of his money or property. In many jurisdictions, such an arrangement is termed a conservatorship.

Several guardianship models have been proposed. In California, regional centers have been created with a wide variety of functions, one of which is carrying out guardianship plans. Currently, the state is also experimenting with a somewhat different plan, a system of "legal advocacy" which would incorporate but go beyond guardianship. The advantage of this structure is the independence of the advocate and the willingness and ability of the advocate to organize political and community support programs on behalf of the retarded. Another model is that of a professional "ombudsman." This person would operate within and outside of institutions for the retarded and would be given added potency by virtue of a quasiofficial role as liaison to the courts and social agencies.

THE CRIMINAL JUSTICE SYSTEM AND RETARDATION

In addition to the problems raised in the civil law area, the mentally retarded individual presents considerable problems for the criminal justice system. The two most common issues are the competency of the person to stand trial and his criminal responsibility. These problems are complicated by the fact that legally there is often an assumption that mental retardation and mental illness are the same.[18] In the U.S. Supreme Court case of *Jackson v. Indiana*,[19] a retarded 27-year-old deaf mute was charged with two minor robberies. The question of his competency to stand trial was raised. He was examined by two psychiatrists in his home state of Indiana, who found that he had the mental age of a preschool child. They concluded that he was not capable of understanding the charges against him or of aiding his attorney in his defense. Because of this, the trial judge found him incompetent and ordered him committed to a state institution until the state's Department of Mental Health could establish that he was competent. There was testimony, however, to the effect that Jackson could never be brought to a state of competency. The Supreme Court of Indiana affirmed the trial court's decision. However, on appeal, the U.S. Supreme Court found unanimously that the case represented an unconstitutional deprivation of the rights of the defendant. The court noted that an institutional commitment under these circumstances could impose, in effect, life-long confinement in the institution. It was ruled that the defendant could only be held for a "reasonable time" during which it could be determined whether or not he could obtain competency through available treatment or rehabilitation. If he could not, he must be released or an independent proceeding must be conducted to commit him civilly.

In a 1966 survey[20] of retarded prisoners, the issue of competency to stand trial was not raised in 92 percent of their convictions. Most, if not all, jurisdictions have no systematic procedure for testing the intelligence of an accused before or during the trial, thus leaving detection of his mental retardation to chance. Unless his clinical or other records are brought into court or he behaves in a bizarre manner, it is unlikely that a retarded defendant will have his competency questioned. Finally, the distinction between competency to stand trial and criminal responsibility is often confused. The main test for criminal responsibility is the capacity to appreciate the criminality of his act at the time of the crime. Competency requires that at the time of the trial a person must have the ability to understand the nature of the criminal proceedings and be able to rationally assist counsel in his defense. A retarded person may have some ability to distinguish the criminality of a criminal act, but such ability is not a guarantee that he possesses mental capacity to stand trial. As long as these two issues are confused, there will always be the danger that the retarded will be tried and convicted without having his competency to stand trial determined.

With respect to criminal responsibility, some psychiatrists contend that a retarded adult with a mental age of 10 ought to be judged with the same standards that would be applied to a 10-year-old child in a juvenile proceeding. Nevertheless, the courts generally do not accept this idea for the retarded, regardless of mental age. Davidson[21] noted the court's view that when a man reaches physical maturity, the presumption is that he possesses the capacity to commit a crime, and it is for the defendant to overcome that presumption.

RETARDATION AND DANGEROUSNESS

Along with the issues of the retarded in the criminal justice system is the question of their capacity for antisocial behavior (e.g., just how dangerous are the retarded?). It is generally agreed that there is a relatively higher proportion of the retarded in correctional institutions. This has contributed to a negative stereotype which assumes that retardation itself precipitates antisocial behavior. In fact, however, there are many other reasons to account for the relatively higher number of retarded in the prison population. In a study of retarded defendants, 59 percent pleaded guilty compared with less than 10 percent of the nonretarded.[22] The retarded also waived their right to counsel and jury trial far more often than the criminal with average intelligence. Finally, reduction of charges is less frequent with the retarded. In 88 percent of convictions, no appeal of judgment or sentence was made. The characteristic passivity of many retarded persons appears to be matched by passivity in the legal advocacy on their behalf

Outside of correctional institutions, there is no evidence to indicate that the retarded are any more dangerous than the rest of the population. In a follow-up study[23] of 348 severely retarded adults who had attended classes for the trainable retarded in New York City, only 2 percent had been involved in offences against property or person. Another study quoted in the same report described 265 persons with IQs between 45 and 75, who lived in a single community in Connecticut. This study concluded that these people were socially adequate and self-supporting and in "no sense" presented a serious threat to the safety of society.

In summary, there is no proof that the retarded represent any significant danger to society, and those officials connected with the administration of their legal rights in the criminal justice system should keep this fact in mind.

REFERENCES

1. American Psychiatric Association: *Diagnostic and Statistical Manual of Mental Disorders.* ed. 2. Washington, D.C., 1968, p. 14.
2. Stone, A. A.: *Mental Health and the Law: A System in Transition.* NIMH Center for Studies of Crime and Delinquency, Rockville, Maryland, 1975, p. 124.
3. *Spangler v. Pasadena City Board of Education,* 375 F. Supp. 501 (D.C. Cal 1970).
4. *Mills v. Board of Education of the District of Columbia,* 348 F. Supp. 866 (D.C. C. 1972).
5. *Pennsylvania Association for Retarded Children v. Pennsylvania,* 334 F. Suppl. 1257; 343 F. Supp. 279 (E.D. Pa. 1972).
6. Turnbull, H. R., III, and Turnbull, A. P.: Deinstitutionalization and the Law. *Ment. Retard.* 13(2):14–20, 1975.
7. Kay, H. H., et al.: Legal Planning for the Mentally Retarded: The California Experience. *Cal. Law Rev.* 60:438–529, 1972.
8. Greenblatt, M.: Class Action and the Right to Treatment. *Hosp. Comm. Psychol.* 25(7): 449–452, 1974. (See also Greenblatt, M.: *Psychopolitics.* Grune & Stratton, New York, 1978.)
9. *Ricci v. Greenblatt,* Civil Rights Action No. 72-469 F, (D. Mass. 1972).
10. Greenblatt, op. cit., p. 452.
11. Ibid.

12. *Wyatt V. Stickney*, 344 F. Supp. 387 (M.D. Ala. 1972).
13. *New York Association for Retarded Children v. Rockefeller*, 357 F. Supp. 752 (G.D. N.Y., 1973).
14. Kay, op. cit.
15. Ibid., p. 475.
16. Cooke, R. E.: Ethics and Law on Behalf of the Mentally Retarded. *Pediat. Clin. North Am.* 20(1):259–268, 1973.
17. *Wade v. Bethesda Hospital*, 40 U.S. Law Week 2165 (D.C. S.D. Ohio, 1971).
18. Curran, W. J.: Competency of the Mentally Retarded to Stand Trial: New Rules from the Supreme Court. *N. Engl. J. Med. 287* 1184–1185, 1972.
19. *Jackson v. Indiana*, 92 S. Ct. 1845 (1972).
20. Marsh, R. L., et al.: The Adult MR in the Criminal Justice System. *Ment. Retard.* 13(2):21–25, 1975.
21. Davidson, H. A.: *Forensic Psychiatry*. Ronald Press, New York, 1952.
22. Kay, op. cit., p. 475.
23. Robinson, H. B., and Robinson, N. M.: *The Mentally Retarded Child*. McGraw-Hill, New York, 1965.

ADDITIONAL READING

Begab, M., and Richardson, S.: *The Mentally Retarded and Society*. University Park Press, Baltimore, 1975.

Blatt, B., and Kaplan, F.: *Christmas in Purgatory*. Yale University Press, New Haven, 1966.

Farber, B.: *Mental Retardation: Its Social Context and Social Consequences*. Houghton Mifflin, Boston, 1968.

Kindred, M. (ed.): *The Mentally Retarded Citizen and the Law*. Free Press, New York, 1976.

Symposium: Mentally Retarded People and the Law. *Stanford Law Rev.* 31(4):541–829, 1979.

CHAPTER 38

Harold W. Demone, Jr. is Dean and Professor of Social Work in the Graduate School of Social Work of Rutgers, the State University of New Jersey. He has served as Commissioner of Alcoholism for the Commonwealth of Massachusetts, and as Executive Director of the Division of Alcoholism of the New Hampshire State Department of Health. Until 1977, Dr. Demone was Executive Vice President of the United Community Planning Corporation of Boston. He has been a member of the Massachusetts Governor's Committee on Law Enforcement and the Administration of Criminal Justice, and is the author of several books and over 40 papers on alcoholism. Dr. Demone serves on a number of national boards in the field of alcoholism treatment and rehabilitation.

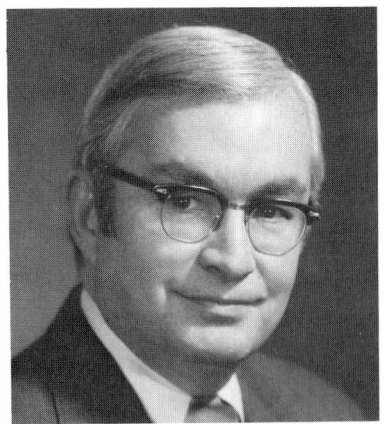

ALCOHOLISM AND ALCOHOL ABUSE

Harold W. Demone, Jr., Ph.D.

HISTORICAL PERSPECTIVE

It is clear that alcohol has played a role in man's development for millions of years. Roueche even suggests that in the Neolithic Period agriculture "may have sprung from a desire to assure a regular supply of alcohol."[1] At the least, it can be posited that a desire for alcohol complemented the need for assured sources of food in the development of organized agriculture.

Just as alcohol and agriculture are inseparably interrelated, so are alcohol and other significant social institutions: government, law, religion, and medicine. Early religions frequently cited the role of alcohol in their practices and ritual. References to wine in the Bible and in ancient Greek literature are numerous. It has been suggested that alcohol's "baffling nature frightened man into his first stumbling steps toward systematized religion."[1]

In his review of 125 preliterate societies, Horton[2] found that alcohol was commonly used in 80 percent of the studied groups. In about half the societies, men and women seemed to drink equally, or were free to drink in this manner without cultural disapproval. In the remainder the women definitely drank less. In about 80 percent of the societies, men and women drank together on many or most occasions.

Moderate drinking as we understand it was rare, drinking to excess being characteristic of primitive peoples. In two-thirds of the societies, intoxication brought about aggression in the males. Actually, these primitive groups were quite permissive about aggressive acting-out behavior, suggesting that they recognized the social utility of catharsis of aggression.

Despite positive sanctions, excessive drinking seldom interfered with necessary social and economic activities. Alcoholism was rare. Beverage alcohol for the preliterate was used for conviviality and to enhance social relations, not as a means of meeting life's problems.

In *Varieties of Religious Experience,* William James wrote, ". . . the sway of alcohol over mankind is unquestionably due to its power to stimulate the mystical facilities of human nature usually crushed to earth by the cold facts and dry criticism of the sober hour . . . the drunken consciousness is one bit of the mystic consciousness, and our total opinion of it must find its place in our opinion of the larger whole."[3]

More immediately germane, but not necessarily more important, are the actions of government to deal with the use and misuse of beverage alcohol. In England, an "Act for the Encouraging of the Distillation of Brandy and Spirits from Corn" was instituted in 1690 and was extraordinarily successful. Output doubled in 25 years; in 40 years, it increased 11 times. In the opening session of the first Federal Congress in 1789, an act placing a tariff on spirits was passed.

Our own country has gone through its share of legal machinations in its effort to deal sensibly with the excesses associated with beverage alcohol. Ordinarily, we seem to focus on one approach at a time: legal, moral, punitive, or therapeutic. The Prohibition era of 1920 to 1933 was preceded by two narrowly averted national prohibitions in the previous century as the individual states attempted to cope with the various and sundry problems related to alcohol abuse.

It has been suggested that the conflict about what should or should not be done with respect to alcohol and its use may well have been more destructive than the problem of alcoholism itself. "The problem is seen in sanitary codes, zoning regulations, traffic laws, educational requirements, welfare and penal legislation, medical administration, supervision of federal wards, maritime jurisdictions, military activities, veterans' affairs, and even budgets for diplomats . . . ."[4]

Our most recent tactics have been principally therapeutic in orientation, beginning in 1933, following the repeal of the Volstead Act. There have been private programs and research efforts, state-level treatment and rehabilitation programs, and most recently Federal Government programs in the field.

Because of the current interest in decriminalization, I will begin with a discussion of this subject. I will also review a variety of other legal and policy issues, including the rights of alcoholics, taxation, health insurance, driving while intoxicated, laws regarding the sale and consumption of beverage alcohol, laws requiring teaching about alcohol, advertising, and other pertinent issues. Seldon D. Bacon, recently retired director of the Rutgers University Center of Alcohol Studies, was fond of stating that there are more pages of federal rules and regulations on alcohol than on any other subject with the possible exception of money and the rights of the individual. I doubt that Bacon has ever perused the thousands of feet of shelf space necessary to store the regulatory provisions regarding alcohol, but his point is well taken. We are terribly invested in this beverage, and since laws and law violations are highly correlated, there must be extensive violations of the laws and regulations controlling alcohol use in this country.

THE CRIMINAL LAW AND INTOXICATION

In 1606, public intoxication was made a criminal offense in England. This legal orientation, brought to the American colonies by early settlers, remained substantially intact until 1966. The behaviors covered by the criminal laws included public intoxication, drunkenness, habitual or common drunkenness, vagrancy, loitering, and drinking in public. A series of state court cases and lower court decisions in the Federal Courts found public drunkenness statutes unconstitutional as "status crimes." However, the U.S. Supreme Court, in *Powell v. Texas*,[5] refused to follow this line of cases, and a divided court held such a statue to be a valid exercise of the police power.

Attention was then turned to reforms in the legislatures rather than in the courts. Hawaii became the first state whose legislature abolished public intoxication laws, although they relied heavily upon commitment procedures already contained in their mental health laws as a substitute for both criminal procedures and voluntary treatment measures. By 1971, North Carolina, the District of Columbia, Maryland, and several other states had eliminated public intoxication as a crime. Parallel to the states' efforts and following the Crime Commission reports, various drafting teams proceeded to prepare models of uniform legislation governing intoxication and alcoholism. In 1971, the National Conference of Commissioners on Uniform State Laws adopted a Uniform Alcoholism and Intoxication Treatment Act. A policy statement in the law enunciated the following: "It is the policy of this state that alcoholics and intoxicated persons may not be subjected to criminal prosecution because of their consumption of alcoholic beverages but rather should be afforded a continuum of treatment in order that they may lead normal lives as productive members of society."

In Boston, arrests for public intoxication went down 30 percent between 1969 and 1973. The following year, the first under decriminalization, 39 percent fewer people were taken under protective custody for public intoxication. Under one rubric or another, formal police-inebriate contacts went down more than 50 percent in a 6-year period.

Clarke[6] reports that by January 1974, of 38 states responding to a questionnaire, 30 had a statutory provision permitting involuntary treatment and commitment; in 28 states the provision was in use. Of the 19 states replying to the question, 13 stated that decriminalization was moderately to extremely effective.

A typical response was that of Minnesota. The state legislature removed public drunkenness as a criminal offense in 1971. The statute mandated 25 detoxification centers, not affiliated with hospitals, for initial medical treatment, diagnosis, counseling, and referral as necessary. The staffing patterns provided for a registered nurse as the supervisor, alcoholism technicians (abstaining alcoholics) for initial evaluation and care, with a physician on call.[7]

One thoughtful review of the decriminalization of public drunkenness was conducted by Rubington.[8] The general assumption of those promoting decriminalization was that inebriates would come under less frequent contact with the criminal justice system. However, public intoxication, even independent of the criminal statutes, remains a police problem since it is often offensive in public, and the police are expected to maintain order on the streets.

The current ideology is one of rehabilitation, presumably under the management of the medical care system. The terms "disease and illness" are used frequently to describe alcoholism. In fact, an analysis of the detoxification programs, an essential element of the decriminalization process, shows that they are generally operated by nonmedical practitioners. Physicians act as consultants on a client basis, but not on therapeutic, structural, or organizational issues. Outpatient medical clinics have more of a medical orientation, but former alcoholics and social workers do the bulk of the staffing, and their views are not always consistent with those of physicians. New cadres of treatment personnel are emerging (often called alcoholism counselors) with their own ideology and values.

Morale among staff is a significant problem. Abstinence as a goal and success criterion, and the failure of a large proportion of the clients to achieve it, has a damaging effect on the staff. Recidivism is often seen as a personal failure by the clinic staff.[9]

LEGAL RIGHTS OF ALCOHOLICS

Although much progress has been made in clarifying the role of the alcoholic with respect to public intoxication and commitment for treatment, many other human and legal rights have yet to be clarified. Is alcoholism a legitimate defense for commission of a crime? Can it be used to mitigate or reduce the seriousness of the charges? Other areas needing clarification include employment, domestic relations, public assistance, health insurance, and occupational licenses.

Plaut[10] related alcohol and crime in four ways: (1) the immediate effects of alcohol use can lead to a criminal act by removing sufficient inhibitions so that a person may behave in a manner not usually within his behavior patterns; (2) criminal activity may be seen in illegal efforts to obtain beverage alcohol; (3) drinking or drunkenness may be associated with criminal behavior; and (4) the prolonged effects of many years of heavy alcohol use may be indirectly related to crime because of the individual's reduced capacity to hold a job. He may then begin to associate with people holding more permissive attitudes toward law-violating behavior.

CIVIL COMMITMENT PROCEDURES

In his 1966 comparative review of American state laws, Curran found involuntary commitment provisions for alcoholism in all 50 states.[11] In 36 of the states the procedures were specific for alcoholism as distinct from mental illness. The range of commitment periods was from 30 days to an indefinite confinement until "cured." His study reported upon a great variety of statutory definitions of the condition, from no definition to such phrases as "loss of control over alcohol," to "habitual use," "danger to public morals, health, safety or welfare," and "inability to manage one's affairs."

Curran identified two polar views in the laws at that time: one which allowed the use of involuntary commitment only as an extreme measure when the person was found dangerous to the public safety, and one which advocated early intervention to force treatment when some noticeable harm, social or physical, had occurred to the individual as a result of his or her drinking.

Well over 30 states have adopted the Uniform Alcoholism and Intoxication Treatment Act which defines an alcoholic as:

> ... a person who habitually lacks self-control as to the use of alcoholic beverages, or uses alcoholic beverages to the extent that his health is substantially impaired or endangered or his social and economic function is substantially disrupted.

A brief analysis of key features of the model act which reflect the current view about civil commitment is given below.

Voluntary treatment is strongly reinforced (Section 10). Even if the patient leaves the treatment program against medical advice, assistance must be given in securing transportation and shelter.

Protective custody is carefully delimited (Section 12). A person appearing to be incapacitated by alcohol must be taken into protective custody by the police or an emergency service patrol and brought forthwith to an approved public treatment facility for emergency treatment. If none is available, he must be taken to an emergency medical service customarily used for persons who are incapacitated. Protective custody is not an arrest, nor shall any record or entry be made to that effect. A person admitted under this provision cannot be held longer than 48 hours without consent or additional civil procedures.

Section 13 provides for an emergency commitment for those "incapacitated by alcohol;" for example, someone who threatens suicide or is likely to inflict physical harm on another. Refusal to accept treatment does not meet these criteria. The commitment can be initiated by a certifying physician, a spouse, a guardian, or relations of the person, or by any other responsible person. In addition to detailing the supporting fact, a physician must certify and support the facts in the certificate. A physician employed by the admitting facility or state division may not be the certifying physician.

No person can be detained under emergency commitment longer than 5 days, although another 10 days is possible if a petition for involuntary treatment has been filed and the petition has yet to be heard.

Involuntary commitment of alcoholics (Section 14) is permitted only if the alcoholic exhibits cognitive deficiencies and is so debilitated that confused thinking exists not only with respect to the alcohol problem, but in other areas as well. Mere custodial care is prohibited. The law requires "adequate and appropriate treatment." Automatic discharge at the end of 30 days is provided unless a court order is secured for a recommitment for a further period of 90 days. Only two recommitment orders are permitted.

Section 37 repeals all state criminal statutes under which drunkenness is the gravamen of the offense, except for driving under the influence of alcohol and the sale, consumption, purchase, possession, or use of beverage alcohol at stated times or by a particular class of persons.

In less than a decade the movement to eliminate the crime of public intoxication and to constrain the use of civil control measures became fully mature. The several court cases already referred to were highly significant to this development. The Highway Safety Act of 1966 and the Economic Opportunities Act of 1967 foreshadowed Presidential messages in 1967 and 1968 which articulated a new view of alcohol addiction and challenged the use of criminal statutes. The Federal Alcoholic Rehabilitation Act of 1968 became the first of a series of rapid developments as Congress began to spell out a new national policy. The states as well began to act during this same time period. The District of Columbia, Maryland, North Dakota, Connecticut, Florida, and Massachusetts all made significant changes in their legal procedures dealing with alcoholism. Thirty-two states have met the provisions of the federal law sufficiently to qualify for special federal grants to implement new programs of treatment and rehabilitation.

DRIVING WHILE INTOXICATED

It is estimated that more than half of the individuals involved in fatal automobile accidents have significant amounts of alcohol in their bloodstreams.[12] In addition to the 28,000 lives lost each year, alcohol-related accidents cause injuries to approximately half a million people with a price tag of more than one billion dollars for property damage, insurance costs, and medical insurance.

Just as the mid-1960s became the turning point in the utilization of criminal and civil law with respect to public intoxication and alcoholism, so too it inaugurated the era in which we seriously challenged the underlying premises associated with drinking and driving. Challenged were the following hypotheses: (1) despite laws to the contrary, traffic deaths would continue to rise; (2) the legal processes would not or could not be used effectively to deal with intoxicated drivers; and (3) "normal drinkers" were the principal cause of the drinking driving problem. Currently, we lean toward other premises, that problem drinkers are a significant cause of highway accidents, and that the problem is one of social health rather than a purely legal matter.

The new approach has stimulated a variety of experiments. Most notable are those of the United States Department of Transportation in its Alcohol Safety Action Program (ASAP). In these demonstrations, the drinking driver is referred to a rehabilitation program. Two systems have developed: prosecutors or presentence and probation personnel make the referral in one system; in the other, the judges will make individual decisions.[13] The typical, required rehabilitation course has four 2½-hour sessions, 1 week apart. The participants are taught about the seriousness of drunken driving, problem drinking, and the skills necessary to drive. The fourth session is directed toward a discussion of individual plans to avoid future drunken driving.

ENFORCEMENT OF DRUNK-DRIVING LAWS

The problems of enforcement of drunk-driving laws involve three types of issues: technological, administrative, and legal. The technological issues range from the value and comparability of breath, blood, and urine samples to the technology of measuring blood-alcohol levels. Complementary is the issue of the level of alcohol in the blood relative to impairment of driving skills and judgment.

Administrative issues range from what tests should be used to when the tests should be administered (e.g., whether to all traffic violators or to those selected by law-enforcement officers).

Among the legal questions still under debate are the adequacy of the various court procedures for identifying problem drinkers; what charges should be made, including driving while unfit because of alcohol; specific penalties versus judicial discretion; the validity of implied consent laws; and what the punishment should be. Alternative punishments range from warnings, fines, and required education to required voluntary service, revocation of driving licenses, and imprisonment.

For physicians a special problem has developed. Should they report patients who are drinking and driving? This issue is rooted in the confidentiality of the physician-patient relationship. What criteria can physicians use if they are to report? When is level of alcoholic impairment a clear traffic hazard? Are black-outs a sufficient justification? These issues have yet to be resolved under our new approaches to preventing highway traffic accidents caused by problem drinkers.

ALCOHOL BEVERAGE CONTROL LEGISLATION

Although every nation has laws regarding the use of beverage alcohol and the variety of circumstances surrounding it, we know very little about the effect of these various statutory systems. The best single publication on the subject is by Wilkinson.[14] I will make reference to it a number of times in this section.

Our beginning will be 1933, the year following repeal of Prohibition. The federal government and the state governments, along with counties, cities, and towns all over the country enacted a variety of regulatory structures. Although changes have occurred since 1933, they are mostly cosmetic and have not significantly affected the principal thrust of the immediate post-Prohibition legislation. Legislation on alcohol use and related problems have been based on opposing assumptions: (1) all alcohol use problems are interrelated, and (2) they are all entirely separate. Most of the prevailing legislation was written in substantial cooperation with the distillers and brewers. The industry also developed its own self-regulation code. The goal was to prevent another Prohibition, to disassociate the alcohol beverage industry from its previous reputation, to anticipate new attacks from the "dries," and to prevent even more stringent control measures. The laws are of great variety and coverage. They include tax provisions on sales; fair trade price controls; public drinking establishment regulation; off-site drinking establishment regulation; age of the consumers; sex of the consumers; number of drinking establishments according to population; distance of establishments from churches, schools, hospitals, railway stations and housing developments; prohibition of sale on Sundays; who can be portrayed in advertising; what can be said in advertising; the media to be used for advertising, and so on. It is obvious that we have a crazy patchwork quilt of laws, regulations, and practices. If these regulatory programs have any effect on drinking, they would seem to be in the direction of moderation rather than excess, for this was one of the original purposes of the control laws. At the federal level, the principal responsibility for liquor industry regulation is assigned to the Alcohol, Tobacco and Fire Arms Division of the United States Treasury Department. As with the rest of the Treasury Department, its principal interests are in collecting taxes and secondarily in protecting the consumer from inadequate merchandise and misleading labeling and advertising. Beverage taxes vary substantially, distilled spirits having the highest rate and wine having the lowest. State and local governments often add their own tax levies. The industry, especially the distilled spirits sector, feels that the taxes on their beverage are grossly excessive and are constantly pressing for reduction. In fact, the current system does give us a natural experiment and could be said to encourage the consumption of lower-proof beverages, although systematic research about whether altering taxes will in fact bring about changes in drinking behavior has not been done.

The federal government is also interested in separating producers, distributors, and retailers in the interest of free competition. Most control on advertising is directed toward the old-time liquor ads which stressed the nutritional and health values of beverage alcohol.

The states vary principally as to whether they are monopoly or nonmonopoly states. At last count, 18 states were monopoly states. In these states, public agencies operate all retail sales outlets. In noncontrol states, the government does not operate any of the industry itself. It is possible in a monopoly state to sublease some of the responsibilities to private industry. In no state does the public own and operate facilities for the manufacture of alcohol.

Typically, each state has an Alcohol Beverage Control (ABC) agency. Their principal function is to manage the various laws and regulations and to grant retail and wholesale licenses. As noted earlier, no significant changes have occurred in these laws since they were first enacted. Everyone in the alcohol beverage industry from producer to retailer must obtain a license. The numbers of outlets are controlled on some sort of population base in order to limit the number of establishments in any neighborhood.

Often in conjunction with the police, the ABC agencies have the responsibility of enforcing the laws and regulations regarding the trade. Specifically, they are concerned with advertising, the sale of the beverage to minors, the sale to habitual drunkards, etc. Another grouping of responsibilities has to do with public morals. The ABC agencies have the responsibility to police bar girls, prostitutes, and floor shows in connection with the sale and consumption of beverage alcohol.

For the most part, this regulatory system of the alcohol beverage industry has little relation to public health education or prevention of alcoholism.

In addition to the legal controls, the industry has developed a variety of written and unwritten procedures which it applies throughout the trade. The most widely known example has to do with liquor advertising on radio and television. The federal government does not fully control such advertising, instead the industry has taken on this responsibility itself.

The industry itself is separated by the type of beverage manufactured. For the most part, the distillers, brewers, and vintners all function independently of each other. The wine makers identify with agriculture and are seen as part of the American agricultural industry. The brewers remind us that their beverage is moderate and even has some food value, while the distillers are constantly on the defensive. For such a large-scale, complex industry, it is remarkable how little enlightened interest is manifested. On the most nominal level possible, the industry participates in programs which may help to control the excessive use of alcohol, but they have failed to take advantage of the many opportunities they have to show a proactive rather than a reactive stance. They still seem to operate as if this were the century preceding 1933, when Americans saw the control of alcohol excesses as a function of alcohol availability and believed that the most effective way to deal with the problem was to forbid the sale and consumption of all alcoholic beverages. Although more than a generation has passed since then, the industry still has a knee-jerk reaction to any kind of criticism or suggestion that there may be regulatory and statutory ways of controlling where alcohol is sold, how it is sold, its proof, and its other components which might in fact have some positive relation to reducing alcohol-related problems.

ALCOHOL EDUCATION IN THE PUBLIC SCHOOLS

Between 1844, when the Oregon Territory adopted a state constitution which was the first to prohibit the sale of alcoholic beverages, and the repeal of the federal prohibition amendment in 1933, repressive legislative action was common in the United States. One such wave of activity occurred during the period 1870 to 1900, when the public schools were drawn into educational programs concerning alcohol and narcotic use. Some of these laws specified the grades and the number of hours and pages to be devoted to the subject. The goal was usually total abstinence and the elimination of the alcohol beverage industry. This wave of attention in the public schools was followed by a similar flurry of activity in the 1920s. The writers of these statutes meant what they said. Local school committee members in New Hampshire were liable to a fine if the state alcohol education requirements were not completely followed in the curriculum. Nearly all of the states still have such statutory requirements. Some amendments have been adopted which alter the basic thrust of these proposals to bring them more in line with contemporary public health education principles. As a case in point, a physiology and hygiene textbook of 1885 concluded its chapter on alcohol by describing it as a powerful drug which causes narcosis and a substantial proportion of crime and poverty. Medical complications were described, including Bright's disease, softening of the brain, stomach ulcers, indigestion, arteriosclerosis, and blindness. The book's focus was clearly physiologic. Current activities generally follow the view of the World Health Organization, which states, "Education must be scientifically sound and built on current attitudes and understanding of the people to be educated."

Interest in controlling the excesses associated with beverage alcohol through education of the young has not dissipated. Unfortunately, research has not been conducted to determine whether alcohol education programs have a significant effect. The findings of current studies show no change in behavior as a consequence of educational intervention.

OTHER ISSUES OF INTEREST

Even though the topics already discussed are those of major significance to those specializing in legal medicine and the allied forensic sciences, we would be doing an injustice to the field of alcoholism and alcohol problems if we did not at least suggest some of the other related issues.

Insurance

Currently, 16 states have mandated the inclusion of alcoholism treatment in group health insurance policies in one form or another. These developments reflected the general dissatisfaction with the continued discrimination against alcoholics by the insurance industry. In 1964, the Blue Cross Association of America recommended that its various affiliates cover alcoholism. Eight years later, in 1972, only one-third of the most widely held contracts included alcoholism in the category of other illnesses. Similarly, in 1972, of 278 commercial health insurance policies, 22 specifically excluded alcoholism, and only 45 policies (16 percent) were nondiscriminating.[15]

Medical Assistance

Considerable state-level activity (e.g., in Arizona and Minnesota) is taking place with respect to legislation which provides that an alcoholic will not be denied medical assistance payments because of his illness or condition.

Supplementary Security Income

The Social Security Amendments of 1972 (PL 92-603) included provisions which required that alcoholics must undergo approved treatment in order to qualify for supplementary security income for the aged, blind, and disabled.

Industrial Alcoholism Programs

A number of American companies, with the full cooperation of organized labor, have developed alcoholism programs for their employees. More recently, several state legislatures have taken the position that state employees should have the same right to alcoholism treatment as they do for other illnesses or conditions. In all of the above, an alcoholic employee can still be dismissed if he or she cannot properly function on the job.

In June 1971, a Presidential order was issued requiring that alcoholics be rehabilitated as fully as possible before discharge from the Armed Forces. The Army developed a 30- to 60-day rehabilitation program. Those alcoholics who seem motivated and improve can remain in the Army and continue in a long-term treatment program. Those who fail to meet the above conditions are given an honorable discharge and referred to the Veterans Administration. Treatment teams are deployed worldwide.[16]

Funding Treatment Programs

In addition to, or in place of, support from general revenue, there is increasing interest in earmarked taxes for alcoholism prevention and treatment programs. One approach is to take a percentage of the state revenues from liquor sales and/or taxes and apply them to the rehabilitation programs via a special account. Another model would use the fines imposed for various crimes in a set-aside system for various alcoholism treatment and rehabilitation programs.

Clients' Bill of Rights and Grievance Procedure

In Wisconsin, a public-interest law firm recently established a program to remove the barriers which hamper the reintegration of the alcoholic into society. In addition to community education, advocacy, and research, the law firm has joined with the state in developing an 800-page manual, "Advocacy for Reintegration," including a clients' bill of rights and a grievance procedure to implement it.

CONCLUSION

In a recent review of human service trends in the mid-1970s, I suggested that a better understanding of the human services industry could be achieved by an analysis of evolving ideologies and social values, emerging technologies, changing administrative patterns, and modified program patterns.[17] These topics are equally applicable to the changes occurring in alcoholism and alcohol abuse programs.

The fundamental characteristics of a society are evident in the values and assumptions by which it determines what is right and wrong and how it will help or punish its citizens. Specific social values differ in stability over time and in the degree of popular acceptance. Despite the homogenizing effects of improved means of transportation and communication, heterogeneous populations, personal values, personal interest, and different life styles persist. The preferences and assumptions of one group may be in direct conflict with those of others. The tortuous shift in legal procedures for managing the manufacture, sale, and consumption of alcoholic beverages is one example. The shift in legal procedures dealing with the public intoxicant, the alcoholic, and the drunken driver are additional examples.

The historical analysis presented in this chapter was designed to underline the tenuousness of many of our values. They clearly change over time in relation to the shifting dominance exercised by various societal groups.

Another set of forces affecting the current approaches to alcoholism and alcohol problems is our increasing level of technological sophistication. After nearly a half century of increasingly intensified research, new standards of human service care are becoming established in alcoholism. They then become the yardstick against which all relevant programs are assessed. Technological innovations are generally applauded for the more effective care which they make possible and for their alleviation of human distress. When widely applicable, they enhance such current social values as equity of care, personal choice, decriminalization, deinstitutionalization, civil rights, and equal protection.

A third set of forces affecting current alcoholism programming is changing administrative procedures. Developments in accountability, evaluation, management, and planning are highly relevant to all human service ventures, and the continuing success of any, and all, are significantly dependent on the ability of the policymakers and managers to integrate contemporary administrative procedures. An ideal human service model should be consistent with the ideologies and social values dominating the contemporary social scene and should be built upon the technologies and administrative practices being injected into human service practices.

REFERENCES

1. Rouche, B.: *The Neutral Spirit: A Portrait of Alcohol.* Little, Brown, Boston, 1960.
2. Horton, D.: The Functions of Alcohol in Primitive Societies. *Q. J. Studies Alcohol,* 4:199–320, 1943.
3. James, W. H.: *The Varieties of Religious Experience: A Study of Human Nature.* Longmans, Green, New York, 1902.
4. Straus, R., and Bacon, S. D.: *Drinking in College.* Yale University Press, New Haven, 1953.
5. *Powell v. Texas,* 392 U.S. 514 (1968).
6. Clarke, S. G.: Public Intoxication and Criminal Justice. *J. Drug Issues* 5:220–232, 1975.
7. Garber, J. D., Dolander, E. V., and Dexter, J. D.: Alcoholic Detoxification: A One-Year Experience. *Minnesota Med.* 57:143–145, 1974.
8. Rubington, E.: Top and Bottom: How Police Administrators and Public Inebriates View Decriminalization. *J. Drug Issues* 5:412–424, 1975.
9. Gottheil, E.: Poor Morale in Treatment Personnel. *Alcohol Health Res. World* 5:20–25, 1975.
10. Plaut, T. A.: Summary of Conference. *Alcohol, Alcoholism and Crime.* Commonwealth of Massachusetts, Chatham, 1962, pp. 116–124.
11. Curran, W. J.: Civil Commitment of Alcoholics: A Legal Survey, in *National Conference on Legal Issues in Alcoholism and Alcohol Usage.* Boston University Law-Medicine Institute, Swampscott, Mass., 1966, pp. 36–70.
12. *Alcohol and Health.* First Special Report to the U.S. Congress from the Secre-

tary of Health, Education and Welfare, National Institute on Alcohol Abuse and Alcoholism, Washington, D.C., 1971.
13. Scrimgeous, G. J.: ASAP and the Courts: Learning from Experience, the Problems of Systems Interface. *J. Drug Issues* 5:248–254, 1975.
14. Wilkinson, R.: *The Prevention of Drinking Problems.* Oxford University Press, New York, 1970.
15. Insurance Coverage for Alcoholics in Treatment: Goals and Progress. *Alcohol Health Res. World* 5:2–7, 1975.
16. Ruben, H. L.: Rehabilitation of Drug and Alcohol Abusers in the U.S. Army. *Int. J. Addiction* 9:41–55, 1974.
17. Demone, H. W., Jr., and Schulberg, H. C.: Human Service Trends in the Mid-1970s. *Social Casework* 56:268–279, 1975.

CHAPTER 39

Charles P. O'Brien is Professor of Psychiatry at the University of Pennsylvania Medical School, and is Director of the Drug Treatment and Research Center at the Philadelphia Veterans Administration Hospital. Dr. O'Brien received his undergraduate and medical degrees, as well as a doctorate in neurophysiology, from Tulane University in New Orleans. He is a Fellow of the American Psychiatric Association and a member of the Psychiatric Research Society, the American College of Neuropsychopharmacology, and the Group for the Advancement of Psychiatry.

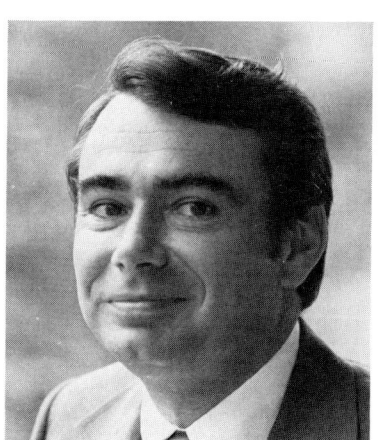

George E. Woody is Associate Clinical Professor of Psychiatry at the University of Pennsylvania Medical School, and is Assistant Director of the Drug Treatment and Research Center at the Philadelphia Veterans Administration Hospital. Dr. Woody is a graduate of Amherst College and Temple University Medical School, and is a member of the American Psychiatric Association, the American Association for the Advancement of Science, and the Society of Biological Psychiatry.

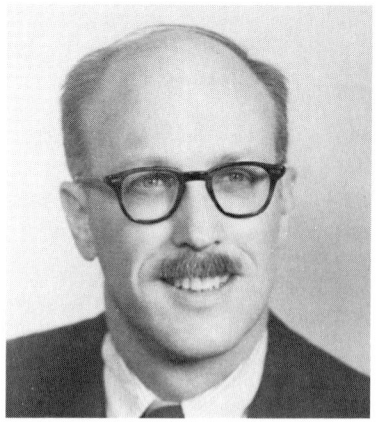

DRUG ABUSE TREATMENT PROGRAMS

Charles P. O'Brien, M.D., Ph.D., and
George E. Woody, M.D.

DEFINITIONAL CONCEPTS

Drug abuse is a complicated phenomenon involving social, psychological, medical, legal, and moral issues. Effective treatment programs should provide a wide range of services to respond to the many problems found among drug abuse patients. The clinical picture of drug abuse exists along a continuum from occasional or controlled use to excessive or compulsive use. The severity of the problem will depend on many factors including the type, frequency, and dose of drug used; the emotional stability of the user; the setting in which the drug is used; and the degree to which drug use disrupts the user's ability to function in his family and in society.

The terms drug abuse and addiction have been used to mean many different things. Medically useful drugs can be used improperly or excessively, and this may be termed abuse, even in the absence of addiction. The use of nonmedically useful or illegal drugs is usually called abuse, even if the use is moderate and leads to no medically defined hazard. It should be noted that use of illegal drugs, even occasionally, may be a medical hazard because of variations in dosage, impurities, or unknown substances in the drug used. The term addiction should be limited to the situation in which drug use has become compulsive and the individual's life is largely built around securing an adequate supply of the drug.

Addiction consists of two components: physical dependence and psychological dependence. Physical dependence is a biological phenomenon which depends on the type, dose, and duration of drug use irrespective of personality factors. A withdrawal syndrome will occur in a physically dependent person if the drug is abruptly withdrawn. The withdrawal symptoms are usually opposite to the effects of the drug itself. For example, opiates constrict the pupils and cause constipation; during withdrawal there is pupillary dilatation and diarrhea. With stimulants, withdrawal effects are more subtle and consist of lethargy and depression. Physical dependence may occur during legitimate medical treatment and does not, by itself, constitute addiction. The presence of psychological dependence, in addition to physical dependence, is required for the diagnosis of addiction.

Psychological dependence refers to a compulsive need for a drug in order to maintain a state of well-being, and it can occur in the absence of physical dependence. The speed and readiness with which physical dependence occurs depends on the type of drug involved. Even if physical withdrawal signs do not occur when the drug is unavailable, the psychological and social disruption may be so severe that for all practical purposes addiction is present.

> **PSYCHOACTIVE DRUG CLASSIFICATION**
> Sedatives
>   Sleeping pills (barbiturates and others)
>   Minor tranquilizers (diazepam and others)
>   Alcohol
> Stimulants
>   Amphetamines, methylphenidate
>   Cocaine
> Opiates
>   Heroin, methadone, morphine, etc.
> Hallucinogens
> Marijuana
> Major tranquilizers (chlorpromazine and others)
> Antidepressants
>   Tricyclics (imipramine and others)
>   Monoamine oxidase inhibitors
> Antimania drugs
>   Lithium

Treatment of the physiologic aspects of addiction is often difficult but is only part of the problem. The nonmedical aspects are perhaps even more complicated and usually require special attention. These include loss of job, involvement in crime, medical complications, and disturbances of personal and psychological adjustment. Treatment programs should employ, or have a working relationship with, professionals specializing in helping patients with problems in these areas. This group of specialists would include physicians, psychotherapists, social workers, vocational counselors, nurses, pharmacists and legal-aid consultants.

PATTERNS OF DRUG ABUSE

Sedatives

The sedative group consists of sleeping pills, minor tranquilizers, and alcohol. These drugs depress the nervous system, eventually causing sedation. Depending on the dose and the previous experience (tolerance) of the user, there may be a period of excitation before sedation. This is described as pleasant or as a "high." As with all drugs, the effects of sedatives vary according to individual differences, the setting in which the drug is used, and the expectation of the user. These drugs all interact with one another and with drugs in other categories which also have sedative effects. This additive interaction often results in accidental overdoses. Another factor which leads to accidental overdose among experienced users is that as tolerance develops, a larger dose is required to produce a "high," but the dose which produces depression of vital functions (overdose) increases relatively little. The margin of safety becomes quite narrow. This effect sometimes leads to inadvertent overdoses in patients who are using large quantities of sedatives.

SLEEPING PILLS

Sleeping pills are widely prescribed for the treatment of insomnia. While they do temporarily relieve this symptom by shortening the time required to fall asleep and increasing the total time asleep, tolerance rapidly develops to these effects. Chronic users of sleeping pills often have poor sleep patterns in spite of the use of the pills. If they attempt to stop the medication abruptly, severe problems in falling asleep can be expected, and fitful sleep, often with nightmares, will occur. In a sense, these drugs create a form of dependence by suppressing normal sleep patterns (slow wave and dreaming sleep). Unless the drugs are withdrawn gradually, the dreaming stage of sleep (rapid eye movement or REM sleep) will rebound, producing a sleep disturbance that may be worse than that for which the sleeping pill was initially prescribed.

Many patients take sleeping pills legally for years without realizing that they are drug-dependent. Some increase the dose gradually and develop obvious abuse problems. Most continue a moderate dose taken at bedtime and assume that they are cursed for life with insomnia.

Insomnia usually is a sign of some underlying problem, often a depression, which may need specific treatment. Treating the insomnia as an illness instead of as a symptom leads to abuse problems. Sleeping pills should only be taken on a short-term basis, and nondrug treatments should be considered in their place. Sleep disturbances caused by depression will often respond to psychotherapy or to tricyclic antidepressant medication.

MINOR TRANQUILIZERS

Minor tranquilizers (e.g., diazepam, oxazepam, chlordiazepoxide, and meprobamate) have many properties in common with members of the sedative category. The benzodiazepine family (including diazepam among others) is the newest and most popular. They are prescribed as antianxiety agents, but diazepam also has anticonvulsant activity (when used intravenously) and muscle-relaxing properties. They are used in so many situations that diazepam is the most commonly prescribed drug in America in any category, and chlordiazepoxide is third.

The great popularity of the benzodiazepines attests to their rewarding or positive-reinforcing effects. Stated simply, most people *like* the feelings produced by diazepam and similar drugs. Abuse problems can occur because patients may take more than the amount prescribed, and they may wish to continue taking diazepam for long periods of time. There is also a tendency among patients to "loan" these drugs to family members and friends. Since patients take them so readily, there is some tendency for physicians to prescribe minor tranquilizers in situations where other less pleasant medication may be more effective, as for example, in easing depression.

Despite the tendency to overuse of benzodiazepines, physical dependence is uncommon. Only at high doses (100 mg per day and more) do clear physical withdrawal symptoms occur. Withdrawal effects are similar to those seen with sleeping pills. They range from increased nervousness and tremulousness at the mild end to epileptic seizures at the severe end.

Benzodiazepines are much less likely than other sedatives to cause a fatal overdose. Large doses have been taken in suicide attempts, but fatalities have not been reported. When taken in combination with other sedatives such as alcohol or sleeping pills, benzodiazepines add to the toxicity of these other drugs, and serious overdoses can occur.

ALCOHOL

The most commonly abused drug throughout the world is alcohol. Up to 10 million Americans are estimated to have drinking problems. It is important that the diagnosis of alcohol abuse not be limited to late-stage alcoholics with severe and long-standing physical and social problems. Alcoholic drinking patterns often begin at an early age, and treatment is considered to be more effective when instituted early.

Alcohol is a sedative which depresses the nervous system and adds to the effects of other depressants such as tranquilizers or sleeping pills. Most drug overdoses involve combinations of alcohol and other drugs. Some are purely accidental and occur when individuals who have been drinking alcohol routinely ingest their regular dose of prescribed medication. The amount of alcohol may be the same as that which they have taken many times before. The prescription medication (e.g., sleeping pill or tranquilizer) may also be in a moderate dose which has been effective for the patient in the past. Nevertheless, when the two drugs (alcohol and sedative-type prescription drug) are ingested together, a serious and potentially lethal overdose can occur. The mechanism of this interaction appears to be simply an additive one and is dose-dependent. Thus a low dose of tranquilizer and a low dose of alcohol may cause only minimal effects. Even if low doses are taken initially, problems may still occur, because the first doses of alcohol may impair judgment and cause an individual to continue drinking even though he has been warned to take only one or two drinks while on the medication.

An extraordinary, idiosyncratic reaction called pathological intoxication also may occur with alcohol ingestion. After a relatively small dose of alcohol (1 to 3 drinks), susceptible individuals exhibit marked changes in behavior, usually extreme aggressiveness or assaultiveness. The condition may last for about 1 to 2 hours, and the individual typically has amnesia regarding this period.

Stimulants

AMPHETAMINES

Amphetamines and amphetamine-like drugs are used most frequently as an aid to weight reduction. While they diminish the appetite and cause weight loss, tolerance is such a prominent feature of these drugs that the weight loss is usually transient. Many obese individuals, however, learn to like the alerting and energizing effects of amphetamines. These patients pressure the physician to continue the use of amphetamines, or, failing that, they shop around for physicians who will freely prescribe them.

Dependence on amphetamines consists of a compulsion to ingest the drug and a feeling of depression and fatigue if the drug is not obtained. The mental depression seen after chronic amphetamine use appears to be related to a biochemical change in the brain as determined by metabolic studies. The depression can be long-lasting and may require treatment with antidepressant medication.

In addition to dependence, amphetamine users run the risk of direct toxic effects. The stimulant effects produce hypertension and sleeplessness. Psychosis may occur in susceptible individuals at moderate doses. At higher doses, psychosis becomes almost certain, even in normal subjects. The user progresses through stages of sensitivity to people in the environment, to suspiciousness, to referential thinking, and on to paranoid delusions and auditory hallucinations. Violent behavior is a common occurrence in acute amphetamine toxicity.

While the value of amphetamines in obesity treatment is doubtful, there is clear evidence that stimulants (e.g., amphetamine, methylphenidate) can be useful for treating two less common disorders. One is hyperkinetic syndrome of childhood. In this condition, stimulants have so-called paradoxical effects causing slowing of motor activity and increases in attention span. This condition is sometimes misdiagnosed, and great care must be exercised to restrict its use to those hyperactive children who actually fit the diagnostic criteria. The second disorder is narcolepsy or compulsive sleep attacks. This is a relatively rare condition, but it usually responds well to stimulant treatment. Amphetamines are not recommended in the treatment of depression, owing to the dangers of dependence, although some clinicians attest to their value in geriatric populations.

COCAINE

The effects of cocaine are in general similar to those of the other stimulants. The drug was at one time widely used as a local anesthetic in dental; ear, nose and throat; and ophthalmologic procedures. While cocaine has been largely replaced by newer drugs for medical uses, its popularity as a recreational drug is on the rise in the United States. Small quantities of cocaine powder may be "snorted," and absorption is rapid via the nasal mucous membranes. The user gets a prompt but transient feeling of excitation and euphoria.

The toxic effects and dependence liability of stimulants have been described above. When used intravenously, high doses of cocaine may also cause apparent convulsions. Cocaine's effects fit into the stimulant category, but dosage is usually quite low due to high costs, and physical dependence is not found. Withdrawal depression, therefore, is not usually seen. Nevertheless, regular cocaine users show a strong compulsion to obtain the drug, even at great personal and family sacrifice. Abuse is sometimes seen among middle-class business and professional people who become involved with cocaine and spend all their available funds to obtain supplies of the drug. Cocaine should clearly be considered to have a high addiction potential.

Opiates

Opiates are medically indicated for the treatment of pain. While the term narcotic has a broad legal meaning, medically it refers only to opiate-type drugs. This category includes morphine, heroin, methadone, codeine, and other related drugs. Opiate effects are many and varied. They include reduction in pain sensation within the central nervous system, a feeling of euphoria, and changes in the levels of several important hormones. Opiates appear to exert their effects because of their chemical similarity to natural substances called endorphins. The opiate drugs activate receptor sites normally occupied by the natural opiates or endorphins.

As with other drugs, the effects of opiates vary considerably with the expectations and experience of the user. They produce excellent analgesia and a state of relaxation in most patients suffering from severe pain. Some, however, feel nauseated and consider the experience unpleasant. In progressively higher doses a dreamlike state is produced. Very high doses can lead to coma and death from respiratory failure. With repeated doses, tolerance to opiate effects occurs, and higher doses are required to obtain a particular effect. Long-term use of opiates appears to produce no serious toxic effects. Hormonal changes occur, but these are reversible. The major toxic problems related to opiates are caused by shared needles, contaminated drugs, and poor hygiene. High rates of infection, especially hepatitis and poor nutritional status, are common among street addicts.

Physicians who prescribe opiates for the relief of pain are justifiably concerned about producing addiction. A distinction must be made, however, between addiction and physical dependence. Physical dependence is a biological phenomenon which will occur in humans or animals who are given significant doses of opiates for several days. The degree of physical dependence depends on dose and duration of treatment. Addiction, as described earlier, implies the presence of psychological dependence with a compulsion to obtain the drug in order to achieve a desired mental state. Physicians can reduce the likelihood of psychological dependence by retaining control of the medication and by determining that it is being used strictly for relief of pain. In patients with severe chronic pain requiring opiates, physical dependence is inevitable and this should not necessarily be considered addiction.

The euphorogenic properties of opiates give them a high addiction liability. Individuals may take them to relieve dysphoria (depression or other unpleasant mood states) or to produce a "high." The most publicized opiate addicts are heroin addicts who frequently commit crimes in order to support their habit. The cost of street heroin is extremely high. A small "bag" (about 100 mg of substance) usually contains less than 2 mg of heroin, although this varies with locale and number of "middle-men." The remainder of the bag is adulterant, usually inactive and often contaminated. Thus the actual physical dependence of most street addicts is fairly low. Even those who spend $50 to $100 per day on heroin are receiving only a small amount of the drug.

Once an individual is dependent on opiates, he will experience withdrawal symptoms if he does not get the drug regularly. Since heroin has a relatively brief duration of action (3 to 4 hours), it must be injected two to four times per day. Withdrawal symptoms include craving for the drug, nausea, restlessness, muscle aches, tearing of the eyes, yawning, vomiting, and diarrhea. If not treated with an opiate, these symptoms gradually worsen over 24 to 36 hours and then gradually improve over the next 3 to 5 days. Opiate withdrawal is quite unpleasant, but in contrast to withdrawal from sedatives, it is not medically dangerous.

Hallucinogens

Hallucinogenic drugs can produce distortions of reality at very low doses. Sensations may be heightened, and there may be a feeling of clarity or insight about past life experiences or the current environment. A variety of perceptual changes occur and these are usually visual, producing mixtures of colors and distortions of shapes. This state may be perceived as pleasant, but in some individuals it becomes terrifying. The effects of street hallucinogens are unpredictable, owing to variations in dose and in the chemical constituents ingested. Most drugs currently sold on the street as hallucinogens actually contain phencyclidine.

Phencyclidine (or PCP) was developed as an anesthetic but was found to have unpredictable effects on humans. Until recently it was used in veterinary medicine. PCP purchased on the street is either smoked or ingested. It causes both stimulant and hallucinogenic effects. The result is pleasant to some users but frightening to others. Psychotic episodes with violence have been reported, and PCP-induced psychosis has been used as a legal defense. The drug has not been studied under controlled conditions, however, and at present the relative importance of pre-existing personality factors in determining the response of the user is unknown. The role of PCP-like compounds which frequently are found in street samples is also unknown.

Marijuana

More than 36 million Americans are estimated to have used marijuana. It affects several organ systems, most notably the brain. A feeling of euphoria and relaxation typically occurs. When used alone, sedation is more pronounced, but when used in groups, spontaneous laughter often occurs. Tolerance and mild dependence are possible but very unlikely in the doses smoked or ingested by American users.

While occasional use of marijuana can hardly be called abuse in the medical sense, certain individuals will have adverse reactions. In high doses, frank hallucinations, delusions, and paranoid feelings can occur. Sensitive individuals, particularly persons recovering from a mental illness, may become paranoid after a relatively low dose.

Another adverse effect of marijuana use that has been reported involves daily use of the drug accompanied by neglect of constructive activities. This has been called the "amotivational syndrome," but there is no real evidence that this condition is caused by marijuana use. Rather it is probable that heavy marijuana use is just one more symptom in a troubled individual.

Most scientific issues concerning marijuana have tended to become politicized. This is unfortunate because it obscures the facts and leads to misinterpretations, especially in regard to the toxicity of marijuana. All drugs are toxic at some dose, and this dose varies according to the susceptibility of the user. Most studies have found marijuana to have a relatively low toxicity, but this does not mean that it is nontoxic.

Major Tranquilizers

Major tranquilizers have distinct neurochemical and behavioral effects which are quite different from those of minor tranquilizers. These drugs are indicated for the treatment of psychosis. They generally do not cause effects interpreted as pleasant and thus they have virtually no abuse potential.

Antidepressants

Tricyclic antidepressants (e.g., imipramine, amitryptiline, and doxepin) combat the depressive syndrome and produce gradual changes in mood.

They are not stimulants such as amphetamines or cocaine, and thus they are rarely abused. There have been occasional reports of drug abusers who take episodic high doses of amitryptiline to get "high." This antidepressant has sedative-like properties which are often regarded as unpleasant rather than desirable effects.

Monoamine oxidase inhibitors (MAO-I) drugs (e.g., tranylcypromine and phenelzine) have different neurochemical effects from the tricyclic antidepressants. These drugs produce some stimulation, but they are much more subtle than amphetamine effects. The MAO-I drugs are also rarely abused.

Lithium

Lithium carbonate is an important drug for the treatment of mood swings in manic-depressive illness. It has both antimanic and antidepressant activity in appropriate individuals, but its direct subjective effects are not considered pleasant. Consequently it is not used excessively or for recreational purposes.

Tobacco

Cigarette smoking should be considered in a discussion of drug abuse. There is evidence that heavy smokers become tolerant to nicotine and develop a mild degree of physical dependence. Although the physical dependence is mild, the degree of addiction is severe. Each puff results in the absorption of a bolus of nicotine into the blood via the lungs and quickly to the brain. The habit in a smoker of one pack per day, therefore, is reinforced about 200 times each day, while a typical heroin habit is reinforced only one to three times per day. The relapse rate after treatment for cigarette addiction is about the same as that for heroin addiction.

METHODS OF TREATMENT

There are many treatments for drug abuse, and each generally involves a combination of several interventions. The treatment chosen depends on the kind of drug, the motivation of the patient, the facilities available, the complications that have resulted from addiction, and practical issues such as where the patient lives and whether he or she is employed. No treatment has yet been found that has a high probability of curing drug addiction, but several can attenuate it or interrupt its course. Most treatments can benefit some addicts. Some treatments are more popular and thus applicable to larger numbers of patients than others. Different therapies often emphasize different goals. For example, therapeutic communities usually aim for total abstinence and are intolerant of continued addiction, while methadone programs generally aim for social rehabilitation even though the patient may continue to be addicted.

The recent expansion of treatment facilities has allowed more patients to be helped by increasing the amount of therapy available and by providing new options that can engage patients who previously refused therapy. Each different therapeutic approach usually involves one major and several minor goals and interventions. Regardless of their orientation, most programs have a considerable amount of structure. For example, rules of conduct are emphasized, and patients are expelled from the program if the rules are broken. Treatment methods are usually directed at the drug of abuse and or at the complications of addiction. Major treatments for the drug of abuse include detoxification, psychotherapy (group, family, or individual), and pharmacotherapy. Treatments for complications include social work services, medical consultation, legal advice, and vocational rehabilitation.

Treatment for Narcotic Addiction

Narcotic addiction is the drug problem that has received the greatest amount of attention and the most active public support. Perhaps this is because narcotic addiction develops in young, healthy people and because it usually progresses rapidly with serious consequences to the addict and to society. This is not said to minimize the damage done by other types of drug abuse, but to emphasize the extremely serious and destructive course that narcotic addiction takes.

The single treatment that has had the greatest impact on narcotic addiction is *methadone maintenance.* This treatment substitutes one opiate (methadone) for another (usually heroin). Well-run methadone programs dispense methadone in the context of other services such as psychotherapy, social work, medical consultation, vocational counseling, and legal assistance. These programs are usually highly structured with written policies for standards of conduct, take-home methadone doses, clinic hours, sign-in procedures, periodic medical examinations, unannounced urine tests, and rigid pharmacy-dispensing procedures including direct observation of patients while they ingest their daily dose of methadone. Treatment results vary, but most programs can demonstrate that patients who continue in methadone treatment have a marked decrease in heroin use, a decrease in criminal activity, an increase in employment, and improvement in personal adjustment. These results have been observed in studies using historical controls as well as in studies employing random assignment of matched addict patients to treatment groups.

Methadone programs do, however, have a great many problems. One of the most serious is the intentional diversion of legally prescribed medication into street sales. This occurs as a result of dispensing methadone to patients for ingestion outside the clinic, the so-called take-home dose. This practice is followed as a necessity or a convenience for patients who are preselected for satisfactory compliance with program rules and goals. Selection reduces but does not eliminate the risk of diversion. Many clinics are open 7 days per week and are very restrictive regarding take-home doses. Nevertheless, a certain amount of diversion nearly always occurs when methadone is allowed to leave the clinic. The alternative, requiring daily attendance at clinic regardless of personal circumstances, eliminates diversion but can be inconvenient, especially for patients who are working and must travel long distances. A long-acting form of methadone (LAAM) that suppresses narcotic withdrawal symptoms for 48 to 72 hours is currently under development and, if shown safe and effective, can help to eliminate diversion.

A second major treatment approach to narcotic addiction is *detoxification.* This consists of a reduction in narcotic dosage over a period of 1 to 3 weeks. It is usually performed on an inpatient unit, but it can be done in clinics as well. A few patients can have long-term benefits from detoxification, but most relapse within 2 months after discharge.

Results of detoxification may be improved by treatment with a *narcotic antagonist* such as naltrexone. This is an orally effective, long-acting drug that blocks the effects of narcotics for 48 to 72 hours. It can only be given after the patient is successfully detoxified, as it will cause a withdrawal reaction if it is given when the patient is physiologically addicted. Patients taking naltrexone cannot become addicted, and they rarely use narcotics. The major problem with narcotic antagonist treatment is that patients often discontinue it and resume drug use within a few days. Naltrexone is not physiologically addicting, and it does not produce a euphoria. Therefore it has considerably less "binding" power than methadone. At present, longer-acting forms of naltrexone are being investigated. If they can be developed, patients can be protected for weeks or months. This should lengthen remissions and give treatment staff time to work with patients who have mixed feelings about stopping their addiction. Moreover, experiments are underway to identify reinforcements (e.g., small amounts of money or special privileges) which will encourage patients to attend clinic and continue taking naltrexone.

A third major treatment for narcotic addiction is the *therapeutic community*. This is a long-term inpatient program that relies heavily on group therapy, group support, and confrontation techniques. It seeks basic changes in the attitudes and life styles of addicted patients. Patients must be detoxified before entering most of these programs. Treatment lasts from 4 to 24 months, and patients who complete the entire program, especially the longer ones, usually do very well. Some studies have shown that even patients who drop out early show significant reductions in post-treatment drug use and illegal activities as well as improvements in personal and vocational adjustment. Therapeutic communities do have notable disadvantages. They are expensive to operate and do not attract large numbers of patients. Most addicted patients lack the motivation to become involved in intense, long-term, drug-free treatment; others are working or have family obligations and thus cannot enter the program. Therapeutic communities are useful for a relatively small number of patients, and selectivity in referral is essential. Patients who have failed in other treatments or who request long-term, inpatient therapy should be considered for a therapeutic community. Patients with significant degrees of multidrug abuse are probably treated more effectively in such programs that on an outpatient basis.

Treatment for Dependence on Sedatives, Minor Tranquilizers, and Alcohol

Drugs in this class that are abused include barbiturates that are used as nighttime sedatives (e.g., Seconal and Nembutal) and nonbarbiturate sleeping pills such as methaqualone (Quaalude), ethchlorovinyl (Placidyl) and glutethamide (Doriden). Alcohol may be included here since it produces a similar type of dependence and withdrawal reaction. Benzodiazepines such as chlordiazepoxide (Librium) and diazepam (Valium) are included here for the same reason as alcohol. As described earlier, benzodiazepines are among the most widely prescribed drugs in the world. They definitely have an abuse potential and can be toxic, especially if used in combination with other sedative or depressant drugs.

Treatment for addiction to any of these drugs begins with detoxification. Unlike narcotic addiction, there is no maintenance drug such as methadone that can be used. Abrupt withdrawal can result in very serious complications, as described earlier. Detoxification is usually done in a hospital under close observation. During detoxification, the addicting drug itself or a substitute (such as phenobarbital) is given in gradually decreasing doses. Detoxification must proceed slowly and can take 3 to 4 weeks. Occasionally, detoxification can be accomplished in outpatient clinics but only by highly experienced personnel.

Some recent work has shown that alcoholics can be detoxified successfully in an outpatient program that uses intensive supportive psychotherapy. However, most clinicians recommend inpatient treatment for alcoholics experiencing detoxification. After detoxification, patients are referred to outpatient follow-up. This may be an intensive program such as that available in a day hospital. Here the patient participates in a structured program that includes group and individual therapy and which meets 5 days per week. Some programs provide sleeping quarters where patients live in the treatment facility. Those who are working leave during the day and return in the evening. There is usually a limit to the time patients can stay in these programs. Partial hospitalization programs for alcoholics are often termed "half-way houses" because they serve as a transition between care in a hospital and fully independent living in the community. Other follow-up programs include group or individual psychotherapy given one to three times per week. Some alcoholics do well in Alcoholics Anonymous, while others are helped by disulfiram (Antabuse) therapy. Disulfiram is a drug that interferes with the metabolic breakdown of alcohol. It stops the degradation of alcohol by the liver, and this results in the accumulation of acetaldehyde, a noxious metabolite of ethanol. Patients who drink alcohol while taking antabuse will produce acetaldehyde and quickly develop anxiety, sweating, headaches, a rapid pulse, and abdominal cramps. This reaction can be fatal to individuals who have heart problems or other serious medical conditions. Thus medical evaluation is necessary before starting disulfiram therapy. Other patients can be referred to a therapeutic community following detoxification where therapy is identical or similar to that described above for narcotic addiction. In fact, some centers combine alcoholics, sedative abusers, and narcotic addicts in the same basic program.

Treatment for Stimulant Abuse

The most commonly abused stimulants are amphetamines, methylphenidate (Ritalin), and cocaine. Stimulant addicts, especially amphetamine abusers, usually take the drug in spurts rather than continuously. They take high doses for several days or weeks, then discontinue it and resume use again at a later time. This pattern is unlike addiction to narcotics or sedatives where the patient takes the drug continuously for months or years. Stimulant addicts commonly develop marked psychopathology while using high doses, and their life style usually becomes chaotic. They have "speed runs" during which they take intravenous injections round the clock, eat very little, and get very little sleep. During this time they lose weight and often develop anemia or infections such as bronchitis or pneumonia. The depression that results from abrupt withdrawal often is accompanied by suicidal ideas or attempts. As with sedative addiction, the first step in therapy is detoxification, and this is usually done in a hospital. Antianxiety medication is often helpful during the first few days. Patients must be observed closely for the development of suicidal behavior during detoxification. The depressive syndrome may be prolonged and require antidepressant medication. Withdrawal is complete in 3 to 5 days, and patients are then discharged to outpatient therapy. Half-way houses, outpatient clinic treatment, or referral to a therapeutic community are usually recommended following detoxification, as in the case of sedative addiction.

Treatment for Hallucinogen Abuse

Hallucinogen abuse is a less frequent but potentially quite serious problem. Hallucinogens include LSD, mescaline, peyote, and PCP (phencyclidine). Physiologic dependence on these drugs probably does not occur, but psychological dependence does. Patients usually seek therapy for treatment of adverse reactions rather than for treatment of abuse of the drug itself. Panic attacks, depression, and schizophrenic episodes are the most common adverse effects. These reactions are best handled by a combination of reassurance, rest, close observation, and talking, a method known as "talking the person down." This process will sometimes consume 12 to 18 hours. Low doses of antianxiety drugs are sometimes used, and benzodiazepines (such as diazepam, 10 or 20 mg, taken orally) are the drugs of choice. Hospitalization sometimes is necessary for treatment of very severe reactions. Schizophrenia can be precipitated by hallucinogenic drugs, and there have been cases of prolonged schizophrenic episodes following their use.

Phencyclidine (PCP) is a combination hallucinogen and stimulant that produces special problems in treatment. It is a very dangerous drug which can provoke prolonged psychoses as well as depression and extreme anxiety. Large doses are available on the street, and they may lead to coma and death. The treatment of the psychotic reaction is similar to that for adverse reactions to LSD. Prolonged hospitalization may occasionally be necessary.

Treatment for Marijuana Abuse

Marijuana is a weak hallucinogen and a mild sedative. Though commonly used, it results in few medical or psychological complications that require treatment. Chronic bronchitis has been associated with heavy marijuana smoking. Any adverse psychological effects, when they occur, are similar to those seen with hallucinogens, and the treatment for them is identical to that used for adverse reactions to other hallucinogenic drugs.

As noted earlier, there have been reports of an amotivational syndrome in chronic users who consume large amounts of marijuana. This consists of fatigue, lack of ambition, and inactivity. There is a controversy over whether this is a drug effect or a pre-existing personality trait found in this particular group of people. Physiologic dependence can occur but only at intake levels that are higher than those commonly found. Marijuana users rarely seek help in drug abuse treatment programs. People who do seek such help often have marked psychiatric problems which are probably not caused by marijuana use, but which may be accentuated by heavy use and by a disorganized life style. Such patients are usually hospitalized for detoxification and then referred to an outpatient, drug-free treatment program.

Treatment for Inhalant Abuse

Inhalant abuse involves the deliberate use of industrial solvents that are present in paint thinners, model airplane glue, fingernail polish, lighter fluid, spot remover, and other products. This problem appears to be limited to the very young (10 to 15 years), probably because these substances are cheap and easily available. The usual procedure is for the user to inhale fumes from a cloth or plastic bag that has been soaked with the inhalant. A plastic bag containing the substance is often placed over the mouth and nose, and several deep breaths are taken, a practice known as "huffing." Sometimes fumes are inhaled directly, such as taking the cap from a gasoline tank and sniffing the air in the spout. Inhalant abuse is very dangerous as it can cause severe damage to the kidneys, liver, bone marrow, and nervous system. Sudden deaths, most likely due to cardiac arrhythmias, have been reported. Accidents due to poor judgment and asphyxiation have also occurred. Very little is known about treatment for this problem. Patients are usually taken to their family doctor or to a mental health clinic where they are encouraged to stop. There are few organized therapeutic programs for inhalant abuse, and very little work has been done to develop adequate treatment.

OVERVIEW OF ANCILLARY SERVICES

Most drug programs utilize several ancillary services in addition to detoxification and pharmacotherapy. Medical consultation is essential as all types of drug abuse can lead to physical illnesses. These illnesses vary according to the drug of abuse and the way it is taken. For example, heroin addicts develop cellulitis and hepatitis from infections introduced by intravenous use. Alcoholics commonly develop cirrhosis of the liver and gastrointestinal bleeding. Cigarette smokers are vulnerable to emphysema, chronic bronchitis, and carcinoma of the lungs.

Specialized psychological treatment services are also necessary. Many addicts have psychiatric problems, the most common probably being mixed states of anxiety and depression. Psychotherapy (individual, group, or family), psychotropic drugs, or a combination of these can usually be of help. Some addicts have psychoses and should be treated with major tranquilizers or lithium. Psychiatric consultation is essential in these cases. Care must be taken to avoid prescribing psychotropic medicines which can be abused, such as diazepam or sedative hypnotics. Some programs have used biofeedback or transcendental meditation as primary treatments for drug abuse or as ancillary treatments for anxiety and/or depression in patients who are also addicted. These treatments are acceptable to many drug-dependent patients, and improvement often results. Nonspecific effects may play a large role, but these treatments appeal to many therapists because they are nonpharmacologic.

Most programs use vocational counselors because unemployment appears to accentuate drug problems and is common among abusers. Legal services are also used, especially in narcotic addiction programs where most patients have engaged in criminal activity.

Family therapy may be especially useful in some cases. Addiction sometimes appears to be maintained by pathologic relationships among family members. For example, parents may unconsciously encourage the continuation of narcotic addiction in one of their children because it keeps the family focused on the child's problems, thereby allowing them to avoid confronting other issues. Skillful interventions in such a dynamic system may be of great help. However, this kind of therapy is complicated and requires specialized training.

Many forms of behavioral treatment have been tried for addictions.

Contingency management has been used widely and is probably effective. It involves an explicit description of specific behaviors that must be accomplished in order to produce certain rewards. For example, patients may be given take-home doses of methadone if they have a job and if their urine tests are free of illegal drugs, or they may get a free meal if no alcohol is measurable on their daily breathalyzer test. Contingencies must be tailored to the individual patient, his circumstances, his strengths, and his weaknesses, in order to avoid setting goals that are unrealistic. Legal pressure is sometimes used via probation or parole officers in a contingency management system. Patients can be released from jail upon the condition that they engage in certain therapy programs. They must also show that it is helping them by producing urine tests that are free of illegal drugs.

Systematic desensitization, covert conditioning, and aversive conditioning have been investigated in experimental programs, but they have not yet been developed into therapies that can be used routinely in general treatment facilities.

CONFIDENTIALITY IN DRUG-ABUSE TREATMENT

Confidentiality is essential for all medical treatment, and this includes therapy for drug dependence. Many patients in drug programs have engaged in criminal activities and are very concerned that any statement they make during therapy remain confidential, particularly statements regarding crimes committed prior to entering treatment. Many patients do not want certain family members to know that they have a drug problem. Other patients are working for employers who are intolerant of drug use and who might discharge them if they knew of their drug problem. For these reasons, patients are very hesitant to engage in therapy programs if they feel that the information they give is not kept strictly confidential. In recognition of these and other issues, state and federal laws have been enacted to insure confidentiality. Federal law stipulates that anyone working in a federally funded program who violates confidentiality regulations may be fined $500 on the first offense and up to $5,000 for a second offense. In addition, federal funds can be withdrawn from the program in such cases. These laws help to insure that confidentiality is maintained and, in doing so, both staff and patients are protected.

Confidentiality laws are complicated, and the *Federal Register* contains detailed regulations which are updated periodically. Generally, no information can be released without the patient's written consent. No blanket consent form can be used; rather, the specific information to be released must be specified in writing and signed by the patient. The only exception is for patients who sign a release of information prior to entering a program as part of a court-stipulated settlement for criminal behavior. These laws apply to everyone (including medical personnel), except in certain medical emergencies or pursuant to an appropriate court order.

If information is to be given to a probation officer, employer, or social agency, the patient must sign a consent form authorizing the program to give the specific information requested. If the patient does not agree to the release of that information, it must not be given. Requests for information are very common in drug programs located in large urban areas because many patients enrolled in them are in contact with legal and social agencies. Some of the most difficult issues arise in connection with police and probation officers. These authorities occasionally press the program for information regarding the patients' status or progress. Since this information may be used to investigate charges, to support an arrest, or as a ground to revoke probation, it is extremely important that the program be absolutely firm in obeying the confidentiality regulations. Callers seeking information (without the patient's consent) should be politely refused and told of the confidentiality requirements, including any fine that can be imposed. This response should be given even to the simplest request for information, such as, "Is Mr. Jones in the program now or has he ever been?" The reminder about confidentiality almost always results in cooperation and helps to insure good working relationships between legal agencies and treatment programs.

Confidentiality laws should be explained to patients at the time they enter treatment. This explanation should include a description of procedures to follow if they wish information to be released and the safeguards that the program takes to insure maintenance of confidentiality. Good judgment is necessary and helpful in cases presenting as medical emergencies. For example, telling the methadone dose to a physician who is preparing a patient for emergency surgery is essential and necessary for good treatment. Other practical situations may include giving the patient's methadone dose to a prison nurse who is trying to find out what to prescribe for a patient who has been arrested and is on the detoxification unit.

When rules have been developed and treatment staff have gained experience in implementing the rules and the procedures necessary to insure compliance with them, confidentiality is rarely an issue. Inservice training sessions on confidentiality procedures are essential for the development of uniform program policies to insure compliance. These sessions should include clinic secretaries as they often are the first contact that outside agencies have with the program, and they must be alert to comply with regulations. Most clinics safeguard the confidentiality of records by storing clinic files in a locked room and labeling each patient record "Confidential Patient Information."

TRENDS IN DRUG ABUSE

Opiate addiction in one form or another has been a problem in the United States for over a hundred years. Alcohol abuse antedates recorded history. It is unlikely that the underlying problems of drug abuse can be solved; they are more in the category of symptoms of individual and social problems than specific medical conditions.

There is no evidence that drug abuse, in general, is decreasing, although it is continually changing in character. Heroin abuse wanes while minor tranquilizer use increases. New chemicals such as phencyclidine are discovered by the recreational user population. Old chemicals such as amyl nitrate are discovered by new populations. We can expect this process to continue, and we must have treatment facilities ready to respond to the inevitable problems that can arise due to the abuse of these substances.

ADDITIONAL READING

Garner, G. W.: *The Police Role in Alcohol-Related Crises.* Charles C Thomas, Springfield, Ill., 1979.

Glasscote, M. A., et al.: *The Treatment of Drug Abuse: Programs, Problems, Prospects.* American Psychiatric Association, Washington, D.C., 1972.

Jaffe, J.: Drug Addiction and Drug Abuse, in Goodman, L.S., and Gilman, A. (eds.): *The Pharmacological Basis of Therapeutics.* ed. 5. Macmillan, New York, 1975.

Kuehle, J. C., Mendelson, J. H., Davis, K. R., and New, P. F. J.: Computed Tomographic Examination of Heavy Marijuana Smokers. *J.A.M.A.* 237:1231–1232, 1977.

O'Brien, C. P., Wesson, D. R., and Schnoll, S. H.: *Diagnosis and Evaluation of the Drug-Abusing Patient for Treatment Staff Physicians.* Medical Monograph Series, vol. 1, no. 1. National Drug Abuse Center, Arlington, Va., 1976.

Peterson, R. C. (ed.): *Marijuana Research Findings: 1976.* NIMH Research Monograph Series, no. 14. DHEW Publication (ADM) 78–501, Washington, D.C., 1977.

Richards, L. G., and Bevens, L. B. (eds.): *The Epidemiology of Drug Abuse: Current Issues.* NIMH Research Monograph Series, no. 10. DHEW Publication (ADM) 77–432, Washington, D.C., 1977.

CHAPTER 40

Jonathan O. Cole is Staff Psychiatrist at McLean Hospital in Belmont, Massachusetts, as well as Lecturer in Psychiatry at Harvard Medical School and Consultant in Research at Boston State Hospital. He is former Superintendent of Boston State Hospital, as well as former Chief of the Psychopharmacology Research Branch of the National Institute of Mental Health in Bethesda, Maryland. Dr. Cole also served as Professor of Psychiatry and Chairman of the Department of Psychiatry at the Temple University School of Medicine in Philadelphia. He has received the Hofheimer Prize for Research of the American Psychiatric Association, and the Paul Hoch Memorial Award for Distinguished Service of the American College of Neuropsychopharmacology. Dr. Cole has published over 100 papers and articles in the field of psychiatric treatment with special emphasis on drug therapy.

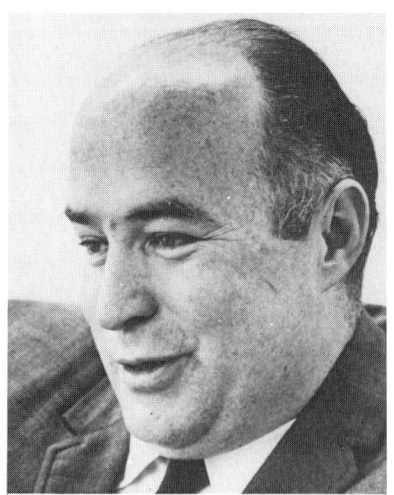

PSYCHOACTIVE DRUGS

Jonathan O. Cole, M.D.

ANTIPSYCHOTIC DRUGS: BENEFITS AND RISKS

The discovery of the first potent antipsychotic drug, chlorpromazine (Thorazine), developed as a super-antihistamine for use in surgery, is well described by Swazey.[1] The drug effected a dramatic change in psychiatric treatment for schizophrenia which is difficult to appreciate at this distance when one usually sees drug failures on the chronic wards of psychiatric hospitals.

Over the years many controlled studies have confirmed that chlorpromazine is quite effective in ameliorating all symptoms of schizophrenia—delusions, hallucinations, thought disorder, excitement, withdrawal, retardation, anger, and bizarre behavior. Crude improvement rates in newly admitted patients run about 75 percent for chlorpromazine and 25 percent for placebo. Placebo patients get even sicker, while chlorpromazine patients do not.

When patients are released as improved, maintenance chlorpromazine prevents relapse in about 55 percent over a 2-year period, while only 15 percent of placebo patients remain intact for that period. Of a group of patients who had adjusted for 2 years in the community, 66 percent relapsed within a year after chlorpromazine was finally stopped.

There are some excellent general reference works on psychoactive drugs. *The Handbook of Psychiatry Therapy*,[2] edited by Shader, is a multiauthored text covering a wide range of topics from emergency room management of overdose patients to a detailed description of drug metabolism, as well as the clinical handling of standard psychiatric syndromes and appropriate drug and nondrug therapy. Hollister's book, *Clinical Use of Psychotherapeutic Drugs*,[3] is a comprehensive text by an internist with 25 years of experience as a clinical investigator and expert in psychopharmacology.

Two review articles by Davis[4] are also recommended because of their coverage of prolonged maintenance drug therapy in the community with schizophrenic and depressed patients.

For medicolegal purposes, I will deal mainly with the problems in the use of these psychoactive drugs. Of primary importance is the fact that these drugs leave most patients improved but not entirely well. Most schizophrenics were socially impaired long before frank psychosis appeared, and they often remain odd, unsuccessful, and inept. Second, the antipsychotic drugs, especially the more sedative ones such as Mellaril and Thorazine, but even long-acting Prolixin injections, are experienced as unpleasant by patients. Some of this is a feeling of numbness and unpleasant sedation; some is a muscular discomfort merging into restless jumpiness known technically as "akathisia," a neurologic side effect. Some patients prefer these drugs as sleeping pills at bedtime, but patients rarely feel "good" on them. Patient compliance in pill-taking is therefore a problem. Many patients never seem to learn that every time they stop taking medication, they relapse and return to the hospital. Part of the problem is that almost no patient relapses the first week after the drug is stopped. Hogarty's calculation[5] is that about 10 percent of patients suffer relapse each month during the first year off the drug; thus there will be about 30 unrelapsed patients out of 100 at this rate at the end of the year.

In the early phases of treatment some patients experience pseudoparkinsonism and briefly, very early in the first few days on the drug, dystonia. None of these side effects is dangerous, and about half of the patients never experience them. Dystonia, pseudoparkinsonism, and akathisia can generally be relieved by adding antiparkinsonian drugs or by lowering the dose. These effects, it is important to note, and the early sedation usually disappears after the first few weeks of medication.

Some other side effects—constipation, blurred vision, and skin rash—seem minor. Agranulocytosis is very rare (1 in 5,000) and occurs chiefly in older patients in the first few weeks of therapy. Leukopenia is more common. Jaundice is rare (1 in 300 to 400 on chlorpromazine and less on other drugs) and benign. Breast-swelling occurs in a few patients. Impotence is common in males on Mellaril and occasionally is seen resulting from other drugs.

The worst side effect in such treatment is tardive dyskinesia—late-appearing abnormal movement—usually manifested by chewing movement, tongue-writhing, and occasional tongue protrusion, lip-smacking, choreiform minor movements of fingers and toes and sometimes of the larger extremities, and trunk movements.[6] Up to 50 percent of long-term chronic patients show this side effect to some extent, but the reactions are almost always mild and usually do not bother the patient, though they may seem rather odd to observers. The condition is related to drug exposure in a general way; all antipsychotic drugs now available in the United States probably can cause it. I have never observed the condition in patients less than 3 months on antipsychotic drugs. The condition tends to disappear over months or years if the antipsychotic drug can be stopped. Unfortunately, there seems no way to avoid a risk of this condition and still treat schizophrenia adequately.

The risk-benefit ratio is still in favor of the antipsychotic drugs for schizophrenia and for the rare depressions and anxiety states which fail to respond to other classes of drugs.

The most serious problem in this field lies in the area of personality-character disorders. Since this is a key interface between law and psychiatry, we will return to this subject after covering other drug classes.

ANTIDEPRESSANT DRUGS

Antidepressant drugs fall into two groups: the tricyclics and monoamine oxidase inhibitors. Both are more effective than placebo but have a slow onset of action of from 7 to 28 days. The tricyclics sedate some patients and agitate others before depression begins to lift. They often cause a dry mouth. Less common side effects are blurred vision, trouble passing water, tremor, and constipation. To complicate matters, depression itself often causes these same symptoms. Occasionally they cause memory difficulty, delirium, or precipitate manic psychosis. The drugs can be used to commit suicide.

Lithium carbonate can be used to cure mania and to prevent future episodes in patients who have recurring periods of mania and depression (bipolar manic depression) and in patients who experience depression only (unipolar manic depressives). The drug does not usually alleviate the depression itself if given during its course.

Lithium's side effects—tremor, diarrhea, nausea, and urinary frequency—are dose-related. Since lithium blood levels are not difficult to measure, patients are easily monitored. At very high blood levels (over 2.0 mg) patients experience ataxia, confusion, and eventually coma. Some patients obtain a therapeutic lithium blood level (about 1.0 mg) on two pills a day, and others require 12 pills a day (600 vs. 3600 mg) to attain the same blood level. If we could as easily measure blood levels on all similar drugs, we would probably find similar individual differences. This probably explains why some schizophrenics do well on 200 mg of chlorpromazine a day, while others need 2,000 mg. The dosage ceilings given in the package inserts for most drugs are usually based on ignorance. The company (which wishes to avoid product liability) and the Food and Drug Administration (which wishes to avoid congressional criticism) collaborate to keep the recommended dosage down. It is sometimes desirable and necessary to go above the recommended ceiling in individual treatment-resistant patients. When this is done cautiously, it is as safe as most medical procedures and may be much safer than letting the patient remain seriously mentally ill.

ANTIANXIETY DRUGS

Antianxiety drugs come in two general classes: the hypnosedatives and the autonomic sedatives. The hypnosedatives can be used in higher doses as sleeping pills and in lower doses as daytime sedatives to relieve anxiety. They all can produce physical dependence. The older ones, except the benzodiazepines, can be used to commit suicide. The benzodiazepines are safer in terms of suicide risk, somewhat more effective in relieving anxiety, and are generally longer-acting. Therapeutic effects may last many hours after a single dose, which makes them useful in treating withdrawal symptoms in alcoholics. Side effects are mainly sedation and, less commonly, malcoordination and/or ataxia. Like alcohol, they can impair driving. However, in low doses in careful people this usually is not a problem. They may disinhibit some neurotic patients, allowing them to express anger or aggression. This could conceivably unleash criminal behavior in much the same way alcohol can, but it does not seem to be a common problem in practice.

The autonomic sedatives are more like the antidepressants and antipsychotics, both of which can improve anxiety when given at low doses. They cause a less pleasurable sedation and do not tend to disinhibit behavior. They are more likely to cause autonomic side effects, such as dry mouth, and are somewhat less effective than the benzodiazepines.

STIMULANTS

Despite their abuse in the form of "speed," amphetamines are clearly safe and effective in hyperkinetic children who show overactivity and short attention span both in school and at home. Seventy percent of such children improve to some extent, and perhaps 30 percent are very markedly helped. The one long-term follow-up study suggests that amphetamine therapy in childhood is not associated with drug abuse later in life. In low doses these drugs avert fatigue and improve concentration. In very high doses they can produce a psychosis often indistinguishable from paranoid schizophrenia except that it remits in a few days when the drug is withdrawn. Depression occurs when amphetamine-addicted patients "crash" (stop taking drugs), and violent behavior sometimes occurs when people are high on speed, some of this reaction being secondary to drug-induced paranoid delusions.

Low-dose stimulants or stimulant-like drugs are used to reduce appetite and may help for 3 months or more. In controlled studies patients on such a drug lose a pound or so a week more than do patients on placebo. Fenfluramine is more sedative than stimulant and may have the lowest abuse potential in the group, but is LSD-like at very high dosage (20 pills or more).

DRUGS IN CHILDREN

In schizophrenic children and young adolescents, antipsychotic drugs are well tolerated and often reduce disturbed, hyperactive behavior. Patients are helped to adapt to special schools but are not usually "normalized." The prescribing of stimulants in hyperkinesis is almost completely restricted to children. Both the condition and the drug effect and need may disappear in the early teens.

Amphetamines may cause anorexia and a probably temporary reduction in weight in many children. Occasional studies show a slowing of general growth over 6 months to a year, but others fail to confirm this. The latter result seems to legitimate risk if the child is much better behaviorally while on the drug. Children don't get "high" on the drug and may even appear sadder after the initial dosage. Imipramine, an antidepressant, has been shown to help children with very severe school phobias. Barbiturates and benzodiazepines sometimes cause excitement or behavior disorders in children.

DRUGS FOR IMPULSE OR ANTISOCIAL DISORDERS

It would be very helpful for psychiatrists, for correction officials, and probably for the patients and/or offenders if there were a safe and reliable drug which would suppress or control impulsive, antisocial behavior. The behaviors involved include aggressive assault (1) from brutal attack to biting or surreptitious hitting or strangling, provoked or totally unprovoked; (2) from self-destructive behavior (wrist-slashing is commonest, but burning and eye-gouging also occur) to escape or running away; (3) from uncontrolled teasing or obnoxious behavior to impulsive breaking or throwing of objects; and (4) from nondirected tantrums to petty, purposeless thievery. When such behavior occurs in the clinical context of schizophrenia, depression, or mania, the psychiatrist can treat the major disorder with reasonable expectation that the antisocial symptom will improve along with the underlying disease. When, as is often the case, there are unclear hints of schizophrenia or depression and the main problem is one of poor ego strength or life-long maladjustment, even though the overt acts may appear self-defeating and without direct or secondary gain to the patient, it is difficult to find a drug to treat this often desperately serious condition.

Two kinds of drug treatment are possible: preventive therapeutic treatment and crisis management (e.g., the application of drugs to make the patient generally more stable and able to cope without exploding or "acting-out" his impulses, and drugs to terminate wildly excited outbursts). The only reliable evidence of drug efficacy relates to a special subgroup of emotionally unstable patients who act as though their mood center were swinging around uncontrollably. Such patients may be suicidally unhappy at one time and giddy and high-spirited two hours later, unpredictably and without evidence that their mood changes occurred in response to any external event. On the basis of only a few studies, such patients respond to Mellaril, an antipsychotic, with increased mood stability. They also tend to stabilize on lithium carbonate. There is limited evidence, including one controlled study in institutionalized juvenile delinquents, suggesting that lithium may also have a general ameliorative effect on impulsive assaultive behavior in inmates of prisons and psychiatric patients.

Many impulse-disorder patients have evidence of brain injury, either at birth or at a later stage. Those with temporal lobe epilepsy may respond to Tegretol and others occasionally to other anticonvulsants, though the evidence for any real effect from diphenylhydantoin (Dilantin) is very weak.

It is conceivable that stimulants or antidepressants might help in some patients. Some early work on d-amphetamine in hyperkinetic syndrome was done in institutionalized, adolescent delinquents.

The drug class most widely used in aggressive, unstable, impulsive, hostile, explosive patients and prisoners is the antipsychotic group. In animals, these drugs decrease activity and response to environmental stimuli. The same effects may occur in impulse-disorder patients, although evidence from well-controlled studies is lacking. Probably these drugs work in some such patients and not in others. The use of drugs in these patients when they are very explosive becomes a crutch and an alternative to, or accompaniment of, physical restraint or seclusion.

As a crisis response to a violent outburst which continues for minutes and hours, oral or, more often, intramuscular antipsychotics are used. Chlorpromazine, in doses between 25 and 100 mg, is often chosen because of its acute sedative effect. The patient may well fall asleep in 20 minutes and remain asleep for several hours. He may also be weak and dizzy because of a drug-related drop in blood pressure and generally will not feel like further fighting or yelling. It remains unclear whether low doses of nonsedative antipsychotics would be more effective for this purpose. If fluphenazine or haloperidol is effective in calming the patient without knocking him out, it would argue that this approach is more rational. If these less sedative drugs are not effective, one could argue that intramuscular sodium amobarbital (Amytal), a short-acting barbiturate, would fully sedate a violent patient faster (3 to 5 minutes) and with fewer side effects.

I know of no controlled or even comparative studies of different approaches to the short-term control of the impulsive, nonpsychotic patient who is temporarily wildly excited. One approach might be to try intramuscular chlorpromazine, intramuscular Amytal, and placebo on a comparative basis for short-term (e.g., 12-hour) efficacy. Other nondrug approaches range from talk to confrontation by a large number of large staff members, to open or locked seclusion, to mechanical restraint, to therapeutic wrestling to the floor by a kindly but overpowering counselor.

All of these options carry risks. Patients and inmates of correctional institutions burn to death or commit suicide, even in well-monitored seclusion rooms, and break bones or lacerate flesh in or out of restraint and sometimes injure others in the process. I doubt that there is any safe, humane way to handle unreasoning violence. By the time full violence has erupted, it may not make much difference whether the violence was totally autochthonous or in reaction to the "unreasonable" behavior of a prison guard.

In some crises, if measures are not taken, the patient and others can be seriously injured. Drugs become a reluctant option. In some circumstances, particularly group violence or riots, Mace may be a more honest form of behavior control than chlorpromazine. I strongly believe that intramuscular medication should be used only in patients or prisoners who have been evaluated by a psychiatrist who judges this alternative to be the appropriate treatment for their condition or temporary state.

To make matters worse, it may now be impossible to study treatment or control approaches to violent behavior. Research is currently banned in most prison systems, and it is admittedly difficult to obtain free and informed consent from someone who is exploding with anger. Both drugs and behavior modification have become abhorrent concepts to many very vocal critics who see no value in any such modalities. Perhaps the recent balanced assessment of psychosurgery, its benefits as well as its risks, is a sign that reason is beginning to prevail over subjectivity in these important areas.

DRUGS AND CRIMINAL RESPONSIBILITY

There is concern in legal areas over the problem posed by artificial sanity. A patient, grossly psychotic because of schizophrenia, commits a murder. When caught, he is incompetent to stand trial and therefore cannot be tried. Three months later, after drug treatment, he is no longer insane and is competent to stand trial, but looks so normal that he is not likely to be found not guilty by reason of insanity.* On the other hand, leaving a patient somewhat psychotic in order to persuade a judge or a judge and jury that he was severely ill at the time of the crime seems clinically unethical for the treating physicians. As a solution to this dilemma, the Group for the Advancement of Psychiatry (GAP) has suggested taking videotapes of the patient's behavior and mental status early in his treatment and close to the time of the alleged crime.[7]

Although there is a conflict in the court cases to date, it would seem just and sensible for all concerned that defendants who are rendered com-

---

*In such a case, the Supreme Court of the State of Washington reversed a conviction. *State v. Murphy,* 56 Wash. 2d 761, 355 P. 2d 323 (1960).

petent to stand trial by medication with psychoactive drugs should be accepted for trial by the courts.[8] It is in the best interest of the defendant to stand trial rather than to languish indefinitely in a hospital or other institution awaiting a trial which may never take place. With the extensive use of such drugs to treat patients in the community, drug treatment of defendants should not be considered unusual or unnatural. As the GAP report points out, it is likely that many of the other persons involved in the trials, including jurors, judges, and attorneys, will be found to have been treating themselves with such drugs.[9]

REFERENCES

1. Swazey, J.: *Chlorpromazine: The History of a Psychiatric Discovery.* M.I.T. Press, Cambridge, Mass., 1974.
2. Shader, R.: *Manual of Psychiatric Therapeutics.* Little, Brown, Boston, 1975.
3. Hollister, L.: *Clinical Use of Psychotherapeutic Drugs.* Charles C Thomas, Springfield, Ill., 1973.
4. Davis, J.: Overview: Maintenance Therapy in Psychiatry: I. Schizophrenia. *Am. J. Psychiatry* 132:1237–1245, 1975; Davis, J.: Overview: Maintenance Therapy in Psychiatry: II. Affective Disorders. *Am. J. Psychiatry* 133:1–13, 1976.
5. Hogarty, G.: Temporal Effects of Drug and Placebo in Delaying Relapse in Schizophrenic Outpatients. *Arch. Gen. Psychiatry* 34:297–301, 1977.
6. Cole, J., and Gardos, G.: Psychopharmacology Update: Tardive Dyskinesia. *McLean Hosp. J.* 1:155–166, 1976.
7. Group for the Advancement of Psychiatry, Committee on Psychiatry and Law: *Misuse of Psychiatry in the Criminal Courts: Competency to Stand Trial.* Vol. 8, Report No. 89, 1974.
8. *State of Louisiana v. Hampton,* 225 La 399, 218 La 2d 311 (1971).
9. Op. cit.

CHAPTER 41

Norman E. Zinberg is Associate Clinical Professor of Psychiatry at Harvard Medical School and Staff Psychiatrist at the Cambridge Hospital. He is also on the clinical psychiatric staff at Children's Hospital Medical Center and Peter Bent Brigham Hospital, and is Psychiatrist-in-Chief at the Washingtonian Center for Addictions in Boston. Dr. Zinberg is a faculty member of the Boston Psychoanalytic Institute, and is a featured columnist for *The Boston Globe.* He has served as Senior Consultant to the Drug Abuse Council in Washington, D.C., and has conducted extensive research in the field of drug use. Dr. Zinberg is currently working on studies of nonmedical drug use and controlled use of illicit drugs.

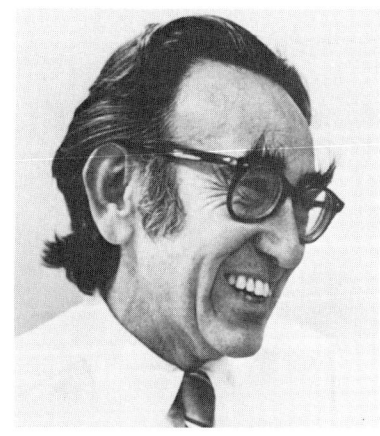

Risa Glaubman Dickstein is Chief Counsel of the New York State Commission on Investigation. She served as a constitutional lawyer with both the Legal Action Center and the New York Civil Liberties Union. Ms. Dickstein is former Director of Planning for the Heroin Research and Rehabilitation Program of the Vera Institute of Justice in New York.

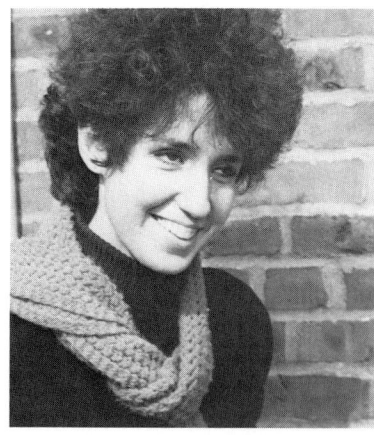

PRESCRIBING CONTROLLED SUBSTANCES: PHYSICIANS' RIGHTS AND RESPONSIBILITIES

Norman E. Zinberg, M.D., and
Risa G. Dickstein, J.D.

A variety of conflicting factors influence and shape the physician's decision to prescribe drugs for a patient: choices among drugs, patient demands and expectations, and government agencies and their regulations. Increasingly, physicians must face moral and legal issues, unknown a decade ago, for which professional education may have left them quite unprepared. The problem becomes more acute when the drugs involved are psychoactive—licit or illicit—and nonacute needs or maintenance factors are at issue.

In this chapter we will discuss two related areas of concern to physicians: the legal context within which they must decide whether or not to continue a patient on a psychoactive drug, and the conceptual difficulties that they must face in carrying out their professional duty to separate recreational use from medical use and both of these from drug abuse.

This chapter will focus primarily on usual medical practice rather than on the specific problems faced by drug treatment professionals (i.e., physicians who specialize in the treatment of addicts and operate within the public sector and under a specific regulatory structure [see Chapter 39]). It is our contention that such practitioners are outside the mainstream of traditional practice and as a group function differently in the prescribing situation. Our discussion of methadone maintenance, because of the number of patients involved and the symbolic and wide-reaching effect of overregulation in that area, will be the one exception. We will also discuss the ways in which conflicts about the moral and legal concerns about psychoactive drugs have interfered with the clinical relationship between doctor and patient, and indeed, constitute a salient area of struggle that affects the entire problem of legal regulation of medical practice.

A lengthy description of the many factors that characterize the two underlying social models—the legal model and the medical model—is beyond the scope of this chapter. Nevertheless, the following useful distinctions can be made. The medical model focuses on the patient, his needs, and the factors that caused the problems he displays; the goal is to treat the patient's disease, and the medical professional's expertise is directed toward that end. The legal model focuses on the public policy implications of an individual's acts, subordinating the individual's needs to those of the community; the goal is to evaluate the individual's behavior only to determine what should be done with him in order to protect the community. In the legal model, individual rehabilitation is not central. Thus, when a prohibited drug is taken illegally, the medical model examines the reasons behind the behavior and attempts to deal with its causes and prevent its repetition; the legal model examines the act in order to determine its effect upon society, disregards the cause of the behavior, and is disinterested in noncriminal justice concerns other than the traditional ones that would prevent its repetition.

It is difficult to understand the interaction between the medical model and the legal model in this country. Nor is it immediately apparent why the legal model has seemed to prevail. Physicians, ostensibly, have been reluctant to give up their role in the drug-use decision. In some cases, however, they have allowed their role to be distorted by ignorance, not only from outside the profession, but also within it. The legal system is, arguably, in control as the source of legitimacy by such acts as granting physicians licenses to practice. The medical profession has further endorsed those powers by overtly supporting and implicitly colluding with the law enforcement agencies that now go much further in regulating specific prescribing practices. The interplay of these issues raises fundamental questions concerning the proper allocation of responsibilities for the therapeutic decision to prescribe a drug susceptible to abuse and for controlling drug abuse.

THE LEGAL CONTEXT: REGULATING THE FREEDOM OF PHYSICIANS TO PRESCRIBE

Viewed historically, legal regulation of the prescribing physician is relatively recent. Controls that confront the doctor today were not operative before the First World War. Simplistic definitions of "healthy" and "natural" were used; recreational drug use was not a culturally recognized concept; bioethical issues were not subject to public debate; and for all drug-related disorders, abstinence was the publicly accepted treatment model.

Before 1914, the responsible physician's job was to recommend a particular drug, state its proper use, and monitor the patient's self-administration. The passage of the Harrison Narcotic Act marked the first serious effort apart from a few local statutes to change an environment in which drugs were available, free of legal controls.*

---

*The Harrison Act, enacted in 1914, required that all persons who import, manufacture, sell, deal in, dispense, or otherwise distribute narcotic drugs register with the Secretary of the Treasury and pay an occupational tax. It also required that any transfer of narcotic drugs be made on a special Treasury order form, with exceptions for physicians who dispense narcotics to patients in the course of professional practice only. (See Uelman, G. F., and Haddox, V. G., *Drug Abuse and the Law,* West Publishing Co., St. Paul, Minn., 1974.)

Previously, the physician had not been held responsible for drug misuse or for any attendant law enforcement duties (e.g., reporting requirements). Physicians, often poorly educated, overprescribed psychoactive drugs, especially narcotics, and opiates were a prime ingredient in many patent medicines.[1] It was the outcry resulting from this excessive use of narcotics that began the move toward greater legal control.

After 1914, the physician's freedom to prescribe was curtailed by legislation, court decisions, and administrative fiat; in fact, administrative interpretations of the legislation and judicial decisions limiting medical prescribing of certain drugs were more restrictive than the laws on which they relied. The Treasury Department acted as the major enforcer of the law that had criminalized addicts and addiction-related activities, as well as the doctors who prescribed for them. Doctors encountered severe penalties for continuing the old, free-style practice: between 1914 and 1933, 25,000 doctors were arrested for supplying opiates, and 5,000 of them actually went to jail.[2]

The Harrison Act Prosecutions

The early 1920s witnessed the first of a series of Harrison Act prosecutions which were aimed at doctors who prescribed maintenance doses of narcotics to addicted patients. In the approximately half-dozen Harrison Act cases that reached the United States Supreme Court, guidelines were formulated that strictly limited what could be *legally* construed as "medical acts" undertaken in the course of "professional treatment." The Supreme Court made it clear that addicts could not be treated as "patients" unless the treatment was abstinence, the course of professional practice could not encompass drug maintenance, and doctors had lost their traditional freedom to make therapeutic decisions based solely upon medical considerations, independent of law enforcement concerns. The following quotation from *Webb v. United States*,[3] affirming the conviction of a physician, is illustrative:*

> If a practicing and registered physician issues an order for morphine to a habitual user thereof, the order not being issued in the course of professional treatment in the attempted cure of the habit, but being issued for the purpose of providing the user with morphine sufficient to keep him comfortable by maintaining his customary usage, is such an order a physician's prescription . . . ? [To] call such an order for the use of morphine a physician's prescription would be so plain a perversion of meaning that no discussion of the subject is required.

The legal concepts that developed in this period have left a legacy for the practice of medicine that makes physicians anxious about prescribing

---

*See also *Jin Fuey Moy v. United States* (254 U.S. 189 [1920]), in which the Supreme Court equated physicians who prescribed maintenance doses of morphine with drug traffickers:

> Manifestly the phrases 'to a patient' and 'in the course of his professional practice only' are intended . . . not to extend it to a sale to a dealer *or a distribution intended to cater to the appetite or satisfy the craving of one addicted to the use of the drug*. A 'prescription' issued for either of the latter purposes protects neither the physician who issues it nor the dealer who knowingly accepts and fills it. [emphasis added].

narcotics to this day. This is not to say that all, or even most, physicians would like to return to the pre-1914 situation. Many were relieved by a series of rules that seemed to free them from concern with opiate addicts and with the less competent members of their own profession. Doctors' use of the legal profession in this way, to help solve—or institutionally fail to solve—social problems, is not uncommon.[4,5] Even in cases that involve analgesics, for example, this concern sometimes causes physicians to prescribe the least possible dose which, in turn, frequently results in unnecessary suffering. This anxiety is so marked that it carries over to treatment of terminal cases: physicians whose clinical judgment is ordinarily impeccable have been known to prescribe virtually homeopathic doses of opiates to patients with terminal cancer. When asked whether they might not increase the dosage to prevent pain, the physicians have replied that they were afraid the patient might become addicted. Doctors are completely unaware of the extent to which they suffer from the medical profession's history of involvement with opiates and the inadequacy of their medical education. The average medical education has often included actual misrepresentation and exaggeration of the harmful and dependency-inducing effects of opiates and a pronounced but unconscious moral bias against the use of drugs that are, in some instances, used responsibly in a recreational context.

A panel on "The Education of Medical Students and House Staff in Substance Abuse" was held at the 1976 National Drug Abuse Conference in New York. The panelists (Drs. Barry Stimmel, Ed Wolfson, and Robert B. Millman) are in the forefront of such medical education and indicate this by the extent to which they present their material in an enlightened, objective, and humane way. Nevertheless, without exception, their instruction focuses on the so-called hard cases. Inevitably there are discussions of heroin addiction, barbiturate addiction, alcoholism, and all the other destructive consequences of drug use. The panelists admitted that no sessions are offered on the range and quality of drug use, none on how use can be controlled, none on the potential psychological or social benefits of such use, or even on therapeutic possibilities, or on the role of the doctor in controlling use of illicit drugs.

The Harrison Act decisions firmly established the predominance of the legal model: the law (not the doctor or the patient) has the power to define appropriate medical decisions. Power to regulate medical prescribing was—and continues to be—extended. The law determines who is and who is not a patient, which drugs do and do not have a "current medical use," and what is and is not a "prescription" issued in the course of professional practice. A 1977 decision concerning the prescribing power of physicians is illustrative. In *Whalen* v. *Roe*,[6] the United States Supreme Court upheld the New York State law requiring that any doctor who prescribes "Schedule II" drugs must also provide patient-identifying information to the government so that it can be encoded in a central computer. The Court stated that when drug prescribing was involved, the doctor-patient relationship did not constitute a "zone of privacy" deserving constitutional protection. Thus the Supreme Court reaffirmed the absolute power of the government to control which drugs can be prescribed, what dosage limits can be set, and what information about the doctor-patient relationship must be provided and therefore can be used for prosecution of doctor and patient. The Court's language in this case clearly reflects the same attitudes that prevailed in the Harrison Act cases:

Nor can it be said that any individual has been deprived of the right to decide independently, with the advice of his physician, to acquire and use needed medication. *Although the State no doubt could prohibit entirely the use of particular Schedule I drugs, it has not done so.* [emphasis added]

The Court felt no need to justify the legal control over the doctor's right to prescribe. It concluded, "It is, of course, well settled that the State has broad police powers in regulating the administration of drugs by the health professions."

The Medical Community's Response to Legal Regulation

The medical profession readily accepted the legal, regulatory approach that began with the Harrison Narcotic Act. Organized medicine responded by abdication.* Thus, for example, in the period 1919 to 1923, when the 44 medically administered opiate maintenance clinics were closed by bureaucratic fiat, the medical profession made no attempt to enter into a discussion of the quality of medical care—despite the fact that some clinics, such as the one in Shreveport, Louisiana, were effective and not poorly run. The medical profession permitted the closings without protest.[7]

In order to explain the response of the medical profession, it is necessary to consider several factors: post-First World War attitudes, perceived benefits to the profession, and an implicitly held allopathic definition of health.

POSTWAR ATTITUDES

This chapter has focused on the legal events precipitated by the Harrison Act. In addition, an underlying moral attitude prevailed. As much as the regulations themselves, this attitude helps to explain contemporary medical practices and the dominance of the legal model. The language used in

---

*The totality of abdication can be seen by the 1924 statement of the American Medical Association. In June 1921, the Committee on Narcotic Drugs of the Council on Health and Public Instruction of the American Medical Association recommended that

> ... the American Medical Association urge both Federal and State governments to exert their full powers and authority to put an end to all manner of so-called ambulatory methods of treatment of narcotic drug addiction, whether practiced by the private physician or by the so-called 'narcotic clinic' or dispensary *(Proceedings of Boston Session,* Minutes of the Seventy-second Annual Session of the American Medical Association, held at Boston, June 6–10, 1921: Report of Committee on Narcotic Drugs of the Council on Health and Public Instruction. *J.A.M.A.* 76:1696–1671, 1921).

This resolution was adopted in 1924 by the House of Delegates of the American Medical Association. As recently as June 1963, the American Medical Association, in a joint statement with the National Research Council, reaffirmed the viewpoint that the complete withdrawal of narcotic drugs is the only acceptable treatment for addicts, stating that "continued administration of drugs for the maintenance of addiction is not a bona fide attempt at cure, nor is it ethical treatment except in a few unusual circumstances" (Council on Mental Health, American Medical Association: Narcotics and Medical Practice. The Use of Narcotic Drugs in Medical Practice and the Medical Management of Narcotic Addicts. *J.A.M.A.* 186:976–978, 1963).

early decisions, such as *Webb* v. *United States,* cited earlier, reveals a moralistic distaste for addicts and a startling ignorance about different drug-taking behaviors. This approach persists in present case law.*

In the leading case in the 1920s under the Harrison Narcotic Act, *United States* v. *Behrman,*[8] the case credited with putting an end to the narcotics maintenance clinics that had been functioning nationwide, the Court described the addict as having a "weak and perverted will" that required the "gratification of a disease appetite."

Cultural and social upheavals following the First World War reinforced the powerful puritan morality of the American mainstream. Their effects were also felt in medicine, inhibiting any inclination among doctors to struggle for greater autonomy in prescribing drugs. Following the Flexner Report in 1910, vituperatively critical of medical education and its reliance on proprietary medical schools, the medical profession itself was struggling to regain moral, intellectual, and academic respectability.[9]

The Harrison Narcotic Act and subsequent regulations came in on a backlash against postwar excesses—a backlash that equated strength with righteousness and power with abstention. This attitude is still prevalent today: Klerman has characterized it as "pharmacological Calvinism."[10] Before the Harrison Act, drug-dependent people were commonly seen as anything from eccentric to diseased. By the postwar years, dependency had come to signal distinct weakness of character: the very notion that a drug was illicitly used and "dependency-producing" evoked images of dope fiends and depravity.

PERCEIVED BENEFITS TO THE MEDICAL PROFESSION

Individually, doctors appeared to go along with the law enforcement approach. It allowed them to reject "clients" whom they found neither attractive nor amenable to the professional services that they offered (and for which they expected to be paid). In addition, it permitted them to punish two categories of unpopular doctors: "bad" doctors who sold prescriptions, and unconventional doctors who, interested in drug research and nonabstinence-based treatment methods, wanted to "treat" addicts. Just how thoroughly the medical profession wanted to divest itself of any involvement with drug use, once the issue of moral responsibilities had been raised, can be seen in the case of marijuana. Only one influential physician, Dr. William C. Woodward, legislative director of the American

---

*In *Robinson* v. *California* (370 U.S. 660, 1962), Justice William O. Douglas, in his concurring opinion, gave this myth-ridden and questionable description of the physical effects of drug addiction:

> To be a confirmed drug addict is to be one of the walking dead . . . the teeth have rotted out; the appetite is lost and the stomach and intestines don't function properly. The gallbladder becomes inflamed; eyes and skin turn a bilious yellow. In some cases membranes of the nose turn a flaming red; the partition separating the nostrils is eaten away; breathing is difficult. Oxygen in the blood decreases; bronchitis and tuberculosis develop. Good traits of character disappear and bad ones emerge. Sex organs become affected. Veins collapse and livid purplish scars remain. Boils and abscesses plague the skin; gnawing pain racks the body; nerves snap; vicious twitching develops. Imaginary and fantastic fears blight the mind and sometimes complete insanity results. Oftentimes, too, death comes—much too early in life . . . Such is the torment of being a drug addict, such is the plague of being one of the walking dead.

Medical Association, protested the removal of cannabis preparations from the pharmacopoeia in 1937,[11] and spoke out against the lurid testimony of Harry B. Anslinger, Director of the Treasury Department's Bureau of Narcotics, who urged the classic law-enforcement approach: a ban against the drug and a higher budget for his agency to enforce the ban.

ALLOPATHIC DEFINITION OF HEALTH

The medical profession subscribes to the allopathic definition of health, which sees the use of chemicals as acceptable only if they are needed to return a dysfunctional individual to normal productive functioning. They are generally opposed to chronic drug use (maintenance) because it presupposes that no return to "normal" (abstinent) functioning is possible, and they also oppose recreational drug use because the potential users are regarded as healthy.* Medical commitment to the allopathic view explains some conduct regarding narcotic control that otherwise appears inexplicable. For example, Musto[12] describes the testimony that occurred during the 1924 Congressional Hearings on prohibiting heroin manufacture. Dr. Dana Hubbard, Director of Public Health Education of New York City's Health Department, declared, "the heroin question is not a medical one, as heroin addicts spring from sin and crime." Musto goes on to say, "these statements [by doctors] were inaccurate and misleading, which is especially disturbing in light of the fact that one would expect the medical profession to be well informed." There is one additional reason that recreational drug use in frowned upon: it leaves the physician out of the transaction entirely.

Two Examples of Medical/Legal Cooperation and the Consequences

The predominance of the legal model, even with acceptance from the medical profession, has not worked smoothly. In this section we consider the problem raised by the development of "schedules" as an attempt to limit doctors' powers to prescribe but still allow them to maintain their function as the only legitimate source of chemical treatment. In addition, we consider methadone maintenance in order to determine whether the present approach, dominated by law enforcement, can accommodate a broad-scale, medically dominant, viable chemical maintenance program.

SCHEDULES

Legal classification of drugs by Food and Drug Administration (FDA) schedules has been adopted at virtually all levels of government. In spite of its considerable problems, this approach is a clear improvement in that schedules at least acknowledge differences among drugs rather than treating all drugs as identical.

Presently, at the federal level, there are five schedules that classify many, but not all, mood-altering drugs on the basis of the "abuse potential" of each. Schedule I includes drugs that have a high potential for abuse and no currently recognized medical use in this country (e.g., heroin, mari-

---

*Alternate consciousness-seeking is not considered legitimate use of a chemical (Zinberg, N.E.: *Alternate States of Consciousness.* Free Press, Riverside, N.J., 1977).

juana, and psychedelics). Schedule II covers drugs with a high abuse potential but with some currently accepted therapeutic use (e.g., other opiates, amphetamines, and most barbiturates). Schedules III and IV each contain drugs with progressively lower potentials for abuse and physical or psychological dependence (e.g., empirin with codeine, paregoric in Schedule III, and paraldehyde and Valium in Schedule IV). Schedule V contains drugs that "might" induce limited psychological or physical dependence (e.g., cough syrups with codeine). Basically, Schedules I through IV regulate the prescriber. Limitations on Schedule V drugs are aimed at the general public rather than the physician, so that buyers must be over a certain age and pharmacies must keep a "log book" of users' names.

The chief drawback to the scheduling method is that it rationalizes myths about drugs, carrying into the 1970s the idea developed in case law 50 years ago that certain drugs have "no accepted medical use," and ignoring the extensive, successful medical use of heroin in England and Europe. It also prevents any public consideration of heroin as a "mere drug" with potential for good or ill that can be judged entirely on rational grounds, liberated from the mythic, moral preoccupation exemplified by the language of *Robinson v. California*.[13] The schedules enforce the supremacy of the legal model, even going so far as to determine the conduct of drug research: the FDA is empowered to decide when a drug can be used experimentally and when it moves from one schedule to another. Any suspicion of illegality puts the matter of drug prescribing into the hands of a law enforcement agency. Currently, this is the Drug Enforcement Administration, the most recent of the bureaucratic reorganizations of the former Federal Bureau of Narcotics.

By placing heroin, cocaine, and marijuana in Schedule I, the classification also perpetuates the concepts of "high abuse potential" and "no medical use," and the practice of making nonmedical, law enforcement judgments about the traditional psychoactive drugs. They, in turn, act to justify ignorant attitudes such as the one expressed by the Supreme Court in *Whalen v. Roe*,[6] discussed above.

> The New York statute classifies potentially harmful drugs in five schedules. Drugs, such as heroin, which are highly abused and have no recognized medical use, are in Schedule I; they cannot be prescribed. Schedules II through V include drugs which have a progressively lower potential for abuse but also have a recognized medical use. Our concern is limited to Schedule II, *which includes the most dangerous of the legitimate drugs.* [emphasis added]

The schedule method also interferes with the doctor-patient relationship, severely restricting the participants in their drug-use decisions. The stated purpose of the schedules is to permit and monitor proper medical use while attempting to deter nonmedical abuse. Far from freeing doctors from regulation, the impact of scheduling appears to be going the other way. It is particulary interesting that very little legislation has been directed at imposing manufacturing quotas on pharmaceutical companies. Almost all of the legislation has imposed regulation on medical practice.

Drugs may be and have been rescheduled since the last scheduling legislation in 1970. Here, too, when it comes to drugs in illicit use, there is evidence that the FDA reacts readily to social and political pressures and has difficulty maintaining an objective stance. When methaqualone was first introduced into this country, for example, it was placed in

Schedule IV. By then it was already well known in England and Europe as a drug of abuse.[14] Its manufacturers pressed successfully to have it available and then began an extensive advertising campaign. When the drug began to be used illicitly in this country and social fears built up, the FDA overreacted and reclassified the drug in Schedule II.

Reclassifications are usually aimed at reducing rather than increasing accessibility. Thus several drugs have been moved from Schedule IV to Schedule II, causing clinical problems, or from Schedule IV to III, and several previously unscheduled drugs have been placed in Schedule V. Ultimately, the standard itself—abuse potential—is so problematic that it is almost useless in actual practice. Although the medical profession's collusion in developing the "scheduling structure" has reinforced the physician's position as the sole legitimate source of drugs in society at large, it has eroded the physician-patient relationship and impeded progressive prescribing practices.

METHADONE MAINTENANCE

Methadone maintenance programs are generally recognized as the most successful treatment plan for heroin addicts. A 1976 study conducted by the Drug Abuse Council, Inc., found that "in most programs retention rates for one year remained about 50 percent; there was also a reduction in antisocial activities, improvement in general psychological functioning and a reduction in the extent of use of heroin or other drugs."[15] Considering that a high percentage of heroin addicts are in their early twenties, have few marketable skills, limited education, and no established work patterns, a remarkably high number of them are able to function effectively on methadone in job-placement or job-training activities.[16]

Despite recognition of its effectiveness and consistent governmental support for these programs from the federal and local agencies concerned with drug abuse treatment, methadone remains the most restricted licit drug in the country; its restrictions reflect the antimaintenance morality described earlier and the continued potency of "pharmacological Calvinism," mentioned earlier.

It is informative to examine when and why society expands and then contracts possibilities for maintenance. Initially, methadone treatment was a purely medical construct. It treated what Dole and Nyswander[17] (initiators of the methadone maintenance model) saw originally as a true metabolic dysfunction. Their treatment model was grounded in a therapeutic relationship between the counselor/doctor and the addict/patient which Dole and Nyswander decided was at the heart of the social rehabilitative process. Essentially, therefore, the therapists were little interested in the patients' drug intake which, of course, was the chief legal concern. They wanted, rather, to know how the patients were working, how they were functioning socially and psychologically, and what problems were actively interfering with their capacity to function.

This clinical point of view made the methadone maintenance program vulnerable to takeover by law enforcement. Excessive optimism about what methadone maintenance could accomplish also generated unrealistic expectations, and backers of the plan underestimated the antimaintenance attitudes in the country. Thus they oversold their program to the public, both as a cure for addiction and as a means of ameliorating the social ills—such as crime—associated with addiction. By suggesting that methadone maintenance treatment of addicts was comparable to using insulin and digitalis on the chronically ill, they troubled those who saw methadone as simply another addictive drug. In a desire to expand these programs, methadone proponents regarded as irrational and thus minimized public fears about the ethnic and racial nature of the treatment populations and the "diversion" problems that resulted in the creation of a volatile black market in methadone (some percentage of which came from government-sponsored programs).

At the same time, social forces with an investment in abstinence were not silent. The maintenance modality assumes implicitly that abstinence is not effective for all patients. True or false, that assumption challenges more than scientific issues—it rejects social values that pervade the American attitude toward addiction and life. Abstinence is consistent with that attitude; maintenance is not. Opponents of maintenance pointed out that despite the substantial allocation of resources to treatment programs, addict crime was still very much with us. As a related matter, these groups organized support within the drug treatment community by appealing to the abstinence modalities and encouraging facile political equations regarding drug substitution therapy and genocide.

In fact, the relationships between the drug-free programs, frequently staffed by ex-addicts with long criminal records, and law enforcement groups became so complex that several prominent proponents of drug-free modalities testified in favor of the punitive New York State 1973 Drug and Sentencing Law. By far the most severe in any state, they make lifetime parole mandatory upon conviction. Law enforcement measures such as these diverted both money and public support from treatment programs. Their proponents emphasized the failure of *all* treatment methods and argued that since most addicts "did not want to be cured," they should be imprisoned. That any treatment advocates supported such measures indicates the wide bitterness and fear that abstinence advocates felt about any chemical maintenance program.*

Finally, the medical profession itself was deeply divided about its role in methadone programs. Although medically developed and controlled, the programs were atypical in that they were not cure-oriented, did not involve traditional manageable patient populations, and embroiled the medical profession in conflicts with its usual public supporters (e.g., community groups and local law-enforcement representatives).

The current scenario for methadone maintenance is not unique: it was previously enacted between 1918 and 1924 on a smaller scale and was aimed at the opiate maintenance clinics.[7] In both instances the pattern has been the same. At the beginning a chemical substance that appears to help addicts function is introduced into medical use. Regulations initially introduced to aid patients (to assure actual delivery of treatment, quality control, and evaluation of the operation) become the vehicle by which opponents of maintenance attack the programs. At this turning point the counteruse of regulations has a dramatic impact on treatment and reduces its effectiveness. Next, the use of the "treatment substance" itself is called into question, and finally the maintenance program is discontinued.[18]

With the opium clinics, we saw the cycle completed and the clinics closed. With the methadone clinics, the cycle has just reached the mid-

---

*The failure of the harsh law approach has been carefully documented by the Drug Law Evaluation Project of the Association of the Bar of the City of New York; see *The Effects of the 1973 Drug Laws on the New York State Courts,* New York, 1976.

point, where overregulation imposes generalized legal rules that go beyond the goal of insuring quality control for patients and instead insure that the legal regulatory agency, rather than the physician/patient, is at the center of the treatment transaction.

In July 1976, Dole and his associates[19] released a study suggesting that if present trends continue unchecked, methadone programs are endangered entities. They concluded,

> Those of us who have witnessed the development of frustration and cynicism in physicians, nurses, counsellors, and patients tend to attribute the decline in morale during the past five years to the heavy handed regulations which dictate every detail of medical practice.

The study includes the following examples of overregulation: eleven distinct agencies have jurisdiction over methadone programs, and at least five of these regulate all details of the treatment; full compliance with the explicit regulations would, by the authors' estimate, require 185 percent of a physician's time, 165 percent of the nurse's time, and 125 percent of the counselor's time; over three-quarters of the mandated time is for paperwork, meetings, and inspections. Dole and his colleagues go on to recommend that:

> . . . appropriate agencies sponsor pilot clinics in which a competent staff is permitted to exercise *normal freedom of medical judgment in the treatment* of addicts, with the result to be evaluated by independent observers not connected with the agencies . . . This much is clear: until some simple, permanent cure for addiction is discovered, governmental agencies should try to make the best possible use of the treatments that are available.[20] [emphasis added]

The inexorable transformation of clinic staff into drug-supply regulators and their increasing involvement with regulatory agencies more than with patients again highlight the problem with the dominant legal/medical hybrid. This model of regulatory control clearly finds the concept of maintenance difficult, forces continued reliance on the law enforcement approach, and minimizes the role of the physician as therapist.

If organized medicine were to accept the concept of maintenance as a legitimate medical treatment, it would have the influence to insist that policy decisions about maintenance be based on evaluations of the results of programs, scientifically judged, and not on legally enforced moral judgments that disapprove of drug substitution per se. If the concept is not accepted, the cycle of the opium clinics will be repeated, and the efficacy of methadone and the social rehabilitation context within which it should be used will be totally undermined.

SEPARATING MEDICAL USE, ABUSE, AND RECREATIONAL USE: THE DOCTOR'S ROLE AS PRESCRIBER

The physician in practice, in addition to being asked to prescribe drugs for the relief of clearly defined medical syndromes, is faced with the fact that more than half of his patients present with complaints such as tension, anxiety, and depression. The physician wants to alleviate secondary symptoms of patients suffering from known conditions and also offer something to those whose discomfort, although emotional in origin, is no less painful. Even when such patients use psychoactive drugs regularly because the drugs are prescribed, they are not traditionally thought of as addicts (although recently law enforcement has attempted to track them through drug use "registers").

The physician who makes the decision to prescribe psychoactive drugs for members of his normal patient population faces several problems. First, there are conflicting schools of medical thought concerning such prescribing practices. Second, physicians have had unfortunate experiences with "cure-all" psychoactive drugs during the past half century. Third, concepts that purport to describe drug use issues objectively turn out upon examination to be less than objective. Concepts such as "tolerance," "drug abuse," and "quantity as a measure of abuse" do not help the physician to function in a moral culture that has assigned him the role of isolating medical use from the enormous social problem labeled "drugs." Although they are of course interrelated, we will discuss the three problems separately.

Conflicting Schools of Medical Thought

The so-called mystification school contends that psychoactive drugs are extensively overused and, as a result, individuals in our society have come to rely on drugs to deal with usual, everyday situations rather than develop their capacity to cope. The mystification school points to drug advertising as an example of this trend: a distraught housewife is urged to take a pill so that she will get through her ordinary day, or a youngster anxious about beginning at a new school is told to quell that anxiety with a capsule.[21]

The other school, spearheaded by Balter and associates[22] from the National Institute of Mental Health, contends that, generally speaking, psychoactive drugs are underused.[23,24] This school points to data from a variety of sources that report high rates of distress from psychological symptoms in general medical populations, and their work suggests that only a small portion of these patients receive prescriptions for psychoactive medication. Moreover, this school contends that when these drugs are prescribed, physicians tend to be conservative about their indication, dosage, and duration of use. Most physicians probably fluctuate between these extremes, although the Balter group's analysis is consistent with the historical development of medical prescribing habits and the explicit legal consequence of excessive or otherwise incorrect prescribing.

The conflict is often exacerbated by the patient's own belief that he should overcome his emotional difficulty rather than be pampered by medication. As a result, patients often end up being inadequately treated for a condition seen as largely psychological in order to avoid the stigma of emotional weakness. These patients do not ask for anything for their "nerves," and the physician does not suggest medication. On the other hand, when the same physicians are asked for such medication, they often betray their discomfort by finding it difficult to refuse: "Ya gotta help me, Doc. I can't afford to lose my job" or "get into trouble at school" or "not take care of the kids" are requests that lead not only to inappropriate prescribing, but also to excessive refills.

The legal system reinforces this practice: the scheduling approach impresses the physician with the extent to which his treatment of such conditions is legally regulated. Thus the legal system "punishes" treatment of emotional distress but does not, to the same extent, interfere in the treatment of physical disease. Our legal system is based on concepts that reward "coping" and excuse misbehavior on physiological but not emotional grounds.

Unfortunate Experiences with Cure-All Psychoactive Drugs

Specific experiences with "cure-all" psychoactive drugs over the past half century have turned out to be problematic. During the past 60 years, physicians have again and again found a medication that they have thought might help. Once convinced that a certain drug "works," many doctors quickly begin to prescribe it, and often overprescribe it, because of both patient demand and pharmaceutical house pressure.* Only later does the medical community find that this drug has potent, noxious side-effects including the producing of dependency as a result of continuous and increasing dosage.† Incursion from law enforcement groups only serves to complicate the picture further. Thus the physician is placed in a bind where he is hampered by inadequate scientific data, influenced by drug manufacturers, and monitored by both medical and legal institutions deeply distrustful of medical prescribing in therapeutic situations that are not clearly defined.

The history of amphetamine prescribing demonstrates the interplay of several of these factors. Amphetamines were first synthesized in 1887, but their pharmacologic properties were not studied at that time. Some 40 years later the substance was rediscovered, and it was found that the original compound (Benzedrine) and its even more active dextro-isomer (Dexedrine), when taken orally or inhaled, markedly alleviated fatigue and created euphoric confidence and alertness. A pharmaceutical manufacturer acquired patents for these drugs and quickly convinced medical practitioners of their unique and remarkably therapeutic applications, ranging from use as nasal decongestants to antidotes for depression and appetite suppressants. The drugs proved extremely attractive to the medical profession which has, historically, been exceptionally receptive to medications that "make people feel better."[25] This receptivity led to problems of overprescribing. However, the data on these drugs were remarkably flimsy. Later studies found that amphetamine use carried with it many serious contraindications. Many physicians then became uncertain

---

*In addition to patient demand and pharmaceutical house pressure, there are groups of physicians who become enthusiasts about a particular drug's properties and prescribe it unceasingly. Many physicians who were not "fat" doctors (i.e., specialists in helping patients lose weight through drugs and diet who run a virtually illicit trade) fell into that trap with amphetamines in the 1950s and well into the 1960s, long after underground newspapers were running full-page headlines declaring that "Speed Kills." Today Valium commands many similar enthusiasts. A very few such enthusiastic doctors can give out a great quantity of drugs under these circumstances, particularly when their reputation for prescribing attracts a specific clientele. All too often, however, they give them to the wrong people.

†During the 1920s, before their toxicity was fully acknowledged, bromides became extremely popular as tension-relievers, both over the counter and upon prescription. Then the barbiturates and amphetamines took center stage, followed by meprobamate and our current host of minor tranquilizers led by Librium and Valium.

about their ability to control their patients' use of the drugs. Almost all of the serious amphetamine problems seen before 1963 were iatrogenic,[26] and even after 1963, patients continued to surface whose doctors had accepted their patients' hopes that slimness and happiness came from more and more of those pills. Often these patients were sent to psychiatrists by the physicians who had been prescribing large doses of amphetamines for years. The patients were distraught and without exception sought to dissociate themselves from the "hippie," the illicit drug user. "I have a large house and four kids to take care of. I need those pills to do a good job, not for fun," one woman said after being refused a prescription when the physician found that her daily dose exceeded 100 mg (at least ten times the recommended dosage).[27]

When rescheduling went into effect in 1974, amphetamines were placed in Schedule II with the understanding that severe hyperactivity in children and actual narcolepsy were the only accepted clinical indicators for prescribing the drug. Here again the legal mechanism was wheeled into place and directed at the prescribing process and the doctor. Again uncertainty within the medical profession led to abdication of responsibility. For now another group of patients began to appear in psychiatrists' offices. Unlike the woman described above and thousands of others whose use had become excessive and psychologically disorganizing, this group had used from 5 to 15 mg of amphetamines daily for years without increasing their dose. They had severe symptoms of fatigue, lassitude, and disorganization if they did not take what could legitimately be called their maintenance dose, but few if any physicians would continue to prescribe for them.

This clinical problem continues to exist for an identifiable portion of the general patient population because, although there are substitutes available for many regulated psychoactive drugs (e.g., barbiturates), there are no equivalent stimulant substitutes. A recent description in a daily newspaper of the situation of the daily, controlled amphetamine user resulted in hundreds of supporting letters from just such people.[28] Invariably the story was the same: after years of prescribing these low doses of amphetamines, physicians regretfully told their patients that they could no longer prescribe for them. A few letters from physicians told the same story from the other side. These doctors felt that they had been deprived of a legitimate medical function.* Only through medical education and consistent and intelligent self-regulation can the physician reassert his right to prescribe or not prescribe for specific acute conditions.

---

*In addition both doctors and patients became reluctant either to accept or to admit to receiving amphetamines, even under legitimate circumstances. In examining the problem in the context of prescribing for hyperactive children, a recent paper had this comment on the negative effects of regulation:

> ... The drugs used [amphetamines] are strictly regulated by laws which require central recordkeeping by government agencies of all prescriptions written, a fact of no minor significance in this day of computer data retrieval and unwarranted government surveillance of the activities of private citizens. If parental fears of stigmatizing children do have any justification, then professionals have important soul-searching to do about the facile use of treatment procedures which carry such implications (Weithorn, C.J., and Ross, R.: Stimulant Drugs for Hyperactivity: Some Additional Disturbing Questions. Unpublished manuscript, 1975, p. 8).

Difficulties with Drug Abuse Concepts

Physicians, while considering their rights and responsibilities concerning psychoactive drugs, run into the problem of distinguishing medical use from abuse. The entire concept of drug abuse is both recent and ambiguous. It does little to clarify issues of dependency for the physician or the public.[29]

Nevertheless, the need to differentiate use from abuse is legally mandated and arises both when physicians prescribe drugs and when patients request their counsel about drug use and experiences. A research project on controlled illicit drug use has begun to collect case reports on how doctors respond when asked for information about how to use drugs safely. They tend to respond by warning of the drugs' illegality and potential for gross harm, even when they are being asked about marijuana.[30] Rarely do they volunteer reasonable information about safeguards. Consider this case:

> A young-looking, previously perfectly healthy, 68-year-old man had an episode of dizziness and vagueness. He did not faint, but the experience disturbed him enough that he arranged for a thorough physical checkup. The doctor reported cheerfully that in fact the man was in unusually good shape for his age, and a thorough workup had found no cardiac or cerebral difficulties. After some hesitation, the patient said he had a question. He told the doctor that he had been using cocaine approximately once a week for 25 years, that he enjoyed this occasional use, and wondered if it were all right to continue. Obviously taken aback by the acknowledgment of chronic illicit drug use by a prominent, respectable individual, the doctor responded sharply by saying, 'Don't you know that's against the law?' 'Of course,' responded the patient. 'I can take no medical responsibility for your condition if you continue to use such drugs,' the doctor said definitively, and offered an opinion that the patient would be taking a great risk. The patient finally asked the physician if he actually knew what the effects of cocaine use might be, to the great annoyance of the physician. They parted; the patient had received no useful information, only the sense that he would mistrust his physician in the future.

Obviously, decisions about illicit drugs often reflect moralistic rather than scientific values. Yet even the most objective physician is placed at a disadvantage. In this day of the dominance of the legal model and in the absence of consistent scientific leadership, the physician finds that values have been placed on certain drugs which may or may not agree with his, and that intrude into his relationships with his patients and his ability to obtain objective data on drug use.

One clinical example concerns a doctor who began to prescribe methaqualone when it was still unscheduled and found it a satisfactory sedative for a patient's occasional periods of insomnia. The patient, though reporting concern about becoming dependent, in fact did not increase the dosage and did not use it every night for prolonged stretches. Knowing his patient, the physician had few worries about dependency. He was more concerned that the patient might not take the medication when needed and be caught in a cycle of increasing sleeplessness. This regimen was working well until methaqualone was reclassified up to Schedule II, which requires extensive reporting, and maintenance is not an accepted principle. (The reclassification was not based on judgments about patients like this one, but on the interest in methaqualone expressed by many teenagers who claimed it gave a potent high.) The next time the doctor saw the patient he prescribed the Schedule IV sedative, Dalmane, which proved unsatisfactory. Then he tried Valium, also a Schedule IV drug, which did not work well. The physician readily admits that in his best clinical judgment he should continue to prescribe methaqualone, although he says that all this jockeying around has created so much anxiety about drugs in the patient that he doubts whether he can reestablish the old, easy relationship that allowed the patient to take a drug comfortably.

Addiction issues are far more idiosyncratic than the morally based legal scheme would have one believe, but the physician must function within all of its restrictions. Thus he relies on traditionally accepted drug abuse indicators, such as "tolerance" and "quantity of drug consumed," that are both unscientific and diversionary—they shift the focus away from the important issue: the meaning of the drug use behavior for the user.

The idea that tolerance is created by drug use is well accepted, and the traditional definition codified by the World Health Organization (WHO) defines tolerance as "a tendency to increase the dose."[31] Our experience and a review of the literature lead us to conclude that tolerance does not follow the classical view of straight-line increase of dosage, and even in cases where it does appear, it is unclear whether it is a function of physiologic tolerance or other factors.

The WHO definition implies several things that may not be true: first, that the user *must* use more of the substance involved in order to achieve the *same* effect and, second, that without a period of abstinence, the development of tolerance is irreversible and will lead to (infinite) increases in dosage. It is impossible for users of any of the drugs ordinarily associated with abuse to continue to increase their doses and get what they want from the drug, or indeed to survive.

Supporters of a simplistic view of tolerance frequently point to the heroin addict as proof that "given the opportunity, junkies would take as much dope as they could."[32] However, the empirical evidence is much more complex. The heroin user's increased use appears to be cyclical, and the addict appears to be able to cope with a stabilized dose despite intermittent periods of heavy use. A typical and very common example is an addict who has developed the habit of using heroin four or five times a day. He acquires a bit of cash, makes a good buy, and suddenly becomes a dealer. With all that dope and money around, his habit increases rapidly: within two weeks he can easily be shooting up 10 or 12 times a day. But by the time he reaches that level, he has exhausted both his capital and his business initiative. He is back on the street, and back to injecting heroin four or five times a day. Is he deriving the same effect that he did before his period of heavy use? He may not know. We surely do not know.

Cases in which the law tries to make "quantity of drug consumed" the crucial indicator of when drug use becomes drug abuse suffer from a similar problem (although this construct is an improvement over earlier, more rigid notions that regarded *any* use of certain drugs as abuse per se). Thus, for example, most statutes dealing with narcotics regulation focus in great detail on the amounts that may be prescribed, possessed, or sold. Quantity, although important for the physician to monitor, is not terribly helpful because it shifts the focus of attention away from the quality of the using experience. It is this latter factor that matters most in "controlled use," the goal which should be posited for our narcotics laws and policies.*

Such value-laden concepts divert physicians, patients, and criminal justice professionals from developing viable methods for dealing with detrimental drug use. Labels such as "drug abuser" penalize the users of certain drugs (or of certain amounts of drugs) and cut them off from consistent educational patterns of proper use and from systematic, viable social sanctions. For example, if a patient (or doctor) is convinced that tolerance to marijuana is inevitable and that ever-increasing dosages will be required, he will not be able to aid others in developing a stabilized use pattern that can be integrated into his life with a minimum of disruption (such as use of marijuana on special occasions). If a physician is convinced that drugs can truly be arranged according to how benign or harmful they are, he will be unable to advise patients in ways that minimize harmful effects, even for drugs associated with causing them. There is now abundant evidence that it was the adoption of the counterculture's suggestion, "Only use at a good time, in a good place, with good people," that reduced the noxious sequelae of psychedelic drug use so prevalent during the mid-sixties.[33,34]

The term "drug abuse" and its constituent elements do not aid the doctor in his role as adviser or prescriber. Moreover, the term has complicated and obfuscated scientific research which should be a vehicle for the development of appropriate forms of controlled use. A moral and not a scientific concept, the term has actually contributed to drug problems.

CONCLUSION

Our survey of the legal context in which the physician carries out his duties shows an inherent tension between the legal model and the medical model. What seems like underregulation when judged against the *general* decision-making function implied in the role of law can appear to be overregulation to the clinician primarily concerned with making a highly *individualized* decision. In the best of all possible worlds, the physician who makes the prescribing decision would take into account what he has learned about drugs, including their potential to induce dependency. From all this he would try to make as highly individualized a decision as possible, fitting the right drug to the described condition in a particular person—and the better he knows the person, the more individualized the decision would become. Unfortunately, no physician prescribes in this utopian way.

Some improvements may still be implemented. To modify those regulations that hamper the physician's capacity to deal with the idiosyncratic suffering of individuals—for example, those who may want a minimal daily dose of amphetamines—requires either creating so many exceptions

---

*For example, quantity is not definitive in deciding when a person qualifies as a user rather than just a "taster." Apart from the most extreme examples where quantity results in an utter breakdown or overdose, sheer quantity does not add to our understanding of drug-using behavior. Even Alcoholics Anonymous, in its 12-question pamphlet on drinking habits, "Is A.A. For You?" puts such questions as, "Have you taken a morning drink during the past year?" and "Have you missed time from work because of drinking?" The pamphlet concludes that four or more "yes" answers are needed to indicate a drinking problem, and only one of the 12 questions is directly addressed to the quantity of use.

as to make the regulation meaningless or doing away with a control mechanism needed to protect society. From the medical model standpoint, the general rules of law are both too scattered and too rigid for good clinical practice.

Although our overall contention is that the medical profession, especially in the matter of psychedelic drugs, has abdicated its responsibility to a large group of patients, few—Thomas Szasz[35] is the notable exception—would say that there should be no regulations at all. At times the legal model does defer to the medical model: a driver involved in an automobile accident after ingesting a dose of Valium is far less likely to be criminally prosecuted if he turns out to be sensitive to a *prescribed* dose than if he has taken the drug illicitly and recreationally.

Despite these exceptions, the medical profession has long been fearful of taking a strong stand about substances that are used medically and recreationally. When the Harrison Narcotic Act was passed in 1914, the provision that allowed physicians to treat addicts was expressly eliminated, and the medical profession made no outcry. England, by contrast, was dealing with the problem at the same time, and there an organized medical profession demanded and received, by way of the Dangerous Drugs Act of 1920,[36,37] the right to treat addicts medically. Although it is an overstatement, some authorities suggest that our entire narcotics muddle might not exist if the medical profession in the United States had reacted differently.[38,39]

But it is no exaggeration to say that a decade later few if any physicians rose to protest the closing of the morphine maintenance clinics between 1918 and 1924. Recent, careful, historical research indicates that the charges of inefficiency and corruption were received in a moral climate which equated abstinence with virtue and which continues to plague methadone maintenance today. The Treasury Department's Narcotic Division was overzealous both in prosecuting offenders and arranging for publicity about the dangers of the clinics to justify its zeal. Narcotic agents were also assiduous in their search for physicians who dispensed narcotics: DeLong[40] suggests that 50 percent of the first cases prosecuted were physicians, which undoubtedly helped to intimidate the profession. The charges of inefficiency were occasionally true, but many clinics, such as that of Dr. Willis P. Butler in Shreveport, Louisiana,[41] were well run and successful; his virtual persecution by bureaucratic authorities received considerable attention, but no public official or unofficial medical support. Rather than abandon doubtful clinics, it would have been more logical for various official medical organizations—hospitals, medical schools, boards of health, and local medical societies—to step in and reform the clinics in order to keep available to patients an important service.

In 1936, when the Treasury Department's Federal Bureau of Narcotics (reorganized in 1930 from its former Narcotic Division) moved to declare war on marijuana as a dangerous, dependency-producing drug (incidentally, reversing its own previous stand), only one physician rose to protest. Dr. William C. Woodward, legislative counsel for the American Medical Association, estimated that it would cost American physicians one million dollars per year to comply with the legislation. He also indicated that he thought marijuana was not necessarily a very harmful drug and that, in the long run, legislation would not suppress its use.[42] His argument seems even more cogent today, but at the time he received no support.

Physicians must be aware of the general medical ambivalence about dealing with psychoactive substances and the people who use them. For it is this ambivalence and the resulting inaction that have permitted—even encouraged—distinct inroads into prescribing autonomy to the detriment of clinical interaction. Perhaps more important, they have resulted in inadequate medical education. Concepts mentioned earlier, such as tolerance, habituation, dependency, craving, continue to have currency despite the growing awareness that they tell us little.

Almost all medical school courses about psychoactive drugs (including alcohol, when there is such a course) concentrate on the hard cases. They present heroin addiction, barbiturate addiction, and alcoholism, but nothing about controlled use. Their either/or view of these drugs accurately reflects the prevailing medical view and leaves doctors quite unprepared to deal with the majority of drug situations which predictably are in the middle. The way in which doctors think about illicit drugs affects the way they consider licit psychoactive substances. It is easy to see how a physician, unfamiliar with and excessively concerned about illicit drug use, would be defensive and overcareful in prescribing licit psychoactive drugs, or overinvolved and anxious when he does. All too often physicians find themselves overprescribing or underprescribing, sounding too shrill in their warnings to experimenting young people, or reluctant to ask questions that might induce patients to inquire about unfamiliar issues.

Medical ambivalence has also generated professional resistance to certain kinds of patients: drug users make physicians feel ignorant and are often difficult to handle; physicians are also uneasy when they must rely on law enforcement agencies to handle these problems for them. Yet physicians have such people as patients and will continue to have them, probably in increasing numbers. Doctors, if they are to do their job, cannot simply dislike addicts, dislike prescribing certain drugs that are potentially intoxicating, dislike keeping patients on drugs that only maintain and do not cure an underlying condition, or dislike discussing, individually and reasonably, recreational or illicit drug use with patients.

It is not good medicine when doctors fall back on a morally based "party line" and tell patients that what they are doing is against the law when it is true but irrelevant, or that it will harm them when the doctors do not know that it will. Whether the drug concerned is licit or illicit, doctors should examine carefully what degrees of use are reasonable and controlled.

If doctors accept the concept of controlled illicit drug use and purvey information and advice on successful use, it means recognizing that all drug use is not concerned with prescribing the drugs themselves. This recognition both reduces the doctors' domain by removing some drugs from their direct control and increases it by permitting them a larger counselor role. However, eventually this changed perception will increase the tension between an individualized medical model and a general legal regulatory model and will be hard for organized medicine. It means a complete reversal of the 1924 and 1963 positions described earlier.

If doctors were to begin seeing their roles with all of these substances in a much broader way, they probably would want to reclaim ground lost to law enforcement agencies. Consider heroin as an example. Heroin could well be a useful analgesic for the physician's armamentarium. Certainly, protecting methadone maintenance as a viable modality might lead to a call for heroin induction clinics (which would begin by giving patients heroin, then move to injected methadone, and finally to oral methadone) or even for heroin maintenance clinics. The fact that we have not tried even one small experimental heroin induction clinic in the past eight years of our national struggle with heroin addiction can only be attributed to a persistently moral, abstinent, and law enforcement-oriented social climate. Two or three small heroin induction or maintenance clinics would teach the medical profession a great deal about how patients do respond to heroin under controlled conditions and enable physicians to study how it is used. The chief advantage of such clinics, however, would be the symbolic acceptance of heroin as simply a drug to be worked with for better or worse. The medical profession's lack of support for such experiments helps to keep heroin as a cryptically evil drug that cannot even be studied or researched.

It will require major readjustments in the thinking of many if doctors are to realize that the drug issue is a major area in which they can begin to actively address the problem of ever-increasing regulation of medical practice. If they do not face the drug issue and participate to a greater extent than at present, it is certain that legal model restrictions will continue to grow, and the dilemma that doctors are only beginning to recognize as a problem for clinical practice will become far worse.

REFERENCES

1. Musto, D. F.: *The American Disease: Origins of Narcotic Controls.* Yale University Press, New Haven, 1973.
2. DeLong, J. V.: Treatment and Rehabilitation, in *Dealing with Drug Abuse, A Report to the Ford Foundation.* Praeger, New York, 1972.
3. *Webb v. United States,* 249 U.S. 497 (1919).
4. Zinberg, N. E., and Lewis, D. C.: Narcotic Usage. I. A Spectrum of a Difficult Medical Problem. *N. Engl. J. Med.* 270:989–993, 1964.
5. Lewis, D. C., and Zinberg, N. E.: Narcotic Usage. II. A Historical Perspective on a Difficult Medical Problem. *N. Engl. J. Med.* 270:1045–1050, 1964.
6. *Whalen v. Roe,* 45 U.S.L.W. 4166 (February 22, 1977).
7. Waldorf, D., Orlick, M., and Reinarman, C.: *Morphine Maintenance: The Shreveport Clinic, 1919–1923.* Publication SS-1. The Drug Abuse Council, Inc., Washington, D.C., 1974.
8. *United States v. Behrman,* 258 U.S. 280 (1922).
9. Bunnell, K. P.: Liberal Education and American Medicine. *J. Med. Ed.* 33:319–340, 1958.
10. Klerman, G. L.: Psychotropic Hedonism vs. Pharmacological Calvinism. *Hastings Center Rep.* 2:1–3, 1972.
11. Grinspoon, L.: *Marihuana Reconsidered.* Bantam Books, New York, 1971, pp. 24–26.
12. Musto, D. F.: An Historical Perspective on Legal and Medical Responses to Substance Use. *Villanova Law Rev.* 18:808–811, 1973.
13. *Robinson v. California,* 370 U.S. 660, 664–665 (1962).
14. Falco, M.: *Methaqualone: A Study of Drug Control.* Publication FS-6. The Drug Abuse Council, Inc., Washington, D.C., 1975.
15. Bourne, P. G.: *Methadone: Benefits and Shortcomings.* Publication MS-12. The Drug Abuse Council, Inc., Washington, D.C., 1975, p. 3.
16. *Proposal for the Use of Diacetyl-Morphine (Heroin) in the Treatment of Heroin Dependent Individuals.* Vera Institute of Justice, New York, 1972.
17. Dole, V. P., and Nyswander, M. E.: Heroin Addiction—A Metabolic Disease. *Arch. Intern. Med.* 120:19–24, 1967.
18. Zinberg, N. E.: The Crisis in Methadone Maintenance. *N. Engl. J. Med.* 296:1000–1002, 1977.
19. Dole, V. P., et al.: *A Survey of Paperwork in Methadone Clinics.* The Community Treatment Foundation, New York, 1976, p. 11.

20. Ibid., p. 12.
21. Lennard, H. L., et al.: *Mystification and Drug Misuse*. Jossey-Bass, San Francisco, 1971.
22. Balter, M. B., and Levine, J.: Character and Extent of Psychotherapeutic Drug Usage in the United States. Proceedings of the Fifth World Congress of Psychiatry, 1971. *Excerpta Medica*, Amsterdam, 1973.
23. Manheimer, D. I., et al.: Popular Beliefs and Attitudes about Tranquilizers. *Am. J. Psychiatry* 130:1246–1253, 1973.
24. Mellinger, G. D., et al.: An Overview of Psychotherapeutic Drug Use in the United States, in Josephson, E., and Carroll, E. E. (eds.): *Drug Use: Epidemiological and Sociological Approaches*. Hemisphere Publishing Corporation, Washington, D.C., 1974.
25. Zinberg, N. E., and Robertson, J. A.: *Drugs and the Public*. Simon & Schuster, New York, 1972.
26. Grinspoon, L., and Hedblom, P.: *The Speed Culture: Amphetamine Use and Abuse in America*. Harvard University Press, Cambridge, Mass., 1975.
27. Zinberg and Robertson, op. cit.
28. Zinberg, N. E.: Forum/Drugs. *The Boston Globe*, April 25, 1976.
29. Zinberg, N. E., Harding, W. M., Apsler, R., and Barry, M.: What is Drug Abuse? *J. Drug Issues* 8:9–35, 1978.
30. Zinberg, N. E., Jacobson, R. C., and Harding, W. M.: Social Sanctions and Rituals as a Basis for Drug Abuse Prevention. *Am. J. Drug Alcohol Abuse* 2:165–181, 1975.
31. Eddy, N. B., Halbach, H., Isbel, H., and Seevers, M. H.: Drug Dependence: Its Significance and Characteristics. *Bull. WHO* 32:721–733, 1965.
32. Smith, D. E., and Gay, G. R. (eds.): *"It's So Good, Don't Even Try It Once": Heroin in Perspective*. Prentice-Hall, Englewood Cliffs, N.J., 1972.
33. Weil, A.: The Natural Mind: A New Way of Looking at Drugs and the Higher Consciousness. Houghton Mifflin, Boston, 1972, pp. 166–172.
34. Zinberg, N. E.: *"High" States: A Beginning Study*. Publication SS-3. The Drug Abuse Council, Inc., Washington, D.C., 1974.
35. Szasz, T.: *Ceremonial Chemistry: The Ritual Persecution of Drugs, Addicts and Pushers*. Anchor Press/Doubleday, Garden City, N.Y., 1975.
36. Zinberg and Robertson, op. cit.
37. Judson, H. F.: *Heroin Addiction in Britain*. Harcourt Brace Jovanovich, New York, 1974.
38. Helmer, J.: *Drugs and Minority Oppression*. Seabury Press, New York, 1975.
39. Musto, *The American Disease*, op. cit.
40. DeLong, op. cit.
41. Waldorf, Orlick, and Reinarman, op. cit.
42. Grinspoon, op. cit.

CHAPTER 42

Amiram Elwork is Assistant Professor of Psychology at the University of Nebraska–Lincoln. A graduate of Temple University and the University of Nebraska, Dr. Elwork is a member of the American Psychological Association, the American Psychology-Law Society, and the American Association of Correctional Psychologists. He has also served as a consulting editor of *Law and Human Behavior*.

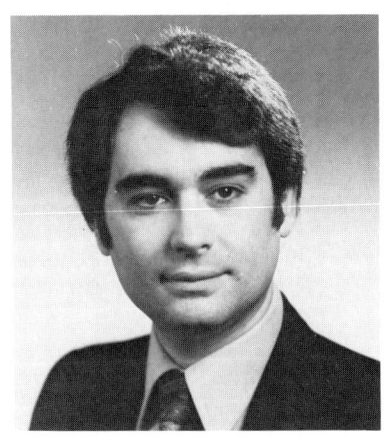

Bruce Dennis Sales is Associate Professor of Psychology and Law and Director of the Law-Psychology Graduate Training Program at the University of Nebraska–Lincoln. He is a member of the American Psychological Association and has served on its Task Force on Legal Action. He has also chaired the American Bar Association's Behavioral Sciences Committee and is former President of the American Psychology-Law Society. Dr. Sales is editor of *Law and Human Behavior* and has edited several books on the psychology of the legal process and the criminal justice system.

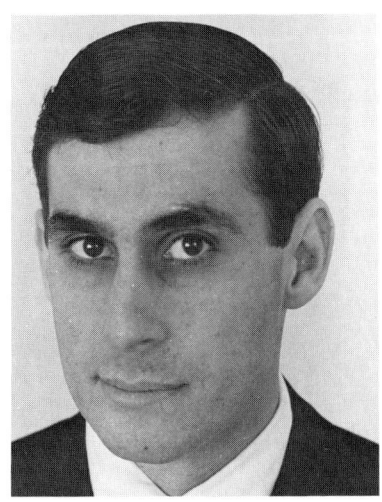

THE JURY AND TRIAL PROCESS: PSYCHOLOGICAL PERSPECTIVES*

Amiram Elwork, Ph.D., and
Bruce Dennis Sales, Ph.D., J.D.

In a democracy, law represents the people's attempt to achieve justice by agreeing on a set of behavioral norms and rules. "Every law, every court decision, and every administrative procedure has an underlying set of assumptions about how people act and how their actions can be controlled."[1] Since lawyers are not scientifically equipped to study those assumptions, behavioral scientists have a unique contribution to make in this area. The interface of law, psychiatry, and psychology, in particular, and of law and behavioral sciences, in general, can help in achieving justice by making laws, court decisions, and administrative procedures conform to empirically derived knowledge about human behavior.

Because one of the most visible dispensaries of justice is the courtroom trial, it has become a central focus of psycholegal research. In his classic book, *On the Witness Stand,* Hugo Munsterberg first proposed in 1908 that "the mental life . . . plays too important a role in court procedure to reject the advice of those who devote their work to the study of these functions."[2] One would have thought that this proposal of "marriage" would be readily accepted and "consummated," but it was not to be so.[3] Wigmore, the noted legal scholar, responded with criticism of psychologists for not really having the strong empirical evidence that Munsterberg alluded to, or at least for not publishing it in legal journals.[4] What should have started in an atmosphere of collaboration began in an atmosphere of antipathy. As a result, the net gains of psycholegal research on the trial process over the past half century have been far below its potential.

In the last few years, however, there has been an encouraging rise in interest and research on the jury and trial processes with articles appearing in both behavioral science and law journals. This has led to a sudden accumulation of findings that deserve review.

---

*During the interval of time that was required to prepare this book, a number of articles appeared which dealt with the jury and trial process. Although they could not be included, these recent articles do not affect any of the substantive points made within this chapter.

ALTERNATIVE APPROACHES TO ORGANIZING RESEARCH

Organizing information is a partially subjective process in which the author attempts to conform to the dictates of logic and to the needs of the audience. However, there are numerous audiences and several different ways that research on the jury and trial processes could be logically organized, including organization by psychological theories and phenomena and by legal theories and issues.

Some researchers use the trial as just another situation to test the basic tenets of a theory of human behavior or to generalize a psychological phenomenon. For example, according to social judgment theory, many of our social attitudes which seem independent are really determined by judgmental contrasts made against some other attitude which is used as a reference point.[5] This phenomenon, known as the contrast effect, was recently extended to a simulated legal setting. Pepitone and DeNubile[6] demonstrated that simulated juries judged a given crime's severity by making comparisons with a preceding judgment of another crime.

Although this type of study may document important facts about the underlying dynamics within a trial, this information is secondary to the avowed purpose of the research, which is to study psychological phenomena and to test psychological theories. If this logic were extended to a review chapter, its organization would emphasize the psychological concerns with section headings such as "The Effect of Social Desirability in the Courtroom."

Another approach at organization, namely, by legal theory and issue, should be more relevant to the forensic specialist since this approach emphasizes studying the trial to specifically learn more about its dynamics and not simply to test the applicability of a particular theory of human behavior in a new situation. The logic of this orientation suggests that section headings should be determined by legally relevant topics with all research pertinent to that topic included, regardless of the psychological-theoretical perspective. This chapter adopts the legal orientation.

We will first present a brief description of the typical trial, followed by a review of the psycholegal research on each of the major topics within the trial process. The reviewed findings will be evaluated from a legal perspective.

CIVIL AND CRIMINAL TRIAL PROCEEDINGS

Our American trial system is designed to resolve two types of controversies, issues of fact and issues of law. For example, when someone is charged with breaking a law and refutes the charge, the controversy may either be over a legal issue, such as whether or not the language of the statute is constitutional, or over a factual issue, such as whether or not it was the defendant who committed the crime. Conflicts over fact and law can occur in either civil or criminal cases. Charges of crime are formally viewed as violations against the public as well as the individuals involved. Civil cases, on the other hand, arise solely to resolve disputes among the parties. The goal of criminal cases is to protect the public and to punish and/or rehabilitate the guilty. In contrast, the emphasis in most civil cases is on compensation to the injured party.

The first decision that a defendant and his lawyer must make in a criminal proceeding is whether to plead guilty or innocent to the charges.

This decision is influenced by an assessment of the probability of being acquitted and by the seriousness of the penalty for the charge. Quite often a bargain is reached between the opposing attorneys, assuring a guilty plea to a lesser charge. Kalven and Zeisel reported that "of the major crime controversies that reach the stage of formal prosecution and are not dismissed, three-fourths are disposed of without trial"[7] because of guilty pleas. Given that a defendant chooses to plead innocent, the next decision he must make is whether to have a jury or bench trial (i.e., trial by a judge). Often this decision is made for strategic reasons. For example, the attorney knows that the presiding judge has been lenient in the past on defendants in similar cases; thus he requests a bench trial.

When a jury trial is chosen, the next step is to select jurors from a larger number of prospective jurors. This process is called the *voir dire,* and its purpose is to weed out unqualified or biased individuals. During this process, prospective jurors are acquainted with the nature of the case and are asked a number of questions by the judge or attorney on a variety of issues that have bearing on the litigation. The judge must then excuse those jurors who are unsuitable to serve because they run afoul of any one of a number of statutory prohibitions (e.g., inadequate comprehension of English, blatant prejudice toward or against one side). The attorneys may also excuse a limited number of jurors without stating a reason to the jury or the judge. The first process is known as excusing for cause, while the second is referred to as exercising peremptory challenges.

After the jurors are chosen, the judge gives preliminary instructions describing the role and duties of the judge, jury, and attorneys. The judge also instructs the jury on their conduct outside the courtroom, such as avoiding the influence of the news media and not discussing the case with others. After the preliminary instructions, the attorneys may make opening statements, outlining the evidence that will be presented. They are not allowed, however, to draw inferences or use argumentation in order to convince the jury. The prosecuting or plaintiff's attorney goes first, while the defense attorney sometimes postpones his opening statements until after the prosecution has presented its entire case.

After opening statements, the prosecution begins the presentation of evidence. Each witness is first directly examined by the prosecuting attorney and then cross-examined by the defense attorney. When the prosecution is finished presenting its case, the defense then presents its evidence. This time the defense attorney directly examines each witness, and the prosecutor cross-examines. Both sides are given ample opportunity to present rebuttal testimony. Throughout these proceedings the judge will rule on what testimony is admissible. When both sides have rested their cases, they present closing arguments, which focus on the factual issues. The attorneys often use emotionally persuasive tactics in order to sway the jury or judge to a favorable verdict for their side of the case.

Following closing arguments, the judge instructs the jury. These instructions, or the jury charge, are given in order to equip the jury with the specific legal criteria by which they must weigh the evidence during deliberation to reach a verdict.

The order of the proceedings in civil cases is very similar to that of the criminal case. The parties engage in pretrial negotiations to see if a settlement can be worked out and thus avoid the necessity of a trial. If an agreement cannot be reached, then the trial is undertaken. In civil cases, however, the jury, if a trial by jury is chosen, will decide not only which party was liable, but also the amount of financial damages to award. This is dissimilar to the criminal case in most jurisdictions in which the jury determines guilt, while the judge does the sentencing.

REVIEW OF RESEARCH FINDINGS

The Adversary Process

Any discussion of the American trial system must begin with its central feature, the adversary process. In our system of justice, a lawyer's duty is to represent his client to the best of his ability. This means that he must present the case that is most favorable to his client and not necessarily one that best represents the complete truth. Although he cannot lie, he can selectively present facts or argue for interpretations of law that would be more favorable to his cause. If both lawyers do this, justice may emerge as a balance between the opposing forces. The judge and the jury are the impartial determiners of where that balance lies.

In a series of studies, Thibaut and Walker[8] tried to demonstrate the effect of the differences between the adversary legal system of our country and the inquisitorial type of legal system which prevails in many other countries. The main difference between these systems is that in the inquisitorial system attorneys are sworn to find the truth and remain free of personal interest on either side of a quarrel (court-centered), while in the adversary process they are sworn to protect their client to the best of their ability (client-centered). The design of these studies was to give volunteer law students either client-centered instructions or court-centered instructions and to observe how a simulated case would be built and argued. Although this research has been criticized for being too simulated,[9] its results can be cautiously generalized to the real courtroom situation. Based upon the results of these studies, Thibaut and Walker concluded that the type of system makes a major difference in the psychological atmosphere it creates in the courtroom. Specifically, the adversary system emphasizes the fact that there are at least two sides to every story. This emphasis, in turn, helps the judge and jury suspend judgment whenever any testimony is given. This effect is crucial when the judge or jury is biased in any way because it indirectly makes them more aware of the possibility of bias in themselves.[10] Furthermore, Sears[11] suggests that people who sit in judgment prefer to make judgments after hearing both sides of a story. Thus the adversary system is more apt to instill in its participants a satisfied feeling that fairness has been achieved. Indeed, subject-defendants felt that the adversary system gave their side a greater opportunity for their case to be presented.[12]

The type of system can also make a difference in the enthusiasm with which attorneys search for evidence.[13] The results of several studies suggest that court-centered attorneys stop searching for evidence as soon as they are satisfied with their own assessment of a case. In contrast, client-centered attorneys continue to search until favorable evidence is discovered. Thus a client-centered attorney will tend to present a better case for the party whose position is least supported by the evidence.[14]

It should be noted that the adversary system is often misunderstood and subjected to opinionated comments. Critics point to examples of dishonesty in the courtroom and argue that the adversary process promotes an atmosphere in which lawyers and their clients are bound to distort and misuse the truth. Unfortunately there is no research on this point and we must also speculate. Since the word "truth" contains dual meanings,[15] when we determine that someone is telling the truth, we may mean it in the sense of "honesty" or in the sense of "accuracy." The dishonesty of some participants in the courtroom is not inherent in the process. In fact, cross-examination tends to discourage dishonesty. It is the accuracy of testimony, on the other hand, that the process appears to distort. The lawyer for a given side will only allow his witness to testify to those facts that are supportive of his position. Furthermore, when conflicts arise, even "honest" men can be "inaccurate" since their testimony is shaped by their interests, values, personalities, and backgrounds.[16] How people perceive this process and how this affects their attitudes and behaviors when interacting within it are important questions that researchers need to address. It is too often the case that uninitiated scientists become disillusioned and hostile after their first court appearance in an adversary proceeding.

Finally, some psychologists have studied the adversary process not to learn more about our system of justice, but rather to use it as a standard against which to compare the scientific method. For example, Levine[17] argues that the adversary process operates in the same manner as the scientific method. Scientific theories like the lawyer's perception of truth and the presentation of his argument are also partly shaped by interest, values, personalities, and backgrounds.[18] Convincing the scientific community into believing in a theory is not much different than convincing a jury into believing one version of a case. The ".05 significance level" in science is as arbitrary as the point beyond which reasonable doubts are dropped in law. Thus Levine suggests that scientists might do well to adopt the adversary process in evaluating scientific theories and "facts." A similar approach has been suggested in relation to educational administration.[19]

The Jury

THE KALVEN AND ZEISEL STUDY

When a jury trial is available, a basic question that the lawyer must ask is, "How will a judge and jury differ in their verdicts in this case?" The answer to that question will determine whether or not to choose a bench or jury trial. *The American Jury,* by Kalven and Zeisel,[20] was one of the first attempts to answer aspects of this question. By mail questionnaires trial court judges were asked to report, for cases tried before them, how the jury decided the case and how they would have decided it, had it been tried before them without a jury. The judges were also asked to give some descriptive and evaluative material about the case, the parties, and counsel.[21] In this manner these researchers tried to measure the magnitude and direction of disagreements between judge and jury.

They found that out of their sample of 3,576 criminal cases, judge and jury would have agreed 78 percent of the time. The juries were more lenient than the judges would have been in 19 percent of the cases, while the judges would have been more lenient than the juries in 3 percent of the cases. "Thus," the researchers found, "the jury trials show on balance a net leniency of 16 percent. This means that in the cases which the defendant decides to bring before the jury, on balance, he fares better 16 percent of the time than he would have in a bench trial."[22]

Contrary to the authors' assertion, we still cannot conclude that juries are generally more lenient than judges, since the decision to have a jury trial is not a random event. Kalven and Zeisel used a sample of jury trials only. These cannot be used to answer any questions about the total universe of trials, which includes the set of bench trials, since there is no way of knowing whether the results indicate a general magnitude and direction of judge-jury disagreements as contended, or whether they indicate the extent to which lawyers made the right decision when they opted for a jury trial in a particular case. What would be needed is jury decisions on a sample of previously held bench trials.

Even if we could have chosen between one of the two alternative explanations, neither would be extremely helpful to a lawyer wanting to decide how to choose in a specific instance. The important question is what are the characteristics of the case that would cause a judge or jury trial to be more advantageous? Kalven and Zeisel present some data that are helpful in answering this question. In their study they also asked judges for other types of descriptive and evaluative information concerning the reasons they gave for the judge-jury disagreement.

In over 79 percent of the disagreement cases, judges reported evidence factors as being at least part of the explanation for the disagreements. Typically, by evidence factors is meant that the evidence on both sides of a case was very close or ambiguous. Judges reported perceiving that jurors had a higher threshold of doubt than they did when the facts were not clear-cut. In addition, judges reported that jurors were more willing to rely on their sentiments and values as a basis for decision when the facts were not absolutely clear. Thus the closeness of evidence was not so much a cause for judge-jury disagreements as it was a condition in which other extraneous variables gain importance. For example, judges reported that when the evidence was very close, a defendant with no prior record stood a better chance with a jury. On the other hand, some judges reported that in close cases defendants with a previous record stood a better chance with them than with the jury. Thus the credibility of the defendant was a stronger variable with the jury than with the judge when the evidence was close.

In 50 percent of the disagreement cases, judges reported that the jury's sentiments on the law were at least partially responsible for the disagreements. Generally, what these judges perceived was that juries were less apt than they to stick to the letter of the law and more flexible when special circumstances were present.

This finding is important to the defense attorney who argues that although his client did break the law, it should be excused because of extenuating circumstances. The extreme example of this class of arguments is the insanity defense. In such cases a judge is under more pressure than a jury to adhere to strictly legal criteria. Unlike the jury, whenever a judge deviates from previously established legal criteria, he is in effect setting new legal precedents. With that in mind, and the fear of being overturned by higher courts, judges tend to be more cautious about excusing a defendant on the grounds of extenuating circumstances. Jurors, on the other hand, feel less pressure to adhere to the letter of the law. The conditions which illustrate this phenomenon are all characterized by the jury's feelings that in addition to what the law provides, justice should serve to restore equity.[23]

Sometimes jurors will bring in a more lenient verdict than a judge when they feel that a defendant has been punished enough, either from time spent in jail awaiting trial, or from life itself. Kalven and Zeisel quote from one of the judges' reports in an income tax evasion case to illustrate this point:

> Defendant did not testify but the evidence shows that, during the years in question, his home burned, he was seriously injured and his son was killed. Later he lost his leg, his wife became seriously ill and several major operations were necessary. About three years before the trial, his wife gave birth to a premature child which was both blind and spastic. These, however, are only a portion of the calamities the defendant suffered during the years he failed to file his income tax return.[24]

The jury found the accused not guilty. It should be noted that a judge feels less restricted in determining a sentence, and in hard-luck cases may suspend a sentence. However, when the evidence is clear, a judge is less likely than a jury to bring in a not guilty verdict, no matter what the circumstances.

Judges also reported that in some cases jurors are more apt to be lenient if they feel that it would be unjust to place all of the blame on the defendant when it should be shared. That is, jurors are more apt to apply their own standard of equity when the law does not provide for it.[25] For example, there are certain kinds of unpopular laws which jurors are less likely to enforce than judges. These are best exemplified by violations of liquor or gambling laws. The justification that jurors might feel when they are lenient is that from time to time these laws are violated by everyone, and it is inequitable to single out particular defendants for punishment.

Another possible condition for jurors being more lenient than a judge is when an accomplice to the crime has escaped punishment or when the victim is seen as a contributing factor to the crime, even though criminal law is not concerned with contributory fault.[26] Rape cases are an example. Whereas the law only deals with the issue of consent at the moment of intercourse, a jury has more of a tendency than a judge to take into account a woman's sexual history and conduct prior to the alleged rape. Jurors are more apt to place themselves in the situation of the defendant and ask whether they would have acted in the same way. When jurors are convinced of contributory fault, they do not necessarily consider the defendant innocent. They are simply more apt to feel that the defendant deserves a lesser sentence or charge. In cases where they are given a chance to convict a defendant on a lower charge, they will do so. In those cases where they are not allowed to lower the charge, they sometimes will acquit, especially when the evidence is close. Again, it must be emphasized that a judge may lower a defendant's sentence in such cases, but is less likely than a jury to acquit the defendant of the charge.

Judges also reported that jurors are prone to be lenient when they feel that the punishment is too severe. For example, jurors are apt to be lenient when they feel that the wrong that was done was a trivial one, and either the victim suffered no loss or the victim was more than adequately compensated. Sometimes this occurs when a crime is committed against a victim for whom the jury feels little compassion, as in a case of a victim with a police record, or a victim who is of a socioeconomic or ethnic group against which the jurors are prejudiced. This is especially likely to occur when the evidence is close.

Finally, it should be noted that there are some offenses about which jurors are likely to be more strict than judges, even when the evidence is close. These usually involve crimes for which the jury feels there is little chance of reparation, as in narcotics cases or sex crimes against children.

Although evidence factors and sentiments on the law account for or are conditions under which most of the judge-jury disagreements occurred in the Kalven and Zeisel sample, other less powerful variables often interact with one or both of the major variables. As was stressed earlier, evidence factors and sentiments on the law cause jurors to vacillate on a verdict. The following variables have been reported as being important in that they tend to determine the final outcome of vacillations.

In 22 percent of the disagreement cases, judges reported sentimentality for the defendant as one of the important determinants of judge-jury disagreements.[27] More specifically, judges reported that certain personal characteristics (e.g., being crippled, elderly, or a widow), certain occupations (e.g., servicemen, clergymen), certain family characteristics (e.g., pregnant wife, children), and certain courtroom impressions (e.g., attractiveness, remorse, crying) had an effect on jury leniency. On the other hand, less favorable characteristics (e.g., undignified occupations, repeated divorces, arrogance) have been reported as being responsible for more strictness from a jury than a judge. These characteristics will be used by jurors in order to assess a person's credibility and/or worthiness. In turn, such an assessment might affect a jury that is vacillating on a verdict because of evidence factors or sentiments on the law.

In 5 percent of the cases in which there were judge-jury disagreements, judges reported that they knew facts that the jury did not know.[28] It is sometimes true that even though the judge and jury are together in the same courtroom, they may not be dealing with the same case. For example, when a defendant does not take the stand, the law provides that the prosecution cannot reveal certain events in the defendant's past, such as the defendant's prior police record, the defendant's withdrawal of a guilty plea, or the defendant's refusal to take a lie detector test. Thus the jury will never know the information to which the judge may be privy. It is easy to see that especially when the evidence is close, this type of evidence can make a tremendous difference in establishing a defendant's credibility and in determining a decision.

In 8 percent of the disagreement cases, judges reported the impact of lawyers as one of the important determinants of judge-jury disagreements.[29] That is, the judges felt that at times the jurors were swayed by the attractiveness of a lawyer or his oratory skills during summation. Apparently, what these judges noted was that especially in cases where there are juridic vacillations, lawyers can have an impact in convincing a jury, whereas a judge is more apt to be resistant to external persuasion.

In the past few years there has been other research[30] which relates to the topics discussed by Kalven and Zeisel. We have reviewed the Kalven and Zeisel study separately because it is unique in several ways. First, it attempted to measure how extraneous variables affect jurors differently than judges. Secondly, it reviewed actual cases and actual judges. In contrast, the studies discussed below were all done by simulation, mostly with college students acting as jurors. To this extent, their reliability is limited.

THE SEVERITY OF THE PUNISHMENT AND THE CRIME

The law differentiates between degrees of criminality (e.g., first-degree murder vs. second-degree murder) and prescribes different penalties for each. The jury in most jurisdictions is supposed to be concerned with the question of guilt or innocence and not with the possible penalties that may ensue from a finding of guilt. Several researchers, however, have suggested that jurors do concern themselves with the penalties of a guilty verdict.[31] Jurow[32] found that people who had scruples about capital punishment sometimes would rather set a guilty person free than send him to his death. Vidmar[33] demonstrated in one simulation that when subjects were given a choice of first-degree murder or not guilty, 54 percent chose not guilty. In the same fact situation, when the defendant was charged with manslaughter, 92 percent of the subjects opted for a guilty verdict, even though the facts did not justify the different finding. Hester and Smith[34] reported similar results but found an interaction with the heinousness of the crime. That is, subjects were more prone to find a defendant guilty, regardless of the penalties, when the crime was more shocking. Several other studies[35] have also shown that the worse the consequences of an accident, the greater the responsibility assigned to the wrongdoer.

Characteristics of the Defendant

PSYCHOLOGICAL ATTRACTIVENESS

Several studies have manipulated the psychological attractiveness of the defendant to determine what effect this variable has on juror decision-making. Psychological attractiveness is defined by characteristics of the defendant that make him more or less attractive to the juror (e.g., family man, good job—attractive; prior record—unattractive). These studies show that subject jurors are less certain of a guilty verdict and will suggest lower prison sentences when the defendant is psychologically attractive.[36] These findings, however, must be carefully interpreted. For example, Griffitt and Jackson[37] used a rating scale for certainty of guilt (1, definitely guilty; 7, definitely not guilty). The mean ratings for defendants with similar versus dissimilar attitudes to those of the subjects were 2.66 and 2.25. These differences in certainty of guilt were statistically significant but not realistically significant. The same criticism can be made about the other studies cited above. Thus, in a real-life situation where a judgment of guilt or innocence has to be made, such small differences in certainty would not be predictive. From the Kalven and Zeisel study, we have learned that psychological attractiveness is probably only important in cases where the evidence is not strong enough to sway the jury in one direction or the other. Nevertheless, most of the simulated studies done in recent years have used cases where the fact situations were very clear. Doob and Kirshenbaum's study was an exception.[38]

This research is problematical in that it fails to apply to courtroom realities, which is a reflection, in part, of a lack of familiarity with courtroom procedures on the part of the behavioral scientists. For example, why have jurors decided sentences when in most jurisdictions in this country it is done solely by the judge? Even if we consider this research to be more of a simulation of a judge's role than a juror's, it still does not address itself to courtroom realities. The results in the Landy and Aronson study[39] were interpreted as a demonstration that perhaps jurors (or judges) are *inappropriately prejudiced* by the personal characteristics of defendants in deciding on sentences. The reality, however, is that a judge is legally given discretion in sentencing so that he may weigh how his sentence will best protect society from further harm by the convicted person. Thus the circumstances of a case and a defendant's previous record are appropriately weighed in making this decision. As one metropolitan judge explained to us, with each violation the severity of his sentence increases. Thus it is appropriate for different people committing an identical crime to receive different sentences.

By looking at the information given to the subject-jurors in the Landy and Aronson study, we can infer that relevant factors entered into their decision-making. In the stories presented, the attractive defendant was described in such a way as to leave the impression that he was less of a threat to repeat a serious offense than the unattractive one. The attractive defendant was described as a respectable citizen who, out of mourning and loneliness for his recently deceased wife, got drunk prior to his negligent automobile homicide. He had no previous criminal record, and he was injured himself as a result of the accident. Everything about the attractive defendant suggests that his crime was a one-time occurrence with a low probability of being repeated. On the other hand, the unattractive defendant was described as a less than dependable person who did have a previous criminal record, including a previous drug violation. Since the negligent homicide was partially caused by drunken driving, the previous drug violation along with the rest of the description led to a conclusion that this defendant did present a threat to society in the future. Thus Landy and Aronson's subjects acted responsibly in assigning higher sentences to the less reliable defendant, while holding both defendants equally guilty.

Since the role of a jury in a criminal trial is to decide only on the guilt or innocence of a defendant, researchers should turn away from using prison sentences as a dependent measure. In addition, more studies should be done simulating civil cases where jurors are allowed to determine the amount of compensation due the plaintiff.

PHYSICAL ATTRACTIVENESS

Another characteristic of the defendant that will make him more or less psychologically attractive is his physical appearance. It has been shown that subject-jurors are prejudiced by the physical characteristics of a defendant. Efran[40] found that subjects evaluated physically attractive defendants with less certainty of guilt than in the case of less attractive defendants. Similarly, Dion[41] demonstrated that adults tend to view transgressions by unattractive children as more serious than transgressions by attractive children. Sigall and Ostrove,[42] however, found that when a crime (e.g., embezzlement) was facilitated by physical attractiveness, the more attractive defendant, as opposed to the less attractive defendant, was dealt with more severely by subjects acting as jurors.

These findings might be explained by the fact that physically attractive people tend to be judged as being more credible.[43] This type of judgment might disappear, however, once people know each other. That is, before we know a person, we are apt to make judgments on the most available information, such as physical attractiveness. In a real courtroom situation, however, a jury may get to know a defendant beyond his physical characteristics. For example, the emotions that a defendant might exhibit while on the stand will communicate many things about the defendant's credibility and worth[45] and will allow jurors to know the defendant at a deeper level than his physical characteristics might first project. Thus it is difficult to know whether these simulated studies can be generalized to an actual courtroom situation since they did not use real trials, or videotaped trials, but only presented selected subject-jurors with a written description of the evidence and a photograph of the defendant.

Size of Jury and Decision Rules

SIX- VERSUS TWELVE-MEMBER JURIES

Because of mounting backlogs, our court system has been increasingly slower in its ability to provide a speedy trial. The problem has reached the point where some defendants actually spend more time in jail awaiting trial than serving their sentences if they were found guilty. Many critics have argued that the jury trial is a major cause of backlogs and delays.[45] It takes more time to select a jury and to await a jury's deliberations than it takes to conduct a bench trial. In addition, jury trials cost the taxpayer much more money. Thus critics have suggested the abolition of the jury trial, at least in civil cases.[46] Others counterargue that representatives of the community should take part in our courts no matter what the cost.[47]

As a compromise, several states have adopted laws allowing six-member instead of twelve-member juries. This practice created a tremendous amount of controversy in legal circles.[48] Eventually, the practice was appealed to the U.S. Supreme Court. In *Williams v. Florida*,[49] the Supreme Court held that six-member juries in criminal cases were constitutional since there was no evidence that juries of different sizes would make any difference in verdicts. In *Colgrove v. Batin*,[50] the Supreme Court held that six-member juries were constitutional in civil cases and cited four "empirical" studies showing that there was no difference between the verdicts of six- and twelve-member juries.[51]

Some commentators have questioned the validity of these studies and disagreed with the Supreme Court's decisions.[52] Two of the studies cited by the Supreme Court were done by comparing the outcomes of cases with six- and twelve-member juries; no significant differences were found.[53] Unfortunately, these comparisons were not done between equivalent cases, which makes their conclusions questionable. For a lawyer, the choice between six- and twelve-member juries is seldom a random one. Where the number of jurors is optional, a lawyer will generally ask for a twelve-member jury in more difficult cases. Another of the studies cited by the Supreme Court did a comparison of outcomes of cases in a county that had switched from twelve- to six-member juries.[54] The conclusion was that there were no major differences. Unfortunately, the two sets of cases compared were not equivalent.[55] In streamlining their court systems to six-member juries, the county had also installed new arbitration procedures which changed the nature of the cases that came to court. In addition, because of an inflationary economy, there were difficulties in comparing monetary awards for the two time periods. The Kessler study,[56] cited by the Supreme Court, was an experiment using a taped mock trial and students as jurors. Kessler came to the conclusion that there were no major differences between six- and twelve-member juries. Diamond,[57] however, has pointed out that the evidence in this mock trial was so heavily weighted to one side that it would take much larger samples to demonstrate differences.

It is our conclusion that there are no clear data to resolve the issue of whether or not there is any difference between six- and twelve-member jury trials. We do believe that larger groups are more likely to represent varied perspectives.[58] Thus twelve-member juries are more likely to represent varied opinions on a case than six-member juries. We also believe that the more people there are in a minority faction, the more resistant to change that minority becomes. Asch[59] demonstrated that a lone person can be much more easily persuaded by a group than when that person has an ally. Since twelve-member juries are more likely to have a larger number of dissenters, it is possible that minority positions in a twelve-member jury are more resistant to consensual persuasion than in six-member juries. Thus it has been suggested that twelve-member juries are more susceptible to becoming hopelessly divided or "hung." What this means, from a defendant's point of view, is that when the facts of a case are against him, a twelve-member jury may be more advantageous because it is more likely to be "hung," while a six-member jury would be better when the evidence favors the defendant since it is less likely to be "hung." Valenti and Downing[60] tested these hypotheses and did find strong support for the first prediction, but weak support for the second. Unfortunately, even this study is inconclusive because jurors were limited on the amount of time that they could deliberate, and this could account for the differences in the numbers of "hung" juries. Perhaps it takes longer for twelve-member juries to deliberate than their six-member counterparts.[61]

UNANIMOUS VERSUS NONUNANIMOUS VERDICTS

The decision rule that governs a jury's verdict has also created a recent controversy. In two separate cases,[62] the U.S. Supreme Court ruled that jury verdicts need not be unanimous. This decision was based upon the assumption that nonunanimous verdicts will make no difference in the way jurors reach their decisions. To date, the evidence is inconclusive.

SUGGESTIONS FOR FUTURE RESEARCH

Part of the problem in demonstrating the effects of the size of the jury and the decision rule is that the impact may not be equally present in all types of trials. The discussion below will illustrate this point. Before we begin, however, the reader must be acquainted with a few basic principles in probability.

The probability that an event will occur in a certain way is "the ratio of the number of ways in which that favored way can occur to the total number of ways the event can occur."[63] For example, when a single coin is flipped in the air, it has a .50 probability of landing on either side. If we flip two coins together, one of the following possibilities will result: (a) HH, (b) HT, (c) TH, or (d) TT. Thus there is a .50 probability of getting one head and one tail, a .25 probability of getting two heads, and a .25 probability of getting two tails. There is a mathematical way of deriving these probabilities, known as a binomial expansion. For two coins the probabilities are derived from the following equation: $(1/2 + 1/2)^2 = 1/4 + 1/2 + 1/4$. For six coins the equation is $(1/2 + 1/2)^6$, and for twelve coins the equation is $(1/2 + 1/2)^{12}$. If we were dealing with unfair coins, so that each coin had a .25 probability of landing on heads and a .75 probability of landing on tails, then our predictions for six and twelve coins would be given by the following two equations: $(1/4 + 3/4)^6$ and $(1/2 + 3/4)^{12}$. Essentially, what we have done in Tables 42-1 and 42-2 is to solve these kinds of equations, as explained below.

Even though we cannot cite conclusive data, it seems reasonable to predict that twelve-member juries are more likely to have dissenting votes before deliberation.[64] We can estimate this difference between the six- and twelve-member juries in the following way. Let us compare five potential fact situations, of varying *unfavorable* weight for the defendant, as in Table 42-1. In one extreme case the evidence is such that only five out of 100 jurors would vote for a guilty verdict prior to deliberation, while on the other extreme the evidence is such that 95 out of 100 jurors would vote guilty prior to deliberation. If we considered the number of guilty–not guilty votes before deliberation as being a binomial distribution, the probabilities for unanimous and diverse opinions for six- and twelve-member juries can be calculated by a binomial expansion as presented in Table 42-1.[65]

As can be seen from this table, the probability of dissenters is consistently higher in twelve-member juries than in six-member juries. This may or may not make a difference in the final outcome of a particular case, but the least that can be said is that a twelve-member jury is more likely than a six-member jury to come to a verdict in light of having considered varying opinions during deliberations. Whether or not the number of dissenters in a jury is going to make any difference in the final outcome of a case will depend upon the fact situation of a case, all of the extraneous variables we have already discussed, and the resistance of the dissenters to being persuaded.

If it does make a difference, from Table 42-1 we can predict that the difference will appear in the form of a higher number of "hung" juries. Although Diamond[66] suggests that researchers use close cases to demonstrate these differences, from Table 42-1 we would suggest the opposite. That is, it is when the evidence is strong in one direction or the other that there is a greater probability of finding more dissenters in a twelve-member jury than in a six-member jury. Since the probability of "hung" juries under these conditions is low, large samples will have to be used before the differences become statistically testable. These methodological problems become compounded when the effects of the size of the jury are tested along with the effects of unanimous versus nonunanimous instructions, as discussed below.

TABLE 42-1. Probability of a Juror Reaching a Guilty Verdict Before Deliberation as a Measure of the Strength of the Case*

	.05		.25		.50		.75		.95	
Number of jurors	6	12	6	12	6	12	6	12	6	12
Probabilities for:										
Unanimous guilty opinions	.0000	.0000	.0002	.0000	.0156	.0002	.1780	.0317	.7351	.5404
Diverse opinions	.2649	.4596	.8218	.9683	.9688	.9996	.8218	.9683	.2649	.4596
Unanimous not guilty opinions	.7351	.5404	.1780	.0317	.0156	.0002	.0002	.0000	.0000	.0000

*Table shows probabilities of getting unanimous and diverse verdict opinions before deliberation in six- and twelve-member juries, given different conditions of evidence strength.

It would seem logical to assume that when a jury has no need to be unanimous, its members are not as likely to spend as much time and energy on dissenters as it would have to if unanimity were necessary. Upon analyzing this issue more deeply, however, researchers may find that this assumption is too simplistic. Nonunanimous versus unanimous conditions are not as likely to be direct and sole causes for differences in deliberations or verdicts as they are to be conditions which interact with other variables. For example, it is possible that the strength of jurors' convictions may interact with the decision rule requirements. Thus, when the majority on a jury panel is strongly convinced of its position, it is likely to spend little time with dissenters unless it has to. On the other hand, when the majority is not strongly convinced of its position, the decision requirements may make little difference during deliberations. In attempting to demonstrate the effects of decision requirements on deliberations, researchers would have a higher probably of success with trials in which the evidence seems weighted in one direction or the other.

Demonstrating the effects of the nonunanimous rule on the final verdicts presents a problem because verdicts result from predeliberation opinions in interaction with that which transpires during deliberation. Thus the ability to predict the effects of nonunanimous instructions on verdicts depends, to some extent, on our ability to predict its effects on deliberations. However, if we assume that all the variables that go into deciding a case interact and result in a certain probability that a juror will vote one way or the other, then we can make certain predictions.

If we consider the number of guilty and not-guilty votes as being a binomial distribution, the probabilities for unanimous and two-thirds majority votes and for six- and twelve-member juries can be calculated by a binomial expansion, as in Table 42-2 below. Please note that in Table 42-1 we were considering the probabilities of predeliberation votes, while here we are considering postdeliberation votes.

Each juror's final vote will depend on the fact situation of the case, all the extraneous variables discussed above, and his or her resistance to persuasion. As can be seen from Table 42-2, when all of these variables combine in such a way as to make the probability of a juror's vote very high in one direction or the other, the nonunanimous instruction is bound to make little difference in the final verdict. This, of course, says

TABLE 42.2. Probability of a Juror Voting for a Guilty Verdict After Deliberation as a Measure of the Strength of the Interaction of All Variables that Go into Deciding a Trial*

	.05		.50		.95	
Size of jury	6	12	6	12	6	12
Probabilities for:						
Unanimous guilty verdict	.0000	.0000	.0156	.0002	.7351	.5404
At least two-thirds majority guilty verdict	.0001	.0000	.3282	.0727	.7374	.5426
Unanimous not guilty verdict	.7351	.5404	.0156	.0002	.0000	.0000
At least two-thirds majority not guilty verdict	.7374	.5426	.3282	.0727	.0001	.0000

*Table shows probabilities of getting unanimous and two-thirds majority verdicts after deliberations in six- and twelve-member juries, given different conditions of the strength of the case.

nothing about the instruction's effects on deliberations, which in turn do affect verdicts. In contrast to the extremely strong or weak case, when the probability of a juror's vote is extremely close in one direction or the other, the nonunanimous instruction is much more likely to make a difference, especially in the smaller-sized jury. In such a situation, the chance that a six-member jury will reach a unanimous verdict is only 1.6 percent, and thus it is very likely that such a jury will be "hung." Under the same conditions, however, there is a 33 percent chance that a jury would be able to reach a verdict if given a nonunanimous instruction. One could argue that the chances for acquittal or conviction are equal, and therefore the condition does not prejudice the jury in one direction or the other. In response, however, it can be pointed out that under these conditions a defendant's acquittal or conviction would be solely left up to chance, and that is not the intention of the law.

Please note that the figures given in Tables 42-1 and 42-2 would be predictive only under the conditions specified and should not be used as predictions about the real population of trials. Since we do not know how many real trials fall under any of the conditions specified, we cannot make absolute predictions about the impact of the size and the unanimity requirements of jurors upon deliberations or verdicts. The figures we gave, however, should help a researcher to identify and use the type of trials that have the highest probability of being affected by the size of the jury and the decision rule.

We believe that the size of the jury will have its greatest probability of affecting the number of "hung verdicts" under conditions where the evidence is strong in one direction or the other. Unanimity requirements will have the greatest probability of affecting deliberations when the majority of jurors have very strong opinions about the case at bar. On the other hand, unanimity requirements have the greatest possibility of affecting the final verdicts when the probability of a juror's vote in one direction or the other is extremely close, especially in a six-member jury.

The Voir Dire

Voir dire is the French term used in law to refer to the process of selecting a jury out of a group of prospective jurors. Its purpose is to insure that a jury is composed of a representative sample of the community, and that it is composed of people competent to render a fair and impartial verdict.[67] During the voir dire procedure the judge and/or lawyers ask the prospective jurors (the venire) for personal information (e.g., occupation, marital status) and question them on a variety of issues that relate to the case. The judge and each lawyer are allowed to challenge the acceptability of the jurors questioned. There are three types of challenges: a challenge of the array, a challenge for cause, and a peremptory challenge.

A challenge of the array is a challenge of the entire venire on the grounds that it is not representative of the community. By law a jury is supposed to be representative of cross sections of the community.[68] For example, in a 1940 Supreme Court decision, *Smith v. Texas*,[69] the Court ruled that Smith had been denied equal protection under the Fourteenth Amendment because black jurors in the community had been kept off grand juries. In reality, however, few juries are truly representative of the community. Businessmen and professionals often avoid jury duty by arguing that it would create too much hardship on themselves, their families, and their employers. It can be fairly said that very often the only people who serve on juries are those who cannot evade it. Thus a disproportionate number of jurors are housewives, retired people, and lower or lower-middle income people.

A challenge for cause may occur when it is argued that a particular juror is unable to render a fair and impartial verdict. Reasons for such a challenge are usually enumerated by statute (e.g., a prospective juror does not speak English or is blatantly prejudiced toward one side). In some situations, the task of arriving at a competent as well as representative jury panel may be mutually exclusive, so that when one is completely achieved, the other is sacrificed.[70] For instance, in *Witherspoon v. Illinois*,[71] the Supreme Court overturned a death penalty verdict and ruled that since jurors who had expressed "qualms" about capital punishment had been disqualified, Witherspoon was convicted by a jury more prone to convict than a representative jury would have been. Thus there are limits to how far either challenge can be pressed. In any case, the judge rules on these two types of challenges.

There is one more type of challenge—the peremptory one. Each lawyer is allowed to remove a limited number of jurors without giving any reason for it. Because their peremptories are limited, lawyers try to use them strategically. Experienced trial lawyers take great pride in their ability to select a jury,[72] and legal journals are filled with quick lessons in this art.[73] Most of these lessons are based on personal experiences, and many times that is the best teacher of all. In the last few years, however, a number of social science researchers have attempted to develop and demonstrate empirically more effective ways of conducting the voir dire.

It should be noted in passing that not all lawyers believe in the voir dire as an effective method of screening,[74] even though there are some data suggesting that it is effective in selecting an impartial jury. Many lawyers have a fatalistic attitude and feel that the replacement for a challenged juror may not be any better. Thus some lawyers use the voir dire as a method of indoctrination.[74] Very little empirical psycholegal research has been done on the effectiveness of the voir dire in indoctrinating a jury.

CONDUCTING THE VOIR DIRE

The effectiveness of the voir dire should be determined by the social situation in which it is conducted. It normally takes place in the courtroom in the presence of the judge, lawyers, witnesses, other jurors, and the public. Two types of questioning techniques are used. Some questions are asked of an entire venire at the same time (e.g., Do any of you think that you will have difficulty rendering a fair and impartial judgment on Miss Smith because she is a prostitute?). Other questions are directed toward individual jurors in the presence of the rest of the venire.

There are several reasons why it is reasonable to assume that neither type of questioning technique is optimally effective in eliciting honest answers. First, it is important to understand the forces of conformity acting upon each of the prospective jurors. They are thrust into an unfamiliar environment with a group of strangers and thus may well be threatened by it. Such a situation will tend to elicit conformity on the part of each juror.[75] Especially in a threatening situation, it is unlikely that a juror will reveal his true feelings when a question is asked of the entire venire at once. Nor will a juror be prone to discredit himself when asked a direct question in front of all of these other people. Thus bringing in jurors as a group will tend to exert social pressures to give socially desirable responses. Perhaps one way to reduce these pressures is to remove jurors from the group settings and question them individually.

In many jurisdictions it is up to the judge to decide whether he, the lawyers, or both will conduct the voir dire. For the sake of saving time, the judge often decides to conduct it himself.[76] There is reason to believe that this practice is also *less* than optimally effective in eliciting honest and relevant answers.

One argument is that the judge is not as familiar with all of the issues that will be brought up during the course of the trial as are the lawyers who have prepared their cases. Thus, as questioning proceeds, judges are less likely to probe indepth areas that may indeed be relevant for determining the competency of a juror. Gutman[77] suggests that attorneys should conduct the voir dire as a matter of constitutional right.

Another argument that has been used is that lawyers are more likely than judges to elicit honest responses because of their strikingly different roles. A judge has a certain role to play, that of an impartial person, and this will tend to limit the kinds of questions that he can ask, the way in which he can ask them, and the way in which a juror perceives him. It is much more likely that a juror will be able to hide his true feelings when answering questions posed by this neutral figure than when posed by the attorneys. Lawyers, in contrast, are expected to play adversary roles and as adversaries can and will ask jurors more poignant questions in a more aggressive manner. They are perceived as more threatening by the juror. This tension should aid the elicitation of more honest answers.

WHAT TO LOOK FOR DURING THE VOIR DIRE

The suggestions we have made above were directed toward eliciting more honest responses from jurors. Besides the direct responses of jurors, there are other variables which might predict a juror's ability to render an impartial judgment. These variables include a juror's personality, demographic characteristics, and nonverbal responses to direct verbal questions. If paid attention to, these variables may make peremptory challenges more effective.

Personality

It would stand to reason that a juror's personality might have an effect on the way he interprets the evidence and renders a judgment. In recent years, several researchers have attempted to demonstrate that jurors with authoritarian personalities will tend to be more harsh on defendants than jurors with less authoritarian tendencies.

In two simulated studies by Gladstone[78] and Thayer,[79] in which attempts were made to find differences in punitiveness between high and low F-scale student respondents, the results were negative. However, in two other similar studies by Friend and Vinson[80] and by Mitchell and Byrne,[81] it was found that authoritarians were inclined to punish defendants more severely. Perhaps the reason for these mixed results is that all four of these studies were conducted with college students as subjects. The college student population is a somewhat homogeneous group with less extreme authoritarian tendencies than the population at large. Other studies have been made with the population at large as subjects, and in these cases the results have been somewhat clearer.[82]

Demography

Jurors' demographic characteristics have been suggested as factors predictive of their level of participation during deliberations, of the criteria that they will use in deciding on a verdict, and of their final verdicts. These characteristics include age,[83], sex,[84] occupation,[85] education,[86] religious affiliation,[87] and socioeconomic status.

We hesitate to delineate the specific findings since they would only apply to the specific cases and may not be generalized. For example, Snortum and Ashear[88] found that males were more punitive toward the defendant in rape cases. As another example, Becker and associates[89] found Catholics to be more punitive on the issue of euthanasia. Unfortunately, we cannot take these findings as a basis for determining how males or Catholics would judge a defendant in most other types of cases.

In recognition of the fact that demographic characteristics cannot be generalized too far as predictors, Schulman helps lawyers during jury selection by collecting attitudinal data on the specific issues in the case from a representative sample of the population from which the jury was drawn.[90] With this information, Schulman can demonstrate the prejudice and bias of the various demographic groups and subgroups with respect to issues within the case at hand. This information can then be compared to the demographic characteristics of the prospective jurors. In contrast to the difficulty that a lawyer would have in gathering information about a juror's personality, each juror's demographic characteristics are traditionally asked for and easily accessible during voir dire.

Nonverbal Cues

Recently, social scientists have suggested that nonverbal cues be used during the voir dire to determine a juror's acceptability.[91] This information can be used by lawyers in determining whether jurors are more favorably disposed to one side or the other. Sales and Suggs are currently testing the validity of such a method, but no data have been published to date.

It is reasonable to assume that when a juror lies, or when he does not favor a lawyer or his client, he is likely to feel at least slightly more anxious than he normally would, and this in turn will manifest itself in paralinguistic and kinesic behavior. Paralinguistic behavior includes such variables as breathing rate, pauses, speed of speech, and stuttering. Kinesic behavior includes such variables as facial expressions, body position, and hand movements. There is a great deal of literature that delineates the specific paralinguistic and kinesic behaviors that can be expected when a person is anxious as a result of the fact that he is lying or is not receptive to some other person in the situation.[92] From this literature, it would stand to reason that peremptory challenges of jurors could be made much more selectively if lawyers or their assistants were trained to observe nonverbal cues. This level of analysis has the particular advantage of not requiring any changes in the voir dire process.

Sequestration

To guard against higher court appeals on the grounds that trial publicity has made it impossible for a jury to reach an impartial decision, the trial judge sometimes sequesters the jury. Such actions are usually taken only in extraordinary cases which have received a great deal of mass-media publicity. The effects of sequestration have not yet been fully studied, but three generalizations are offered here.

The most obvious effect of sequestration is that it insulates jurors from information in the media. It is commonly believed that such information will affect a jury's verdict. Indeed, several researchers have suggested that trial publicity can color jurors' evaluations of the evidence and can affect a jury's verdict.[93] Trial publicity will especially affect a jury's verdict when the evidence presented in a trial is weak[94] and/or when the publicity is strongly damaging.[95] Sequestration is designed to insure that a defendant will be tried only on the evidence presented in the courtroom.

The second reason for sequestering a jury is that it protects jurors from being influenced by family, friends, and public opinion.[96] It is logical to assume that social interaction with people outside the jury might weaken a juror's ability to remain impartial, and from that point of view sequestration may have positive effects. However, there is a possibility that sequestration can affect the interaction of jurors in detrimental ways. Janis,[97] for example, has suggested that isolated groups often begin to live in a world of illusions about morality, invulnerability, and unanimity. Cohesiveness sometimes becomes such an overwhelming goal that extreme conformity can result. How would this affect a person's constitutional right to a fair trial? Unfortunately, there is no empirical research on the social and psychological effects of sequestration on jurors.

Deliberations

Very few researchers have been able to study the process that takes place in an actual jury room.[98] One of the finest attempts at reproducing what occurs during deliberations is included in Rita James Simon's book, *The Jury and the Defense of Insanity*.[99]

Among the topics discussed in the literature on jury deliberations is the relationship between a juror's characteristics and the kind of participation that can be expected from that person. For example, James[100] reported in 1959 that males particpated more actively than females. (It should be noted that this finding may not be applicable today.) Hawkins[101] reported that dissenters on a jury panel tend to be very talkative because they are forced to clarify their position to the rest of the jurors. Bevan[102] found that an autocratic as opposed to a democratic foreman was effective in leading jurors to quicker decisions. Kessler[103] has provided a useful review of this literature.

Individual indications of predeliberation attitudes* generally determine postdeliberation jury verdicts.[104] Several studies, however, have suggested that deliberations have a tendency of shifting verdicts toward greater leniency.[105] One explanation for this tendency is that it may be easier to convince dissenters to vote for a not guilty verdict than for a finding of guilt. That is, in giving in to the rest of the group, jurors might feel less anxiety about letting a guilty defendant go free than about convicting an innocent person. Thus not guilty verdicts may not always be as unanimous as they seem.

There is evidence, on the other hand, that when a jury does bring in a guilty verdict, its individual members actually increase their negative

---

*These occur when juries take a vote as soon as they sit down after hearing the case and before they begin to discuss the case.

evaluations of the defendant.[106] One possible explanation for this is that jurors feel a tremendous amount of anxiety in bringing in a guilty verdict and seek social validation from each other before doing so. In convincing each other that they are doing the right thing, they actually increase their negative evaluations of the defendant and thus feel less anxious about deciding on a guilty verdict.

The Judge

Although the judge is at least as important as the jury in the trial process, relatively little psycholegal experimental attention has been paid to his work. This may be due to the fact that it is difficult to get judges to participate in experimental studies. It is equally problematic to attempt to simulate their behavior. What little research has been performed is anecdotal, and thus this section will discuss only those topics that have been shown to be open to experimental investigation.

Throughout a trial, the judge is responsible for instructing the jury on various topics. These instructions may be broken down into instructions that describe the role of the jury, the role of the judge, and instructions about the substantive law that must guide the jury in weighing the evidence in reaching a decision. The latter is also called "the charge to the jury" at the end of the evidence.

When people drawn from the jury pool first enter the courtroom, they usually have very little idea about what is expected of them. The purpose of the first two types of instructions is to inform the jurors of what role they and the judge should play in the trial. These preliminary instructions will include such things as the jurors' conduct during the trial, their need for impartiality, and their duties as triers of fact. Similarly, it is important that the jurors fully understand the role of the judge during the proceedings. They must be informed of his duty to make decisions as to the appropriate law controlling the case, his duty to instruct the jurors as to the law that they must apply to the case, and his general responsibility for the conduct of the entire proceeding.

Substantive instructions, or the charge to the jury, are given at the very end of a trial's proceedings after the closing arguments. The purpose is to state the law that governs the case. These instructions define legal terms and explain how jurors should apply the law in interpreting the facts and in reaching their verdict.

An example of one of these instructions is presented below. Before reading it, however, imagine yourself an average juror sitting and listening to a complete charge to a jury for as long as an hour or two. Would you be able to comprehend, remember, and apply the law it contains?

> A person furnishing or leasing an article to another for compensation owes a duty to such person to whom the article is supplied and to all others whom the supplier should expect to use the article with the consent of the person to whom furnished or who may be endangered by its probable use, to exercise ordinary care to see that the article, when furnished, is in a reasonably safe condition to avoid injury to such persons, and to see that such article is free from defect of which he had knowledge, or should have had knowledge, or which he could have discovered by reasonable inspection or by such simple and available tests as to its condition as the intended use would normally suggest, unless: (1) the person so furnishing had reasonable cause to be-

lieve that the user would discover the defect and realize the danger, or (2) the person so furnishing used reasonable care to warn the user of the dangerous condition. [*Nebraska Jury Instructions*, 11.01]

It should not come as a surprise that several researchers have found that jurors are often confused by jury instructions.[107] The problem of the use of incomprehensible language in the judge's charge to the jury has been analyzed by Sales, Elwork, and Alfini.[108] In reviewing the available psycholinguistic knowledge, these researchers have outlined many of the variables that should be controlled in writing more comprehensible instructions.

Not only have judges failed to take steps to insure that their instructions are phrased in clearer language, but they have also failed to consider other factors which could have an effect upon the jurors' understanding of their duties and of the applicable law. For the most part, these factors are procedural in nature. For example, consider the timing of presentation of the instructions. The prevailing practice is to instruct the jury on the law at the close of the case; that is, after argument and just before the jury retires to deliberate. This practice has received criticism in that it is believed to lead to juror confusion.[109] Would not the jury be better able to weigh the evidence if they were instructed on the applicable law prior to the presentation of the case?

The presentation of instructions to jurors at the end of a trial is psychologically suspect for two reasons. First, it assumes that the jurors have perfect memories and that once charged with instructions, they can selectively recall and evaluate all of the appropriate evidence. In addition, it assumes that until the instructions are given, the jurors will passively listen to all of the evidence without evaluating it. Neither of these assumptions is supported by research literature.[110]

What about the manner of presenting the instructions to the jury? In most jurisdictions, the judge reads the instructions to the jury. Commentators have discussed the efficacy of allowing the jury to take copies of the judge's instructions into the jury room.[111] If the charge is long, as is often the case, is the average juror expected to remember all the critical points of law? One way to increase the probability that jurors will comprehend and remember instructions would be to present them in written form as well as orally. The longer and more complex the jury instructions, the more justification there is for presenting them in written form. Several jurisdictions allow the judge to comment on the evidence or to summarize it. The various approaches may have differential impact on a juror's decision-making ability to reach a verdict on the basis of the evidence presented at the trial and in light of the law. To the best of our knowledge these procedural variables have never been studied, although the potential for differential impact on the ultimate result of the trial is obvious.

Similarly, how effective are a judge's instructions to a jury to disregard certain testimony? The few studies that have been done have yielded mixed results.[112] It seems reasonable to predict that the effectiveness of this type of instruction will depend a great deal on the relevance of the deleted evidence. A previous arrest record on similar charges, for example, is one kind of evidence that can be devastating to the defendant's credibility. It is doubtful that once such information is introduced a judge's instruction to ignore it could be followed.

Another important duty for a judge in a criminal trial is sentencing. Within certain limitations, a judge has a great deal of discretion in imposing a sentence, although he should consider the nature of the offense, the character of the defendant, and the public interest involved.

One of the most common criticisms of criminal sentencing is the wide disparity that often occurs in sentencing defendants who have committed similar crimes.[113] Several researchers have found statistically significant disparities in sentences given to defendants of different races and socioeconomic status.[114] As Howard has observed, "Judges, like all other human beings, are products of their experiences. The way they think, their value systems and defenses come largely from society and its influence on them."[115] Thus it is not surprising that some of the same prejudices that exist in our society are reflected in judges' sentencing.

The Lawyers

After participating in the voir dire, each lawyer's task is to present the case for his client. The presentation can be divided into three parts: the opening statement, the presentation of evidence, and the closing argument. In the opening statement, the lawyer attempts to outline the evidence he intends to present. In presenting this evidence, the lawyer's task is to examine favorable witnesses and to cross-examine unfavorable ones. Throughout all of this, the lawyers are in a constant battle to present strong evidence that will withstand cross-examination and to undermine the evidence presented by the opponent. When the evidence is close, as it often is, the battle results in the jury's swaying back and forth on their opinions of the guilt or innocence of the defendant.[116] By the time all of the evidence is presented, however, many jurors will have made their decisions. A jury is likely to favor the side whose evidence outweighs the other's in either quality or quantity.[117]

After the testimonial evidence is completed, the closing arguments are the lawyers' final opportunity to convince the jury. Whereas during the presentation of evidence both lawyers are restricted to factual information, the closing arguments are intentionally argumentative.[118] Furthermore, in the closing arguments, the lawyers are permitted to address the jury directly, draw inferences, express opinions, and use all of their persuasive skills to convince the jury to accept their position. Although there is a great deal of psychological literature on persuasion techniques, very few psycholegal researchers have applied their findings to the courtroom situation. The only applications we have found have dealt with suggestions concerning the way lawyers should organize and argue their case.[119]

The order in which the evidence and the arguments are presented in a trial is set by law. The prosecution (or plaintiff) presents its evidence first; when the time comes for closing arguments, however, the order is reversed. Since the defendant is presumed to be innocent, the prosecution has the burden of proof and thus is given the advantage of the last word. These legally set orderings have recently come under analysis by several researchers.

Walker, Thibaut, and Andreoli[120] have conducted a simulated study in which they attempted to determine whether presenting evidence first or second in an adversary situation has an advantage in convincing the jury. They found that the side presenting second has a distinct advantage. One explanation for this is that in an adversary system the jurors are keenly aware that each bit of evidence is carefully selected to present a favorable impression. It has been shown that when a person expects to hear a different version of a story, he tends to suspend judgment of the first version until all sides are heard.[121] It is this "suspension of commitment" that may explain the findings of Walker, Thibaut, and Andreoli.

It would seem then that the defense, in presenting its evidence second, has the advantage in convincing a jury. The experiment, however, had a significant flaw. Unlike a real trial, both sides of the case were permitted to present their witnesses without being cross-examined. As Lawson argues, the fact that in a real trial every witness can be cross-examined may in fact substantially reduce any advantage in going first or second.[122]

Walker, Thibaut, and Andreoli also tested the effect of presenting the strongest evidence first or last (anticlimactic versus climactic order). Their finding was that the climactic order is more effective in convincing a jury. This order is especially effective for the prosecution and less effective for the defense. That is, the accusing side is especially advantaged by building a climactic case because of the emotionality it is bound to elicit.

Unfortunately, the same major flaw we mentioned before also stands in the way of making this experiment convincing on the matter of the effectiveness of a climactic order. It is possible that cross-examination has the tendency of wearing away the effectiveness of a climactic order of presentation.

The effect of the order in which closing arguments are presented is another area which needs study. As mentioned earlier, the prosecution has the last word under the assumption that this order is advantageous. In reviewing the literature on persuasion techniques, Lawson[123] has suggested that the evidence is not so clear-cut as to require the conclusion that it is advantageous to be either first or second in closing arguments. He maintains that the extent to which a listener already holds opinions on a topic will affect whether the order of arguments will make any difference in the final outcome. Several researchers have found that when a person is not already predisposed to one side or the other, the side that is first in attempting to convince that person will have better success than subsequent attempts, even when the person expects more than one persuasive argument.[124] To the extent that some jurors will not have come to conclusions on their own, these experiments suggest that it is the defense and not the prosecution that has the advantage in closing arguments. It is naive, however, to assume that most jurors will not have opinions of their own, regardless of the instructions they receive from the judge. People who already have opinions of their own on a topic may be very resistant to being persuaded solely because of the order of presentation of the arguments.[125] Thus, until there is direct psycholegal research on this matter, we cannot conclude that the order in which arguments are presented affects the final outcome of a trial.

As Lawson has noted, the trial advocate is always confronted with the dilemma of whether to limit his communication to strictly supportive material or to anticipate in an attempt to demolish his opponent's argument before it is raised.[126] The one-sided versus two-sided argument has never been empirically studied in the courtroom situation. Nevertheless, since the general topic has been the subject of a great deal of psychological research, certain conclusions can be offered.

In previous psychological research, two-sided arguments have been found to be consistently more effective than one-sided presentations. One of the main strengths of a two-sided argument is that it tends to deal with, and therefore offset, counterarguments to the one being advocated.[127] Another of its strengths is that it tends to attribute fairness and thoroughness to the persuader.[128] Two-sided arguments are especially effective with people who are initially opposed to the view being proposed.[129] Since these are the people that need to be persuaded, two-sided arguments should be used all of the time. In addition, a two-sided argument should also be more effective in making the fact-finders more resistant to persuasion by the opposing attorney.

The Witness

Of all the areas of psycholegal research, the area of witness testimony has had the oldest tradition.[130] In 1904, Beecher outlined the directions that he felt this line of research should take. The object of evidence, he stressed, is to establish truth. But truth has a dual meaning. There is truth in the sense of sincerity and truth in the sense of accuracy. Courts have always been concerned with insuring sincerity by having witnesses take an oath and by enforcing strict penalties for perjury. The growing use of technological methods such as lie detectors has been another major step in insuring sincerity. Unfortunately, courts have not been as concerned with insuring the accuracy of testimony. This lack of concern and the fact that psychologists could make a major step in insuring accuracy were the major themes in Munsterberg's book, *On the Witness Stand*. Nevertheless, as Wigmore[131] has pointed out, psychologists of that time did not have the strong empirical evidence necessary to convince courts to follow their direction. In the past few years psycholegal researchers have begun to amass evidence specifically directed toward demonstrating the problems with courtroom testimony.[132] We will outline this research and present its major themes.

Courts have functioned under the assumption that being sincere was equivalent to telling the truth, as if witnesses are capable of perfect perception, recollection, and articulation.[133] The major themes of psycholegal research on testimony have dealt with demonstrating human limitations in these three abilities.

The fallibility of human perception and memory are due to internal as well as external factors. By internal factors we refer to those physiological and psychological states and events that determine a person's perception and memory. By external factors we refer to the environmental variables which affect a person's perception and memory.

INTERNAL FACTORS

There are obvious internal factors limiting perception and memory, such as the age and health of a witness. We will not discuss these, however, but instead focus upon less obvious factors that have been neglected by courts.

One of the internal variables that is responsible for inaccuracies in testimony is the expectation that people bring to any situation. For example, there have been several reports of situational expectancies determining perceptual experiences. Sommer[134] reported a case of a hunter who mistook another hunter for a deer and shot him. At the trial, the police reconstructed the scene and reported that under similar visibility conditions it was unlikely that anyone could have made the mistake the defendant was claiming. The major variable missing from the police reconstruction was the fact that whereas the police expected to see a man, the defendant expected to see a deer.

It has been suggested that psychologists be allowed to aid courts in determining the reliability of testimony.[135] There is precedent for this in Great Britain, where a psychologist was called to help in the defense of an "indecent acts" trial.[136] The defense attorney argued that the only reason the police had perceived what they thought were indecent acts by the defendants was that the complaining neighbors had labeled them as such, and that this labeling in turn determined the arresting policemen's perceptual expectations and experience. In aiding the court, the psychologist performed an experiment in which three sets of people with varying expectations were asked to look at the same pictures. The experiment demonstrated that those people who expected to see indecent acts did so with a greater frequency than those people who did not have those expectations.

In addition to situational expectancies, more permanent aspects of a person's personality will also determine a person's perceptual experiences. Marshall,[137] for example, found that punitive people (e.g., authoritarians) had greater correct recall of the details of a simulated kidnapping scene than a comparable nonpunitive group. One explanation for this is that punitive people are more expectant of malice from others and therefore are more alert to threatening situations. Along the same lines, Allport and Kramer[138] found that anti-Semitic individuals could identify Jews from non-Jews more frequently than the population at large. In another experiment, Allport[139] demonstrated how stereotyping can lower a person's ability to perceive and remember correctly. Subjects were asked to look at a drawing of people in a subway train, which included a black man standing next to a white man who was holding a razor. When asked which man held the razor in his hand, half of the subjects incorrectly reported that it was the black man.

The most striking example of the courts' neglect in insuring accuracy and the courts' concern with insuring sincerity is their treatment of hearsay evidence given under conditions of emotional stress. Normally, hearsay testimony is not allowed as evidence because it does not insure against insincerity on the part of the person being quoted, since that person is not in court to be cross-examined and viewed by the jury. One exception to this rule is the "spontaneous exclamation." That is, hearsay is allowed if it can be shown that the person being quoted was under enough emotional stress to say things "spontaneously" without the ability or will to edit his utterances for the listener. The assumption is that under emotional stress people tell the truth (in the sense of sincerity). There is little psychological evidence to support this assumption. Even if it were true that people are most sincere under conditions of emotional stress, the rule on spontaneous exclamations ignores evidence that emotional stress tends to limit perceptual and memorial accuracy.[140]

To some extent emotionally significant events do tend to arouse perceptual acuteness and do tend to make memories more vivid. However, there is a point beyond which emotional arousal begins to narrow observation and distort memory. Under extreme states of emotional arousal, a person becomes very concerned about himself and is therefore less capable of perceiving or remembering details about the environment.[141] Such events as robberies, accidents, and murders are the kinds of emotionally upsetting events that make eyewitness testimony extremely unreliable. For example, Hutchins and Slesinger[142] did an experiment in which several confederates were asked to stage a fight in one of their classrooms. After the fight, students were asked to give reports on what had occurred. The results showed that those students who were most upset by the incident gave the least accurate description of what happened.

EXTERNAL FACTORS

There are many external factors which will tend to limit a witness' perceptual and memorial accuracy. Perceptual accuracy will be affected by such factors as exposure time, distance, lighting and noise conditions, and movement and speed of the phenomena being observed.[143] The characteristics of the object of perception will also affect accuracy. Action events, for example, will be perceived much more accurately than the background (e.g., noise, crowd) in which they occur. The extent to which things are perceived will affect the extent to which they are remembered. In addition, memory will be affected by the time lapse between the perception and occasion on which it is recalled.

The general unreliability of human voice and face identification has been established empirically in the laboratory.[144] For example, several laboratory studies have demonstrated an average 30 percent error rate in tasks where people were shown faces for a brief period of time and then after a few days were asked to recognize the faces they had seen previously.[145] In addition, several researchers have demonstrated that recognition rates are not the same for all types of faces. For example, white subjects have been shown to be more able to recognize white faces than Oriental or black faces.[146]

Whereas the subjects in the above experiments knew that they would be quizzed later, real-life witnesses are seldom aware while they are witnessing a crime that they will later be asked to recall events and identify people. It has been shown that when people are aware that they will be asked to reconstruct events they are witnessing, they tend to perceive and remember those events much more clearly than if they are not aware of their future roles.[147]

Although eyewitness testimony has been shown to be inaccurate, it tends to be the strongest and most acceptable kind of evidence. Why is it that these supposed inaccuracies seldom become apparent in court? There are several reasons, but the main one is that the witnesses themselves are unaware of their own misrepresentations, thinking that sincerity is all that is necessary to telling the truth. With the passage of time, everyone has a tendency to begin forgetting the details of what was witnessed. Very often, however, our minds unintentionally fill in the gaps with memories of other experiences[148] or other people's recollections of the same events. For example, while the courts have often been concerned with the effects of trial publicity on jurors, little has been said on the effects of trial publicity on the witnesses. It has been shown, however, that after a time people do begin to confuse their memories of newspaper reports with their own first-hand memories of events.[149] The more a witness repeats a story, as is the case during preparation for a trial, the more that witness is likely to believe it himself.

Investigation techniques by police have also been criticized for causing distortions in eyewitness testimony, as in the case of lineup identifications. Lineups are social-psychological situations with many biasing factors. Typically a witness is placed in a situation where everyone expects and wants the witness to identify the criminal. Since a cooperative witness is very much influenced by these social pressures and wants to be cooperative, such pressures tend to make it likely that someone will be identified. Police practices in choosing lineup participants also have been criticized for biasing eyewitness identification. Doob and Kirshenbaum[150] reported a study in which it was demonstrated that although witnesses may not remember the details of the physical characteristics of a suspect, in lineups they will choose people who best approximate those features they do remember. Thus, when a witness describes the criminal as being tall, the police should not select a lineup of five men who are short and one man who is over 6 feet tall.

ARTICULATION

Given that there are limitations to human perception and memory, information can also be distorted in the way that it is communicated. The questions that lawyers ask of a witness will definitely affect the accuracy of that witness' testimony. As early as 1909, Whipple demonstrated how questions by lawyers could affect the accuracy of testimony. On one extreme, a lawyer can ask a witness to give a free narrative account of what he knows. On the other extreme, the lawyer can prearrange very specific questions with which to interrogate the witness. A free narrative has the advantage of being less suggestive, but is likely to elicit irrelevant testimony. Prearranged interrogatory questions have the advantage of keeping a witness on track, but the disadvantage of being very suggestive.

Several researchers have studied how the specificity of questions lowers the accuracy of a witness' testimony.[151] In one laboratory experiment, subjects were asked to watch a short film of an auto accident and later were asked questions about what they had seen.[152] Some subjects received implicative questions such as, "Did you see *the* broken headlight?" Other subjects were asked more disjunctive questions such as, "Did you see *a* broken headlight?" The results showed that subjects who were asked implicative questions were more likely to report having seen something, whether or not it was in the film. In another similar experiment, Loftus and Palmer[153] found that subjects gave higher estimates when asked "About how fast were the cars going when they *smashed* into each other?" than when they were asked "About how fast were the cars going when they *hit* each other?" It has also been demonstrated that suggestive questioning affects not only the actual answers that subjects give, but also their own memorial representations of the witnessed events. Even when biased questions do not affect the witness' testimony, they do significantly affect jurors' interpretations and reconstructions of the testimony.[154]

SOME FINAL CONSIDERATIONS

Psycholegal research, like all research, has suffered from methodological problems. Some of these have been discussed within the body of this chapter. They are sufficiently important, however, to warrant addressing these concerns again. In the past, researchers on the trial process have been broadly criticized on three counts:[155] (1) they have often misunderstood the legal adversarial system; (2) they have often engaged in research which failed to conform to legal realities; and (3) they have often come to unjustified and overgeneralized conclusions.[156]

The first criticism, that psycholegal researchers have often misunderstood our adversarial system, is self-explanatory. The quality of any researcher's work will be partially determined by his ability to appreciate the system that he is studying. This means that he must seek the help of people versed in the law to help him to identify the issues in need of study. Unfortunately, there is still a great deal of antipathy between social scientists and people in the legal system. If advancement is to occur, this communications gap must be closed.

The communications gap has caused many psycholegal researchers to conduct studies which failed to take account of legal realities. In addition, since much psycholegal research has been performed primarily to test a psychological theory, legal realities often suffer. Purely psychological research, however, can be made legally relevant, thus resulting in double gains.

One only has to look at a typical psycholegal experiment to realize why the third criticism, reaching unjustified conclusions, has a great deal of merit. Researchers on the trial process have often turned to the use of simulations of an actual trial. Simulation is often a very effective technique. Some of the simulations have, however, been grossly inadequate and have thus greatly limited the validity of the findings. A typical experiment starts out with the experimenter advertising on the campus for volunteer college students to act as jurors. These students are then directed as to the time and the classroom in which the experiment will be conducted. Upon arrival they are given a short written summary of the "evidence" in the case, followed by a questionnaire, the content of which depends upon the experimenter's interests.

In doing such research the experimenter needs to ask himself many questions. For example, is the sign-up method equivalent to the voir dire in a real case? Can students represent average jurors who are older and less educated and who often have more disparate attitudes and beliefs? Does the atmosphere of a classroom provide a sufficiently realistic environment? Does the short written summary of a case adequately simulate the complexity of the evidence, the credibility of the witnesses, the demeanor of the attorneys, the judge, and the litigants? Does the use of a questionnaire to probe responses adequately reflect the decision-making processes of the jurors during deliberation?

In the past few years there has been an upsurge in the number of researchers who have taken the external validity problem more seriously and have attempted to correct for it by using videotapes of full trials and by using jurors drawn from the actual jury population. There are times when less realistic simulations are appropriate. For example, if a researcher is studying the visual field that a juror has from a jury box, the concerns raised above would be of no real consequence. Even when the concerns are applicable, it may be appropriate to perform less representative simulations as pilot studies.

Finally, it should be noted that external validity may be impossible to attain in psycholegal research on the jury and trial processes due to ethical limitations. External validity could only be adequately achieved by conducting the research within the confines of an actual trial or deceiving the juror-subjects into believing that they were participating in an actual trial.

No matter how characteristic the simulation, it still differs from an actual trial since the juror-subjects know that it is an experiment. This knowledge may affect their decision processes. Thus, to insure complete external validity, researchers may be tempted to deceive the subjects. This could be done by conducting the experiment in a vacant courtroom, using jurors actually called for jury duty that day, and employing either professional actors to re-enact the case or a videotape of a real or simulated case. This solution seems ideal, at least superficially. Unfortunately, deception requires debriefing, and debriefing will create a situation where henceforth those jurors and others who hear about it will be suspicious of whether they are participating in an actual trial or in an experiment. This doubt may affect their deliberations and thus prejudice the right to a fair trial. We must therefore caution researchers not to use deception in circumstances which may corrupt the very system they wish to study.

REFERENCES

1. Special Commission on the Social Sciences of the National Science Board: *Knowledge into Action: Improving the Nation's Use of the Social Sciences.* National Science Foundation, Washington, D.C., 1969.
2. Munsterberg, H.: *On the Witness Stand.* Doubleday, Page, New York, 1908, p. 117.
3. Greer, D. S.: Anything But the Truth? The Reliability of Testimony in Criminal Trials. *Br. J. Criminol.* 11:131–154, 1971.
4. Wigmore, J. H.: Professor Munsterberg and the Psychology of Testimony. *Illinois Law Rev.* 3:399, 1909.
5. Sherif, C. W., Sherif, M., and Nebergall, R.: *Attitude and Attitude Change: The Social Judgment-Involvement Approach.* W. B. Saunders, Philadelphia, 1965.
6. Pepitone, A., and DiNubile, M.: Contrast Effects in Judgments of Crime Severity and the Punishment of Criminal Violators. *J. Personality Social Psychol.* 33(4):448–459, 1976.
7. Kalven, H., Jr., and Zeisel, H.: *The American Jury.* Little, Brown, Boston, 1966, p. 17.
8. Thibaut, J., and Walker, L.: *Procedural Justice: A Psychological Analysis.* Lawrence Earbaum Associates, Hillside, N.J., 1975.
9. Brett, P.: Legal Decision-making and Bias: A critique of an Experiment. *U. Colorado Law Rev.* 45:1–24, 1973.
10. Thibaut, J., Walker, L., and Lind, E. A.: Adversary Presentation and Bias in Legal Decision-making. *Harvard Law Rev.* 86:386–401, 1972.
11. Sears, D. O.: Opinion Formation and Information Preferences in an Adversary Situation. *J. Exp. Social Psychol.* 2:130–142, 1966.
12. Walker, L., LaTour, S., Lind, E. A., and Thibaut, J.: Reactions of Participants and Observers to Modes of Adjudication. *J. Appl. Social Psychol.* 4:295–310, 1974.
13. Thibaut and Walker, op. cit., chap. 3.
14. Lind, E. A., Thibaut, J., and Walker, L.: Discovery and Presentation of Evidence in Adversary and Nonadversary Proceedings. *Michigan Law Rev.* 71:1129–1144, 1973; Lind, E. A.: The Exercise of Information Influence in Legal Advocacy. *J. Appl. Social Psychol.* 5:127–143, 1975.
15. Beecher, F.: Evidence versus Psychology. *Canadian Law Times* 24:195–200, 1904.
16. Bazelon, D. L.: Psychiatrists and the Adversary Process. *Sci. Am.* 230(6):18–23, 1974.
17. Levine, M.: Scientific Method and the Adversary Model. *Am. Psychologist* 29:661–675, 1974.
18. Maslow, A. H.: *The Psychology of Science.* Henry Regnery, Chicago, 1969; Rychlak, J. F.: *A Philosophy of Science for Personality Theory.* Houghton Mifflin, Boston, 1968.
19. Wolf, R. L.: *The Application of Select Legal Concepts to Evaluation Research.* Unpublished doctoral dissertation, University of Illinois, Urbana, School of Education, 1973.
20. Kalven and Zeisel, op. cit.
21. Ibid., p. 45.
22. Ibid., p. 59.
23. Mysliwiec, S. R.: Towards Principles of Jury Equity. *Yale Law J.* 83:1023–1054, 1974; Savitsky, J. C., and Sim, M. E.: Trading Emotions: Equity Theory of Reward and Punishment. *J. Communication* 24:140–147, 1974.
24. Kalven and Zeisel, op. cit., p. 305.
25. Mysliwiec, op. cit.

26. Kalven and Zeisel, op. cit., chap. 17.
27. Ibid., chaps. 15, 30.
28. Ibid.
29. Ibid.
30. Brooks, W. N., and Doob, A. N.: Justice and the Jury. *J. Social Issues* 31(3):171–182, 1975.
31. Goldman, J., Maitland, K. A., and Norton, P. L.: Psychological Aspects of Jury Performance. *J. Psychiatry Law* 3:367–379, 1975.
32. Jurow, G. L.: New Data on the Effect of a "Death Qualified" Jury on the Guilt Determination Process. *Harvard Law Rev.* 84:567–611, 1971.
33. Vidmar, N.: Effects of Decision Alternatives on the Verdicts and Social Perceptions of Simulated Jurors. *J. Personality Social Psychol.* 22:211–218, 1972.
34. Hester, R. K., and Smith, R. E.: Effects of a Mandatory Death Penalty on the Decisions of Simulated Jurors as a Function of Heinousness of the Crime. *J. Crim. Justice* 1:319–326, 1973.
35. Chaikin, A. L., and Darley, J. M., Jr.: Victim or Perpetrator: Defensive Attribution of Responsibility and the Need for Order and Justice. *J. Personality Social Psychol.* 25:268–275, 1973; DeJong, W., Morris, W. N., and Hastorf, A. H.: Effect of an Escaped Accomplice on the Punishment Assigned to a Criminal Defendant. *J. Personality Social Psychol.* 33(2):192–198, 1976: Walster, E.: Assignment of Responsibility for an Accident. *J. Personality Social Psychol.* 3:73–79, 1966; cf., Shaver, K. G.: Defensive Attribution: Effects of Severity and Relevance on the Responsibility Assigned for an Accident. *J. Personality Social Psychol.* 14:101–113, 1970.
36. Fishman, L., and Izzett, R. R.: The Influence of a Defendant's Attractiveness and Justification for His Act on the Sentencing Tendencies of Subject-Jurors. Paper presented at Midwestern Psychological Association Meeting, 1974; Friend, R. M., and Vinson, M.: Leaning Over Backwards—Jurors' Responses to Defendants' Attractiveness. *J. Communication* 24:124–129, 1974; Griffitt, W., and Jackson, T.: Simulated Jury Decisions: Influence of Jury-Defendant Attitude Similarity-Dissimilarity. *Social Behav. Personality* 1:1–7, 1973; Izzett, R. R., and Leginski, W.: Group Discussion and the Influence of Defendant Characteristics in a Simulated Jury Setting. *J. Social Psychol.* 93:271–279, 1974; Kaplan, M. F., and Kemmerick, G. D.: Juror Judgment as Information Integration: Combining Evidential and Nonevidential Information. *J. Personality Social Psychol.* 30:493–499, 1974; Landy, D., and Aronson, E.: The Influence of the Character of the Criminal and His Victim on the Decision of Simulated Jurors. *J. Exp. Social Psychol.* 5:141–152, 1969; Mitchell, H. E., and Byrne, D.: Minimizing the Influence of Irrelevant Factors in the Courtroom: The Defendant's Character, Judge's Instructions, and Authoritarianism. Paper presented at the Midwestern Psychological Association Meeting, 1972; Mitchell, H. E., and Byrne, D.: The Defendant's Dilemma: Effect of Juror's Attitudes and Authoritarianism on Judicial Decisions. *J. Personality Social Psychol.* 25:123–129, 1973; Nemeth, C., and Sosis, R. H.: A Simulated Jury Study: Characteristics of the Defendant and Jurors. *J. Social Psychol.* 90:221–229, 1973; Reynolds, D. E., and Sanders, M. S.: The Effects of Defendant Attractiveness, Age, and Injury on Severity of Sentence Given by Simulated Jurors. Paper presented at Western Psychological Association Meeting, 1973; Sigall, H., and Landy, D.: Effects of the Defendant's Character and Suffering on Juridic Judgment: A Replication and Clarification. *J. Social Psychol.* 88:149–150, 1972.
37. Griffitt and Jackson, op. cit.
38. Doob, A. N., and Kirshenbaum, H. M.: Some Empirical Evidence on the Effect of S.12 of the Canada Evidence Act Upon an Accused. *Crim. Law Q.* 15:88–96, 1972.
39. Griffitt and Jackson, op. cit.
40. Efran, M. G.: The Effect of Physical Appearance on the Judgment of Guilt, Interpersonal Attraction, and Severity of Recommended Punishment in a Simulated Jury Task. *J. Res. Personality* 8·45–54, 1974.
41. Dion, K.: Physical Attractiveness and Evaluation of Children's Transgressions. *J. Personality Social Psychol.* 24:285–290, 1972.

42. Sigall, H., and Ostrove, N.: Effects of the Physical Attractiveness of the Defendant and Nature of Crime on Juridic Judgment. *Proc. 81st Annu. Convention Am. Psychol. Assoc., Canada* 8:267–268, 1973.
43. Widgery, R. M.: Sex of Receiver and Physical Attractiveness of Source as Determinants of Initial Credibility Perception. *West. Speech Communicator* 38:13–17, 1974.
44. Savitsky and Sim, op. cit.
45. Rosenblatt, J. C.: Should the Size of the Jury in Criminal Cases be Reduced to Six? An Examination of Psychological Evidence. *Prosecutor* 8:309–314, 1972.
46. Landis, B.: Jury Trials and the Delay of Justice, in Winters, G. R. (ed.): *The Jury*. The American Judicature Society, Chicago, 1971.
47. Kreindler, L. S.: The Jury System in Court Cases, in Winters, G. R. (ed.): *The Jury*. The American Judicature Society, Chicago, 1971.
48. Diamond, S. S.: A Jury Experiment Re-analyzed. *U. Michigan J. Law Reform* 7:520–532, 1974; Pabst, W. R.: What Do Six Member Juries Really Save? *Judicature* 57:6–11, 1973; Valenti, A. C., and Downing, L. L.: Differential Effects of Jury Size on Verdicts Following Deliberation as a Function of the Apparent Guilt of a Defendant. *J. Personality Social Psychol.* 32:655–663, 1975; Zeisel, H., and Diamond, S. S.: Convincing Empirical Evidence on the Six Member Jury. *U. Chicago Law Rev.* 41:281–295, 1974.
49. 399 U.S. 78, 1970.
50. 413 U.S. 149, 1973.
51. Bermant, G., and Coppock, R.: Outcomes of Six and Twelve Member Jury Trials: Analysis of 128 Civil Cases in the State of Washington. *Washington Law Rev.* 48:593–596, 1973; Kessler, J. B.: An Empirical Study of Six and Twelve Member Jury Decision-making Processes. *U. Michigan J. Law Reform* 6:712–734, 1973; Mills, L. R.: Six-Member and Twelve-Member Juries: An Empirical Study of Trial Results. *U. Michigan J. Law Reform* 6:671–711, 1973; Stoever, W.: *A Comparison of Six and Twelve Member Juries in New Jersey Superior and County Courts*. The Institute of Judicial Administration, New York, 1972.
52. Diamond, op. cit.; Zeisel and Diamond, op. cit.
53. Bermant and Coppock, op. cit.; Stoever, op. cit.
54. Mills, op. cit.
55. Diamond, op. cit.
56. Kessler, op. cit.
57. Diamond, op. cit.; Davis, F.: *Inside Intuition*. New American Library, New York, 1975.
58. Hare, A. P.: Interaction and Consensus in Different Sized Groups. *Am. Sociol. Rev.* 17:261–267, 1952; Zeisel, H.: The Waning of the American Jury. *Am. Bar Assoc. J.* 58:367–370, 1972.
59. Asch, S. E.: Effects of Group Pressure Upon the Modification and Distortion of Judgments, in Cartwright, D., and Zander, A. (eds.): *Group Dynamics*. Row-Peterson, Evanston, Ill., 1953.
60. Valente and Downing, op. cit.
61. Zeisel, H.: What Determines the Amount of Argument per Juror? *Am. Sociol. Rev.* 28:279, 1963.
62. *Apodaca v. Oregon* 406 U.S. 404, 1972; *Johnson v. Louisiana* 406 U.S. 356, 1972.
63. Guilford, J. P.: *Fundamental Statistics in Psychology and Education*. McGraw-Hill, New York, 1965.
64. Zeisel, H.: And Then There Were None: The Diminution of the Federal Jury. *U. Chicago Law Rev.* 38:710–724, 1971.
65. Guilford, op. cit., p. 120; Selby, S. M.: *Standard Mathematical Tables*. Chemical Rubber Co., Cleveland, 1967, p. 528.
66. Diamond, op. cit.
67. McCart, S. W.: *Trial by Jury: A Complete Guide to the Jury System*. Chilton Books, Philadelphia, 1964; Tate, E., Hawrish, E., and Clark, S.: Communication Variables in Jury Selection. *J. Communication* 24:130–139, 1974.
68. Robinson, W.: Bias, Probability and Trial by Jury. *Am. Sociol. Rev.* 15:73–78, 1950.

69. 318 U.S. 128, 1940.
70. Jurow, op. cit.; Erlanger, H. S.: Jury Research in America: Its Past and Future. *Law Society Rev.* 4:345–370, 1970.
71. 319 U.S. 510, 1968.
72. Tate, Hawrish, and Clark, op cit.
73. Adkins, J. C.: Jury Selection: A Series—an Art? a Science? or Luck? *Trial* 5:37–39, 1968–1969; Katz, L. S.: The Twelve Man Jury. *Trial* 5:39–40, 42, 1968–1969.
74. Broeder, D. W.: The Voir Dire Examination—An Empirical Study. *S. Cal. Law Rev.* 38:503–528, 1965.
75. Hardy, K. R.: Determinants of Conformity and Attitude Change. *J. Abnormal Social Psychol.* 54:289–294, 1957; McGhee, P. E., and Teevon, R. C.: Conformity Behavior and Need for Affiliation. *J. Social Psychol.* 72:117–121, 1967; Sarnoff, I., and Zimbardo, P. G.: Anxiety, Fear and Social Affiliation. *Abnormal Social Psychol.* 62:356–363, 1961; Schachter, S., *The Psychology of Affiliation.* Stanford University Press, Stanford, Cal., 1959.
76. Levit, W. H., Nelson, D. W., Ball, V. C., and Chernick, R.: Expediting Voir Dire: An Empirical Study. *S. Cal. Law Rev.* 44:916–995, 1971.
77. Gutman, S. M.: The Attorney-Conducted Voir Dire of Jurors: A Constitutional Right. *Brooklyn Law Rev.* 39:290–329, 1972.
78. Gladstone, R.: Authoritarianism, Social Status, Transgression and Punitiveness. *Proc. 77th Annu. Convention Am. Psychol. Assoc.* 4:287–288, 1969.
79. Thayer, R.: Attitude and Personality Differences Between Potential Jurors Who Could Return a Death Verdict and Those Who Could Not. *Proc. 78th Annu. Convention Am. Psychol. Assoc.* 5:445–446, 1970.
80. Friend and Vinson, op. cit.
81. Mitchell and Byrne, op. cit.
82. Centers, R., Shomer, R., and Rodrigues, A.: A Field Experiment in Interpersonal Persuasion Using Authoritative Influence. *J. Personality* 38:392–403, 1970; Crosson, R. F.: An Investigation into Certain Personality Variables Among Capital Trial Jurors. *Dissertation Abstracts* 27:3668B–3669B, 1967; Snortum, J., and Ashear, V.: Prejudice, Punitiveness, and Personality. *J. Personality Assessment* 36:291–296, 1972.
83. Sealy, A. P., and Cornish, W. R.: Jurors and Their Verdicts. *Modern Law Rev.* 36:496–508, 1973.
84. James, R.: Status and Competence of Jurors. *Am. J. Sociol.* 64:563–570, 1959; Snyder, E.: Sex Role Differential and Jury Decisions. *Sociol. Social Res.* 55:442–448, 1971; Strodtbeck, F., and Mann, R.: Sex Role Differentiation in Jury Deliberations. *Sociometry* 29:3–11, 1956.
85. Nemeth and Sosis, op. cit.; Reed, J. P.: Jury Deliberations, Voting and Verdict Trends. *Southwest. Social Sci. Q.* 45:361–370, 1965; Simon, R. J.: *The Jury and the Defense of Insanity.* Little, Brown, Boston, 1967; Strodtbeck, F., James, R., and Hawkins, C.: Social Status in Jury Deliberations. *Am. Sociol. Rev.* 22:713–719, 1957.
86. James, op. cit.; Nemeth and Sosis, op. cit.; Reed, op. cit.; Simon, op. cit.
87. Becker, T. L., Hildum, D. C., and Bateman, K.: The Influence of Juror's Values on Their Verdicts: A Court and Politics Experiment. *Southwest. Social Sci. Q.* 46:130–140, 1965.
88. Snortum and Ashear, op. cit.
89. Becker, Hildum, and Bateman, op. cit.
90. Kairys, D., Schulman, J., and Harring, S. (eds.): *The Jury System: New Methods for Reducing Prejudice: A Manual for Lawyers, Legal Workers and Social Scientists.* National Jury Project and National Lawyers Guild, Philadelphia, 1975.
91. Nieremberg, G. I., and Calero, H. H.: *How to Read a Person Like a Book.* Simon & Schuster, Richmond Hill, Canada, 1973, pp. 157–160.
92. Davis, F.: *Inside Intuition.* New American Library, New York, 1975; Eisenberg, A. M., and Smith, R. R.: *Nonverbal Communication.* Bobbs-Merrill, Indianapolis, 1971; Ekman, P., and Friesen, W. V.: *Unmasking the Face.* Prentice-Hall, Englewood Cliffs, N.J., 1975; Strongman, K. T.: *The Psychology of*

Emotions. Wiley, New York, 1973; Weitz, S. (ed.): *Nonverbal Communication.* Oxford University Press. New York, 1974.
93. Bird, C.: The Influence of the Press Upon the Accuracy of Report. *J. Abnormal Social Psychol.* 22:123–129, 1927.
94. Sue, S., and Smith, R. E.: How Not to Get a Fair Trial. *Psychology Today* 7:86–90 1974; Sue, S., Smith, R. E., and Caldwell, C.: Effects of Inadmissible Evidence on the Decisions of Simulated Jurors: A Moral Dilemma. *J. Appl. Social Psychol.* 3:345–353, 1973.
95. Hoiberg, B. C., and Stires, L. K.: The Effect of Several Types of Pretrial Publicity on the Guilt Attributions of Simulated Jurors. *J. Appl. Social Psychol.* 3:267–275, 1973; Sue, S., Smith, R. E., and Gilbert, R.: Biasing Effects of Pretrial Publicity on Judicial Decisions. *J. Crim. Justice* 2:163–171, 1974.
96. Schulman, J., et al.: Recipe for a Jury. *Psychology Today* 6:37–44, 78–84, 1973.
97. Janis, I. L.: *Victims of Groupthink.* Houghton Mifflin, Boston, 1972.
98. Kessler, J. B.: The Social Psychology of Jury Deliberations, in Simon, R. J. (ed.): *The Jury System in America.* Sage Publications, Beverly Hills, 1975.
99. Nemeth and Sosis, op. cit.
100. James, op. cit.
101. Hawkins, C.: Interaction Rates of Jurors Aligned in Factions. *Am. Sociol. Rev.* 27:689–691, 1962.
102. Bevan, W., et al.: Jury Behavior as a Function of the Prestige of the Foreman and the Nature of His Leadership. *J. Public Law* 7:419, 1958.
103. Kessler, op. cit.
104. Stone, V. A.: A Primacy Effect in Decision-making by Jurors. *J. Communications* 19:239–247, 1969.
105. Davis, J. H., et al.: The Decision Processes of 6 and 12 Person Mock Juries Assigned Unanimous and Two-Thirds Majority Rules. *J. Personality Social Psychol.* 32:1–14, 1975; Izzett, R. R., and Leginski, W.: Group Discussion and the Influence of Defendant Characteristics in a Simulated Jury Setting. *J. Social Psychol.* 93:271–279, 1974; Rumsey, M. G., and Castore, C. H.: The Effects of Defendant's Character and Group Discussion on Individual Sentencing Judgments. Paper presented at the Midwestern Psychological Association Meeting, 1974.
106. Simon, R.: Use of Semantic Differential in Research on the Jury. *Journalism Q.* 45:670–676, 1968.
107. Forston, R. F.: Judges' Instructions: A Quantitative Analysis of Jurors' Listening Comprehension. *Today's Speech* 18:34–38, 1970; O'Mara, J.: The Court's Standard Jury Charge—Findings of a Pilot Project. *Pa. Bar Assoc. Q.*, January 1972, pp. 166–175. Sigworth, H., and Henze, F.: Jurors' Comprehension of Jury Instructions in Southern Arizona. Unpublished report prepared for the Committee on Uniform Jury Instructions of the Supreme Court of the State of Arizona, 1973.
108. Sales, B. D., Elwork, A., and Alfini, J.: Are Jury Instructions Understandable? Paper presented at the meeting of the American Psychology-Law Society, 1975; Sales, B. D., Elwork, A., and Alfini, J.: Improving Jury Instructions, in Sales, B. D. (ed.): *Perspectives in Law and Psychology. Vol. I: The Criminal Justice System.* Plenum, New York, 1977.
109. Prettyman, D.: Jury Instructions—First or Last? *Am. Bar Assoc. J.* 46:1066, 1960; Smith, G. P. II: Orthodoxy versus Reformation in the Jury System. *Judicature* 51:344–346, 1968.
110. Sales, Elwork, and Alfini, "Improving Jury Instructions," op. cit.
111. Cunningham, T. J.: Should Instructions Go Into the Jury Room? *Cal. State Bar J.* 33:278–289, 1958.
112. Sealy, A. P., and Cornish, W. R.: Juries and the Rules of Evidence. *Crim. Law Rev.* April 1973, pp. 208–223; Smith and Gilbert, op. cit.
113. Korbakes, C. A.: Criminal Sentencing: Is the Judge's Sound Discretion Subject to Review? *Judicature* 59:112–119, 1975; Korbakes, C. A.: Criminal Sentencing: Should the Judge's Sound Discretion be Explained? *Judicature* 59:184–191, 1975.
114. Bullock, H. A.: Significance of the Racial Factor in the Length of Stay of

Prison Sentences. *J. Crim. Law Criminol. Police Sci.* 52:411–415, 1961; Hagan, J.: Extralegal Attributes and Sentencing: An Assessment of a Sociological Viewpoint. *Law Society Rev.* 8:357–383, 1974; Howard, S. C.: Racial Discrimination in Sentencing. *Judicature* 59:120–125, 1975; Nagel, S. S.: Disparities in Criminal Procedure. *UCLA Law Rev.* 14:1272–1305, 1967; Thornberry, T. P.: Race, Socioeconomic Status, and Sentencing in the Juvenile Justice System. *J. Crim. Law Criminol.* 64:90–98, 1973.

115. Howard, op. cit.
116. Weld, H., and Danzig, E.: A Study of the Way in Which a Verdict is Reached by a Jury. *Am. J. Psychol.* 53:518–536, 1940; Weld, H., and Roff, M.: A Study in the Formation of Opinion Based upon Legal Evidence. *Am. J. Psychol.* 51:609–628, 1938.
117. Calder, B. J., Insco, C. A., and Yandell, B.: The Relation of Cognitive and Memorial Processes to Persuasion in a Simulated Jury Trial. *J. Appl. Social Psychol.* 4:62–93, 1974.
118. Lawson, R. G.: The Law of Primacy in the Criminal Courtroom. *J. Social Psychol.* 77:121–131, 1969.
119. Blunk, R. A., and Sales, B. D.: Persuasion During the Voir Dire, in Sales, B. D. (ed.): *Psychology in the Legal Process.* Spectrum Publications, New York, 1977; Lawson, op. cit.; Lawson, R. G.: Relative Effectiveness of One-Sided and Two-Sided Communications in Courtroom Persuasion. *J. Gen. Psychol.* 82:3–16, 1970; Thibaut and Walker, op. cit., chap. 7.
120. Walker, L., Thibaut, J., and Andreoli, V.: Order of Presentation at Trial. *Yale Law J.* 82:216–226, 1972; Thibaut and Walker, op. cit., chap. 7.
121. Luchins, A. S.: Primacy-Recency in Impression Formation, in Hovland, C. I., et al. (eds.): *The Order of Presentation.* Yale University Press, New Haven, 1957.
122. Lawson, op. cit.
123. Ibid.
124. Lana, R. E.: Familiarity and the Order of Presentation of Persuasive Communications. *J. Abnormal Social Psychol.* 62:573–577, 1961; Luchins, op. cit.; Luchins, A. S.: Definitiveness of Impression and Primacy-Recency in Communications. *J. Social Psychol.* 48:275–290, 1958.
125. Hovland, C. I., and Mandell, W.: Is There a Law of Primacy in Persuasion? in Hovland, C. I., et al. (eds.): *The Order of Presentation in Persuasion.* Yale University Press, New Haven, 1957; Hovland, C. I., Campbell, E. H., and Brock, T.: The Effects of Commitment on Opinion Change Following Communication, in Hovland, C. I., et al. (eds.): *The Order of Presentation in Persuasion.* Yale University Press, New Haven, 1957; Lund, F. H., The Psychology of Belief. IV. The Law of Primacy in Persuasion. *J. Abnormal Social Psychol.* 20:183–191, 1925.
126. Lawson, op. cit., p. 3.
127. Lumsdaine, A. A., and Janis, I. L.: Resistance to Counterpropaganda Produced by One-sided and Two-sided Propaganda Presentations. *Public Opinions Q.* 17:311–318, 1953; McGuire, W. J.: Inducing Resistance to Persuasion, in Berkowitz (ed.): *Advances in Experimental Social Psychology.* Vol. I. Academic Press, New York, 1964.
128. Chu, G. C.: Prior Familiarity, Perceived Bias, and One-sided versus Two-sided Communication. *J. Exp. Social Psychol.* 3:243–254, 1967.
129. Chu, op. cit.; Insco, C. A., One-sided versus Two-Sided Communications and Countercommunications. *J. Abnormal Social Psychol.* 65:203–206, 1962; Hovland, C. I., Lumsdaine, A. A., and Sheffield, F. D.: *Experiments on Mass Communication.* Princeton University Press, Princeton, N.J., 1949; McGinnies, E.: Studies in Persuasion. III. Reactions of Japanese Students to One-sided and Two-sided Communications. *J. Social Psychol.* 70:87–93, 1966.
130. Beecher, op. cit.; Munsterberg, op. cit.; Whipple, G. M.: The Observer as Reporter: A Survey of the Psychology of Testimony. *Psychol. Bull.* 6:153–170, 1909.
131. Wigmore, op. cit.
132. Buckhout, R., Eyewitness Testimony. *Sci. Am.* 231:23–31, 1974; Downing, J.

D. S.: Inaccurate Perception and Evidence in Court. *New Law J.* 122:600–602, 1972; Goldstein, A. G.: The Fallibility of the Eyewitness: Psychological Evidence, in Sales, B. D. (ed.): *Psychology in the Legal Process.* Spectrum Publications, New York, 1977; Greer, op. cit.; Levine, F. J., and Tapp, J. L.: Psychology of Criminal Identification: The Gap from Wade to Kirby. *U. Pa. Law Rev.* 121:1079–1131, 1973; Lezak, M. D.: Some Psychological Limitations on Witness Reliability. *Wayne Law Rev.* 20:117–133, 1973.
133. Marshall, J.: *Law and Psychology in Conflict.* Bobbs-Merrill, Indianapolis, 1966.
134. Sommer, R.: The New Look on the Witness Stand. *Canadian Psychologist* 8:94–100, 1959.
135. Lezak, op. cit.
136. Haward, L. R. C.: The Reliability of Corroborated Police Evidence in a Case Flagrante Delicto. *J. Forensic Sci.* 3:71–81, 1963; Haward, L. R. C.: Some Psychological Aspects of Oral Evidence. *Br. J. Criminol.* 3:342–360, 1963; Haward, L. R. C.: Psychological Experiments and Judicial Doubt. *Bull. Br. Psychol. Soc.* 17:54–64, 1964.
137. Marshall, op. cit.
138. Allport, G. W., and Kramer, B. M.: Some Roots of Prejudice. *J. Psychol.* 22:9–39, 1946.
139. Marshall, op. cit.; Buckhout, op. cit.
140. Gardner, D. S.: The Perception and Memory of Witnesses. *Cornell Law Q.* 18:391, 1933.
141. Buckhout, op. cit.
142. Hutchins, R. M., and Slesinger, D.: Some Observations on the Law of Evidence. *Columbia Law Rev.* 28:432–440, 1928.
143. Buckhout, op. cit.; Marshall, op. cit.
144. Buckhout, op. cit.; Goldstein, op. cit.; Greer, op. cit.; Levine and Tapp, op. cit.; Marshall, op. cit.
145. Goldstein, op. cit.; Shepard, J. W., and Ellis, H. D.: The Effect of Attractiveness of Recognition Memory for Faces. *Am. J. Psychol.* 86:627–634, 1976; Shepard, J. W., Derogowski, J. B., and Ellis, H. D.: A Cross Cultural Study of Memory for Faces. *Int. J. Psychol.* 9:205–211, 1974.
146. Elliott, E. S., Wills, E. J., and Goldstein, A. G.: The Effects of Discrimination Training on the Recognition of White and Oriental Faces. *Bull. Psychonomic Soc.* 2:71–73, 1973; Malpass, R. S., and Kravitz, J.: Recognition for Faces of Own and Other "Race." *J. Personality Social Psychol.* 13:330–335, 1969.
147. Munsterberg, op. cit., pp. 49–51; Stern, W.: The Psychology of Testimony. *J. Abnormal Social Psychol.* 34:3–20, 7–17, 1939.
148. Greer, op. cit.; Marshall, op. cit.
149. Bird, op. cit.
150. Doob, A. N., and Kirshenbaum, H. M.: Bias in Police Lineups: Partial Remembering. *J. Police Sci. Admin.* 1:287—293, 1973.
151. Marquis, K. H., Marshall, J., and Oskamp, S.: Testimony Validity as a Function of Question Form, Atmosphere and Item Difficulty. *J. Appl. Social Psychol.* 2:167, 186, 1972.
152. Loftus, E. F.: Reconstructing Memory: The Incredible Eyewitness. *Psychology Today* 8:116–119, 1974; Loftus, E. F., and Zanni, G.: Eyewitness Testimony: The Influence of the Wording of a Question. *Bull. Psychonomic Soc.* 5:86–88, 1975.
153. Loftus, E. F., and Palmer, J. C.: Reconstruction of Automobile Destruction: An Example of the Interaction Between Language and Memory. *J. Verbal Learning Verbal Behav.* 13:585–589, 1974.
154. Kaspryzk, D., Montano, D. E., and Loftus, E. F.: Effects of Leading Questions on Jurors' Verdicts. *Jurimetrics J.* 16:48–51, 1975.
155. Greer, op. cit.
156. Meehl, P. E.: Law and the Fireside Inductions: Some Reflections of a Clinical Psychologist. *J. Social Issues* 27:65–100, 1971; Zeisel, H.: Reflections on Experimental Techniques in the Law. *J. Legal Studies* 2:107–124, 1973.

CHAPTER 43

A. Louis McGarry is Professor of Clinical Psychiatry at the State University of New York at Stony Brook and Director of the Division of Forensic Services at the Nassau County Medical Center in East Meadow, New York. A graduate of Harvard College and Boston University Medical School, he is a Fellow of the American Psychiatric Association and a member of the Committee on Psychiatry and Law of the Group for the Advancement of Psychiatry. Dr. McGarry is a former Associate Clinical Professor of Psychiatry at Harvard Medical School. He has also served as Assistant Commissioner of Mental Health for Legal Medicine in the Massachusetts Department of Mental Health and as Associate Professor of Legal Psychiatry in the Law-Medicine Institute at Boston University. The author of numerous professional papers and monographs, Dr. McGarry is former Chairman of the Editorial Board of the *Massachusetts Journal of Mental Health* and is currently a member of the Editorial Board of *Psychiatric Opinion*.

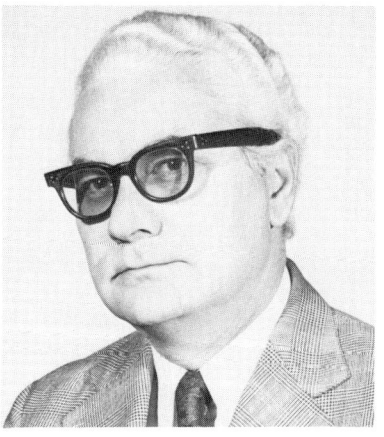

William J. Curran is Frances Glessner Lee Professor of Legal Medicine at Harvard University and Chairman of the State Medicolegal Investigation Committee of Massachusetts. Professor Curran writes regularly for the *New England Journal of Medicine* and teaches at the Medical School, Law School, and School of Public Health at Harvard. He was formerly Robert R. Utley Professor of Legal Medicine and Director of the Law-Medicine Institute of Boston University. He also served as Assistant Professor of Law and Government and Assistant Director of the Institute of Government at the University of North Carolina. Professor Curran is the author of several books in the medicolegal field including *Law, Medicine and Forensic Science* (with E. D. Shapiro); *Trauma and the Automobile; The Doctor as a Witness;* and *Medicolegal Proof in Litigation*. He is an Associate Editor of the *American Journal of Law and Medicine* and was formerly Medicolegal Editor of the *Massachusetts Law Quarterly*.

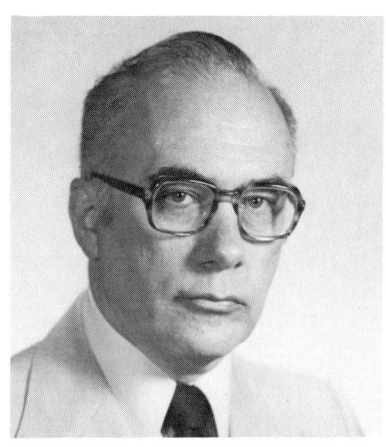

COURTROOM PRESENTATION OF PSYCHIATRIC AND PSYCHOLOGICAL EVIDENCE*

A. Louis McGarry, M.D., and
William J. Curran, J.D., LL.M., S.M.Hyg.

STATE OF THE ART PROBLEMS

The most serious problem for courtroom presentation of psychiatric and psychological evidence is the inherent uncertainty of the field itself. We do not have objective biochemical measures of behavioral and mental disorders. There is often a confusion between findings and opinions in the evaluation of an individual patient. Genuine disagreement between experts is not uncommon, even in such fundamental areas as the diagnosis of a mental illness or, even more so, its prognosis. The "battle of experts" in the courtroom is thus found more frequently in issues of psychiatry and psychology than in other forensic scientific fields.

Some commentators have observed, however, that psychiatric testimony, particularly where special psychological standards are not imposed and where the psychiatrist can offer an unrestricted clinical judgment, is no more intuitive and judgmental than that of a surgeon. In an interesting query, Diamond and Louisell also added the dimension of the complexity of the trial itself as a factor:

> Might not the generalization be made that the more difficult the trial situation, the more controversial the issues to be resolved, and the more uncertain the balance of the evidence, the more likely the expert testimony, be it surgical, medical, pathological, criminalistic or ballistic, will approach the subjective, intuitive quality of the psychiatrist's expertise. . . ?[1]

---

*This chapter was supported in part by Grant No. R01 MH25955 from the Center for Studies of Crime and Delinquency of the National Institute of Mental Health.

This wise observation may well explain the depth of disagreement in forensic scientific testimony in such diverse situations as the Jack Ruby trial and the Sirhan Sirhan trial concerning criminal responsibility, the Howard Hughes will contest involving questioned documents, and the Northeast Airlines case involving forensic pathology and conscious pain and suffering before death.

There are some excellent general reviews of expert psychiatric testimony[2] and of the functions of forensic psychiatrists and psychologists in court.[3] There are also some useful publications of psychiatric testimony, both from actual cases and from mock trials involving well-known trial attorneys and expert witnesses.[4]

JUDICIAL AND LEGAL PRACTICES

The difficulties for presentation of behavioral science testimony are also compounded by certain judicial and legal practices and prejudices as follows:

1. The judicial rulings that many of the behavioral issues are matters of common knowledge and not subject to expert evaluation.
2. The growing hostility of some legal and civil rights groups toward psychiatry.
3. The tendency of courts to assume that all psychiatrists are "expert" in all forensic psychiatric subjects.

Common Knowledge

In a number of areas of behavioral or mental-status evaluation, the American law has held that laymen can offer opinions based upon common knowledge.[5] Courts and learned commentators have expressed the view that expert opinion is of no greater, and sometimes *less*, value than the testimony of someone who knew the person well,[6] or of a lawyer who knows the legal rules applicable to the situation,[7] or of a trial judge. In a famous opinion passed down a half century ago, Chief Justice Charles Rugg upheld the determination by a trial judge of a defendant's criminal responsibility based upon the judge's observation of the defendant in the courtroom and under direct and cross-examination. He concluded,

> The judge may well have been able to form a judgment as to legal responsibility of the defendant for crime, based upon common sense inferences and intelligent observation, more reliable as a practical guide to accomplishment of justice than refined distinctions and technical niceties of alienists and experts in psychopathic inferiority.[8]

The Chief Justice here displayed some of the distrust and hostility toward psychiatrists (then called "alienists") which we still see in the later decades of the century. His mention of "refined distinctions" and "technical niceties" reminds one of common criticisms of *lawyers*, another highly suspect group, perhaps even more than of psychiatrists.

In practice, it is often true that intelligent and observant laymen can form quite reliable opinions of the mental capacity of individuals. The situations where expert psychiatric and/or psychological evaluation is most clearly demanded will arise when the individual has a definite psychological disturbance or illness, often of a subtle nature, which specifically affects or determines his behavior in the given, legally related situation. We should note also that the fact that psychiatrists and psychologists are *trained observers of human behavior* makes them valuable evaluators of human interaction, even where the circumstances do not demand expertise in mental illness as such.

Legal Hostility

Currently, there is a definite and overtly expressed "antipsychiatry attitude" among many younger lawyers trained in American law schools in recent years. The emphasis on civil rights is very strong in current law school education. Courses on criminal law, Constitutional law, and psychiatry and law emphasize the weaknesses in psychiatric testimony and evaluation and stress the damage done to the civil rights of criminal defendants and mental patients in the past due to psychiatric evaluations. There is also a strong disenchantment with the effectiveness of psychiatric treatment, especially with efforts to change or control behavior.

The "antipsychiatry attitude" can also be found among the judiciary and is especially evident in recent decisions imposing very strict standards for commitment of the mentally ill.[9]

Weak Standards for Testimony

The courts, while suspicious of psychiatric testimony in general, set few if any standards on what qualifications a physician or a psychiatrist should meet in order to give an opinion on such matters as criminal responsbility and capacity to stand criminal trial. These psycholegal issues assume legal as well as psychiatric knowledge. They are complex matters which require a high degree of emotional security on the part of the expert to deal with the issues. This emotional security, coupled with knowledge of the interrelated legal and psychological standards to be applied, can be gained only with training and experience in forensic psychiatry. Nevertheless, the courts continue to exhibit great latitude in allowing physicians, even without general training in psychiatry let alone forensic psychiatry, to offer expert opinions in these fields. The result of this looseness of courtroom standards is inadequate psychiatric testimony, much of it transparently incompetent and highly vulnerable to savage destruction on cross-examination. The entire field of forensic psychiatry is thus subject to ridicule, owing to the assumption that the performance of these inadequate witnesses is typical of all forensic psychiatric evaluation methodology.

We should note before closing this section that the courts have been much more cautious about admitting the testimony of psychologists on issues of mental illness and mental capacity. Until recent years, the tendency was to admit clinical psychological evidence only as supportive of "medical" testimony on a mental condition. The psychologist was allowed to state his findings (often more objective than anything offered by the psychiatrist), but not to disclose any complete opinion on diagnosis.[10] Now, however, the courts have recognized the qualifications of clinical psychologists, especially those with doctorates, to offer both findings and opinions in areas of their specialization.[11] The courts have not, however, laid down special qualifications for forensic psychological evaluations any more than they have done so for forensic psychiatric testimony.

GENERAL AND SPECIAL EVALUATIONS

Psychiatrists and psychologists are called to give evidence or to prepare reports on two types of legal cases. The first requires presentation of general clinical materials. No special legal rules apply to the situation, and the report or evidence will rarely differ significantly from any other clinical presentation. This type of evidence is most commonly given in personal injury cases and workers' compensation litigation and in other claims for insurance benefits. Domestic relations and child custody matters are similar, though greater sophistication is probably required of the practitioner to understand the issues before the family and probate courts than in personal injury or insurance claims cases. Clearly distinguishable from these, however, are the special circumstances of legal matters which are not within the common experience of practitioners and which require the application of specific legal standards of behavior. On the civil side these include the mental capacity to make a will, to execute a contract, to marry, and to manage one's business affairs. On the criminal side these issues will be of criminal intent, criminal responsibility, and mental capacity to stand trial. In between these classifications will be found evaluations for involuntary commitment and for the release of mental patients and mentally retarded persons. Though clearly a part of clinical practice, these latter areas contain quite specific legal standards often closer to the criminal law model than the civil law system.

Other chapters in this text will be found to deal with psychiatric and psychological tesimony in many of the areas outlined above. Special attention has been given to the situations where clinical and legal standards are mixed. In our further discussion in this chapter, we will point to these distinctions frequently. It is our position that specialized training and experience are especially required for involvement in the second type of litigation which is the type we refer to as essentially psycholegal in content.

TESTIMONIAL PRESENTATION

Practical Suggestions

We would like to offer in this section some practical advice based upon the experience of both authors in over two decades in the medicolegal field.

We would begin with the observation that there is no substitute for basic intelligence and clinical competence. This will be particularly true in the rare situations where a courtroom appearance is necessary. Most reports for lawyers and courts do not involve actual court testimony. Nevertheless, every report required for a legal evaluation should be prepared as if litigation and a contest of the report could be expected. The clinician should be ready to defend every finding and conclusion in the report on clinical and scientific grounds. He should be aware of professional and scientific viewpoints which might differ from his and should be familiar with the latest scientific literature in relation to the subject involved. As was pointed out in Chapter 30, the clinician should be very clear about what *questions* are being asked by the lawyer or the legal tribunal. Analysis of the questions is greatly aided by experience; the lawyers and even the courts often express themselves in obscure terms—sometimes intentionally. Moreover, the overt questions may not fully reveal the underlying interests of the interrogators. When the clinician suspects that this may be the case, he should seek further information about the circumstances of the referral.

Prior to a court appearance, the clinician should review his report and his clinical records, if any, quite thoroughly. The testimony should be based essentially upon the report. This will be especially important if both parties have had access to the report, as is often the case today in both civil and criminal matters. Any deviation of significance (and even of slight detail) from the report may be brought out in testimony and will then need to be explained. This places the witness on the defensive and makes him seem uncertain; it adds confusion to the testimony. It is not only the opposing counsel who may be confused. The counsel calling the witness also bases his direct examination on the report. If no pretrial conference is arranged, or if it becomes impractical or impossible, the counsel calling the witness will base his questions on his own recollection of the report. Deviations from the report can "throw off" the questioning lawyer and result in a lack of coordination between interrogator and witness, an undesirable situation on direct examination.

Pretrial Preparation

We suggest, of course, that pretrial consultation between counsel and his witness should take place in all possible situations. Most of the serious problems in expert-witness presentation can be traced to inadequate pretrial preparation between the witness and the counsel. As our experience grows, we are more and more convinced of this observation.

The witness and counsel should go over the substance of the *actual questions* and the *expected answers* thoroughly. There should be no surprises on direct examination. This does not mean that the witness is rehearsed; nor does it mean that counsel puts words in the expert's mouth. In fact, the witness should resist this approach firmly. The questions belong to the lawyer; the answers must be those of the witness. Any amount of courtroom experience will prove this maxim. The witness must stand or fall, ignominiously, on the soundness of the responses given on the stand. Many lawyers will try to shape the answers of the expert. There are two levels at which this may be attempted, one more dangerous than the other. The first relates to form, the other to substance. The interrogator may try to discourage the witness from being too loquacious, or circumloquacious, on the witness stand. All lawyers (and judges, too) prefer direct, clear, and relatively short answers, even to the most complex of questions. They are inclined to become impatient with attempts to qualify an answer or to volunteer observations that they consider irrelevant or unnecessary to the issues at hand. Some witnesses are better than others at serving these ends of efficiency and dispatch in court. However, the witness should be himself, be comfortable in the style of his answers, and should resist too aggressive coaching on style. Again, courtroom experience generally helps expert witnesses to cut down on overlong answers. Much of the reason for them is nervousness which causes overcompensation in wordy explanations. Experience often proves, however, that the extra information or opinion volunteered beyond the question is the weakest part of the testimony and the most subject to challenge on cross-examination. This is due to the fact that it generally goes beyond the report and was not well-prepared and thought through beforehand. As a general rule, the witness should *not volunteer information* beyond the scope of the question asked.

Attempts to shape the *substance* of an answer are of a different order. The lawyer may say, "That's not what I want (or need), Doc." This is always a danger signal. If the lawyer is merely seeking to make the answer relevant and responsive to the question, it is a proper correction. It is not proper if the lawyer is seeking a different and more favorable answer on his client's behalf. Sometimes, the expert witness becomes too caught up in the gamesmanship of the case, too involved in the partisan aspects of the litigation. He then listens to this sort of admonition and, without perhaps realizing it, reshapes his testimony to fit the lawyer's strategy, or what he often calls "the theory of the case." When the witness resists, the lawyer will often retreat to the position that he is only suggesting the "form" of the answer. If the expert resists further, counsel has the choice of accepting the answer or *not asking the question* on direct examination. If the latter course is selected, the interrogator usually expects that the witness will not volunteer his unfavorable material in answer to other related questions.

Reasonable Certainty of Conclusions

We noted earlier that a major weakness in behavioral science areas is the lack of objective proofs. This results in placing a high value on clinical opinions or conclusions and the firmness with which they are stated and held. If the psychiatrist or psychologist cannot offer his opinion within reasonable medical or psychological certainty and be able to support it with historical data from the patient and clinical observations, if made, his answer to the key question "Have you an opinion?" should be "No, I do not." Some courts will allow a "clinical impression" to be placed in the record, implying a lesser degree of certainty. Unless opposing counsel is somnolent, this hedging will be objected to and usually will be stricken. In Chapter 29, Dr. Modlin makes some useful suggestions on these issues in civil law litigation.

Psycholegal Issues and Ultimate Questions

We spoke earlier of the "psycholegal" issues put to behavioral science clinicians. In these situations, the witness is being asked to answer what is legally called a mixed question of fact and law, of finding and opinion. (In Chapter 27, Seymour Pollack refers to this whole area as "fact-finding" in the sense that it contributes to the factual part of the case before a jury.) Under the rules of evidence, the witness should be asked the specific questions which make up the legal standard. In a will-capacity case, for example, these questions would be: Did the testator know the nature and extent of his property? Did he know the natural objects of his bounty (i.e., his family or close friends)? Did he understand the disposition under the will or the estate plan? Did he appreciate these elements in relation to each other and form an orderly, rational plan for his will? Moreover, in a practical sense, did he understand that the instrument he was signing was a legal will embodying these objectives? The answer to all of these questions must be positive to support a finding of competency.[12] For the psychiatrist or psychologist, the last proposition is very important since it synthesizes the earlier foundation questions into the action, the human behavior, on which the witness is expected to be an expert observer. In many jurisdictions, the witness cannot be asked to answer "the ultimate question" of whether the testator had or did not have the mental capacity to make a will. To allow such testimony, these courts assert, is to "invade the province of the jury." The more modern rule, however, favored by nearly all legal commentators, is that an answer to the ultimate question is helpful to the jury which can accept it or reject it.[13] The most noted of the legal scholars on evidence law, Dean John Wigmore, always pungent in his comments on evidentiary decisions he did not favor, was especially critical of this exclusionary rule. He asserted that it was "so misleading as well as unsound that it should be repudiated. It is a mere bit of empty rhetoric."[14] McCormack, another commentator, says that the rule is unduly restrictive.[15] In Chapter 27, Dr. Pollack supports the answering of "ultimate questions" by psychiatrists as an aid to jury understanding.

In essence, the ultimate question is a synthesizing proposition, like the last question on testamentary action quoted above. It appears in every case where the issue turns on the "mental capacity" to perform a legally significant activity. An especially important and often misunderstood area is mental capacity (or mental fitness) to stand criminal trial. The particular functions required for such an activity are not a part of the common knowledge of most psychiatrists and psychologists who do not work in court settings. In a research project that both authors participated in a few years ago, the first year of the study was spent by the research team in examining court practices in different types of cases and in interviewing court personnel, lawyers, prosecutors, and defendants. As a result of this research, we found that an expert, forensically trained psychiatrist or psychologist on the issue of criminal-trial competency should have the following specialized knowledge and skills: (1) working knowledge of the criminal justice system; (2) adequate professional and interpersonal skills in interviewing and eliciting relevant, legally oriented data from defendants who are mentally ill or retarded; (3) adequate knowledge of, and skill in, application of the legal criteria for competency; and (4) proper professional credentials to assure expert credibility in court.[16] The behavioral science clinician is, of course, expected to be particularly skilled in the second criterion as it applies to mentally ill or retarded persons. Only the forensically trained expert can qualify on the third criterion, which requires legal knowledge.

The foundation elements for mental competency to stand criminal trial in the United States can be expressed in these questions: Does the defendant understand the criminal charges against him? Does he have the intelligence and contact with reality to assist his counsel in his own defense? Some jurisdictions add: Does the defendant appreciate his peril (i.e., does he understand and feel emotionally the danger he faces of being convicted as a criminal, having a criminal record, and paying the penalty of a fine or a term in jail or prison)?[17]

The psychiatrist or psychologist will be expected to answer these questions in terms of the current mental capacity of the party when examined, but he may also be asked in a report to the lawyer or the court whether or not psychiatric treatment of a short- or long-term variety would be likely to render the party competent. A mere refusal on the part of a defendant to cooperate with the court or his lawyer does not make him incompetent. If a person displays, due to a depression, a desire to be found guilty and be punished, this depression does not itself make the defendant incompetent. It has been our experience that many, if not most, mentally disturbed and psychotic persons are competent to stand trial, unless their psychosis detaches them so much from personal reality or so severely distorts the court and legal reality that they cannot meet the criteria given above. Failure to meet any one of the required elements would result in a finding of lack of mental competency.

As mentioned in other chapters, psychiatric and psychological criteria, checklists, and instruments have been prepared by our research group[18] and others[19] for use in testing defendants in criminal trial competency. Unlike criminal responsibility, which is nearly always a jury issue, the question of criminal trial competency is most frequently a pretrial issue for the judge.[20] Because of this, the issue is often disposed of in psychiatric reports or an informal, largely *ex parte* hearing in court. In the past, the courts have been prone to rely on a brief report by a psychiatrist or observational hospital that the defendant is "incompetent and irresponsible criminally." The grounds for the opinion are often not given, or if they are, the finding is that the defendant is psychotic and a fit subject for mental hospitalization. The courts have too readily and uncritically accepted these conclusions from professional consultants and hospitals that were unaware or disregarding of the legal requirements for either condition. Thomas Szasz has compiled a revealing book on famous determinations in these fields where ignorance or prejudice played a part in the psychiatric determinations.[21]

The area of criminal responsibility also contains legal standards which must be fully understood and accepted by the psychiatrist or psychologist if he or she is to provide proper testimony in court on this issue. This subject is discussed by Dr. Roth in Chapter 28 and by Dr. McGarry in Chapter 30. Dr. Pollack (in Chapter 27) deals with the ethical aspects of providing testimony on criminal responsibility.

Manner and Style of Giving Evidence

General advice concerning the manner and style of presenting expert testimony, including psychiatric testimony, has been offered by one of the authors[22] and by others.[23] Suggestions will be found in other chapters in this section and also in Chapters 17 and 56, which discuss courtroom presentation.

All forensic science expert witnesses must strive to achieve respect, understanding, and credibility in court. They must give the appearance, the aura, of being independent, nonpartisan scientists or clinicians. As Dr. Pollack puts it in his chapter, ". . . the appearance and projected image of neutrality, impartiality, and objectivity are as important as the authentic characteristics." Another experienced forensic psychiatrist, Bernard Diamond, has expressed his doubts about impartial expertness in legal psychiatry areas,[24] but the concept continues to be greatly important to the establishment of respect and credibility, whether the witness is called as an "impartial expert" by the judge, or is called by either side in the trial itself.

The appearance of impartiality is best achieved by the witness who treats both lawyers (on direct and cross-examination) with the same professional courtesy and distance, or avoidance of undue familiarity. Especially on cross-examination, the witness should resist sparring or debating with the lawyer.

Personal appearance is probably not as important as it was in the past. The reaction of juries to witnesses is highly unpredictable (see Chapter 42). Nevertheless, attorneys are still prone to advise "experts" who seek to gain the jury's respect to dress somewhat conservatively: this means a business suit or sport coat (not too flamboyant) and slacks, a shirt and tie (in colder weather, at least), and clean shoes for the male witness, and a two- or three-piece suit with a skirt (not slacks) or a conservative dress for the female expert witness. Age can make a difference. The younger person is apt to wear somewhat more informal clothes and to assume a more casual style. The key is being oneself; an abrupt change in personal appearance and dress can adversely affect the composure of the witness, expert or not.

It is of utmost importance to speak clearly, distinctly, and loudly enough to be heard and understood. The female witness with a thin, reedy voice has the greatest trouble here, but many males also have trouble projecting their voices. Some accent, either regional or foreign, is generally not a handicap if the meaning is clear enough and the witness speaks slowly and distinctly. In fact, an accent is often an advantage, since the jury and the court are apt to listen more closely and attentively. The witness should pause before answering questions, especially on cross-examination, to allow time to reflect on the answer and to allow any objection to be made to the question. If the questions are not understood, the witness can ask clarification or a repeat of the question. Often the "repeated question" is not the same as the first. If the witness is bothered by this, he or she should call attention to the difference.

Expert witnesses are often especially bothered by being asked to answer a question "yes" or "no." This generally happens only on cross-examination. Most judges today will allow experts to resist the categorical reply and to explain their answer, especially if the witness turns to the judge and says "May I explain my answer, your honor?"

The most effective behavioral science experts in the courtroom, in our view, are those who do not retreat from the use of scientifically accurate terms but who can interpret them in common human correlates which a jury or a judge can relate to and understand. For example, one of the authors testified in the case of a highly compulsive woman with an exaggerated need for control who had been subjected to a terrifying automobile accident when a large truck, out of control, bore down on her while she was stopped, waiting for a light to change—a situation thoroughly out of her control. Although the woman was not physically harmed, it was Dr. McGarry's view that she had been severely psychologically traumatized. Subsequent to the accident, after two days of free-floating anxiety, she developed the very curious symptom of being unable to have a spontaneous bowel movement and was forced to remove fecal matter with a gloved hand. In relating what he perceived as the dynamics of this case, Dr. McGarry analogized that the symptom was an unconscious effort to bind her anxiety by symbolically displacing the out-of-control accident scene to a totally controlled bodily function, where ordinarily one has to "lose control" by relaxing the anal sphincter. In this case, damages were, in fact, awarded. Also effective is the use of literal quotes from the examined person or from records illustrative of clinical points that have been made in the testimony.

The Vulnerability of the Professional Narcissist

Mental health experts, particularly when they are physicians, are not accustomed to having their authority challenged. Doctors' orders are absolute. It is, therefore, especially vexing for expert psychiatric witnesses to be subjected to cross-examination. For the inexperienced witness, the adversary process becomes a revelation when he sees the opposing attorneys, who have been tearing at each other and at each others' witnesses all morning, amiably having lunch together. In the cross-examination process, counsel often seeks to prick the narcissism of the witness, to provoke his sense of entitlement to respect and authority. Once such narcissism is breached, the witness can resemble a pompous leviathan provoked to indiscretion and extremities. Conversely, the expert who despite baiting and provocation answers questions with good will and accuracy, and who does not make statements that he cannot defend, will survive and prosper under such attack.

Techniques of Cross-Examination

There are many techniques used in cross-examination, all designed to diminish the strength or credibility of the direct testimony.[25] It is important to know that counsel, in cross-examining, is usually limited to the content of the direct testimony. It is the responsibility of the counsel who called on the expert for direct testimony to object to excursion into content not covered in the direct examination. This offers little protection in actuality, however, and the expert must anticipate, at times, the most vigorous, searching, and wide-ranging attack on his competency, honesty, and motivation. If the purpose of such an attack is understood and if it is borne with equanimity, the experience can be very positive.

Cross-examination is by no means always vigorous and challenging, but the expert must be prepared for it. The techniques utilized when cross-examination is vigorous are many and are intended both to disconcert the witness and to discredit his testimony. When voluminous records are involved, a not uncommon technique is for the cross-examiner to require that the expert witness find the documentation for a statement he has made. What then follows with an inexperienced witness as he searches for the documentation—aware that he is delaying the proceedings—is that counsel will ask still another question of the witness. This can be most disconcerting, and it is intended to be. The experienced witness, however, will not permit himself to be flustered, but rather will take the time required to answer one question at a time. If there is any uncertainty in the mind of a witness regarding a question put to him by counsel, it is proper and appropriate for the witness to ask for clarification or repetition of the question.

Another cross-examination technique consists of questions which are asked with an accelerating rhythm such that a further question is asked before a prior answer is completed. Accommodating to such a technique can lead to confused testimony and diminished credibility. The experienced witness will not permit himself to be manipulated in this fashion. He will calmly answer the question in his own time and then ask for a repetition of the next question, if necessary, before going forward unhurriedly to answer subsequent questions.

Some counselors are fond of using hypothetical questions, and these are a proper mode of inquiry. The expert witness should be sure, however, that he fully understands the question before answering. Again, it is acceptable and appropriate for the witness to ask for clarification so that he knows exactly what is being dealt with. This can prove difficult when counsel has included an overly complex set of facts in the hypothetical question.

Although not out of the question, it is quite risky for a mental health professional to arrive at an expert opinion solely by observing courtroom behavior and testimony, basing his opinion on such observations. In such situations, the questions and areas covered are in the hands of others. The observable behavioral data will vary widely in richness and detail and, in our experience, most often are inadequate to permit arrival at defensible expert opinion. Valid data from historical or other sources are usually required before an opinion could be risked.

Psychiatrists can be in difficulty during cross-examination in attempting to defend a diagnosis of a functional mental disorder. The cross-examiner may attempt to force the witness into providing objective findings of the condition. He may ask, "Well, Doctor, can't you tell us what this disease is without merely describing the symptoms?" A particularly effective use of this technique can be found in the trial of Alger Hiss, an alleged Soviet spy who had worked for the State Department in World War II and in the years following. The chief prosecution witness was Whittaker Chambers. The defense presented rebuttal evidence by a psychiatrist that Chambers was a psychopathic personality whose testimony should not be believed. The expert's opinion was shaken by his apparent inability to provide objective criteria of the disease, as he was able to provide for pneumonia. The cross-examiner, Thomas Murphy, kept pressing the witness to "define" psychopathic personality. The witness would try, but kept reverting to a description of its symptoms. The fact that the witness formed his opinion solely by observing Chambers in direct and cross-examination at the trial also weakened the credibility of his diagnosis.[26]

Examinations for Purposes of Litigation

Psychiatrists and psychologists are often retained by the lawyers or the courts to examine a person for purposes of a civil lawsuit or a criminal trial. In the civil cases, the psychiatric or psychological evaluation is not essentially different than other medical or forensic scientific examinations. There is no confidential relationship in such an examination, since it does not concern treatment. The interview or testing with psychological instruments is entirely voluntary. Where the examination is conducted for the benefit of the party at the request of his or her own attorney, the psychiatrist or psychologist must guard against accepting self-serving statements at face-value. Outright malingering is sometimes attempted with the hope that the clinician will believe (or at least not challenge) the story and relate it in court. On the other hand, if the psychiatrist or psychologist is conducting the examination for the opposite party, other precautions must be taken. The party can be expected to be guarded or even hostile in replies. Psychological testing is often refused entirely because of fear that the results can be distorted. The lawyer for the party generally insists on being present during the examinations. Some consultants, being unaccustomed to having third parties sit in on clinical interviews, may refuse to conduct the evaluation or will perform only a cursory interview. In some situations, the psychiatrist or psychologist who insists on a private examination will be allowed to conduct it, either because the lawyer is inexperienced, or because he is very confident of his client's performance, or because the insurance company refuses to agree to a favorable settlement without the private evaluation. The lawyer who is willing to go to trial may still refuse a private examination which he feels is against his client's best interests.

In criminal cases, a psychiatrist, and less often a psychologist, may be assigned by the court to examine a defendant regarding competency to stand trial and/or criminal responsibility. In these cases, the examiner is performing a service for the court and is an *agent* of the court, as Dr. Pollack has noted in his chapter. The examination is not confidential, and the defendant cannot be required to cooperate or to answer any of the questions. The psychiatrist or psychologist should introduce himself to the defendant and explain the circumstances of the examination and appointment by the court. The defendant should be told that he does not have to submit to the examination or to answer any questions. The defendant can have his attorney present. If the examiner wishes to record the interview orally or on videotape or film, the permission of the defendant and counsel must be obtained. If the recording is to be used in court, it is advisable to gain the court's permission in advance to make the recording for possible use by either party at the trial. Many states provide by statute or case law that any statements made concerning the alleged crime which are self-incriminatory cannot be admitted at the trial, even though the defendant provides them to the examiner voluntarily during the interview. The latter exclusion can generally be waived by the party if he intends to admit committing the act, but to defend on the basis of criminal irresponsibility due to mental illness.

The Presumption of Soundness of Mind and the Burden of Proof

One of the common errors of the behavioral science clinician who is not familiar with legal evaluations for the courts is to assume that doubts should be resolved in favor of psychiatric or psychological treatment if the party would seem at all likely to benefit from such treatment. The legally inexperienced clinical evaluator may be inclined to believe the story received about the crime in a police report accompanying the "order" for the examination. Such examiners may assume the individual's contradictions of the "official version" of the crime to be a clinical sign of delusion or a lack of "cooperation" with the examiner. Each of these tendencies must be avoided.

The clinical examiner is required by law to assume that the party is of sound mind, within normal limits, in *all* legal situations, civil or criminal. The assumption of soundness of mind continues to exist until relevant and legally admissible evidence is produced to rebut it. In most instances, the presumption is rebutted by a preponderance of the evidence, but proof of the existence of a mental illness beyond a reasonable doubt is the rule in involuntary commitment in a few American jurisdictions. The U.S. Supreme Court has required "clear and convincing" proof, but not proof beyond reasonable doubt, in civil commitment. The prosecution in a criminal case must prove the defendant to be of sound mind regarding criminal responsibility beyond a reasonable doubt as soon as any evidence of lack of mental soundness is pleaded or presented by the defense. If no defense on this issue is alleged or presented, the prosecution can rely on the general presumption of soundness of mind, and the court will receive no evidence from either the prosecution or the defense on the issue.

In some of the situations above, the expert witness will be asked to provide an opinion on an ultimate issue in accordance with the burden of proof, such as being asked if he or she has any reasonable medical (or psychological) doubt about it. In most cases, however, the medical witness is answering factual issues which, in most jurisdictions, are supportable on the basis of *reasonable certainty*—medical, psychological, or scientific. The fact that the behavioral scientist relies on relatively less objective proofs than would satisfy a physical scientist can be taken into consideration in the determination of *reasonable* psychiatric or psychological proofs. In most situations, the witness can base an expert opinion (such as on a causal relationship) upon the weight of reasonable probabilities. This is not mere "speculation," but a clinical-scientific assessment of the factors involved. On the other hand, a conclusion based only on a possibility of its validity is not enough to support reasonable certainty or any required burden of proof. However, on cross-examination, an expert who has offered a positive opinion based on reasonable medical or psychological certainty can admit without hurting his positive opinion that remote possibilities do exist that could contradict his conclusion.

ILLUSTRATIVE TESTIMONY

The examples of a report and testimony here presented were taken from the same case. The names of the participants have been changed. Otherwise, the material is from the public record and is unedited, except for dates which are omitted. As in the Alger Hiss trial noted earlier, the defense attempted to challenge the credibility of a key prosecution witness on the basis that he was "a pathological liar." Again, the psychiatrist based his evaluation in part on observing the witness in his testimony in court in the particular case. He did not personally conduct a psychiatric examination of the witness, but had available to him extensive, prior psychiatric records of the witness. The witness had a history of psychiatric illness and a long criminal record.

The report of the psychiatrist called by the defense appears first, followed by his testimony, both direct and cross-examination. The dangers of cross-examination on *symptoms* of mental disturbance, here pathological lying, are again displayed. The witness is questioned about current diagnostic concepts and about his own prior writings in the field. It can be expected that skilled cross-examiners will review all of the witness' prior published papers and even his prior courtroom testimony in similar cases. The witness should always review his own prior experience and papers and be ready for such inquiry. If the witness usually appears only for the defense (or the prosecution) in criminal matters, he may expect this to be brought out and his bias questioned. Often there is little that can be said in rebuttal of these challenges; the best countermove is to try to make oneself more available to the other side in future cases. The witness should respond that he or she is available to both sides and that the testimony is always unbiased. This answer should be given forthrightly and without too much heated resentment at the challenge.

After the testimony of the expert witness for the defense (here called Dr. Austin), the direct evidence of a prosecution's rebuttal expert witness is presented in full. There was no cross-examination. The rebutter was careful to stay within scientific areas and not to contradict the other expert personally. He did not volunteer material but answered the questions conservatively.

The prosecution's expert had the advantage of conducting a psychiatric examination of the person involved (here called Mr. Dingman). Since Mr. Dingman was a witness for the prosecution, it would be expected that such an examination would be permitted by the prosecution itself. It could also be expected that the prosecution (and the witness himself) would refuse an examination by the defense psychiatrist. It should be noted that the psychiatrist for the prosecution also sat in the courtroom and observed Mr. Dingman in his testimony. This psychiatrist was asked to state his "observations" of Mr. Dingman "as he testified." In a quite noncommittal response, he answered, "They were quite consistent with and confirmatory of my observations during my psychiatric examination [of a few days before]." No further questions were asked on this matter at this point, even though this doctor (here called Dr. Cermesoni) had not offered any diagnostic evaluation of Mr. Dingman as yet; he had only offered his findings on a simple mental status examination without offering a diagnostic impression or opinion. Later, when he provided his diagnosis, he was again cautious and conservative, asserting that "a *fairly characteristic* life style and pattern *emerges* of an antisocial personality disorder with adult situational reactions" (emphasis added). The prosecuting attorney then returned to the issue of Mr. Dingman's testimony. He asked the expert if, from the point of view of psychiatry, a definitive and conclusive method existed for determining whether the witness, Mr. Dingman, was or was not "telling the truth during the course of his testimony." The prosecution's expert answered "no." He offered a clear and understandable explanation. The style of the witness' direct testimony rendered him much less vulnerable to damaging cross-examination than the more venturesome, combative, loquacious psychiatrist or psychologist who believes that elaborate explanations are protective.

Psychiatric Report to the Court on the Credibility of Witness Albert Dingman

by Stephen Austin, M.D.

To the Justices of the Honorable Court:

At the request of counsel for each of the Respondents in the case before this Honorable Court, I have undertaken extensive review of available material on the background of one Albert Dingman.

The material reviewed includes the following items:

[Extensive prior psychiatric record cited.]

In addition to a close reading of the above noted items, I was personally in Court . . . and closely observed Albert Dingman as he testified both in direct and in cross-examination. As a result of all of the foregoing, I have no difficulty in arriving at an opinion as to the diagnosis of Albert Dingman.

I diagnose this individual as an antisocial personality and pathological liar.

The mental disease or defect is synonymous with sociopathic personality, psychopathic personality, constitutional psychopathic inferiority, and moral insanity.

All of those latter terms have been historically applied to what is now entitled antisocial personality. The condition has also been referred to and categorized as moral agenesis, inadequate social deviant, and inept social deviant. Each of the conditions referred to after my primary diagnosis of antisocial personality is simply a different name by which the same psychiatric disease was known at differing points in time. I arrived at my diagnosis by reason of the following:

1. The background of his antisocial behavior dating back to the age of 15;
2. His record of family conflict and, particularly, conflict with his father;
3. His inability to adjust to social, scholastic, familial, occupational, institutional, and Armed Service situations;
4. His confirmed and repetitious criminal activity commencing at an early age, that criminal activity taking the form of larcenies, swindles, and extortions and, in at least one instance, perjury, all of these offenses requiring successful and convincing fabrication;
5. His glib, cunning, and sometimes evasive manner while furnishing testimony in this Court;
6. His claim of feigning psychiatric symptoms in order to obtain self-serving results while in the United States Army and Federal custody;
7. His revelation of hallucinatory experiences to Doctor Sallinger and the nature of those experiences; and
8. The history of psychiatric care, treatment, and diagnoses relating to the subject.

The disease from which Mr. Dingman suffers is characterized in him by a marked lessening of natural and normal inhibitions against falsely testifying and narrating.

It is further characterized in him by a compulsive resort to fabrication.

In addition, he suffers from a general deficiency or defect in conscience.

My diagnosis is fortified by clear indications both by way of review of material and my personal observation of a malformed and malfunctioning superego.

In my opinion this disease raises a very serious question of the credibility, reliability, and believability of a narration or even testimony furnished by the patient in any given set of circumstances.

Very truly yours,

Stephen Austin, M.D.

Direct and Cross-Examination of Dr. Austin

Stephen Austin—Sworn

Direct Examination

Q [by Mr. Kranz]: Your name, sir?
A: My name is Dr. Stephen Austin.
Q: And, sir, did you offer the report which is in evidence before the Court?
A: Yes, I did.
Mr. Kranz: Your witness.

Cross-Examination

Q [by Mr. Grey]: Dr. Austin, do you have a copy of your report in front of you?

A: Yes, sir, I have it here.
Q: And do you have your diagnosis on page 3: antisocial personality and pathological liar?
A: Yes, sir.
Q: Now, let me ask you this basic question. Is pathological liar an addition to the diagnosis of antisocial personality or is it one facet or ingredient of an antisocial personality?
A: It is one facet or ingredient. It's one specific type of antisocial personality.
Q: So that pathological liar doesn't add anything to the basic antisocial personality diagnosis?
A: It makes it clearer as to which aspect we are referring to in this matter.
Q: Now, am I right in thinking that the lying which takes place in the so-called antisocial personality is lying for the purpose of advancing the person's concept of his own best self-interest?
A: That is correct, sir.
Q: And you recognize, do you not, that lay people have an idea of what is a pathological liar? That's a lay term, isn't it?
A: Do I recognize—
Q: Yes.
A: —that lay people have an idea—
Q: Yes, of what pathological liar means.
A: Yes, I think they do.
Q: And, as a matter of fact, pathological liar is exclusively a lay term. It is not used in the modern nomenclature of your profession, isn't that right?
A: It is excluded from the latest *Diagnostic and Statistical Manual of Mental Disorders,* that is true, but it does occur in previous editions.
Q: And in your own book on clinical psychiatry, the phrase pathological liar is not used, is it, Dr. Austin?
A: Not in the third edition, but it appears in previous editions.
Q: Well, if it's now out of both the current nomenclature and your current edition, it means it's a term that has ceased to have significance for ongoing definitions in psychiatry, doesn't it?
A: Not necessarily, sir.
Q: Well, does the concept of pathological liar mean that the person has to lie even when it's against his own interest?
A: No, sir.
Q: So we may exclude, therefore, from the concept of pathological liar any notion of compulsive lying under any and all circumstances by the individual in question?
A: I wouldn't say that such a person would lie under any and all circumstances, no, sir, but usually would lie when it would serve his own purpose.
Q: And we may reject from the term pathological liar any notion that the person is under an obsession to lie any and all times and under any and all circumstances, may we not, Doctor?
A: You mean compulsion, not obsession, I think, if I may correct you.
Q: Yes.
A: But in terms of the sense of your question, that is correct. It is possible for a pathological liar to tell the truth.
Q: Now, can you tell me why you saw fit to introduce into this diagnosis of an antisocial personality the additional phrase pathological liar if the term has gone out of current semantics in the profession?

A: Yes. Because I feel that the problem that is before us here does not involve whether he commits crimes or not. In other words, we are not here trying to figure out if he is now guilty of swindling or if he is guilty of any other particular felony; but the issue here, as I understand it, is essentially the truthfulness of his accusations and of his statements; therefore, I took the liberty of resurrecting this term because of its descriptive importance in this particular matter. I feel it hits the nail right on the head.
Q: Well, you didn't think, Doctor, that people reading this report might think that pathological liar meant someone who had to lie under any and all circumstances, did you, by any chance?
A: No, sir.
Q: You didn't put it in here, in other words, for coloration?
A: No, sir.
Q: Do you regard this diagnosis, antisocial personality, as the diagnosis of a mental illness?
A: Yes, it is.
Q: In the current nomenclature of your profession, is there not an overall definition of what is called mental disorder?
A: Yes.
Q: And under mental disorder there are things that are described as mental illness, are there not?
A: Could you refresh my mind on this please?
Q: Well, I think you might refresh my mind on it.
A: I have a copy of *DSM* here, too.
Q: Well, I wish you would refer to it.
A: To what are you referring, please?
Q: I am referring to the overall terminology which is under the heading of the diagnostic nomenclature, 'List of Mental Disorders,' and their code numbers.
A: Yes, sir. That's on page 5.
Q: Yes. That's the total overall category, isn't it?
A: That's correct.
Q: Now, under that category, do you recognize that there is a category known as mental disease?
A: You will have to point this out for me. As far as I am aware, they are all mental diseases.
Q: Well, Doctor, do you recognize a distinction between a psychosis and the diagnosis of antisocial personality?
A: Yes, I do recognize that there is a difference in diagnosis between psychosis and antisocial personality.
Q: And a psychosis would come under the category of a mental disease, would it not?
A: Yes. So does an antisocial personality.
Q: You consider that that is also a mental disease?
A: Yes, sir.
Q: Well, now, in the case of a psychosis, where is the root of the difficulty?
A: In a psychosis the usual difficulty involves the person's contact with reality, and this is usually disturbed.
Q: And in the case of the antisocial personality I think you say someplace in your report that it has something to do with the superego?
A: Yes, sir. It has to do with the superego or conscience or the individual sense of morality or his sense of right and wrong, as contrasted with a psychotic individual, where contact with reality would be lost.

Q: So there is a difference between the psychotic individual who has lost contact with reality and the antisocial personality?
A: Yes, there is a difference. But I am not sure which direction you are going in.
Q: Doctor, may we agree that a deficiency in the superego is not to be equated with a psychosis?
A: Yes, sir, we can agree on that.
Q: Now, this superego is a conscience or monitoring factor, as I understand it, in psychiatric language?
A: That is correct, sir.
Q: And you also speak of something which you call the ego?
A: Yes, that is correct.
Q: And also the id?
A: That is also correct.
Q: And in general, is the id the source of impulses; the superego, the monitoring or conscience factor, and the ego, the executing psychic instrumentality?
A: Yes, in a general way.
Q: Now, all of these phenomena—ego, superego, and id—are terms referred to in a certain school of psychiatry, are they not?
A: Yes, sir.
Q: And it is what one might describe as a working psychiatric series of postulates, isn't it?
A: Yes, that is correct, sir.
Q: You never see in any tangible forms the superego itself, do you?
A: No, sir.
Q: And you never see the ego itself or the id itself?
A: No, you're absolutely right.
Q: Now, when you say, on page 5 in your report to the Court, that your diagnosis is fortified by clear indications, both by way of review of material and by personal observation of a malformed and malfunctioning superego, you don't mean to give the Court the impression that you have actually observed Dingman's superego, do you?
A: No, sir.
Q: What you mean is that you made certain observations as to events in his testimony, or as described in his testimony, which caused you to believe that he had a malformed superego, isn't that right?
A: That is precisely what I said.
Q: And in the course of his testimony, he described his perjury in a certain instance, did he not?
A: I believe it was referred to, yes.
Q: And you believed that, didn't you?
A: I think I was inclined to, yes. There are some times when it was sort of hard to figure out whether he was telling the truth or whether he was lying; but that I tended to believe.
Q: And when he described his activities as a swindler, again there was a situation where you tended to believe him, didn't you?
A: Yes, I did. There was confirmatory evidence in those cases.
Q: And when he described his feigning certain psychiatric symptoms at certain periods, you tended to believe that he actually did feign those symptoms?
A: I am just not sure. There are some antisocial personalities who do have psychotic episodes in which they can have hallucinations, but the nature of his hallucinations were such that I tended to believe they were lies.

Q: So as he described certain symptoms, certain past activity, certain lying, certain swindling, certain episodes of conflict in his life, you tended to believe him, didn't you?
A: Some of the conflicts I believed. When he told lies about certain things, I believed them, yes, sir.
Q: You believed he was lying when he said he was lying?
A: I believed so, yes, sir.
Q: And, therefore, on page 5 of your report, when you speak of 'a compulsive resort to fabrication,' once again we ought to have in mind your earlier testimony about how you define a pathological liar, had we not? You didn't mean to suggest here, when you used the 'compulsive resort to fabrication,' that he would lie under any circumstances other than those when he thought it was in his best interest?
A: I believe I made it clear that a pathological liar can tell the truth and that it is difficult to know when he is lying and when he is telling the truth, but that if he's got—if you've got a choice of believing him or not, I would view his statement with suspicion, and I would prefer to have outside evaluation of what he is saying before I would accept his statements as being true. And if you compare him, the pathological liar, with a normal person, I think his tendency—the tendency of the pathological liar to lie—is much greater than that of a normal person. So that I am skeptical of what he said.
Q: Doctor, this phrase, 'compulsive resort to fabrication,' might connote that you meant that under any and all circumstances he had an irresistible, an uncontrollable impulse to lie, and that you did not mean?
A: No, sir. There are times when he can tell the truth, that's right.
Q: You also referred in your report to what you regarded as his glib, cunning, and sometimes evasive manner while furnishing testimony in this Court, did you not?
A: Yes, I did sir.
Q: And would you agree that other competent psychiatrists, making observations with respect to his manner, when he was testifying, might disagree with those characteristics?
Q: Yes, they might.
Q: Now, in the last paragraph of your report, you say that his disease raises a very serious question of the credibility, reliability, and believability of narration. Those three words are all synonyms for the same thing, aren't they?
A: I think they have slightly different shades of meaning.
Q: Well, would you tell us what they are?
A: Yes. I think a thing is believable if it is within the level with which people usually associate believable things. I think a thing is a reliable statement, on the other hand, which is one upon which you can place reliance. It is not merely that you believe it, but that you can rely upon it, and you can take further action based upon it. So that I think there is a difference between a thing being believable and a thing being reliable. My understanding of the general word credibility is that it includes both the term competency and something more than competency. Competency means the ability to perceive and to recollect and to recite what you have seen and what you recall. But I think credibility involves the trustworthiness of the truthfulness of that statement. It involves the individual's—a consideration of the individual's morality, of his sense of right or wrong, his appreciation of an oath, his deterrence not to lie, and his tendency to lie. I think that these are three different terms. And that is why I included them.

Q: Have you reviewed the direct testimony of Dr. Bolster and Dr. Cermesoni?
A: Yes, I have.
Q: And do you agree with them that the present-day science of psychiatry offers to a Court no infallible index of the credibility, reliability, and believability of a witness, even one who suffers from a sociopathic personality, in fact?
A: I missed your adjective. Could I have the question repeated?
Q: Do you believe that present-day psychiatry furnishes to a Court no infallible yardstick with respect to whether or not a given witness suffering from an antisocial personality problem is in a given situation telling or not telling the truth?
A: Yes, I agree with that, sir.
Mr. Grey: Thank you very much.
Mr. Kranz: No further questions.
Mr. Holder: I have no questions.
Chief Justice Ames: You may step down, Doctor.
The Witness: Thank you.
[Witness excused.]

Direct Testimony of Dr. John P. Cermesoni

Q: What is your name?
A: John P. Cermesoni.
Q: Where do you live?
A: 10 Ashmont Road, Pully, Vermont.
Q: What is your profession?
A: I am a doctor of medicine who specializes in psychiatry.
Q: Will you give the court an outline of your professional education, qualifications, and experience?
A: This outline is contained in the curriculum vitae which is attached as Appendix 1.
Q: At the request of Special Counsel in this case, did you examine one Albert Dingman?
A: I did.
Q: When did you make this examination?
A: On Sunday evening, between the hours of 4:30 and 6:00 p.m.
Q: Who was present at this examination?
A: Myself, Dr. Bolster, Mr. Grey, Mr. Konrad [co-counsel], and Mr. Dingman.
Q: What was the purpose of the examination as you understood it?
A: The purpose of the examination, as I understood it, was to make psychiatric observations and such conclusions as were within the range of reasonable medical certainty relating to the following three areas:
   (1) The presence or absence of mental illness or mental disorder in Mr. Dingman at the time of examination and his testimony;
   (2) The nature and extent to which any such mental illness or disorder if found would impair his competency to testify as a witness;
   (3) The nature and extent to which psychiatric observations and conclusions could contribute to the court's weighing of the credibility of Mr. Dingman's testimony in these proceedings.
Q: At the time of the examination, what material pertaining to Mr. Dingman's psychiatric history had you examined?
A: [Extensive clinical records cited.]

Q: What other materials pertaining to Mr. Dingman had you examined?
A: I had read through the transcript of his testimony before a certain Subcommittee of the United States Senate, and had also been furnished, by counsel, with copies of the Information with respect to Mr. Regan and Mr. Esposito.
Q: Did you at that time have the Probation Records?
A: No. These were furnished by counsel at a later date.
Q: Will you state the observations which you made of Mr. Dingman at the interview?
A: [Mental Status]

[*General Description*]

Mr. Dingman proved to be an obese, well-groomed, highly articulate, somewhat fatigued and subdued but highly alert and reflective man. He adopted what I would characterize as a weary 'noblesse oblige' attitude in which he implied that we were naive amateurs in understanding what he referred to as the 'milieu' of organized crime and the area of illegal high-finance manipulations. Mr. Dingman is a highly cynical man. Nevertheless, toward the end of the interview, in the context of discussing the impact of his most recent incarceration on his wife and children, I had the impression that Mr. Dingman was close to tears. It should be noted that his father died about two months before this examination.

[*Perceptions*]

Normal; no illusions or hallucinations were noted.

[*Associations*]

Normal; no looseness of associations, tangentiality, circumstantiality, or concreteness was noted.

[*Thought Content*]

Normal; no delusions or slips were noted.

[*Affect*]

Normal; subdued but appropriate. No significant depression or elation was noted. The range of affect was somewhat constricted in that he sometimes showed smiling affect, but it was rather faint and controlled.

[*Memory*]

Normal; unusually precise with an apparently excellent memory for both recent and past events.

[*Orientation*]

Normal; oriented as to time, place, and person.

[*Intelligence*]

Normal; highly intelligent.

[*Behavior*]

Abnormal by history in a social sense. Mr. Dingman has a number of convictions for fraud and forgery and one for perjury. During the examination he was courteous and appropriate. No tics or unusual mannerisms were noted.

[*Speech*]

Normal; flow of speech and syntax normal. Vocabulary excellent; articulate and precise.

[*Insight and Judgment*]

Normal. He observed that he had psychiatric 'problems' which he summarized as follows: 'I took too many risks I didn't have to take.'

Q: Were you in the courtroom during the entire period of Mr. Dingman's testimony before the court?

A: Yes.
Q: And did you observe Mr. Dingman as he testified?
A: Yes.
Q: And will you state what your observations were of Mr. Dingman as he testified?
A: They were quite consistent with and confirmatory of my observations during my psychiatric examination . . . .
Q: Is 'mental illness' a term which has an accepted meaning in the medical-psychiatric profession?
A: Yes.
Q: What is the meaning of the term 'mental illness'?
A: I am guided by the most recent articulation of mental illness promulgated in the regulations of the Vermont Department of Mental Health. It is consistent with the definition of 'psychosis' in the *Diagnostic and Statistical Manual of Mental Disorders* of the American Psychiatric Association. Although the Vermont definition is articulated in the context of the basis for involuntary commitment, I accept it for broader usage. It states:

> 'For purposes of involuntary commitment mental illness shall mean a substantial disorder of thought, mood, perception, orientation, or memory which grossly impairs judgment, behavior, capacity to recognize reality, or ability to meet the ordinary demands of life . . . .'

Q: Is there also a condition known to psychiatry as 'sociopathic' or 'antisocial personality'?
A: Yes.
Q: What is the generally accepted meaning of that term in psychiatry?
A: This term is reserved for individuals who are basically unsocialized and whose behavior pattern brings them repeatedly into conflict with society. They are incapable of significant loyalty to individuals, groups or social values. They are grossly selfish, callous, irresponsible, impulsive, and unable to feel guilt or to learn from experience and punishment. Frustration tolerance is low. They tend to blame others or offer plausible rationalizations for their behavior. A mere history of repeated legal or social offenses is not sufficient to justify this diagnosis.
Q: Will you differentiate between 'mental illness' and the condition known as 'antisocial personality'?
A: 'Antisocial personality,' along with the other personality disorders, is characterized by an ingrained, usually life-long, dysfunctional style of coping with the challenges of living. The disorder is a persistent and consistent dysfunctional part of the psychological equipment of the individual. 'Mental illness,' on the other hand, represents an often episodic and, from a psychological point of view, more severe period of dysfunction or disease with characteristic patterns of symptoms which are most often time-limited with treatment.
Q: On the basis of your examination of the material pertaining to Mr. Dingman's psychiatric history which was made available to you and which you have listed in your answer to a preceding question, were you able, within reasonable medical certainty, to form an opinion as to his mental and psychiatric condition as of [current date]?
A: Yes.
Q: What is that opinion?
A: In my opinion, a fairly characteristic life style and pattern of behavior emerges of an antisocial personality disorder with adult situational depressive reactions.

Q: Did you observe any evidence of mental disease or illness during your examination of Mr. Dingman?
A: No.
Q: Did you observe any evidence of mental disease or illness during your observation of him during his court testimony?
A: No.
Q: Does the diagnosis of sociopathic or antisocial personality make it probable that the person so diagnosed will lie on any and all occasions?
A: No.
Q: Will you explain the reason for that answer?
A: He will lie when it suits his self-serving purposes. He will tell the truth when it serves his self-serving purposes.
Q: Are you able to give this Court, from the point of view of psychiatry, in large measure, a definitive and conclusive method of determining whether or not the witness Dingman was or was not telling the truth during the course of his testimony?
A: No. In psychiatry, in large measure, we have to rely on the frequent testing of reality external to what our patients tell us in order to illuminate distortions and misperceptions, both deliberate and unconscious, on the part of our patients. To a certain extent, common sense helps us to clarify distortions, but confirmatory history from other sources is frequently necessary. It is relatively rare that we can ascertain within reasonable medical certainty from interview alone, for example, whether or not a patient is malingering.
Q: Are you able to form an opinion as to the mental and psychiatric condition of Albert Dingman as of the fall of [12 years previously]?
A: Yes with respect to the presence of antisocial personality disorder; no with respect to an intervening mental illness.
Q: Will you give us the reasons why you were not able with reasonable medical certainty to form an opinion as to Mr. Dingman's mental and psychiatric condition as of the fall of [12 years previously]?
A: In my opinion, the recorded data do not permit an opinion within reasonable medical certainty at this distant point in time without the opportunity of having examined Mr. Dingman at that time. I did not find the recorded observations in the record . . . to be persuasive of a mental illness, certainly not within reasonable medical certainty. I believe Mr. Dingman to have been consistently an antisocial personality for the past 25 years. Whether an intercurrent illness intervened in his life in [12 years before] I cannot say.
Q: Assume that as of [12 years previously] a complete psychiatric examination of Mr. Dingman led to a diagnosis of schizophrenic reaction, schizoaffective type with obsessive-compulsive features, were you able to determine from your observations and examination of Mr. Dingman whether or not there were symptoms of that condition existing as of the time of your examination?
A: Yes.
Q: What is the opinion?
A: Symptoms of a schizoaffective illness were not present.
Q: What are the bases for that opinion?
A: None of the characteristic clinical symptoms seen in a schizophrenic illness, such as loose or illogical associations, inappropriate or blunted affect, odd mannerisms, concreteness of thinking, or bizarre behavior, was observed during my examination or my observations during his testimony. Neither were the mood disturbances of pronounced elation

or depression present which would support a schizoaffective diagnosis.

Q: Assume that this man, in [12 years before], had a schizophrenic reaction, schizoaffective type with obsessive-compulsive features. On the basis of the history which you have and your observations and examination, do you have an opinion as to whether or not, as of [the current date], there was a remission of that condition?

A: Yes.

Q: Again, what are the reasons for that opinion?

A: If it had ever occurred, it was no longer present.

REFERENCES

1. Diamond, B. L., and Louisell, D. W.: The Psychiatrist as an Expert Witness: Some Ruminations and Speculations. *Michigan Law Rev.* 63:1335–1346, 1965.
2. Dieden, J., and Gasparich, S. M.: Psychiatric Evidence and Full Disclosure in the Criminal Trial. *Cal. Law Rev.* 52:543–560, 1964; see also, *Effective Utilization of Psychiatric Evidence,* Practicing Law Institute, New York, 1970.
3. Pollack, S.: Psychiatric Consultation for the Court, in Mendel, R., and Solomon, P. (eds.): *The Psychiatric Consultation.* Grune & Stratton, New York, 1968; Diamond, B. L.: The Fallacy of the Impartial Expert, *Arch. Crim. Psychodynamics* 3:221–230, 1959; Guttmacher, M.: What Can the Psychiatrist Contribute to the Issue of Criminal Responsibility? *J. Nerv. Ment. Dis.* 136:103–110, 1963; Dershowitz, A. M.: Psychiatry and the Criminal Process: A Knife That Cuts Both Ways, *Judicature* 23:101–120, 1973; Cooke, G.: *The Role of the Forensic Psychologist,* Charles C Thomas, Springfield, Ill., 1979.
4. *Examination of Medical Experts,* Matthew Bender, New York, 1968; *Effective Utilization of Psychiatric Evidence,* op. cit.
5. Cleary, E. W.: *McCormick's Handbook of the Law of Evidence.* ed. 2. West Publishing Company, St. Paul, Minn., 1972; Allen, R. C., Ferster, E. Z., and Weihofen, H.: *Mental Impairment and Legal Incompetency.* Prentice-Hall, Englewood Cliffs, N.J., 1968.
6. *In Re Keidaisch's Will,* 13 N.Y.S. 255 (1918); *Dossenbach v. Reidhar's Executrix,* 245 Ky. 449, 53 S.W. 2d 731 (1935); *In Re Lawrence's Will,* 59 N.Y.S. 174 (1936); *Cundick v. Broadbent,* 383 F. 2d 157 (10th. Cir. 1967); Note, *Am. Law Reports,* 2d 40:15 et seq., 1955.
7. Rosenberg, A. H.: Competency to Stand Trial: Who Knows Best? *Crim. Law Bull.* 6:55–65, 1970.
8. *Commonwealth v. Devereaux,* 257 Mass. 391, 153 N.E. 881, 1926.
9. *Lessard v. Schmidt,* 349 F. Supp. 1078 (E.D. Wisc. 1972); *In Re Bailey,* 482 F. 2d 648 (D.C. Cir. 1973); *Suzuki v. Quisenberry,* 411 F. Supp. 1113 (D. Hawaii 1976).
10. *Dobbs v. State,* 191 Ark. 236, 85 S.W. 2d 694, 1935; *People v. Spigno,* 156 Cal. App. 2d 279, 319 P. 2d 458, 1957.
11. *Sandow v. Weyerhauser Co.,* 449 P. 2d 426, Oregon, 1969; reprinted in Curran, W. J., and Shapiro, E.D. (eds): *Law, Medicine and Forensic Science.* ed. 2. Little, Brown, Boston, 1970, pp. 324–328.
12. Strout, A. R.: Some Problems in the Trial of a Will Contest. *Baylor Law Rev.* 7:121-135, 1955.
13. Norwell, J.A.: Invasion of the Province of the Jury. *Texas Law Rev.* 31:731–749, 1953.
14. Wigmore, J. H.: *Evidence,* ed. 3. Little, Brown, Boston, 1949, p. 17.
15. Cleary, op. cit., p. 27.
16. McGarry, A. L., et al.: *Competency to Stand Trial and Mental Illness.* Monograph Series, Crime and Delinquency Issues, National Institute of Mental Health, DHEW Publication No. (HSM) 73-9105, Washington, D.C., 1973.
17. Rosenberg, A. H.: Competency for Trial: A Problem of Interdisciplinary Communication. *Judicature* 53:316–321, 1970.

18. Lipsitt, P. D., Lelos, D., and McGarry, A. L.: Competency for Trial: A Screening Instrument. *Am. J. Psychiatry* 128:105–109, 1971; McGarry, et al., op.cit.
19. Robey, A.: Criteria for Competency to Stand Trial: A Checklist for Psychiatrists. *Am. J. Psychiatry* 122:616–622, 1965; Bukataman, B. A., Foy, J. L., and DeGrazia, E.: What is Competency to Stand Trial? *Am. J. Psychiatry* 127:1225–1229, 1971.
20. Matthews, A. R.: *Mental Disability and the Law.* American Bar Foundation, Chicago, 1970.
21. Szasz, T. S.: *Psychiatric Justice.* Macmillan, New York, 1965.
22. Curran, W. J.: *Tracy's the Doctor as a Witness.* ed. 2. W. B. Saunders, Philadelphia, 1965.
23. Stryker, L. P.: *Courts and Doctors.* Macmillan, New York, 1932; Simpson, K.: *A Doctor's Guide to Court.* ed. 2. Butterworth, London, 1967; *Effective Utilization of Psychiatric Evidence,* op.cit.
24. Diamond, op.cit.
25. Watson, A.S.: Untying the Knots: The Cross-Examination of the Psychiatric Expert Witness, in *Examination of Medical Experts.* Matthew Bender, New York, 1968; Rothblatt, H. B.: The Preparation of the Psychiatric Defense and the Direct Examination of the Psychiatric Witness. *Legal Med. Ann.,* 1971, pp. 450–468.
26. *U.S. v. Hiss, trial transcript,* Criminal No. C128-402, U.S. District Court of So. Dist. of N.Y., November, 1949; reprinted in part in Curran, W.J. (ed.): *Law and Medicine.* Little, Brown, Boston, 1960, pp. 577–582.

ADDITIONAL READING

Curran, W.J., and Shapiro, E.D. (eds.): *Law, Medicine, and Forensic Science.* ed. 2. Little, Brown, Boston, 1970; Supplement, 1974.

Ennis, B. J., and Litwack, T.R.: Psychiatry and the Presumption of Expertism: Flipping Coins in the Courtroom. *Cal. Law Rev.* 62:693–752, 1974.

Ewalt, J.R.: Mental Competency, in Houts, M. (ed.): *Courtroom Medicine.* Matthew Bender, New York, 1960.

Hirschfield, A.H., and Behan, M.D.: The Psychiatrist and the Defense Counsel. *Ins. Counsel J.* 32:215–220, 1965.

Katz, J., Goldstein, J., and Dershowitz, A.: *Psychoanalysis, Psychiatry and Law.* The Free Press, New York, 1967.

MacDonald, J. M.: *Psychiatry and the Criminal.* ed. 3. Charles C Thomas, Springfield, Ill., 1976.

Roberts, L.M.: Some Observations on the Problems of the Forensic Psychiatrist. *Wisc. Law Rev.* 25:240–267, 1965.

Stein, J.: Mental Competency and the Law. *Med. Trial Tech. Q.* 10:155–180, 1964.

Watson, A.: Communication Between Psychiatrists and Lawyers. *Int. Psychiatric Clin.* 1:186–193, 1964.

PART 5 THE FORENSIC SCIENCES

CHAPTER 44

Joseph L. Peterson is Associate Professor and Director of the Center for Research in Criminal Justice at the University of Illinois, Circle Campus. He is the former Executive Director of the Forensic Sciences Foundation, Inc., of Rockville, Maryland, and also served as Director of the Criminal Justice Center at John Jay College of Criminal Justice in New York. He has been the project director of Federally supported research on physical evidence collection and utilization. A graduate of Carthage College and the University of California at Berkeley, Dr. Peterson is a Fellow of the American Academy of Forensic Sciences and a member of the California Association of Criminalistics and the Northeastern Association of Forensic Scientists.

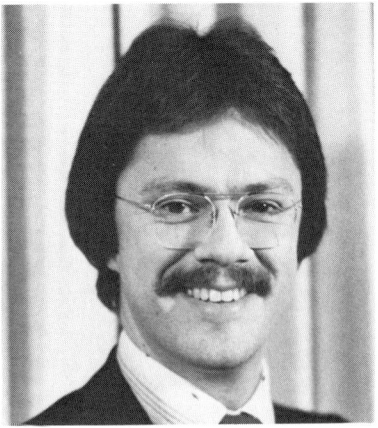

THE TEAM APPROACH IN FORENSIC SCIENCE

Joseph L. Peterson, D. Crim.

Forensic science is the application of science to the purposes of justice and thus functions within a legal environment unique to most natural and behavioral sciences. Due to the interdisciplinary nature of the forensic sciences and their position within the legal system, the need for cooperation and teamwork is essential for optimal productivity.

The necessity for teamwork in the forensic sciences is exhibited at two levels. First, the forensic scientist must routinely work with forensic scientists of various other scientific disciplines in the investigation of a criminal matter or civil dispute. It is not uncommon for a single incident to yield a number of different evidence types, which then dictates the summoning of various kinds of expertise. Furthermore, a single item of evidence may potentially reveal information which can only be elicited by the combined examination of several different scientists.

Secondly, the need for teamwork, cooperation, and communication extends outside the scientific realm into the areas of law enforcement and civil concerns such as insurance, environmental protection, emergency room services, and the investigation of mass disasters. The forensic scientist functions primarily in a reactive mode, responding to the requests of various investigative personnel to aid in the examination of physical evidence, to provide the interpretation of scientific data, and to present his findings in such a manner that they will be used in the best interests of justice and society.

This chapter will examine and discuss how and why the forensic scientist must cooperate with the other scientific and nonscientific professionals that he encounters during the course of an investigation. It will identify those areas in which communications often become strained and where cooperation sometimes breaks down completely. Recommendations will be advanced for reducing barriers to communication and cooperation, which would lead to the more effective utilization of the forensic sciences.

Initially, the primary scientific disciplines which are routinely involved in a forensic investigation will be identified. Each of these disciplines is founded in a natural or behavioral science which may be applied to legal problems (see Fig. 1-1, p. 3). While most full-time forensic scientists operate within federal, state, or local laboratories, many scientists are private examiners or work on a part-time basis, primarily as consultants, while regularly employed by an academic institution.

Following this brief introduction to the forensic science disciplines is an outline of the important characteristics of the legal system which influence its acceptance of scientific evidence in court cases. Basic differences exist in philosophy and decision-making practices between those in legal and law enforcement positions and those in the scientific community. Such conflicts help to explain why close teamwork among scientists and attorneys or police officers is often difficult. The impartial, objective, and technical fact-finding methods of the scientist are sometimes incompatible with the more subjective modes of inquiry employed by the legal investigators, the result being two adversaries with the ultimate goal of justice sometimes obscured.

A third section in this chapter will describe the evidence utilization process, identifying key points at which teamwork and cooperation are essential. Because the scientist primarily operates within the laboratory, the initial recognition and preservation of physical evidence is usually carried out by a citizen or police officer. The products of the scientist's examinations are in the form of written reports and scientific opinions which, again, are ultimately used by nonscientists. Because the forensic scientist functions within an adversary environment, he must take great care to insure that his examinations receive proper interpretation and appropriate weight in court.

The final section of the chapter will summarize the primary problem areas which impede forensic teamwork.. In order to ameliorate these problems, the greatest attention should perhaps be focused on proper training of personnel and the opportunity to exchange information among the respective counterparts. Additional requirements include the need for a logical organizational structure for the laboratory and its users, proper management-reporting procedures, and the support of the chief policymakers within the laboratory's jurisdiction.

FORENSIC SCIENCE SPECIALTY AREAS

Forensic science is the study and application of science to the processes of law involving the scientific examination and evaluation of evidence. The field encompasses several areas of expertise which, if properly utilized, can contribute much to the investigations of both civil and criminal cases. These areas include:

1. *Criminalistics,* wherein evidence such as bloodstains, glass, soil, clothing, and firearms is compared, identified, individualized, and interpreted and, on the basis of this interpretation, the facts surrounding an event at the time that it occurred may be reconstructed.
2. *Forensic pathology.* The forensic pathologist investigates and interprets injury and death resulting from violence or occurring suddenly, unexpectedly, or in an unexplained manner. The forensic pa-

thologist, in his examination of the body, also serves to collect physical evidence which will undergo examination by toxicologists, criminalists, and other forensic scientists.
3. *Forensic toxicology.* The toxicologist performs analytical studies of the hazards and harmful effects of such external substances as poisons, drugs, pollutants, and potentially toxic chemicals which may be introduced into living systems.
4. *Forensic anthropology,* which involves the use of standard physical anthropological techniques to identify skeletal or otherwise unidentifiable remains. The physical anthropologist is routinely involved in mass disaster investigations in the identification of human remains.
5. *Forensic dentistry.* Often working closely with the forensic pathologist and physical anthropologist, the forensic dentist or odontologist examines and evaluates injuries to the teeth, jaws, and oral tissues and examines dental remains for the purpose of victim identification. He also examines bite marks in cases of homicide, child abuse, and sexual assault to provide identification of a suspect.
6. *Questioned documents examination.* The questioned documents examiner is involved in the scientific examination of handwriting, typewriting, printing, ink, paper, or other aspects of a document for the purpose of determining various legal questions asked about the document in civil or criminal cases.
7. *Other forensic science specialties,* which include voiceprint examination, polygraph technology, and related police science specialties such as fingerprinting and ballistics.

THE ADVERSARY SYSTEM OF JUSTICE

The laws of science which serve as the basis for all scientific inquiries are fundamentally different from those laws which govern society. Natural science laws, experimental and empirical methods of inquiry and examination, the requirement of objectivity, and the pursuit of truth all form the basis for scientific findings. For the scientists, the manner of approaching a problem is just as important as the end product itself.

The civil and criminal law reflects the progression of society's values and mores, and therefore is constantly changing. The aim of the law and accompanying procedures is properly described as "the just resolution of human conflict."[1]

Our American system of justice places responsibility upon the adversaries in the litigation to present the relevant facts and hopefully to determine the truth. However, in reality, the adversary system very often undermines the pursuit of truth with the opposing sides seeking to win at all costs without obligation to reveal information which may be detrimental to their case or their clients' best interest.

> ... the lawyer aims at winning in the fight, not at aiding the court to discover the facts. He does not want the trial court to reach a sound educated guess if it is likely to be contrary to his client's interests.[2]

On the contrary, the scientist should have no personal stake in the outcome of a civil or criminal case. The scientist's expertise is in the application of science to a legal controversy and the proper interpretation of scientific findings, while the expertise of the attorney is as much based upon his abilities as an *advocate* as it is on his proficiency in gathering facts. The attorney is representing the interests of one side in a case and is the key spokesman for that position only (see Chapter 2).

The law functions to bring cases to a satisfactory resolution. Charges are filed and a decision must be forthcoming—innocence or guilt. Although there are many shades of gray as to what constitutes "proof" or "reasonable doubt," the court is required to make a black and white decision based upon the evidence presented. Accordingly, the attorney will press a witness to take a firm stance regarding the content of the testimony in order to weigh the balance of evidence in his client's favor.

Unfortunately, for the attorney, the scientist's conclusions often cannot be stated in unequivocal terms. The state of the art of the analysis being performed may only allow a conclusion such as: "The evidence is found to be *consistent* with materials of known identity." The scientist can only infrequently state that evidence *absolutely* connects a suspect with an offense or victim or indicates that the alleged offender was responsible for the crime.

The scientist can make his strongest statements regarding the *exclusion* of certain evidence from consideration (e.g., the evidence hair is totally inconsistent with the hair of the suspect and therefore could not have originated from that source). This type of information which may exonerate the defendant may not be presented by the prosecution in court; however, it may be brought out by the defense through discovery or upon cross-examination.

Affirmative statements by the forensic scientist, with few exceptions, are statements of probability. Examinations may show that there is a high probability that two objects have a common origin, although there always remains the possibility that the objects did not share a common source. Statements made in probabilistic terms must be translated into layman's language so that the judge and jury can consider them in the context of the legal case (see Chapters 55 and 56).

At other times, the physical evidence in a case is inconsistent with other circumstantial or eyewitness accounts. The court then is faced with the dilemma of explaining the inconsistency or compromising either set of testimony.

The law also struggles to keep scientific testimony in its place, giving it proper weight but always reserving the right to temper it or perhaps eliminate it from consideration altogether. Courts and juries reserve the right to disregard scientific evidence in any given case and thus to maintain the upper hand in the application and administration of law.[3]

What these previously stated conditions tell us is that the law and science have several fundamentally different premises in their philosophies, objectives, and methods of inquiry. The individuals within the science and law professions have undergone years of education and training, both philosophically and in practice, in their chosen fields and work within quite different professional environments with their own respective peer groups and professional associations.

The classical stereotyping of scientists and attorneys does have some validity, for the two fields will attract different types of individuals into them at the outset. With few exceptions, the attorney is much more verbally adept than the scientist. Nevertheless, both must use this skill to communicate in the courtroom setting. Although it is most assuredly an important professional requirement, "forensics," or the art of debating, is not a strong feature in the public role of many forensic scientists. Most scientists would be more comfortable expressing their findings through written reports or through a lecture in a classroom atmosphere. The adversary setting is frustrating to the forensic scientist because he often cannot handle the attorney's firing-line approach which may prevent him from communicating his findings to the best of his ability with the appropriate explanations and qualifications.

While alternatives to our present system of justice and means for introducing scientific findings into a case have been proposed, major changes in the near future are unlikely. These fundamental differences between the legal and scientific professions have been discussed because they unquestionably influence the level of teamwork possible. The adversary system of justice often makes the attorney and the scientist unlikely teammates, particularly when conflicts arise with regard to service for the accused in a case. While teamwork among the police and prosecution has the greatest potential at present, the forensic scientist must strive to serve all parties in the resolution of a legal conflict.

FORENSIC SCIENCE INVOLVEMENT

While the forensic sciences become involved in a wide array of criminal and civil cases, this chapter will, for the purposes of illustration, focus upon their role in criminal cases. The need for teamwork in the utilization of the forensic sciences can be best illustrated by examining a case as it progresses from its commission on through the investigation and adjudication processes. As we examine the progressive stages in a criminal investigation during which one or more of the forensic science disciplines become involved, the need for teamwork and cooperation will become very evident as police investigators, scientists, and attorneys all play important roles in determining whether evidence will yield its potential information.

A study in 1969 set out to determine the level and types of physical evidence at crime scenes which was worthy of preservation, collection, and scientific examination.[4] Of the 749 felony crime scenes investigated by the study team, 88 percent were judged to have potentially valuable physical evidence. Of these cases, however, only four resulted in evidence being collected and routed to the crime laboratory for examination. This project also resulted in the development of a decision-making model for conceptualizing and identifying those important decision levels which constitute the investigative process and particularly the search for physical evidence. Figure 44-1 depicts these decision points and illustrates the "funneling" effect which accounts for the great majority of physical evidence being screened out of the investigation before it even reaches the attention of the laboratory examiner.[5]

Initial Police Response

Following the commission of a crime, it is the police officer's responsibility to respond to the suspected criminal incident and to determine how the event will be handled. In cases involving serious personal injury or substantial property loss, the officer has little opportunity to exercise discretionary powers, which in less serious situations may mean that the incident is not written up or handled through formal channels. The official police guidelines, the seriousness of the suspected offense, the cap-

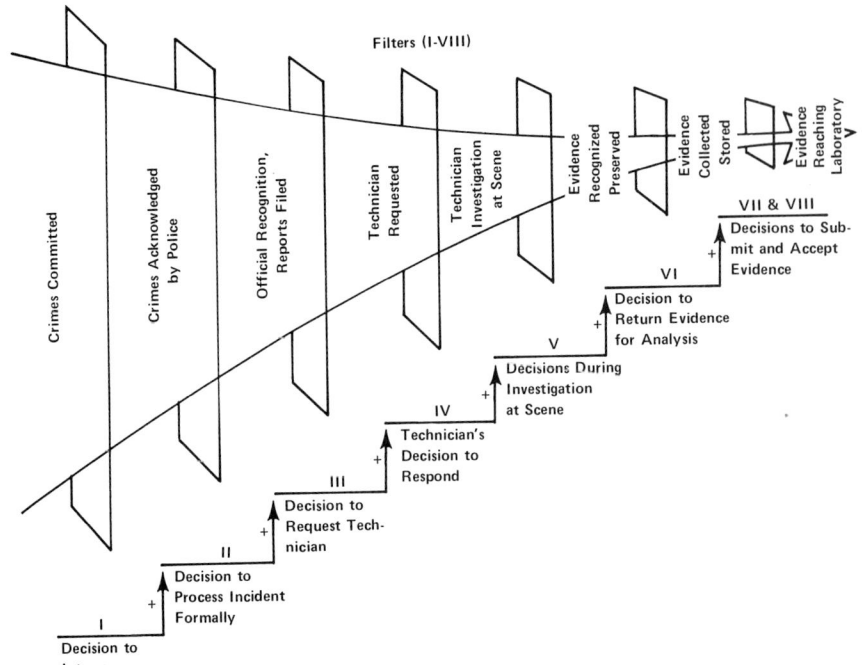

FIGURE 44–1. The screening of evidence. Plus signs indicate positive decisions.

ture of the suspect, and the presence of physical evidence which clearly substantiates the claims of a victim or eyewitness all influence the police officer's decision to process the case formally.

The Investigation

As the investigation of the case is launched, a number of decisions will be made which influence subsequent forensic scientific inquiries. Depending once again on the seriousness of the crime and other circumstances of the case, various professionals will become involved.

THE DETECTIVE

Most serious felonies will receive some type of follow-up investigation by a detective; however, contrary to popular belief, the detective usually devotes only superficial attention to most cases, and of the cases which are investigated, they typically receive less than one day's effort. The 1975 Rand study, *The Criminal Investigation Process*,[6] found that detectives spend most of their time on paperwork, often devoting more time filing the required postarrest forms than in identifying the suspect in the first place. This same research project found that of cases that are cleared, most are the result of immediate apprehensions of suspects at the scene by patrol officers or through information identifying the felon supplied by the victim or eyewitness. Except in the most extraordinary cases, the detective, because of an extensive backlog of cases awaiting his attention, rarely devotes more than superficial attention to physical evidence at the crime scene. If a thorough investigation for evidence is to take place, it is usually the result of the arrival at the scene of a trained evidence technician.

THE EVIDENCE TECHNICIAN

Forensic scientists and police officers concerned with the effective utilization of physical evidence recognize that the success of an evidence program hinges upon the quality of crime-scene investigation procedures. Many investigations have been bungled and crucial information lost due to the destruction of physical evidence at the scene which, after undergoing scientific examination, could have led to the successful clearance of the case. As Parker has observed, "The initial steps in the investigation of a suspected criminal violation can easily nullify any possible help by scientific personnel."[7] Combined dependence upon the patrolman, detective, and forensic scientist to investigate crime scenes for physical evidence often results in disjointed and inadequate investigations. The evidence technician, or crime-scene search officer, is a specialist who is trained in the recognition, gathering, and preservation of physical evidence from crime scenes and ideally can devote his total attention to this function. With the proper training, equipment, and supplies, and with proper supervision, the evidence technician can dramatically improve the quality and completeness of investigations for physical evidence. Still, all efforts to improve and expand evidence collection activities must be matched with a commensurate improvement in evidence examination capabilities. Evidence collection and analysis resources must be developed together in a balanced fashion if they are to be effective in the field.

THE CRIMINALIST

The criminalist, that forensic scientist who devotes his attention to the examination and evaluation of physical evidence by application of the natural sciences, is called to the scene only in major cases. It is often stated that the forensic science laboratory is responsible for insuring the proper collection and submission of physical evidence from the crime scene to the laboratory. However, a shortage of criminalists compared with a high volume of cases requiring laboratory analysis usually precludes the criminalist from investigating all but the most serious scenes. This condition further underscores the need for well-trained and equipped evidence technicians who can assume major responsibility for crime-scene investigations.

One of the most valuable services the criminalist can provide is in the training of evidence technicians and all other police personnel who become involved in investigative work. The criminalist must take an active role in the training of police officers and civilians in procedures to follow in gathering and preserving physical evidence and in marking evidence properly to maintain the chain of custody. The criminalist must also take the time to evaluate the quality of all evidence and reports submitted to the laboratory by field personnel and provide prompt feedback to these individuals, detailing both the positive and negative aspects of their work.

THE MEDICAL EXAMINER

In many jurisdictions around the country, the law dictates that the medical examiner or coroner is in control of a crime scene involving a death. Policies and procedures must be established with the local police department and crime laboratory insofar as which individuals are to be notified in the event of a suspicious or unattended death and the authority and responsibilities of the various parties involved. A well-trained and experienced forensic pathologist at the scene can be of great assistance to the criminalist or evidence technician in assuring that the body is properly preserved and handled; that the scene itself is protected from intrusions by unauthorized family, police, and press; that all necessary photographs and sketches are made; and that all potentially valuable evidence is recognized, collected, and marked by the appropriate officials.

The information to be derived from a proper scene investigation can be of considerable assistance to the forensic pathologist in his procedures with respect to the autopsy of the deceased, in determining the cause of death, and in forming other opinions concerning how the death occurred, be it accidental, suicidal, or homicidal.

If one or more of the above individuals is called, teamwork and coordination of their efforts are critical. However, even prior to their arrival, the police officer has the very important responsibility of preserving and protecting the crime scene.

PRESERVATION

If there is a single area where inadequate measures most often lead to evidence being contaminated or destroyed, it is in the preservation of the scene. The patrol officer must initially secure the cooperation and assistance of victims and witnesses to remain outside the scene and not to disturb any of its aspects. Even more difficult is the requirement to keep other police officers away from the scene and from altering the physical environment. There is a strong temptation for police officers to want to view the scene first-hand and to search out physical evidence themselves.

Except in cases involving personal injury where immediate first aid and medical assistance to a victim must be administered, all unauthorized police *must* be prevented from entering the crime-scene area. This requirement for both quick and firm action by the patrol officer must be covered in official departmental policies and stressed in the academy and in-service programs. Under no circumstances should officers of higher rank than the patrol officer guarding the scene be permitted to use their authority to gain entrance into a secured crime scene.

THE SEARCH FOR EVIDENCE

Although a supervising sergeant or detective will have the responsibility for coordinating the entire investigation, the crime-scene search officer or evidence technician should have responsibility for the preservation, development, and collection of physical evidence at the scene. Under no circumstances should other police officers be allowed to disturb the position or status of objects at the crime scene. While the technician must establish a good working relationship with other police personnel so that all potential evidence is recognized and preserved, the technician should make the final decision in determining whether particular items are worthy of collection. This authority is important since the technician will be called on to testify in court and to attest to the fact that materials submitted as evidence to the laboratory were submitted in the same condition as when the police arrived at the scene and that the chain of evidence has been preserved.

In cases where a criminalist or representative of the coroner or the medical examiner's office is summoned, they must all work closely with the evidence technician in the search of the crime scene. Where crime-scene specialists have the proper training and experience, the forensic scientist should not take control of the investigation, thereby indicating a lack of confidence in that officer's abilities. Situations under which technicians should be notified must be covered in considerable detail during meetings between police and laboratory personnel, as well as in department policy manuals and in training classes for detectives and crime-scene search officers. Except in particularly serious crimes, which will receive the attention of the media, or death investigations where the presence of a coroner or a medical examiner is mandated by law, the experienced crime-scene search officer is just as qualified as the forensic scientist to conduct the crime-scene search for physical evidence.

Where the forensic scientist is involved in the search of the crime scene, he and the police investigators need to coordinate their efforts closely. The scientist will have the added ability to provide some immediate feedback to investigators regarding the significance of particular physical evidence. The preliminary field examination and interpretation of evidence may provide investigators with valuable leads. Confirmation of such, however, must await subsequent laboratory examinations of evidence.

Particularly complex scenes involving large quantities of evidence will require the continued assistance of police officers for many hours or possibly for days. Where the crime scene is out-of-doors, efforts to preserve the scene will require police assistance in barring other police, media representatives, or the public from disturbing it.

Routing Evidence for Analysis

Evidence collected by the crime-scene specialist or others will often be stored in a police property store room until a detective makes an official request to the laboratory for a scientific examination. The criteria by which the investigating officer makes his decision to request an analysis are influenced by the seriousness of the case, his success in other parallel areas of the investigation, the availability of a suspect with whom evidence may be compared, and the detective's overall assessment of the potential value of the evidence awaiting analysis.

There are two often countervailing factors to be considered: on the one hand, there is the tendency of the detective to not want unnecessarily to overburden the laboratory with evidence which will probably not yield positive information; on the other hand, there is the fact that evidence often does not reveal its true value until after examination. Some detectives are reluctant to utilize the forensic laboratory unless all other aspects of the investigation have failed. Detectives also retain negative feelings from encounters with laboratory personnel wherein they have received criticism for submitting too much evidence for analysis or from situations in which they have been rebuffed for trying to pressure the laboratory for a rapid examination in order to apprehend a suspect.

This interface between detectives and laboratories must receive priority attention in order that a positive relationship, one in which both parties acknowledge that cooperation is essential, may develop. Regular meetings and workshops involving laboratory personnel and investigators are mandatory. The underlying philosophy, though, should be to encourage investigators to submit evidence, even when in doubt.

Receipt of Evidence by the Laboratory

Another problem which affects the interface between investigators and the laboratory involves the integrity of the evidence submitted for analysis. The packaging, labeling, and preservation of the evidence must meet or surpass minimum standards developed by the laboratory to insure that the evidence has not been altered, contaminated, or misplaced from the time the materials were collected in the field to the point at which they are examined by the scientist in the laboratory.

The legal requirements for insuring the chain of custody must also be satisfied. To meet these standards, the evidence gatherers must be informed and instructed as to the scientific and legal requirements for preservation of the evidence. They must also be provided with the necessary equipment, containers, supplies, and report forms in order to accomplish these tasks. Guidelines for procurement of these supplies should emanate from the scientific laboratories.

It is essential that the laboratory make the crime-scene search officers feel that they are part of the total forensic team. This entails regular communication with, and feedback to, the officers regarding their performance in the field. With regard to the preservation of evidence, the laboratory must inform investigators when collection efforts fall below accepted standards. The forensic scientist must take the time to explain how these shortcomings may be corrected and why. Similarly, scientists should attempt to supply positive feedback to the officers in situations where exceptionally fine work has been accomplished in the field. The value of continuous feedback will be discussed in more detail in a later section.

Teamwork Within the Laboratory

The late Dr. Paul L. Kirk, Professor of Criminalistics at the University of California at Berkeley, one of the pioneers in the field of forensic science, was a staunch proponent of the "generalist" approach to the examination and interpretation of physical evidence. It was his philosophy that the criminalist should be proficient in the examination of all forms of physical evidence including blood, hair, glass, paints, soil, fibers, and other forms of trace material. It was under the tutelage of Dr. Kirk that many of the criminalists who now staff and direct crime laboratories in California and throughout the country received their training.

California remains the single largest jurisdiction in the nation in which the generalist approach is still widely practiced. Within the past decade, most forensic science laboratories have developed into large scientific operations which have become increasingly specialized. As the development of sophisticated laboratory techniques and instrumentation continues, the need for natural scientists who have advanced knowledge and experience in special scientific areas, and in their application to physical evidence, will become more pressing. Even those who still consider themselves generalists within crime laboratories must regularly interact with the specialists. With the advancement of new techniques and procedures, it is important that each analyst recognize his own scientific limitations and be able to locate and call upon experts who can offer specialized assistance.

Allocation of Laboratory Resources

A single case brought to a laboratory for analysis frequently contains a variety of physical evidence, including firearms, documents, bloodstains, impressions, hairs and fibers, and latent fingerprints. As such evidence enters the laboratory, it must be routed through a criminalist who has breadth of knowledge and experience. He must have the ability to recognize the specific forms of evidence present so that he may send the evidence to the appropriate section and individual within the laboratory with the qualifications to examine it. He must also have the ability to recommend the proper *order* in which the evidence should be examined. A single item may contain several types of evidence and would have to be routed through several sections of the laboratory. The order of the examinations must be arranged so that each analysis will not interfere with those tests which may follow. Each individual examiner must be alerted that subsequent examinations may be performed so that his protocol preserves any remaining evidence.

A large, complex case will frequently require a conference of all examiners before, during, and after the analyses. Such conferences provide an opportunity for all the evidence and examination results to be discussed and interpreted. Such "brainstorming" sessions will yield theories and alternatives for the proper interpretation of the evidence. The various examiners in the laboratory unquestionably form the critical elements of a team effort with regard to the interpretation of the evidence.

Coordination with Other Examiners

There are three primary evidence examination units within the present structure of criminal investigations: the crime laboratory, the medical examiner's office, and the latent fingerprint examination unit (or ID unit). While the latent print section, which constitutes a crucial element of the total evidence utilization process, is positioned within some forensic laboratories, most of them are located outside the laboratory proper and within the local law enforcement agency.

The lines of communication between the crime laboratory, the latent fingerprint section of the police department, and the police officers themselves are crucial. Evidence technicians and laboratory analysts must recognize the potential value of latent prints and those evidence items upon which such prints may be present. Very early on in the total examination process, latent prints must be searched for on evidence which will undergo other types of scientific examination in the laboratory.

The interface between the medical examiner's operation and the crime laboratory is more complex. The body of the victim of a murder, suicide, or accident initially comes under the jurisdiction of the medical examiner. While the body and related tissue and body fluids will be handled by the pathologist and toxicologist, associated clothing, weapons, and other possessions will most likely be transferred to the crime laboratory for examination.

Far in advance of any case coming into these offices, the representatives or the heads of the crime laboratory and medical examiner's office should meet to discuss their philosophies and capabilities in the various examination areas. The two must coordinate their operations to avoid duplication of effort and also to insure that no areas are overlooked. Each program should develop its own character and scientific resources and capabilities. The examination of clothing and wounds for the presence of gunshot residue, the typing of blood and body fluids, or the interpretation of blood splatters will, in some jurisdictions, be handled by the medical examiner's office and in others by the crime laboratory. The line of demarcation is not as important as the clarity of the division of effort. The forensic laboratory which assumes responsibility for the analysis of a particular evidence type must possess the equipment and scientific capabilities to perform the necessary work.

Special Outside Expertise

In some situations the local forensic laboratory will not have the capability to examine particular evidence types or to perform specialized tests. In such circumstances, the laboratory should secure outside consultation. Many forensic scientists are reluctant to examine evidence which has already been analyzed by another laboratory. However, in situations where superior capabilities exist outside the confines of the local laboratory, forensic scientists must make efforts to secure such assistance. Special assistance may be available at a state or federal laboratory, a private research laboratory, or at a neighboring college or university facility.

The medical examiner and forensic toxicologist form a close partnership in most death investigations. However, in situations of dismemberment, fire, explosion, or severe decomposition, the pathologist may be required to call in the services of a physical anthropologist or forensic dentist. Because there are very few such specialists with forensic experience, the medical examiner or crime laboratory may be forced to search beyond the local community for assistance. At present, knowing where to look for special assistance usually comes through personal contacts in such associations as the American Academy of Forensic Sciences. With the advent of certification in specialized forensic fields such as forensic anthropology and dentistry, however, the ability to identify those individuals with the requisite training and experience will become easier.

Communicating Results to Users

The next step in the processing of physical evidence by the forensic laboratory is the prompt feedback of results to the police investigator. Although many laboratories are faced with overwhelming caseloads and have a long backlog of cases awaiting analysis, the team approach requires that they make every effort to provide rapid feedback.

Investigators voice two primary criticisms of forensic science laboratories: the "turn-around time" from the submission of evidence to the receipts of results is excessively long; and the results, when they are returned, are either negative or, at best, ambiguous or inconclusive. From the laboratory's perspective, police detectives are often a nuisance, expecting immediate, positive analysis on evidence which is contaminated or which has remained in a property storage area for months. For the team to function properly, there must exist mutual respect and understanding of the other's job and circumstances. This can only come about through knowledge of the other's operations and through regular communication.

The Southwestern Institute of Forensic Sciences at Dallas is making increasing use of the computer in various areas of operation, including the communication of laboratory results to users. The results of autopsies and scientific analyses of evidence are fed into the computer for storage and for rapid retrieval, not only by laboratory scientists, but by other users as well. The police and courts, by feeding the appropriate case number into their own computer terminal, can retrieve the laboratory results on that particular case within a matter of seconds. The scientific data together with the investigative information gathered by the police can provide the interested party with a complete and up-to-date summary of all available evidence.

Results, although only preliminary in nature and based on presumptive tests, may be communicated to the investigator verbally. This should be followed up by a complete written report after the completed examination. Results, both positive and negative, must be communicated as quickly as possible to investigators since they may be critical in the clearance of a particular case.

A negative response to a detective, or a response which discredits a theory formed by the detective implicating a particular suspect, may strain relations between the police and the laboratory. This leads to a particularly important point: the forensic scientist must be careful not to allow his desire to become a strong team member to cloud his impartiality as a scientist. He should not become emotionally involved in a case or identify too closely with the efforts of the investigator which might influence his interpretations of scientific examinations. He must possess the courage and high ethical standards to be able to interpret the evidence as he sees it, even if it weakens or destroys a detective's case against a suspect. In such a situation, the detective, whose mission is to identify and arrest suspects, may question the loyalty of the forensic scientist as a trusted "team member." Only through periodic conferences and the exchange of information and philosophy can the detective come to understand the role of the forensic scientist. While it is the detective's job to be suspicious and to gather evidence against a particular individual (sufficient to secure an indictment or information), the forensic scientist must be more conservative and use total objectivity in his assessment of the evidence.

Preparing a Case for Court

Physical evidence and the results of scientific examinations are often decisive in determining whether the weight of the evidence will support an indictment against a suspect. One problem which exists within our justice system is the incongruity between the requirements to make an arrest and the requirements to make a formal charge against an individual. In very simplistic terms, the major responsibility of the police officer stops upon arrest. All too often the quality of the case will not support a formal charge, let alone a conviction. It is in this context that the forensic scientist can contribute essential information to insure that the decision to charge is proper and supportable.

Prosecutors view scientific evidence as the crucial link which holds the case together and often provides the degree of proof required for a conviction. This is based upon their knowledge that judges and juries view scientific evidence very carefully and place considerable weight and confidence in the findings of the forensic scientist.

Forensic scientists have the requirement of insuring that the prosecutor understands the true significance of the evidence. The scientist should be prepared to advise what this expert opinion will be on aspects of the evidence. He must advise attorneys of any doubts or uncertainties he has with regard to evidence which potentially links the suspect with the victim or crime scene. More intensive discussions and preparation of specific areas of questioning should take place during subsequent sessions prior to actual trial.

The Defense Attorney as a Team Member

The forensic scientist must view the defense attorney as a potential member of the team with whom he should share information and offer assistance. In most jurisdictions, the written reports of the forensic scientists are available for review by the defense attorney through discovery motions. In others, this is a regular procedure, with or without a discovery.

Unfortunately, many forensic scientists view the defense lawyer only as an adversary who will subject them to cross-examination, question their scientific qualifications, and try to find a flaw in their scientific procedures and interpretation of the evidence. In many jurisdictions, such confrontations are avoided and less hostility results because of a closer relationship from the outset between the laboratory and the public defender's office and defense counsel.

The forensic science laboratory should set out to educate regularly active defense attorneys just as it tries to educate the prosecuting attorneys. Tours should be conducted through the laboratories, and the capabilities and limitations of all tests and equipment should be covered in considerable detail. By such education, the defense attorney will view the laboratory as it really is—an impartial scientific operation—not as an adversary or a source of unintelligible scientific information aligned with the prosecution. In actual cases, defense attorneys should be encouraged to discuss the evidence prior to courtroom presentations. They can be advised as to how the expert will testify and why. Many laboratories have found that such procedures reduce suspicion and hostility, and streamline the total scientific utilization process.

In circumstances where the defense elects to call in its own scientific expert, the government's forensic scientist should make every possible effort to cooperate. However, the laboratory must exercise reasonable caution and security measures with regard to the physical evidence and its examination by outside experts. Where possible, communication among such experts prior to the adjudication of the case to clarify or resolve any scientific differences should be attempted. Individual laboratories must formulate their own policies concerning the use of laboratory space and equipment by outside experts.

Pretrial Conferences

While ongoing dialogue between the forensic scientist and prosecuting attorneys is necessary, it is particularly important for the scientist to meet with the attorney immediately prior to cases which are about to be adjudicted. If there is a complaint which occurs most often in laboratories when speaking about relationships with the prosecutor's office, it concerns the absence of communication prior to trial. Without such conferences, attorneys often do not gain a clear understanding of the significance of the findings developed by the laboratory. In addition, they will not have the benefit of discussing and clarifying the limitations of the laboratory examinations as, for instance, in cases where evidence at the scene is "consistent with" evidence from the suspect but is by no means "individualistic," as in the case where a latent print matching the suspect's is recovered.

Such pretrial conferences may reveal particularly useful information which may be used during plea-bargaining situations. Once again, if evidence is generated which clearly indicates the presence of the suspect at the crime scene or having contact with the victim, this information may lead to a guilty plea. Such evidence certainly is in the best interests of justice for it leads to a verdict and disposition which reflect the actual events and involvement of the suspect in the criminal incident.

Presentation of Evidence and Testimony

If the courtroom can be viewed more as a fact-finding effort to establish truth rather than as a game field in which adversaries match wits and strategies, then this is the ultimate example of teamwork in which the forensic scientist may participate. The forensic scientist, as an expert witness, acts to educate the court, judge, and jury in the scientific procedures he or she employed to examine the evidence and expresses an opinion concerning the meaning and implications of that evidence. The prime objective of the expert must be to convey his testimony to the judge and jury in a way which is understandable and which reflects, as nearly as possible, the weight which, in the expert's opinion, it properly deserves. The expert has no stake in the outcome of the case, only insuring that his examination and findings are properly understood and considered by the triers of fact.

Administrative and Financial Issues

It is comparatively easy to discuss the desirability of forensic science "teamwork," but it is more difficult to identify measures which need to be taken to improve this spirit of cooperation and exchange of information. Teamwork is defined as "cooperative effort by the members of a team to achieve a common goal." In this example, the common goal must be to bring the guilty to justice and to exonerate the innocent.

Unfortunately, there are aspects of our present system of criminal justice which impede the teamwork which is essential to the full and equitable utilization of the forensic sciences. For purposes of summary, these most pressing problem areas are identified as follows:

1. *Budgetary support.* The most common problem plaguing forensic science laboratories today is that of inadequate budgets. This situation leads to many conditions which impede effective teamwork, including insufficient staff, inadequate facilities, and equipment.
2. *Training programs.* Nonexistent or inadequate training programs for police and legal representatives result in these critical "users" not knowing the actual capabilities and limitations of the forensic science laboratories. Without such basic information, such users will be reluctant to cooperate with the laboratory and to seek assistance in the investigation and adjudication of cases.
3. *Organizational impediments.* Forensic laboratories often occupy an inferior position within the parent agency, which leads to poor com-

munication between the laboratory and the commanders of other divisions of the agency and outside users.
4. *Management information.* Teamwork is dependent upon effective communication techniques. Verbal communication alone cannot be relied upon to satisfy information transfer requirements. Written procedures and computer capability must be established which facilitate information transfer to and from the laboratory and provide for prompt feedback of results to interested parties.
5. *Competition.* The crime laboratory and the medical examiner's office in many communities have poor relations and often compete with each other for funds. Close working relationships are essential, and consolidation of operations into a single laboratory should be explored. The Southwestern Institute of Forensic Sciences at Dallas has both the medical examiner's office and the forensic laboratory within a single administrative unit under the direction of the Chief Medical Examiner. The Dallas approach should be examined carefully by other jurisdictions around the country as one alternative to maintenance of two separate laboratory organizations.
6. *Periodic briefings.* The laboratory should hold regularly scheduled briefings with police and legal representatives to review current practices and problem areas. These regular sessions will also give the laboratory the opportunity to provide such users with information on new or updated techniques and breakthroughs in ongoing investigations.

REFERENCES

1. Cowan, T. A.: Decision Theory in Law, Science, and Technology. *Science* 140:1065, 1963.
2. Frank, J.: *Courts on Trial.* Atheneum, New York, 1963, p. 85.
3. Mumford, M.: Disregard of Scientific Proof by Juries. *J. Crim. Law Criminol. Police Sci.* 41:325, 1950.
4. Parker, B., and Peterson, J. L.: *Physical Evidence Utilization in the Adminstration of Criminal Justice.* LEAA Grant No. NI–032. U.S. Department of Justice, Washington, D.C., 1972.
5. Peterson, J. L.: *Utilization of Criminalistics Services by the Police.* U.S. Government Printing Office, Washington, D.C., 1974, p. 12.
6. Greenwood, P., and Petersilia, J.: *The Criminal Investigation Process. Vol. I: Summary and Policy Implications.* LEAA Grant No. 73–NI–99–0037–G. The Rand Corporation, Santa Monica, Cal., 1975, pp. vi–vii.
7. Parker, B.: Science and Crime. *Technol. Rev.* 70:10, 1968.

CHAPTER 45

Larry B. Howard is Director of the Georgia State Crime Laboratory and Assistant Professor of Clinical Pathology at Emory University in Atlanta. He is past President of the American Society of Crime Laboratory Directors, Inc., and past Vice President of the American Academy of Forensic Sciences. Dr. Howard is a member of the American Academy of Forensic Sciences and the Southern Association of Forensic Scientists, and is on the Board of Trustees of the Forensic Sciences Foundation, Inc., and the American Board of Forensic Toxicologists.

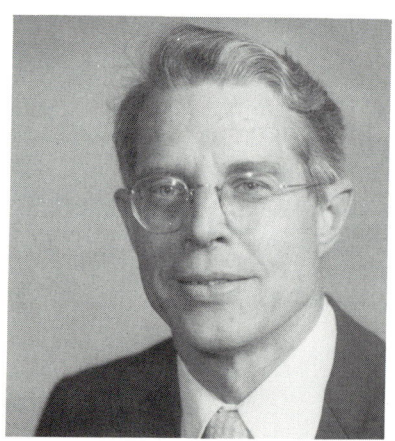

ORGANIZATION OF A CRIME LABORATORY

Larry B. Howard, Ph.D.

DEFINITIONS AND MISCONCEPTIONS

The term "crime laboratory" is sometimes misused, often as a status symbol for the purpose of acquiring funds, legitimizing a closet operation, or providing increased prestige on the witness stand. The usual police fingerprint or photography laboratories do not constitute crime laboratories, any more than the possession of a uniform makes one a police officer.

As an illustration, many years ago I wished to visit the crime laboratory in a large western state. I was told, however, that this would be impossible since each individual police agency had its own crime laboratory. Further investigation showed no evidence of the application of forensic science at any level. This situation has since been corrected, but only because here, and in many other places, the drug abuse explosion forced the development of a laboratory.

A crime laboratory is an organizational unit composed of university-level individuals, educated in the natural sciences and trained in the forensic sciences. Their mission is the examination of physical evidence and the submission of their conclusions to the criminal justice system. It should be noted that the responsibilities for prosecution and the administration of justice lie elsewhere.

Crime laboratory development has been associated with many pioneers and a few charlatans always ready to take financial advantage of a new field. Some of the latter, well equipped with the latest vocabulary but little else, are still with us today. Their court appearances are disproportionate to their numbers because of the shopping techniques used by some defense attorneys. The forensic sciences are by nature applied sciences, and instant expertise, even by presentation of advanced academic credentials, is questionable.

Crime laboratories in the United States are a relatively recent development, most having their beginnings after 1930. In spite of or because of this, there is an amazing volume of diverse opinion as to how a crime laboratory should be constituted and administered. No crime laboratory should ever be initiated without the advice of an experienced crime laboratory scientist. No single system is uniformly "correct."

NEED FOR A CRIME LABORATORY

Factors influencing the need to establish a new laboratory are multiple and often complex. Almost certainly a few partial services will already be established. Population, population density, crime index, and police population[1] will determine caseload and have all been properly used as a basis to justify a new laboratory facility. Justification to local political interests is based on the rights of constituents to timely, complete evaluation of the scientific aspects of criminal charges. The ratio of cases submitted to a local laboratory is approximately 25:1 over those submitted to a remote facility.[2]

SERVICE FEATURES

Both the type of laboratory services and the number of laboratory personnel vary within wide limits in response to population, area, and jurisdiction. Obviously the full-service laboratory offers a marked increase in efficiency over a number of partial-service laboratories. A full-service laboratory or laboratory system should offer the following specialties:

1. Crime scene evaluation;
2. Document examination;
3. Drug identification;
4. Firearms and toolmarks identification;
5. Implied consent;
6. Latent prints;
7. Photography;
8. Serology;
9. Toxicology;
10. Trace evidence.

Crime Scene Evaluation

Crime scene evaluation is an area of great controversy and variation. Certainly any system that gets the job done right is acceptable. Unfortunately, no system anywhere in the United States has achieved perfection or near perfection in crime scene evaluation. This is, without a doubt, the weakest link in our criminal justice system, and unfortunately it is also the starting point of the evidence chain. Our police investigating system is generally weak, ill-trained, and ego-armored in this one area. In death cases, body focusing by medical examiners, trained to look at bodies, often overlooks other evidence. Every error, omission, or artifact at the beginning creates vacuums or distortions as the evidence or lack of it moves through the system. The recent increase in the number of crime scene schools is a step in the right direction. These comments are not original or meant to be particularly profound. Few in the criminal justice community would refute them. The best solution is some form of supervision or participation by the laboratory scientists who process the evidence. There is a clear advantage in the use of physical evidence, mission-oriented specialists. This may take the form of specially trained police investigators, latent print examiners, or actual participation or a participation option by crime laboratory personnel. Conversely, crime scene training is mandatory for all forensic scientists with the possible exception of those who specialize in drug identification. This training includes the examination of hit-and-run vehicles. For the reader's reference, a thorough crime scene search, with a two-man team, requires a minimum of 4 hours and may take several days.

Document Examination

Document examination services include comparison of signatures; typewritings; restoration of charred documents; identification of photocopies and inks; and detection of erasures, tracings, and forged forms. Training is extensive because a pertinent academic course does not exist.

Drug Identification

Most laboratories are relatively strong in the area of drug identification. Chemists are essential in that identifications based solely on color tests are worthless. The laboratory should have the capability not only to recognize the common drugs of abuse, but also to identify new drugs as well as binders, diluents, traces of base chemicals, and intermediates present in the mixture. Good instrumentation is an absolute necessity, and access to sophisticated instrumentation is desirable.

Firearms and Toolmarks

The matching of bullets, cartridge cases, toolmark striae, and approximation of muzzle to target distances are standard examinations for crime laboratories. Additional services should include muzzle velocity measurements, trajectory projections, and identification of powder and powder residues. Examination of explosive residues is an optional but desirable capability.

Alcohol Level Evaluation (Informed Consent Laws)

The purpose of alcohol level evaluation is to detect intoxicated drivers through analysis of appropriate specimens. Setting standards for training and checking the operation of instrumentation for in situ analysis of breath samples of alcohol are included in the program. Since alcohol will only be positive in approximately 75 percent of traffic arrests, toxicologic analysis of blood and urine may be included or referred to a separate section, such as toxicology.

Latent Prints

A latent print team may or may not be separated from the regular fingerprint classification section. If these personnel perform crime scene examinations, a close working relationship with the laboratory provides a broader-based training, minimizes errors, prevents collection of inappropriate objects, and inhibits destruction of potential evidence. A good latent print team at the scene will solve many cases and prevent an often perfunctory examination for prints by police officers in a hurry.

Photography

The photographic division, an essential part of any crime laboratory, is sometimes placed under its principal user, the document section. This service differs from the usual police photography in the inclusion of special techniques using infrared and ultraviolet light and the preparation of court exhibits by photomicroscopy.

Serology

The serology section primarily identifies and classifies blood and seminal stains. Dried blood stains are examined for the ABO, MN, Rh antigens, polymorphic enzymes, and blood proteins such as hemoglobin and haptoglobin. It is now possible to determine the sex of the victim and the presence of certain drugs. ABO antigens and certain enzymes can often be identified in seminal and other body fluids by serologic procedures on a routine basis. Interpretation of blood splatter patterns can be included if the serologist wishes to be included on the crime scene team. The laboratory work is tedious and there are serious pitfalls.

Toxicology

Toxicology is discussed elsewhere and in most crime laboratories is combined with implied consent and/or drug identification.

Trace Evidence

Trace evidence evaluation requires the most scientific versatility of all. Services should include examination and comparison of paint chips and smears, hairs, glass, soils, wood, volatile accelerants, fibers, particulates, safe insulation, and other miscellaneous types of evidence. Depending on philosophy and available talent, this section may be combined with the firearms division. This combination is very useful but can only be readily accomplished if the firearms examiner is scientifically trained. In addition, lack of training in physics limits the examiner's usefulness in ballistics cases. Classically, ballistics is defined as expertise in bullet trajectory, muzzle velocity, and bullet penetration.

ORGANIZATIONAL CONSIDERATIONS

Hierarchy

For highest quality work in a large laboratory, the specialty areas discussed above may be subspecialized and staffed by individuals with slightly different education, ability, and training. Ideally, smaller laboratories should be backed by larger laboratories with specialists in the appropriate areas. Work quality and accessibility, not political entity (i.e., city, county, state, and federal), should be the controlling factor in referring work upward or laterally. The headquarters laboratory should process a varied caseload of its own for maximum utility and to supply a research base and capability. Many state systems are organized with one large central laboratory supporting several smaller regional laboratories that in turn support smaller branches. Approximately 90 percent of the work received by the branches can be successfully completed locally. No laboratory should be staffed by less than two scientists if a wide spectrum of examinations is to be attempted. These two individuals should have different emphasis in their training, best determined by case-type frequency and usually consisting of familiarity with drugs and/or toxicology and trace evidence and/or firearms. In-depth expertise in serology, handwriting, and toxicology should await expansion of caseload or be located at the next highest echelon. Nothing should prevent even the highest echelon from referring cases to other experts or consultants. Concordant analytical results from unassociated laboratories are a potent factor in disqualifying dishonest experts. The strong uniformity of good opinion was recently demonstrated in the re-evaluation of firearms identification data in connection with the assassination of Senator Robert F. Kennedy.

Accessibility

Human nature responds to convenience. The number of cases submitted by jurisdictions located more than 70 miles from the laboratory drops off rapidly with distance. Although most police departments operate around the clock, the officers work shifts. Strict adherence to a 40-hour laboratory schedule discourages submissions from distance and from shifts discordant with laboratory hours. In a large laboratory, it is relatively easy to stretch the working day to 12 hours by staggering work hours. Availability at other times can be arranged "on call." The proper examination of difficult evidence is a perfect example of an efficient feedback system. Other than speed and the vast increase in evidence evaluated, one of the greatest justifications for a local crime laboratory is the ease of multiple-stage analysis with intervening police feedback, impossible with more remote facilities. A personal acquaintance between the investigator and laboratory personnel accelerates call and feedback, appreciation of mutual problems and cooperative crime scene investigation, and also instills mutual confidence.

Utility

Although crime laboratories usually cannot specifically tie in suspects until they have been identified by investigation, continuing evaluation of physical evidence from any incident sets limits and directions for the investigator. Police and judicial efficiency is markedly handicapped by lack of timely scientific information. However, new crime laboratories should not be expected to have a marked effect on the crime rate since they only help to identify criminals and have no direct control over causation and incarceration. Since calling the crime laboratory requires an extra step, many easy cases are completed without scientific assistance.

Police Sophistication

Some police departments are progressive and receptive; others are stagnant and rigid. Habit, trust, and ego play a strong part in the proper use of a crime laboratory. Since most evidence examinations must originate from the police, their attitude will make or break the laboratory. Social status factors may be even stronger if the laboratory is part of the police department. This is one reason why the laboratory's scientists should be included in all possible police training programs. Better officers will use a *good* crime laboratory. In some instances, it may be necessary to give promotion points on laboratory usage. No police department can be exemplary unless all investigative tools are in use. On the other hand, a forensic scientist can easily destroy his usefulness by supercilious behavior when he forgets that he is only one cog in the machinery.

Integration

Efficiency demands that as many forensic services as possible be combined in one laboratory. Loss of efficiency is secondary, not only to duplication of space, records, and instrumentation, but also to the necessity of splitting evidence for distribution to various laboratories and to confusion generated by the conflicting rules and egos of the heads and scientists of different divisions. Laboratories probably should not be organized under more than one government entity or across political boundaries unless there is a permanent statutory source of funding. Several experiments with federal funds in this direction have been unsatisfactory. Occasionally, partial services can be supplied by private laboratories.

Parent Organization

The choice of parent organization is relative. All governmental agencies at all levels present both advantages and disadvantages. Certainly there is little advantage in sowing crime laboratory seed in a barren plot. The spirit of the laboratory is investigative, not prosecutive or regulatory. Therefore, a practical case can be made for including the laboratory in the major police organization in the area to be served at a state, county, or city level. However, working for a police organization does not insure freedom from "result pressure" and allows some susceptibility to innuendo of prejudice by the defense. However, any department or division that shows an inclination to place low-level personnel in charge of the laboratory for promotional purposes or for any other reason should be avoided at all costs. The higher the laboratory director in the organization, the greater the potential of the laboratory. Division status is preferable. Overlying layers of civil servants or police personnel serve only to attenuate the rising thrust of scientific innovation and need. Sworn or unsworn status is immaterial as long as all personnel, including the director, are scientifically trained. A mixture of sworn and unsworn personnel is a constant source of friction. The crime laboratory is almost never a sufficiently large entity to stand efficiently on its own. Logistics, personnel, and building maintenance are best shared as part of another entity. However, the budget *must* be planned and earmarked exclusively for the laboratory. Years of unsatisfactory experience with attempted pirating of laboratory funds by other departmental divisions have soured the author forever on the concept of budget sharing.

Laboratory Size and Sophistication

There are no restrictions except a minimum population to support a small, two-man laboratory. The number of police officers and the crime rate can also serve as a basis. The population will determine the final potential, while the number of active police officers will be more closely correlated with current potential. An average of 2.5 cases per officer per year can be expected.[3] One drug chemist can be supported by an urban population of from 50,000 to 100,000. A combination trace evidence, firearms, and crime-scene expert can handle approximately double this population. Variables include population density, utilization, court appearances, training assignments, and overtime or compensatory time policies. A larger caseload permits more scientific specialization of the staff and a better and more complete array of instrumentation. The knowledge and techniques of forensic science are progressing rapidly. It is impossible for one or two individuals to be fully knowledgeable and competent in all areas. Much sophisticated instrumentation is either very expensive or is used only sporadically. Large state and federal laboratories have unique opportunities to develop rare but essential specialties through application or research positions. The availability of the rapid response of this special group of forensic scientists to crises cases, adverse testimony, unexpected defenses, and a host of other problems will enhance the reputation and spectacularly add to the value of the laboratory. The need for a laboratory may be based on the need for one or more functions listed under laboratory services. The services may be currently completely lacking or inadequate. It is important that initial planning include all needed services; otherwise the final product is likely to have a patchwork appearance. In addition, the choice of a director will be determined by the areas of expertise to be included.

Director

Once the decision is made to construct a new building or alter an existing one, a laboratory director should be employed. Contrary to popular opinion, personnel lacking crime laboratory experience, regardless of their adminstrative talents, architectural ability, educational level, university appointment, or police experience, cannot, by themselves, adequately design a structure of maximum utility. This is not an implication that good ideas on the building of a crime laboratory are limited to crime laboratory scientists. It does mean that predictive ability on idea desirability is highly correlated with experience. In this respect, the American Society of Crime Laboratory Directors have access in their membership to a major portion of crime laboratory expertise to be found in this country.

The director must be a scientist who possesses at least a Bachelor of Science degree, has bench and courtroom experience in one or preferably several areas, and shows some administrative and political ability. A law degree is an added, but secondary, attraction. Care is the watchword since the world is full of good scientists who lack adminstrative talent and personability.

PHYSICAL FACILITY

Needs relating to the physical facility vary somewhat according to laboratory coverage, association, parent or sister organization, size, type of caseload, and complexity. Certain structural needs are, however, universal.

The most efficient building plan is two-story with a foundation adequate to allow future vertical expansion. When funds are short and future expansion inevitable, space for elevator shafts is included in the original structure. Placement of the building on pylons will allow the addition of one more floor without disruption of function and replacement of the roof. No laboratory should be located in a basement because of the effect of humidity on instrument function and the possibility of flooding.

An efficient laboratory requires approximately 350 square feet of working space per person. One must remember, however, that this is only 65 percent of the total space required, since storage, lavatories, closets, maintenance facilities, and accessible raceways for plumbing and electrical lines require more room. (Plumbing or electrical lines must never be buried in a concrete floor.) Design for space need is based on a 20-year staff and case projection. These predictions are most accurate for multidiscipline laboratories because errors tend to cancel each other. The typical crime laboratory case and/or work growth curve is helpful in this regard. Most laboratories show an initial spurt, a plateau or decrease, a slow increase, a rapid increase and, with maturity, a less precipitous but gradual increase. Unfortunately, this can be altered by many factors, not the least of which are legislative changes, addition of new services, and laboratory salesmanship. Potential use of laboratory services is markedly in excess of any current laboratory workload. Current limiting factors include space limitations, high personnel workloads, case backlogs, lack of funds for training in additional specialties, and especially loss of time due to multiple court appearances fostered by a minority of defense attorneys who confuse justice with delay, trial longevity, and misdemeanor civil rights issues.

Comment is also appropriate on the general outline of the laboratory. The new Ontario Laboratory, for example, designed an efficient floor plan separating sections by floors where appropriate and using a rectangle within a rectangle arrangement. The space in the outside rectangle is reserved for laboratory and office space and the inside rectangle for instrumentation. A continuous hall separates the two areas.

Some architectural provision must be made for the inevitable requests for tours and their management. Tours represent an inconvenient, but absolutely necessary, aspect of crime laboratory public relations. The FBI solved this problem, to their satisfaction, by designing wide halls and providing large "look in" windows in the various section areas. Hall design should include space for evidence exhibits or interesting case sequences. Moreover, the laboratory director can save considerable time by limiting tours to students of at least the tenth grade level.

Every large laboratory needs a small kitchen to help host the inevitable social functions associated with laboratory administration. This facility is also a definite advantage to both the employer and employee since it is convenient for employees to eat lunch and have their coffee "on the job." At the same time personnel are more accessible to the client. A location near the conference room or library is desirable.

Location

Obviously the structure needs to be centrally located in the service area and as near as possible to the courts. Minimum lead time for testimony will save both the taxpayer and the laboratory considerable money and time. All sections with the exception of toxicology can expect to spend approximately 20 percent of their time in court. Insistence that the crime laboratory scientist be present during the whole trial process is, in most cases, an inexcusable abuse of public money. Subtle pressures, such as a laboratory time allocation for a jurisdiction, can be brought to bear on flagrant violators. Cooperation at every level has to be reciprocal. Some states have eliminated nearly all court appearances by crime laboratory personnel through legislation allowing court use of laboratory reports. This does not abridge constitutional guarantees, if the defense attorney retains subpoena rights. Location near the appropriate police academy facilitates the training so necessary to the proper use of the laboratory. Sensitive instrumentation demands a site as free as possible from sources of ground and air vibration.

Laboratory Systems

SECURITY

Laboratory records, evidence, and chemical standards must be maximally protected against theft, fire, accident, loss, and vandalism. Stolen records or evidence are worse than useless since the theft not only lessens the weight of evidence against the accused, but gives the defense attorney a wedge in attacking the competence of the investigation. In addition, laboratory records can be used for all kinds of blackmail, including unethical use in political races. Drug evidence quite obviously has value other than the evidentiary. We can record two attempts to steal and destroy incriminating evidence over the last 25 years. One of these was successful and involved the theft of a laboratory vehicle.

The first line of defense is a high, barbed-wire, capped fence, a night watchman, and a building tall enough to make roof access difficult. It follows that the planting of trees immediately adjacent to the building should be prohibited.

The second line of defense is a combination of a good lock and deadbolt system. The number of outside doors should be minimal and all but one or two deadbolted at night. The deadbolted doors also serve to minimize false alarms through the actions of careless employees. Window-concealing shutter systems that might allow unobserved building access are to be avoided. Adequate outside illumination is a desirable supplement. Nonopening windows are recommended, although they present problems during air-conditioning failures and with odor retention.

The third line of defense is a double alarm system. The current best available, but not always adequate, defense consists of magnetic switches on all windows that open, and all outside doors and inside doors to key areas such as those for storage of records and evidence. (Bathrooms need to be vented, not windowed.) High windows prevent identification of possible targets by outside observation. Vibration sensors should be added to evidence and record rooms. Tape circuits may be placed on nonopening windows. The two systems are routed separately to an alarm box in a facility manned on a 24-hour basis, such as a police radio room. The frequency of false alarms in the system mandates an auditory alarm in the laboratory loud enough to notify laboratory personnel when they inadvertently set off the system. A television security system is particularly advantageous for monitoring entrances in smaller laboratories when the scientific staff is absent in court or processing crime scenes. Complete TV coverage is too expensive and poses a possible morale problem.

For fire protection, sprinkler systems are often erratic and may be activated in the absence of flames. Certain laboratory systems or instrumentation may be irretrievably damaged by false alarms. High-voltage electrical fires may be explosively catalyzed by water. The clever arsonist may turn off the water before setting fire to a building. We intend to try a combination of a smoke detector and limited sprinkler system, wherein the latter will not function unless the former is activated. A complete carbon dioxide or halogenated hydrocarbon system is the best.

EMERGENCY POWER SYSTEM

Temporary power loss can damage computerized record systems, necessitate extensive recalibration of some types of instrumentation, such as nuclear magnetic resonance (NMR), and shut off essential refrigeration. The latter is critical since lightening, the usual cause of power failure, reaches peak intensity during the hot summer months. Most police systems and/or National Guard facilities have auxiliary generators that are automatically activiated in emergencies. Tie-ins are desirable.

COMMUNICATIONS

Nothing is more detrimental to efficient laboratory function than an inadequate communications system. Information is our life blood; with it we flourish; without it we hibernate. An approximate rule of thumb is one outside telephone line for every five scientists. Telephones need to be convenient to work areas and must be supplemented by a PA system that can be activated both by microphone and by telephone. For federal, state, or regional systems, a WATS line is desirable. The FBI is currently activating the Crime Laboratory Information System (CLIS). Space for a computer terminal or arrangements for access to a terminal should be planned.

PARKING FACILITIES

Sooner or later, every new public facility seems to get caught in the parking crunch. The laboratory plans must include enough parking for the anticipated staff level at the end of the projected period, as well as the number of assigned laboratory vehicles and an approximate 50 percent buffer. A convenient zone close to the main entrance is set aside for users only. Planners or politicians may argue about furnishing free parking space to employees. However, this is one of many fringe benefits that can be offered to attract competent employees. Civil service salaries are often an insufficient attraction. Poor crime laboratories do not just happen; they were organized that way.

AIR CONDITIONING AND HEATING

Instrumentation is usually more sensitive than the scientist. Many instruments function well only within a narrow range of humidity and temperature. High temperature, high humidity, a high concentration of particulate matter, and proximity to chemical fumes are destructive. Instrumentation and chemical laboratories must be separated. In northern climates, air conditioning is still essential because of the beneficial effect on air quality. A large cooling and heating system must be designed which is capable of generating positive air pressure in many areas of the laboratory, carrying away excess heat generated by instrumentation and burners, and countering outside hot or cold air return from the hood vents. Air flow in the system outside the working space must be ducted and filtered to minimize particulate, fume, and odor retention. Photography must have a separate system because of special temperature requirements and the constant surfeit of acid fumes.

PLUMBING

Plumbing needs are relatively simple but very important. All laboratory sinks *must* have duriron or glass drains. Use of septic tanks necessitates at least a limestone filter tank. Dilution tanks are installed as needed.

LABORATORY FURNISHINGS

For laboratory furnishings, hard-wood or metal construction is acceptable. Metal does not warp in case of leaks and is easier to match when replacing parts. One of the most important choices the laboratory director will make is that of the bench top. I hesitate to recommend a specific material since advances in this area are rapid. However, the best grade of chemically inert material will save money in the long run. There is nothing wrong with the time-honored method of testing the chemical resistance of small block samples of the manufacturer's line with every chemical in sight. The testing procedure should not omit the effect of the local water and impact resistance. Similar criteria apply to the tops and lining of the hoods. Teflon-coated fan blades are desirable. Explosion-proof motors will be needed in some hoods. Some thought needs to be given to the areas downwind from the hood vents. Acid condensation nuclei are common under conditions of high humidity. The quadrilateral between the scientist's work area, desk, instruments, and telephone is a prime determinant of efficiency. Many supply companies offer combination benchwork that includes both desk and laboratory space in the same furniture unit. These are not only utilitarian, but are well accepted by most scientists.

All floors should be covered with a good grade of chemically resistant tile. A soft surface serves to decrease leg fatigue, and portions of floor can easily be repaired after the inevitable accident. It is wise to order excess tile at the time of the original installation to insure availability of a matching pattern for repairs. Rugs in administrative offices are aesthetic, noise-reducing and add insulating qualities. Dust control is aided by washable wall tile, which tends to be expensive. Accoustical ceiling tile adds little to the cost. Potential plumbing and electrical connections need be available to all offices in case of needed conversion to laboratory space.

EVIDENCE ROOMS

The design of an evidence room is relatively simple. Windows should not be provided, and a location remote from an outside wall is desirable. A reinforced roof, particularly in a single story of a multiple occupancy building, is a must. The walls are to be shelved with continuous numbered cubicles of convenient size, approximately 3 feet deep, 2 feet high, and 4 feet wide. Aisles need to be approximately 4 feet wide. There is no prohibition against single or double tiers in the center space. If firearms evidence is to be stored here, one end is equipped with a pegboard for hand guns and rifle racks. A solid, reinforced door and frame with a high security lock should be installed. We also recommend reinforced walls of cement block.

The number of evidence rooms is a function of laboratory size and organization. In medium-size or large laboratories, separation of criminalistics and drug identifiction sections is not only efficient, but also more acceptable to the courts. Size will depend both on policy as to storing evidence and on caseload. The evidence room will never be big enough.

GAS AND VOLATILES

It is often impossible to arrive at an arrangement that is completely satisfactory both to the safety people and the operation of the laboratory. Everyone recognizes hydrogen and acetylene as the two gases with the greatest explosive hazard. Isolation of all gas cylinders in a separate building sounds marvelous but increases the probability of leaks due to the length of the associated plumbing. Placing a conduit around this plumbing reduces the chances of filling the wall spaces with gas, but also insures a passage for escaping gases into the building. The best system we have seen consists of a short transfer system from an outside wall storage rack for individual cylinders. A tank with a water trap in the same location for liquid nitrogen is an option for the nitrogen supply. Security considerations may require limited access to this area. A vented storage room for volatiles should be constructed with a blow-out ceiling or wall.

EMERGENCY EQUIPMENT

It is doubtful that there is an active chemist in the country with at least 20 years experience who has never been faced with a chemical or thermal emergency in the laboratory. Minimum injury is assured by ready access to safety equipment, including eye baths, emergency showers, fire extinguishers, fire blankets, and respirators. A special note is appropriate on attempted flushing of corrosive fluids from the eyes. The victim has a reflex and voluntary tendency to hold the lids tightly closed. The best eye bath in the world is useless unless the lids are pulled open for cleansing.

Special Sectional Needs

ADMINISTRATION

In terms of laboratory administration there are many options, depending on size and preference. The lobby needs to be big enough to orient a normal-size tour (up to 30 individuals), include adequate seating for other visitors, have access to restrooms and closet space, and be contiguous with the evidence receiving rooms. A single entrance from this area to the laboratory proper can be equipped with a buzzer-operated door with a small window. One or more evidence reception rooms can be added as needed. These rooms can be separated from the lobby by a half-height partition topped with a counter. The top half can be equipped with sliding glass partitions for security and noise control. A separate entrance into the evidence reception room from the laboratory proper expedites efficiency. (This assumes that scientists are receiving their own evidence.)

1. Lobby	600 square feet
2. Evidence reception area(s)	200 square feet
3. Director's and assistant director's offices	290 square feet
4. File room	
5. Administrative assistant's office (optional)	170 square feet
6. Computer room (optional)	200 square feet
7. Library and conference room	430 square feet
8. Secretarial office(s)	120 square feet
9. Kitchen	110 square feet
10. Supply room(s) for supplies, volatiles, laundry	
11. Lecture room (optional)	1200 square feet
12. Mail room and loading dock	70 square feet
13. Janitorial room	50 square feet

The size of the file and computer rooms is dependent on caseload and method and time retention of case record storage. If the caseload exceeds 10,000 per year, computer storage of most records can be considered. Most computers have special operation temperature parameters, may require subfloor wiring (sunken or raised floor), and must have their own unique electrical circuit. When the caseload exceeds 30,000 per year, any other method is inefficient. When the annual caseload exceeds or is anticipated to exceed 4,000, large rotating files make more efficient vertical utilization of space than do file cabinets. If decisions of this type are not made early, one will incur increased costs, for disassembling and assembling of rotary files or the tearing down of walls will be necessary. Plans should also be made to store records on microfilm after approximately two years, regardless of the system used.

A combination conference room and library is a must for every crime laboratory. A larger room permits sectional training and seminars. Failure to provide appropriate reference books, field-related periodicals, and abstracts insures a low level of proficiency. Only acquaintance with the literature, personal contact with other forensic scientists, seminars, and constant contact with users and crime scenes can prevent the forensic scientist from going stale. Thus administrators must choose early between a laboratory staff that dutifully grinds out routine results and an enlightened, enthusiastic group full of new suggestions, ideas, and methods of analysis.

Items 1 through 7 above need to be clustered centrally in the area of the lobby. The use of an administrative assistant is also a function of caseload and the scientific and administrative abilities and responsibilities of the director and assistant director.

A secretarial office-supply receiving room should be located conveniently near the storage room and loading dock. There is no substitute for designated responsibility in this area. Leaving this type of record-keeping to the nearest warm body is often a disaster.

TRACE EVIDENCE AND FIREARMS

The diverse and complex nature of trace evidence and firearms units will require more space per person (i.e., 500 square feet) than any other section of the laboratory. Another office may be added for the section secretary. The decision to create a shared sectional secretarial office (e.g., with the serology unit) or to combine it with that of the section head is a matter of personal preference. Privacy, however, is desirable. Desk space for the working criminalist is most efficiently supplied in the various working areas. This tends to encourage various desirable subspecializations by different staff members.

1. Supervisor's office	280 square feet
2. Evidence examining room	750 to 1500 square feet
3. Arson laboratory with arson evidence storage room	600 square feet
4. Garage for examination of vehicles	1250 square feet
5. Shower and toilet	
6. Firearms examination room with shoot tank	500 to 900 square feet
7. Energy-dispersive x-ray room	250 square feet
8. Spectrograph room	250 square feet
9. Research laboratory	180 square feet
10. Atomic absorption instrument room	180 square feet
11. Research laboratory office	180 square feet
12. Voiceprint room	100 square feet
13. X-ray diffraction instrument room	180 square feet
14. Small storage room	

Separation and analysis of arson residues is a dirty job. Specimens generate dust or are soaked with water and/or various combustible and volatile constituents. Separation from the rest of the section guards against contamination. This room should be equipped with benchwork along two sides, a gas chromatograph, required distillation apparatus, and a hood. Storage of arson evidence requires special conditions because of bulk and the presence of flammable components. A small, vented (with fan), adjacent 10- by 15-foot evidence room with cement floor, drain, and metal shelves should be constructed with the usual security door.

Criminalistics evidence is often large and bulky or voluminous. These items require a large, flat, clean surface for gross and low magnification and/or fluorescence examination. A large central table, bench space along both sides with knee space, several stereoscopic microscopes, at least one with a long boom, and a sink and a hood at one end are minimum requirements.

Examination of vehicles or other large evidence is unsatisfactory outside the laboratory, even with the assistance of the nearest convenient garage. Problems include artifactual contamination, sun, rain, wind, inadequate lighting, poor security, and a sore neck for the examiner from extended periods of hypertension. The laboratory garage equipped with slightly raised cement strips for the wheels solves all these problems. The next best solution is a floor pit. The examination is conducted on a mechanic's cart in a comfortable, supine position. Examination by fluorescent light is facilitated. Examination of the vehicle in this manner insures that no new surfaces are contacted by foreign objects (suspension points are still the tires). Serial number restorations can be conducted here as well. A floor drain insures a potentially clean room. Air conditioning and heat are supplied.

Place a bench with drawers across one end of the garage for minor mechanical manipulations necessary in the examination of cars and other large physical evidence objects. Drawers with locks or hasps for appropriate tools are included. A restroom opening off the garage with shower, large laundry tub, wash basin, and drainboard provides clean-up of analysts and evidence. Anyone who considers this a frill has never examined a vehicle trunk or other large container for physical evidence from which a decomposing body has been removed. Preliminary examination of burned debris may also take place here.

The firearms examination room requires benchwork with drawers along one side and benchwork with bins with lock hasps along another. An ammunition cabinet or locker, a device for measuring land and groove width, and a stereoscopic microscope for identification of trace evidence or bullets are other essentials along with the comparison microscope. Placement of the bullet recovery tank is always a problem. In our experience, a water tank is essential. The cotton box was adequate only until the introduction of the "Saturday night special." In warm climates, the tank can be placed outside, much to the relief of the other building occupants. In less ideal climates, the tank goes inside near the examination room, separated by an acoustically muffed door, walls, and ceiling. There is no surer prescription for two black eyes than to be caught looking through a binocular microscope when a large-caliber weapon is discharged nearby. We prefer a vertical water tank similar to the one in use by the Maryland Crime Laboratory. A small aperture in the top and a little distance to the water level minimizes the shower potential. (Ear protection is *essential*.) An accessible gate valve on the bottom, a drain, and a removable top for personnel entry are standby items for the inevitable emergency. Bullet recovery is effected through the top by a hollow metal mesh cylinder, closed at one end, inserting into the bottom drain. This is pulled to the top by a chain, preferably through a separate top slot, to minimize "chain shots." Access to a bullet trap for range estimation is both a convenience and a safety measure.

The spectrograph room should be vented and equipped with a small fan and vent, dark room plumbing, a 220-volt outlet, and a film viewer, in addition to the spectrograph. Separation from other instrumentation is advisable because of smoke from instrument operation. Atomic absorption instrumentation requirements are similar. One 220-volt outlet and three 110-volt sources are required. The x-ray diffractometer requires filtered cold water and a 220-volt source. Proper shielding eliminates radiation danger. Installation with other instruments is not prohibited. These days, however, most personnel prefer not to work near a radiation source. Benchwork is arranged so that samples may be prepared while sitting. Access to a dark room, cabinet storage for accessories, and file space need to be provided. Some may question the use of a spectrograph if energy-dispersive x-ray analysis or scanning electron microscopy is available. This criticism is partially valid. However, the spectrograph shows several orders of sensitivity higher than either instrument. Laser excitation can be focused on very small areas. Systems with several regional laboratories can vary major instrument purchases to gain maximum total capability.

Every large laboratory needs a research or application division in the criminalistic area, provided that someone is available with the experience and background to make it work. Problem-solving is an integral part of every area of forensic science.

Scanning electron microscopy and energy-dispersive x-ray have added a complete new dimension to criminalistics. Use of the former is probably the method of choice in identifying firearms residues. Unfortunately, high magnification is irrevocably associated with smaller fields. Therefore, valuable time can be wasted unless the significant targets or particles can be located by other means. The potential, however, is clearly defined. At this magnification, every possible step must be taken to exclude extraneous dust from the air. Water, a 220-volt outlet, and at least three 110-volt outlets must be supplied. Benchwork is supplied as needed for sample preparation. A computer with its unique wiring requirements is an essential part of the system.

DRUG IDENTIFICATION

A "normal" drug load per year for one scientist is approximately 800 cases. Maximum efficiency in drug analysis is provided by individual laboratories housing two scientists. There is minimum conversation, near maximum security, minimum movement, and efficient usage of the hood and sink placed at opposite ends. Floor and wall cabinets are built in. Built-in locks or at least hasps for the bin-type floor cabinets (for preanalysis evidence storage) are utilitarian. Most glassware is stored in the wall cabinets. Bench-top gas and electrical outlets every 3 or 4 feet, in addition to those in the hood, are standard. Ever mindful of security, and chain of custody requirements, each laboratory door lock should be unique. Sloping tops on wall cabinets minimize dust accumulation. Low-power visual examinations, chemical analysis, and thin-layer chromatography can all be conducted in these laboratories.

1. Chemistry laboratories	250 square feet per scientist
2. Mass spectrometer laboratory	250 square feet
3. NMR laboratory	192 square feet
4. Supervisor's office	275 square feet
5. Secretarial office	150 square feet
6. Instrument rooms (2)	
7. Computer terminal room	192 square feet
8. Research laboratory	250 square feet
9. Crystal laboratory (optional)	150 square feet
10. Drug standards locker	
11. Plant room (greenhouse equivalent)	100 square feet

In general, expensive instruments should be housed in individual laboratories. Instrument security is better served and special training easier to conduct. Two 220-volt and six 110-volt outlets should be furnished for each room. If the gas chromatograph mass spectrometer is to be complemented by a computer, a depressed floor for necessary wiring (with emergency drain) may be more aesthetic than a raised floor. A sink is convenient. Narrow temperature and humidity parameters argue against vents or hoods and for separate thermostats.

Other instrumentation is housed in two instrument rooms. One contains the gas and liquid chromatographs, and the other the fluorometer, infrared and ultraviolet spectrophotometers, balances, and polarimeter. Electrical outlets must be plentiful. A sink and hood are useful.

An extremely practical arrangement for the gas chromatographs in the instrument room is that used by Dr. Narish Jain in Los Angeles. He has aligned them in a U-shaped configuration. The analytical side faces outward into the room. The electrical and gas connections are made from a manifold on the inside of the U. Individual gas control valves are provided for each instrument. The two limbs of the U are wide enough to permit easy entry to the back side of all instruments. Maintenance problems are markedly attenuated. Scales used to weigh dusty materials such as marijuana should not be placed in the instrument rooms.

If there is extensive reliance on microcrystal tests, a separate laboratory with a stereoscopic and polarizing microscope is advisable. Two microscope stands, a sink, a hood, and floor and wall cabinets are also recommended. In small laboratories, or laboratories only occasionally using crystal confirmation, the polarizing microscope in trace evidence technology will serve.

If space permits, a research laboratory in which one or more scientists can work on unidentified sample components, new analytical methods, or applications of new instruments pays off in many ways. Separation serves to isolate "research" physically and psychologically from everyday casework.

Research is not for everyone. Nevertheless, it is not and should not be degree-controlled. A Ph.D. researcher, however, can neutralize and even reverse the academic advantage of an "ivory tower" defense witness.

Available drug and botanical standards are the resources of every good drug identification laboratory. The responsibility of keeping standards up to date and the timely replacement of deteriorating samples are important factors.

A small greenhouse, using artificial or natural light, is not an extravagance. The submission of seeds or immature plants for identification is common, and identification and insurance of fertility may await development of a viable plant or even final classification from the flower.

Finally, this section accounts for a good proportion of the total laboratory load. If computerized records are developed, computer generation of drug reports with standardized forms is a relatively simple and desirable procedure.

SEROLOGY

The serology section will ordinarily handle 3 to 5 percent of the caseload. The timing of the creation of one or more full-time serology positions is difficult. A full-time serologist, performing quality work, can complete 180 cases per year. However, foresight in planning for this special area will save lost motion, tempers, and time. In common with drugs and committed to the philosophy that a supervisor should spend part of his time working on cases, the supervisor's office may be combined with a secretarial office, and/or the latter separated and shared with another section.

1. Supervisor's office — 180 square feet
2. Secretarial office
3. Electrophoresis room — 350 square feet
4. Analytic serological laboratory — 500 square feet for two scientists
5. Dark room — 180 square feet
6. Research laboratory — 250 square feet
7. Walk-in refrigerator — 200 square feet
8. Walk-in hood
9. Store room

In this section, separation of the major analytical functions of electrophoresis and serology follows a natural cleavage. One of the specialty rooms, preferably that of analytical serology, should be large enough and equipped to facilitate examination of large items of clothing and bedding.

The electrophoresis laboratory should have direct access to the serology laboratory. It should be equipped with a walk-in refrigerator and dark room. At the other end of the serology laboratory, a large, walk-in hood should be located to circulate warm, dry air for drying and/or temporary storage of wet or large objects. Warm, moist, or wet conditions accelerate protein denaturation and preclude accurate identification of blood factors. These laboratories, including outlets inside the refrigerator, require more power than any other section. Offices and a research or applications laboratory should be placed opposite the electrophoresis laboratory. The rapid development of new technology in serology provides a strong argument for a research laboratory. This technology must be tested, validated, and modified before use in the laboratory. The opposing expert witness problem is with us in every area.

Serologic laboratory furniture consists, in part, of a large center examination table, benchwork all around, interrupted by microscope tables and desks. Wall cabinets for glassware are added as needed. A scrupulously clean laboratory with washable ceramic tile walls adds immeasurably to the accuracy of results. Temperature, dust control, and a method of sunlight screening are all highly desirable. Gas connections are less numerous than in drug laboratories.

DOCUMENTS

The two major and rather unique requirements of the documents section are noise control and good access to northern light. Document examiners spend most of their working time at their desks. One document examiner, working full time, can handle 500 cases per year. Noise generation from the secretary's office prohibits combination with the scientific offices. Document cases are rarely combined with services other than photography, and the creation of a small but separate evidence room, adjacent to the secretary's office, is convenient and serves to reduce surplus courtroom conversation on chain of custody. The examining rooms serve as staff offices and should never house more than two examiners. Each has a wide examining table or bench extending across one side. The laboratory room is equipped with benchwork along one side, a fuming cabinet with hood, standard laboratory plumbing, and a large, centrally located examining or exhibit table.

1. Section supervisor's office — 250 square feet
2. Secretarial office and evidence storage — 260 square feet
3. Examining room — 200 square feet
4. Laboratory — 400 square feet
5. Dark room — 100 square feet

Special instrumentation designed to measure luminescence and fluorescence and a photocopy setup are included in the dark room. The latter can be moved to the laboratory photography space, provided that it is contiguous with the document section. A standard floor and wall strip electrical supply is usually sufficient.

PHOTOGRAPHY

An office in the darkroom complex, but without other technical function, serves for "photo job" conferences and provides space for case negatives, miscellaneous filing space, and film storage. The subdividing of the remaining space into work units is somewhat arbitrary and based on what is estimated as an average need. The complex requires heat and humidity controls independent of the main laboratory system with separate thermostats in each room. An active, multispeed light-tight exhaust system keeps chemical fumes (e.g., acetic acid) at acceptable levels. Plumbing is complex with heating/cooling elements designed for precise control of water temperatures in each major dark and print room. Control of water quality may require filters and selective use of deionized water, as well as pressure-volume control. Electrical demand is heavy with 110- and 220-volt requirements in both wall and floor sockets. A separate circuit is recommended for the complex. Dust-repellent floor tile and nonreflective walls and ceilings with infrared shields are a must. Two walls of wood and two of nonpermanent carpet screen are recommended.

1. Office — 175 square feet
2. Microfilm — 165 square feet
3. Studio — 320 square feet
4. Refrigerator and supply storage
5. Document dark room — 110 square feet
6. Color process dark room — 200 square feet
7. Black and white process dark room — 165 square feet
8. Print and copy room — 300 square feet
9. Latent print dark room — 110 square feet

The same accessory lines (e.g., vacuum) available to the rest of the laboratory are made available to at least one photography room. All sinks should be of stainless steel. Earlier mention was made of noncurrent record storage by microfilm. Simultaneous processing and storage are best provided in this complex.

"IMPLIED CONSENT" ALCOHOL AND DRUG TESTING

There is much variability in the enforcement of "drunk driving" statutes. The most important variable—workload—will depend on legislation, inclusion of fatalities, type (if any) of breath program, degree of coverage of other drugs, and access to other body fluids. In our jurisdiction, approximately 75 percent of all cases tested by any method are positive for alcohol. In 60 percent, the alcohol level is above the prima facie limit. This should *not* be interpreted to show that either 25 or 40 percent of those arrested are not driving under the influence.

1. Blood alcohol laboratory — 300 square feet
2. Toxicology laboratory — 300 square feet
3. Store room — 200 square feet
    - chemicals
    - breath instrument parts
4. Office and secretary's office — 180 square feet
5. Cold room — 200 square feet
6. Lecture room (optional) — 1,250 square feet

Our toxicologists find drugs in over half of the alcohol negatives and in many of those with low alcohol levels. Admissions or evidence of marijuana use are common both with and without alcohol. At this point, the only impediments to analysis of body fluids for marijuana are financial and political. Allegations that marijuana does not affect driving ability, based on equivocal results in simulated driving test experiments, are contrary to field studies and experience.

The purpose of these comments is only to portray the variability inherent in any implied consent program. It is clear, however, that in most good laboratories, with adequate funds, this function is large and complicated. It may include:

1. Comprehensive analysis of blood, breath and urine specimens.
2. A viable quality control program.
3. Constant evaluation of new breath-test instrumentation.
4. Organization, scheduling, and teaching of training courses at both the initial and refresher level for breath-test operators.
5. Supervision of a team of breath-test field supervisors.
6. Maintenance of breath-test instruments.

Administrative procedures require a considerable amount of the supervisor's time. Conferences and phone calls are frequent. Therefore, it is not advisable to combine this office with a secretarial office. School scheduling requires a great deal of the secretary's time.

The blood alcohol laboratory will also require a built-in desk because of the large amount of associated paperwork. Most blood alcohols are now processed by instrumentation incorporating gas chromatograph analysis with some type of automatic sampling and/or reporting system. It is well to decide on the anticipated instrumentation so the benchwork can be designed for maximum utility. The number of electrical and gas outlets will hopefully exceed actual need because of unpredictable location requirements. A hood, benchwork and wall cabinets, and the usual gas connections are included.

The separate toxicology laboratory has the same general requirements as the drug laboratories except that more space per scientist is needed. Modification of shape, bench height, and desk space is dependent on techniques and types of body fluid analysis. The enzyme-multiplied immunoassay technique (EMIT) and radioimmunoassay (RIA) should be considered. The EMIT technique can be modified for blood analysis. Thin-layer techniques are the method of preliminary analysis in most laboratories.

Under most circumstances, other necessary instrumentation will be found in the drug identification instrument rooms. Access to a mass spectrometer is mandatory for unequivocal identification of some drugs present in minute amounts.

Regardless of the breath instrument chosen, breakdown is inevitable. All supervisory personnel must be able to effect at least minor repairs. There is no substitute for a stockroom of instrument parts.

The cold room serves, among other things, to store blood samples and urines. Joint capacity with serology saves on space and frustration when trying to locate samples.

For purposes of space-need calculation, it is impractical to save any biological sample for more than a year. The lecture room answers the breath test operator training space requirement if another facility is not available. Efficiency requirements necessitate a design suitable for both lecture and instruction in instrument operation. Therefore, desk top design, individual access to electricity and plumbing, and general access to the various gas lines available in the other laboratories are important considerations.

LATENT PRINTS

Physical location of the latent prints division adjacent to the photography laboratory is an obvious advantage. The supervisor's office may be combined with the secretary's office unless separate evidence reception is planned for this section. Caseload in latent prints is high enough to qualify for computer terminals into both the fingerprint and record system. In our experience, these two systems are usually not compatible within the same computer setup. This question, however, needs to be re-examined.

1. Supervisor's office — 250 square feet
2. Secretary's office — 150 square feet
3. Chemical laboratory — 150 square feet
4. Fingerprint powder laboratory — 150 square feet
5. Examining room(s) — 150 square feet
6. Evidence room — 200 square feet

The small laboratory for chemical development of prints is equipped much as other laboratories. The hood with exhaust is particularly important. Sink and benchwork complete available wall space. One wall-length wall cabinet is usually sufficient.

A separate fingerprint powder processing laboratory limits the inevitable fingerprint "dust" to one area of the section. A fan and vent are required. Bench space with cabinets across one end of each office is useful for sorting and/or examining evidence. A shower for "dusty" fingerprint examiners is not a luxury.

PERSONNEL

The staff is the backbone of the crime laboratory. It is no surprise that the secretarial staff, appropriately recruited and administered, determines the efficiency of the laboratory.

Attainment of scientific competence is more complicated. High-level forensic science is one of the great challenges to the scientific community. The scientist who knows the most about the least is useless in this field. A solid background of scientific knowledge, ability to apply this knowledge to ever-changing and unpredictable situations, arduous training, long hours, inquisitiveness, oral and written communication skills, and thoughtful attention to observed details and/or related information from all possible sources contribute to defining the professional.

When organizing a new laboratory, the first step in building a good staff is the acquisition of an experienced scientist (not a technician) in each skill area. The second step is the setting of qualifications under a civil service umbrella. (Hopefully this step minimizes political hiring and establishes uniformity.) With the exception of several special areas to be listed later, no scientific position should be set up with less than a natural science (B.S.) degree requirement. Most forensic science is based on chemistry with some additional course work in physics and biology. Only serology permits the reversal of the biology and chemistry concentration. This point is made because biology majors often avoid chemistry courses. These graduates are rarely acceptable as laboratory staff. (If the reader wishes to disagree, let him imagine himself challenged as a biology major in a drug identification case on the witness stand by a Ph.D. in chemistry.) Exceptions to this rule include document, latent print, and firearms examiners. Scientists holding M.S. degrees generally complete their forensic training phases more rapidly. The minimum number of salary levels in all sections without supervisory responsibility is three. A level consists of an entry step plus annual increments. In this day and age, increments only keep pace with inflation. Motivation to excel is best supplied by aspiration to higher pay scales.

Scientific Classifications

Crime Laboratory Scientist I. This position requires a B.S. degree and serves primarily as a training position. Eligibility for promotion to the next level begins after one year.

Crime Laboratory Scientist II. Direct entry requires an M.S. degree. A journeyman level exists for trained candidates with a B.S. Promotion eligibility for all employees to the next higher level begins after two years. Ph.D.-level candidates without experience are usually recruited in the middle of this grade.

Crime Laboratory Scientist III. This position requires some further education or training as well as evidence and practice of advanced skill.

Crime Laboratory Scientist IV. This position requires a B.S. degree plus five years' experience in criminalistics or an allied field. Levels consist of section supervisory, research scientist, and outstanding scientist grades. In addition to supervisory responsibility, the wide IV availability gives goals to personnel who have outstanding research or other scientific talent. The limited number of supervisory slots should not be a bar to promotion of deserving scientists. It will serve to keep valuable and talented personnel who would otherwise be siphoned off by other laboratories.

Documents. The same levels apply. A scientific degree is not required, but is useful. Artistic talent is valuable. A degree completion that correlates with the development of a good document examiner is not available. The specialty is unusual in that it is both an art and a science. No salary penalty is justified when a proficient examiner lacks a scientific degree.

Latent Prints. Although no degree is required, a minimum of one year of college, including English and Chemistry, is an advised requirement. Three levels are advised (Latent Print Examiner I, II, and III) with a fourth as supervisor. A lower range than that of crime laboratory scientist series is competitive.

Photography. Good forensic photography requires more expertise than most other photographic positions. A good basic background, special training, ingenuity, and the demonstrated ability to produce quality work of great variety for use in court and training combine to require a favorable salary.

Administrative Assistant. This position is open to graduates of the Crime Laboratory Scientist III series. Administrative, writing, and budget preparation talent is required. Lack of scientific training markedly decreases usefulness. Need is proportional to laboratory size as well as the scientific duties required of the assistant director and director.

Assistant Director. Candidates must have earned an advanced degree or equivalent and have five years' experience in a crime laboratory.

Director. Candidates must have an advanced degree or equivalent plus six years' experience.

For the protection of both the employee and the employer, each level of each section and all others must have a job description. This should be signed by both the employer and employee. Merit boards will, with reason, reject level changes based on longevity alone. Professional personnel evaluation consultants can do more harm than good. Their personnel often consist of social scientists trying to equalize the world. Their personnel salary formulas are subject to the same judgment criteria as other evaluations without the inclusion of reality.

Salaries. New laboratories have to pay more to get experienced scientists. Comparison of scientific jobs will show that the competency, responsibility, versatility, and communication skills requirements of the crime laboratory scientist are considerably above average for the scientific community, provided that the job is being properly performed; salary levels should reflect this. There is no substitute for satisfactory quality-assurance programs to indicate the caliber of laboratory work. The American Society of Crime Laboratory Directors is in the process of developing a Crime Laboratory Accreditation Program. Mediocre salaries insure mediocre staff that in turn insures mediocre performance, in turn insuring mediocre justice. The politician complaining about the lack of proficiency or competency in his area's crime laboratory has usually gotten exactly what he paid for!

PROCEDURES

Evidence Handling

The transfer of evidence from the police officer to a responsible scientist or evidence technician must be fully recorded in terms of submitting officer, case officer, suspect or victim's name, jurisdiction, date, description of evidence, and services requested on a standard form. (Fig. 45-1). A unique case number is affixed to the form and sequentially numbered case items. (For this purpose a case involves victims and/or suspects involved in a specific incident.) The master evidence sheet is "filed," and a duplicate accompanies the evidence to the scientist's bench or storage area. Each service requires a duplicate sheet. To insure accurate evidence tracking in the latter, the sequential transfer of case material from one scientist to another is recorded on the master sheet by the initials of the recipient. Removal of the evidence from the laboratory for any reason is duly recorded by the dated signature of the recipient, including the courts. Return of evidence by certified or registered mail requires retention in the file of the signed receipt form. There is a great diversity of philosophy on

```
                                        E.C. _____ C. _____
                                        CASE _____
DATE RECEIVED _____ 19 _____ TIME _____ RECEIVED BY _____
VICTIM _____ SUSPECT _____
COUNTY _____ CITY _____
OFFICERS _____
RECEIVED FROM _____ REMARKS _____
OF _____
SERVICES REQUESTED _____
DESCRIPTION OF EVIDENCE _____



                                        DISPOSITION OF EVIDENCE
                                        Returned to _____
                                        By _____
                                        Date _____
GBI-024 (2/75)                          Destroyed _____
```

FIGURE 45-1. Record of evidence received by the crime laboratory.

the disposition of evidence once evaulated. There is no right or wrong answer. Three choices are apparent:

1. Returning the evidence to the officer;
2. Retaining the evidence in the laboratory;
3. An intermediate solution.

The first solution absolves the laboratory of all responsibility other than testimony. This is convenient for the laboratory but requires all police departments to have secure evidence rooms with a responsible evidence technician so that changes in employment status prior to court will not jeopardize custody. The chances for drug evidence to go astray is markedly increased in proportion to the number of custodians.

Laboratory retention of the evidence leads to more effective testimony but gives rise to a host of bookkeeping and space headaches. In addition to file records, an evidence book should be kept for each major evidence room. It lists the bin location of evidence in every case and must be signed and dated by the laboratory scientist removing evidence from this room. The result is a double recording of evidence removal. It is, of course, the procedure, not the exact form, that is important. An evidence card can be sent to the case officer with the report or at a later time. The returnable card asks him to indicate the disposition of the evidence over his signature and states that unless the card is returned, the evidence will be destroyed within 60 days. Approximately twice a year the evidence is inventoried, and cards or lack of cards determine the fate of the evidence. This process is much more easily carried on by a computer. However, cards should not serve as a substitute for judgment.

In the intermediate system evidence is either returned or destroyed after a specified period of approximately two years. Fatal bullets in homicides are never destroyed. All possible evidence is sealed in bags by initialed evidence tape that must be destroyed to remove.

Records

CASE RECORDS

Case record numbers can be referenced by a simple annual card index file. Where the laboratory serves several police jurisdictions, two sets of color-coded cards are kept, one alphabetically arranged by suspect or victim names, the other by county and date of receipt. All cards show case type, date submitted, and police agency in addition to the number.

CASE NUMBER	SERVICES	COUNTY	DATE RECEIVED	DATE ALL SERV. COMP.	DATE TYPED

DPS-314(12/72)

FIGURE 45-2. Sequential case tracking record.

It is suggested that case records themselves be kept in file for approximately two years. Our practice has been to purge all negative and misdemeanor cases and microfilm the remaining at that time. Microfilm is active for 10 years before permanent storage.

Data from which the reports are derived are kept in individual notebooks by the individual scientists. A sequential case tracking record (Fig. 45-2) on a clipboard is useful, particularly when the laboratory has many multiservice cases. This serves as a quick case-status reference for both the secretarial and professional staff. With computerized records both systems are combined, with only occasional or unusual cases requiring hard copy-filing. This is accomplished through standardized forms for all sections. A minicomputer on the premises with disc drive in duplicate is in use in some laboratories. The system is fast and will work at night preparing reports.

WORK RECORDS

Adminstrative efficiency and budget preparation require monthly and annual workload and caseload reports (Tables 45-1 and 45-2). Caseload is not an adequate measure of workload because of the variability in multiservice and multi-item cases in addition to the increasing amount of casework input in part associated with the evolution of the forensic sciences. Therefore each scientist in each area records in his monthly report not only his caseload, but also the number of items tested and the number of tests performed. In addition, some jurisdictions require greater scientific proof of identity than others. For example, it is our understanding that after some very dubious testimony by a mass spectrometer expert in Minnesota, that state now requires a mass spectrometer analysis on all drugs, including marijuana. It is unfortunate that theory, rather than chemical identity, was accepted by the court. Regrettably, many defense experts would rather talk than work.

Operating Procedures

This section could also be titled "preventive medicine." Certain crime laboratory operations cause frustration so frequently that the wise administrator formulates equitable and useful rules effective on opening day. They will generally be part of the laboratory's operating procedure manual.

Travel. The circumstances under which employees may recover travel expenses from the laboratory budget must be explicit. The administrator can cover himself by adding the phrase "at the discretion of the Director." Mileage allowable, costs per meal, and allowable costs for motel accommodations are placed in writing. The circumstances and authorizations for travel inside or outside laboratory jurisdiction may be added as well.

Work Time. The issues of credit and debit of compensatory time and overtime are troublesome. The minimum allowable time credit increment (5 minutes or 30 minutes) must be reasonable and consistent. A good understanding or rule is needed as to allowable working hours.

News Releases. Police officers and district attorneys are very sensitive about news releases from the laboratory. The case does not belong to the

TABLE 45-1. Monthly Activity Report—Crime Laboratory (Total System): October*

Service	Cases Received During Month†	Cases Carried Over From Previous Month	Cases Completed During Month	Active Cases End of Month	Percent Increase/ Decrease Over Previous Month	Total Cases Year to Date
Pathology	31	21	27	25	+29	135
Handwriting	212	87	234	65	−6	860 (6)
Criminalistics	383 (40)‡	177 (22)	389 (39)	171 (23)	−3	1466 (278)
Serology	85 (16)	45 (21)	77 (10)	53 (27)	+6	352 (65)
Drug Identification	1205 (18)	284 (9)	1213 (22)	276 (5)	+8	4590 (69)
Toxicology	132 (91)	126 (24)	136 (101)	122 (14)	−11	597 (426)
Photography	(9)	(4)	(9)	(4)	+125	1 (38)
Latent Fingerprint	180 (49)	37	173 (49)	44	−15	653 (208)
Implied Consent	712 (154)	20 (108)	706 (159)	26 (103)	−5	2810 (695)
Total	2940 (377)	797 (188)	2955 (389)	782 (176)	−1	11,464 (1785)

*Implied consent training—number of sessions: four refresher courses and two regular intoximeter courses; number of law enforcement agencies served: 255.

†Scientific cases only; not entire caseload.

‡Represents section examinations which are a second service on otherwise tallied cases.

TABLE 45-2. Performance Report—Georgia Bureau of Investigation: Crime Laboratory

Program Name Measures	Actual Annual Measure (FY 77)	Projected Annual Measure (FY 78)	Program Expenditures	
			(77)	(78)
Drug identification 4-4			342,121	Decrease because of branch laboratory activity
Submissions	10,618	9,000		
Court appearances (% submissions)	4	4		
Time available for research	50 hrs/wk	50 hrs/wk		
Number of "hits" (% submissions)	93	93		
Submissions per scientist	757	650		
Cost per submission	$32.00	$30.00		
Overtime	445	450		
% Cost	18	16		
% Personnel	19	20		
Scientific turnaround time (% over 10 days)	11	8		

laboratory. Investigators are very sensitive to "their" publicity. Permission from the officer is good public relations. The rule should be, when in doubt, don't!

Other Procedures. Other important or emotional issues include private cases and remunerative defense work, procedures in vehicle accidents, determination of testifiers, carrying of firearms, access to reports, telephone reports, drug evidence destruction, sick leave, and the inevitable lie detector test for both new and established employees.

TRANSPORTATION

Vehicles are required for courts, crime scenes, and breath-testing supervision. Any individual whose duties require 20,000 miles or more of travel per year should be assigned a car on a permanent basis. Advantages include better car care, savings on equipment wear in packing and unpacking, and efficient travel scheduling. To the staff, car assignments should justify placing them on 24-hour call. The remaining vehicles, including those for rotating call, are placed in a car pool. The type and vintage of the cars the laboratory receives are a good indication of the value their parent department places on laboratory services. Low evaluation means low morale and low work output. In high-mileage situations, car leasing is a very attractive possibility. This is especially true when purchasing practices force acceptance of low bids, regardless of maintenance cost and downtime.

Some laboratories prefer crime-scene vans; others prefer station wagons. This preference is often a reflection of the average distance to be traveled versus carrying capacity. Crime-scene vehicles need positraction.

COST

Construction costs for a laboratory range from $55 per square foot to in excess of $100. The cabinet work is included and constitutes about $20 per square foot. Operating costs vary somewhat but average about $55 per case. Salaries will constitute 75 percent of the laboratory budget. When budgets are cut, great difficulty is experienced in reducing expenses without eliminating staff positions. Most new laboratories are constructed with local money and equipped with funds from the Law Enforcement Assistance Administration (LEAA). LEAA sometimes supports the staff for a brief period.

It would appear that the "new look" at LEAA will consist of support solely for law enforcement improvement projects. Thus new crime laboratories or crime laboratory improvement projects should still receive funds. However, if liberal philosophy prevails, "criminal improvement projects" may provide the profession with more active criminal clients but little or no money.

In this regard, there is some agitation to provide a separate system of crime laboratories for the defense. This is quite a compliment to the effectiveness of existing crime laboratories. The purpose of the second system would be to neutralize the first so that cases would be decided on witness and argument.

APPENDIX

Suggested Major Instrument List	*Current Approximate Cost (to show magnitude only)*
Light Microscope	$ 4,000
Petrographic microscope	$ 4,000
Stereoscopic microscope	$ 1,000
Spectrophotometers	
Infrared with accessories and diamond cell	$25,000
Ultraviolet (visible with accessories)	$12,000 to $15,000
Fluorometer	$13,000
Atomic absorption	$35,000
Nuclear magnetic resonance	$25,000 to $35,000
X-ray diffractometer	$40,000 to $50,000
Spectrograph	$40,000
Gas chromatograph	$15,000 to $48,000
Pyrolysis attachment	$ 2,500
Mass spectrometer	$70,000 to $170,000
Scanning electron microscope	$60,000
Energy-dispersive x-ray	$60,000
Ballistics microscope	$18,000
Blood alcohol analyzer (automated)	$25,000
Enzyme-multiplied immunoassay	$15,000
Radioimmunoassay	$24,000
Liquid chromatograph	$10,000

REFERENCES

1. Joseph, A.: Study of Needs and Development of Curricula in the Field of Forensic Science. Crime Laboratories: Three Study Reports. LEAA Project Report, Washington, D. C., April 1968.

2. Benson, W. R., Story, J. E., and Worley, M. L.: Systems Analysis of Criminalistics Operations. Final Report, Midwest Research Institute Project No. 3333-D, LEAA Grant NI-044, U.S. Department of Justice, Washington, D. C., June 1970.
3. Gunn, J. W., and Frank, R. S.: Planning a Forensic Science Lab, in Peterson, J. L. (ed.): *Forensic Science Scientific Investigation in Criminal Justice,* AMS Press, New York, 1975. pp. 289–300.
4. Field, K. S.: Quality Assurance through Proficiency Testing and Quality Control Programs, in Fox, R. H., and Wynbrandt, F. H. (eds.): *Crime Laboratory Management Forum,* Forensic Science Foundation Press, Rockville, Maryland, 1976.

CHAPTER 46

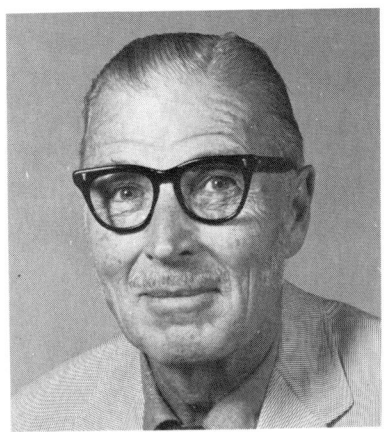

Morton F. Mason is Professor of Forensic Medicine and Toxicology at the University of Texas Southwestern Medical School at Dallas. Dr. Mason is former Director of the Dallas City–County Criminal Investigation Laboratory. He is a Past President of the American Academy of Forensic Sciences and is a Director of the American Board of Forensic Toxicology. Dr. Mason has published a number of papers and articles in renal physiology, liver physiology, forensic chemistry, and analytical and forensic toxicology.

QUALIFICATIONS AND TRAINING FOR FORENSIC TOXICOLOGY

Morton F. Mason, Ph.D.

GENERAL QUALIFICATIONS

In the staffing of a laboratory unit undertaking forensic toxicologic examinations, questions often arise concerning desirable qualifications of the individuals selected to engage in such activities. Two kinds of personnel are mostly involved: supervisory and technical. Occasionally others must be considered, including secretaries, especially for reasons of confidentiality and technique in handling office or telephone inquiries, and janitorial and dishwashing employees, especially if they have access to the laboratory facility at hours when no supervisory, technical, or secretarial personnel are present.

The initial step in any consideration for employment is to obtain verified information regarding the personal character of the subject. Has he ever been arrested for other than a traffic violation (and not too many of these)? Has he produced documentation of his academic and previous employment experience? If he has had military service, does he have an honorable discharge? Has he been considered reliable by previous employers, if any? Has he established an acceptable work output and attendance record? Has he any disqualifying habits such as a drinking or drug abuse problem? Can he be trusted not to disclose confidential information? Has he any record of a treated disorder of mentation? Is he reasonably compatible with co-workers? An employer with knowledge of defects of the applicant in respect to these matters may choose to overlook them in individual instances for a variety of reasons; however, to hire an employee without making these kinds of inquiries is to invite disaster.

The mandatory qualifications of supervisory and purely technical personnel differ by virtue of the forensic features of their activities. The adjectival meaning of the word forensic is not strictly limited. For the present purpose it may be taken that in order for an activity to be forensic, the following noun must be one which enables the combination to involve provision of evidence accompanied by explanation and intepretation in, to, or for courts of law or other law-enforcing components of the legislative, judicial, or executive branches of government.* In the case of toxicology this limits the forensic qualifications to knowledge regarding kinds of chemical structures which, in quantities which are relatively small compared to those incidentally entering a living organism, usually exert deleterious effects (i.e., "poisons").

The character and depth of special knowledge required includes important structural features and properties (biochemistry); means of identifying, isolating, and quantifying such substances (analytical toxicology); having information regarding the nature of their deleterious effects; the amounts or concentrations required to have effects ranging from disability to death (pharmacology); and, to a limited degree, the chief features of the macro- and microstructural changes in organs or tissues which may result (pathology).

In most jurisdictions in the United States supervisory personnel may give evidence regarding the findings of technical personnel, provided that it is shown that the manual features of the examinations were done under a loosely interpreted meaning of the phrase "supervision and control" of the supervisor, although this is not always the case. In addition admissibility may depend upon the supervisor's showing that the technical workers in question have had the education and experience necessary for obtaining the findings, or the bench worker himself occasionally may be called into the witness box so that judge and jury may directly form an opinion.

It is mandatory that supervisory personnel have special knowledge which is demonstrable during witness qualification by a review of curricula vitae, past experience and, preferably, publications of work which either advance understanding in some portion of their field or otherwise demonstrate extensive information, especially information relevant to explanation and interpretation of the immediate matters about which testimony is to be given.

FORENSIC PATHOLOGISTS

In the case of a pathologist, the possession of a degree of Doctor of Medicine and licensure in a given state are usually sufficient legally to qualify him as a witness to give evidence regarding toxicologic findings. For many years, however, resident training in forensic pathology has been available, and at the present time most medical examiners are certified in forensic pathology by the American Board of Pathology. Many of their assistants, in turn, receive the training necessary to be eligible for certification. In small or inadequately funded units in some jurisdictions, the forensic pathologist may also participate in the bench performance of toxicologic examinations and may have acquired special knowledge essential for its forensic presentation. However, in recent years, the combination of caseload, administrative responsibilities, and the technical expansion of the informational base of forensic toxicology has made many forensic pathologists prefer to delegate all matters having to do with toxi-

---

*A commonly accepted, simple definition of forensic toxicology is the study and practice of the application of toxicology to the purposes of the law.

cology to supervisory persons with advanced, specialized academic training in forensic toxicology or established competence through self-training in the course of their experience. The former group, holding a doctorate in forensic toxicology or analytical toxicology, is increasing in number, and it is likely that the latter group will gradually decrease or disappear.

TECHNICIANS

The technician is not required to exhibit extensive knowledge, but he must be able to show that he has had the education, training, and experience to justify the presumption that his findings are reliable. Moreover, he must have kept records which enable him to state precisely what instructions he received to undertake the various manipulations in the examinations he made and how he conducted these. Hence, in employing a technical worker, it is highly desirable that he has had college or university training leading to a B.S. degree in chemistry, physics, or biology. In the absence of such formal training, he needs to have had considerable experience in analytical chemical work to justify the presumption of reliability of his findings.

While not generally obligatory, it is advantageous and preferable for the technical worker to obtain recognized credentialing by meeting the formal requirements of one of five certifying or accrediting organizations: the Registry of American Technologists (ASCP), the American Society for Medical Technology, the American Board of Bioanalysts, the National Registry in Clinical Chemistry, and the American Board of Forensic Toxicology (ABFT). Although no special emphasis is given to forensic toxicology in all but the last of these organizations, the meeting of their requirements assures a sufficient background such that chemical, pharmacological, pathological, and medical matters encountered in day to day work do not remain completely unfamiliar or incomprehensible to the technician performing toxicologic analyses.

The curricula vitae of technical applicants rarely include outstanding academic records. Subjects with exceptionally high grade averages usually make professional or graduate school training the next step in their careers.

ACADEMIC PROGRAMS

The reasons for the relative scarcity of academically trained forensic toxicologists are mostly related to the failure of forensic toxicology, medicolegal pathology, and the forensic sciences generally to achieve a standing in Academia comparable with that seen in many European universities during the nineteenth and twentieth centuries. In the United States a kind of stagnation set in, consequent to the absence of interest in course presentations and the lack of funding for training programs at undergraduate, graduate, and postdoctoral levels. Toxicology was absorbed into, and then essentially neglected by, most departments of pharmacology in other than matters having directly to do with animal and human clinical drug toxicity and a few other facets having little or no forensic relevance. Exceptions included a medicolegal department at Harvard University, the School of Criminology at the University of California at Berkeley, and, in a more restricted scope, the Biochemistry Department at the Indiana University Medical Center, where special emphasis was given to forensic toxicology by Dr. R. N. Harger.

The report of a Presidential Commission during the mid-1960s pointed strongly to the lack of adequate information regarding the toxicity of a large number of new chemicals being employed in industry, and the absence of described methods of detection, quantitation, and isolation of many of these from materials of body origin.[1] Very shortly this resulted in federal funding of activities such as toxicology training centers at several universities; a broadening of grant support of toxicologic research projects by divisions of the Public Health Service and subdivisions of the Department of Health, Education and Welfare; and the creation of the Law Enforcement Assistance Administration and other authorizations under the Omnibus Crime Act. Of considerable importance was the establishment of "Toxline," "Medline," and "Chemline" computerized information storage and retrieval systems at the National Library of Medicine from which it is now possible to obtain by telephone summaries of information and literature references regarding rare or unfamiliar compounds, as well as common ones, within a few minutes.

In spite of these encouraging developments, educational programs are relatively sparse in respect to the educational needs of the criminal justice system imposed by the increasing use of forensic sciences in law enforcement as both population and total incidence of crime increase, along with competition for services of the analytical toxicologist by a variety of governmental regulatory agencies. A recent survey of the availability of formal education in the forensic sciences, which contains a roster of institutions, addresses, courses offered, and degrees obtainable, shows that there are still only a few advanced degree programs in forensic analytical toxicology.[2]

SUPERVISORY QUALIFICATIONS

Assessment of qualifications of an individual for a supervisory position in forensic toxicology in the absence of specific academic training (i.e., an advanced degree in analytical or forensic toxicology) is best made on the basis of such criteria as validation of information in his curriculum vitae and contact with previous and present employers regarding the character and quality of his bench and forensic experience. Although not yet an absolute requirement, it is desirable that the subject possess a doctorate (see below) in a natural science, preferably in chemistry, physics, or biology, or more recently in analytical forensic toxicology. It is also desirable that several years of his previous laboratory experience have been in association with, or under the supervision of, a well-recognized individual or department involved with forensic toxicology. For example, a number of older forensic toxicologists had their only direct training in analytical toxicology during a period of participation in the day to day work of the toxicology laboratories of the Office of the Medical Examiner for the Borough of Manhattan, under the supervision of Alexander Gettler. An alternative is a briefer period of such association together with several years of self-learning that has become recognized as adequate by established forensic toxicologists.

A further desirable qualification is creativity which may be manifested not only by authorship or co-authorship of publications in scientific journals, but also by teaching activities; appearance and presentation of papers at national, sectional, or local meetings; and even opinions based upon conversations with peers which have given evidence of the presence of an active and inquiring mind. Usually these characteristics are found in individuals who have already become members of the chief professional society representing their professional interest—in the U.S. this is the American Academy of Forensic Sciences—or are eligible to do so.

Following creation of the Public Health Service and, especially, the Department of Health, Education and Welfare, it became apparent that substantiation of competence might soon be required for individuals holding supervisory positions in local, state, or federal agencies, or in privately owned laboratories performing services for which payment in part or whole came from the federal government. In addition evaluation of the laboratory unit may become subject to scrutiny by mandatory participation in proficiency testing at a state level, a federal level, or both, and by other means. Since some jurisdictions, notably New York, had already formalized certain requirements for clinical chemistry laboratories,[3] and agencies such as the Center for Disease Control were formulating proficiency testing plans, it seemed desirable to establish certification programs in the forensic sciences which would provide substantiation of competence analogous to that offered by the various medical specialties, thus lessening the extent and possibly the inflexibility which might attend precipitous federal intervention. After some inquiry and study, a formal request to implement certification under the aegis of the American Academy of Forensic Sciences, operating through its research and educational arm, the Forensic Sciences Foundation, Inc., was approved in 1974. The original plan which involved a single certifying body for the Academy Sections proved unacceptable at the time, and the seven individual sections (other than Pathology/Biology) were authorized to proceed individually to formulate their requirements and to fulfill the legal requirements for operation of a certification program as required by the state in which it is incorporated.

BOARD CERTIFICATION

The American Board of Forensic Toxicology, Inc., was established in 1975 and immediately entertained applications for certification.* All applicants are required to pass a written examination if they meet the other requirements of education and experience. The former includes an earned Doctor of Philosophy or Doctor of Science degree in one of the natural sciences from an accredited institution (in most instances one recognized by the Regional Accrediting Commissions of the U.S. Office of Education) or from one whose pertinent programs in natural science (e.g., chemistry) were at the time so recognized, or recognized by other institutions, at the discretion of the Board. In addition the applicant must have had adequate undergraduate and graduate training in biology, chemistry, and pharmacology or toxicology which shows 32 semester hours of chemistry or the equivalent and which includes courses in inorganic, organic, analytical, and physical chemistry.†

The latter includes at least three years of full-time (or the equivalent in part-time) experience in forensic toxicology acceptable to the Board and acquired after receiving the doctoral degree. The experience may include

---

*The American Board of Forensic Toxicology, Inc., c/o The Forensic Sciences Foundation, Inc., 11400 Rockville Pike, Suite 515, Rockville, Maryland 20852.
†Recognition and allowance are made for instances where analytical chemistry has been abolished as a separate formal course and integrated into other course presentations.

postdoctoral education and training in toxicology or closely related disciplines, practice, research, teaching, administration, or combinations of these. At least one year of such experience must have been acquired during the five years preceding the date of application, and the applicant must be engaged in the practice of forensic toxicology at the time of application. Experience must be documented as professional activity in keeping with the concept that forensic toxicology is the study and practice of the application of toxicology to the purposes of the law.

The requirement of an earned doctorate and postdoctoral experience described above has been waived through December 31, 1979, provided that the applicant possesses an earned baccalaureate degree in one of the natural sciences from an institution acceptable to the Board *and* at least six years of full-time post-baccalaureate experience (or the part-time equivalent thereof) in forensic toxicologic activity acceptable to the Board (which may include graduate education deemed acceptable).

It is likely that, except under exceptional circumstances, it will soon be considered an administrative impropriety to employ a supervisory forensic toxicologist not certified by the American Board of Forensic Toxicology.

It is an advantage if the supervisory forensic toxicologist selected, but already employed, comes from a jurisdiction formally or informally related to a medical school or health science center where he has had the opportunities of participation in academic matters including research, teaching, and administration. This preferably has entailed appointment on a visiting or part-time basis to an academic department—usually pharmacology, chemistry, biochemistry, or pathology. It assures against the insidious decrement in knowledge, interest, external communication with peers, and the appearance of boredom which are the almost inevitable consequences of isolation. If the position in question is not already so related, it is well worthwhile to attempt to make some arrangement if there is a suitable institution within a reasonable distance (e.g., 50 to 100 miles).

With the qualifications described, the governmental or private unit undertaking forensic toxicology may expect that the supervisory toxicologist will exhibit capability and reliability in exclusion of toxic agents or their detection and quantitative determination in specimens submitted to him with a degree of expertise approved by his peers. He should be able to understand and interpret forensically the significance of toxicologic findings to a depth and extent deemed competent by his peers and consonant and compatible with the "state of the art" and the limitations of certainty at the time. He should be agreeable to obligatory proficiency testing programs and arrange an internal one which is part of the daily or weekly operation of the laboratory.

An especially important obligation of the supervisory forensic toxicologist is to allocate an appropriate amount of the bench-performance time of technical workers to proficiency testing and in-house quality control. The time allotted may be expected to range between 10 and 15 percent in laboratories expecting to maintain consistent competence. External proficiency testing, as mentioned before, is likely to be imposed on all laboratories receiving payments for services to governmental agencies, to be followed by performance grading which may determine whether the laboratory will continue to be licensed to perform the tests they offer. The individual states are expected to follow with regulation of *all* laboratories providing services to the public.

Early published and unpublished reports of results of proficiency testing for various drugs and heavy metals by forensic and clinical chemistry laboratories revealed deficiencies fully justifying obligatory programs in the public interest.[4]

LABORATORY QUALITY CONTROL MEASURES

In many, if not most, laboratories a proficiency test specimen is identified as such upon presentation to the technical personnel performing the analysis. Thus it is given special attention, and the results obtained throw little light upon the day to day competence of the laboratory. The specimen is best handled as an ordinary, routine submission with the specified analyses requested, or a case history may be composed which points to the items which should be sought.

Numerous descriptions of quality control programs have appeared in journals, such as *Clinical Chemistry*, over the past 10 to 15 years. A recent book dealing in part with this matter, sponsored by the American Public Health Association, has been prepared.[5]

The proper arrangement of quality control procedures and interpretation of data accumulated, as well as the understanding of reports dealing with proficiency testing, require an understanding of elementary statistics and represent another qualification for the forensic toxicologist.

To realize such expectations over a significant period of time imposes obligations and responses by the employing unit. These comprise budgetary arrangements which include adequate provision of supplies; modern, sophisticated equipment; space; and secondary personnel sufficient for the workload anticipated. Appropriate conditions of employment having to do with salary; subsequent salary adjustments for all personnel; hours; specifications for 24-hour service, if imposed; vacation time; sick leave; availability of medical service, if any; conditions of tenure, if any; and retirement must be clearly delineated.

In addition, provision should be made for subscription by the unit to a few "key" journals and support for attendance of supervisory toxicologists at meetings. Presence at two or three meetings might well become a condition of acceptance of employment. Moreover, in light of the continuing growth in complexity and utility of instrumentation and in forensic toxicologic knowledge, funds should be available for attendance at occasional "short courses" or "workshops" arranged by technical societies or private, commercial, or governmental agencies, which often provide important continuing education that may materially improve the subsequent performance of the laboratory personnel in dealing with new problems or old ones which have hitherto vexed the toxicologist and his associates.

A clear understanding must exist regarding the expectation that the supervisory toxicologist will engage in some form of creative activity, either individually or collectively with other members of the laboratory unit. The time and support necessary for this activity is to be administratively arranged. Such creative activity includes research in one of its various forms, internal and (if available) external teaching, invited external technical speaking presentations, demonstrations or seminars, and limited public relations appearances at professional business clubs.

Suitably disposed, these matters provide a stability and professional attitude essential to high-quality performance, which in turn assures its enthusiastic acceptance by the components of the system of justice or other agencies which may be incidentally served.

EXPERT QUALIFICATIONS AND TESTIMONIAL ISSUES

In the case of the already established forensic toxicologist, his forensic capabilities usually can be evaluated by telephone or by written communication with persons who have dealt with him both as colleagues and as opponents in courts or other settings in which advocacy is integrally involved in the search for truth. Glaring deficiency as a witness entails sufficient risk to the effectiveness and reputation of the unit to exclude an offer of employment.

The forensic toxicologist, like other forensic scientists, is properly concerned only in the validity of his findings, his interpretation of their meaning, and the degree of their certainty when he is retained by one side in the role of an adversary. He is in the difficult position of avoiding participation in advocacy, indeed, in rare instances to the point of consciously or unconsciously presenting and defending his evidence more for the purpose of influencing the final verdict than establishing truths. One way to minimize bias and enhance detachment from advocacy is to insist upon a pretrial conference on the evidence he is to present. At this time he can insist that defects bearing on the weight of his evidence are not to be concealed and that findings failing to substantiate the case of the side he is representing be brought out during direct examination. Failing in this, he may take care to blurt them during subsequent direct or cross-examination.

Avoiding either intentional or, more likely, unintentional advocacy is not easy, particularly in instances where the witness is always representing one side (e.g., the state in criminal cases). Thus his own position in his unit or the standing of the unit in the law enforcement community may be endangered or lessened by insistence upon dealing with his findings without regard for the effects that these may have upon the ultimate verdict, especially when he has been asked specifically to respond with slanted (not perjured) answers and to omit items in replies which might lead to discovery by the adversaries of matters which weaken rather than strengthen the impact of his findings.

The behavior of forensic toxicologists in effectively giving evidence can range from a soft-spoken or even somewhat halting manner to a firmly aggressive demeanor accompanied by a loud or truculent voice. This matters little so long as the overall attitude conveys the impression of truthfulness. It is important for the witness to avoid any trace of evasiveness, especially in trying to sidetrack a direct, true answer that might diminish the weight of evidence that he or others have given. Garrulousness lessens the impact of evidence upon a jury.

Especially undesirable are attempts at humor, for in instances where penalties upon conviction are severe, some jurors are deeply offended by any departure from a serious attitude. Humor is best left to counsel, and the witness will do well to respond in a reasonably restrained and dignified manner.

It is very important during direct or, especially, cross-examination to respond without hesitation, "I do not know," or "I do not remember," or "I would have to refresh my mind by examining the records" when one of these is a true and appropriate answer. To attempt to create the impression of knowledge not actually demonstrable is risking what it deserves—further entrapment by a knowledgeable examiner, confusion, and unintentional falsity in answers, leading to impeachment of credibility—which may be brought up again and again in related kinds of cases.

The appearance of a witness affects the acceptance of his evidence by more than an occasional juror, although perhaps to a lesser extent than was the case prior to about 1960. It must be remembered that strong prejudice created in the mind of a *single* juror may determine a verdict. Thus extremes are to be avoided, and the advice given by one of Shakespeare's characters—"Neat, but not gaudy"—is good advice today.

Almost all of the perils and discomforts of the witness stand can be avoided by adhering strictly to the truth, stated simply and directly; by having at hand all necessary records of examinations made to be freely scrutinized by opposing counsel if he so desires; and by prior refreshing of the information base involved in supporting the interpretation and conclusions presented. In the training of a modern forensic toxicologist, he should be required to observe procedure in court, as well as the performances of experienced, capable, and even inept witnesses, in order to confirm for himself the appropriate features he wishes to incorporate into his own subsequent appearances.

Toxicology, as one of the prime disciplines in the forensic sciences, is changing very rapidly. The information and instrumental explosion and the appearance of relevant immunologic and isotopic techniques along with computerized data processing have forced rapid change and growth of capability and sophistication comparable to that realized in medicine and surgery following the Second World War.

What was a relatively primitive applied science three decades ago is now far advanced, but along with this development has come a greatly increased operational cost. Many medicolegal jurisdictions have been unable, for various reasons, to provide the funds needed to take advantage of these advances. Thus it is that modern analytical forensic toxicologic services are mostly confined to large urban centers, with many of the less populated jurisdictions being limited to the capabilities of 25 years ago. The features of the advances are here for all to see, but the problem of making them available to citizens in all communities remains unsolved.

REFERENCES

1. Report of the President's Science Advisory Committee: The Handling of Toxicological Information. U.S. Government Printing Office, Washington, D.C., 1966.
2. Field, K. S., Lipskin, B. A., and Reich, M. A.: *A Survey of Educational Offerings in the Forensic Sciences.* vol. 1. National Institute of Law Enforcement and Criminal Justice, Washington, D.C., 1977.
3. Commission Rules, Regulations and Sanitary Code Pertinent to Clinical Laboratory Personnel and Operations. Article V, Title 5, *Laboratory Act of 1965,* State of New York.
4. Identical Memoranda, No. 1–4. Center for Disease Control, Atlanta, 1968–1972; Proficiency Testing, Toxicology, Drug Abuse Survey 1. Center for Disease Control, Atlanta, 1972; Blood-Alcohol Proficiency Test Programs. Interim Report No. DOT-TSC-NHTSA-74-5. Technical Information Service, Springfield, Va., 1975.
5. Inhorn, S. L. (ed.): *Quality Assurance Practices for Public Health Laboratories.* American Public Health Association, Washington, D.C., 1978.

CHAPTER 47

James C. Garriott is Chief Toxicologist at the Criminal Investigation Laboratory of the Southwestern Institute of Forensic Sciences at Dallas. He is also Assistant Professor of Forensic Science at the Southwestern Medical School of the University of Texas Southwestern Medical School at Dallas. A graduate of the University of Louisville and Indiana University Medical Center, Dr. Garriott is a member of the American Academy of Forensic Sciences, the American Chemical Society, the American Association for the Advancement of Science, and the International Society of Toxicology.

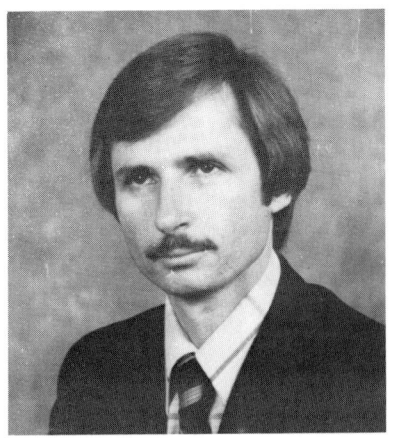

FORENSIC TOXICOLOGY: GENERAL CONSIDERATIONS

James C. Garriott, Ph.D.

The advancements in toxicology in the last ten years have been legion. Application of modern and highly refined instrumental capabilities to the field of forensic toxicology, as well as the advancement of knowledge about the effects of drugs and other toxic agents, their metabolism and distribution after both therapeutic and overdose administration, and under conditions of both tolerance and intolerance, have made us capable of very thorough toxicologic evaluation of autopsy and clinical specimens. This is, of course, dependent upon the cooperation of the submittor (who must supply the necessary specimens and adequate information) and individual laboratory expertise.

It is safe to state that virtually any case involving drug or common poison toxicity can be detected and evaluated if one has the proper resources available. In addition, it is feasible to determine whether an individual is taking adequate therapeutic doses of prescribed medication, is taking psychoactive drugs for purposes other than therapeutic, is a drug addict, or is abusing various nonmedicinal chemicals. No one can deny, however, that there remain some limitations to what can be done in even the most modern laboratory. These will be discussed separately.

The sources of submissions to the forensic toxicologist include primarily medical examiners (or other pathologists involved in the performance of autopsies for forensic purposes), law enforcement agencies and courts, drug addiction treatment agencies, and hospitals. The medical examiners or pathologists must determine the presence (or absence) of drugs or exogenous chemical substances for the proper assessment of the cause and manner of death in autopsy cases. The law enforcement agencies request the identification of confiscated substances to find out whether the individuals investigated have broken the law by illegal possession or sale of proscribed and controlled substances or have been operating a motor vehicle while intoxicated with alcohol or controlled substances. Hospitals often need to know the nature and quantity of toxic or drug substances ingested for the proper evaluation and treatment of overdose or poison victims, as well as blood concentrations of some drugs administered for therapeutic purposes, to determine proper individual dosage. Since the forensic laboratory is well equipped for these analyses, and some hospital intoxication cases may have some legal involvement, the forensic toxicologist often performs these "clinical" analyses.

The extensive use of toxic agents for pest control and exposure to industrial chemicals can lead to intoxications in workers or laymen exposed to these agents. The toxicologist is often called on to perform analyses on body specimens for detection of these pesticides, heavy metals, or any of a wide spectrum of toxic substances.

Litigation may occur in any of these types of cases as a result of criminal prosecution for improper use of these agents, or from civil matters involving insurance claims, or compensation sought for injuries suffered from exposure to toxic substances. Thus the toxicologist must be prepared to fulfill the total obligations his work may entail.

The first consideration should be to establish a chain of custody for all specimens submitted by law enforcement agencies or any cases deemed likely to involve legal proceedings. These items should be stored in locked compartments or under such conditions that the toxicologist can affirm that the specimen could not have been adulterated while under his purview. Perishable items or body tissues should, of course, be maintained under refrigeration or frozen to prevent deterioration of contents.

The analyses should be carried out with the utmost care and with the consideration that the analyst may have to testify under oath as to his results. This entails a thorough understanding of the methods used in the analysis, as well as the accurate identification and quantitation of the agents in question. It is usually essential that the identification made be confirmed by more than one type of analysis. Thus it is often desirable to use one or more procedures to "screen" for the presence of a large number of agents. This may involve the use of semispecific color or crystal tests, thin-layer chromatography, ultraviolet spectrophotometry, or gas chromatography. When these tests indicate positive results, a more specific analysis should be performed. Whether the procedures used involved wet chemistry manipulations, chromatography, or the highly sensitive and specific mass spectrometry, the toxicologist should know the limitations and capabilities of the procedure and should satisfy himself that the results he reports are accurate. He should never draw nonanalytical conclusions in his written reports. He may, however, offer his expert opinion on any of his results or on their interpretation to the extent of his expertise.

For example, he may have unequivocally established that a specimen contained cocaine and accurately quantitated this substance. He cannot, however, identify the substance as the dextrorotary isomer, the active form of the drug, unless he has performed additional optical rotation studies to determine this property.

As with any expert witness in the courts, he should always be prepared to refuse testimony when requested to enter areas outside of his professional expertise, or, if opinionated on the subject, to clearly state the extent of his qualifications in the particular area and qualify his answer as an opinion.

LABORATORY CONSIDERATIONS

Conventional Equipment and Methodology

The usual spectrum of instrumentation in today's toxicology laboratory includes various combinations of the following: thin-layer and/or paper chromatographic equipment, ultraviolet and visible spectrophotometry, infrared spectrophotometry, fluorescence spectrophotometry, atomic absorption spectrophotometry, emission spectrography, gas chromatography, and, increasingly, gas chromatography interfaced with a mass spectrometer, high-pressure liquid chromatography, and radioimmunoassay equipment.

For principles and general capabilities of each, the reader is referred to several published volumes dealing specifically with analytical toxicology.[1,2,3] Many laboratories performing drug detection assays utilize only thin-layer chromatographic techniques and ultraviolet and visible spectrophotometry, along with certain wet chemical procedures and color reagents or crystallography. Using these techniques alone, it is possible to identify the vast majority of drugs and toxic products that might be encountered in the evaluation of autopsy or clinical specimens, assuming adequate extraction and purification techniques and comparison of results with known standards. Most substances cannot be detected in blood specimens by these methods, however, because of the small quantities present, and most could not be detected in any biological specimens, excepting urine, in quantities present after therapeutic administration. Accurate quantitation cannot be accomplished by these techniques for most compounds. Exceptions to this are the barbiturates,[4] glutethimide[5] (as a decomposition product), propoxyphene[6] (as a derivative), salicylates, quinine, chlorpromazine, caffeine, diphenylhydantoin[7] (as a derivative), and a few others, for which specific procedures exist for accurate quantitation by ultraviolet spectrophotometry.

If these agents are present as single agents and other interfering substances are not present, adequate quantitation can be accomplished by ultraviolet spectrophotometry. Ultraviolet absorption spectra are not entirely specific since there are often several related compounds that have similar spectral absorbance patterns. Derivatization, such as is done with propoxyphene and diphenylhydantoin, increases the probability of specificity. With the barbiturate group, qualitative confirmation of the actual derivative involved must be accomplished by use of another separation technique, such as thin-layer chromatography. Table 47-1 lists those common compounds which have been identified in blood samples using ultraviolet spectrophotometry combined with thin-layer chromatography as a screening procedure and extracting blood at pH 6.0 with chloroform.

Thin-layer chromatography can be used to separate and identify many drug and toxic substances and can be advantageously utilized in conjunction with ultraviolet spectrophotometry. For example, the scan solution with its absorption characteristics can be re-extracted with an organic solvent and applied to a thin-layer chromatogram. This technique could serve to confirm positive findings by the ultraviolet technique or to identify the barbiturate derivative detected by ultraviolet spectrophotometry. Conversely, an extract from urine, for example, could be applied to the thin-layer plate in large quantity, the plate developed, and the "bands" eluted to be scanned in the spectrophotometer for more specific identifi-

TABLE 47-1. SUBSTANCES DETECTABLE IN BLOOD BY ULTRAVIOLET SPECTROPHOTOMETRY COMBINED WITH THIN-LAYER CHROMATOGRAPHY

Acidic Drugs

Acetaminophen	Ethamivan
Acetazolamide	Hydrochlorothiazide
Aminophylline	Phenols and cresols
Barbiturates	Phenylbutazone
Chlorothiazide	Salicylamide
Chlorpropamide	Salicylic acid*
Chlorzoxazone	Sulfadiazine
Coumadin	Sulfisoxazole
Diphenylhydantoin	Thiopental
Dramamine	Tolbutamide

Neutral and Weak Basic Drugs

Meprobamate†	Diazepam‡
Ethinamate†	Glutethimide
Carisoprodol†	Methaqualone
Caffeine	Phenacetin

Basic Drugs

Chlordiazepoxide	Nicotinamide
Chloroquine	Quinine and quinidine
Chlorpromazine‡	Thioridazine‡
Methapyrilene‡	

*Salicylates must be extracted at pH 2.
†Identified by thin-layer chromatographic analysis of the neutral extract; spray furfural; hydrochloric acid.
‡Detected by ultraviolet spectrophotometry in blood after overdose only.

cation. Some agents, such as carbamates, can be quantitated with reasonable accuracy by thin-layer chromatography, due to the sensitivity of the color development reaction with the mixture of furfural and hydrochloric acid.

In the modern toxicology laboratory, application of gas chromatography, spectrofluorimetry, and gas chromatography interfaced with mass spectrometry has extended our capabilities to the ability to identify and quantitate single-drug and toxic agents, as well as mixtures of many agents present in biological specimens after ingestion of either therapeutic or overdose quantities. Due to the increased specificity, greater sensitivity, and better separational capabilities over spectrophotometric or thin-layer techniques, as well as moderate cost, gas chromatography is regarded as the most useful tool for the identification of most drugs and toxic organic compounds. As can be seen in Table 47-2, a large number of drugs or toxic agents can be detected using gas chromatography, if one chooses the proper columns and temperature conditions for each group of substances. Agents listed in Groups I and II have all been detected in blood by gas chromatography, using 1-chlorobutane as the extracting solvent and flame ionization detection.[8] Suggested systems are given for each group of agents (see Table 47-3).

The identification features of gas chromatography consist of retention times of the agents in question, as indicated by the time required for the substance to pass through the column under a given set of conditions. This time factor is determined by the physical and chemical qualities of the column material, the temperature of the columns, the flow rate of the carrier gas, and the size and reactivity of the molecule of the substance being analyzed. The detection of the substance as it comes off the column

TABLE 47-2. DRUGS AND TOXIC AGENTS DETECTED BY GAS CHROMATOGRAPHY

Group I: Basic Drugs Detected in Blood by Gas Chromatography

Generic Name	Trade Name
Amitriptyline	Elavil
Benzphetamine	Didrex
Bromodiphenhydramine	Ambenyl
Brompheniramine	Dimetane
Chlorpheniramine	Multiple preparations
Cocaine	
Codeine	Multiple preparations
Cyclizine	Marezine
Demethyldiazepam	Clorazepate
Diethylpropion	Tenuate
Diphenhydramine	Benadryl
Desipramine	Norpramin
Diazepam	Valium
Doxepin	Sinequan
Flurazepam	Dalmane
Hydroxyzine	Atarax, Vistaril
Imipramine	Tofranil
Lidocaine	Xylocaine
Meperidine	Demerol
Mepivacaine	Carbocaine
Methadone	
Methyprylon	Noludar
Methapyrilene	Multiple preparations
Methaqualone	Quaalude
Methylphenidate	Ritalin
Nikethamide	Coramine
Nortriptyline	Aventyl
Orphenadrine	Norflex
Oxazepam	Serax
Oxycodone	Percodan
Pentazocine	Talwin
Phencyclidine	
Prilocaine	Citanest
Procaine	
Promethazine	Phenergan
Proparacaine	
Propoxyphene	Darvon
Propanolol	Inderol
Racemorphan	d-Dromoran
Trihexylphenidyl	Artane

Group II: Basic Drugs Detected by Gas Chromatography

Generic Name	Trade Name
Amphetamine	Dextro- or dl-amphetamine
Chlorphentermine	Pre-Sate
Clortermine	Voranil
Fenfluramine	Pondimin
Methamphetamine	Desoxyn
Mephentermine	Wyamine
Methoxyphenamine	
Nicotine (urine)	
Phendimetrazine	Plegine
Phenethylamine	Decomposition product
Phenmetrazine	Preludin
Propylhexedrine	Benzedrex inhaler

TABLE 47-2. *Continued*

Group III: Alcohols	
Methyl alcohol	n-propyl alcohol
Ethyl alcohol	Acetone
Isopropyl alcohol	

Group IV: Volatile Substances Detected by Gas Chromatography	
Methane	Ethyl acetate
Ethane	Diethyl ether
Propane	Carbon tetrachloride
Acetaldehyde	Benzene
Freon 12	Methyl ethyl ketone
Freon 11	Methylene chloride
Methanol	Ethylene dichloride
Ethanol	Trichloroethylene
Acetone	1,1,1-Trichloroethane
Isopropanol	Toluene
Chloroform	Paraldehyde
	Trichlorethanol

*See also Table 47-3.

by various types of detectors, some more sensitive for certain entities than others, can add to the specificity and sensitivity of the analysis. For example, the halogenated hydrocarbons, such as benzodiazepine tranquilizers, trichlorethanol, and chlorinated hydrocarbon pesticides, can be detected with much greater sensitivity with the electron capture detector than with the more conventional flame ionization detector.

It must be borne in mind, however, that the retention time is a nonspecific parameter for identification of unknown substances. One may only presume a substance is present when the retention time on a single column corresponds with that of the known compound. The specificity may be greatly improved by analysis on additional columns under different conditions. The use of other identification features, such as thin-layer chromatography, infrared spectrophotometry, and ultraviolet spectrophotometry, can be used in conjunction with gas chromatography to confirm the tentative identification. For forensic purposes, it is desirable to utilize at least two parameters for identification of unknown substances. Identification by certain instruments, such as mass spectrometry and infrared spectrophotometry, however, can usually stand alone.

The mass spectrometer is probably the most specific and most useful tool to confirm the identification of small quantities of unknown compounds as detected on the gas chromatograph. Thus a compound appearing as a peak on the gas chromatogram after extraction from a blood sample can usually be identified by obtaining the mass spectrum or fragmentation pattern, enabling one to confirm the molecular structure. Reference data are available for mass spectral identification of over 450 drugs and metabolites.[9] Since mass spectra can be obtained even with low nanogram quantities, it has been of great value for identifying drugs or metabolites when only trace quantities are present. Moreover, when numerous peaks and interfering substances are present as the result of putrefaction, mass spectrometry can enable one to "sort out the maze" and identify these peaks as drugs, metabolites, or putrefactive products.

Specimens

Although certain specimens should always be available for toxicologic studies, the final choice of specimens to be submitted to the toxicology

TABLE 47-3. GAS CHROMATOGRAPHIC CONDITIONS

Group I and II Drugs

Columns: 6 ft × 2 mm i.d. packed with
a. 3% OV-1 on 80/100 mesh Chromosorb, W, A/W DMCS
b. 3% OV-17 on 80/100 mesh Chromosorb W A/W DMCS
c. 5% Apiezon L, 5% KOH on 80/100 mesh Chromosorb G, A/W, DMCS
d. 2.5% SE-30 on 80/100 mesh Chromosorb, G, A/W DMCS (Column a could be substituted for this column.)

Operating Conditions:
Gas Flow Rates
  Nitrogen (carrier gas): 30 ml/min
  Hydrogen: 30 ml/min
  Air: 240 ml/min
Column Temperature
  Columns a and b: Programmed at 8° min, from 174° to 270°; final temperature held for 8 min.
  Column c: Programmed at 8° min from 110° to 190°; initial temperature held for 2 min, and final temperature held for 4 min.
  Column d: Programmed at 8° min, from 130° to 190°; initial and final temperature held for 4 min.

Group III Drugs

Column: 6 ft × 2 mm i.d.
e. Porapak Q 80/100 mesh, detector F.I.D.

Operating Conditions:
Gas Flow Rates
  Nitrogen (carrier gas): 20 psi
  Hydrogen: 16 psi
  Air: 6 psi
Column Temperature
  150°C

Group IV Drugs

Columns: 3 ft × 2 mm i.d. packed with
f. Porapak Q 80/100 mesh, detector F.I.D.
g. 15% FFAP on 60/80 mesh Chromosorb W A/W, detector—electron capture

Operating Conditions:
Gas Flow Rates
  Nitrogen (carrier gas): 20 psi
  Hydrogen: 10 psi
  Air: 6 psi
Column Temperature:
  Column f: 150°C
  Column g: 125°C

---

laboratory is dependent upon the capabilities and routine procedures in use by the laboratory. Table 47-4 lists types and suggested quantities of specimens to save. It is futile and impractical to request that all of these specimens be saved in each case requiring toxicologic testing. Many cases can be adequately evaluated merely by blood testing, provided that the laboratory uses techniques which can recover and quantitate drugs in blood in quantities to be expected after therapeutic dosage. It is dangerous to rely on this specimen entirely, however, no matter what the laboratory's capabilities. A trace quantity of a substance detected in blood cannot usually be confirmed. The minimum of specimens to be saved for an adequate toxicology workup include the following: blood, liver, stomach content, bile, and urine when available.

The blood can be analyzed for almost all toxic and therapeutic substances, so at least 30 ml should be available. The concentrations of drugs

TABLE 47-4. SUGGESTED AUTOPSY SPECIMENS AND QUANTITIES TO BE SUBMITTED FOR TOXICOLOGIC EXAMINATION

Specimen	Minimum Amounts	Indications
Bile	All available	Valuable in narcotic poisonings
Blood	As much as possible 20–30 ml	For all types of determinations
Brain	100 gm	Desirable for Flurazepam (Dalmane) Diazepam (Valium)
Fat	200 gm	For insecticides and other fat-soluble drugs (Thiopental)
Hair	About 0.5 gm	Chronic (not acute) arsenic poisoning
Fingernail clippings or whole nails	As much as possible.	Chronic arsenic poisoning
Intestinal contents	30 gm	In instances in which poison presumably was taken orally.
Kidney	1	For all types of poisoning, especially heavy metals, narcotics
Liver	200 gm	For all types of poisoning, especially heavy metals, alkaloids
Lung	1	For inhaled poisons, Propoxyphene (Darvon), synthetic narcotics
Muscle	200 gm	In instances in which internal organs are badly putrefied
Spinal fluid	All available	All types of poisonings when blood is not available
Stomach contents	All available	In instances in which poison presumably was taken orally
Urine	All available	Valuable in nearly all types of poisonings
Vitreous humor	From both eyes (about 5 ml)	Most drugs; alcohol

or toxic substances in blood are the most meaningful of those in any of the specimens, and, consequently, efforts should be made to quantitate these substances. It may be more practical to use urine or stomach contents to qualitatively identify or confirm these substances, but blood concentrations should then be obtained.

The liver concentrates most drugs and toxic substances, and it is here that they are metabolized. In an overdose, very high concentrations of substances often may be detected in the liver. For example, propoxyphene may be present in liver at a concentration of 40 or more times than in blood after an acute overdose.

The stomach content is of primary value for estimating the quantity ingested in acute overdoses, and qualitatively in identifying substances which have been recently ingested. The equivalent of ten doses of pentobarbital remaining in the stomach, plus a high blood concentration of this drug, is certainly good evidence for drug ingestion with suicidal intent, whereas a very low concentration in the stomach content with a minimally toxic blood concentration may indicate accidental overdosage, especially when coupled with a drug abuse history.

Some drugs and toxic agents are concentrated in the bile. Of great importance toxicologically is the storage of morphine and other opiate alkaloids in bile prior to excretion. In an individual using opiates chronically, large concentrations may be detected. Up to 50 $\mu g/ml$ or more of morphine may be present in a heroin addict, while 220 $\mu g/ml$ has been detected after a morphine overdose in a child.[10] It should be noted, however, that the concentration in bile is of no value in interpreting toxicity, since it represents metabolized drug that may have been taken up to several days prior to death.

Brain tissue is frequently saved for toxicologic testing, presumably because of the known pharmacologic activities of toxic agents at this site. In fact, however, brain tissue does not accumulate most drugs, and the concentrations usually are found to be less than those present in blood. Exceptions are certain lipophilic agents such as the benzodiazepines, benzene and derivatives, and cocaine, which accumulates in the brain to a concentration slightly higher than that found in blood. The concentrations found in blood, however, may be used more reliably to assess pharmacologic activity. After many reports of distribution studies of drugs including this organ, it is doubtful that any useful information can be gained from analysis of this specimen.

Adipose tissue may be of value in special types of cases. Certain drugs and pesticides accumulate in adipose and may be detected where absent or in low quantities in other specimens. Over 90 percent of a dose of thiopental is accumulated in the fat within 3 hours.[11] Chlorinated hydrocarbons and other pesticides also accumulate in fat. For chronic exposure to lipophilic agents, fat tissue should, therefore, be analyzed.

Metals which combine with sulfhydryl groups accumulate in skin, hair, and nails, and relatively high concentrations of arsenic can be found in hair after arsenic intoxication. What is often overlooked, however, is that arsenic is also present in clearly abnormal concentrations in whole blood and urine in clinical circumstances, or in liver or kidney and blood at autopsy, when the victim has been exposed to toxic quantities of arsenic. The hair and nails retain their arsenic until cut, and, therefore, prior exposure to arsenic can be affirmed by analyzing several sections of hair. The time factor could conceivably go back for many months, depending on the length of the individual's hair. The history of exposure to arsenic over this period of time could thereby be elicited.

Small intestinal contents can be analyzed if no stomach contents are present, or to assist in evaluation of the estimated dosage taken. In a few cases involving gastrectomy or partial gastrectomy, the intestinal contents have yielded large quantities of drugs after overdose, when little or none was present in the stomach. Lung tissue accumulates lipophilic drugs and inhaled substances.

Agents such as propoxyphene are found in very large quantity in lung tissue after overdose, and drugs taken by injection accumulate rapidly in the lung. Other than the large quantity sometimes present, no particular advantage is apparent for analyzing this specimen. Muscle tissue may be analyzed in place of internal organs when the latter are badly putrefied. Drug concentrations here would be expected to be low, however, and found concentrations would be difficult to evaluate for lack of data.

Spinal fluid is probably equivalent to blood for evaluation of many drugs. Unfortunately, it is seldom available for toxicologic analysis, and, consequently, little is known about drug levels to be expected in this specimen after therapeutic administration or overdose.

Urine is a convenient specimen to analyze for drugs or toxic substances in the living patient as a urine specimen of sufficient volume can usually be obtained on request or by catheterization. In the autopsied individual, however, its availability is unpredictable; and urine may or may not be present in the bladder, depending upon circumstances of death. When available, drugs can usually be easily detected in this specimen. Protein binding factors are not in effect, making extraction of drugs simpler than in other body specimens, and drugs and other toxic agents are often concentrated in urine. The disadvantages and limitations, however, are several. Some drugs (e.g., morphine) must be hydrolyzed for complete recovery from urine. The concentration of agents found in urine is usually of no significance in evaluating the quantity ingested or the toxicity, since urinary concentration factors sometimes lead to large quantities, even after therapeutic administration. Some drugs are present only as metabolites in urine, owing to extensive body metabolism and low water solubility. Virtually no diazepam is detectable in urine, even after overdose. Cocaine is excreted unchanged only to the extent of 1 to 9 percent, depending on pH, with the remainder being excreted as the metabolite benzoylecgonine[12] (see Table 47-5). In drug addicts or individuals who are drug-tolerant, the ratio of the drug metabolite excreted to that of the unchanged drug may be much greater than in a nontolerant individual. This has been observed with methadone and propoxyphene.[18,19]

The eye fluid, "vitreous humor," has undergone recent study in toxicologic investigation of drug overdoses. It has been found that most drugs pass through the eye membrane and may be found in varying concentrations in vitreous humor. Indeed, some agents such as alcohols, paraldehyde, ethchlorvynol, and barbiturates may be found in greater concentrations in vitreous than in blood at equilibrium (completion of distribution).[20,21] It may be of value to estimate the time between drug administration and death by comparing the concentration in vitreous humor with that in blood. In cases where blood is not available, such as in exsanguination, it may be of great value in estimating the blood concentration of the agent in question.

Thus there are a variety of specimens that can be used for toxicologic analyses. Those intended for routine and special circumstances should be chosen on the basis of laboratory capabilities and resources. If the workload is such that time cannot be spent to extract body organs and obtain distribution on certain cases, it serves little purpose to save all the specimens listed in Table 47-4. If laboratory personnel are interested in further knowledge of drug methodology and distribution, most of these specimens must be available.

It should always be remembered in forensic toxicology, however, that after the body is autopsied and released, it is, for all practical purposes, too late to obtain additional specimens, and questions may forever remain unanswered. How many times does a routine blood screen for drugs in a "signout" of death from natural causes turn up a potentially lethal concentration of a drug? On more than one occasion this has happened to the complete astonishment of the pathologist and investigators. When little or no metabolite is detected, the questions that remain unanswered in-

TABLE 47-5. EXCRETION OF DRUGS IN URINE (PERCENT OF DOSE)

Drug	Unchanged	Metabolites	References
Morphine	1	60	13
Demerol	5	57	13
Pentobarbital	1	32	13
Chloral hydrate	0	87	13
Meprobamate	12	50	13
Chlordiazepoxide	1	49	13
Diazepam	0	71	15
Diphenylhydantoin	0	64	12
Pentothal	0.3	10–25	10
Propoxyphene	3	20	14
Amphetamines	30	60	16
Chlorpromazine	1	80	17

clude the following: Could the blood specimen accidentally have been contaminated by stomach contents? Could diffusion have occurred from the stomach? Could there have been a mix-up in blood specimens? In cases where no other specimens were saved and questions concerning drug use were turned up through subsequent information, these must remain unanswered.

It is, therefore, recommended that a minimum of three specimens (blood, liver, and gastric content) be saved on all autopsied cases under medicolegal investigation, even though it may not be necessary to analyze each specimen. Vitreous humor or urine may sometimes be substituted for the latter two, or collected for supplemental analysis.

Handling and Storage of Specimens

Ideally, the medical examiner or his agent should deliver the specimen to the toxicology laboratory with the pertinent information supplied on a transmittal form. Specimens from other agencies for forensic purposes should be delivered in a manner such that a chain of custody can be established for court purposes, if necessary. This can be accomplished by use of a form or letter with a brief description of specimens and signatures of transmitting personnel. If delays are involved, tissue should be frozen and fluids refrigerated at about 4°C. Upon receipt by the laboratory, the date received, types and quantities of each specimen, and the person receiving the specimens are recorded. Again, all tissue samples should be maintained in a frozen state and liquids refrigerated until analyzed and subsequently until destroyed.

Presuming early analysis and reporting to the submittor, specimens should be retained for a minimum of 6 months. At the end of that period of time, a listing of cases 6 months old may be circulated to the submittors and permission sought to discard them. It should be remembered that, due to frequent delays in our legal proceedings, some cases may be heard in court several years hence, and at that time additional questions concerning toxicologic results may require further analyses. These possibilities should be anticipated for those special cases and these specimens retained until the case in question is closed.

Toxicology Screening

One of the limitations or "pitfalls" of toxicology is the use of proper methodology and "screens" for the agents sought. It should be understood at the outset that there is no single screen that can detect all or even a majority of toxic agents. Thus we must define our parameters and know what we can detect and how much or how little when we perform a given procedure. A negative result after a thin-layer screen on a urine sample from an autopsy case does not mean that no toxic agent was present. In order to perform a valid toxicologic interpretation of an autopsy case involving potential drug abuse, for example, we must look for acidic, basic, and neutral drugs in blood and/or tissues; opiate narcotics, by specific techniques; alcohols; other volatile substances; and, if indicated, certain specific toxic agents such as cyanide or toxic metals. To do this one must employ several analytical approaches. Tables 47-1 and 47-2 divide into analytical categories most of the drug and chemical agents encountered in biological specimens. Table 47-1 lists those agents which have sufficient absorbance in ultraviolet light to be measured in blood by spectrophotometry, after extraction with chloroform at pH 6, and partitioning into acidic, basic, and neutral fractions. Acidic drugs were removed from chloroform with 0.45 N NaOH, basic drugs with 0.2 N H_2SO_4, and the neutral and weak basic drugs remain in the chloroform phase. This does not include a few, such as propoxyphene, which can be measured directly by ultraviolet spectrophotometry, but must be derivatized prior to analysis.[6] Of this group, meprobamate does not have sufficient ultraviolet absorbance for detection, but can be detected in a chloroform residue of the neutral phase by its characteristic reaction with furfural-hydrochloric acid, and glutethimide is detectable by a specific procedure. Details of an ultraviolet screening procedure for this group of drugs have been described by Jatlow.[22] Salicylic acid cannot be detected in low quantities unless the blood is adjusted to a pH of 2.0 prior to extraction. Drugs listed in Table 47-2 are detectable in therapeutic concentrations in blood when measured by gas chromatography. This entire list consists of substances identified in blood after extraction with 1-chlorobutane. Most of the compounds in this list do not have sufficient absorbance in ultraviolet light to be detected by that technique in the concentrations normally found in biological specimens. The gas chromatographic conditions used are specified in Table 47-3.

Group III (Table 47-2) consists of the lower alcohols. Since ethyl alcohol is present in varying concentrations in a very large percentage of drug deaths and deaths from a variety of other causes, a procedure to screen for this group should be utilized in any toxicologic evaluation of an autopsy case, as well as in most clinical cases and in all cases that involve driving under the influence. Many procedures are published for ethyl alcohol, including headspace and direct injection gas chromatography, enzyme-spectrophotometric assays, and oxidation techniques.[23,24] For medicolegal purposes, the most desirable is gas chromatography in which specificity can be ascertained.

Group IV (Table 47-2) consists of other volatile components which can be detected most conveniently by a blood headspace injection on the gas chromatograph. For some of the halogenated compounds (trichlorethanol and Fluothane) it is necessary to use other columns and the electron-capture detector (see Table 47-3).

Table 47-6 consists of a group of drugs not detected well by either ultraviolet spectrophotometry or gas chromatography, unless certain preparatory procedures are followed. They are unique in that they are present to a large degree in urine, bile, or tissue as a conjugate with glucuronic acid. Therefore, a preliminary hydrolysis step must be carried out to be able to extract these quantitatively. Analysis can then be accomplished by thin-layer chromatography or gas chromatography. A scheme for detection of this group of drugs by thin-layer chromatography has been presented by Parker and Hine.[25]

Utilization of screens to detect the agents described in Table 47-2 will probably satisfy the requirements for 98 percent of the autopsy cases involving death from toxicologic circumstances. Those agents not included

TABLE 47-6. NARCOTICS

Morphine	Oxycodone (Percodan)
Codeine	Dihydromorphine
Nalorphine	Dihydrocodeinone
Hydromorphone (Dilaudid)	

in the groups above can usually be evaluated by the use of specific procedures for the agent in question.

The question of heavy metals can usually be resolved by a Reinsch test[26] which will detect arsenic or mercury when present in toxic quantity, or by atomic absorption assay for the specific method in question. It is rare that these agents are involved as a cause of death without specific history or pathologic indications of their presence. Abnormal exposure to metals, however, is an increasingly frequent phenomenon in our industrialized society, and, in some areas, a more comprehensive screening for metals may be desirable. The emission spectrograph and energy-dispersive x-ray are instruments capable of detecting a wide spectrum of metals in biological samples.

Cholinesterase-inhibiting agents, such as organic phosphates, are indicated, when present, by performing a cholinesterase activity test on serum or blood. If this is abnormal, specific testing by gas chromatography for organic phosphate or carbamate pesticides should be carried out. More exotic but important poisons, such as cyanide, fluoride, or phosphorus, must be assayed for specifically in cases suspected of these types of poisoning. Carbon monoxide exposure is usually detected by measurement of the carboxyhemoglobin content of the blood, although carbon monoxide can be measured directly by gas chromatography. Spectrophotometric techniques are reliant on the differential spectrum between oxyhemoglobin, carboxyhemoglobin, and reduced oxyhemoglobin. More rapid measurement can be accomplished by use of the carboximeter.[27]

Incidence of Agents Detected in Chemical-Involved Deaths

A recent year's tally of drug and chemical deaths may serve to illustrate the incidence of drugs detected in autopsy cases, as well as the most frequent sources of these deaths (see Table 47-7). In this jurisdiction the first five leading agents are consistent from one year to the next in single-agent-caused deaths. These include carbon monoxide, narcotics, barbiturates, propoxyphene, and ethyl alcohol. Mixed drug intoxications are the most common source of chemical deaths in this jurisdiction. Thus one must be prepared to perform as comprehensive a drug screen as possible to detect the variety of agents that may be involved and to evaluate the concentrations found as to their relative pharmacologic and toxicologic actions on the body.

Limitations in Toxicologic Analyses

A few compounds present analytical problems not yet solved in most laboratories. These consist of drugs which are therapeutically effective and even toxic in very low concentrations; those which may be rapidly metabolized to polar metabolites, making extraction difficult; and a host of biological toxins and venoms which may be proteinaceous in nature and cannot be separated from body tissues. One answer to the detection of these compounds is the use of immunoassay procedures. For example, digoxin and other digitalis glycosides, therapeutically effective at blood concentrations of 2.0 to 4.0 ng/ml, are below detection limits for gas chromatography. They can, however, be detected and reliably quantitated by radioimmunoassay.

The nonmedicinal but popular street drugs, lysergic acid diethylamide and cannabis components, also cannot be detected in biological speci-

TABLE 47-7. DRUG AND CHEMICAL DEATHS—1976*

CO (accident)	19
CO (suicide)	11
Ethanol	16
Narcotics (heroin)	4
Heroin and other drugs	10
Morphine and codeine	1
Propoxyphene	7
Barbiturates	4
Gases (propane, 2; methane, 1)	3
Amitriptyline	2
Doxepin	2
Imipramine	2
Salicylate	2
Arsenic	1
Meprobamate	1
Paraldehyde	1
Propylhexedrine	1
Quinidine	1
Strychnine	1
Volatiles	
Freons 11 and 12	1
Trichlorethanol and trichlorethylene	1
Spray paint	1
Miscellaneous agents†	4
Mixed drug intoxications	21
Total	117

Incidence of Drugs Involved in Mixed Drug Intoxications

Diazepam	7
Propoxyphene	6
Amitriptyline	4
Codeine	4
Ethanol	4
Amobarbital and secobarbital	3
Meperidine	3
Methaqualone	3
Phenobarbital	3
Chlordiazepoxide	2
Flurazepam	2
Glutethimide	2
Methapyrilene	2
Pentazocine	2
Pentobarbital	2
Thiopental	2
Thioridazine	2
Trichlorethanol	2
Salicylate	2
Butalbital	1
Dihydrocodeinone	1
Dilaudid	1
Diphenhydramine	1
Doxepin	1
Ethchlorvynol	1
Imipramine	1
Hydroxyzine	1
Meprobamate	1
Phenyltoloxamine	1

* Data courtesy of Dallas County Medical Examiner's Office.
† These included one instance each of ingestion of cleaning fluid containing benzalkonium chloride, and ethyldimethyl benzylammonium chloride, ingestion of colchicine, and one instance of injection of magnesium sulfate.

mens by conventional methodology. However, radioimmunoassay procedures now exist which permit detection of these agents in biological specimens. On a practical level, however, it must be recognized that the commercially available kits for these assays are expensive and have a limited effective life. Thus, if one is requested to run an LSD assay only rarely, the expense per test might be prohibitive.

Diphenoxylate is a commonly used antidiarrheal medication having narcotic-like properties. Effective doses are in the range of 2 mg, and the parent drug rapidly breaks down into polar metabolites.[28] No adequate method for detecting this compound in biological specimens is yet available.

Disulfiram is another compound which is extremely difficult to document in biological specimens. A published procedure relying on a color reaction may be adequate for tentative identification in urine, but interferences prevent its use for other specimens.[29] A technique using cathode ray polarography has been reported, but this instrument is not readily available to the toxicologist.[30] Considering the broad spectrum of potentially toxic agents including biological venoms and toxins, as well as quaternary bases which can be potent paralytic agents, there are many toxic agents which even the most advanced toxicology laboratory is not equipped to detect in biological specimens. Thus, although circumstances in which these may occur are probably rare, this must be recognized as a deficiency in the usual "complete" toxicology workings of an autopsy.

INTERPRETATION OF TOXICOLOGIC RESULTS

Inherent Factors

The interpretation of positive toxicologic findings and quantities must rely on certain pre-existing factors.

TOLERANCE

Perhaps the most important consideration in evaluation of drug levels in biological specimens is the degree of drug tolerance of the individual. This has become very evident in recent years as more and more data are accumulated on individuals taking drugs regularly as opposed to those who don't. Cross-tolerance among certain groups of drugs may occur, so that an alcoholic, for example, can tolerate larger quantities of most drugs than can a nonalcoholic. Thus ethanol and various barbiturates, when consumed habitually, stimulate their own metabolism and that of various drugs in man. In addition, the neurologic tolerance of individuals who take alcohol or depressant drugs regularly is enhanced so that they are able to ingest much larger doses of drugs and achieve higher blood concentrations than those who are nontolerant. This fact is exemplified in a study of some individuals who were arrested for driving under the influence of drugs or were killed in motor vehicle crashes (see Table 47-8).[31,32] Each of these cases had high or potentially lethal concentrations or combinations of drugs as determined by drug analysis on blood samples. They are obviously individuals with a high degree of drug tolerance, as these drug concentrations are often associated with coma or death. Likewise, blood concentrations of methadone are usually in the same range for fatalities from overdose as the "therapeutic" range for those on methadone treatment.[33] Doses up to 120 mg per day may be taken by tolerant

TABLE 47-8. CASES OF DRIVING UNDER THE INFLUENCE OF DRUGS

Case	Age/Race/Sex	Drugs	Blood Concentrations	Behavior and Additional Information
1	36 w/m	Propoxyphene Pentazocine Amitriptyline	2.8 µg/ml 2.3 µg/ml 1.2 µg/ml	Fatality in motor vehicle accident
2	43 w/m	Meprobamate	43 µg/ml	Mental confusion; slow, erratic driving; faulty judgment
3	29 w/m	Pentobarbital	8.0 µg/ml	Erratic driving; multiple accidents; lack of responsible action
4	24 b/m	Pentobarbital	12.6 µg/ml	Methadone patient; bad perception; vehicle accident; excited
5	18 w/m	Secobarbital	10.5 µg/ml	Vehicle accident; disoriented
6	21 w/m	Chlordiazepoxide	26.3 µg/ml	Vehicle accident; uncoordinated; mental confusion
7	17 w/m	Alcohol Amobarbital and secobarbital	100 mg/100 ml 12.9 µg/ml	Vehicle accident; erratic driving; mental confusion; poor coordination
8	42 w/m	Chlordiazepoxide Secobarbital	11.7 µg/ml 15.6 µg/ml	Very erratic driving; reduced sensory perception; reduced coordination
9	23 b/m	Methaqualone Amobarbital and secobarbital	1.4 µg/ml 11.2 µg/ml	Vehicle accident; incoherent; resisted arrest
10	22 w/m	Alcohol Methaqualone Pentobarbital Amobarbital and secobarbital	60 mg/100 ml 0.9 µg/ml 15.4 µg/ml Trace (1.0 µg/ml)	Driving 70 mph in 30-mph zone; erratic driving; impaired perception; possible marijuana use; needle tracks on arm; uncooperative

individuals or drug addicts, whereas 40 mg or less may be a lethal dose in a nontolerant individual.

SYNERGISM

Another important factor in interpretation of individual drug levels is the synergistic interactions among drugs. This effect may be defined as the combined action of several drugs exerting a greater effect than the sum of the drug actions if present separately. This may result from several factors. Chief among these is the inhibition of metabolism of one by the other as a result of competition for metabolizing enzymes. This results in higher blood levels and longer half-lives, thus enhancing and prolonging the effect of the drug. Another effect elicited by alcohol and possibly other agents is an improved absorption of one drug by another. Thus blood levels of diazepam were nearly double in subjects 1 hour after dosing when the drug was taken in combination with 1 ounce of 100-proof alcohol.[34] Often, in drug intoxication deaths, several drugs may be detected in concentrations which, alone, may represent therapeutic quantities. In combination and in circumstances of low drug tolerance, however, they may be lethal.

CONDITION OF THE INDIVIDUAL

The pathologic circumstances or state of health of the individual, as well as age and body size, must also be taken into consideration. A child under

2 years of age has not yet fully developed the drug-metabolizing enzymes of the liver and does not yet have an effective blood brain barrier. He is thus much more susceptible to the effects of most drugs. An older individual with compromised cardiovascular system or with reduced lung capacity because of pulmonary disease may be much more susceptible to toxic effects of drugs which depress the respiratory centers.

INHERENT TOXICITY OR POTENCY OF DRUG IN QUESTION

The toxicity of the found drugs must always be taken into consideration. The "therapeutic index," or the ratio of the toxic to the effective dose of a drug, indicates the relative toxicity of these drugs. Thus some may be ingested in doses many times that of the therapeutic dosage and never cause a lethal reaction. With others, such as propoxyphene, however, as few as eight or ten therapeutic doses (65 mg) may be lethal.

Therapeutic and Toxic Concentrations of Drugs and Poisons in Blood

The blood concentrations following in Table 47-9 may be used as guidelines in assessing the found values, but each drug and each individual case must be considered separately. The maximum therapeutic concentrations are those to be expected after ingestion of the "oral dose" given, or after the highest expected doses to be taken for therapeutic purposes. For carbon monoxide, toxic metals, and other nontherapeutic poisons, maximum "nontoxic" exposure concentration in blood is given when known. A drug overdose can usually be evaluated by determining the relationship of the found concentration to the therapeutic range of concentrations; however, the toxicity of the individual drug will determine its significance. For example, diazepam and chlordiazepoxide are drugs prescribed and used as frequently as barbiturates and propoxyphene. Serious overdoses from the former drugs, however, are not common. Even after ingestion of large quantities of diazepam or chloridazepoxide, death from overdose of these agents alone is extremely rare, whereas propoxyphene and the barbiturate group are the leading cause of drug deaths in many localities. For these "rarely lethal" agents, the lethal concentrations, if given, are speculative but based on values obtained after severe clinical overdoses.

For some agents, no data were available to assess values for lethal concentrations. For those which act as depressants, the blood concentration at the induction of coma is regarded as potentially lethal, since difficulties such as obstructed respiration can lead to death in comatose individuals. The coma-producing blood concentration and lethal concentration will, of course, be higher in the addict or regular drug user.

Stability of Toxic Substances in Blood or Other Biological Specimens: Artefactual Circumstances

Another factor which one must consider in interpreting toxicologic results is the validity of the test result. The following factors may need to be considered, depending on the agent in question:

1. *Extraction efficiency.* Does the extraction procedure recover all or most of the agent present, and have recovery experiments been

TABLE 47-9. THERAPEUTIC AND TOXIC CONCENTRATIONS OF COMMON DRUGS AND POISONS*

	Oral Dose (mg)	Maximum Therapeutic Concentrations in Blood ($\mu g/ml$)†	Approximate Lethal Concentration in Blood ($\mu g/ml$)
Acetaminophen	325–2600	30.0	300.0
Aminophylline	500	6.0–12.0	50.0
Amitriptyline	50 t.i.d.	0.08	1.5–2.0
Amphetamine	5–30	0.02–0.10	10.0
Arsenic	"Normal"	0.07	0.70
Barbiturates			
Slow-acting (Phenobarbital)	600	25.0	75.0
Rapid-acting (Secobarbital)	100–200	2.0–4.0	10.0
Intermediate-acting (Amobarbital)	600	4.0–8.7	30.0
Pentothal	Peak anesthetic	30.0–50.0	—
Boron	"Normal"	0.8	40.0
Bromides	"Normal"	50.0	1000.0
Caffeine	300	5.0	150.0
Carbamazepine	5–20 mg/kg/day	1.4–12.0	—
Carbon monoxide	"Normal" smoker	7% carboxyhemoglobin saturation (maximum 13%)	50% carboxyhemoglobin saturation
Carisoprodol	350 t.i.d.	1.0–5.0	30.0
Chloral hydrate	1000	10.0‡	100.0‡
Chlordiazepoxide	150/day	10.0 1.0–2.0	30.0
Chlorpromazine	1000/day	1.0	5.0
Chloroquine	300	1.5	—
Chlorzoxazone	1000	10.0–20.0	—
Cocaine	1.5 mg/kg (intranasal)	0.3	7.0
Codeine	15	0.03	5.0
Cyanide	—	—	5.0
Diazepam	40/day	1.0	20.0
Digoxin	0.25/day	0.7–2.0 ng/ml	10 ng/ml
Digitoxin	0.20/day	10.5–30 ng/ml	34 ng/ml
Diphenylhydantoin	600	10.0–20.0	50.0–100.0
Diphenhydramine	400	1.0	10.0
Doxepin	75–150/day	0.3	7.0
Ephedrine	45 mg/day	0.1	—
Ethanol	1 oz. (2 oz whiskey or 2 bottles beer)	50.0 mg/100 ml	400.0 mg/100 ml
Ethchlorvynol	200 1000	2.0 14.0	100.0
Ethinamate	1000	5.9	—
Fluoride	10	0.4	2.6
Flurazepam	90/day	0.01	2.0
Glutethimide	1000	7.5	20.0
Halothane	1% anesthetic gas	150.0	—
Hexachlorophene	None	None	10.0
Hydrocodone	10	0.02	0.2
Hydroxyzine	75–400/day	—	6.0
Imipramine	300/day	0.6	2.0
Isopropanol	—	—	150 mg/dl
Ketamine	175 mg (IV)	1.0	—
Lead	Normal max.	0.6	1.0
Lidocaine	50–100 (IV)	2.0–10.0	50.0
Lorazepam	2	0.02	—
Meperidine	100 (IM)	1.1	5.0
Meprobamate	400 1200	5.0 20.0	100.0
Mercury	Normal max.	0.02	3.00

TABLE 47-9. *Continued*

	Oral Dose (mg)	Maximum Therapeutic Concentrations in Blood ($\mu g/dl$)†	Approximate Lethal Concentrations in Blood ($\mu g/dl$)
Methadone	(Tolerant) 40–120 (Nontolerant) 10	0.01	0.1–1.0
Methamphetamine	5–10	0.04	1.0
Methanol	—	—	80.00 mg/100 ml
Methapyrilene	25	—	12.0
Methaqualone	500	5.0	20.0
Methylphenidate	20	0.04	—
Methyprylon	300	10.0	50.0
Morphine	10 (IV)	0.08	0.5
Nicotine	"Normal" smoker	0.30	5.0
Orphenadrine	60	—	4.0
Paraldehyde	10 ml (IM)	77.0	500.0
Pentazocine	50	0.5	3.0
	45 (IM)	0.15–0.30	
	24 (IV)	0.15–0.30	
Phencyclidine	—	—	0.5
Phenylbutazone	400/day	50.0–150.0	—
Primidone	250–1500/day	2.0–19.0	50.0
Procainamide	1000–4000/day	4.0–8.0	12.0
Propoxyphene	130	0.12	2.0
Propoxyphene (maintenance)	800	1.00	2.0
Propranolol	80	0.03–0.020	10.0
Propylhexedrine	By inhalation	0.01	1.0 (IV)
Quinidine	600	3.0–6.0	—
Quinine	1000	2.0	10.0
Salicylate	1000	100.0	500.0
Strychnine	—	—	2.0
Theophylline	500	6.0–12.0	—
Thioridazine	50–800/day	2.3	5.0
Tolbutamide	1000–2000	50.0–100.0	640.0

*Adapted from Baselt, R. C., Wright, J. A., and Cravey, R. H.: A Compendium of Therapeutic and Toxic Concentrations of Toxicologically Significant Drugs in Human Biofluids, *J. Anal. Toxicol.* 1:81, 1977; Garriott, J. C., personal observations; McBay, A. J. (Office of the Medical Examiner, Chapel Hill, N.C.), personal communication; and Registry of Human Toxicology, Data on Fatal Cases, 1969–1976. Data compiled by the Toxicology Section of the American Academy of Forensic Sciences.
†To Convert to mg/dl (mg %), divide concentration in $\mu g/ml$ by ten. Thus, 20 mg/ml = 2 mg/dl.
‡Trichloroethanol.

carried out? Many drugs are protein-bound, and selective pH extraction or hydrolysis may be necessary for good recovery.

2. *Has there been deterioration in the sample?* Certain drugs deteriorate in whole blood. An example of this is shown in Table 47-10. Chlordiazepoxide deteriorated to about one-sixth of its original concentration in a whole blood sample kept under refrigeration (at 3° C) for 18 days. In 4 days, it had deteriorated to one-half of its original concentration. The concentration in the serum sample, on the other hand, remained unchanged. Observations with ten other basic drugs after adding them to whole blood, maintaining under refrigeration and analysis at 7, 30, and 120 days, however, indicated that they were relatively stable (see Table 47-11).
3. *Putrefactive changes.* The effect of various stages of putrefaction on drug concentrations in autopsy specimens is largely unknown. Drug concentrations, when found in decomposing bodies, cannot

TABLE 47-10. CHLORDIAZEPOXIDE IN BLOOD AFTER A CASE OF OVERDOSE*

Day	Chlordiazepoxide Concentration ($\mu g/ml$)		
	0	5	19
Whole blood	—	9.6	3.3
Serum	2.09†	—	21.7

*A 42-year-old man was admitted to the hospital with an overdose of drugs. The emergency toxicology laboratory detected 20.9 $\mu g/ml$ of chlordiazepoxide in a serum sample taken on admission. The blood samples were taken at autopsy the following day, then retained for analysis at the specified interval.
†Ethyl alcohol concentration: 220 mg/100ml.

be compared with those present at the time of death, and it may only be surmised that a certain loss had occurred as a result of bacterial action. Many are of the impression that toxicologic studies on putrefied bodies are futile. It is certainly true that the decomposing proteins and fats and their products complicate the picture extensively for the toxicologist. However, it may be untrue that many drugs readily decompose along with the body tissues. Some drugs may be stable even after complete skeletonization of the body. Bösche reports isolation of glutethimide and amobarbital in the soil underneath the skeleton of a man who overdosed with these drugs and was found in the woods 6 months after death.[35] In eight autopsy cases in which barbiturates were found and quantitated on initial analysis, the bloods were allowed to decompose for 14 days by remaining untreated at room temperature in the laboratory. All of the bloods had obvious decomposition changes as indicated by their offensive odor. On reanalysis (all analyses were performed using gas chromatography) 7 and 14 days later, no losses of barbiturates had occurred in any of the specimens. The barbiturates studied were pentobarbital (18.6 $\mu g/ml$ and 3.6 $\mu g/ml$); phenobarbital (13.6 $\mu g/ml$); amobarbital and secobarbital mixture (14.9 and 12.5 $\mu g/ml$; 1.3 and 4.9 $\mu g/ml$; 1.9 and 6.7 $\mu g/ml$, respectively, in three cases); and butabarbital and secobarbital mixture (7.1 and 15.9 $\mu g/ml$), respectively.[10] The badly decomposed body of a young woman was found in a shallow grave on a lakeshore in the summertime. She had last been seen alive 3 months previously. No cause of death could be deter-

TABLE 47-11. STABILITY OF DRUGS IN WHOLE BLOOD UNDER REFRIGERATION*

	Drug Concentration (Time 0)	Drug Concentration ($\mu g/ml$) Measured		
		(7 Days)	(30 Days)	(120 Days)
Meperidine	1.00	0.94	0.95	0.86
Propoxyphene	1.00	0.93	0.94	0.81
Codeine	1.00	0.96	0.89	0.82
Methaqualone	1.00	0.99	1.00	0.85
Doxepin	1.00	0.88	0.90	0.75
Diazepam	1.00	0.97	0.99	0.87
Diphenhydramine	1.00	0.96	0.93	0.88
Amitriptyline	1.00	0.91	0.92	0.77
Pentazocine	1.00	0.88	0.82	0.82
Flurazepam	1.00	0.93	0.93	0.78

*The drugs were added to separate, untreated whole blood samples as 1.0 mg/ml solutions of their salts in ethanol to contain 1.0 μg of drug per milliliter of blood. Analyses were performed by gas chromatography at 7, 30, and 120 days after preparation. Values given are the average of two gas chromatographic analyses. Samples were stored at 4°C.

mined at autopsy, although a history of drug use suggested involvement of drugs. Since no blood remained, the liver was subjected to toxicologic screening. Meperidine and its major metabolite, demethylmeperidine, were detected by gas chromatography and their identification confirmed by mass spectrometry. The quantity of meperidine found was 56 µg/gm. The kidney also contained 13.6 µg/gm, and 53.1 mg were detected in the stomach contents. The quantity of ethyl alcohol in the liver was 30 mg/100 ml.[10]

The Exhumed Body

The exhumed body presents a variety of problems to be dealt with when toxicologic analyses are required. The legally buried body has usually been embalmed prior to burial. The embalming fluid consists mostly of formaldehyde, although other aldehydes, phenols, various esters, and other volatile substances such as methanol or ethanol may be present. The chief consideration in evaluating the embalmed body toxicologically is that much of the blood has been replaced with this fluid, which penetrates the organs and almost all other parts of the body, "fixing" the tissues by reaction with proteins. This process delays the decomposition processes considerably, so that the features and organs may remain essentially intact for many months if the body was well embalmed.

The fixative process makes drugs more difficult to extract, and some may actually be chemically altered by the process. However, the embalming itself should not preclude the performance of a good toxicologic examination. The primary differences between embalmed bodies and nonembalmed bodies are the absence of a valid blood sample to work with and the unreliability of quantitative data from organ analyses due to fixation.

Volatile substance examination is impaired by the presence of methanol and formaldehyde. However, if one can exclude the presence of ethyl alcohol in the embalming fluid (getting a sample of fluid from the funeral director), he can perform an alcohol analysis on vitreous humor (if the eyeball has not collapsed) or on heart blood or spleen which may not have been penetrated completely by the embalming fluid as well as the other organs. If much time has elapsed, or if warm temperatures have expedited decomposition, eye fluid will not be present, and more advanced changes may have taken place. The heart blood (if present), the liver, or the kidney may be analyzed for alcohol. If putrefactive changes have taken place, however, postmortem production of alcohol may have occurred, invalidating the results of the analysis.

If the liver or other organs are recognizable, it may be possible to detect many drugs if they had been present initially. Barbiturates (e.g., secobarbital, amobarbital, and pentobarbital) seem to be relatively stable and detectable at least 3 to 6 months after burial if they were initially present in high concentrations. Where dehydration has occurred, one must use caution in evaluating the concentrations found. The apparent concentration may be double or triple the actual concentration at death, due to loss of weight by dehydration. Presuming that the drugs were stable under these conditions, the apparent concentration per weight unit would, therefore, increase.

It is impossible to say when complete loss or degradation of drugs occurs and which are the most stable, due to lack of controlled studies on such cases. However, it may be assumed that the acidic and neutral compounds (e.g., barbiturates and glutethimide) are more stable than the basic drugs. Many of the products of decomposing tissue have properties resembling basic drugs, making their separation and identification more difficult. One must be aware of these products if he is searching for drugs in putrefied tissue. The well-known decomposition product, β-phenethylamine, resembles amphetamine and even propoxyphene in its ultraviolet absorbance spectrum. A fine study on many of the interfering products commonly found in autopsy tissue was performed by Kaempe.[36] Use of these data may serve to identify many of the products inevitably found. In the experience of the author, β-phenethylamine, nicotinamide, tyramine, and phenylacetic acid are often encountered in putrefied tissue.

It is well known that heavy metals are stable indefinitely. Death from arsenic intoxication, once a not infrequent means of homicide, has been demonstrated by analysis of bodies years after burial. If arsenic poisoning has occurred, high concentrations of arsenic will be detected in all parts of the body. Hair and nails will often yield very high concentrations if the poisoning was chronic. In fact, an analysis of a sample of Napoleon's hair, collected after his death in 1821, revealed a pattern of abnormal arsenic exposure when analyzed by neutron activation analysis in 1962.[37]

Ethyl Alcohol

Ethyl alcohol is not only the most commonly involved agent in drug intoxications, but it is the only drug for which well-defined laws exist, attempting to curtail its use by motor vehicle drivers. Thus the forensic toxicologist must be capable of measuring blood concentrations accurately, and be prepared to testify in court on the results of his analyses, as well as on the pharmacology and toxicology of ethyl alcohol.

In deaths from alcohol intoxication, blood concentrations usually exceed 400 mg/100 ml. There appear to be some circumstances, however, in which the individual has suffered acute alcohol intoxication to the point of irreversible brain damage, yet survives long enough to metabolize much of the circulating blood alcohol. In these circumstances, vitreous humor and urine analysis may provide useful information.

The urine alcohol concentration correlates well with that of the blood (when the urine concentration is multiplied by 0.7) at the time the urine is being formed.[38] In cases involving coma, however, urine may remain in the bladder for several hours, and at the time of death, it may contain many times the concentration of alcohol found in the blood, thereby providing an indication of the blood concentration at some earlier time.

The vitreous humor concentration of ethyl alcohol follows that in the blood, but exhibits a lag time for equilibrium to occur with the blood. Therefore, up to about an hour after ingestion of alcohol, the blood concentration will be higher than that in vitreous humor. After that period of time, the vitreous concentration exceeds that of blood. At equilibrium, the blood/vitreous humor ratio would be expected to be around 0.79, based on the water content of each fluid.[39,40] Found comparisons usually substantiate this ratio. The lag period required to re-equilibrate with the circulating blood often leads to much higher alcohol concentrations in the vitreous humor.[41] When this occurs, it may be assumed that the blood concentration had earlier been that high (if the vitreous concentration is multiplied by 0.80).

Table 47-12 lists some examples of cases of death from ethyl alcohol

TABLE 47-12. ETHYL ALCOHOL OVERDOSE FATALITIES: COMPARISON OF BODY FLUID CONCENTRATIONS

	Ethyl Alcohol Concentration (mg/100ml)			
A/R/S	Blood	Vitreous Humor	"Corrected" Value*	Urine
65 w/f	540	310	250	—
41 w/m	380	470	370	500
39 n/m	280	360	290	400
48 w/m	370	420	340	—
49 w/m	280	410	330	—
	(Isopropanol 110)	(Isopropanol 150)		
37 w/m	400	510	410	50
19 w/m	340	280	220	—
49 w/m	460	530	420	—
42 n/m	550	600	480	630
64 w/m	500	590	470	490
16 w/m	450	510	410	470

*Expected blood concentration if distribution were at equilibrium, obtained by usine a correction factor of 0.80 to account for the higher water content in vitreous humor.

intoxication, comparing blood and vitreous humor concentrations. In most of these cases, the vitreous alcohol concentration is greater than that of the blood, indicating distribution equilibrium of alcohol in the body, or, if much greater than the blood alcohol concentration, indicating that the person was in the postabsorptive phase of alcohol intoxication and had metabolized at least some of the alcohol from the blood. In those cases in which the blood alcohol is greater than that of the vitreous humor, the individual would have been in the preabsorptive phase, or would have ingested some alcohol within the 1- to 2-hour time period prior to death.

One of the problems involved with interpretation of postmortem alcohol concentrations is the question of postmortem production of alcohol as the result of putrefaction. One way of substantiating the found blood alcohol is by the analysis of vitreous humor and urine. These specimens are protected from putrefactive processes for a longer period of time and do not contain much glucose, which is the source of endogenous alcohol in the blood.

It has been reported that bacterial action of putrefying blood can produce up to 200 mg/100 ml of ethyl alcohol.[42] Most early reports of high quantities produced in this manner, however, were based on nonspecific oxidation analyses for alcohol. By gas chromatographic analyses, quantities of up to 60 mg/100 ml were produced in 48 hours in human tissue media.[42] The quantity produced may be dependent upon the glucose content of the blood and the types of bacteria present. In the experience of this author, quantities greater than 60 mg/100 ml are rarely encountered due solely to postmortem production, and any greater than 120 mg/100 ml is assumed to have resulted from premortem ingestion. Alcohol that may be present in the stomach at death may diffuse into surrounding tissues and fluids. Little, if any, however reaches the heart blood by this means.[43] A real danger, however, exists from faulty collection processes. If blood is taken by cardiac puncture from outside the chest wall, the collector may inadvertently puncture the stomach, or withdraw pericardial fluid or chest fluid which may contain higher concentrations of alcohol than were present in the blood at the time of death because of diffusion from the stomach. In cases where doubt exists, the values obtained should be substantiated by analysis of vitreous humor and urine.

In blood collected from living individuals or nonputrefied autopsy cases, the alcohol remains stable for long periods of time (6 months or longer) if the blood is treated with a preservative such as sodium fluoride. One report claims no change after 3 years.[42] A reanalysis of blood samples from autopsy cases 7 months after the initial analysis revealed no change in most from the original values.[10] The bloods had been collected in "red-top" vacutainers, without preservative, and maintained under refrigeration at 4° C during this period of time (see Table 47-13). Alcohol analyses were performed, using a modification of the method of Jain.[44] Three of the nine cases showed some decrease in blood alcohol concentrations, but in only one case was this greater than 20 mg/100 ml. In this case (No. 3, Table 47-13), two antemortem blood samples were available from the same individual (a motor vehicle accident victim). These decreased 57 and 22 mg/100 ml respectively in the 8-month period of refrigeration. In this case, the blood and vitreous humor tubes had been opened after collection, and evaporation losses may have resulted. In those cases where vitreous humor or urine samples were available for reanalysis, one of the four vitreous humor samples showed some decrease in alcohol content, and the single urine analyzed showed a decrease of 86 mg/100 ml. No explanation for this observation is apparent, although bacterial contamination of these samples at autopsy may be more likely than contamination of blood samples taken from the heart.

Narcotics

Narcotic overdose cases present some special problems to the toxicologist, of both an analytical and interpretive nature. Heroin abuse is a predominant problem in many major cities, owing to its strongly euphoriant properties. The depressant effect of the narcotic drugs on the respiratory system leads frequently to overdose. This group of drugs, therefore, is a major

TABLE 47-13. REANALYSIS OF BLOOD SAMPLES FOR ETHYL ALCOHOL AFTER STORAGE*

		Initial Autopsy		Reanalysis
	Date	Ethanol (mg/100 ml)	Date	Ethanol (mg/100 ml)
1. Blood	7-3-76	116	2-10-77	109
2. Blood	7-3-76	227	2-10-77	239
3. Blood (1)	7-4-76	165	3-17-77	108
Blood (2)	7-4-76	81	3-17-77	59
4. Blood	7-4-76	323	2-10-77	318
Vitreous	7-4-76	322	2-10-77	322
5. Blood	7-4-76	105	2-10-77	108
Vitreous	7-4-76	92	2-10-77	66
			3-2-77	45
6. Blood	7-5-76	18	2-10-77	17
7. Blood	7-6-76	267	2-10-77	248
Vitreous	7-6-76	345	2-10-77	353
8. Blood	7-8-76	23	2-10-77	21
Vitreous	7-8-76	35	2-10-77	36
9. Blood	7-17-76	274	2-10-77	268
Urine	7-17-76	276	2-10-77	184
			3-2-77	190

*Blood, urine and vitreous humor samples were stored in untreated vacutainer tubes under refrigeration at 4°C during the time intervals indicated. Results are the average of two gas chromatographic analyses.

source of drug deaths. The medicolegal assignment of death from heroin use is based on a combination of pathologic findings at autopsy, historical circumstances, and toxicologic results. Needle puncture sites on the body, lung edema, and certain microscopic changes in the lungs are usually observed, but not always. In deaths occurring soon after injection and with obscure injection sites, none of the above may be present. Morphine can be detected in the blood in at least 61 percent of heroin overdose fatalities, however, and probably in all deaths occurring within a short time interval after injection. The actual concentration of morphine in the blood is probably of little significance in evaluating the role of heroin in the death, since blood concentrations in heroin addicts who died from traumatic injuries closely paralleled those dying of heroin overdose.[45] Morphine is detected in the bile or urine in about 90 percent of these cases, although in a few circumstances these specimens may be negative. When the individual dies within minutes after injection, no morphine may be present in these specimens, if the individual had not used heroin within the previous few days or more preceding death. Morphine is present in organs, especially kidney and liver, if death occurred from intravenous heroin overdose, even if absent from bile or urine.[46] The kidney concentration after acute intravenous overdose of heroin is usually 1.5 μg/ml or greater.[47]

In many of these cases, other drugs or alcohol are found in addition to morphine. In 78 percent of heroin overdose cases occurring over the last 3 years in Dallas County, other central depressant drugs or alcohol were detected in addition to morphine; 28 percent of the cases had alcohol detected, and 50 percent had other drugs. These included methaqualone, diazepam, pentobarbital, amobarbital and secobarbital mixture, dilaudid, meperidine, ethchlorvynol, codeine, phencyclidine, and meprobamate. It would appear that the concomitant use of other drugs may play a significant role in the etiology of heroin overdose.

REFERENCES

1. Sunshine, I. (ed.): *Handbook of Analytical Toxicology.* Chemical Rubber Company, Cleveland, 1969.
2. Clarke, E. G. C.: *Isolation and Identification of Drugs.* Pharmaceutical Press, London, 1969.
3. McFadden, W. H.: *Techniques of Combined Gas Chromatography/Mass Spectrometry: Applications in Organic Analyses.* Wiley, New York, 1973.
4. Goldbaum, L. R.: Determination of Barbiturates. *Anal. Chem.* 24(10):1604–1607, 1952.
5. Goldbaum, L. R.: Determination and Distribution of Doriden. *J. Forensic Sci.* 7(4):499–503, 1962.
6. McBay, A. J., Turk, R. F., Corbett, B. W., and Hudson, P.: Determination of Propoxyphene in Biological Materials. *J. Forensic Sci.* 19(1):81–88, 1974.
7. Wallace, J. E.: Microdetermination of Diphenylhydantoin in Biological Specimens by Ultraviolet Spectrophotometry. *Anal. Chem.* 49(6):552–59, 1966.
8. Foerster, E., Hatchett, D., and Garriott, J. C.: A Rapid, Comprehensive Screening Procedure for Basic Drugs in Blood or Tissue by Gas Chromatography. *J. Anal. Toxicol.* 2:50–55, 1978.
9. Finkle, B. S., Foltz, R. L., and Taylor, D. M.: A Comprehensive GC/MS Reference Data System for Toxicological and Biomedical Purposes. *J. Chromatogr. Sci.* 12:304–328, 1974.
10. Garriott, J. C.: Unpublished data.
11. Brodie, B. B., et al.: The Fate of Thiopental in Man and a Method for Its Estimation in Biological Material. *J. Pharmacol.* 98:85–96, 1950.

12. Fish, F., and Wilson, W. D. C.: Excretion of Cocaine and Its Metabolites in Man. *J. Pharm. Pharmacol.* 21 (Suppl.):1355–1385, 1969.
13. Smith, R. L.: Drug Metabolism and Forensic Toxicology. *J. Forensic Sci.* 7:71–85, 1967.
14. Amundson, M. E., Johnson, M. L., and Manthey, J. A.: Urinary Excretion of d-Propoxyphene Hydrochloride in Man. *J. Pharm. Sci.* 54(5):684–686, 1965.
15. Schwartz, M. D., et al.: Metabolism of Diazepam in Rat, Dog and Man. *J. Pharmacol. Exp. Ther.* 149(3):423–435, 1965.
16. Dring, L. G., Smith, R. L., and Williams, R. T.: The Metabolic Fate of Amphetamine in Man and Other Species. *Biochem. J.* 116:425–435, 1970.
17. Clarke, op. cit., p. 257.
18. Nash, J. F., et al.: Quantitation of Propoxyphene and Its Major Metabolites in Heroin Addict Plasma After Large Dose Administration of Propoxyphene Napsylate. *J. Pharm. Sci.* 64:429–433, 1975.
19. Garriott, J. C., Sturner, W. Q., and Mason, M. F.: Toxicological Findings in Six Fatalities Involving Methadone. *Clin. Toxicol.* 6(2):163–173, 1973.
20. Sturner, W. Q., and Garriott, J. C.: Comparative Toxicology in Vitreous Humor and Blood. *Forensic Sci.* 6:31–39, 1975.
21. Felby, S., and Olsen, J.: Comparative Studies of Postmortem Barbiturate and Meprobamate in Vitreous Humor, Blood and Liver. *J. Forensic Sci.* 14(4):503–514, 1969.
22. Jatlow, P. I.: UV Spectrophotometry for Sedative Drugs Frequently Involved in Overdose Emergencies, in Sunshine, I. (ed.): *Methodology for Analytical Toxicology.* CRC Press, Cleveland, 1975, p. 414.
23. Jain, N. C., and Cravey, R. H.: Analysis of Alcohol. 1. A Review of Chemical and Infrared Methods. *J. Chromatogr. Sci.* 10:257–262, 1972.
24. Cravey, R. H., and Jain, N. C.: Current Status of Blood Alcohol Methods. *J. Chromatogr. Sci.* 12:209–218, 1974.
25. Parker, K. D., and Hines, C. H.: Manual for the Determination of Narcotic and Dangerous Drugs in the Urine. *Psycopharmacol. Bull.* 3(3):18–43, 1966.
26. Gettler, A. O., and Kaye, S.: A Simple and Rapid Analytical Method for Hg, Bi, Sb and As in Biological Material. *J. Lab. Clin. Med.* 35:146–151, 1950.
27. Williams, L. A.: Carbon Monoxide, Type A Procedure; Freireich, A., et al.: Type B Procedure; Finkle, B.: Type C Procedure, in Sunshine, I. (ed.): *Methodology for Analytical Toxicology.* CRC Press, Cleveland, 1975, pp. 64–71.
28. Karim, A., Ranney, R. E., Evensen, K. L., and Clark, M. L.: Pharmacokinetics and Metabolism of Diphenoxylate in Man. *Clin. Pharmacol. Ther.* 13(3):407–419, 1972.
29. Tompsett, S. L.: The Determination of Disulfiram (Antabuse Tetraethyl Thiuram Disulphide) in Blood and Urine. *Acta Pharmacol. Toxicol.* 21:20–22, 1964.
30. Porter, G. S., and Williams, A.: The Determination of Low Concentrations of Disulfiram by Cathode Ray Polarography. *J. Pharm. Pharmacol.* 24 (Suppl):145, 1972.
31. Garriott, J. C., and Latman, N.: Drug Detection Cases of "Driving Under the Influence." *J. Forensic Sci.* 21(2):398–415, 1976.
32. Garriott, J. C., DiMaio, V. J. M., Zumwalt, R., and Petty, C. S.: Incidence of Drugs and Alcohol in Fatally Injured Motor Vehicle Drivers. *J. Forensic Sci.* 22(2):383–389, 1977.
33. Segal, R. J., and Catherman, R. L.: Methadone—A Cause of Death. *J. Forensic Sci.* 19(1):64–71, 1974.
34. Hayes, S. L., Pablo, G., Radomski, T., and Palmer, R. F.: Ethanol and Oral Diazepam Absorption. *N. Engl. J. Med.* 296(4):186–189, 1977.
35. Bosche, J., and Burger, E.: Schlafmittelnachwies am Skelett und im Erdreich nach einem halben Jahr Liegezeit im Wald. *Arch. Kriminologie* 153(1,2):36–41, 1974.
36. Kaempe, B.: Interfering Compounds and Artifacts in the Identification of Drugs in Autopsy Material, in Stolman, A. (ed.): *Progress in Chemical Toxicology.* vol. 4. Academic Press, New York, 1969, pp. 1–54.
37. Smith, H., Forshufuud, S., and Wassen, A.: Distribution of Arsenic in Napoleon's Hair. *Nature* 194:725–726, 1962.

38. Heise, H. A.: Concentrations of Alcohol in Samples of Blood and Urine Taken at the Same Time. *J. Forensic Sci.* 12(4):454–462, 1967.
39. Hentsch, R., and Muller, H. P.: Tierexperimentelle Untersuchungen über die Konzentration von Peroral Zugefuhrtem Athanol im Blut und Glaskorper. *Arch. Klin. Exp. Ophthal.* 168:330–334, 1965.
40. Felby, S., and Olsen, J.: Comparative Studies of Postmortem Ethyl Alcohol in Vitreous Humor, Blood and Muscle. *J. Forensic Sci.* 14(1):93–101, 1969.
41. Audrlichy, I., and Pribilla, O.: Vergleichende Untersuchung der Alkoholkonzentration im Blut, der Glaskorperflussigkeit, der Synovialflussigkeit und im Harn. *Blut Alkohol* 8:116–121, 1971.
42. Blackmore, D. J.: The Bacterial Production of Ethyl Alcohol. *J. Forensic Sci. Soc.* 8(2–3):73–78, 1968.
43. Plueckhahn, V. D.: The Evaluation of Autopsy Blood Alcohol Levels. *Med. Sci. Law* 8:168–176, 1968.
44. Jain, N. C.: Direct Blood Injection Method for Gas Chromatographic Determination of Alcohols and Other Volatile Compounds. *Clin. Chem.* 17(2):12, 1971.
45. Baselt, R. C., et al.: Acute Heroin Fatalities in San Francisco. *West. J. Med.* 122(6):455–458, 1975.
46. Garriott, J. C., and Sturner, W. Q.: Morphine Concentrations and Survival Periods in Acute Heroin Fatalities. *N. Engl. J. Med.* 289:1276–1278, 1973.
47. Johnston, E. H., Goldbaum, L. R., and Whelton, R. L.: Investigation of Sudden Death in Addicts with Emphasis on the Toxicologic Findings in Thirty Cases. *Med. Ann. D.C.* 38:375–380, 1969.

CHAPTER 48

William T. Lowry is Chief of the Regulated Substances Section of the Southwestern Institute of Forensic Sciences and is Assistant Professor of Pathology at the University of Texas Southwestern Medical School at Dallas. Dr. Lowry, who holds degrees from East Texas State University and Colorado State University, is a Fellow of the American Academy of Forensic Sciences and the American Institute of Chemists and is a member of the American Academy of Clinical Toxicology and the International Association of Forensic Toxicologists. He has authored a textbook in forensic toxicology in addition to numerous professional articles and papers.

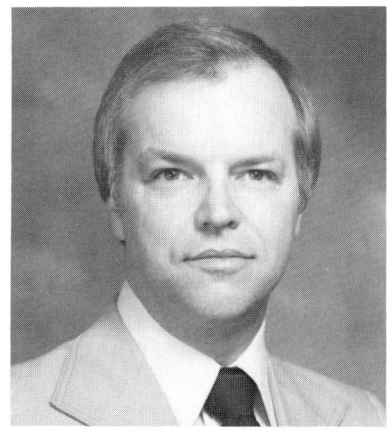

SPECIALTY AREAS OF FORENSIC TOXICOLOGY

William T. Lowry, Ph.D.

In today's society with constant exposure to foreign chemicals such as industrial wastes, food additives, pesticides, fertilizers, cosmetics, drugs, and other general air and water pollutants, the importance of toxicology is rapidly increasing. It is well understood that chemical compounds vary in their hazard to man, domestic animals, and other living members of the environment.

While practically all materials can be toxic under the proper conditions, the interpretation of their effects under normal conditions of use is extremely important when criminal or civil litigation is pending. Thus the applications of the specialty areas of toxicology, such as clinical, environmental, industrial, and veterinary, in legal problems are quite numerous. From this it is obvious that the term forensic toxicology is much broader in scope than the generally accepted concept involving the application of toxicology in the medicolegal investigation of death.

TOXIC SUBSTANCES

The toxicity of a chemical substance is the property of that substance which has injurous effects upon a living organism. As a general principle, all substances have the potential to be toxic to all living things. However, the individual susceptibility of each species to the substance varies. Susceptibility varies with such factors as age, sex, state of health, rate of dosage, and diet. Therefore, the evaluation of toxicity data must take these factors into account in addition to the route of administration and the time of frequency of exposure. For the forensic toxicologist, the primary concern is for those chemical substances which are or could be damaging to humans in amounts that ordinarily occur or might occur in the everyday living environment, such as industrial, medical, or scientific environments. It is from these settings that legal actions are most likely to arise.

TOXICITY AND HAZARD RATINGS

The toxicologist must bear in mind the difference between the "toxicity" rating and "hazard" rating.[1] A substance could possibly have a high toxicity rating and a low hazard rating. The hazard rating is simply a measure of the likelihood of damage to humans working with or around the substance in question. In most cases, though, highly toxic materials such as arsenic and mercury are generally considered very hazardous as well. Thus, when highly toxic and highly hazardous substances are subject in a legal action, the forensic toxicologist realizes that the chance for injury is great. He must do everything possible to establish the facts in the case in order that the truth be determined through a legal mechanism.

A knowledge of toxicity, an ability to evaluate health hazards, and a knowledge of regulations are the basic attributes of a forensic toxicologist. When evaluating a case, the primary goal is to determine the probability that a hazardous situation did exist.

When evaluating toxicity, external factors must be taken into account. These can be classified in three groups that influence biologic response: (1) those related to the poison, (2) those related to the exposure situation, and (3) those related to the subject.[2] The subject-related group can be subdivided into those that are inherent, or a part of the subject, and those that are external to the subject but are a part of his environment. The external environmental factors include the chemical environment, the physical environment, and the social environment. These external environmental factors are only capable of influencing toxic response when they produce some type of internal modification in the biologic system.

ENVIRONMENTAL FACTORS AFFECTING TOXICITY

The three physical environmental factors are considered to be temperature, pressure, and radiation. The concentration of a specific toxic agent or its metabolites in the biologic system is influenced by the processes and is to some extent temperature-dependent. Both increased and decreased environmental temperatures have been shown to influence toxic responses in animals and in man.

The study of the effects of increased and decreased barometric pressure on the toxicity of drugs and other chemical agents has been advanced through space medicine. There has been fairly extensive investigation on the effect of increased environmental pressure on divers. In addition, cases of barometric pressure variation on the pharmacologic and toxic effects of an agent have been attributed to changes in the environmental oxygen tension, rather than to a direct pressure effect. However, there are exceptions such as the effects produced under these conditions by morphine, chlorpromazine, amphetamine, and meperidine.[3] In general, severe pressure changes are likely to produce variable degrees of stress, which in turn can influence the toxic response. It may be difficult, however, to separate the effects of the physical environment on the toxic response from the general effects of the toxic agent.

Hyperbaric oxygen exposure has also been used in the treatment of poisoning by carbon monoxide, cyanide, and barbiturates and has been recommended for use in the management of other types of acute poisoning. It has also proven to be a useful tool for enhancing the tumoricidal activity of radiation. There has been relatively little attempt to investigate the effects of ionizing radiations on the response of biologic systems to toxic agents. However, since radiation exposure is known to affect blood-tissue barriers, to modify enzyme systems, and to produce disturbances in the normal excretory patterns of numerous species, including man, it is reasonable to expect that such exposure would be capable of influencing the distribution, metabolism, and excretion of at least some drugs and toxic agents. These effects, in most cases, are relatively small in magnitude.

The CNS stimulant group appears to produce a significant change in response to radiation exposure. The toxicity of both amphetamine and pentylenetetrazol has been shown to increase in irradiated animals. In contrast, the toxicity of barbiturates and other CNS depressants is decreased; there is no change in the analgesic effect of the narcotics, and there is little significant change in either the toxicity or the analgesic produced by the antipyretic analgesics.

Environmental chemicals are capable of influencing toxic response in several ways. Two factors are related specifically to the formulation and administration of the specific substances. Chemical substances in the environment may have the ability to influence the biologic system in such a way that its susceptibility to toxic agents is altered. For example, chemical agents may produce changes in metabolism by means of induction of the liver microsomal enzyme system. In addition, environmental chemical substances may alter the receptor sites in the biologic system as well as changing the absorption, distribution, and excretion of the substance.

In test situations it has been shown that the manner in which an animal or biologic specimen responds to a toxic agent is influenced by the immediate exposure situation as well as by the way in which it is housed, fed, and generally treated prior to exposure.

Toxic exposures are seldom limited to single agents. They usually involve mixtures of potentially injurious substances with unknown concomitant action upon the body. To add further complications, one must consider work conditions such as heat, humidity, vibration, noise, and severe exertion. Any or all of these factors may alter the response resulting from a particular exposure.

A recent review points out that it is "highly unlikely that a single scientifically sound level for all inorganic compounds in air can be established from the data at hand."[4] Since arsenical compounds, which vary in oxidation states and complexes, vary in toxicity, it is also reasonable to assume that other chemical elements behave similarily. Thus, when considering forensic aspects, the variable of toxicity must be taken into account.

The following considerations in determining the probability of a cause-effect relationship between illness and environmental/chemical substance factors should serve as basic guidelines in a thorough forensic investigation:

1. Analysis of the person's medical, personal, family, and occupational history.
2. Thorough physical examination and clinical evaluation (analysis of signs and symptoms).
3. Laboratory evaluation (analysis of clinical chemistries and clinical toxicology tests).

THE FORENSIC TOXICOLOGIST AND EVIDENTIARY RESPONSIBILITY

The field of forensic toxicology encompasses a wide spectrum of specialty areas in toxicology. Of particular importance is the fact that the forensic toxicologist must be aware of the physiologic effects of a multitude of potentially hazardous compounds; the regulations controlling these substances; the potential litigation which may arise from other aspects, such as the identification and quantification of exposure levels; the application of realistic methods of evaluating the living and working environment; and the application of factual information to the law.

The forensic toxicologist must have a broad knowledge of chemistry, especially of those aspects dealing with the analysis of trace quantities of materials.

The forensic toxicologist is concerned as well with the actual collection, preservation, and analysis of evidence. The forensic toxicologist who collects samples for evidence must have a complete understanding of the chain of custody of evidence to assure that the sample which is taken will be admissible in a court of law. In addition, he must insure that the sample collected is of adequate size to allow accurate determination of the contaminant in question. All sampling equipment and reagents must be appropriate for the task at hand, and the presence of possible significant interferences must be properly noted at the time of collection of the sample. The specialist in toxicology must understand not only the application of toxicologic information to legal problems, but also the variables affecting the toxicity of various substances.

The principal function of the forensic toxicologist is to evaluate alleged hazardous situations based on as many facts as can be determined and present these facts for legal interpretation. No single individual is an expert in all aspects. An ability to adapt training and experience to new situations and to seek out expert assistance when required is important for a total functional team in this small but viable profession.

When poisoning is suspected by any party, legal action may follow. In today's society this practice is increasing. Notes must be made at any time the case is evaluated or investigated, always noting date, time, and all the pertinent observations. Photographs are a valuable resource. Careful records indicate conscientious work and will be favorably received in court. When poisoning is a possibility, the forensic toxicologist must be prepared to gather all facts possible to support any opinion he may render.

A forensic toxicologist's integrity, if not previously established, may well be put to the test when he is called to testify in legal proceedings. Professional ethics are clear and must be strictly followed. The forensic toxicologist should welcome the fact that other professional people may be brought in to testify. Their testimony will probably carry a weight equal to his own if they are indeed professional. The forensic toxicologist appears in court to establish fact as an unbiased expert and not as an advocate for a particular party.

The forensic toxicologist appearing as a witness needs only to be honest, accurate, and complete concerning the questions asked. In this way he will not become confused if badgered by an attorney. An expert witness assumes major responsibilities and must prepare carefully for his appearances in court. To be worthy of his title, he must have had enough experience to permit him to derive logical conclusions from the facts in the case.

SPECIALTY AREAS OF FORENSIC TOXICOLOGY

There are many specialty areas that may be properly included within the operational field of forensic toxicology. To be considered in this chapter are:

1. Clinical toxicology,
2. Environmental toxicology,
3. Industrial toxicology,
4. Veterinary toxicology,
5. Worker's compensation,
6. The Occupational Safety and Health Act (OSHA),
7. Product labeling,
8. Product liability,
9. Food additives,
10. Environmental regulations,
11. Drug regulations,
12. Plant toxins,
13. Insect and animal toxins,
14. Microbiological toxins,
15. Mycotoxins.

Clinical Toxicology

Clinical toxicology is an area of medical science which deals with human diseases caused by, or associated with, abnormal exposure to chemical substances.[4] The degree of toxicity is directly related to the quantity within the system and the route of administration. The clinical toxicologist has the responsibility to obtain scientific information regarding biological interactions to assist in predicting the immediate as well as long-term effects on a patient of a particular chemical substance.

The clinical toxicologist may become involved in legal matters through the science of toxicology when a patient is examined because of a work-related chemical exposure, home-related accidental exposures such as pesticides in home-grown vegetables accidently contaminated by a neighbor, or even attempted homicide. The pending legal actions may be apparent at the onset, but, in most cases, these will not come about until a much later date. Each instance is unique, and the event must be documented by clinical and laboratory means to provide the facts in order that, at a later date, legal interpretation may be accomplished. Acute intoxication in an emergency room does not often occur at a time or place prepared for an investigational approach beyond the most basic clinical means. Interpretation is complicated by uncertainties as to substances involved, time of exposure, and clinical complications. In such situations the need for immediate treatment may cause lack of documentation which may be needed in the future if legal actions are taken.

That the clinical toxicologist must be aware of potential legal involvement is obvious. The results of investigations of the toxicologist must be translated into terms that will be meaningful, not only to the clinician, but also to the legal community. The experience with human intoxication must be well documented in order that the data will be sufficiently valid to allow a meaningful interpretation.

In many cases in an emergency room setting, the physician may be faced with the situation in which the symptoms and signs presented by a patient do not suggest a diagnosis. In addition, the physician may be faced with the absence of a definite history of the patient, or altered facts given by a friend of relative of the patient. The possibility of poisoning should always be considered in situations in which diagnosis presents a difficult problem. Since a knowledge of the sources, actions, and therapy of every known poison is an impossibility, the emergency room physician often has to rely upon a toxicologist for assistance. From the moment the physician decides to request the toxicologic analysis he must insure that his record of the case is meticulous in detail. Since the emergency room physician's time is severely limited, a preprepared toxicology request form will be extremely beneficial. An example of such a form is shown in Figure 48-1.

In a major hospital setting which sees the majority of emergency poisoning cases, a 24-hour toxicology service should be an integral part of the laboratory activities. Generally, the analytical problems that confront the toxicologist in the identification of poisons are twofold: (1) the quantity of sample is usually limited, and (2) the presence or absence of a large number of chemical substances must be determined. Thus it is most important that the toxicologist be provided with as much data and history as possible in order that he may select a more appropriate test for the first procedure to be employed. A preprepared toxicology request form will greatly enhance the probability that more data will be supplied by the physician.

Environmental Toxicology

The term environmental toxicology refers to the application of toxicology to organisms other than man and domestic animals. Owing to terminological confusion, environmental toxicology has been subdivided into toxinology, ecological toxicology, and wildlife toxicology.[5]

Toxinology refers basically to toxins produced by living organisms which are dangerous to man. Among these are poisonous plants, the venom of snakes, spiders, bees, etc., and bacterial and fungal toxins.

Ecological toxicology is the study of all toxins produced by living organisms and of the ecological relationships made possible by these poisons. In a broad sense this includes man's use of poisons and his defenses against them.

Wildlife toxicology involves the study of the effects of toxins of any origin on wildlife, in the same context in which veterinary toxicology is related to domestic animals.

In the overall context, however, one can relate the science of environmental toxicology to forensic toxicology through the regulatory aspects of the Environmental Protection Agency, including the Clean Air Act, the Resources Conservation and Recovery Act, the Federal Water Pollution Control Act, the Federal and Environmental Pesticides Control Act, and the Toxic Substance Control Act. The latter legislation has an overlapping relationship to industrial toxicology as well.

A full understanding of toxicology must involve knowledge of the problems produced by chemicals or from physical forces, which have real or potentially injurious effects, resulting from violation of the above legislation and regulations adopted under the authority of these laws. In this respect, the term forensic toxicology is applicable to the environmental toxicology field where both criminal and civil actions are commonly involved in regulatory efforts.

DALLAS COUNTY HOSPITAL DISTRICT
Dallas, Texas

DEPARTMENT OF PATHOLOGY

TOXICOLOGY REPORT

Name ____________________

Address ____________________

Birthdate ____________________

Classification ____________________

OP ☐ ER ☐ IP ☐ Admit ____________________

Date: ____________________ Time: ____________________

CLINICAL HISTORY (Pertinent information must be included):

☐ Non-emergency Drug level	☐ Coma	☐ Irrational Behavior (Hallucinatory)
☐ Emergency overdose	☐ Convulsion	☐ Other ____________

Specimen: A ☐ Blood B ☐ Urine C ☐ Gastric Contents

☐ Alcohols (A)*	-------	☐ Glutethimide (A) 0.05–0.20	-------
☐ Amitriptylene (Elavil) (A) <0.100**	-------	☐ Lead (24 hr Ur. or A)	-------
☐ Amphetamines (A or B) <0.010	-------	☐ Post Chelation Treatment	-------
☐ Arsenic (24 hr Ur. or A)	-------	☐ Mercury (24 hr. Ur.)	-------
☐ Post-Chelation Treatment	-------	☐ Post-Chelation Treatment	-------
☐ Barbiturates (A)		☐ Methaqualone (Quaalude) (A or B) .20	-------
Long acting – 0.5–2.80	-------		
Short acting – 0.05–0.20	-------	☐ Morphine or Heroin (Overdose) (A + B)	
☐ Cholinesterase Activity (A)	-------	☐ Opiate Narcotics (Non-emergency) (B)	-------
☐ Chlordiazepoxide (Librium) (A) 0.1–0.20	-------	☐ Phenothiazines (A or B) 0.10	-------
☐ Diazepam (Valium) (A) 0.02–0.20	-------	☐ Propoxyphene (Darvon) (A)	-------
☐ Diphenylhydantoin (A) 0.8–1.50	-------	☐ Salicylates (A or B) 5–10	
		☐ Volatiles (Other than Alcohols)	-------
☐ Ethchlorvynol (Placidyl) (A) 0.50	-------	☐ Other ____________	
☐ Ethylene Glycol (A)	-------	____________	-------

* PREFERRED SPECIMEN
** THERAPEUTIC BLOOD CONCENTRATION IN mg%

REQUESTED BY____________________

COMMENTS:____________________

TOXICOLOGIST____________________ ANALYST____________________ 658

FORM NO. 55985 (REV. 9/74) MEDICAL RECORD

FIGURE 48-1. Toxicology request form.

Industrial Toxicology

The term industrial toxicology denotes concern primarily for the injurious potentials and the dosage-response relationships of the substances encountered by industrial workers. These include raw materials and intermediates as well as finished products. In the practice of forensic toxicology there is no useful purpose in separating this area from those parts of clinical and environmental toxicology that deal with materials arising from the workplace, such as air and water pollutants, or that are concerned with the possible effects of industrial products upon transport workers and upon the ultimate consumer.[6]

Forensic toxicologic investigations must consider the exposures that are most frequent and most frequently injurious in industry when litigations are pending. Skin contact is the most important route of exposure for industrial toxicologic studies. This is followed by injuries from inhalation. Injuries from swallowing are rare in industry and are seldom accidental in nature.

Toxic effects resulting from occupational exposure may be acute or chronic. An acute exposure is a single, relatively brief exposure to high concentrations. A chronic exposure is caused from prolonged and repeated exposures to small amounts. An acute exposure is most often accidental in nature; however, considering that the employer has little relief from tort liability, the chronic exposure is most often questioned in a court of law as being accidental.

The forensic toxicologist considering industrial problems must keep in mind the effects which the questioned chemical substance may produce as well as every possible external factor and condition having a significant bearing on the case. For opinion purposes, consideration must be given to the possible long-term problems which may result from chemical exposure.

Since the forensic aspects of industrial toxicology only come to light after the fact, the toxicologist must have a detailed and comprehensive study outlined in his mind prior to initiating an investigation. Many of the questions to be answered are general in scope and have been described previously. Additional information should include the following:

1. Does the case warrant a full-scale toxicologic investigation?
2. Is the chemical substance capable of causing toxic injury or causing an aggravation of a pre-existing condition or disease in persons having contact with it by the route, quantity, and frequency alleged in the case?
3. Were other persons exposed to the same substance in the same manner, quantity, and frequency alleged in the case?
4. Do any other persons exhibit toxic symptoms, even in the subclinical state?
5. Are there any data regarding quantities of the chemical substance in air, water, etc., prior to injury date?
6. Do photographs of the area where injury occurred adequately depict the physical environment?
7. Was there any faulty machinery, such as a ventilation hood?
8. What data are needed to bring forth the facts of the case?

It is possible that the conclusion of a comprehensive study would be that the substance was not safely used. Such results should be utilized to establish protocols for use that will reduce exposure and result in safety. It is also possible that the injury was not work-related. These results should reduce further claims and/or legal actions.

The forensic toxicologist in the industrial setting cannot confine himself strictly to the clinical aspects of toxicology. He must be just as concerned with the likelihood that injury resulted from use of a chemical substance in a particular quantity and manner, while keeping in mind the external environmental factors.

The overall goal of the industrial toxicologist is to protect workers from the health hazards of their working environment. The forensic toxicologist in the industrial setting must recognize that there will nearly always be toxic and potentially hazardous materials to be processed or handled. In addition, the employees always have some degree of physical stress such as noise, heat, or radiation. It is his function to determine whether a hazard existed at the time of alleged injury, the degree of that hazard, and the applicable regulatory requirements existing in the knowledge of all regulations involving hazardous and toxic materials.

Veterinary Toxicology

The veterinary toxicologist is primarily concerned with clinical cases of poisoning in the large variety of animals dealt with in veterinary practice. Unlike other areas of toxicology, the veterinary toxicologist must deal with a large number of different species of animals. The basic difference in animals involves physiologic difference in organ size, function, and capability, as well as limitations of tissue activity. The biochemistry of individual tissues in animals varies from species to species. Because of these differences, animal sensitivity and responses to foreign chemicals vary greatly between species. As is the case in other areas of toxicology, the veterinary toxicologist is concerned with variations in external environmental conditions. However, these factors differ greatly from those encountered with humans.[7]

Veterinary toxicology provides a foundation for the development of compounds for therapy as well as for the control of pests, disease, and parasites of plants and animals. Standards and regulations are established regarding safety and are revised as new information is developed concerning the effects upon man, animals, or vegetation.

Standards of safety are developed by comparing economics and/or the degree of injury being treated with the undesirable effects of the proposed compound. When the economic effect is greater than the undesirable or personal injury effects of the chemical, that chemical will be utilized under appropriate restrictions until a safer one can be developed. In some countries it is not uncommon to find livestock producers willing to sustain a low mortality and high morbidity from poisoning by parasiticides in exchange for a reduction of the high mortality to be expected from an injurious disease such as piroplasmosis.[8]

As serious diseases and pests are brought under control, the criteria for safety become more restrictive. In the United States, a livestock producer may bring legal action for damages against a chemical manufacturer if that company's product causes him the slightest real or imaginary damage. In many countries the producers would welcome the same material, together with the risks of using it, without holding the manufacturers responsible for minor damage.

The situation is similar with residues of chemicals in foods. In those countries enjoying a high standard of living with an adequate food supply, the permissible residues are very small. However, in countries with inadequate food supplies, the risk of a higher level of chemical in the diet is preferred to a further restriction of the diet.

Manufacturers have developed extensive programs to investigate all of the potential applications of a new compound in the control of disease, pests, and parasites; however, more governmental regulations are being imposed. With each new regulation comes the possibility of potential legal actions. Thus the development of new compounds and their ultimate application are costly in many ways.

Of special interest to veterinary toxicologists and to certain segments of the public is the occurrence of drugging in horses and dogs for the purpose of shifting the outcome of a race.[9] One example is an adrenalin preparation in oil which is injected into the horse's bloodstream several hours before the race. About half an hour prior to post time, the horse is given a booster shot of amphetamine. This combination has made several 50 to 1–shot horses winners.

Depressants are also used to reduce the performance of a winning horse. The phenothiazine tranquilizers have been quite popular. Scarne[9] has outlined the betting procedure in this type of doping. In an eight-horse superfecta race, four horses are injected with a tranquilizer. Then bets are placed on the other four nondrugged horses, covering all 24 of the possible four-horse combinations. Thus, regardless of the order in which the nondrugged horses finish, the perpetrators are sure of a winning (1-2-3-4) superfecta ticket. Twenty-four different combination bets of $3, for a total of $72, assure a winning superfecta ticket which will almost certainly pay more than $72.

This type of race-fixing is decreasing because screening for drugs in all horses is becoming a routine procedure at the racetrack.

Worker's Compensation

Worker's compensation laws have been designed to protect employees and their families from the risks of accidental injury, death, or disease arising out of, and in the course of, employment. They have been enacted because the common law was viewed as deficient in the protection it afforded employees from the hazards of their work. Under common law, if an employer acted unreasonably and his carelessness resulted in physical injury to one of his employees, the employee could theoretically sue and recover damages from the employer. However, there were means of escaping this tort liability in most cases. The employer had three defenses, known as (1) assumption of the risk, (2) contributory negligence, and (3) the fellow-servant doctrine.[10]

Every state has enacted worker's compensation statutes. These laws vary a great deal from state to state as to the industries that are subject to them, the employees they cover, the nature of the injuries or diseases that are compensable, the rates of compensation, and the means of administration.

Generally, state worker's compensation statutes provide a system of paying for death, illness, or injury occurring during the course of the employment. The three defenses that the employer had at common law are eliminated. The employers are strictly liable without fault.

Most state statutes exclude certain types of employment from their coverage. Primarily these involve domestic and agricultural employees. In the majority of states, the statutes are compulsory. In some states, employers may elect to be subject to lawsuits by employees or their survivors for accidental injuries or death. In these cases, the plaintiff must prove that the death or injury resulted proximately from the negligence of the employer, as at common law, and is not subject to the common-law defenses discussed above. In such a case, there is no statutory limit to the amount of damages recoverable.

Even though the right to worker's compensation benefits is given without regard to fault of either the employer or the employee, employers are not always liable. The legal tests for determining whether an employee is entitled to worker's compensation are simple: (1) "Was the injury accidental?" and (2) "Did the injury arise out of and in the course of the employment?" Worker's compensation laws have been very liberally construed. In recent years the courts have tended to expand coverage and the scope of the employer's liability. For example, courts have ruled that heart attacks are compensable as "accidental injuries," usually under the concept of aggravation of a pre-existing disease.

The system of state worker's compensation laws has been subject to much criticism. The increase in claims as well as challenges in the court have promoted the need for well-documented medical and physical data. Forensic toxicology, through its clinical, industrial, and environmental aspects, is increasing in importance as the quality of administration and investigation of most worker's compensation claims increases.

The Occupational Safety and Health Act

The enactment of worker's compensation and the imposition of employer liability without fault has not eliminated occupational diseases and industrial accidents. To further the goal of ensuring safe and healthful working conditions, Congress in 1970 enacted the Occupational Safety and Health Act (OSHA) under its powers found in the commerce clause.[11]

The quasilegislative powers which this act has delegated to the Secretary of Labor include the authority to set mandatory occupational safety and health standards applicable to business affecting interstate commerce. Pursuant to this authority, the Department of Labor has issued detailed rules and regulations setting forth safety standards for almost every industry.

These rules and regulations originated from numerous sources. When these standards were adopted, they became legislative means to which all employers must conform. While compliance usually has not been difficult for the very large corporation which maintained a substantial staff devoted to safety matters prior to the enactment of OSHA, there have been many problems for the small business and heavy costs involved in compliance.

OSHA inspectors visit the job site and determine whether the health and safety standards adopted by the Secretary of Labor are being met. These inspectors may appear at a place of business on their own initiative, or they may appear as the result of an employee complaint. An employee who believes that a violation of job safety or health standards exists may request an inspection by writing to the Department of Labor. The inspectors have authority to issue citations if they find a violation of the applicable rules and regulations. The great majority of all inspections do result in citations. The employer may be fined up to $1,000 for every citation, but if the employer does not agree that the alleged violation exists, he may appeal to the Review Commission, which will conduct a hearing to determine whether the citation is valid. Decisions of the commission, as well as appeals from rules enacted pursuant to the delegated authority, may be appealed to the circuit court.

An employer who willfully or repeatedly violates the safety and health rules and standards may be penalized up to $10,000 for each violation. The penalty for a simple citation is any amount up to $1,000, and an employer who fails to correct a violation within the period permitted for its correction may be penalized $1,000 for each day the violation continues.

OSHA does not preempt state laws on occupational safety and health. It encourages states to assume responsibility for developing health and safety standards.

OSHA has created several problems for the business community. The burden is placed on the employer to prevent unsafe practices by employees and to discipline workers for noncompliance with safety work rules. An employee may refuse to work in unsafe surroundings. This gives labor unions additional power in dealing with management. The law imposes numerous record-keeping requirements concerning accidental injuries and job-connected health problems. Even though this administrative burden is not great for large businesses, it causes difficulties in obtaining compliance by small businesses. Many of the standards are unclear, and businessmen are often generally confused about what is actually required.

Passage of the Occupational Safety and Health Act and of the Toxic Substances Control Act has drawn attention to the need for good procedures for testing new chemical products in order that the proper safety precautions can be taken during manufacturing processes and they can be safely marketed. Such screening procedures should reduce the probability of withdrawing a product from the market for safety reasons. This latter measure is embarrassing and economically damaging to many producers.[12]

It is an unfortunate fact that too often in the past the effects of exposure to certain chemicals during manufacturing have been first noted in plant employees and not in test animals.

Further evidence leading to increased regulations of industrial chemicals comes from epidemiologic studies of various occupational groups. By comparing the incidence rates for various diseases in these selected groups with the incidence of the general population, areas where the risk is greater than average can be pinpointed.

It is necessary, therefore, to conduct a thorough series of tests for the toxicity of any new substance for which large-scale production is considered. Although such tests are quite expensive, one suit successfully concluded against the company and/or the closure of the plant will make the premarketing testing costs seem like small change.

In a complete evaluation of any substance, acute, short-term, and long-term toxicity tests are necessary. As previously stated, acute toxicity signifies the toxic effects produced by a single short-term exposure or dose of a chemical substance. In acute toxicity testing procedures, varying concentrations usually selected on a logarithmic scale are administered to a selected number of test animals. On the basis of observed mortality at different dose levels, further studies are made to delineate more closely the maximum tolerated dose and the median lethal dose (LD_{50}). The animals are examined carefully for signs of toxicity, and any observed changes in body weight and food intake are noted. Based on the mortality and weight loss in the acute study, three or four levels for a longer test of 4 to 8 weeks can be selected. Groups of animals are administered these selected levels of the test substance during the test period, observed carefully, and at termination examined thoroughly for any adverse effect.

The results of the acute toxicity study provide the basis for selecting levels of the substances to be administered during a long-term or chronic toxicity study. For greater certainty regarding the safety of a chemical, a two-year study in at least two species of animals, usually rats and mice, is considered suitable. Other species such as hamsters, rabbits, dogs, or primates may be employed for special reasons.[13-15] Sequential testing of animal species is presently being evaluated

Under current chronic-toxicity testing requirements, our legislators and regulators, along with public interest groups, are placing heavy burdens on industry without adequate weighing of economic considerations. For example, the information required to protect people who may be exposed to industrial chemicals may, in many cases, be less than that required to protect patients who may receive new drugs. However, toxicity testing protocols are being developed and required following most of the standards promulgated by the Federal Food and Drug Administration (FDA). Most of the information required in this type of study includes the toxicity and/or pathologic changes of the central nervous system, cardiovascular system, respiratory systems, reproductive system, special senses, and composition of blood. Obviously not all chemicals can be tested in such detail for toxicologic effects. Many chemicals can be evaluated for safety if the testing is based on the absence of toxic symptoms, rather than insisting on establishing a specific toxic-exposure level.

The Occupational Safety and Health Administration and the Department of Transportation have specific product labeling requirements based upon the substance's toxicity and/or hazard rating. The basic standards of toxicity ratings, as previously mentioned, follow those set forth by the FDA.

Product Labeling

The Food and Drug Administration of the Department of Health, Education and Welfare regulates hazardous substances intended to be packaged in a form suitable for use in the household.[16] This includes such articles as polishes or cleaners designed primarily for professional use, but that are available in retail stores such as hobby shops for nonprofessional use. Also included are such items as antifreeze and radiator cleaners that, although principally for car use, may be stored in or around dwelling places. The term does not include industrial supplies that might be taken into a home by a serviceman. The size of a container is not the only index of whether the article is suitable for use in or around the household. Consideration is given as to whether under any reasonably foreseeable condition of purchase, storage, or use the article may be found in or around a dwelling.

Under customary conditions of purchase, storage, and use, the required labeling information must be visible, noticeable, and in clear, legible English. Factors affecting a warning's prominence include location, size of type, and contrast of printing against background. Also bearing on the effectiveness of a warning is the effect of the package contents if spilled on the label. Unless impracticable because of the nature of the substance, the label must be of such construction and finish as to withstand reasonable spillage through foreseeable use.

A *highly toxic substance* is any substance falling within any of the following categories:

1. Any substance that produces death within 14 days in half or more than half of a group of white rats, each weighing between 200 and 300 gm, at a single dose of 50 mg or less per kilogram of body weight, when orally administered.

2. Any substance that produces death within 14 days in half or more than half of a group of white rats, each weighing between 200 and 300 gm, when inhaled continuously for a period of 1 hour or less in an atmospheric concentration of 200 parts per million by volume or less of gas or vapor, or 2 mg per liter by volume or less of mist or dust, provided that such concentration is likely to be encountered by man when the substance is used in any reasonably foreseeable manner.
3. Any substance that produces death within 14 days in half or more than half of a group of rabbits weighing between 2.3 and 3.0 kg each, tested in a dosage of 200 mg or less per kilogram of body weight, when administered by continuous contact with the bare skin for 24 hours or less.

The number of animals tested must be sufficient to give a statistically significant result and be in conformity with good pharmacologic practice.

A *toxic substance* is any substance falling within any of the following categories:

1. Any substance that produces death within 14 days in one-half of a group of white rats, each weighing between 200 and 300 gm, at a single dose of more than 50 mg per kilogram, but not more than 5 gm per kilogram of body weight, when orally administered. Substances falling in the toxicity range between 500 mg and 5 gm per kilogram of body weight are considered for exemption from the labeling requirements act. However, it must be shown that because of the physical form of the substances (e.g., solid, thick plastic, emulsion, etc.), the size or closure of the container, human experience with the article, or any other relevant factors, such as labeling is not needed.
2. Any substance that produces death within 14 days in one-half of a group of white rats, each weighing between 200 and 300 gm, when inhaled continuously for a period of 1 hour or less at an atmospheric concentration between 200 and 20,000 parts per million by volume of gas or vapor. Also, substances that produce the same toxicity data at an atmospheric concentration of 200 mg per liter by volume of mist or dust, provided that such a concentration is likely to be encountered by man when the substance is used in any reasonably foreseeable manner.
3. Any substance that produces death within 14 days in one-half of a group of rabbits weighing between 2.3 and 3.0 kg each, tested at a dosage of 200 mg or less per kilogram of body weight, when administered by continuous contact with the bare skin for 24 hours by a specified, approved method.

Again, the number of animals tested must be sufficient to give statistically significant results and be in conformity with good pharmacologic practice.

The inhalation method is indicated for compounds which are gases at ordinary temperatures and pressures or for finely powdered materials capable of being inhaled. By this method the animals are exposed for several hours daily in chambers where a measured amount of the test substance is distributed throughout the air the animals breathe.[13]

The recognition of the association between exposure to noxious gases such as ozone, nitrogen dioxide, and sulfur dioxide; airborne particulates such as silica and asbestos; and the development of respiratory infection has resulted in the use of microbiologic and immunologic parameters to evaluate toxicity.[13-25] The lungs are generally protected from bacterial and viral infection by the interrelationship of the mucociliary, phagocytic, and immune systems. There are methods available to evaluate these defense systems as well as their function as a unit in preventing pulmonary bacterial and viral invasion. The results of these experiments have provided valuable information concerning the toxicity of airborne contaminants.[26-29]

Another example of the need for inhalation testing for product labeling concerns the fluoralkanes because of their use as fire extinguishing agents, aerosol propellants, refrigerants, and solvents. In recent years they have shown an increasing potential for abuse, particularly among drug-oriented youth. A specific fluoroalkane, halothane, has been in common use in most hospitals since 1954 as an inhalation anesthetic.

The fluroalkanes readily diffuse through cell membranes because of their lipid solubility. This results in a highly probable pulmonary absorption of fluoroalkanes. Generally, fluoroalkanes are not pulmonary irritants. In low concentrations acute inhalation is not an unpleasant experience, nor does prolonged exposure result in pathologic change in the upper respiratory tract or lungs.

Clayton reviewed the literature on fluorocarbon toxicity in 1967.[30] Aviado reviewed the toxicity of the fluorocarbon propellants,[31] such as trichlorofluoromethane (CCl_3F), dichlorodifluoromethane (CCl_2F_2), trichlorotrifluoroethane (CCl_2F-$CClF_2$), dichlorotetrafluoroethane ($CClF_2$-$CClF_2$), and chlorodifluoromethane ($CHClF_2$). Fire extinguishing agents include trifluorobromomethane ($CBrF_3$), chlorobromodifluoromethane ($CBrClF_2$), dibromotetrafluoroethane ($CBrF_2$-$CBrF_2$), dibromotrifluoroethane ($CBrF_2$-$CHFBr$), and chlorobromomethane (CH_2ClBr). Underwriters Laboratories developed a simple method for evaluating the relative acute toxicities of the fluoroalkanes. It involves exposing a small number of guinea pigs for up to 2 hours and counting the survivors. From these studies it is evident that the fluoroalkanes are low in the order of toxicity. However, the most important toxicologic effects produced by the fluoroalkanes are on the central nervous and cardiovascular systems. They cause alterations of perception and a reduction in reaction time, and they hinder the ability to concentrate on complex intellectual tasks. The cardiovascular effects are observed as changes in cardiovascular dynamics and the electrical activity of the heart.[32-33]

The central nervous system effects seem to appear at lower levels of exposure than clinically important cardiovascular effects.[34] The manifestations of fluoroalkane toxicity, such as the occurrence of cardiac arrhythmias, have been documented as life-threatening.

Dermal irritation is defined as nonimmunologically mediated dermatitis resulting from contact with a chemical. Recent advances in the understanding of irritant dermatitis are conceptual rather than mechanistic or technical. For cutaneous drugs and consumer products it is realistic to expect that under appropriately exaggerated circumstances all chemicals will cause irritation. A new chemical or product may be compared to a similar agent for which there has been extensive human use. Rather than determining a numerical value with somewhat arbitrary limits for acceptability, the new agent may be given a value equivalent to that of the substance with which it is compared.

Another consideration is that the substance may have a cumulative irritancy potential rather than an irritancy potential from single exposure. When dermatitis develops after repeated exposures of weeks to years, contact sensitization is generally assumed. While sensitization may occur in this situation, cumulative irritancy is even more likely with numerous chemical classes.[35]

For testing skin or eye exposures such as cosmetics and solvents, application to the skin or eyes of test animals by an approved or required procedure is necessary.[17] The term irritant includes primary irritants to the skin as well as substances producing irritation to the eye or mucous membranes. A primary irritant is a substance that is not corrosive, but available data on human experience or testing indicate that it produces irritation to the skin. A substance is an irritant to the eye if the available data on human experience or testing indicate that it produces irritation to the eye.

A corrosive substance is one that causes visible destruction or irreversible alterations in the tissue at the site of contact. A test for a corrosive substance determines whether, by human experience, such tissue destruction occurs at the site of application. A substance would be considered corrosive to the skin if when tested on the intact skin of an albino rabbit by an approved technique, the structure of the tissue at the site of contact is destroyed or changed irreversibly in 24 hours or less. Other appropriate tests should be applied when contact of the substance with other than skin is being considered.

The FDA has specified testing procedures for hazardous substances which must be followed to establish product labeling.[36]

ACUTE DERMAL TOXICITY (SINGLE EXPOSURE)

In acute exposures the agent is held in contact with the skin by means of a sleeve for periods varying up to 24 hours. The sleeve, made of rubber dam or other impervious material, is so constructed that the ends are reinforced with additional strips and should fit snugly around the trunk of the animal. The ends of the sleeve are tucked, permitting the central portion to "balloon" and furnish a reservoir for the dose. The reservoir must have sufficient capacity to contain the dose without pressure. The sleeves are 7 cm in diameter and 12.5 cm long for animals 2.5 to 3.5 kg in weight. The sleeves may vary in size to accommodate smaller or larger subjects. In the testing of unctuous materials that adhere readily to the skin, mesh wire screen may be employed instead of the sleeve. The screen is padded and raised approximately 2 cm from the exposed skin. In the case of dry powder preparations, the skin and substances are moistened with physiological saline prior to exposure. The sleeve or screen is then slipped over the gauze which holds the dose applied to the skin. In the case of finely divided powders, the measured dose is evenly distributed on cotton gauze, which is then secured to the area of exposure.

The animals are prepared by clipping the skin of the trunk free of hair. Approximately one-half of the animals are further prepared by making epidermal abrasions every 2 cm longitudinally over the area of exposure. The abrasions are sufficiently deep to penetrate the stratum corneum (horny layer of the epidermis), but not to disturb the dermis (i.e., not to obtain bleeding).

The sleeve is slipped onto the animal, which is then placed in a comfortable but immobilized position in a multiple animal holder. Selected doses of liquids and solutions are introduced under the sleeve. If there is slight leakage from the sleeve, which may occur during the first few hours of exposure, it is collected and reapplied. Dosage levels are adjusted in subsequent exposures (if necessary) to enable a calculation of a dose that would be fatal to 50 percent of the animals. This can be determined from mortality ratios obtained at various doses employed. At the end of 24 hours the sleeves or screens are removed, the volume of unabsorbed material, if any, is measured, and the skin reactions are noted. The subjects are cleaned by thorough wiping, checked for gross symptoms of poisoning, and then observed for 2 weeks.

PRIMARY IRRITANT SUBSTANCES

Primary irritation to the skin is measured by a patch-test technique on the abraded and intact skin of an albino rabbit, clipped free of hair. A minimum group of six subjects is used in abraded and intact skin tests. Under a square patch such as surgical gauze measuring 1 inch by 1 inch, two single layers thick, 0.5 gm (in the case of solids and semisolids) of the test substance is introduced. Solids in an appropriate solvent are dissolved, and the solution is applied as for liquids. The animals are immobilized with patches secured in place by adhesive tape. The entire trunk of the animal is then wrapped with an impervious material such as rubberized cloth for the 24-hour period of exposure. This material aids in maintaining the test patches in position and retards the evaporation of volatile substances.

After 24 hours of exposure, the patches are removed and the resulting reactions are evaluated on the basis of the designated values given in Table 48-1.

TABLE 48-1*

Evaluation of Skin Reactions	*Value†*
Erythema and eschar formation:	
No erythema	0
Very slight erythema (barely perceptible)	1
Well-defined erythema	2
Moderate to severe erythema	3
Severe erythema (beet redness) to slight eschar formation (injuries in depth)	4
Edema formation:	
No edema	0
Very slight edema (barely perceptible)	1
Slight edema (edges of area well defined by definite raising)	2
Moderate edema (raised approximately 1 ml)	3
Severe edema (raised more than 1 ml and extending beyond the area of exposure)	4

*Federal Register, 29 F.R. 13009, September 17, 1964.
†The value recorded for each reading is the average value of six or more animals subject to the test.

Readings are again made at the end of a total of 72 hours (48 hours after the first reading). An equal number of exposures is made on areas of skin that have been previously abraded. The abrasions are minor incisions through the stratum corneum, but sufficiently deep to disturb the derma or to produce bleeding. The reactions of the abraded skin at 24 hours and

72 hours are evaluated. The values of erythema and eschar formation at 24 hours and at 72 hours for intact skin are added to the values on abraded skin of 24 hours and at 72 hours (four values). The values of edema formation at 24 hours and at 72 hours for intact and abraded skin (four values) are similarly added. The total of the eight values is divided by four to give the primary irritation score.

In general the rabbit assay provides good correlation for man with chemicals.[37] Information for animal use in toxicology studies has been correlated with comparative human and rabbit data.[38]

On a scientific basis, other animals would be adequate. However, the advantages for their use are cost and ease of handling. In addition, the rabbit skin develops erythema and induration that is easily quantitated and is similar to that of man. The guinea pig could be utilized for similar reasons.[39]

It is commonly held that most nonindustrial dermatitis is immunologic in nature rather than caused by an irritant. However, Maibach has evidence that cumulative irritation is much more frequent than contact sensitization.[35] This includes most consumer, skin-care, and cosmetic products.

EYE IRRITANTS

Six albino rabbits are used for each test substance. Animal facilities for such procedures shall be so designed and maintained as to exclude sawdust, wood chips, or other extraneous materials that might produce eye irritation. Both eyes of each animal in the test group must be examined before testing, and only those animals without eye defects or irritation are used. The animal is held firmly but gently until quiet. The test material is placed in one eye of each animal by gently pulling the lower lid away from the eyeball to form a cup into which the test substance is dropped. The lids are then gently held together for 1 second and the animal is released. The other eye, remaining untreated, serves as a control. For testing liquids 0.1 ml is used. For solids or pastes, 100 mg of the test substance is used, except that for substances in flake, granule, powder, or other particulate form, the amount that has a volume of 0.1 ml (after compacting as much as possible without crushing or altering the individual particles, such as by tapping the measuring container) is used whenever this volume weighs less than 100 mg. In such a case, the weight of the 0.1 ml test dose should be recorded. The eyes are not washed following instillation of test material except as noted in Table 48-2.

The eyes are examined and the grade of ocular reaction is recorded at 24, 48, and 72 hours. Reading of reactions is facilitated by use of a binocular loupe, hand slit-lamp, and other indicated means. After the recording of observations at 24 hours, any or all eyes may be further examined after applying fluorescein. For this optional test, one drop of fluorescein sodium ophthalmic solution (U.S.P.) or equivalent is dropped directly on the cornea. After flushing out the excess fluorescein with sodium chloride solution (U.S.P.) or equivalent, injured areas of the cornea appear yellow; this is best visualized in a darkened room under ultraviolet illumination. Any or all eyes may be washed with sodium chloride solution (U.S.P.) or equivalent after the 24-hour reading.

An animal is considered as exhibiting a positive reaction if the test substance, at any of the readings, produces ulceration of the cornea (other than a fine stippling), or opacity of the cornea (other than a slight dulling

TABLE 48-2*

	Exposure Time	Exposure Unit
Erythema and eschar formation:	Hours	Value
Intact skin	24	2
	72	1
Abraded skin	24	3
	72	2
Subtotal		8
Edema formation:		
Intact skin	24	0
	72	1
Abraded skin	24	1
	72	2
Subtotal		4
Total		12

*Federal Register, 29 F.R. 13009, September 17, 1964.

of the normal luster), or inflammation of the iris (other than a slight deepening of the folds or rugae or a slight circumcorneal injection of the blood vessels), or if such substance produces in the conjunctivae (excluding the cornea and iris) an obvious swelling with partial eversion of the lids or a diffuse crimson-red with individual vessels not easily discernible.

The test is considered positive if four or more of the animals in the test group exhibit a positive reaction. If only one animal exhibits a positive reaction, the test is regarded as negative. If two or three animals exhibit a positive reaction, the test is repeated, using a different group of six animals. The second test is considered positive if three or more animals exhibit a positive reaction. If only one or two animals in the second test exhibit a positive reaction, the test must be repeated with a different group of six animals. Should a third test be needed, the substance will be regarded as an irritant if any animal exhibits a positive response.

The method of administration must be thoughtfully selected since it can affect the outcome of chronic toxicity studies. Among these are the age of the test animals, their sex, the species and strain employed, the vehicle, and the diet.

INFORMATION ACCESS

The improper storage or use of toxic or hazardous materials is a prime cause of accidents resulting in injuries to people and property. In the past, information vital to safety was unavailable to the user of these materials, but regulations have been increasingly imposed, describing labeling requirements and imparting concise safety instructions at the point of use of toxic and hazardous materials.

The regulations are changing constantly because of the introduction of products containing new chemicals, new applications of old products, refinement in occupational health knowledge and analytical procedures, and general impact upon the environment and consumer. As a result of this constant change, the forensic toxicologist must have access to up-to-date sources of information in order to maintain accurate knowledge of the regulations with which he is concerned. For labeling, this is essential since accurate application of any labeling system requires careful study of current versions of the rules, possibly involving direct contact with the sponsoring organization. Many of these laws provide substantial penalties for improper labeling of a toxic or hazardous material.

PRODUCT USE

The users of labeling systems may be categorized as manufacturers, shippers, and employers. The manufacturer of a material has the responsibility of complying with all applicable laws and regulations dealing with his product. The same product may be classified as toxic or hazardous for the consumer, requiring one type of label, and nontoxic or nonhazardous for industrial use, requiring different labeling statements.

The shipper must comply with the extensive shipping regulations of the Department of Transportation. International air shipments must comply with the rules of the International Air Transport Association. The employer must be aware of applicable regulations of the Atomic Energy Commission for manmade radioactive materials and of the Department of Labor's OSHA labeling regulations. In addition, state or local occupational laws may require labeling of certain substances in the workplace.[40]

In 1961, the Federal Drug Administration (FDA) initiated a regulation that provided for a package insert to be on or with all prescription drug packages. The initial reasoning was the need to present physicians with accurate information regarding a drug's effects, usage, dosage, and safety apart from that listed in the manufacturer's advertising and promotional literature. This full-disclosure regulation requires that labeling on or within the package from which the drug is to be dispensed bear adequate information for its use. Included in this is the information concerning indications, effects, dosages, routes, methods, and frequency and duration of administration, relevant hazards, contraindications, side effects, and precautions under which practitioners licensed by law to administer the drug can use the drug safely and for the purpose for which it is intended.

The FDA considers the insert to serve two purposes. It is included to alert the physician to the conditions under which the drug is deemed safe and effective for the designated purpose, and it serves to limit the manufacturer in his claims regarding the drug product. Basically, the FDA considers the package insert as part of the labeling of the drug.[41]

This insert has figured in judgments against members of the health care industry and is being used with increasing frequency to determine negligence. However, the physician is not restricted in using the drug only for labeled indications, but he may have to defend against a deviation if a lawsuit is brought against him.[42-43]

Product Liability

One of the consequences of manufacturing or selling a product is the responsibility to a consumer or user if the product is defective and causes injury to a person or property. This responsibility is generally referred to as product liability. A suit for damages for injuries caused by a product may be predicated on the theory of (1) negligence; (2) misrepresentation; (3) breach of warranty, either expressed or implied; or (4) strict liability.[44]

Product liability cases may be brought against manufacturers, sellers, or anyone in the chain of sale. Such cases may be brought by the buyer, by another user of the product, or by some third party whose only connection with the product is the sustaining of an injury caused by it.

The Uniform Commercial Code states that expressed or implied warranties extend to any person who is in the family or household of the buyer or who is a guest in his home, if it is responsible to expect that such person would use, consume, or be affected by the goods. If this person is injured because of a defect in the goods, he may bring an action against the seller. This provision for a third-party beneficiary of a warranty is restricted in that a suit cannot be brought against anyone but the seller. The Code takes a neutral position in other aspects of product liability and makes allowances for case law. The trend of the law on product liability in our society today is clearly in the direction of extending greater protection to consumers.

In a tort action based upon negligence, the action can be maintained by the person who purchased the defective product as well as any person who suffered an injury on account of a defect in the product if the defect was the proximate cause of his injury. The Restatement of Torts (Second), Section 395, states the rule as follows:[44]

> A manufacturer who fails to exercise reasonable care in the manufacture of a chattel which, unless carefully made, he should recognize as involving an unreasonable risk of causing physical harm to those who use it for a purpose for which the manufacturer should expect it to be used and to those whom he should expect to be endangered by its probable use, is subject to liability for physical harm caused to them by its lawful use in a manner and for a purpose for which it is supplied.

The plaintiff must prove by appropriate evidence that the manufacturer was negligent and failed to exercise reasonable care.

Another method by which negligence is established is to prove that the manufacturer violated some statutory regulation in the production and distribution of his product. Most industries are subject to regulations under state and/or federal laws with regard to product quality, testing, advertising, and other aspects of production and distribution. Proof of a violation of a regulatory statute may be sufficient to establish negligence in the case of a manufacturer in such industries.

A more recent development in product liability is the natural extension of the erosion of privity. This is known as the theory of strict liability, and it imposes liability wherever damage or injury is caused by a defective product that is unreasonably dangerous to the user or consumer. The theories of negligence and breach of warranty are becoming less significant in states that have adopted the strict liability theory. Strict liability is a tort rather than a contract cause of action. However, the result is similar to breach of warranty suits in those states that have abolished privity and extended implied warranties to all parties.

The theory of strict liability has been accepted and adopted in the Restatement of Torts if the product is unreasonably dangerous. Under the Restatement, strict liability will be imposed only upon a seller who is engaged in the business of selling an unreasonably dangerous product. The consumer is not required to prove that the seller was negligent. This liability imposed upon a seller has been applied both to personal injuries and to damage to the property of the user or consumer.

The Restatement has other provisions that are related to strict liability. One of these imposes liability upon a seller of goods manufactured by a third person, if he fails to give proper warning that a product is, or is likely to be, dangerous or if he fails to exercise reasonable care to inform buyers of the danger or to otherwise protect them against it. This applies to a product, such as a toxic substance, that may have inherently dangerous properties. A similar duty to give warning applies to the manufacturer. This relates in part to regulations requiring that a warning be placed on a container or label if a product is explosive, poisonous, etc.

The provisions of the Restatement do not have the force of a statute. They are simply an authoritative exposition on the subject. The courts decide cases on the basis of law and facts. As a result, the responsibilities of the forensic toxicologist are greatly increasing.

Food Additives

The Food and Agriculture Organization (FAO) of the United Nations defines a food additive as "a non-nutritive substance added intentionally to food, generally in small quantities to improve its appearance, texture or storage properties."[45] The Food Protection Committee of the National Research Council defines food additives as "substances added to foods either directly and intentionally for a functional purpose, or indirectly during some phase of production, processing, storage, or packaging without intending that it remain in or serve a purpose in the final product."[46] The definition specified in the Food, Drug, and Cosmetic Act is as follows:[47]

> The term 'food additive' means any substance the intended use of which results or may reasonably be expected to result, directly or indirectly, in its becoming a component or otherwise affecting the characteristics of any food (including any substance intended for use in producing, manufacturing, packing, processing, preparing, treating, packaging, transporting, or holding food; and including any source or radiation intended for any such use), if such substance is not generally recognized, among experts qualified by scientific training and experience to evaluate its safety, as having been adequately shown through scientific procedures (or, in the case of a substance used in food prior to January 1, 1958, through either scientific procedures or experience based on common use in food) to be safe under the conditions of its intended use. . . .

Exempt from the category of food additives, as defined in the statute, are: (1) pesticide chemicals in or on raw agricultural commodities, or to the extent that they are used or intended for use in the production, storage, or transportation of any raw agricultural commodity; (2) color additives; (3) substances used in accordance with sanctions or approvals granted before 1958, pursuant to the Food, Drug, and Cosmetic Act, the Poultry Products Inspection Act, and the Meat Inspection Act, as amended and extended; and (4) new animal drugs.[48]

In the 1958 Food Additive Amendment, exceptions were made for all additives that were "generally recognized as safe" (GRAS) because of widespread use in foods. The term "safe" means "that after reviewing all available evidence, including (1) the probable consumption of the substance and of any substance found in or on goods because of its use; (2) the cumulative effect of the substance in the diet of man and animals, taking into account any chemically or pharmacologically related substance or substances in such diet; and (3) safety factors which, in the opinion of experts qualified by scientific training and experience to evaluate the safety of foods and food ingredients, are generally recognized as appropriate in the use of animal experimentation data, the Food and Drug Administration can conclude that no significant risk of harm will result when the substance is used as intended."[49] Proof "beyond any possible doubt" is not required to show that the additive is safe under all conceivable circumstances of use or misuse.

The statute forbids the issuance of a food additive regulation if a fair evaluation of the data fails to establish that the proposed use of the additive will be safe.

However, the statute also included the Delaney clause, which states that "no additive shall be deemed to be safe if it is found to induce cancer when ingested by man or animal, or if it is found, after tests which are appropriate for the evaluation of the safety of food additives, to induce cancer in man or animal . . . ." Several pre-existing food additives have been denied continued use by reason of this principle. One recent example is the 1977 proposed ban of saccharin after 85 years of use.

The provisions of the Delaney clause do not apply to any substance used as an ingredient of feed for animals raised for food production if, under the proposed conditions of use, the substances will not adversely affect animals for which the food is intended and no residue will be found by prescribed or approved methods of examination in any food derived from the animal. From the definition of food additives, one can see the separate classification as intentional and nonintentional food additives. Intentional food additives are substances, either natural or synthetic in origin, which are added to the original food or mixture of foods for a specific purpose. Nonintentional additives are substances which are not present in the food as produced and have not been added to serve a specific purpose in the final product.[49]

Legal intentional additives are those introduced into food through good manufacturing practices in order to improve the nutritive value, facilitate production, or increase acceptability by the consumer.[50]

The primary goal of food additive regulations is to encourage good production practices by preventing the inclusion of harmful additives and/or to maintain any inclusion at a level below what would be considered toxic. This latter point, however, is not exact as understood by the problems in assessing the potential for biologic damage caused by low levels of suspected teratogens, mutagens, and carcinogens which may be present.

Environmental Regulations

All persons are subject to contaminants within the environment in which they reside and work. These contaminants include toxic substances in these surroundings which are affected by the physical properties of the surroundings. Since exposure to the air environment is continuous for all persons, it is the first principal factor to be considered.

The Clean Air Act Amendments of 1970 (Public Law 91-604) require that the Administrator of the Environmental Protection Agency establish ambient air quality standards for pollutants at any location accessible to the public. These standards are generally considered applicable to outside locations, but in some situations the standards are extended within buildings and inclosures. However, the latter extension may overlap regulations set forth by OSHA.[51]

Ambient air quality standards have been set forth for several pollutants under the provisions of the 1970 Clean Air Act Amendments. Two separate standards are defined in the Act: primary standards are intended to protect the public health; secondary standards are intended to protect the public welfare, including protection against damage to buildings, crops, and other vegetation and animal life.

Atmospheric pollution by combustion products (smog) can produce toxicity on a mass scale. The chief components of smog are products of combustion from automobiles, heating fuels, and industrial plants, as well as their photochemical reaction products. There are two general types of smog. Photochemical-oxidant smog is characterized by a high concentration of ozone. It is derived from the photolysis of NO_2 and combination with O_2. The brown color of this type of smog is due largely to NO_2. This type is like that found in Los Angeles. Reducing smog is composed primarily of SO_2 and particulates. This type has been found in London, where a high particulate concentration is present from smoke. However, the prohibition of the use of coal with a high sulfur content virtually abolished the London smogs.[52-53]

Oxides of nitrogen (NO and NO_2) are produced by automobile exhausts as well as by fuels used in heating. In man, respiratory symptoms may develop when exposed to concentrations between 5 and 10 ppm. This is about ten times that found in ordinary photochemical smogs.[54]

Oxides of sulfur (SO_2, SO_3) are generated from fuel oil and petroleum refining processes. Respiratory illness may be associated with levels above 0.05 ppm, while increased mortality is found above 0.2 ppm.[55] Plant life is also affected adversely at these levels.

The particulates in smog may contain significant quantities of asbestos fibers. Asbestos is known to produce lung cancer in those exposed occupationally; however, no data are available to link lung cancer to any kind of air pollution. Cigarette smoking also presents a major environmental hazard of this type.

The characteristics of lead uptake by man from known and suspected environmental sources are a matter of great practical importance, particularly when multiple sources exist or are suspected to exist. Respiratory intake via ambient air and oral intake via food and beverages are the obvious major sources and routes of entry.[56] Lead may also be derived from the combustion of leaded gasolines. Tetraethyl and other alkyl leads are added to fuels in order to permit high compression without knocking. Studies have shown that urban air over a wide area is contaminated with lead in proportion to the density of automobile traffic. Carbon monoxide enhances the difficulties in assessing the possible toxic effects of chronic environmental exposure to a known toxic agent at low levels.

Atmospheric CO is produced primarily by automobiles, and levels fluctuate with conditions conducive to air pollution in general. Ambient levels have rarely exceeded 50 ppm, but are frequently in the 10-ppm range. Exposure in the 10- to 20-ppm range leads to blood levels of 4 to 8 percent carboxyhemoglobin. Cigarette smoking adds very considerably to the CO level. Heavy smokers may reach a blood level of 7 percent or more carboxyhemoglobin.

The Occupational Safety and Health Act of 1970, as previously defined, requires the Secretary of Labor to set and enforce safety and health standards for businesses engaging in interstate commerce. This Act, covering workers and workplaces throughout the nation, includes extensive standards relative to dusts, fumes, mists, and vapors in the working environment. The primary goal of the Act is to provide protection for workers, leaving the Clean Air Act to set appropriate exposure guidelines for the general population.

The goal of the Toxic Substances Control Act (TSCA) is to protect human health and the environment from unreasonable risks. To achieve this goal, TSCA implementation activities emphasize not only control of specific problems under TSCA regulatory provisions, but also use of TSCA authorities to support other governmental and nongovernmental programs to control toxic substances. These programs encompass activities of EPA and other federal and state agencies, activities of environmental and public interest groups and of professional societies, policies of the financial and investment communities, and efforts of individual companies and trade associations.[57]

During the first several years, EPA will give top priority to the following implementation activities:

1. *Establishment and implementation of a premarket review system.* The system will emphasize (a) the responsibility of industry to develop adequate data for meaningful chemical assessments, (b) categorization of new chemicals by broad chemical classes and broad uses with particular attention to those categories of greatest environmental concern, and (c) procedures for rapid decisions and adequate documentation of these decisions.
2. *Establishment of initial testing requirements.* Testing will be required in a hierarchical manner on selected categories of both new and existing chemicals. Industry will be required to develop data concerning both toxicity and exposure and to conduct risk assessments based on these data. Quality assurance of the data that are developed will be stressed.
3. *Regulatory actions to control a limited number of environmental problems associated with existing chemicals.* In addition to early action on polychlorinated biphenyls (PCBs) and selected chlorofluorocarbons, a limited number of serious chemical problems for which adequate data are currently available will be selected for intensive review and for regulatory action as appropriate. Concurrently, a systematized approach for identifying, characterizing, and controlling toxic substances under TSCA will be developed and implemented as rapidly as possible.
4. *Assessment and control of unanticipated problems of urgent concern.* Unexpected problems will inevitably arise, and provisions will be made to respond to such problems without unduly disrupting other priority activities.

In these four priority areas, as well as in other areas, continuing attention will be directed to several concerns. Activities will be oriented to serve the interests of both EPA and other organizations, particularly with regard to data dissemination. Data will be gathered on a highly selected basis to serve specific purposes. Confidentiality aspects will be a major factor influencing data collection, use, and dissemination strategies and activities.

An estimated 1,000 new chemical substances are introduced into commerce each year in addition to the 30,000 or more which are currently used. Assessing and dealing with chemical problems involves the complex tasks of measuring their presence, estimating their effects, and evaluating the economic and social costs and benefits of their use and control

There also exists a wide variety of regulatory authorities and support activities directed to toxic substances at the national, state, and local levels. TSCA is designed to help reduce scientific uncertainties concerning toxic substances while adding protection from unreasonable risks to man and the environment.

TSCA authorizes EPA to obtain information about existing and new chemicals and take appropriate action against those which may present unreasonable risks. Manufacturers or processors of chemicals may be required to conduct tests and submit to EPA data on the effects and behavior of chemicals. EPA must be notified 90 days in advance of the manufacture of new chemicals and supplied with information necessary to evaluate their effects. When necessary, EPA is authorized to take steps to limit manufacturing, processing, use, or disposal of a chemical substance which may present an unreasonable risk.

TSCA contains several explicit authorities to promote better coordination among federal agencies in identifying, assessing, and controlling toxic substances. If the Administrator determines that an unreasonable risk may be prevented or sufficiently reduced under a law not administered by EPA, he will request the relevant agency to evaluate the problem and take appropriate action. Similarly, other laws administered by EPA will be used in preference to TSCA when these authorities can adequately address the problems.

The quality of our water has increasingly been a subject of serious concern. Thus federal, state, and local governments have passed legislation, organized regulatory agencies, and established basic standards. The goal of these programs has been to prevent additional pollution while improving existing quality. The Federal Water Pollution Control Act of 1972 (FWPCA) is the foundation for all water regulations. However, specific requirements and enforcement may vary from agency to agency, depending upon the pollutant, its sources, and/or its location. Therefore, prior to investigating a particular problem, it is wise to determine the responsible agency for contact regarding specific regulations.

The National Water Quality Standards Program was initiated with the passage of the Water Quality Act of 1965. The Water Quality Standards are comprised of use designations for each water body or portion thereof, water quality criteria to support the use designations, and implementation plans for scheduling the construction of the necessary treatment facilities. The designations by water use include protection and propagation of fish, aquatic life, and wildlife (freshwater and marine), and water for public, recreational, agricultural, and industrial supplies. The Water Quality Standards prior to enactment of the FWPCA Amendments of 1972 were applicable only to interstate waters and their tributaries. The Act extends the coverage to include all intrastate waters, and the state standards have since been, or are in the process of being, reviewed accordingly.

The objective of the Act is to restore and maintain the chemical, physical, and biological integrity of the nation's waters. The national goal, Section 101(a) (1), is to eliminate the discharge of pollutants into navigable waters by 1985, with an interim goal, Section 101(a) (2), to attain by July 1983, a water quality which provides for the protection and propagation of fish, shellfish, and wildlife and for recreation in and on the nation's waters.

Section 304(a) (1) of the Federal Water Pollution Control Act Amendments of 1972 establishes and reviews annually water quality criteria on

(1) all identifiable effects of pollutants on human health, fish and aquatic life, plant life, wildlife, shorelines, and recreation; (2) concentration and dispersal of pollutants; and (3) effects of pollutants on biological community diversity, productivity, and stability, including factors affecting rates of eutrophication and sedimentation.

Section 304(a) (2) establishes and reviews annually water quality criteria (1) on the factors necessary to restore and maintain the chemical, physical, and biological integrity of the aquatic environment; (2) on the factors necessary for the protection and propagation of shellfish and fish wildlife for all classes and categories of receiving waters, and to allow recreational activities in and on the water; (3) on the measurement and classification of water quality; and (4) on the identification of pollutants suitable for maximum daily load measurement correlated with the achievement of water quality objectives.[58]

Although there are many factors determining water quality, the following parameters are generally the first to be determined:[59]

pH: A comparative measurement of the acidity-alkalinity relationship. Normal accepted ranges will vary between 6.0 and 8.5.

Total alkalinity: An indicator of aquatic productivity.

Dissolved oxygen: For determining the ability of the water to support aquatic life. Levels in the magnitude of 4 to 5 mg/L are considered satisfactory, whereas near saturation at levels of 8 to 9 mg/L is considered excellent.

Chlorides: The presence of chlorides is related to such factors as highway runoff where the material is used in snow/ice control and in the treatment of sewage.

Temperature: This parameter is determined in conjuction with dissolved oxygen levels. Any serious variations from the local norm can seriously affect resident species and the ecological system.

Biochemical oxygen demand (BOD): This factor represents the organic waste load. Ranges of from 1 to 2 are generally considered satisfactory.

Chemical oxygen demand (COD): This represents the chemical organic load and the oxygen demand of that material. It is an extension of, and is studied with, the BOD level.

Coliform level: This represents the amount of bacteria generated from both the waste of warm-blooded animals and from the soil. Fecal coliform counts serve as an indicator of the level of sewage pollution contributions as they derive primarily from human waste. Although state standards vary, no more than 1000 to 2000 counts per 100 ml are allowed in water that is to be used for swimming activities.

Nitrogens and phosphates: These serve as indicators of eutrophication which is an oversupply of nutrients with a corresponding depletion of oxygen, particularly in the lower levels.

Suspended solids: This is a measure of particles maintained in suspension in the body of water. The greater the number, the greater the turbidity.

Total dissolved solids: This level serves as an indicator of inorganic pollution of which brine might serve as an example.

Once the above parameters are determined, specific substances may be measured which are capable of producing significant toxicity. These chemicals include metals, pesticides, petroleum products, and salts (such as nitrates).

It should be pointed out that the presence of most of the materials and/or conditions just described need not be serious. It is only when the levels exceed certain limitations that they are to be classified as pollutants. In addition, not all are man-produced. For instance, it is known that some species of ducks defecate approximately 12 ounces each day. If a large number are in residence near a small lake, it becomes obvious that nutrient levels will be excessive.

In terms of human influence on water quality, several of our activities are major contributors to high pollution levels. Industrial wastes have long been recognized as significant sources of organic and inorganic chemical substances. Existing regulations limit the discharge of polluting material. Agricultural activities can be responsible for an overabundance of nutrients as well as various pesticides. Sewage treatment facilities have often not been adequate but are currently being upgraded on a rather large scale with the aid of federal funding.

The elevated acidity of many streams as a result of the interaction of sulfur and water has been caused by mining activities. Power plants utilizing water on a once-through cooling cycle discharge a higher temperature effluent than the receiving waters, causing a definite effect on local aquatic life. Highway deicing methods produce measureable amounts of contaminants, and their sources must be identified and cause established.

The effects of pollutants on fish have been comprehensively reviewed annually since 1968 in the *Journal of the Water Pollution Control Federation*. Three critical reviews dealing with pesticides, chemicals, and fish have appeared and are particularly useful.[60-62] Predicting when, where, and to what degree a fish will accumulate a particular chemical is of ecologic and economic importance, and, in cases where litigation has been initiated, forensic importance as well.

The Federal Insecticide, Fungicide and Rodenticide Act (FIFRA), now amended to include nematocides, plant regulators, defoliants, and desiccants, is the jurisdiction of the Environmental Protection Agency. Two major portions of the Act are devoted to defining the classes of pesticides and setting the requirements for proper labeling. In addition, the Act regulates the marketing of these substances.

The Resource Conservation and Recovery Act of 1976 lists criteria for hazardous waste management. The Solid Waste Utilization Act of 1976 proposes that hazardous wastes be managed from their point of origin until their ultimate disposal or storage is an environmentally sound manner. For this purpose the federal permit program was established for the control of hazardous waste disposal, which may be assumed by states with qualified programs.[57]

Solid waste may potentially contain any of the solid materials found in nature as well as many manmade materials. They constitute the most heterogeneous collection of substances possible. Laws and ordinances may prohibit certain materials from being put into the solid waste stream, but these regulations are no guarantee that prohibited substances might not occasionally appear. Domestic refuse has been found to contain many highly toxic substances and disease sources.

Industrial wastes from any one location are usually more homogeneous than domestic refuse. However, the variations of contaminants and properties from one operation to another and from one type of industry to another are numerous.

Solid wastes may be hazardous as generated. They may also subsequently combine to produce secondary hazards. Solid wastes which are dangerous at the point at which they are discarded constitute the most obvious category of hazard. They generally include substances which are toxic to man and/or to organisms beneficial to man. A related but distinct category includes the broad range of wastes which, while not toxic, have the potential of causing injury. An example would be a broken plate glass window. This latter subject will not be discussed further as it is outside the realm of toxicology. However, it is an important and ever-increasing problem which may have a bearing in a forensic investigation.

A wide variety of substances can cause harm or disfigurement either in general or to sensitive individuals. Acids and alkalis are a major problem; although not strictly considered solid wastes, they appear along with other liquid substances in discarded containers. Children have encountered pesticide containers resulting in intoxication and death. Minute quantities of foaming or hardening agents used for plastic resins cause acute reactions in some individuals. Aerosols and petroleum products represent not only a potential fire hazard, but also a toxic hazard if sniffed.[63]

A related category of dangerous solid wastes is that which has the potential for producing disease. Many organisms can cause disease. These are organic in nature and will live on organic refuse. The quantity of organic material necessary to maintain a culture is so small that persons will not be aware of their presence. For example, the culture might be maintained at the tip of a hypodermic needle. The careless discarding of hypodermic needles after use, as into wastebaskets, may result in transferring infection.[64]

When disposed, solid wastes normally are first placed in a container. The wastes are then generally transported by vehicle to a processing stage such as incineration, compaction, shredding, or reclamation. The final product will then go into the environment in solid, liquid, or gaseous form.

During this general sequence of events, nontoxic wastes may become poisonous. Sterile wastes may become capable of transmitting disease. Nonexplosive wastes may cause explosions. In general, wastes which initially had no injury-causing potential may in fact be capable of producing injury and even death.

In the natural environment, especially in warmer temperatures, sterile organic matter such as cooked meat can become a potentially lethal source of toxic or disease-producing organisms. However, the environment is full of bacteria, viruses, and insects awaiting a favorable site on which to multiply. These cultures of potentially disease-producing organisms in solid wastes are generally transmitted by flies and to a lesser extent by rats. However, certain microbes are beneficial to industrial waste treatment. Selective enzymatic degradation of industrial chemicals using specific microbes is becoming an economic and effective method for waste treatment.

Drug Regulations

The Comprehensive Drug Abuse Prevention and Control Act of 1970 consolidated the provisions of the previous laws.[65] The Act classifies controlled substances in one of five possible categories. The classification is based upon the drug's potential for abuse as well as its physiological and psychological effects. The penalties imposed for the various offenses involving these controlled substances are dictated by the schedule under which it is listed.

Drugs which have a potential for abuse are classified according to criteria promulgated by the Act. The Act provides that the Attorney General shall consider the following factors with respect to each drug or substance proposed to be controlled or removed from the schedules:

1. Its actual or relative potential for abuse.
2. Scientific evidence of its pharmacologic effect if known.
3. The state of current scientific knowledge regarding the drug or other substances.
4. Its history and current pattern of abuse.
5. The scope, duration, and significance of abuse.
6. What, if any, risk there is to the public health.
7. Its psychic or physiologic dependence liability.
8. Whether the substance is an immediate precursor of a substance already controlled.

The criteria set forth are used as determinative factors in placing a controlled substance within any of the five schedules.

Schedule I. To be placed in this category, these findings must indicate that:

1. The drug or other substance has a high potential for abuse.
2. The drug or other substance has no currently accepted medical use in treatment in the United States.
3. There is a lack of accepted safety for use of the drug or other substance under medical supervision.

The federal government has defined marijuana as a hallucinogenic substance. This may be compared to those states which still define marijuana as a narcotic drug.

Schedule II. To be placed in this category, the findings must indicate that:

1. The drug or other substance has a high potential for abuse.
2. The drug or other substance has currently accepted medical use in treatment in the United States, or a currently accepted medical use with severe restrictions.
3. Abuse of the drug or other substances may lead to severe psychological or physical dependence.

No controlled substance in Schedule II may be dispensed without the written prescription of a practitioner, except when dispensed directly to an ultimate user by a practitioner other than a pharmacy. However, in emergency situations, drugs in this schedule may be dispensed upon oral prescription of a practitioner. This prescription must be rendered promptly in writing by the pharmacy and filed. No prescription for Schedule II narcotic drugs shall be filled more than 48 hours after the prescription was issued. No drug from this schedule may be refilled. A controlled substance in this schedule shall be distributed by a registrant to another registrant only pursuant to an order form as set forth by federal law.

Schedule III. To be placed in this category, the findings must indicate that:

1. The drug or other substance has a potential for abuse less than the drugs or other substances in Schedule I and II.
2. The drug or other substance has currently accepted medical use in treatment in the United States.
3. Abuse of the drug or other substance may lead to moderate or low physical dependence or high psychological dependence.

Except when dispensed directly to an ultimate user by a practitioner other than a pharmacy, a substance controlled by Schedule III shall not be dispensed without a written or oral prescription of a practitioner. The prescription shall not be filled or refilled more than 6 months after the date issued. It cannot be refilled more than five times, unless renewed by the practitioner. A controlled substance in this schedule shall be distributed by a registrant to another registrant only pursuant to an order form as set forth by federal law.

Schedule IV. To be placed in this category, the findings must indicate that:

1. The drug or other substance has a low potential for abuse relative to the other substances in Schedule III.
2. The drug or other substance has currently accepted medical use in treatment in the United States.
3. Abuse of the drug or other substance may lead to limited physical or psychological dependence relative to the drugs or other substances in Schedule III.

Except when dispensed directly to an ultimate user by a practitioner other than a pharmacy, a substance controlled by Schedule IV shall not be dispensed without a written or oral prescription of a practitioner. The prescription shall not be filled or refilled more than 6 months after the date issued. It cannot be refilled more than five times, unless renewed by the practitioner. A controlled substance in this schedule shall be distributed by a registrant to another registrant only pursuant to an order form as set forth by federal law.

Schedule V. To be placed in this schedule, the findings must indicate that:

1. The drug or other substance has a low potential for abuse relative to the drugs or other substances in Schedule IV.
2. The drug or other substance has a currently accepted medical use in treatment in the United States.
3. Abuse of the drug or other substance may lead to limited physical dependence relative to the drugs or substances in Schedule IV.

The drugs and substances included within this schedule are compounds, mixtures, and preparations containing limited quantities of narcotic drugs and include one or more non-narcotic, active medicinal ingredients so that the mixture or preparation acquires medicinal qualities which are not possessed by the narcotic drug alone.

FRAUDULANT OFFENSES

Fraudulant offenses are classified as follows:

1. To distribute as a registrant a controlled substance classified in Schedule I or II, except by a registrant to another registrant only pursuant to an order form. The order forms are in compliance with federal regulations.
2. To use in the course of the manufacture or distribution of a controlled substance a registration number which is fictitious, revoked, suspended, or issued to another person.
3. To acquire or obtain possession of a controlled substance by misrepresentation, fraud, forgery, deception, or subterfuge.
4. To furnish false or fraudulent material information in, or omit any material information from, any application, report, or other document required to be kept or filed by or under the Controlled Substances Act.
5. To make, distribute, or possess any punch, die, plate, stone, or other thing designed to print, imprint, or reproduce the trademark, trade name, or other identifying mark, imprint, or device of another or any likeness of any of the foregoing upon any controlled substance or container or labeling thereof so as to render the controlled substance a counterfeit substance.

COMMERCIAL OFFENSES

Commercial offenses are classified as follows:

1. For a practitioner knowingly or intentionally to distribute or dispense a controlled substance without proper prescription.
2. For a registrant knowingly or intentionally to manufacture a controlled substance not authorized by his registration or to distribute or dispense a controlled substance not authorized by his registration to another registrant or other person.
3. To refuse or fail to make, keep, or furnish any record, notification, order form, statement, invoice, or information required under the Controlled Substances Act.
4. To refuse an entry into any premises for any inspection authorized by the Controlled Substances Act.

PRESCRIPTION OF NONSCHEDULED DRUGS

The Federal Drug and Cosmetic Act lists the following criteria for classification as a prescription drug:

1. Any drug in a list of named habit-forming drugs.
2. Any drug which because of its toxicity or other potential for harmful effects, or the method of its use, or the adjunctive measures necessary to its use, is not safe for use except under the supervision of a practitioner licensed by law to administer such a drug.
3. Any substance so named as a prescription drug under the new drug provision of the Act as being a component of an approved new drug application.

The third criterion is basically the classification of substances as legend drugs. Significantly, legend drugs are to be dispensed only upon a written prescription written by a practitioner licensed by law to administer such drugs. The law achieves identification of prescription drugs by requiring that the statement "Caution: Federal law prohibits dispensing without prescription" appear on all drugs classified as legend drugs. In addition, if the statement "Caution: Federal law restricts this drug to use by or on the order of a licensed veterinarian, or on his prescription order" is applied, then the drug is a veterinary prescription drug and classified as a legend drug.

Plant Toxins

J. M. Kingsbury has written extensively on the subject of poisonous plants. There is much confusion in the area of plant identification and nomenclature as applied by nonspecialists or by virtue of hybridization. The genus *Cannabis* has recently been the subject of debate as to whether it is mono- or polytypic in nature.[66] In certain localities poison dogwood refers not to a species of *Cornus*, but to poison sumac *(Toxicodendron vernix)*. Deadly nightshade is a common synonym for *Atropa belladonna*; however, this name is often applied to *Solanun dulcamura* in the Pacific Northwest. Moreover, belladonna has been used to designate the *Amaryllis* genus. *Celastrus scandeus,* commonly known as European bittersweet, may be confused with the genus *Euonymus*, also known as bittersweet. The common names elephant's-ear and mandrake have been used interchangeably in referring to certain species within the genera *Caladium, Colocasia, Dieffenbachia, Podophyllum,* and *Mandragora*.

Kingsbury has outlined a variety of compounds produced in, or absorbed by, plants which may cause toxic reactions when ingested by animals:[67]

1. Alcohols
2. Alkaloids
3. Polypeptides
4. Amines
5. Glycosides
    a. Cyanogenetic (nitrile)
    b. Goitrogenic
    c. Irritant oils
    d. Coumarins
    e. Steroids and triterpenoids
       (1) Cardiac
       (2) Saponins
6. Oxalates
7. Resins or resinoids
8. Phytotoxins (Toxalbumins)
9. Minerals
    a. Copper
    b. Lead
    c. Cadmium
    d. Fluorine
    e. Manganese
    f. Selenium
    g. Molybdenum

10. Nitrogen
    a. Nitrites
    b. Nitrates
    c. Nitroses
    d. Gaseous oxides of nitrogen
11. Compounds causing photosensitivity
    a. Primary photosensitization
    b. Hepatogenic photosensitization

It is in this field where the practicing toxicologist can make a contribution to public health and community welfare. The toxicologist may be called upon by the physician, the veterinarian, the poison control center, the layman, or the forensic pathologist.

Many of the most dangerous higher plants are cultivated species which exist in numerous varieties. Those found in any given community will vary according to climate, geography, proximity to certain seed houses and nurseries, and type of agricultural activities. The toxicologist should endeavor to become thoroughly familiar with both the indigenous and cultivated plants of his community.

Insect and Animal Toxins

The Hymenoptera are one of the largest and most highly developed orders of the class Insecta. Included in this order are bees, wasps, hornets, and ants. As members of the phylum Arthropoda, these invertebrates exhibit segmented bodies, jointed appendages, and hard exoskeletons. The venom of various Hymenoptera is a complex mixture of biochemical compounds ranging from simple amines to complicated proteins and enzymes. Because of their painful and sometimes fatal reactions in humans, Hymenoptera venoms are of interest to the toxicologist as well as to the clinician and researcher.[68]

Other orders of insects, some more properly referred to as the class Arachnida, which produce venom harmful to animals by their sting, bite, or secretions, are the Scorpiones (scorpions), Diptera (mosquitoes), Araneida (spiders), Lepidoptera (caterpillars, larvae only), Coleoptera (blister beetles), and Acari (ticks).

Poisonous and venomous animals are widely distributed throughout the animal kingdom. Included are approximately 1,000 species of marine organisms. Like the insects, the animal toxins are complex mixtures which vary considerably in their chemical and pharmacologic properties. Some are proteins or enzymes, while others are amines, quaternary ammonium compounds, mucopolysaccharides, lipids, and saponins. Venoms from animals within a single phylum tend to bear some relationship to each other. This is most obvious at the species or subspecies level and least obvious at the class or order level. Venoms used in offensive activities, as in the gaining of food, have some similar biochemical and pharmacologic properties, as do those used in defense. The toxins from venomous animals differ from the toxins of poisonous animals, even from those animals within the same phylum. Some poisons from one species or genus within a phylum may be similar to, or identical with, those from another phylum.[69]

There now exists no comprehensive classification for venoms or animal poisons. They may be referred to as neurotoxins, hemotoxins, or cardiotoxins, based upon their primary pharmacologic action. However, Oehme and coworkers[70] outlined "zootoxins" for the purpose of basic classification as follows:

1. Protozoa—dinoflagellates (shellfish toxicity);
2. Porifera—sponges;
3. Coelenterata—hydroides, Portuguese man-of-war, jellyfish, anemones, urchins;
4. Echinodermata—echinoderms, urchins;
5. Mollusca—shellfish, snails, octopus;
6. Annelida—segmented worms;
7. Arthropoda—insects, arachnids;
8. Chordata—fishes, amphibians, reptiles, birds, mammals.

Microbiological Toxins

Foodborne disease is an inclusive term for many syndromes. Acute gastroenteritis with sudden onset of vomiting and/or diarrhea and abdominal pain is a condition sometimes accompanied by fever, prostration, shock, or neurologic effects.

Bacterial contamination of food is the most frequent cause of foodborne disease. Many factorial pathogens that are conveyed by foods (e.g., salmonellae, some shigellae, and some enteropathogenic strains of *Escherichia coli*) invade the intestinal mucosa, causing true infection. Others release enterotoxins during growth or lysis (e.g., *Vibrio cholerae,* and some enteropathogenic *E. coli*), or during sporulation (e.g., *Clostridium perfringens*) in the gut. Other bacteria, such as *Clostridium botulinum* and *Staphylococcus aureus,* produce toxins as they proliferate within a food and, when the food is eaten, cause an intoxication.[71]

Verification of a foodborne illness requires the coordinated effort of the attending physician, an epidemiologist, a microbiologist, a toxicologist, and, in some cases, a forensic pathologist. The materials needed for examination may vary between cases, but the following are suggested:[71] (1) leftover food from the incriminated or suspected meal; (2) vomitus and stool or rectal swab from patients (blood serum and feces of patients suspected of having botulism); (3) blood, spleen, liver, and intestinal contents in fatal cases; (4) specimens such as stool blood or nasal, throat, and rectal swabs, or swabs of infected lesions from persons who handled the food; (5) swabs of equipment used to process epidemiologically incriminated foods; (6) portions, scraps, or swabs of raw foods which may have introduced pathogens into the kitchen or plant environments; and (7) when applicable, rectal or cloacal swabs of animals, swabs of animal droppings, or samples or swabs of environmental contacts of animals that may have introduced pathogens into processing plants.

Mycotoxins

Mycotoxins are fungal metabolites which possess toxic properties. These naturally occurring chemical compounds, like the plant and animal toxins, are diverse in structure and biological effect. Some mycotoxins were used originally as antibiotics but have been found unsuitable for therapeutic use because of toxicity. The disease produced by ingestion, inhalation, or other contact with a mycotoxin is called mycotoxicosis.[72]

Wogan[73] has categorized the various known mycotoxins and mycotoxicoses as follows:

1. Only two toxicoses of many are known by virtue of direct evidence of exposure and response to have been caused by mycotoxins. This category would include only ergotism and alimentary toxic aleukia; possibly aflatoxins will be added to the list as additional information becomes available.
2. Some mycotoxins known to be toxic to animals have been identified in human foods by chemical assay. However, little or no direct evidence is available on the extent to which contaminated foods are actually eaten or whether toxic responses are induced in man. This category would include aflatoxins, sterigmatocystin, ochratoxins, patulin, and penicillic acid.
3. A few specific mycotoxins are known to occur in the feeds or forage of domestic animals and to cause toxicity syndromes in them. These agents would present the additional potential risk of human exposure through residues in meat, milk, or eggs. In addition to aflatoxins, ochratoxins, trichothecenes, and zearalenone, this list would include citrinin and sporidesmin.
4. Numerous fungi isolated from human or animal foods can be shown to be toxigenic when cultured experimentally. It is generally unknown whether the potential for toxin production is ever actually expressed. However, in a few instances, specific mycotoxins in this category have been identified (e.g., cyclopiazonic acid, cytochalasin E, rubratoxins, and a butenolide).

There have been many publications and critical reviews on mycotoxins since the early 1960s.[74] The relationship between malnutrition and the toxic effects of mycotoxins has not been established, but there is concern that the two factors may make mycotoxin contamination of foods a particular problem in those areas where protein deficiency is endemic.

The findings that aflatoxins are carcinogenic in nature have caused a few questions as to the effect the Delaney clause may have in the relation to aflatoxins as an indirect food additive.

Since mushrooms are classified as fungi, they should be mentioned since some are more commonly known poison producers. Particularly well known are the deadly *Amanita* and the hallucinogenic *Psilocybe*. Although mushroom consumption is increasing, mycotoxicosis from this source is rare. Most mushrooms eaten today are of the nontoxic species, *Agaricus campestris*, grown commercially under carefully controlled conditions.

REFERENCES

1. Sax, N. I. (ed.): *Dangerous Properties of Industrial Materials.* ed. 4. Van Nostrand Reinhold, New York. 1975, pp. 5–7.
2. Doull, J.: Factors Influencing Toxicology, in Casarett, L. J., and Doull, J. (eds.): *Toxicology: The Basic Science of Poisons.* Macmillan, New York, 1975, pp. 143–146.
3. Doull, J.: The Effect of Physical Environmental Factors on Drug Response, in Hayes, W. J. (ed.): *Essays in Toxicology.* Academic Press, New York, 1972.
4. Pinto, S. S., and Nelson, K. W.: Arsenic Toxicology and Industrial Exposure. Ann. Rev. Pharmacol. Toxicol. 16:95–100, 1976.
5. Comstock, E. G.: Clinical Toxicology, in Casarett, L. J., and Doull, J. (eds.): *Toxicology: The Basic Science of Poisons.* Macmillan, New York, 1975, p. 657.
6. Hayes, W. J., Jr.: *Toxicology of Pesticides.* Williams & Wilkins, Baltimore, 1975, pp. 6–8.

7. Smyth, H. F., Jr.: Industrial Toxicology, in Caserett, L. J., and Doull, J. (eds.): *Toxicology: The Basic Science of Poisons.* Macmillan, New York, 1975, pp. 683–684.
8. Oehme, F. W.: Veterinary Toxicology, in Casarett, L. J., and Doull, J. (eds.): *The Basic Science of Poisons.* Macmillan, New York, 1975, pp. 701–705.
9. Radeleff, R. D.: *Veterinary Toxicology.* Lea & Febiger, Philadelphia, 1964, pp. 29–31.
10. Scarne, J.: *Scarne's New Complete Guide to Gambling.* Simon & Schuster, New York, 1974, pp. 63–66.
11. Corley, R. N., and Robert, W. J.: *Principles of Business Law.* ed. 10. Prentice-Hall, Englewood Cliffs, N.J., 1975, pp. 629–631.
12. Ibid., pp. 803–805.
13. Weisburger, E. K.: Industrial Cancer Risks, in Sax, N. I. (ed.): *Dangerous Properties of Industrial Materials.* ed. 4. Van Nostrand Reinhold, New York, 1975, pp. 274–278.
14. Benitz, K. F.: Measurement of Chronic Toxicity, in Paget, G. E. (ed.): *Methods in Toxicology.* F. A. Davis, Philadelphia, 1970.
15. Magee, P. N.: Tests for Carcinogenic Potential, in Paget, G. E. (ed.): *Methods in Toxicology.* F. A. Davis, Philadelphia, 1970.
16. Weisburger, J. H., and Weisburger, E. K.: Tests for Chemical Carcinogens, in Busch, H. (ed.): *Methods in Cancer Research.* vol. 1. Academic Press, New York, 1967, pp. 307–398.
17. *Federal Register,* 32 F. R. 11322, August 4, 1967.
18. Goldsmith, J. R.: in Stern, A. S. (ed.): *Air Pollution.* ed. 2. Academic Press, New York, 1968, pp. 547–615.
19. Bates, D. V.: Air Pollutants and the Human Lung. *Am. Rev. Respir. Dis.* 105:1–13, 1972.
20. Lillington, G. A., cited in McKee, W. (ed.): *Environmental Problems in Medicine.* Charles C Thomas, Springfield, Ill., 1974, pp. 314–324.
21. Goldstein, E.: Reevaluation of the United States Air Quality Standard for Nitrogen Dioxide. *Rev. Environ. Health.* 2:5–37, 1975.
22. Ramirez, J., and Dowell, A. R.: Silo-filler's Disease: Nitrogen Dioxide Induced Lung Injury. Long-term Follow-up and Review of the Literature. *Ann. Intern. Med.* 74:569–576, 1971.
23. French, J. G., et al.: The Effect of Sulfur Dioxide and Suspended Sulfates on Acute Respiratory Disease. *Arch. Environ. Health.* 27:129–133, 1973.
24. Tepper, L. P., and Redford, E. P.: *Harrison's Principles of Internal Medicine.* ed. 6. McGraw-Hill, New York, 1970, pp. 1322–1327.
25. Selikoff, I. J., Nicholson, W. J., and Langer, A. M.: Asbestos Air Pollution. *Arch. Environ. Health.* 25:1–13, 1972.
26. Dalhamn, T., and Sjoholm, J.: Studies on SO_2, NO_2, and NH_3: Effects on Ciliary Activity in Rabbit Trachea of Single in vitro Exposure and Resorption in Rabbit Nasal Cavity. *Acta Physiol. Scand.* 58:289–291, 1963.
27. Ehrlich, R.: Effect of Nitrogen Dioxide on Resistance to Respiratory Infection. *Bacteriol. Rev.* 30:604–614, 1966.
28. Goldstein, E., Tyler, W. S., Hoepride, L. D., and Eagle, C.: Ozone and the Antibacterial Defense Mechanisms of the Murine Lung. *Arch. Intern. Med.* 127:1099–1102, 1971.
29. Coffin, D. L., and Blommer, E. J.: Acute Toxicity of Irradiated Auto Exhaust. Its Indication by Enhancement of Mortality from Streptococcal Pneumonia. *Arch. Environ. Health.* 15:36–38, 1967.
30. Clayton, J. W., Jr.: The Toxicity of Fluorocarbons. *Fluorine Chem. Rev.* 1:197–252, 1967.
31. Aviado, D.: Toxicity of Propellants. *Prog. Drug Res.* 18:365–397, 1974.
32. Svirbely, J. L., Highman, B., Alford, W. C., and von Oettingen, W. F.: Toxicity and Narcotic Action of Mono-chloro-mono-bromomethane with Special Reference to Inorganic and Volatile Bromide in Blood, Urine, and Brain. *J. Ind. Hyg. Toxicol.* 29:382–389, 1947.
33. Van Stee, E. W., Harris, A. M., Horton, M. L., and Back, K. C.: The Effects of Three Vaporizable Fire Extinguishing Agents on Myocardial Metabolism and

Cardiovascular Dynamics in the Anesthetized Dog. *Toxicol. Appl. Pharmacol.* 34:62–71, 1975.
34. Back, K. C., and Van Stee, E. W.: Toxicology of Haloalkane Propellants and Fire Extinguishants. *Ann. Rev. Pharmacol. Toxicol.* 17:83–95, 1977.
35. Maibach, H.: Cutaneous Pharmacology and Toxicology. *Ann. Rev. Pharmacol. Toxicol.* 16:401–411, 1976.
36. *Federal Register,* 29 F. R. 13009, September 17, 1964.
37. Phillips, L., Steinberg, M., Maibach, H., and Akers, W.: A Comparison of Rabbit and Human Skin Response to Certain Irritants. *Toxicol. Appl. Pharmacol.* 21:369–382, 1972.
38. Marzulli, F., and Maibach, H.: The Rabbit as a Model for Evaluating Skin Irritants: A Comparison of Results Obtained on Animals and Man Using Repeated Skin Exposures. *Food Cosmet. Toxicol.* 15:533–540, 1975.
39. Roudebush, R., Terhaar, C., Fassett, D., and Dzuiba, S.: Comparative Acute Effects of Some Chemicals on the Skin of Rabbits and Guinea Pigs. *Toxicol. Appl. Pharmacol.* 7:559–565, 1965.
40. Lewis, R. J., Sr.: Labeling and Identification of Hazardous Materials, in Sax, N. I. (ed.): *Dangerous Properties of Industrial Materials.* ed. 4. Van Nostrand Reinhold, New York, 1975, pp. 330–339.
41. Rheinstein, P. H.: Drug Labeling As a Standard For Medical Care. *J. Legal Med.* 4:22–24, 1976.
42. Mills, D. H.: Physician Responsibility for Drug Prescription. *J.A.M.A.* 192:116–118, 1965.
43. Hirsh, H. L.: The Medicological Implications of the Package Insert. *Case Comment.* 82:14–19, 1977.
44. Corley, R. N., and Robert, W. J.: *Principles of Business Law.* ed. 10. Prentice-Hall, Englewood Cliffs, N.J., 1975, pp. 337–339.
45. Davis, J. G.: Food Additives: An Introductory Paper on General Problems, in Goodwin, R. W. L. (ed.): *Chemical Additives in Foods.* Little, Brown, Boston, 1967.
46. National Research Council: *Evaluating the Safety of Food Chemicals.* National Academy of Sciences, Washington, D.C., 1970.
47. Federal Food, Drug, and Cosmetic Act, United States Code Title 21 U.S. Government Printing Office, Washington, D.C., 1970.
48. Oser, B. L.: Food Additives, in Sax, N. I. (ed): *Dangerous Properties of Industrial Materials.* ed. 4. Van Nostrand Reinhold, New York, 1975, pp. 299–303.
49. Painter, R. R., and Kilgore, W. W.: Food Additives, in Casarett, L. J., and Doull, J. (eds.): *Toxicology: The Basic Science of Poisons.* Macmillan, New York, 1975, pp. 555–569.
50. Coon, J. M.: Protecting Our Internal Environment. *Ind. Med. Surg.* 39:420–425, 1970.
51. Mahoney, J. R.: The Effects of the Air Environment in Industrial and Residential Facilities, in Sax, N. I. (ed.): *Dangerous Properties of Industrial Materials.* ed. 4. Van Nostrand Reinhold, New York, 1975, pp. 131–134.
52. Morgan, G. B., Ozolins, G., and Tabor, E. C.: Air Pollution Surveillance Systems. *Science* 170:289, 1970.
53. Ayres, S. M., and Buehler, M. E.: The Effects of Urban Air Pollution on Health. *Clin. Pharmacol. Ther.* 11:337, 1970.
54. Ehrlich, R.: Effect of Nitrogen Dioxide on Resistance to Respiratory Infection. *Bacteriol. Rev.* 30:604, 1966.
55. U.S. Department of Health, Education and Welfare: *Air Quality Criteria for Sulfur Oxides: Summary and Conclusions.* Public Health Service Publication No. 5016, U.S. Government Printing Office, Washington, D.C., 1969, pp. 344–844.
56. Hammond, P. B.: Exposure of Humans to Lead. *Ann. Rev. Pharmacol. Toxicol.* 17:197–214, 1977.
57. Stern, L. S. (ed.): *Toxic Materials Reference Service.* vol. 1. Business Publishers, Inc., Silver Spring, Maryland, 1977.
58. 86 Stat. 816; 33 U.S.C. 1314, 1972.
59. Rosen, S. J.: *Manual For Environmental Impact Evaluation.* Prentice-Hall, Englewood Cliffs, N.J., 1976, pp. 56–59.

60. Johnson, D. W.: Pesticides and Fishes—A Review of Selected Literature. *Trans. Am. Fish Soc.* 97:398–424, 1968.
61. Johnson, D. W.: Pesticide Residues in Fish, in Edwards, C. A. (ed.): *Environmental Pollution by Pesticides*. Plenum, New York, 1973, pp. 181–212.
62. Hanelink, J. L., and Spacie, A.: Fish and Chemicals: The Process of Accumulation. *Ann. Rev. Pharmacol. Toxicol.* 17:167–177, 1977.
63. Wolfe, H. R., et al.: Health Hazards of Discarded Pesticide Containers. *Arch. Environ. Health.* 3:45–51, 1961.
64. Wilson, D. G.: Hazards of Solid-Waste Treatment, in Sax, N. I. (ed.): *Dangerous Properties of Industrial Materials*. ed. 4. Van Nostrand Reinhold, New York, 1975, pp. 237–245.
65. 21 U.S.C.A. 801 et seq (1970).
66. Lowry, W T., and Garriott, J. C.: On the Legality of Cannabis: The Responsibility of the Expert Witness. *J. Forensic Sci.* 20:624–629, 1975.
67. Kingsbury, J. M.: *Poisonous Plants of The United States and Canada*. Prentice-Hall, Englewood Cliffs, N.J., 1964.
68. Cavagnol, R. M.: The Pharmacological Effects of Hymenoptera Venoms. *Ann. Rev. Pharmacol.* 17:479–498, 1977.
69. Russell, F. E.: Pharmacology of Toxins of Marine Organisms, in Raskove, H. (ed.): *Pharmacology and Toxicology of Naturally Occurring Toxins*, in *International Encyclopedia of Pharmacology and Therapeutics*. Pergamon Press, Elmsford, N.Y., 1971, pp. 3–114.
70. Oehme, F. W., Brown, J. F., and Fowler, M. E.: Toxins of Animal Origin, in Casarett, L. J., and Doull, J. (eds.): *Toxicology: The Basic Science of Poisons*. Macmillan, New York, 1975, pp. 570–590.
71. Sanders, A. C., Bryan, F. L., and Olson, J. C., Jr.: Foodborne Illness—Suggested Approaches for the Analysis of Foods and Specimens Obtained in Outbreaks, in Speck, M. L. (ed.): *Compendium of Methods for the Microbiological Examination of Foods*. American Public Health Association, Washington, D.C., 1976, pp. 451–461.
72. Rodricks, J. V., and Lovett, J.: Toxigenic Fungi, in Speck, M. L. (ed.): *Compendium of Methods for the Microbiological Examination of Foods*. American Public Health Association, Washington, D.C., 1976, pp. 451–461.
73. Wogan, G. N.: Mycotoxins. *Ann. Rev. Pharmacol.* 15:437–451, 1975.
74. Rodricks, J. V., (ed.): Mycotoxins and Other Fungal Related Food Problems, in Gould, R. F. (ed.): *Advances in Chemistry*. American Chemical Society, Washington, D.C., 1976.

CHAPTER 49

Charles S. Hirsch is Director of Forensic Pathology at the Hamilton County Institute of Forensic Medicine, Toxicology, and Criminalistics in Cincinnati. Prior to assuming his present position, he was Associate Pathologist and Deputy Coroner for Cuyahoga County, Ohio, and Associate Professor of Forensic Pathology at Case Western Reserve University in Cleveland. Dr. Hirsch is Past President of the Cleveland Society of Pathologists and is a member of the Board of Editors of the *American Journal of Clinical Pathology*. He is a diplomate of the American Board of Pathology in anatomic and forensic pathology.

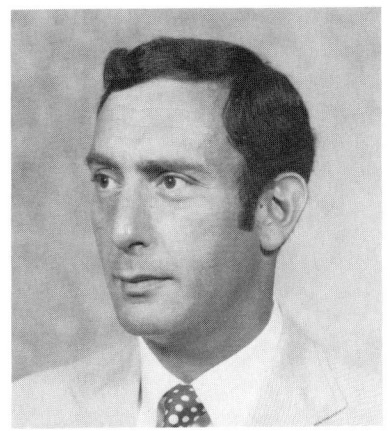

THE ROLE OF THE PATHOLOGIST IN CHEMICALLY INDUCED DEATH CASES

Charles S. Hirsch, M.D.

Day-to-day toxicology in most medicolegal facilities and hospitals involves two different types of professional activity. *Interpretative toxicology* is practiced by the pathologist. He performs the autopsy, collects appropriate biological specimens for chemical analyses, submits these to the laboratory, and receives a report from the chemist. The pathologist arrives at conclusions about the significance of the chemical data when he evaluates them in light of anatomic findings and the available environmental and historical information. The person we call a toxicologist is usually a Ph.D. chemist who actually does the chemical analyses, manipulates dials on the instruments, and produces the data; he practices *analytical toxicology*.

Ideally, the pathologist and toxicologist work harmoniously, know something about each other's business, try to understand mutual problems, and share expertise. Their contributions are interdependent, although their disciplines are as distinct as dachshunds and Great Danes. The toxicologist requires appropriate samples and the insight of anatomical and historical information in order to efficiently focus his analytical procedures. It is naive to believe that every specimen from every autopsy can (or should) be tested for all potential drugs of abuse or poisons. The greater the toxicologist's index of suspicion, and the more specific the information provided him, the greater is his likelihood of identifying or excluding the chemical agents appropriate to the case in question.

On the other hand, the pathologist usually has limited knowledge of analytical toxicology and relies implicitly on data supplied to him by the chemist when evaluating most autopsies. This pertains to the majority of sudden, unexpected deaths due to natural causes, most victims of fatal mechanical trauma, and, of course, all deaths due to chemical agents. Even in nonchemical fatalities, toxicologic findings are required to assist in determining cause and manner of death and to help reconstruct lethal events. Although this chapter deals primarily with the recognition, recording, and interpretation of autopsy observations in chemically induced fatalities, several considerations must be discussed first to place in accurate perspective the interpretations of pathologic findings in deaths caused by drugs.

DEATHS DUE TO NATURAL CAUSES

Fatalities caused solely by disease are classified as natural deaths. When such deaths occur suddenly, unexpectedly, under suspicious or unusual circumstances, in persons thought to have been in good health, or when there is no attending physician to sign a death certificate, the fatality requires some form of medicolegal investigation. Natural deaths comprise approximately two-thirds of the total caseload and one-third of the autopsies in our jurisdiction, figures which probably are representative of most metropolitan areas in the United States.

Factors which bear on the decision whether or not to perform an autopsy on a victim of an apparent natural death include the circumstances surrounding death, the medical history of a disease with lethal potential, and the victim's age. The role of toxicology in evaluating natural fatalities is primarily exclusionary, because no disease renders its victims immune to poisoning and because the anatomic findings seldom stand independent of all other considerations in determining the cause of death.

Autopsy identification of the cause of natural death usually is not a simple matter of finding a single, self-explanatory lesion which is incompatible with continued life. Examples of pathological findings which are incompatible with life include ruptured infarcts of the myocardium, ruptured aneurysms with lethal internal hemorrhage, and spontaneous intracerebral hemorrhages. For practical purposes, such findings explain the cause of death beyond a reasonable doubt, and toxicologic data usually are incidental. Unfortunately, for those who seek pat answers to all problems, these cases account for only approximately 5 percent of sudden, unexpected deaths due to disease.

In the remaining 95 percent, the anatomic findings cannot be competently evaluated without additional information. For example, experienced observers would agree unanimously that extensive atherosclerosis, producing foci of 90 to 95 percent stenosis in more than one coronary artery, is a reasonable explanation for sudden, unexpected death. If a person with severe coronary atherosclerosis were observed by a reliable witness to virtually "drop dead" in his tracks, the arteriosclerotic heart disease would explain the fatality with a probability approaching certainty. However, if the same person with precisely the same heart disease had a history of depression requiring psychiatric treatment and were found dead in bed at home, the anatomic findings might be incidental to an overdose of drugs or some other substance ingested with suicidal intent. Consequently, in the latter instance, the anatomic findings would have to be supported by exclusionary toxicologic studies before they could provide a sound explanation for death. We refer to this as the distinction between "a" cause of death and "the" cause of death.

Another type of fatality due to natural causes requiring toxicologic investigation is typified by epilepsy, a potentially lethal disease which is not structurally demonstrable in many of its victims. Fatal epilepsy is sometimes witnessed, but more often occurs during sleep with the decedent found in bed. A reasonable conclusion of death due to epilepsy rests upon a previously documented diagnosis of this disorder, autopsy exclusion of other anatomically demonstrable causes, and toxicologic study. The chemical data are always important, whether positive or negative. Was the person taking prescribed anticonvulsant medications? Did he take too much? Was he under the influence of ethanol (ethyl alcohol)? Beyond this, the scope of a reasonable toxicologic survey is defined by the person's history, circumstantial data, and the presence or absence of suspicious anatomic findings such as a residue of tablets or capsules in the stomach or acute bronchopneumonia without demonstrable cause.

How much of a toxicologic survey needs to be done in a particular instance is determined by judgment and evaluation of the case in question rather than reference to a standard list of drugs or poisons. Generally, it is reasonable to call a halt to the chemical investigation following exclusion of commonly abused drugs and of substances which were readily available in the decedent's home, place of employment, and social milieu. In the absence of investigative leads which suggest the responsibility of some additional specific chemical agent, further toxicologic studies are little more than blind thrusts with scant likelihood of providing illuminating results.

In summary, a small proportion of sudden, unexpected deaths due to disease are explained completely, without regard to history, circumstances, or chemical studies, by autopsy findings which are incompatible with continued life. Another small percentage of sudden, natural deaths are caused by lethal functional disturbances which are not pathologically demonstrable; epilepsy is the prototype of this class of fatalities. At least 90 percent of medicolegal autopsies on victims of disease show pathologic findings somewhere in between the foregoing two extremes of obviously lethal and anatomically negative. In these instances, the scope of necessary exclusionary toxicologic study is determined by history and circumstances as well as autopsy findings. Finally, in a small percentage of medicolegal autopsies, the cause of death eludes determination despite the best efforts of the pathologist and toxicologist. This is no more than an honest expression of the limitation of our methods and is not indicative of professional incompetence.

DEATHS DUE TO MECHANICAL VIOLENCE

In contrast to natural fatalities, when death is due to mechanical trauma, its cause is incontrovertibly demonstrable by anatomic findings in most instances. Blunt and penetrating injuries can be subtle, but occult, fatal, mechanical trauma is exceptional rather than typical. The role of toxicologic studies in evaluating such deaths, whether they represent instances of homicide, suicide, or accident, is one of helping to determine the manner of death and of reconstructing the fatal episode. The presence or absence of ethanol and other chemical agents frequently is of paramount significance in adjudicating criminal and civil controversies arising from violent deaths.

Whatever the manner of death, the medicolegal evaluation of a violent fatality is incomplete without toxicologic studies. The appropriate scope of such studies varies with a logical consideration of the victim and the history and circumstances surrounding death. An octogenarian victim of a fatal mugging obviously does not need the same chemical workup as a young person who runs naked down the street and then jumps from the roof of the tallest building in town after setting his hair ablaze. As a frame of reference, in our jurisdiction, teenage and adult homicide victims routinely are tested for ethanol, narcotics, and commonly available stimulants, sedatives, and tranquilizers.

DEATHS DUE TO DRUGS

The following sections deal primarily with fatalities involving ethanol and drug abuse. Similar principles apply to other forms of chemical injury, but no attempt is made to provide an encyclopedic discussion of "poisons" in general or of adverse reactions to ethically prescribed medications. In this regard, a poison is defined as a substance (solid, liquid, or gas) which exerts harmful effects by virtue of its chemical action. Adverse reactions to therapeutically administered drugs and chemical substances used in diagnostic procedures run a gamut ranging from anaphylactic or allergic phenomena to toxic damage of organs (e.g., liver and bone marrow) or systems (e.g., immunosuppression).

Types of Drug Fatalities

Regardless of the pharmacologic properties of the abused drug or its route of administration, drug-related deaths can be conceptually arranged into three groups: (1) *primary drug fatalities* are those in which death is due to the toxic or adverse effect of the chemical agent, with or without the contributory influence of pre-existing, unrelated natural disease; (2) *secondary drug fatalities* are those arising from medical complications of drug abuse, such as viral hepatitis and bacterial endocarditis; (3) *drug-associated fatalities* are those caused by homicidal, accidental, and suicidal violence stemming directly or indirectly from activities related to the obtaining and use of illicit drugs.

An abundance of medical literature deals with the morbidity and mortality arising from complications of parenteral drug abuse. However, secondary drug fatalities of this type account for only 5 to 10 percent of the total drug-related mortality, and despite their medicolegal importance, it is unusual for such deaths to become the subject of legal controversy. Primary drug fatalities occur in large numbers and sometimes engender legal controversy when the manner of death is an issue. This usually revolves around the question of accident versus suicide, although considerations of murder and manslaughter sometimes surface in these cases.

Methods of Parenteral Drug Abuse

Parenteral drug abuse takes one of two forms, depending upon the person's intended route of drug administration. Intravenous drug injection commonly is referred to as "mainlining," whereas drug injection without intent to enter a vein is "skin-popping." The latter activity results in either subcutaneous or intramuscular deposition of the chemical agent. Most primary drug abuse fatalities from parenteral injections occur in persons who mainline heroin.

Regardless of the intended route of administration, drugs are prepared for injection in a similar fashion. Illicit drugs are obtained in the form of a powder, tablet, or capsule which the user dissolves in a small volume of water. This is accomplished in any suitable small receptacle such as a spoon or bottle cap. The receptacle is called a "cooker" because it generally is heated over a lighter or match to facilitate dissolution of the substance. Next, the solution is drawn from the cooker into a syringe or eyedropper, frequently with a wisp of cotton serving as a filter over the orifice of the syringe. Most parenteral drug abusers prefer to use eyedroppers rather than standard syringes, because the former are inexpensive, freely obtainable, and easy to manipulate with one hand. The end of the eyedropper commonly is wound with a bit of paper or rubber band to improve the snugness of its fit with the hub of a standard hypodermic needle.

Persons who inject pharmaceutical preparations which are legitimately intended for oral consumption prepare their drug solutions in the same fashion as do heroin abusers. However, aside from its chemical composition, the resulting solution differs because it contains insoluble crystalline debris. Most tablets and capsules contain "filler" material in addition to the active ingredient. Lactose, talc, starch, and cellulose are commonly utilized for this purpose. The proportion of the pharmaceutical preparation which is filler is determined by the quantity and nature of the active ingredient. For example, a 5-grain aspirin tablet may be all or almost entirely acetyl salicylic acid, whereas a tablet containing 5 mg of amphetamine is more than 95 percent filler. Talc, cellulose, and starch are pathologically important fillers because they remain in the tissues and cause characteristic inflammatory reactions.

If the user intends skin-popping, he plunges the needle through the skin in order to make the injection. Thighs are frequent target areas for skin-popping, although some persons bear scars on their trunk, arms, and calves from this practice.

Intravenous needle punctures are facilitated when a tourniquet is fastened above the intended target area to produce venous engorgement. Belts make satisfactory tourniquets, but any encircling band can accomplish the same purpose. Entry of the needle tip into the vein lumen allows flow of blood backward through the needle into the syringe, signaling its location. The tourniquet is then released and the drug-containing solution injected. Following completion of the injection, blood may be aspirated into the syringe and reinjected. This maneuver serves to further extract remnants of drug from the syringe's interior and "verifies" the intravenous route of administration. The primary target areas for mainlining are usually in the antecubital fossae and proximal forearms. As veins become unusable ("burned out"), the person seeks new injection sites on the dorsum of his hands and lower extremities. Some chronic intravenous narcotic addicts are forced to resort to skin-popping because they no longer can find and inject accessible subcutaneous veins.

Autopsy Findings in Parenteral Drug Abuse

SKIN

The skin and subcutaneous tissues provide a high yield of characteristic pathologic findings in parenteral drug abuse. Skin-popping induces foci of subcutaneous inflammation which can be septic, aseptic, or granulomatous. Resolution of the inflammatory reactions causes scarring of the skin and underlying adipose tissue, producing an appearance which ranges from inconspicuous punctate scarring to grostesque deformity. The amount of scar tissue is determined by the irritant quality of injected substances, presence or absence of infection, depth of injection, presence or absence of insoluble debris in the injected fluid, and the person's natural tendency to form scars which can be small or large and pale or pigmented. Hemorrhage is usually inconspicuous or absent from these areas, because vascular perforation from skin-popping is inadvertent and usually involves only tiny vessels.

The dead victim bearing stigmas of skin-popping may be a neophyte to parenteral drug abuse who has not yet progressed to mainlining, or he may be an older addict whose accessible subcutaneous veins are no longer suitable for injections. Allegedly, women are more prone to skin-popping than are men because their subcutaneous veins are not as conspicuous and easy to inject. Tetanus is the only life-threatening complication of parenteral drug abuse which is more frequent in skin-poppers than in mainliners.

Cutaneous and subcutaneous lesions induced by mainlining typically consist of a linear series of punctures over the course of a vein. The associated subcutaneous inflammatory reactions are similar to those in skin-popping but have the added components of perivenous hemorrhage, thrombophlebitis, and phlebosclerosis. Repeated injection of the same vein ensures chronicity of the perivenous inflammation which usually eventuates in scarring and hyperpigmentation of the overlying skin, thus producing the pathognomonic "track" or "tracer" of the mainliner.

Most heroin addicts show a few particles of optically active crystalline material in inflammatory reactions induced by skin-popping or mainlining. However, abundant deposits of crystalline material and resulting foreign body granulomas indicate that the victim injected oral pharmaceutical preparations such as amphetamine, barbiturates, methadone, or pentazocine.

Visceral Changes in Parenteral Drug Abuse

The most common internal pathologic changes from parenteral drug abuse consist of hepatic lymphadenopathy and hepatic portal triaditis. Enlarged lymph nodes at the porta hepatis, adjacent to the common bile duct, and at the pylorus of the stomach frequently measure 3 to 4 cm in greatest dimension. Microscopically, such lymph nodes show nonspecific hyperplasia. Dense lymphocytic infiltrates involve all or almost all of the portal triads, with or without parenchymal pathologic stigmas of viral hepatitis. The hepatic and lymph node alterations are present in most, if not all, persons who chronically practice parenteral drug abuse. However, in and of themselves, these findings are not diagnostic of parenteral drug abuse.

Nonspecific acute pulmonary changes are nearly invariable concomitants of primary parenteral drug abuse fatalities, especially mainlining. Victims who die soon after an intravenous injection show pulmonary edema which frequently is blood-tinged. Ventilatory agitation of edema fluid in the trachea and proximal respiratory passages beats its albumin into a froth which issues from the victim's nose and mouth. Persons who succumb in coma with gradually deepening respiratory depression of a few hours duration may have bronchopneumonia, with or without aspiration of gastric content.

The person who mainlines oral pharmaceutical agents induces highly characteristic pulmonary lesions because each intravenous injection produces a shower of insoluble microcrystalline emboli. The crystals lodge in pulmonary capillaries, eliciting a foreign body, granulomatous reaction. Such granulomas erode the walls of capillaries and coalesce, thereby forming larger and larger granulomas. In extreme instances the lungs have a multinodular, gritty texture, and microscopic examination under polarized light discloses enormous quantities of talc, starch, or cellulose in these lesions. Pulmonary hypertension with right ventricular cardiac hypertrophy (cor pulmonale) is a sequel of extensive microcrystalline pulmonary emboli.

Less common visceral complications of parenteral drug abuse include bacterial endocarditis, which can involve the right or left side of the heart. In the latter instance, septic emboli can lodge in virtually any organ. Cerebral lesions can be localized phenomena, produced by emboli, or can take the form of nonspecific anoxic encephalopathy as a complication of respiratory or circulatory insufficiency following an overdose of, or adverse reaction to, intravenously injected drugs. In rare instances drug abusers transmit malaria and syphilis when they share their paraphernalia.

Drug Ingestion and Inhalation

Characteristic physical signs and pathologic alterations are usually absent when chemical substances are taken orally, smoked, or inhaled ("snorted"). Repeated inhalation of cocaine over a prolonged period causes perforation of the nasal septum in rare instances.

Occasionally the victim of a fatal drug ingestion shows vomitus containing particles of pills or the telltale residue of capsules. Usually, however, such material is observed only in the gastric content. The physical appearance of gastric content in these situations is determined by the color of capsules or tablets consumed, the amount of drug ingested, the decedent's survival interval, and the presence or absence of food. Ingested drugs do not produce gross or microscopic pathologic changes in the stomach unless an undigested bolus of material rests on the gastric mucosa for a prolonged period, in which case it can cause an ulcer. Such a bolus can persist for days in a comatose patient. However, even without a drug bolus, microscopic examination of a sample of stomach under polarized light commonly shows particles of optically active material adherent to the gastric mucosa. Quantitative as well as qualitative analysis of gastric content can help considerably in determining both cause and manner of death.

CASE

A 43-year-old woman with a history of despondency was found dead in bed. Autopsy disclosed no anatomic cause of death. Toxicologic examination showed that her blood contained a toxic but ordinarily sublethal concentration of a sedative. No other chemical agent could be identified. One's doubts about the adequacy of the chemical findings to explain death could be eradicated by knowing that her stomach contained 2 gm of the sedative drug. Furthermore, if the drug had been available to the decedent in the form of 100-mg capsules, the presence of 20 times that amount in the gastric content indicates that she died from the drug ingestion and that the fatality resulted from an intentional self-destructive act.

Autopsy Techniques and Sample Collection in Drug Abuse Fatalities

The autopsy on an alleged victim of drug abuse should always include an examination of the brain and neck organs as well as the thoracic and abdominal viscera. Failure to examine the brain is a serious omission. The cutaneous and visceral anatomic findings and toxicologic data in a drug abuse fatality seldom provide categorical exclusion of a possible intracranial cause of death. For example, intravenous heroin addicts are not immune to berry aneurysms or vascular malformations of the brain which can rupture, causing death which is completely unrelated to the person's addiction. Performance of a complete autopsy provides the most reliable means to establish the cause of death beyond a reasonable doubt and to evaluate the possibility that natural disease played a causal or contributory role.

Appropriate specimen collection is a crucial part of such an autopsy. The type of container used for autopsy specimens varies from one institution to another, depending upon local availability, cost, and personal preferences. At our office, we use 50-ml glass tubes, containing two to four drops of a 30 percent calcium oxalate–1 percent sodium fluoride solution, for blood and urine specimens. We save samples of bile, gastric content, and organs in disposable plastic or paper cartons. In instances of suspected drug-caused deaths, we collect 100 ml each of blood and urine, all of the bile and gastric content, and approximately 250 gm each of liver, brain, lung, fat, and kidney. Each uncontaminated specimen must be placed in a separate container and preserved by refrigeration or freezing.

The sections which follow are examples of autopsy descriptions in typical fatalities from drug ingestion and injection, and contain comments on interpretation of common findings.

GENERAL PULMONARY FINDINGS

Passive hyperemia with edema of the lungs, aspiration of gastric content, and acute bronchopneumonia are common, nonspecific, general pulmonary findings which occur frequently in a variety of natural and violent deaths. Victims of fatal intoxications, regardless of the route of drug administration, usually have pulmonary edema, commonly aspirate gastric content, and often develop acute bronchopneumonia if they lie comatose for more than a few hours prior to death. None of these findings is pathognomonic of poisoning, but the presence of any or all of them should suggest the possibility of a drug-induced death when the autopsy fails to disclose an alternate explanation for their presence.

It is emphasized that the pulmonary findings listed above, in and of themselves, are *incompetent* to explain death. Pulmonary edema and bronchopneumonia do not develop *de novo* as primary causes of death in otherwise healthy persons. These lung abnormalities are common terminating mechanisms of many causes of death and demand causal clarification. In natural deaths, their primary etiology varies from the vulnerability of infancy to the debility of chronic disease or senility, but there always must be an underlying cause.

Similarly, aspiration of gastric content is not a cause of death which competently stands independent of other considerations. A sober, neurologically intact person sitting down to a meal or retiring for sleep is not at any appreciable risk to die from aspiration of a bolus of food or vomitus. Many persons, including infants, regurgitate and aspirate stomach contents in the process of dying (i.e., they aspirate vomitus because they are dying, not vice versa). Consequently, any physiologically deleterious episode of aspiration, whether it be an obstructive, unmasticated bolus of food or finely chewed gastric content, should stimulate a search for an underlying cause. If none is identified, the case should be regarded as unsolved.

DRUG INGESTION

Specific external and internal anatomic findings in deaths due to drug ingestion are governed by the physical nature and color of the pharmaceutical preparation (tablet or capsule), quantity of substance ingested, presence or absence of food in the stomach, and the postingestion survival interval. Vomitus which obviously contains a residue of tablets or capsules in the decedent's mouth or on the face, body, clothing, or bedding may provide an indication of a fatal drug ingestion (Fig. 49-1). Such findings should be described in objective rather than interpretive terms.

For example, the following description might be appropriate for a person who died from ingesting secobarbital capsules (which are red):

> The mouth contains light red, watery fluid in which there are numerous, amorphous, tiny particles of white material. A dried residue with the same appearance extends from the right corner of the mouth across the cheek to the right shoulder. Subsequent internal examination discloses that the stomach contains 300 ml of watery fluid and that a 2.0 × 2.0 × 0.5 cm bolus of gelatinous red and white material is adherent to the gastric mucosa on the greater curvature.

Microscopic examination of sections of stomach under polarized light sometimes shows particles of optically active filler material (e.g., starch, talc, cellulose) adherent to the gastric mucosa in victims of fatal drug ingestion.

When drugs are detected in gastric contents, their quantitative analysis can help establish the minimum number of capsules or tablets swallowed by the victim. Such data are obviously useful in deciding whether or not a given instance of fatal drug ingestion was an intentional self-destructive act. For example, if the hypothetical secobarbital victim previously de-

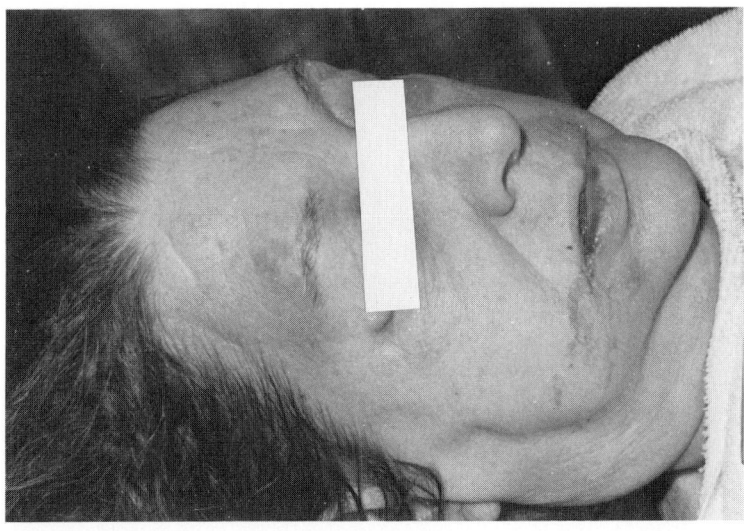

FIGURE 49-1. Residue of capsules at the right angle of the mouth and across the right cheek in a victim of fatal drug ingestion.

scribed had 2.0 gm of the compound in her stomach, one would add at least 20 capsules to the number required to produce the lethal concentration detected in her blood.

One caveat should be mentioned in connection with quantitative analysis of gastric content. Selection of a few suspicious particles for analysis is helpful to the chemist in his attempt to qualitatively determine which drug(s) the decedent took. The gastric content, however, must be homogenized prior to extracting an aliquot for quantitative analysis in order to avoid astronomical distortions of the resulting data.

SKIN-POPPING AND MAINLINING

Autopsy descriptions of cutaneous scars resulting from skin-popping should include a general statement about the size, shape, color, and distribution of lesions. For example:

> The decedent's anterior thighs show numerous (approximately 50), roughly circular, slightly retracted, pale scars measuring between ¼ and ¾ inch in diameter. Incision of representative lesions in each thigh discloses gray-white fibrosis of skin which extends into subcutaneous tissue as deeply as ½ inch. There is no hemorrhage associated with these scars, and there are no subcutaneous abscesses. In addition, each thigh shows a few poorly circumscribed, erythematous patches measuring up to ½ inch in diameter. Two of these on the left side have an overlying, centrally situated, tiny cutaneous puncture.

Microscopic description of lesions should note the character of the inflammatory response and the maturity of collagen in the scar tissue. Examination of such lesions under polarized light provides a means to identify optically active, crystalline filler material, which usually elicits foreign body, granulomatous inflammation. Abundance of crystalline material indicates that the person was injecting solutions prepared from oral pharmaceutical preparations.

Linear scars over the course of subcutaneous veins on the arms, hands, and lower extremities are the hallmark of mainlining. The scars frequently are hyperpigmented and have a superimposed series of punctures. Precursors of such scars are simple cutaneous punctures with or without surrounding hemorrhage and inflammation. If the mainliner makes an attempt to sterilize the needle by flaming it prior to vein puncture, a film of carbonaceous debris is deposited on its surface. Some of the carbon is deposited in the dermis during the ensuing cutaneous puncture, implanting a permanent black dot in the skin ("soot tattooing").

Autopsy of an apparent victim of intravenous drug abuse should include a dissection of the antecubital regions, proximal forearms, and suspicious lesions on the lower extremities (Fig. 49-2A and B). The following example is typical of the characteristic external and internal findings in a victim of intravenous drug abuse:

> Each antecubital region and the volar surfaces and radial borders of the forearms show scars up to 5 inches long and ⅛ inch wide over the course of underlying subcutaneous veins. The scars are slightly darker than the adjacent skin and bear superimposed punctures in many areas. Similar scars are present on the dorsum of the left hand. There are no scars on the legs.

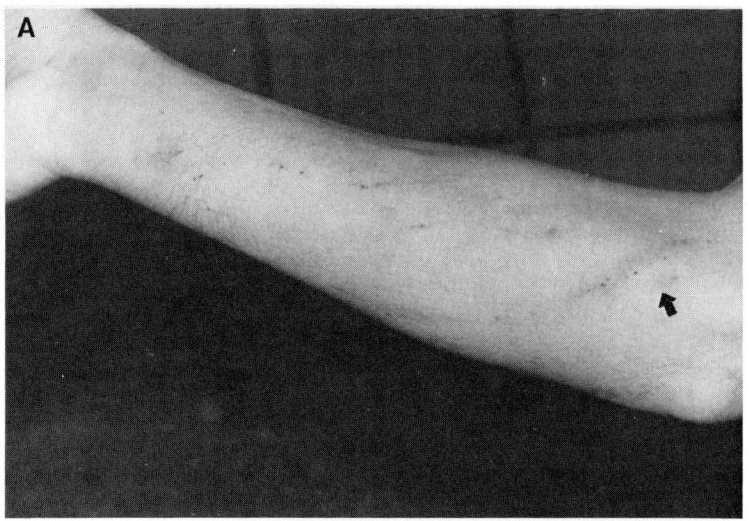
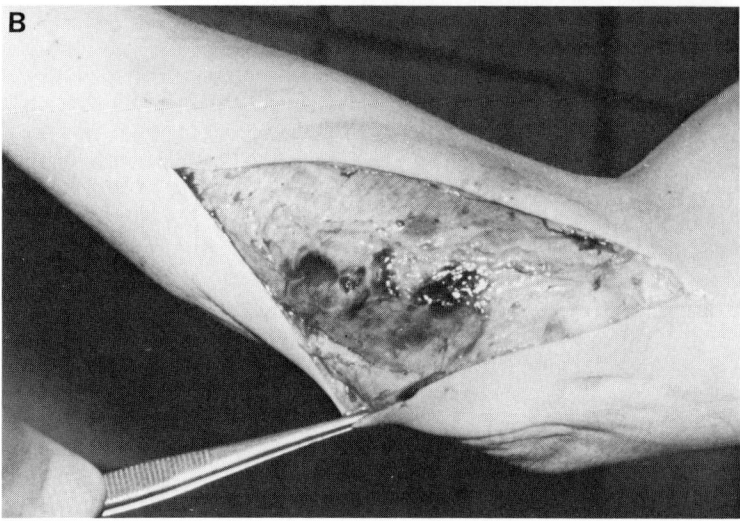

FIGURE 49-2. "Mainlining." *A.* Volar surface of the right forearm showing numerous needle punctures overlying subcutaneous veins. A "track" or "tracer" in an early stage of development is indicated by the linear series of punctures just distal to the elbow (arrow). *B.* Dissection of the same area reveals perivenous hemorrhage and fibrosis.

The flexor surface of each arm is incised from the midbicep to a level approximately 2 inches proximal to the wrist. Skin and subcutaneous tissues are reflected to expose the superficial veins, disclosing extensive perivenous fibrosis and phlebosclerosis. In the left antecubital area, there is a 1-inch focus of dark red-blue perivenous hemorrhage. An ill-defined zone of red-brown, resolving perivenous hemorrhage is located at the proximal aspect of the radial border of the right forearm. The vein in this area contains a grayish-red, obstructive thrombus.

Microscopic examination should include samples representative of the gross pathologic findings. Inflammatory reactions are similar to those induced by skin-popping, and perivenous hemorrhages commonly have

ROLE OF THE PATHOLOGIST

features of recent, resolving, and old extravasations of blood. Caution must be exercised in dating such hemorrhages and inflammatory reactions, because repeated vein punctures in one target area complicate the morphologic picture.

Although most intravenous drug abusers have obvious external stigmas of their habit, conspicuous needle punctures and cutaneous scars are not invariably present. Therefore, the autopsy on a suspected victim of parenteral drug abuse should include a meticulous search for injection sites and dissection of the arms. In some instances there are no demonstrable cutaneous punctures or subcutaneous perivenous hemorrhages.

Typical visceral anatomic findings include the nonspecific pulmonary triad of edema, bronchopneumonia, and aspiration of gastric content; hepatic lymphadenopathy; and hepatic portal triaditis with or without viral hepatitis. Most heroin addicts have a few optically active crystals in their pulmonary capillaries. Abundant pulmonary crystalline emboli result from mainlining solutions prepared from oral pharmaceutical preparations and cause pulmonary hypertension with cor pulmonale.

Toxic and Lethal Drug Levels

Tables listing toxic and lethal ranges of various drug concentrations in blood provide a useful frame of reference and help to place the chemical data from a given autopsy in the perspective of experience (see Table 47-9). However, such tables do not contain "magic numbers" suitable for dogmatic application to individual problems.

At one end of the spectrum, we must consider the effect of tolerance acquired through long-standing abuse of, or addiction to, substances such as barbiturates, amphetamine, and opiates. Tolerance is the phenomenon whereby repeated administration of the same dose of a given drug has a decreasing effect, and when larger quantities of the drug must be administered in order to achieve the effect produced by the original dose. Consequently, some drug-tolerant persons can have high blood concentrations of certain substances, particularly narcotics, without lethal effect. On the other hand, neither ethanol nor barbiturate tolerance produces a marked elevation of the lethal dose.

An individual's drug tolerance cannot be assessed quantitatively on the basis of pathologic changes in organs or in chemical findings. For example, it is reasonable to infer that a decedent bearing stigmas of chronic intravenous narcotism had developed tolerance to opiates, but his degree of tolerance cannot be weighed or measured in objective units after death. In the case of orally ingested drugs, tolerance is evaluated on the basis of history rather than pathologic findings.

At the other end of the spectrum, many victims of drug-caused deaths have lower blood concentrations of the responsible agent(s) than those ordinarily regarded as lethal. Several mechanisms can be responsible for such findings: (1) the decedent may have been unusually susceptible to the deleterious effect of the drug(s) in question; (2) combinations of drugs can interact in an additive fashion; (3) some pre-existing natural disease may have contributed to death; (4) rapid absorption of large quantities of drug can kill prior to complete absorption of all of the substance from the gastrointestinal tract; and (5) normal metabolic degradation of the chemical can reduce its blood concentration during a prolonged survival interval in which respiratory complications and hypoxic encephalopathy maintain coma and act as the immediate causes of death.

In summary, appropriate interpretation of chemical data requires the consideration of autopsy findings, historical information, and environmental evidence. A conclusion that person X died from Y concentration of drug Z must rest upon evaluation and correlation of all of the available findings. No tabular list of data, book, or journal will ever provide an acceptable substitute for the exercise of sound judgment in evaluating the biological significance of toxicologic data in a particular case.

ADDITIONAL READING

Adelson, L.: *The Pathology of Homicide.* Charles C Thomas, Springfield, Ill., 1974. (Detailed chapters on poisons and alcohol.)

A.M.A. Committee on Medicolegal Problems: *Alcohol and the Impaired Driver.* ed. 2. American Medical Association, Chicago, 1973. (General source of information on alcohol pharmacology, toxicology, and testing procedures.)

Baselt, R. C., and Cravey, R. H.: A Compilation of Therapeutic and Toxic Concentrations of Toxicologically Significant Drugs in Human Biofluids. *J. Anal. Toxicol.* 1:81–103, 1977. (Index of therapeutic and toxic concentrations of drugs with extensive bibliography.)

Cherubin, C. E., et al.: Chronic Liver Disease in Asymptomatic Narcotic Addicts. *Ann. Intern. Med.* 76:391–395, 1972. (Various types of hepatitis in narcotic addicts.)

Garriott, J. C., and Sturner, W. Q.: Morphine Concentrations and Survival Periods in Acute Heroin Fatalities. *N. Engl. J. Med.* 289:1276–1278, 1973. (Blood morphine concentrations and pulmonary pathology in heroin fatalities.)

Gross, E. M. (ed.): Symposium on Pathology of Narcotics and Addictive Drugs. *Hum. Pathol.* 3:13–112, 1972. (General coverage of parenteral drug abuse; also contains an article on narcotic "snorting.")

Irey, N. S., and Froede, R. C.: Evaluation of Deaths from Drug Overdose, A Clinicopathologic Study. *Am. J. Clin. Pathol.* 61:778–784, 1974. (General approach to evaluation of drug deaths.)

Kaufman, R. E., and Levy, S. B.: Overdose Treatment, Addict Folklore and Medical Reality. *J.A.M.A.* 227:411–413, 1974. (Complications and artifacts induced by home "treatments" of adverse drug reactions.)

Moritz, A. R., Morris, R. C., and Hirsch, C. S.: *Handbook of Legal Medicine.* ed. 4. C. V. Mosby, St. Louis, 1975. (Chapter on drugs and poisons is a brief survey of the subject, suitable for the nonmedical reader.)

Reiner, N. E., Gopalakrishna, K. V., and Lerner, P. I.: Enterococcal Endocarditis in Heroin Addicts. *J.A.M.A.* 235:1861–1863, 1976. (Infective endocarditis in heroin addicts.)

Spitz, W. U., and Fisher, R. S., *Medicolegal Investigation of Death.* Charles C Thomas, Springfield, Ill., 1973. (General chapters on handling of toxicologic evidence, alcohol, and drug abuse.)

Sturner, W. Q., and Garriott, J. C.: Comparative Toxicology in Vitreous Humor and Blood. *Forensic Sci.* 6:31–39, 1975. (Detection of drugs in vitreous humor.)

Sunshine, I. (ed.): *Handbook of Clinical Toxicology.* CRC Press, Cleveland, 1977. (General source on analytical toxicology which also has therapeutic, pharmacokinetic, excretion and metabolism data on most commonly used drugs.)

Welti, C. V., Davis, J. H., and Blackbourne, B. D.: Narcotic Addiction in Dade County, Florida, an Analysis of 100 Consecutive Autopsies. *Arch. Pathol.* 93:330–343, 1972. (Review of cutaneous and visceral pathologic findings in narcotic addicts.)

Winek, C. L.: Tabulation of Therapeutic, Toxic, and Lethal Concentrations of Drugs and Chemicals in Blood. *Clin. Chem.* 22:832–836, 1976. (Includes heavy metals and chemicals as well as drugs.)

CHAPTER 50

Stanley M. Schwartz is the Forensic Dental Examiner for the Commonwealth of Massachusetts, as well as Associate Professor of Oral Health Service and Head of the Division on Oral Diagnosis at Tufts University School of Dental Medicine. Dr. Schwartz is also a Lecturer in Oral Pathology at the School of Dental Medicine of Harvard University. He is a diplomate of the American Board of Forensic Odontology and of the American Board of Oral Medicine, and is a member of the American Academy of Forensic Sciences, the American Dental Association, the American Academy of Dental Radiology, and the American Academy of Oral Pathology.

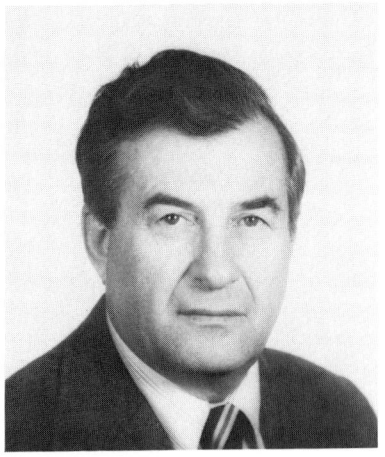

FORENSIC DENTISTRY

Stanley M. Schwartz, D.M.D.

Forensic dentistry contributes to the administration of justice through positive dental identification, encompassing areas of anthropology, anatomy, radiography, pathology, medicine, and clinical diagnosis.[1] The forensically trained dentist or odontologist requires particular expertise in areas of pathology, anthropology, radiology, photography, and a wide range of investigative techniques. The identification of any unknown person is based on thorough investigation backed by extensive clinical experience. Areas of investigation in a given case may include age, sex, race, personal traits, habits, genetic makeup, and medical-dental history. A forensic odontologist can expeditiously assess and properly handle a wide range of relevant dental evidence for utilization by medical examiners, law enforcement agencies, and courts. Charts, radiographs, photographs, and written observations by the forensic dentist may be used as evidence and must be prepared as such in order to be used effectively in court.

The forensic dentist or odontologist is fully recognized in Europe and in Japan as a forensic scientific expert. The specialty has only recently begun to be accepted in the United States, and the number of qualified practitioners is still quite small.[2] In 1969 the American Society of Forensic Odontology was formed. The Odontology Section of the American Academy of Forensic Sciences was established in 1970. Of greatest significance was the organization, in 1976, of the American Board of Forensic Odontology as a certifying board for the field. Currently, however, there are about 40 diplomates of the Board. The American Society of Forensic Odontology has approximately 200 members throughout the United States.

DENTAL IDENTIFICATION: GENERAL PRINCIPLES

Where identification by visual examination or fingerprints fails, due to fire, amputation, or decomposition, a qualified forensic dentist may be able to offer considerable help. A team consisting of a forensic pathologist, a forensic dentist, and trained police investigators should work together for the positive identification of the victim. In cases of mass disaster, such a team effort is usually essential. Stevens indicates that in Great Britain it is routine for a forensic dentist to be a member of the staff at the Accident Investigation Branch of the Department of Civil Aviation.[3] In the United States all diplomates of the Board are formally assigned to medical examiners' offices, law enforcement agencies, or to various branches of the armed forces.

The forensic dentist should be involved in the collection of evidence at the site where the victim or victims are found. Where available, antemortem records belonging to the presumed victims should be collected and examined. A thorough intra- and extraoral examination should be performed by the forensic dentist with the help of charts, photographs, and radiographs. In certain cases it may be necessary to remove the maxilla and mandible from the victim for more thorough examination. The comparison of antemortem charts and postmortem evidence presents many problems ranging from differences in nomenclature to variations in numbering systems. Study of all available data will help to reveal information on the age, sex, race, and habits of the disaster victims as an aid in eventual positive identification.

ANTHROPOLOGY

One of the most important disciplines with which a forensic odontologist interacts is physical anthropology. The well-trained forensic dentist working with an anthropologist and a forensic pathologist can make valid estimations of the age, sex, race, habits, culture, geographic origin, disease status, stature, cause of death, and time of death of the deceased. Skull measurements, suture closing, and fusion of frontal bone halves are some of the facets of physical anthropology which aid the forensic dentist in skeletal studies. Age, race, and sex are the most important areas in dealing with unknown skeletal remains. The site where the body or skeletal remains were found can also be investigated by the dentist and the anthropologist. Site descriptions and photographs are also useful. Brooks describes the mapping of sites.[4] El-Najjar and McWilliams have demonstrated this subject with a typical report to a medical examiner and with advice for courtroom presentation.[5]

AGE DETERMINATION

The examination of teeth as an aid to the determination of age dates from the early nineteenth century in England, when British law decreed that children under the age of 7 were not liable for crimes they committed. Since births were not registered at that time, some means of age determination was necessary in numerous cases involving children. In 1836, Thomason, a forensic medical expert, stated, "If third molars hath not protruded, there can be no hesitation in affirming that the culprit had not passed his seventh year." This statement refers to the first molar of the permanent dentition.

In 1833, Parliament passed the Factory Act, which prevented children under the age of 9 from working and also limited the working hours of children between the ages of 9 and 13. Parents and employers alike tried to evade these regulations. In 1837, a well-known British dentist published a study entitled *The Teeth, A Test of Age,* in which he demonstrated an ability to determine the age of children. His study of 1,000 children concerned itself with eruption patterns. The author, a Dr. Saunders, maintained that the results of his study would reduce the number of illegally employed children.

Forensic dentists can now reasonably estimate age from 13 to 16 weeks in utero and through 14 years of age where the calcification of the permanent second molar usually occurs.[6] At birth, a disturbance occurs in the formation of enamel and dentin. This may be found as a noticeable line, known as the neonatal line, visible only in the microscopic examination of a ground tooth section. If the crown is incomplete, the layers of dentin deposited after birth are measured on either side of the line. Schour and Massler estimate the growth of dentin at approximately 4 μm per day.[7] Determination of the neonatal line is valuable where the question of full-term birth is significant in a particular case (e.g., the issue of live birth versus stillbirth or abortion).

The most reliable chart concerning calcification, eruption, and apex formation was developed by Schour and Massler in 1941, based on the work of Logan and Kronfield in 1933 (Fig. 50-1). The chart begins with the formation and calcification of the central incisors and continues in a regular sequence to the age of 35. Another modification of Kronfeld's work has also been an accepted standard since 1940 (Table 50-1).[8] Although references to calcification date back to 1861, no single method or combination of methods has been found completely accurate.

As the eruption pattern nears completion, age determination becomes increasingly difficult. Guidelines for age determination are hindered for

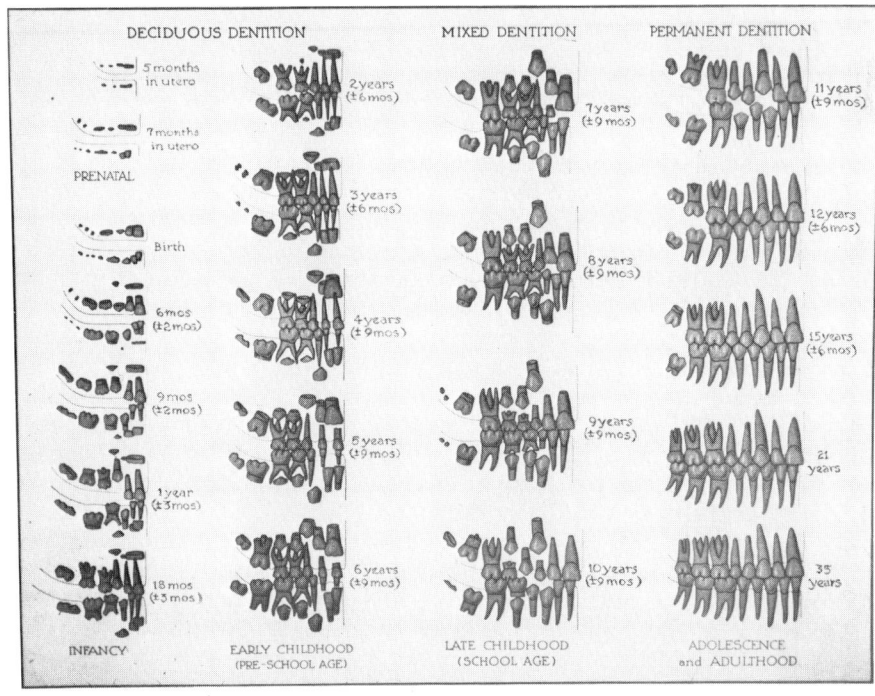

FIGURE 50-1. Development of the human dentition as conceptualized by Drs. I. Schour and M. Massler of the University of Illinois College of Dentistry. (Courtesy of the American Dental Association.)

TABLE 50-1. THE CALCIFICATION OF THE DECIDUOUS DENTITION*

Deciduous Tooth	Hard Tissue Formation Begins* (Fertilization Age in Utero, Weeks)	Amount of Enamel Formed at Birth	Enamel Completed (Months After Birth)	Root Completed (Year)
Maxillary				
central incisor	14 (13–16)	Five-sixths	1½	1½
lateral incisor	16 (14⅔–16½)†	Two-thirds	2½	2
canine	17 (15–18)†	One-third	9	3¼
first molar	15 (14½–17)	Cusps united; occlusal completely calcified plus one-half to three-fourths crown height*	6	2½
second molar	19 (16–23½)	Cusps united; occlusal incompletely calcified; calcified tissue covers one-fifth to one-fourth crown height*	11	3
Mandibular				
central incisor	14 (13–16)	Three-fifths	2½	1½
lateral incisor	16 (14⅔–)†	Three-fifths	3	1½
canine	17 (16–)†	One-third	9	3¼
first molar	15 (14½–17)	Cusps united; occlusal completely calcified*	5½	2¼
second molar	18 (17–19½)	Cusps united; occlusal incompletely calcified*	10	3

*From Kraus, B.S., and Jordan, R.C.: *The Human Dentition Before Birth*. Lea & Febiger, Philadelphia, 1965, pp. 107, 109, 127 (except variation ranges of lateral incisors and canines.
†Variation ranges of lateral incisors and canines from data by Nomata. (Fetal length-to-age conversions were made; no values are available for late onset in mandibular lateral incisors and canines, since all values from Nomata's data are earlier than the mean values from Kraus and Jordan.) Fetal length/age data from Patten, *Human Embryology*, p. 184.

many reasons. For example, eruption has been shown to occur earlier in warmer climates than in cooler ones. Urbanization has also been shown to cause acceleration of the eruption of permanent teeth. Hence available charts of eruption can only be used for a normal child of a particular race, culture, and country. Severely carious or destroyed teeth found in children and adults alike hinder accurate age determination. Changes related to the angle between the body of the mandible and the ramus also occur with age. In children, it is wide; in middle age, it may be almost 90 degrees. When the jaw is edentulous it may become obtuse again. The value of these changes is limited since they may also occur with the loss of teeth, although some changes in the jaw occur only in advanced age or in persons with advanced atrophy. In such cases, the mental foramen is situated near the upper border of the mandible.

In 1950, Gustafson developed a system of age determination using six factors known to change with advanced age.[9] These are attrition, gingival attachment, form of pulp chamber due to secondary dentin deposition, transparency of the root, thickness of the cementum, and apical root resorption. Each of these factors is allotted points, the sum of which is compared with data of teeth with known age. The precise result of this method is dependent on all six factors, as no single factor in itself is a reliable indicator.

In 1957, Clemencon showed that the value of some of Gustafson's indicators of age were exaggerated, and added the value of measuring the diameter of dentinal tubules. Unfortunately, measuring the diameter of tubules is a difficult and time-consuming task. Controlled investigations have been performed using Gustafson's method with results comparable if not identical to those of Gustafson.[10]

Although it is not visible until approximately 30 years of age, root transparency is the most accurate of the factors introduced by Gustafson. The pulp chambers are wide and can easily be seen (Fig. 50-2). With advancing age, the pulp canals are filled with minerals, while the parts of the dentin in which the pulp canals are filled become transparent. The chemistry is controversial, but clinically, transparency is a fact. Before the tooth is extracted, an estimate is made of the condition of the gingivae. Then the extracted tooth is ground down on glass slabs from both sides of the tooth to a thickness of 1 mm. Any bends found in the root warrant an estimation of cementum thickness. The section is further ground to 0.25 mm and embedded in Canada balsam for microscopic examination. These values in combination with the others are calculated on a regression line where each factor is equal in value on a scale of 0 to 3.[9]

Miles has used the same criteria, substituting for the regression line used by Gustafson a multiple regression line where transparency is of a higher value than any of the other indicators.[11] This multiple regression line increases the reliability of Gustafson's method. Obviously the statistical evaluation of more than one tooth in each individual increases accuracy.

Further studies are being undertaken on enzymes as well as on chemical methods demonstrating the increse of mineralization of teeth with age. Nevertheless, at this time, Gustafson's method remains the most reliable determination of age.

RACE DETERMINATION

Teeth exhibit few definite racial characteristics in shape, but many in size, ranging from the larger teeth of the Melanesians, Amerinds, and Eskimos to the smaller teeth of the Lapps and Bushmen. Of course, this is a matter of relative comparison. The shovel-shaped incisor, in its fully developed form, is almost specifically confined to the Mongoloid population (Fig. 50-3). Three major subspecies are recognized: Caucasoids, Negroids, and Mongoloids. The best data available with regard to racial differences are those concerning blacks and whites in the United States.

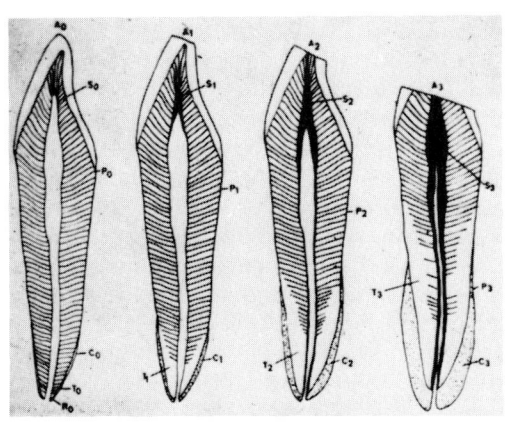

FIGURE 50-2. Root transparency with advancing age. (Reproduced from Gustafson, G.: *Forensic Odontology.* Elsevier, New York, 1966.)

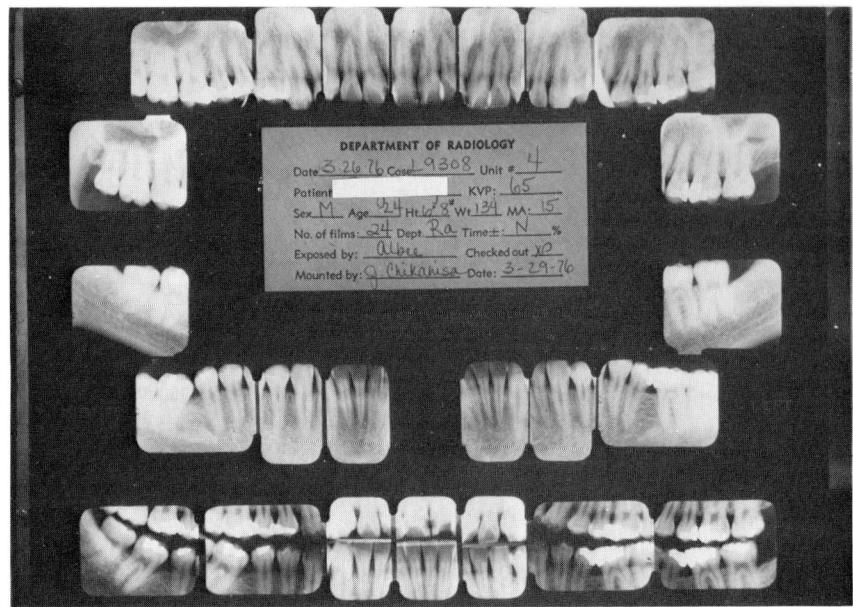

FIGURE 50-3. In a case such as this of unknown skeletal remains, if the anterior upper teeth were seen with the radiolucency apparent in the four incisors, a comparison with antemortem radiographs could be made.

Even for the most skilled physical anthropologist, the remains of a mandible exclusive of teeth are not diagnostic. The skull, however, may be diagnosed with 85 to 90 percent accuracy via morphology and morphometry, and increased to 90 percent via discriminant analysis.

PERSONAL HABITS

One of the most easily recognizable habits with regard to the dentition is smoking. Cigarette smoke marks mainly the lingual (inner) surface of the upper anterior teeth (Fig. 50-4). Pipe smokers are also said to develop oval-shaped notches on the occlusal (biting) surfaces from clenching the pipestem. This pattern may also be found in people who chew cigarette holders. Loss of tooth structure involving the incisal edge may be common to seamstresses, carpenters, cobblers, and others who hold nails or pins between their teeth, as well as to women who open bobby pins with their teeth. Sandblasters and stonemasons suffer abrasions on the labial or occlusal surfaces of their teeth. Musicians may alter the position of their teeth due to mouth formations necessary for playing instruments. This is also true of persons who consume excessive amounts of citrus fruit juices or carbonated drinks (Fig. 50-5). Careful observation of the victim's teeth may reveal the tendency to be right- or left-handed. Dental characteristics regarding diet, occupation, and caliber of dental work may yield information as to the victim's socioeconomic status and possibly his area of residence. The presence of wear facets and carious or restored lesions on the buccal or lingual surfaces of certain teeth may show the wear of removable appliances which may not have been found at the scene. Mutilation of teeth by filing and inlaying with precious metals or stones, not done professionally, may indicate a tribal custom or a cultural

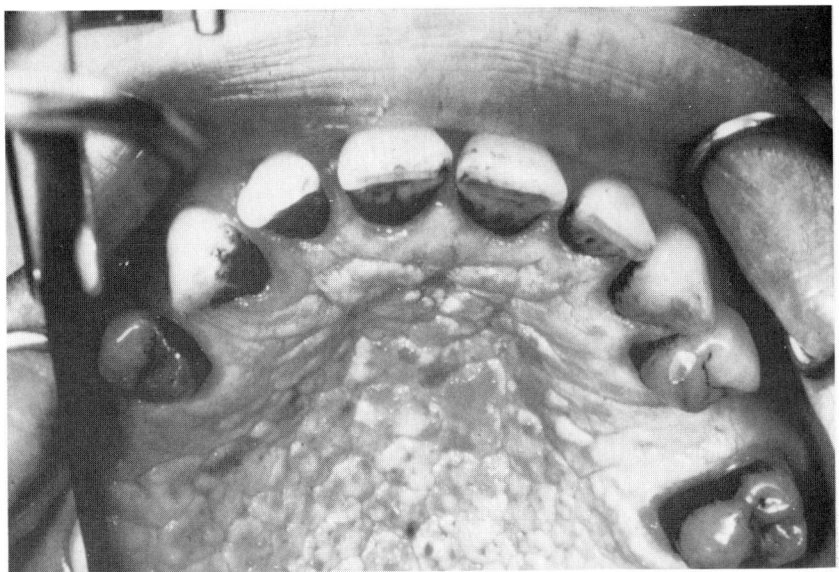

FIGURE 50-4. The palate and inner (palatal) surfaces of the upper anterior teeth, showing tobacco stains caused by the insertion of the lit end of cigarettes into the mouth, a practice known as "reverse smoking." The palate itself has become almost "cooked."

peculiarity. Loss of teeth by brutal methods in puberty or fertility rites or as a symbol of status is also significant. Skulls found in areas of the United States where ancient peoples lived can usually be differentiated from modern skulls by studying nutritional wear patterns, pathology, and anthropometrics.

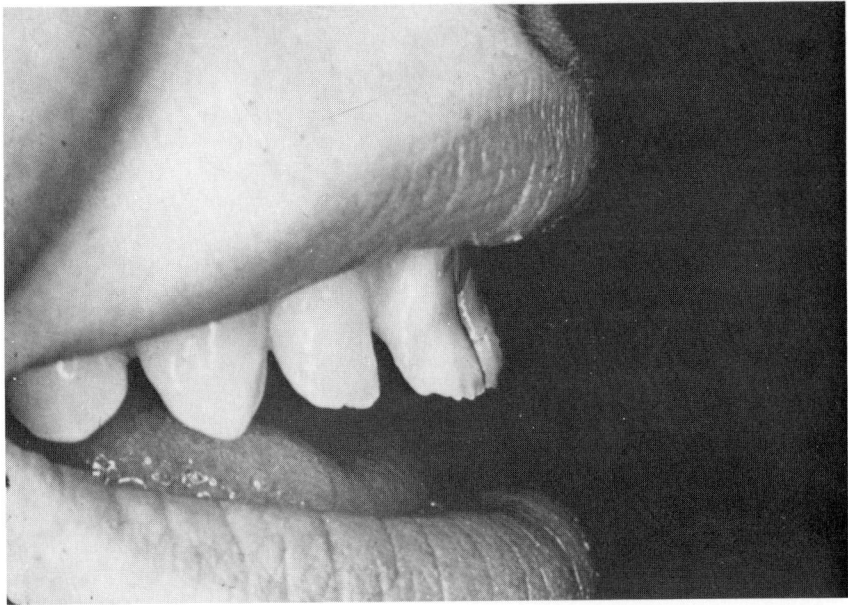

FIGURE 50-5. The teeth of a woman with a history of sucking on lemons. This practice succeeded in dissolving the enamel structure of the two central incisors.

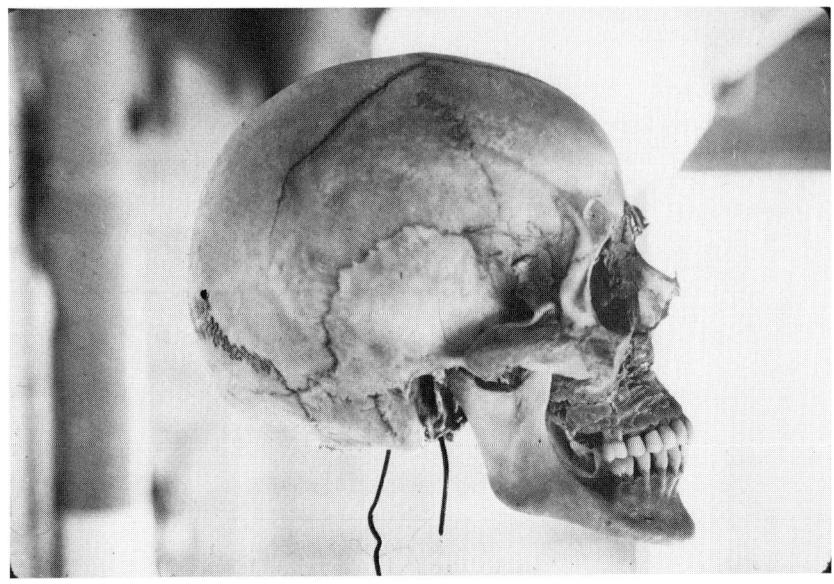

FIGURE 50-6. The skull of an unknown woman found murdered in Provincetown, Massachusetts, in July 1974, and still unidentified. The supraorbital margins, mastoid process, and occipital line are less prominent than in the comparable male skull shown in Figure 50-7.

SEX DETERMINATION

In cases where the full skeleton of the victim is preserved, the determination of sex does not require the expertise of a forensic dentist. The determination of sex by the skull alone, however, is extremely difficult and is basically a matter of relative comparison and anthropometrics (Figs. 50-6 and 50-7).[12]

At the present time the physical anthropologist can successfully determine sex from the skull with 90 percent accuracy, using one of two meth-

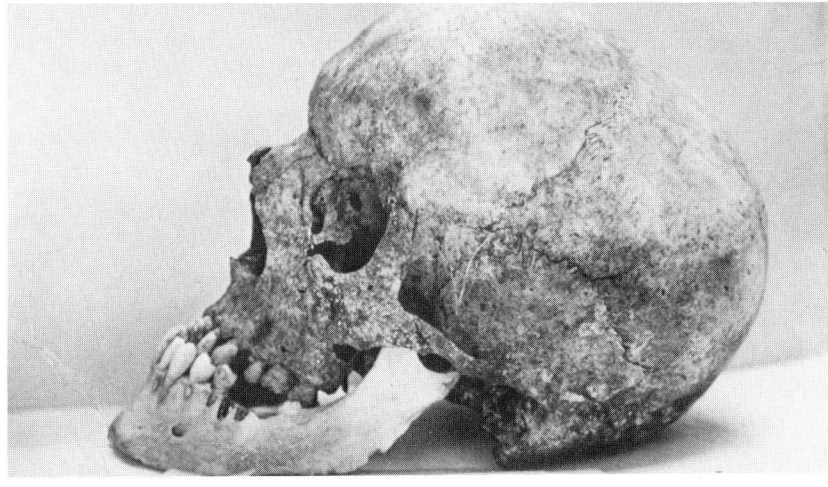

FIGURE 50-7. A male skull showing a prominent mastoid process, supraorbital ridge, and mandible.

ods: descriptive morphology, and mensurational morphology which involves either measurement and proportion or statistical evaluation. A forensic dentist may make use of these methods in addition to clinical experience, radiology, and other measurements. Some radiopacities of the mandible may be associated with the taking of oral contraceptives, thus indicating a female subject.

RADIOLOGIC EVALUATION

It is axiomatic in dental school instruction that radiographs are tools from which dentists can interpret or read results, but not diagnose. For example, one may state that a radiolucent area is seen at the root apex rather than concluding that an abscess is present at the site. However, in forensic dentistry, greater specificity is expected. In comparing antemortem and postmortem radiographs, definite statements as to positive comparison of landmarks, tooth form and shape, bone pattern, and pathologic lesions must be made. An experienced dentist can interpret enough from radiographs to compare such entities as tooth and root forms, restorations, caries, and common landmarks (Fig. 50-8). When restorations are not present in the mouth, conclusions are more difficult, and greater expertise may be required to interpret radiographs. Variations in trabecular bone patterns, stress patterns, anatomic forms, genetic and pathologic changes, and racial characteristics are some of the conditions relied upon for comparison. For example, assume that skeletonized remains are found with a skull but without teeth. Radiographs may be interpreted to show antemortem or postmortem tooth loss; approximate time since extractions, up to about 2 years; and possibilities of pulpal or periodontal disease, in

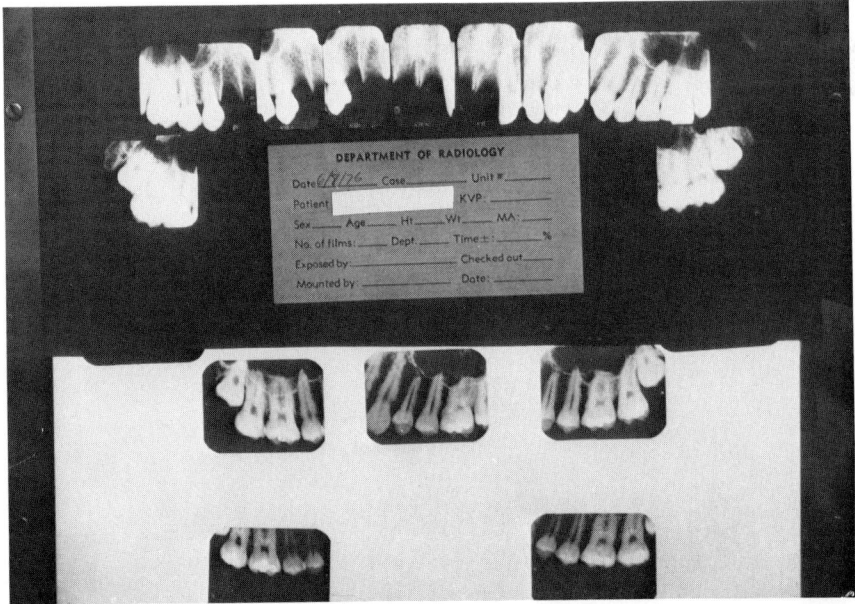

FIGURE 50-8. Skeletonized remains found by fishermen near Gloucester, Massachusetts. Only parts of a skull and upper jaw were present. Police compiled a list of missing drowning victims in the Gloucester area, and postmortem radiographs were made. These films were taken in normal settings; those in the blank area were taken to imitate antemortem films.

addition to evidence as to the extent of destruction relating type of disease and bone reaction to the disease process (Figs. 50-9 to 50-12). Radiographs may also show the possibility of trauma or orthodontic work. Systemic disease such as Cooley's anemia may be evident through radiographs, thus narrowing the field of inquiry to persons treated for that disease, or the possibility that the investigators are dealing with someone of Mediterranean ancestry.

Extraoral films showing anteroposterior, posteroanterior, and lateral views, and all the sinus projections are useful for certain determinations, but since they are taken only very rarely, comparison to antemortem counterparts would be highly unlikely. Panoramic views are more popular, but certainly much less so than intraoral exposures. The value of the panoramic view is shown by Schwartz and Woolridge.[13] In the great majority of dental offices, intraoral films are used extensively.

It is recommended that the forensic odontologist's laboratory have a wide range of radiologic capability. A darkroom with variable safelights, automatic and manual processing tanks, film copy machine, and labeling and storage facilities is required. A portable x-ray machine is desirable, but its use should be confined to work by the forensic odontologist trained in hazards of radiation exposure, electrical shock, and exposure factors. In cases of unknown deceased remains requiring dental identification, complete intraoral surveys and pertinent extraoral views should be performed routinely.

It is fair to state that since x-rays are so well accepted by the courts as evidence, they are the best evidence with which the forensic dentist can deal. This cannot, of course, be the rule in mass disasters. Antemortem radiographs, when available, can be compared since such postmortem problems as loss, breakage, deterioration, color changes, water loss, and

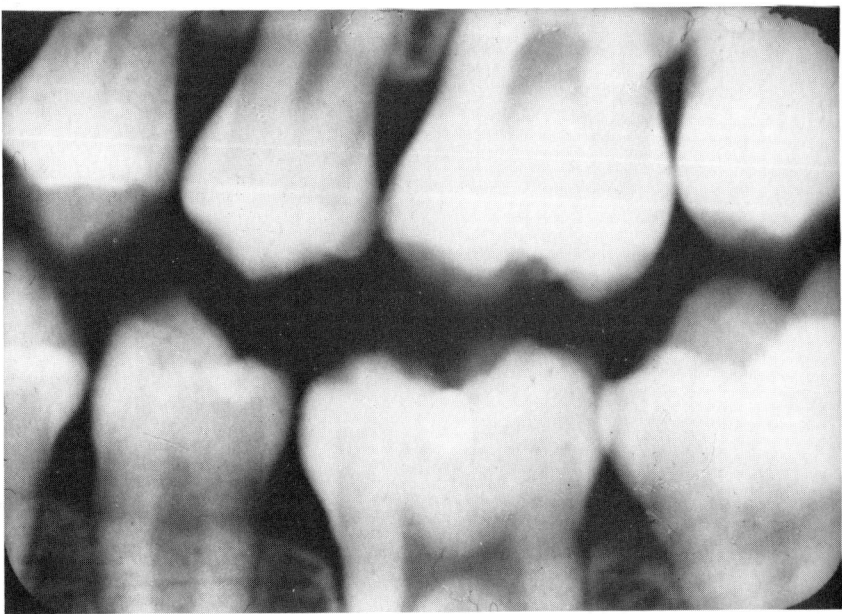

FIGURE 50-9. Left bitewing radiograph. The upper teeth can be compared with those in Figure 50-8. The first bicuspid is tilted palatally, both clinically and on antemortem and postmortem radiographs. Two metallic restorations can be seen in the first molar.

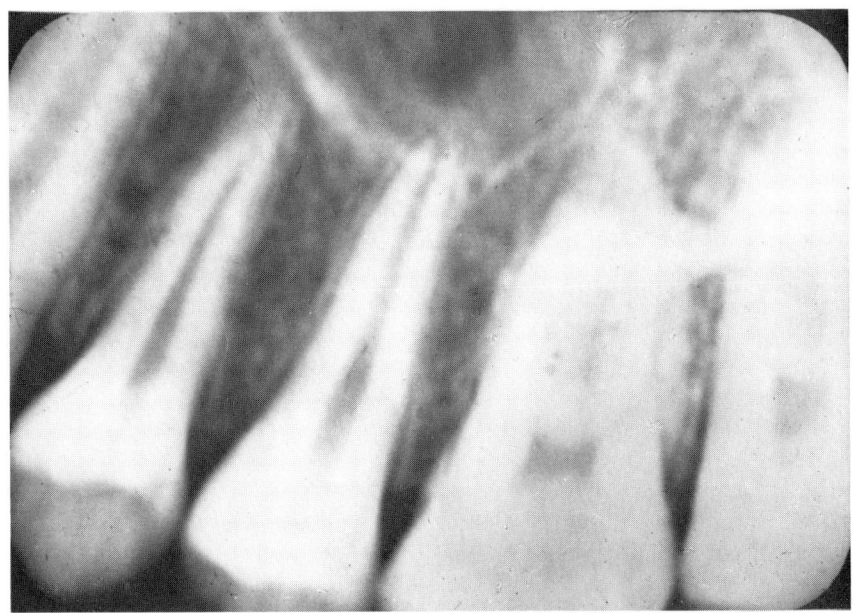

FIGURE 50-10. Periapical view showing a tilt of the first bicuspid, restorations in the first molar, and a large maxillary sinus, all comparable to the postmortem radiographs.

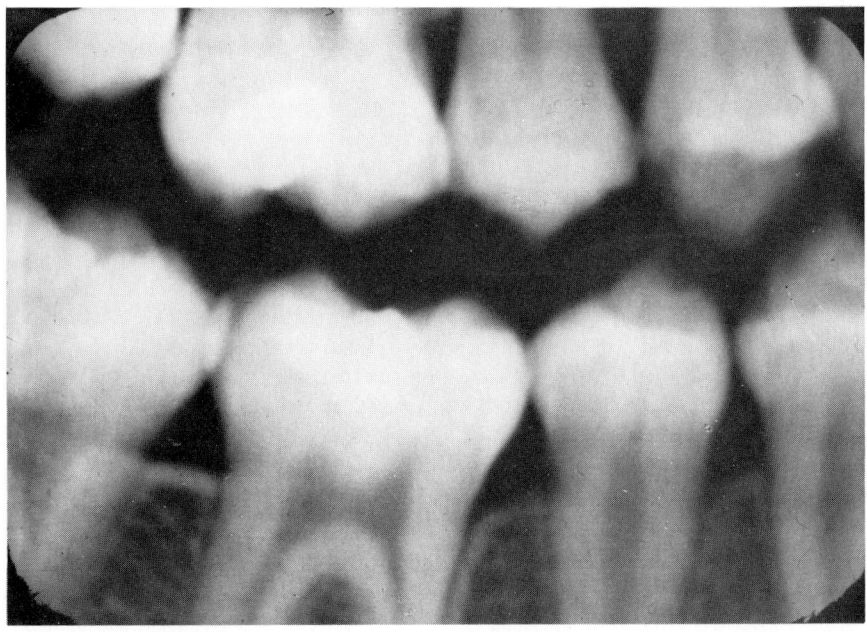

FIGURE 50-11. Right bitewing antemortem radiograph showing a single metallic restoration in the first molar and a palatal tilt of the first bicuspid, comparable to postmortem radiographs.

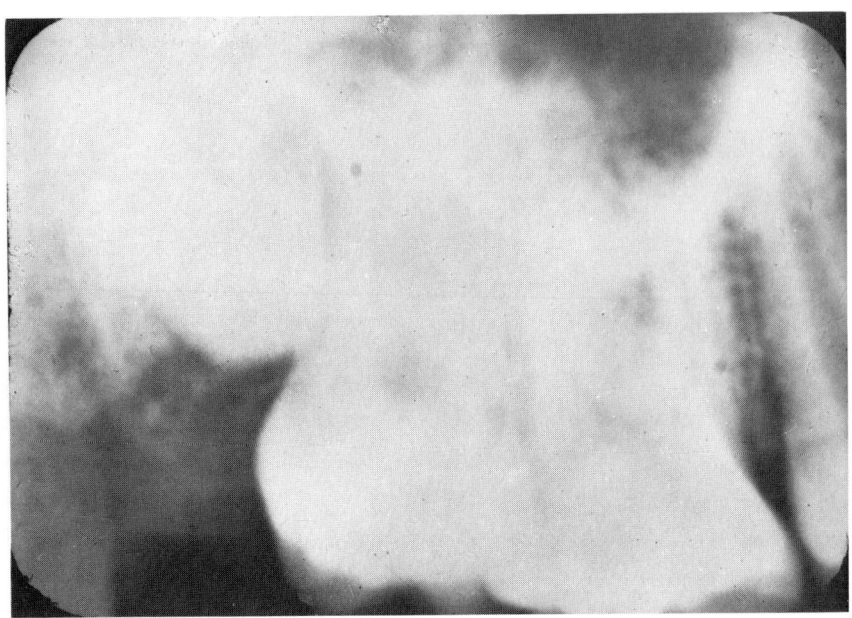

FIGURE 50-12. Right periapical antemortem radiograph showing an unerupted third molar and a large sinus, comparable to postmortem radiographs.

shrinkage will be at a minimum. The previously stated factors can then be compared on the view box side by side or by overlaying one on the other.

In summary, radiographs are indispensable in comparing antemortem to postmortem conditions. Without antemortem records or radiographs determinations of the following are impossible: intracoronal changes or pathology; pulpal changes; pathology; treatment; root variations; the size, shape, position, and nomenclature of certain teeth; bone pattern pathology or variations; landmark variations and foramina; borders; zygoma; and sutures.

EXAMINATION OF SINUSES

A thorough investigation not only of the dentition, but also of the surrounding structures, is necessary in completing the antemortem or postmortem dental examination. The examination and diagnosis of frontal, sphenoid, and maxillary sinuses have been found to be beneficial in matters of identification, although very rarely has positive identification occurred by the use of sinuses alone. The forensic dentist who attempts to include the sinuses in his postmortem dental examination requires extensive knowledge of the anatomy and radiography of the sinuses. Developmental changes and variations as well as regressive changes in old age account for the fact that no two pairs of sinuses are the same. Even the sinuses of monozygotic twins, though similar, are not identical. Rarely are two sides of the same skull symmetrical. Various configurations of sinuses have been classified by type and subtype.

Advanced age brings a thinning of the frontal sinus wall together with an enlargement compensating for the shrinking of frontal lobes. It is well known that the relative geographic position, if not the actual size and shape, of the maxillary sinuses change on intraoral radiographs after tooth extraction in the area. Radiographic changes also occur with inflammatory processes, tumors, and injuries. Identification of skeletal remains can be assured only by comparison, and therefore it is essential that antemortem radiographs be available.

CHILD ABUSE INVESTIGATIONS

The role of the forensic odontologist has expanded with the awareness of the general populace that child abuse knows no racial or economic bounds. All 50 states have enacted laws in response to widespread reports of child abuse. Kempe and Helfer assert that in the United States, 60,000 cases are reported each year.[14]

In 26 states dentists are required by law to report child abuse cases. The dentist who fails to report a case of child abuse is subject to prosecution. The reporter's diagnosis need not be absolute, but he must have "reasonable cause to suspect" that a child's injuries were inflicted by other than accidental means and came as a result of abuse or neglect. Most investigators agree that facial injuries are present in up to 50 percent of child abuse cases. Diagnosis of child abuse begins with a clearly documented history. Any discrepancies or inadequacies must be noted as an important clue to diagnosis. Woolridge cites old, untreated fractures appearing as malpositioned fragments or callous formation, discolored teeth, lip and frenum lacerations, and bruises from falls, blunt instruments, or fists.[15]

Superficial hematomas appear when bleeding has occurred beneath the galea. The hematomas may spread gradually to involve great areas of the scalp in a boggy, fluctuant mass which may extend to eyelids and face, supplying a telltale sign of cranial trauma by the swollen, discolored lids and face. Careful examination, both visual and palpatory, is necessary. Swelling may easily be missed by a generous growth of hair. The appearance of a painless, ecchymotic discoloration in the mastoid area that increases gradually may be indicative of a basal skull fracture. The same lesion may also produce an accumulation of blood behind the eardrum.

In child abuse cases, repeated head injuries are common. However, even a single blow may have serious effects, especially during a period when the brain is developing rapidly. Intracranial hematoma and infection warrant consideration of primary and secondary brain damage. These complications can, of course, be fatal. Shock due to these injuries may compromise the oxygenation of the brain within 1 hour or less. Although this stage may be survived, the brain may still suffer secondary lesions usually associated with intracranial pressure.[16] If coma is prolonged, metabolic imbalance or chest complications may prove fatal, even though the brain lesion may resolve itself.[17]

The forensic odontologist may be called upon in suspected cases of child abuse. He will be basically concerned with the oral manifestations involved. Radiographs are instrumental in various aspects. They may show evidence of deciduous roots forced into developing follicles and teeth driven into bone. Such injury to deciduous teeth may also cause damage to permanent crowns.

Evidence of mandibular fractures in children is often confused by unerupted teeth and the small size of jaws, which limits the areas of bone visible on radiographs. Evidence of fractures is dependent on several details further complicated by definite limitation. For example, fractures may be so oblique that it is impossible for x-rays to pass in the same direction as the line of cleavage.

Upon examination of a child, each injury should be reasonably accounted for and its explanation compatible with the surrounding circumstances. Multiple injuries inflicted by a fall should be in approximately the same stage of healing. Injuries from a genuine accident usually occur on one surface. Unusual burns should be noted and photographs taken whenever possible (Figs. 50-13 and 50-14). Schwartz and Woolridge have extensively discussed the dental aspects of child abuse and their legal implications.[18]

EXAMINATION OF BITE MARKS

The recent introduction of bite marks as a major evidentiary feature in criminal cases brings to light a new approach in the investigation of homicide and battered child deaths. Although bite marks primarily involve the anterior teeth, they may be as individual as fingerprints. They can be found anywhere on the body, though marks on the breasts, buttocks, thighs, back, and arms seem to predominate. Their detail is based on the location and manner in which they were inflicted. From time to time the forensic dentist may be called upon to determine not only to whom the bite mark belongs, but also whether or not the mark was inflicted by a human, an animal, or by mechanical means. In still other cases he may be asked to process information with regard to apparent bite marks on foodstuffs or other objects left by the perpetrator or victim at the crime scene. It is of major importance that police officers be well trained regarding the discovery, significance, fragility, and handling of bite mark evidence, as well as the critical effect of time on human tissue and on the mark itself. The forensic dentist should be called upon for this training.

Levine[19] states that there are two types of marks. The first is the slowly

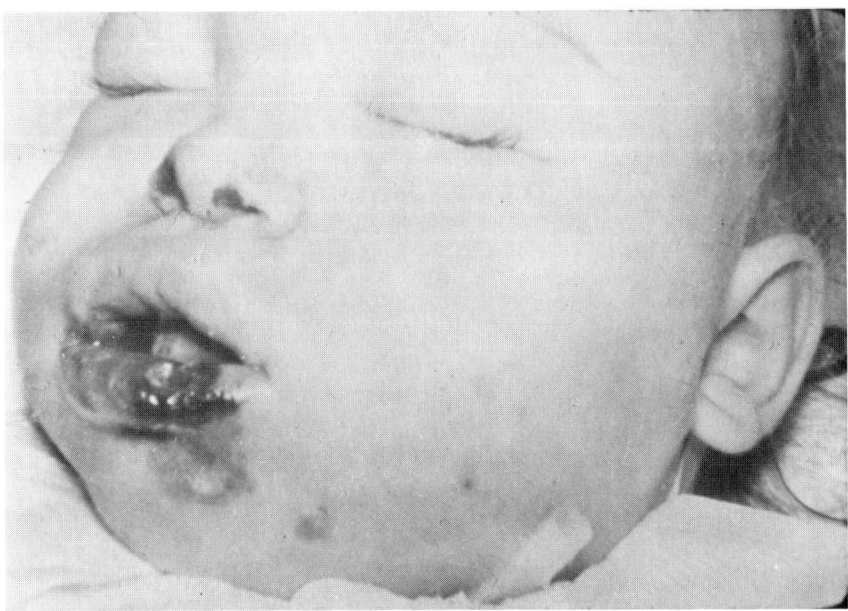

FIGURE 50-13. A 6-month-old child, treated at the Tufts University School of Dental Medicine, who was subjected to repeated beatings by his mother's boyfriend. A cricothyrotomy was performed, and edema and lacerations were treated.

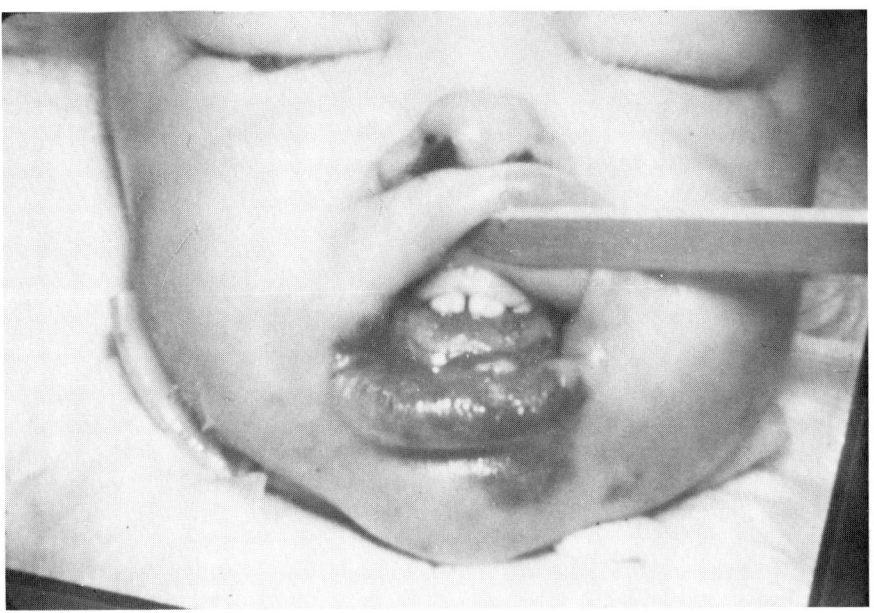

FIGURE 50-14. Another view of the injuries sustained by the child shown in Figure 50-13.

inflicted one with a central ecchymotic area or "suck mark" with a radiating linear abrasion pattern as in a sunburst, most often seen in sexual murders. The second is the attack or defense type most often seen in battered children.

Photographs should be taken in black and white with a 1:1 lens system having the lens as nearly parallel to the bitten surface as possible. A body landmark and a ruler should be included in the photograph for evidentiary purposes. Saliva washings should be taken since most investigators in the field agree that saliva is invariably present. Proof of saliva presence via amylase activity in hydrolyzing a starch substrate is first established. Blood ABO grouping tests are also conducted. Antibodies for AB factors are added for absorption and the elution accomplished with the addition of indicator cells after excess antiserum is washed away. Harvey[20] describes reliable methodology and cites various other useful references.

Impressions can often be taken of bite marks in materials such as foodstuffs, chewing gum, pens, and pencils. Casts can then be made of the teeth involved. If there are suspects, comparisons can be made which may at least place that person at the crime scene. It should be noted that the impressions of the suspect's teeth can be made only with their informed consent or under a court-ordered examination. In battered children, the field of suspects is narrow since the number of persons with access to the child is usually limited. Comparisons can be made via photographs as well as through impressions of human tissue. There are cases in which exhumation has revealed a body with bite marks still utilizable. It is reasonable that dentists, with their extensive training and experience with impression materials, take these complicated impressions.

The bite mark that compares with a suspect's dentition does not, of course, prove commission of the crime. The forensic dentist should maintain his own impartiality on issues of guilt or innocence and testify only on his own expert findings and opinions.

OTHER ISSUES OF DENTAL IDENTIFICATION

The identification of unknown skeletal remains brings into operation the adjunctive investigative capacities of disciplines heretofore considered beyond the province of dentistry. The forensic odontologist has available to him widespread resources in anthropology, pathology, radiology, tool and die marking, ballistics, toxicology, and many other fields. A typical illustration is given below.

A skeletonized body with skull and teeth intact is determined by anthropologic means to be a 19- to 20-year-old white female. Internal and external skull suture lines, bone and joint radiographic and clinical study for growth and development, and comparison to standardized charts for race, age, and gender are undertaken. Size, shape, and configuration of the skull are added to the dental radiographic aging evidence, and a starting point for identification is reached. The dental restorations are studied for manifestations of geographic origin. Unless there is an especially unique type of dental amalgam or tooth-colored plastic, or a porcelain restoration, such remains are clinically nonidentifiable. The use of sophisticated analysis may be beyond the usual medical examiner's office resources, either in funds or expertise. However, a forensic dentist with wide clinical and laboratory experience can at times determine "a school of dentistry" estimate on clinical dental work, such as East Coast or West Coast. He can suggest evidence of industrial hazards peculiar to geographic areas or work places. He can identify dental school treatment and generalist or specialist treatment as well as combinations thereof. He can offer estimates of income or financial status via dental care. The data may provide leads to the provider of the dental care, a step in the direction of identification. A rather nonproductive approach is the publishing of dental charts in dental or police journals. Since dental facilities have numbers of patients totaling in the thousands, it is clearly impossible, except under extraordinary circumstances, for the dentist to effect a postmortem to antemortem dental chart comparison by remembering that he rendered the postmortem charted treatment.

Identification of prosthetic dental appliances such as dentures, removable partial dentures, and orthodontic retainers may seem to be a simple matter. Indeed it would be simple if those restorations were marked. They are not, except in certain circumstances. The armed forces of the United States and the U.S. Coast Guard do mark all dentures with serial numbers and the service branch. Forensic dentists agree that dentures are well preserved in fires, blasts, and drownings, probably due in some part to the insulation of the oral tissues. The first suggestion for effective marking of dentures was made in Europe in 1931, elaborated in Chile in 1947, and at an Interpol conference in South America in 1965. There are several methods in use: (1) engraving by marking the impression; (2) scribing with a dental bur after fabrication, writing on a previously disced surface; (3) placing onion-skin paper bearing the patient's name into the plastic base material on the inner surface; and (4) placing stainless steel with the name typed on it into the inner surface of the base material. The latter system is the most popular.

Pyke[21] observes that the placing of names in dentures may be considered a threat to the privacy of the individual, but proper explanation should help dispel such impressions. There have been efforts to label restorative materials such as on silver amalgam and gold crowns. The use of various marking devices leaves a great deal to be desired when one considers the wear of occlusion, reaction to oral fluids, and chewing habits, all of which can destroy markings. There are also considerable difficulties of processing such markings in dental laboratories.

REFERENCES

1. Gustafson, G.: *Forensic Odontology*. Elsevier, New York, 1966.
2. Woolridge, E. D., Schwartz, S. M., and Riesner, N.: Dental Jurisprudence: An Overview. *Ann. Dent.* 36:81–84, 1977.
3. Stevens, P. J., and Tarlton, S. W.: Medical Investigation in Fatal Aircraft Accidents: The Role of Dental Evidence. *Br. Dent. J.* 120:263, 1966.
4. Brooks, S. T.: Human or Not? A Problem in Skeletal Identification. *J. Forensic Sci.* 20:149–153, 1975.
5. El-Najjar, M. Y., and McWilliams, K. R.: *Forensic Anthropology*. Charles C Thomas, Springfield, Ill., 1978.
6. Miles, A. E.: Dentition in the Estimation of Age. *J. Dent. Res.* 42(Suppl. 1):255, 1963.
7. Schour, I., and Massler, M.: The Development of the Human Dentition. *J.A.D.A.* 28:1153–1160, 1941.
8. Kraus, B. S., and Jordan, R. C.: *The Human Dentition Before Birth*. Lea & Febiger, Philadelphia, 1965.
9. Gustafson, G.: Age Determination in Teeth. *J.A.D.A.* 41:45–54, 1950.
10. Burns, K. R., and Maples, W. R.: Estimation of Age from Individual Adult Teeth. *J. Forensic Sci.* 21:343–356, 1976.
11. Miles, A. E.: The Assessment of Age from the Dentin. *Proc. R. Soc. Med.* 51:1057-1060, 1957.
12. Krogman, W. M.: The Skeleton in Forensic Medicine. *Proc. Inst. Med. Chicago* 16:154–167, 1971.
13. Schwartz, S. M., and Woolridge, E. D.: The Use of Panoramic Radiographs for Comparisons in Cases of Identification. *J. Forensic Sci.* 22:145, 1977.
14. Kempe, H., and Helfer, R.: *Helping the Battered Child and His Family*. J. B. Lippincott, Philadelphia, 1972.
15. Woolridge, E. D.: Significant Problems of the Forensic Odontologist in the U.S.A. *Int. J. Forensic Dent.* 1(2), October 1973.
16. Jennet, B.: Head Injuries in Children. *Dev. Med. Child Neurol.* 14:137–147, 1972.
17. Caffey, J.: The Parent-Infant Stress Syndrome. *Am. J. Radiol. Radium Ther. Nucl. Med.* 114:218–229, 1972.
18. Schwartz, S. M., Woolridge, E. D., and Stege, D.: Oral Manifestations and Legal Aspects of Child Abuse. *J.A.D.A.* 95:586–591, 1977.
19. Levine, L. J.: Bitemark Evidence. *Dent. Clin. North Am.* 21:145–158, 1977.
20. Harvey, W.: *Dental Identification and Forensic Odontology*. Henry Kimpton, London, 1976.
21. Pyke, T.: Personal Identification from Artificial Dentures. *Aust. Dent. J.* 15:495, 1970.

CHAPTER 51

Oscar I. Tosi is Director of the Institute of Voice Identification at Michigan State University. He is also Director of the University's Speech and Hearing Sciences Research Laboratory, and is a member of the Board of Directors of the International Association of Voice Identification. Professor Tosi is a former member of the faculty of the National University of Buenos Aires, where he earned a doctorate in engineering and physics. Dr. Tosi holds a second doctorate in audiology, speech sciences, and electronics from the Ohio State University. He is a member of the American Speech and Hearing Association, the Acoustical Society of America, the International Collegium of Experimental Phonology, and the International Association of Phonetics, and is a consultant to the State Police of Michigan. Professor Tosi has conducted extensive research in voice identification methods, including evaluation of voiceprint technology, under research grants from the Federal Law Enforcement Assistance Administration.

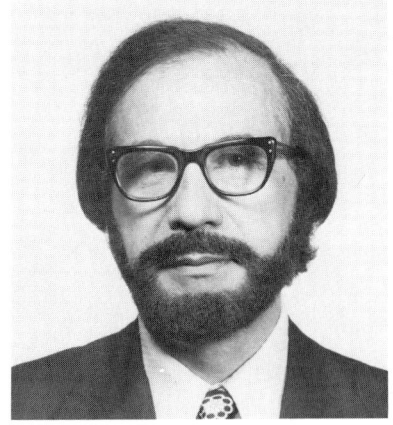

FUNDAMENTALS OF VOICE IDENTIFICATION

Oscar I. Tosi, Ph.D., Sc.D.

Speaker identification has intrigued people since ancient times. One of the oldest reports involving voice identification related to a criminal case of false impersonation is found in the Bible, in Genesis 27:22. Jacob, instigated by his mother, Rebecca, impersonated his first-born brother, Esau, to obtain from their father, Isaac, the rights and assets concomitant with seniority (primogeniture). Isaac was blind and near to death; however, after listening to Jacob, who pretended to be Esau, Isaac stated with no hesitation: "The voice is the voice of Jacob, but the hands are the hands of Esau." Of course, Rebecca very conveniently had previously fitted a fur on the hands, arms, and neck of her favorite son, Jacob. Isaac gave more credit to his tactile perception than to his auditive senses, producing the wrong judgment. A little more credit from Isaac to the reliability of the speaker identification process possibly would have changed the course of history.

During thousands of years people have been identifying speakers through their voices with a great deal of certainty if the listener was familiar with the voice of the speaker. Courts of law in all times and cultures have admitted voice identification evidence as reliable, for what it was worth, in particular cases. Even the identification of a dog through his bark was admitted in an American court in 1861. In this case, *Wilbur v. Hubbard,* the court ruled that if a person can be identified through his voice, the same could be done with the barking of a dog. The owner of the dog, which during the night had killed some sheep belonging to the plaintiff, was condemned to pay damages.

During the many centuries that have elapsed since the case involving Isaac and his sons, no formal study or experiment was done to obtain laboratory data on the reliability of speaker identification. As recently as 1935, the famous Hauptmann trial focused the attention of scientists on this problem. Bruno Hauptmann was accused of kidnapping the son of Charles A. Lindbergh. In court Lindbergh recognized the voice of the defendant Hauptmann as being the voice of the person who demanded a ransom by telephone. On various evidence, a jury found Hauptmann guilty and he was executed. Since this voice identification was one of the main supports for the verdict, controversy was inevitable.

Dr. Frances McGehee, Professor of Psychology at Johns Hopkins University, performed experiments on voice identification designed to bring insight to bear on the reliability of the process. The listeners in this experiment were not experts, and the method utilized was the only one available at that time (i.e., aural identification by long-term memory). In this method the listener stores information on perceptual features of the speaker's voice, such as pitch, melodic pattern, quality, and respiratory group. Recent electronic developments, including the tape recorder, the acoustic spectrograph, and the computer, have introduced other methods of voice identification which will be described in this chapter.

A MODEL OF VOICE COMMUNICATION

Before entering into a description of voice identification methods, it seems convenient to discuss briefly some basic acoustics and theory of voice production. First a cybernetic model of voice communication will be introduced (Fig. 51-1).

Normally, three elements are required for speech-voice communication: the speaker, the transmission medium, and the listener. The box in Figure 51-1, symbolizing the speaker, is further divided into three compartments or levels: (1) the psycholinguistic level where verbal messages are generated; (2) the physiologic or neural and anatomic level where a series of motor pulses are fired to activate the muscular mechanisms of the vocal tract; and (3) the acoustic level where speech waves are formed by proper modulation of the air stream from the lungs. The final product from the speaker's vocal tract is an acoustical wave codified according to a phonetic and linguistic system which varies for each language and dialect.

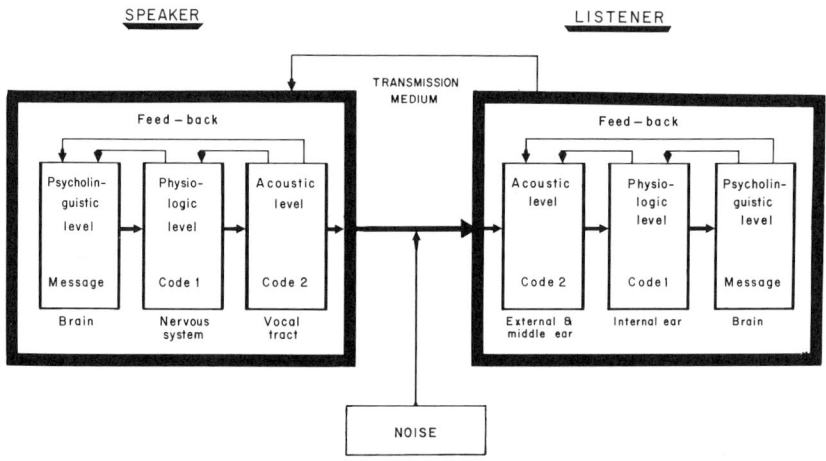

FIGURE 51-1. A cybernetic model of voice communication. This block model portrays three elements of voice communication—speaker, transmission medium, and listener—with the corresponding feedback loops. Speaker and listener blocks are subdivided into three levels: the psycholinguistic, the physiologic, and the acoustic level.

This speech wave (a longitudinal wave) propagates through the medium with a constant velocity in all directions. Eventually, this vibration or speech wave reaches the hearing structures of the listener where the process is inverted in order to decode the original message.

As can be seen from this model, the acoustical signal includes all other levels of speech production in addition to a phonetic content. The speech acoustic signal carries speaker-dependent features that can be used to identify or to discriminate one speaker from another. A critical problem for speaker identification is to detect features that are strongly speaker-dependent. Parameters vary according to the type of method used for speaker identification. Even for subjective methods these parameters are difficult to list. Any listener can identify a familiar voice with great reliability. However, the untrained person would be unable to describe the features used to produce the identification.

METHODS OF VOICE IDENTIFICATION

A description of the different methods that can be used to identify or eliminate an unknown speaker among other known speakers is given below. It should be clear that these methods are not exclusive; they can be used simultaneously.

The methods of voice identification and elimination can be classified into two general groups: subjective methods and objective methods. Subjective methods are those in which identification decisions are produced by the human observer or listener. Objective methods are those in which identification decisions are produced by mechanical or electronic means. Actually, there is a continuum of methods. The aural identification of "living" voices of speakers out of the sight of the listener is the most subjective end of the continuum, and the computer authentication of a speaker whose voice is claimed to be stored in a memory bank of the computer is the most objective end of the continuum.

Typically, all types of aural examination of voices and visual examination of speech spectrograms are considered subjective methods, although the latter is closer to the objective part of the spectrum of methods than the former.

Semiautomatic and automatic methods are considered objective, but the former is closer to the subjective part of the scale than the latter. Whether subjective or objective, voice examinations for legal purposes always require the intervention of an examiner, at least to prepare the samples and to interpret the results from the computer. Computers will perform only according to the instructions and programming produced by a human being.

Tests of voice identification or elimination can be classified into three general groups according to the composition of known and unknown samples: (1) discrimination tests, (2) open tests, and (3) closed tests.

In the discrimination tests the examiner is provided with a known sample. He must decide whether or not both samples belong to the same speaker. Two types of errors can be produced in this test: *false identification*, when the examiner decides incorrectly that both samples belong to the same subject; and *false elimination*, when the examiner incorrectly decides that the samples belong to different persons when they are actually from the same subject.

In the open tests the examiner is given several known samples and an unknown sample. He is told that the unknown may or may not be found among the known speakers. Here the test can yield three types of errors. The first is the error of *false elimination,* when the unknown speaker is among the known speakers but the examiner is unable to match the unknown. The second and third types are errors of false identification which can originate from two possibilities: (1) one of the known speakers is the same as the unknown, but the examiner selects a different one; and (2) none of the known speakers is the same as the unknown, but the examiner decides that one of them was the same as the unknown.

In the closed tests the examiner is told that the unknown speaker is one of the known speakers. Consequently, only one type of error can be produced: the error of false identification.

In the three types of tests discussed above, the examiner may include a confidence rating together with each decision, according to a scale (i.e., (1) almost certain, (2) fairly certain, (3) fairly uncertain, and (4) quite uncertain). These confidence ratings allow the determination of the receiver-operating characteristic described below.

The *number of utterances* refers to the repetitions of the same sample word taken from the same subject. Different utterances of the same word are useful for surveying the range of intraspeaker variation.

Contemporary samples are defined as those utterances of the same words from a speaker obtained during the same recording session. *Noncontemporary samples* are those obtained during different recording sessions. In real-life situations, questioned voices and suspected voice samples are noncontemporary.

Receiver-Operating Characteristic

The receiver-operating characteristic (Fig. 51-2) is a plot of the probability that an examiner will decide "same" when this is correct in a discrimination test involving a scale of confidence ratings against the probability that he will decide "different" when this is not correct. Each point of the receiver-operating characteristic curve represents the cumulative percentage of the correct "same" responses versus the incorrect "same" responses, obtained for each grade of the confidence scale for a given number of tests. Cumulative refers to the summation of percentages of all superior levels of confidence to the one considered at each point of the curve plus the percentages corresponding to that particular level. In general, the larger the area subtended by the curve, the better the discriminating ability the examiner possesses.

To determine the receiver-operating characteristic of an examiner, it is necessary to submit him to a series of tests and to compute percentages as explained. The receiver-operating characteristic of a computer is calculated *a priori* according to the decision algorithm programmed.

It is clear, then, that the receiver-operating characteristic may serve to test the reliability of an examiner or expert witness in voice identification. Rather than try to argue against methods of voice identification I suggest to counselors that they try to establish the reliability of an examiner through his receiver-operating characteristics.

THEORY OF SPEECH PRODUCTION

Sound in general and speech sounds in particular are vibrations of recurrent movements of a body, as for instance, particles of air. The number of recurrences per second is called the frequency of the sound. A human ear

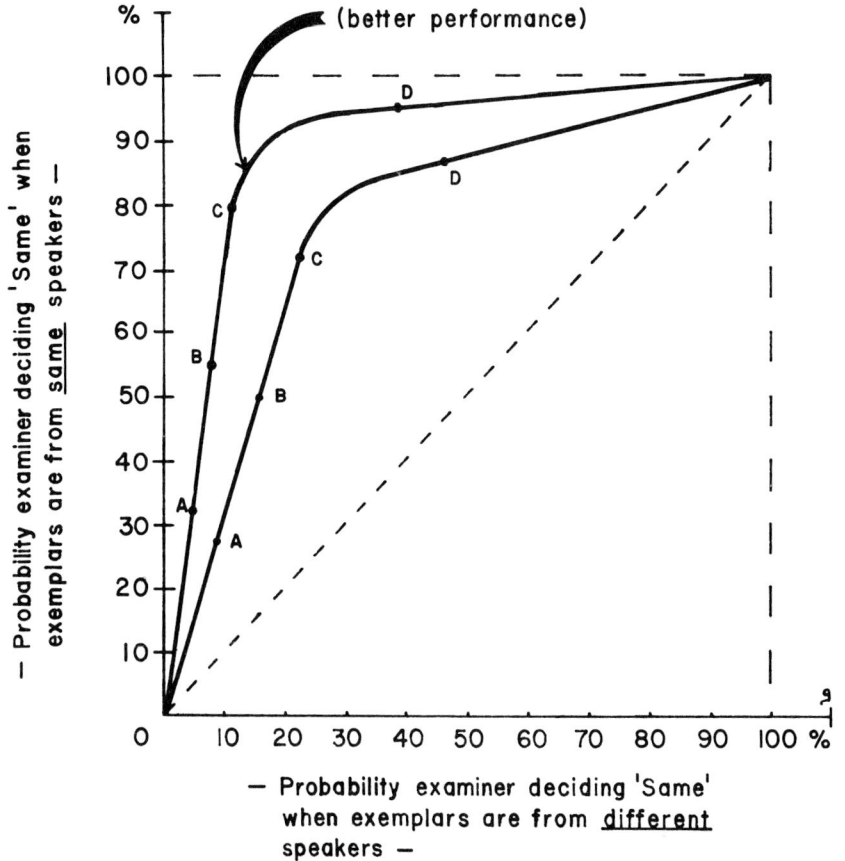

FIGURE 51-2. Receiver-operating characteristic. This curve portrays the probability that an examiner decides same when the exemplars examined correspond to the same speaker versus the probability that the examiner decides same when the exemplars are from different speakers. Points A, B, C, and D correspond to different criteria. The larger the area subtended by the curve, the better the examiner's performance.

in optimal condition can perceive as sound vibrations from 20 to 20,000 cycles or Hertz, provided that the intensity is above a given threshold. The frequency range of speech extends from approximately 100 to 7,000 Hz. The different quality of the sounds depends on a characteristic called spectrum. Since the concept of spectrum is so closely related to the speaker-dependent features of speech, a discussion on sound spectra follows.

Sound Spectra

Sounds can be classified into two groups: simple and complex. A simple sound is produced by a recurrent movement of a body (i.e., a particle of air), called simple harmonic motion (SHM). This SHM is depicted by a sinusoidal wave in a time domain plot, that is, in a graph in which time is plotted on the horizontal axis. On the verticle-axis intensity, amplitude or other parameters of sound can be plotted. The same type of vibration can be expressed in the frequency domain, rather than in the temporal

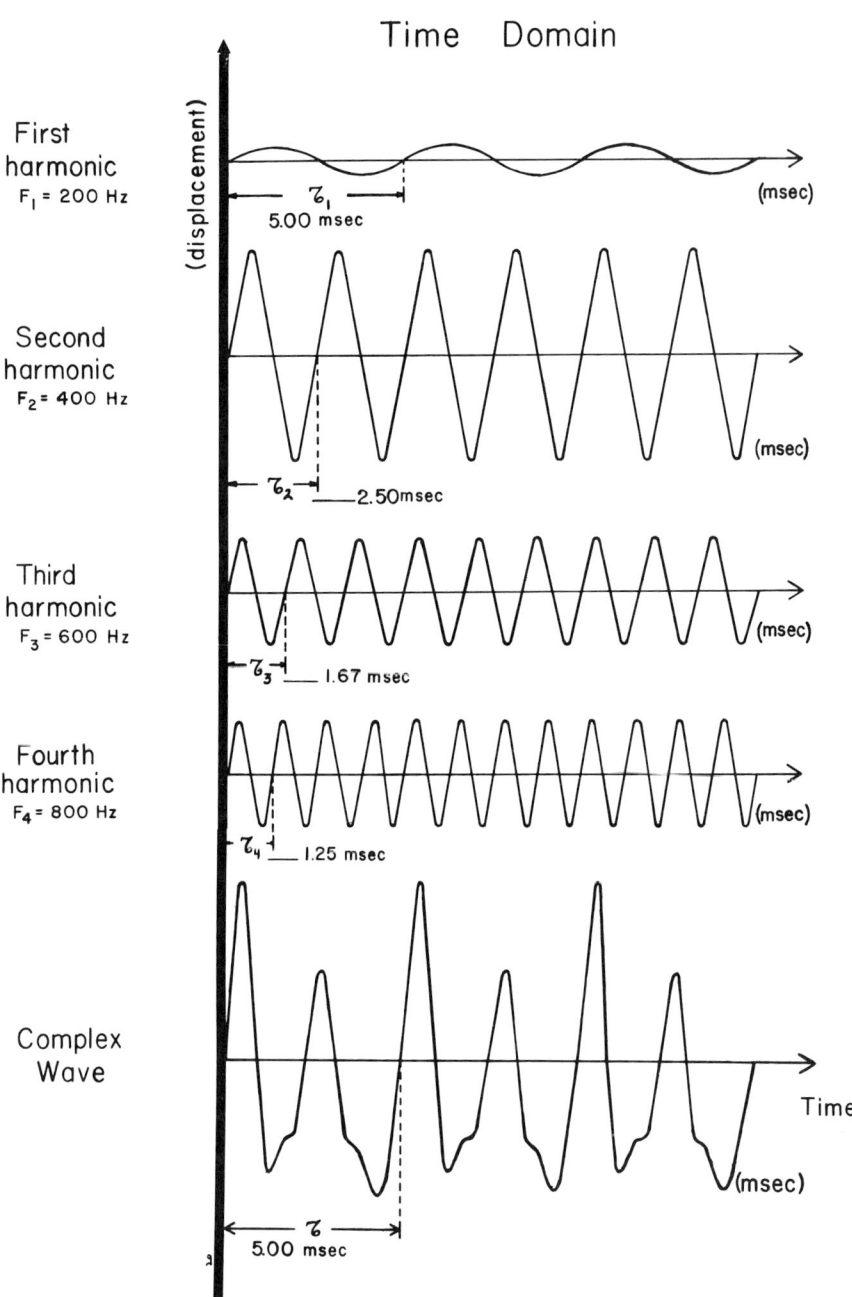

FIGURE 51-3. Fourier analysis of a complex wave on the time domain. A complex wave of period 5 msec (frequency = 200 Hz) is decomposed into four harmonics of frequencies of 200, 400, 600, and 800 Hz respectively.

domain. Frequency domain plot is a graph in which frequency is plotted via the horizontal axis. Intensity amplitude or phase can be plotted on the vertical axis. Since for a constant SHM there is only one frequency of vibration, the frequency domain plot of this sound will consist of only one line at the particular frequency of the sound considered. The length of such a line will portray, according to a graphic scale, the intensity of that sound. A complex sound is one which is not simple, or sinusoidal. The French physicist Fourier discovered in the last century that any complex sound can be decomposed into a set of simple sounds of different frequencies and intensities. As an illustration of this principle, Figure 51-3 shows a complex wave decomposed into four simple or sinusoidal sounds called harmonics. This graph presents the waves in the time domain. Figure 51-4 portrays the same waves in the frequency domain. We can conclude that the spectrum of a complex sound consists of several lines each representing a simple sound or harmonic component of the complex sound. Different shapes of spectrum of a complex sound determine the quality or characteristics of a particular sound. An illustration of different spectra associated with different speech sounds (or phonemes) is presented in Figure 51-5. From an acoustical point of view, to speak means to produce a variable acoustic spectrum correlated with a message through a particular phonetic code or language. This variable spectrum is produced by each talker acting upon his articulators (i.e., mandible, tongue, soft palate) to obtain particular resonances from the primary generators of sound, the glottal vibration and the friction of the stream of air from the lungs. To have resonance at least two acoustic systems are necessary: a source or generator of sound and a resonant system. This latter will amplify some harmonics of the source sound and will dampen some other harmonics, giving to the output-spectrum sound a particular shape. This particular shape of the spectrum of a sound includes both a phonetic content and the individual characteristics of each speaker.

Indeed, the speaker-output variable spectrum of ongoing speech carries not only semantic information, but also speaker-dependent features. Therefore, any method of speaker identification or elimination has to be

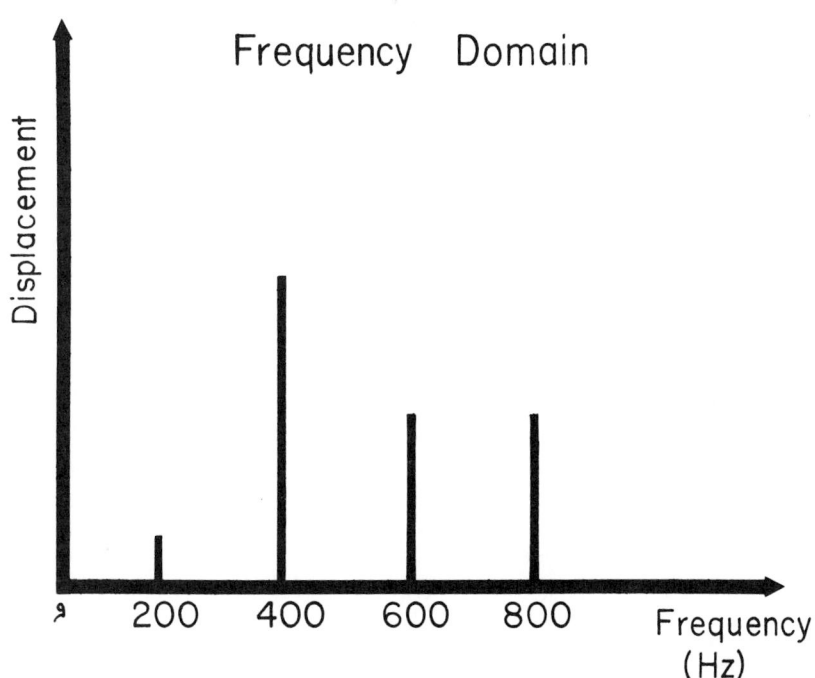

FIGURE 51-4. Fourier analysis on the frequency domain of the wave seen in Figure 51-3.

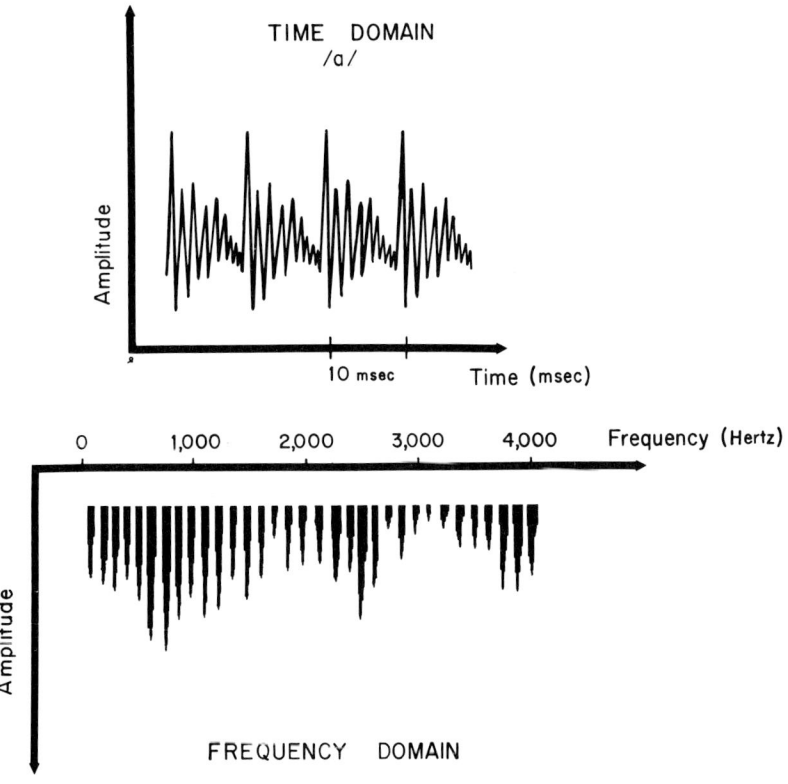

FIGURE 51-5. Complex wave on the phoneme /a/ portrayed in the time domain and in the frequency domain (continuum spectrum).

based in some way on acoustic spectra. Figures 51-5 and 51-6 present spectra of sounds /a/ and /s/ uttered by the author.

As previously discussed, the speaker has available two primary sources of sound to produce speech spectra: the glottal source and the frictional source. These sources can be used successively or simultaneously during ongoing speech according to instantaneous phonetic needs. The use of the glottal source originates the so-called voiced phonemes (vowels and voiced consonants). The exclusive use of the frictional source of sound produces the voiceless consonants.

To establish a phonetic code (i.e., to speak), the spectra of the sources are modified at each instant by resonance in the vocal tract, conveniently shaped by the speaker through the articulatory movements. Each position of the articulators produces the desired phonetic spectrum that conveys a semantic meaning to the listener. In these spectra there are frequency bands of relative higher amplitude called *formants* in the case of vowels. There are also frequency bands of relative higher amplitude in spectra of consonants. The relative position of the center frequency of these bands, their bandwidths, their relative amplitudes, and their transitions determine the different phonetic elements as well as the speaker-dependent features necessary for voice identification. However, these parameters are variable not only among different speakers, but also within the same speaker uttering the same phonetic elements. Coarticulation is one important factor responsible for these variations.

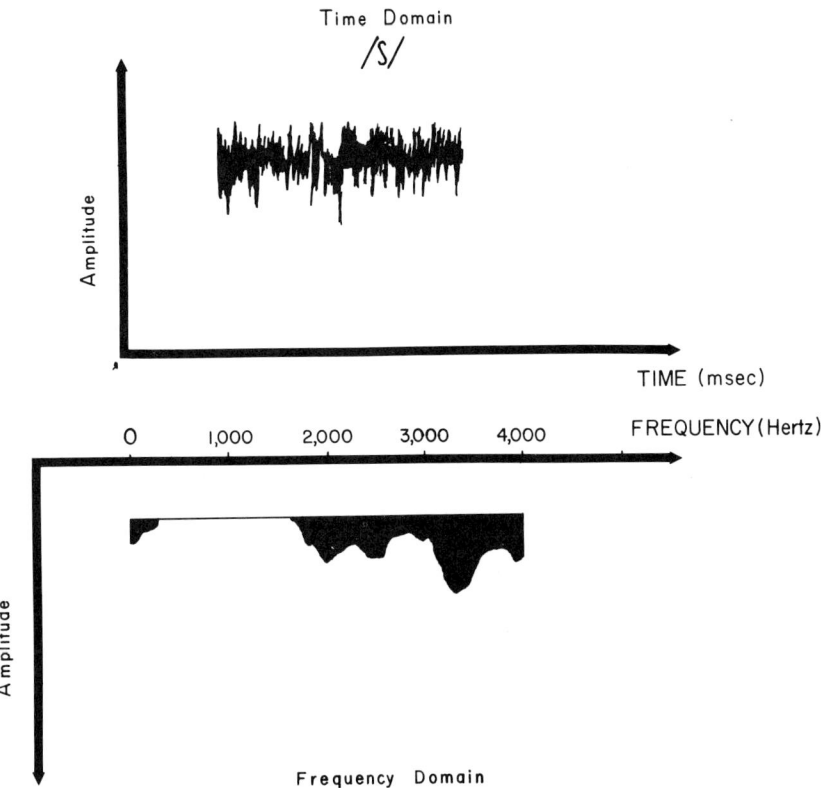

FIGURE 51-6. Complex wave correlated with vowel /a/ in the time domain and in the frequency domain (discrete spectrum).

Frequency range of speech extends from the glottal frequency (average 120 Hz for men and 220 Hz for women) up to about 7 kHz. However, most speech and speaker information is properly conveyed by a restricted range, up to about 4 kHz. Both the glottal spectrum and resonance curves of a vocal tract are dependent on anatomic and organic characteristics as well as on the functional or behavioral process experienced by each person during the learning state of speaking.

Speech Acoustic Parameters and Speaker Variability

The general acoustic parameters of speech are time, frequency, and intensity distribution. Comparisons of these general or derived spectral parameters are the basis of all speaker recognition systems, both subjective and objective. Variation of these spectral parameters depends on phonetic content and speaker individuality. In voice identification tests, the phonetic source of variation can be minimized by limiting comparisons of questioned and known voices by comparing only similar sample sentences produced by the speakers. The problem is that even maintaining a constant text, values of the selected parameters will differ not only among different speakers, but also will vary within the same speaker when different utterances of this same text are compared. The first type of variation is called interspeaker variability; the second type is referred to as intraspeaker variability. Researchers of voice identification have searched for sets of efficient parameters (i.e., parameters that present the least and the most interspeaker variability in all conditions that may occur in normal or even in disguised speech). These efficient parameters are selected according to the particular method of voice identification explored. Optimal selection of parameters for aural examination cannot be adequate for visual examination or for automatic recognition.

One recent study searching for efficient parameters in automatic speaker identification was conducted by Wolf.[1] He selected the following parameters: fundamental frequency at given locations of the sample sentences; amplitude of nasal consonants; moment calculations with frequency band amplitudes of filtered vowels; mean frequencies of formants F1 and F2 in given locations of the sample sentences; spectrum slope at a given location of /u/; and high-frequency spectrum shape at the middle of /s/. Atal[2] selected pitch contours for his method of automatic speaker recognition.

For visual examination of spectrograms, the following parameters are suggested by the author and his associates: mean frequencies and bandwidths of vowel formants; gaps and type of vertical striations; slopes and transients of formants; duration of similar phonetic elements and plosive gaps; energy distribution of fricatives; plosives; and interformant acoustic density.[3]

For aural examination, Holmgren[4] suggests perceptual parameters and voice-attribute rating tests such as pitch, rate, intensity, and quality.

In summary, organic and learned differences are the sources of interspeaker variability. Time elapsed, psychologic and physiologic changes, circadian rhythm, and articulatory dynamics are the sources of intraspeaker variability. Additional variability is introduced by the effect of coarticulation when similar phonetic elements, extracted from different contexts, are compared. More variability is introduced by environmental reverberations, noise, and distortions of the transmission and recording systems. Considering all these sources of variability, there is little hope to develop a method, or even a clustering of methods, that could provide a positive speaker identification in 100 percent of the cases examined, within a legally acceptable rate of error. In many cases, whether the methods used are objective or subjective, the outcome of an honest examination has to be "no decision" one way or the other.

SUBJECTIVE METHODS OF SPEAKER RECOGNITION

Aural Examination of Voices

A listener may use the long-term memory process or the short-term memory process to identify or eliminate an unknown speaker as being the same as a known one. The long-term memory process is utilized when the voice to be identified is a familiar one to the listener. The short-term memory process is employed when the unknown and known voices to be compared are made available to the listener through recordings.

The success of aural recognition based on long-term memory depends on the remembrance or the familiarity of the listener with the questioned voice, the time elapsed since it was last heard, the homogeneity of the "challenging" speaker's group, and the discriminating ability of the listener. The voice sample duration seems not to be critical after 1 second of continuous speech. If a transmission or recording system is used to obtain challenging speakers' voice samples, distortions introduced by such a system may increase the percentage of errors. Filtering below 500 Hz and above 3,000 Hz seems to have no significant influence in the results of tests. This information is important since most voice evidence is obtained through the telephone, which filters harmonics of speech below 150 Hz and above 4,000 Hz. Attempts of the challenging speaker to disguise his voice, or even to use whispered speech, may decrease greatly the correct identification percentages.[5]

The first significant experiment done in the area of aural examination, using the long-term memory process, was performed by McGehee.[6] He used 31 male and 18 female speakers reading a paragraph of 56 words. Apparently, these speakers belonged to a phonetically homogeneous group, all university graduate students. A total of 740 undergraduate students were employed as listeners in this experiment in which live voices were used exclusively. Listeners were divided into 15 panels, each panel participating in at least two sessions. During the first session they listened behind a screen to a speaker reading a paragraph. During the second session, five speakers, including the one from the first session, read the same paragraph. Each listener had to indicate who, among these five speakers, was the one they had heard previously. The second listening session was spaced from 1 day to 5 months from the first one, according to the particular panel of listeners. The mean percentage of correct identifications varied from 83 percent to 13 percent. McGehee also investigated the effect of disguising the voice by changing the pitch, which drastically reduced the percentage of correct identifications. Other findings of this early study were that male and female voices are equally identifiable and that increasing the number of known speakers reduces the percentage of correct identifications. It is noted that all trials of identification were of the closed type and that no recordings were used.

Pollack, Pickett, and Sumby[7] performed an experiment on aural recognition based on long-term memory. All 16 speakers used in this experiment were familiar to the listeners, who performed the so-called speaker-naming tests for groups from two to eight speakers. These authors investigated the effect of several variables on the percentage of correct identifications, namely, duration of the speech sample, filtering, and whispering. Their findings can be summarized as follows: durations longer than 1 second do not improve significantly the percentage of correct identifications, which reached a figure close to 95 percent after this interval of time. Whispered speech reduced by approximately 30 percent the correct identifications with other conditions remaining constant. For low-pass and high-pass filtering, the authors concluded that "over a rather wide frequency range, identification performance is resistant to selective frequency of this type." For this experiment, the authors used a phonetically balanced list of monosyllabic words from the Harvard Psychoacoustic Laboratory.

Bricker and Pruzansky[8] studied the effects of stimulus content and duration on aural speaker identification. They used 16 listeners familiar with 10 speakers, who recorded different materials through high-fidelity equipment. The examiners listened to the tapes through a loudspeaker. The best examiner was able to obtain a 100 percent correct identification when listening to sentences with a mean duration of 2.4 seconds, containing about 15 phonemes. The worst examiner, for the same trials, obtained only 92 percent correct responses. These researchers also ran tests based on short-term memory, including two known subjects A and B to be compared with one unknown X using reversed excerpts. Listeners were not familiar with the speakers. Average results of correct identification in these closed tests reached the 75 percent level.

One of the few studies in aural examination using open trials and short-term memory process was performed by Stevens and associates.[9] In this study the authors attempted to compare results obtained from aural examination and from visual examination of spectrograms using the same materials and the same examiners. They employed 24 highly homogeneous speakers from the point of view of perceptual attributes of speech. All of these speakers recorded twice, 1 week apart, repeating 10 times a reading list of nine words and two short sentences. These materials were dubbed into loops of 4.5 seconds duration, each loop containing two utterances of the same word or one utterance of a short sentence. Spectrograms of these materials were also subsequently prepared. Six examiners performed open and closed tests of speaker identification and elimination with these materials, using separate aural and visual examinations. They did not receive training in either of the two methods. However, they were selected on the basis of their ability to become aurally familiar with an ensemble of six previously unfamiliar voices. All tests included one unknown and eight known speakers. The examiners could listen to the nine tape loops representing these speakers, switching as necessary among the tape-recorded channels.

In all cases the percentages of correct responses were significantly higher for aural examination than for visual examination. For the closed-test types, mean errors yielded by aural examination ranged from 18 percent to 6 percent. Mean errors yielded by visual examination of spectrograms of the same materials ranged from 28 percent to 21 percent. The lower percentages correspond to later tests when some learning effect had obviously interacted with the results. For the open-test types, results were as follows: aural method, 8 to 6 percent error of false identification and 12 to 8 percent error of false elimination; visual method, 4 to 31 percent error of false identification and 20 to 10 percent error of false elimination.

These percentages would appear to be biased, since the examiners had normal hearing and therefore were accustomed to discriminate voices aurally from the early stages of life, but they were not familiar with spectrograms, at least in that they had had no special training. Furthermore, the examiners in this study were selected on the basis of their aural ability, but their ability to match patterns was not tested. Moreover, the lengths of the samples used were inadequately short for spectrographic recognition. In a letter to prosecutor P. Lindhom of St. Paul, Minnesota, Dr. Stevens acknowledged that these factors might be the reason for the high percentage of errors produced in his experiment.

Other conclusions of this study were that (1) some speakers are more difficult to identify than others, even when the experimental speakers are homogeneous from the point of view of the perceptual attributes; (2) there are greater differences in the ability to identify a speaker by listening to front vowels than to back vowels; and (3) longer utterances increase the probability of correct identifications using visual methods.

Other authors have taken a different approach to studying aural identification by trying to determine significant perceptual attributes of speakers' voices in order to create reliable classification scales. Such perceptual scale might help an examiner to perform aural discriminations on a systematic and consistent basis. A classic effort of this type was undertaken by Voiers, who was able to isolate four significant perceptual scales—clarity, roughness, magnitude, and animation—as a means to discriminate among speakers. Holmgren[10] found that pitch, intensity, quality, and rate scales helped to classify the uniqueness of each particular voice. In practical application, however, it was found that the same set of numbers from the four scales might correspond to different voices. Therefore, perceptual scales should be considered only as a helping device for speaker identification or elimination.

In summary, aural examination of voices is the most familiar and natural system of speaker identification and elimination. It is accepted by all courts of law. The expected percentage of error for open tests using the short-term memory process (i.e., listening through recordings to the known and unknown voices) has not been accurately determined by experimentation. It might be as large as 20 percent, according to particular circumstances, especially if the examiner is forced to reach a positive decision in all tests. Distorting or disguising of the voice can increase greatly the expected error percentages.

In spite of the modern trend toward developing automatic systems of speaker recognition, continued research on aural examination is worthwhile. Experimental designs should include open tests, low-quality transmission, recording systems, and background noise to approach real-life situations. Cartridge tape recorders, presently available, are convenient instruments for this type of research.

Visual Examination of Spectrograms

SPECTROGRAPHY

The purpose of speech spectrography is to resolve the complex speech signal into its single components (i.e., to produce Fourier analysis of spectra of speech versus time). This operation was first performed at the turn of the century for sustained vowels. The instrument used in these early studies was the mechanical Henrici analyzer. With such a machine, Black[11] was able to produce tridimensional spectra (intensity, frequency, and time) of the same vowel as spoken by different speakers, plotting harmonic frequencies and corresponding intensities against time.

A spectrograph project was begun in 1941 at the Bell Laboratories by Dr. Ralph Potter.[12] This machine was developed with the primary purpose of helping the military during time of war, and only when World War II was over did the spectrograph become available to speech scientists. The input to the spectrograph is a recorded speech sample limited to segments 2.4 seconds long. The output consists of a graphic display (spectrogram) of frequency-intensity of sound versus time for the sample analyzed. Frequencies are plotted on the vertical axis and time on the horizontal axis. Relative intensities are portrayed by the different degrees of darkness of the patterns produced. In the commercially available spectrographs, there are several options for setting the ranges of frequencies of analysis (60 to 4,000 Hz or 60 to 7,000 Hz, etc.) using logarithmic or lineal scales. The bandwidth of the scanning analyzing filter can be selected at 45 or 300 Hz. In addition, it is possible to obtain bar or contour spectrograms with these machines.

The operation of the spectrograph consists of performing a continuous Fourier analysis of the speech sample at each instant of time. If the narrow-band filter (45 Hz) is selected, the actual Fourier harmonics of the input speech sample are displayed on the spectrograms. If the broad-band scanning filter (300 Hz) is utilized, the formants, rather than the individual harmonics, appear on the spectrogram. These two types of displays are called bar spectrograms. Since the relative intensity of each harmonic or each formant is portrayed by the different degrees of darkness of the patterns produced, and the intensity range of the speech harmonics or formants can be as large as 40 dB, a compressor circuit reduces the intensity of the input signal proportionally to the scanned range of frequencies. The reason for this procedure is to compensate for the reduced dynamic range of the Teledeltos paper (about 10 dB) where the spectrogram is printed, making it possible to record on the paper the weak, higher harmonics or formants of the speech signal.

VOICEPRINT IDENTIFICATION

The original spectrograph design, marketed by Kay Elemetrics, was improved in 1966 by Anthony Presti, an engineer at the Bell Laboratories, who later joined Voiceprint Laboratories, Inc., to market his new, improved spectrograph with the brand name Voiceprint.[13] He also introduced in the machine a display called "contour," where relative intensities are plotted by isobaric lines (contours) at 6-dB steps.

The sound spectrograph or sonograph can be considered a universal instrument for researching and teaching the acoustics of speech or sound in general. In addition, it has practical applications such as improving the speech of deaf persons. In 1944, Gray and Koop found that spectrograms could be applied to identify speakers, since the spectrogram portrays not only the phonetic features of speech, but speaker-dependent features as well. They wrote a report[14] containing their experiences in this field and describing practical means of putting this system into use, including how to train examiners to identify questioned speakers. Gray and Kopp concluded their report with the following paragraph:

> Voice print identification seems to offer possibility of a useful radio intercept feature and one that could be put into use without extensive training or elaborate equipment. As a study of combat conditions in the European and Pacific theatres indicates a need for such identification, it is suggested that a trial voice identification group be established to carry on the work under actual or simulated field conditions to test the conclusions of this laboratory work.

To the best knowledge of this author, such a test was not completed because of the end of the war and the problem of recordings. Tape recorders were not practically developed at that time.

STUDIES BY KERSTA

During the early 1960s, Lawrence Kersta, a staff member of the Bell Laboratories, reexamined the voiceprint method at the request of a law enforcement group. He performed laboratory experiments using spectrograms from five clue words spoken in isolation by an unspecified population.[15] All the tests were of the closed type, using contemporary spectrograms, that is, spectrograms produced from each speaker sample obtained during the same recording session. The maximal number of known speakers in each trial of identification was 12. The examiners were requested to render a positive identification on all cases. These examiners were a group of high school girls trained by Kersta 1 week before the start of the experiment. They worked in pairs. Correct identification in these experiments was better than 99 percent. In the Kersta papers there was no report of significant performance differences among examiners. Homogeneity and number of speakers were not discussed. Other experiments that Kersta performed, such as sorting spectrograms in order to form groups including the same speaker, also showed a high percentage of correct responses.

Kersta became absolutely convinced on the "infallibility" of the spectrograms for identification purposes. In November 1962, he presented a paper before a meeting of the Acoustical Society of America in which he compared the reliability of this method with that of fingerprints.

In 1966, Kersta retired from Bell Laboratories and established his own company, Voiceprint Laboratories, Inc., with the goal of producing spectrographs on a commercial basis. He offered his professional services to identify persons through their voices and to train police officers as speech spectrogram examiners.

The scientific community soon voiced its opposition to Kersta's claims. Experiments were cited which contradicted the extremely high success percentages reported by Kersta. One of the most adamant opponents was Dr. Peter Ladefoged, who published a paper[16] contradicting the statements of Kersta.

STUDIES BY YOUNG AND CAMPBELL, STEVENS AND ASSOCIATES, AND HAZEN

Young and Campbell[17] published a study dealing with closed tests of speaker identification by visual examination of spectrograms. Five talkers uttering two words were used as known speakers in each trial. These researchers used 10 examiners who received a maximum of 2.5 hours of training before the start of the experiment. During this training phase, using one word ("you" or "it") spoken in isolation, the identification success reached a mean of 78.4 percent. During the experimental tasks, spectrograms of the same two words (you, it) were used, but this time they were excerpted from a sentence rather than produced in isolation. The percentage of success decreased to a mean of 37.3. Young and Campbell attribute these differences to the shorter stimulus represented by the excerpted words, as compared with the longer similar words uttered in isolation, and to the coarticulation factors. They recognized, however, that the different experimental approach they took as compared with that of Kersta, the difference in training of examiners, and possible differences in population homogeneity could have accounted for the different score percentages obtained in both experiments.

Stevens and associates[18] produced another experiment using separate aural and visual examination of the spectrogram. Results from this experiment were presented earlier in this chapter in the section of aural examination.

In a published thesis an experiment was reported on speaker recognition using five words physically excerpted from spectrograms obtained from spontaneous speech.[19] Hazen used seven panels of teams of two examiners who received a "few sessions" of training before the start of the experiment. There were different types of tasks to be performed, including absolute identification of elimination of one unknown speaker among 50 known speakers. Hazen forced the examiners to reach a positive decision in the 40 tests performed by each panel. The range of errors ran from 0.00 to 83.33 percent, according to the task and the panel. The error was always larger when comparing words cut off from different speech contexts than when words were taken from the same contexts. Considering the types of errors he obtained, Hazen concluded that identification using speech spectrograms should not be utilized "until sufficient and consistent data are gathered to establish the limits of this technique."

Certainly, this would be a most reasonable conclusion if speech spectrograms by five physically excerpted words were used as the sole means of identification by examiners with no experience who are forced to render a positive decision in 100 percent of the cases examined. On the other hand, it should be pointed out that Hazen's idea of using words from spontaneous speech as opposed to words from reading was an excellent one, since in real-life cases the questioned person indeed uses spontaneous speech. However, to separate these words from ongoing speech spectrograms was not a commendable procedure since it is almost impossible to target the spectrographic boundaries of a word in the condition. Furthermore, transient patterns are speaker-dependent features, and they become lost with this procedure. In addition, 40 trails of absolute identification or elimination per panel (or 280 trials in total) do not constitute an impressive amount of statistical data to substantiate solidly any recommendation.

The merit of Hazen's study is in having reiterated what should not be done with spectrograms, namely, to segment spectrographic patterns of a given word from an ongoing text and to use random contexts for matching techniques.

STUDIES BY TOSI AND ASSOCIATES

To date, the largest study on voice identification and elimination using speech spectrograms has been performed by the author and associates[20] at Michigan State University. This study was made possible through a grant from the U.S. Department of Justice. It was carried on from the beginning of 1968 to December, 1970. This experiment included a total of 34,992 trials of identification and elimination, according to different models, performed by 29 experimental examiners who were trained for 1 month.

Each trial involved up to 40 known voices in various conditions: closed and open trials, contemporary and noncontemporary spectrograms, and nine or six clue words spoken in isolation in a fixed context and in random context. The 250 speakers used in this experiment were randomly selected from a homogeneous population of approximately 25,000 male students at Michigan State University.

The experimental examiners were forced to reach a positive decision (identification or elimination) in each text, taking an average time of 15 minutes. Their decisions were based solely on examination of spectrograms; listening to the voices was discarded from this experiment. The examiners graded their self-confidence in their judgment on a 4-point scale: 1 and 2, uncertain; 3 and 4, certain. Percentage error of false identifications obtained from the forensic models (open test, noncontemporary spectrograms, and ongoing speech texts) tested in this experiment was approximately 6.4. Percentage error of false elimination from these models was approximately 12.7. Kersta's models (closed tests, contemporary spectrograms, and words spoken in isolation) were also tested in this experiment and yielded a percentage error of less than 1. Examiner's answers graded "uncertain" were computed in order to determine the possible percentages that would have been obtained if the examiners had not been forced to reach a positive conclusion in 100 percent of the tests. The computer analysis determined that in this case, percentage error of false identification for the forensic models would have been reduced approximately to 2.4, percentage error of false eliminations approximately to 4.8, and percentage of tests with "certain" answers to 74.

At the same time that the laboratory study was being conducted by the author, a field study was completed at the Crime Laboratory of the Michigan State Police by Lt. Ernest Nash, with the purpose of finding the difference between laboratory conditions and the actual situation a professional examiner encounters when handling forensic situations. This field study included 673 voices involved in actual crime investigations.

After evaluation of laboratory and field conditions, the conclusion was reached that *a combined method of aural and visual examination* of spectrograms can be used in the investigation of a crime if the following standards are maintained:

1. The examiner must be qualified professional trained in phonetics and speech science. A 2-year apprenticeship in field work should be required along with academic training before a voice examiner is qualified professionally.
2. The professional examiner must abstain from offering any positive conclusion when he has the least doubt of the exactness of such conclusion. Since this method is essentially subjective and relies heavily on the expertise of the examiner, prudence should be the cardinal principle guiding the examiner's decisions. The examiner should select among the following alternatives after completing the examination:
   a. Positive identification;
   b. Probability of identification;
   c. Positive elimination;
   d. Probability of elimination;
   e. No opinion one way or the other.
3. The examiner must be entitled to spend as much time and to demand as many voice samples of good quality as he deems necessary to reach a conclusion. Otherwise, he should select alternative decisions such as probability of identification or elimination, or simply no conclusion one way or the other.
4. The sample of the defendant's voice should include the same contextual materials as found in the questioned voice.

In keeping with these standards, the Michigan State Police decided to employ these combined aural and visual methods of speaker identification or elimination, starting in December 1970.

In summary, subjective methods of voice identification or elimination can offer reasonable reliability if the above-listed standards are rigorously maintained. Distortions caused by transmission and recording systems, background noise, or psychologic or physiologic alterations of the speakers will greatly decrease the percentage of cases in which an honest and well-trained examiner could reach a positive identification using these subjective methods. However, the same statement could be applied to objective methods if and when they become sufficiently developed to be applied to forensic cases. The crucial issues in the reliability of subjective methods are the testing of the capability of the examiner and obtaining the examiner's receiver-operating characteristic curve.

Bolt and associates[21] have expressed their opposition to the use of speech spectrograms for legal purposes. Their opinions are most reasonable indeed, if they mean exclusion of aural examination and the reaching of positive decisions in 100 percent of the cases examined, irrespective of the conditions and frequency range of the voice samples, psychologic and physiologic alterations of the speakers, and distortions introduced by the recording and transmission systems and by background noise. These conditions, however, clearly contradict the standards specified by the author and his associates for real-life examinations.

OBJECTIVE METHODS OF SPEAKER RECOGNITION

Both automatic and semiautomatic methods of speaker recognition are considered objective, each according to a different degree of objectivity. These methods are presently in the early stages of development. To date, objective methods are more suitable for speaker authentication or verification in security systems than for speakers identification in legal cases. Automatic systems are available, with a limited (about 10) library of voices, which are able to autheticate a collaborative speaker with an error of the order of 10 percent or even less.

Further development of automatic methods is desirable because of the many assets these methods possess, such as the possibility of producing mathematical specifications of the expected error, the receiver-operating characteristic, and the elimination or great reduction of human bias. Although a human operator is always necessary to prepare the samples and to interpret results from the computer, the necessary skill of such an operator could be reduced to minimal levels, compatible with the characteristics of each particular system. In addition, human fatigue, a factor that may contribute to errors in subjective methods, is nearly eliminated.

Two functional steps are necessary in all automatic systems: (1) extraction of relevant parameters from the questioned and known speaker samples; and (2) consequent decision "same-different" (or "no decision" in some systems), according to rules based on a programmed algorithm. There are two general procedures to complete the first step in automatic or semiautomatic speaker identification: (1) forming a matrix based on the spectra of the common phonetic elements selected; or (2) extracting from these spectra a variety of derived parameters that are considered relevant by each particular experimenter searching for an efficient speaker identification or elimination system.[22]

To complete the second step, rules of decision are programmed. Generally, they consist of comparing statistically the data obtained from the first step after introducing weighing factors, computing Euclidean distances, and so forth. An alternative procedure consists of forming hierarchical clustering groups with the data. The decision algorithm provides a choice of possible responses when comparing a known speaker to the questioned one, such as "same-different-no decision," according to limits of decision arbitrarily set by a programmer.

One problem that plagues most objective systems is the automatic recognition and alignment of the common phonetic elements to the "known" and "unknown" samples which are the sources of the parameters on which to base a decision. The risk consists of false targeting. In this case comparison would be based on different phonetic elements, a method which may greatly hinder the process.

Semiautomatic Systems of Identification

Semiautomatic systems include recognition of the common phonetic elements from samples to be compared by a human operator. An excellent semiautomatic system was produced by scientists from the Stanford Research Institute. In this system the operator observes on a cathode ray tube the sample sentence waves and selects the segments to be analyzed through a display window.

After this selection is made, amplitude spectra of these segments (generally steady portions of a vowel) are obtained and compared with similar ones obtained from other speech samples. Through a special algorithm a decision among the following alternatives is reached: the examined samples were produced by the same speaker; the samples were produced by different speakers; or no decision could be reached one way or the other.

By changing the decision algorithm, percentages of expected errors of false identification, false elimination, and no decision can be produced in known proportion. For instance, to have less than 1 percent chance of error of false identification, the percentage of no decisions has to be as high as 30.

A companion to this study was conducted by Hair and Rekieta[23] in which they performed open tests by automatic means, including 32, 8, and 2 suspects, respectively. The authors claimed a 99 percent accuracy of the system, provided that certain conditions were maintained. Moreover, according to the experimenters, their semiautomatic system of voice identification could be easily implemented for use by law enforcement agencies.

Automatic Systems of Identification

Atal[24] reported the use of pitch contours as an efficient parameter for automatic speaker recognition. Closed tests involving 10 speakers yielded 97 percent correct identification using his method.

Wolf[25] described another automatic system using efficient parameters for voice identification. Correct results from a population of 21 speakers using such a set of parameters, programmed in a computer, reached the 98 percent level in closed tests of speaker authentication.

Su and Fu[26] have published an important study on automatic speaker identification. They based their method on statistical information derived from spectra of nasal consonants, spectra of words excerpted from ongoing speech, and spectra of continuous speech. Spectra of nasal consonants proved to be the best of the three clues for speaker identification, and spectra from excerpted words were the least favorable. Using readings from 10 speakers, 3 female and 7 male, in closed tests of voice identification, they obtained percentages of correct responses from 100 percent to 10 percent, according to the materials and decision algorithms used. In their report, they included a complete review of the available literature on automatic speaker identification up to 1973.

In 1973, during a sabbatical leave spent at the Galileo Ferraris Institute in Turin, the author experimented with choral speech spectra applied to voice identification.[27] This study attempted to eliminate the problem of temporal alignment of common phonetic elements from the unknown and known voices to be compared, as well as to eliminate the requirement demanded by many systems of voice identification of having "known" and "unknown" samples of similar texts. Choral speech is defined as the spectra of mixed temporal segments of different speech produced by the same speaker.

In the Turin study choral spectra of different texts recorded by 20 speakers were compared through a special computer algorithm. The purpose was to test whether or not it is possible to produce reliable discriminations based on relative individual invariances of such spectra, irrespective of text or language used by the speakers. The speakers, 14 male and 6 female, all had education beyond high school, had no noticeable speech defects, and spoke fluent Piamontes, Italian, and French. All were natives of the Piedmont region and therefore had a high degree of phonetic homogeneity. They recorded three times, within 1-week intervals, a 10-minute text in Piamontes, Italian, and French, respectively. Texts consisted of items from two newspapers and a book. Recordings were obtained within a sound-isolated room and using a high-quality recording system.

Recordings of each language were temporarily segmented into 14 parts and dubbed into loops each approximately 20 seconds long, utilizing a Sanborn 3917 FM tape recorder. The mixed output from these loops, played back simultaneously, were re-recorded into an 8-second single loop, obtaining a total of nine of these choral speech loops per speaker. Each loop therefore was defined by speaker, language, and recording session, respectively. Intensity of all loops was adjusted to a common peak value of 25 dB against an arbitrary zero.

Output from this system consisted of 180 choral speech spectra, each representing a speaker, language, and recording session. Range of spectra was from 63 to 6,300 Hz processed through a 1/3 octave filter. Spectra were digitally sampled at every 4/100 octave, obtaining 156 readings of relative decibels versus frequency for each spectrum (Fig. 51-7). These digital data were transferred onto IBM cards and processed through a hierarchical clustering algorithm, implemented on the CDC 6500 computer at Michigan State University.

Hierarchical clustering algorithms provide one way of investigating the following questions:

1. Are the spectra for a particular speaker more similar to one another than to the spectra for other speakers?
2. Are the spectra from one language more similar to one another than to those from other languages?
3. Do the answers to the first two questions remain consistent in time?

Similarity matrices of spectra were computed in this study by two different methods: (1) the sum of absolute differences between energies of corresponding frequencies on all pairs of spectra; and (2) the squared root of the sum of the squared differences between these energies. The hierarchical clustering algorithm translates these similarity matrices into a dendrogram or tree. Cutting the dendrogram at various levels clusters the spectra into groups that enclose the most similar components.

The various methods to cluster these spectra, as described earlier, were explored. In all cases spectra clustered very well according to subject rather than to language or recording session. Errors of clustering or "iden-

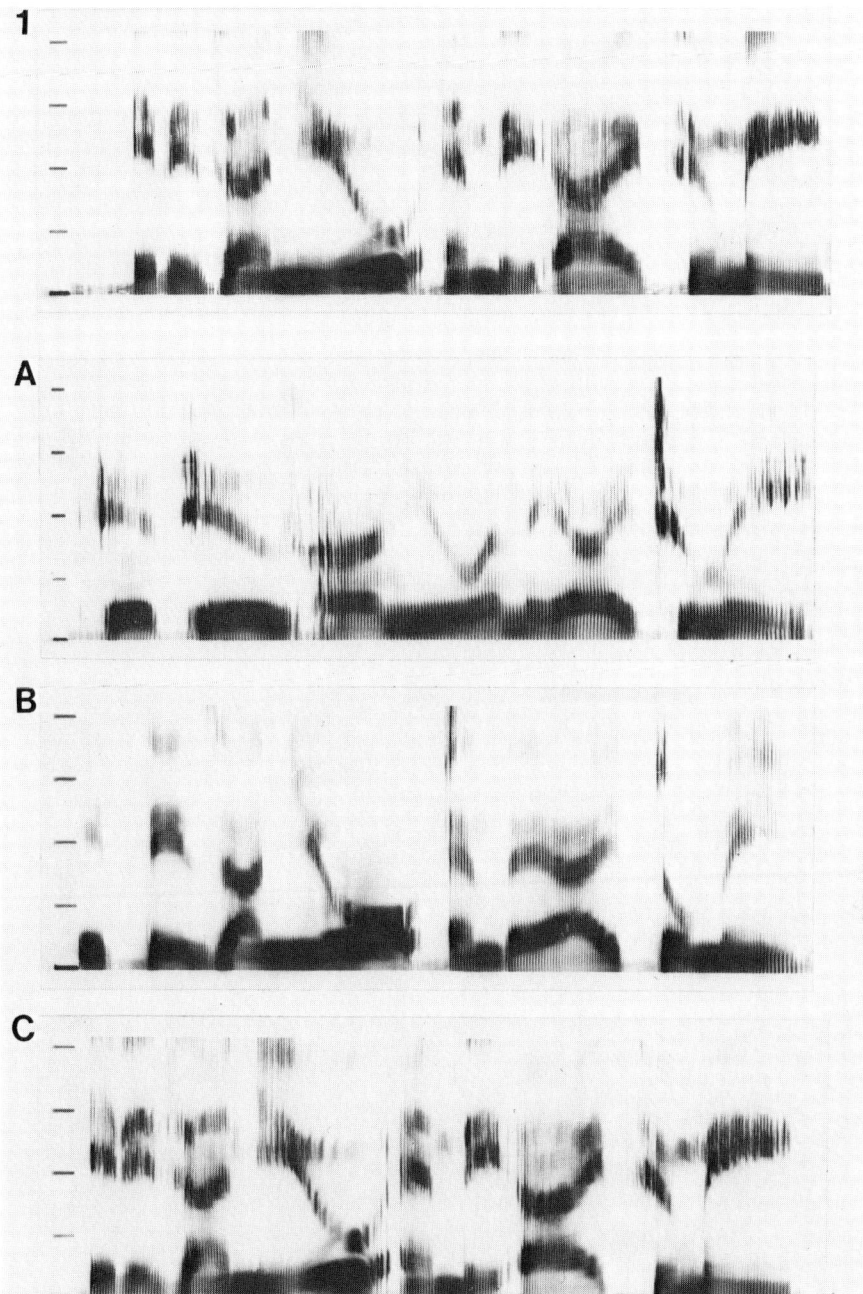

FIGURE 51-7. Spectrograms *A, B,* and *C* correspond to three different persons who have recorded the same sentence. Spectrogram 1 corresponds to person *C* who has uttered the same sentence on a different occasion. Note the spectrographic similarities between 1 and *C,* which do not exist between 1 and *A* or 1 and *B.*

tifying" speakers ran from 30 percent to 5 percent, according to the methods used for cluster and for computing percentages. This finding suggests that each speaker possesses relative invariances in his or her choral spectra, irrespective of the text of language used.

From 1973 to the present more research projects on the objective method of voice identification were conducted by the author and his associates. Procedure to obtain choral speech spectra from the voice samples is now completely automatic, using a special program for the minicomputer PDP 11/40. Multidimensional scaling is used to group the different spectra, to facilitate elimination and identification decisions.[28] In 1978, this procedure was accepted by a court of law in the case of *Indiana v. Weatherford* (C-4116).

LEGAL ACCEPTANCE OF VOICE IDENTIFICATION

With the exception of the decision in *Indiana v. Weatherford*, the only methods of voice identification and elimination accepted as evidence in American courts of law have been the subjective ones, namely, aural and visual examination of spectrograms. Court cases where aural evidence based on the long-term memory process were used are numerous; this evidence is accepted from witnesses "for what it is worth" in each case. In a similar manner, person identification is accepted from any eyewitness. From 1962 to 1970 there were several cases where spectrograms were introduced in court, all by Lawrence Kersta. The bulk of the usage of spectrograms in court, however, has postdated December 1970.

Court Cases from 1970 to the Present

The first case which admitted voice identification evidence based on combined aural and visual examinations of spectrograms was *Minnesota v. Trimble* (1970). In this case of assassination, 12 suspected persons were eliminated by the examiner, Lt. Ernest Nash; Ms. Trimble, a suspect, was identified as being the unknown caller. Expert witnesses for the prosecution were Lt. Nash and the author. The rebuttal expert witness for the defense was Dr. Peter Ladefoged. The defendant admitted that she produced the questioned call.

From the time of this first case to the end of 1976, approximately 75 other court cases in the United States and Canada have included this type of evidence. In most of the cases, identification was offered, but in a few cases the examiners were asked to provide elimination, such as in *U.S. v. Sisco* (1974) and *Florida v. Otero* (1976). The antagonistic party, defense lawyers in most cases, called rebuttal expert witnesses in approximately 30 percent of the cases.

The total number of voices examined by members of the International Association of Voice Identification, to December 1976, was approximately 10,000. In approximately 15 percent of the criminal cases examined, a positive identification of the defendant was offered. In 35 percent of the cases, elimination, or probability of identification or elimination, was reached by the examiner. In the remaining 50 percent, no opinion was reached one way or the other. In many court cases, after examination was performed, evidence was not offered for several reasons, including an admission of guilt by the suspected person.

There have been several State Supreme Court decisions concerning this type of evidence. In 1976, the Supreme Court of California reversed a trial court decision, but did not rule for or against the use of voice identification by speech spectrograms. The reversal was based on lack of proper foundation by the prosecution in the particular case. The Supreme Court of Massachusetts has upheld a guilty verdict based on voiceprint evidence in the case of *Commonwealth v. Lykus*. In February 1977, the Supreme Court of Pennsylvania ruled against use of speech spectrograms in the case of *Pennsylvania v. Toppa*. The Court ruled that the human voice was too variable, owing to the effects of physiologic, psychologic, and enviromental changes, to produce reliable spectrograms and that the scientific community did not support the spectrographic method at that time.

In the opinion of the author, the first holding is a reasonable one. However, when the intraspeaker variations are so great, owing to the factors mentioned in the resolution, the trained examiner will either render no opinion one way or the other, or will offer a false elimination. A positive identification is not possible under these circumstances. The second holding is controversial and not completely clarified. Which persons form the scientific community? Are they the people who practice a given specialty, or those who hold the same degree, in this case a degree in the speech sciences? The author's point of view is that the scientific community is formed by those who practice a given specialty, in this case, voice identification by aural and visual examination of speech spectrograms. At present, there are about 16 professional examiners and 25 trainees in the International Association of Voice Identification. About 20 Ph.D.s and a number of persons with a master's or bachelor's degree in speech sciences, who are knowledgeable about this particular technique, also support the spectrographic approach. It is true that a small group of speech scientists are very active *against* the method and try to attract other colleagues to their side, very often successfully. The point is that in order to give a valid opinion on the validity of the method, it is essential to have practical experience in dealing with it. Most of the opponents lack this type of expertise.

It should be noted that a short time after the Pennsylvania case, the State of Mississippi did accept voice identification evidence in a first-impression case, *Mississippi v. Winton*. In this case, the Court, being aware of the Pennsylvania opinion, held that the method of voice identification by aural and visual examination of speech spectrograms was accepted in the scientific community under the Frye rule, which is discussed later in this chapter. The defense produced two expert witnesses who were adamantly opposed to the use of this method.

In the case there were three persons who were suspected of having made a bomb threat by telephone to an industrial plant. One of them was kept in jail for more than a month on the grounds that one of the calls had been traced to his telephone. Expert witnesses for the prosecution were Lt. Lonnie Smrkovski of the Michigan Department of State Police and the author. These expert witnesses were able to positively eliminate two of the suspected persons, including the one in jail, and positively identify the third suspected person.

Rebuttal expert witnesses for the antagonistic party in court cases dealing with voice identification evidence usually consist of speech scientists who have steadfastly opposed the use of aural and visual examiniation of spectrograms for court purposes. In the opinion of the International Association of Voice Identification, these speech scientists are not qualified as professional examiners in this specialty.

At present there are several laboratories where examination of voices using combined aural and visual examination of spectrograms is offered, namely, the Voice Identification Unit of the Michigan Department of State Police; the Institute of Voice Identification at Michigan State University; the Firearms, Alcohol and Tobacco Administration in Washington, D.C.;

the Miami (Florida) Department of Police; and Voiceprint, Inc., of New Jersey. The FBI also uses this method for investigative purposes, but has not offered the results of these examinations as legal evidence. Recently the FBI requested the National Academy of Sciences to form a committee to study the reliability of the voiceprint method for legal purposes.

This committee was chaired by Dr. Richard Bolt and consisted of nine members representing different specialties within acoustics, speech sciences, and law. The author was one of those nine persons. After two years of deliberations and gathering data, the committee published a report, *Theory and Practice of Voice Identification* (National Academy of Sciences, Washington, D.C., 1979), including four recommendations as follows:

1. *Scientific understanding of voice identification.* We recommend that a mechanism be established to stimulate, guide, and coordinate a broad national program of scientific research on the processes of speech generation, transmission, and analysis as they pertain to the practice of voice identification.
2. *Certification of voice identification examiners.* We recommend that a national mechanism be established to develop objective standards and methods for testing the performance of voice identification examiners and to certify their competence as examiners.
3. *Improvements in methods and training.* We recommend that practitioners of aural-visual voice identification make full use of certain available knowledge and techniques that could improve the voice identification method.
4. *Forensic testimony on voice identification.* We recommend that if evidence on voice identification is admitted in court—and we take no position on admissibility—then the inherent limitations in the method and in the performance of examiners should be explained to the fact-finder, whether the judge or the jury, in order to protect against overevaluation of such evidence.

   The Committee puts great importance on communicating exactly what it means and does not mean by the words inherent limitations. We do not mean that examiners using the present practice cannot correctly identify voices. We do not mean that the errors are 'too great' or that the reliability is 'too low.' What we do mean by inherent limitations relates to the probabilities of error in a given situation and to the degree of confidence with which the probabilities of error can be estimated. All human decisions based on complex data of the sort encountered in voice identification involve some amount of error on a statistical basis. In voice identification, a given decision can incorrectly match two voices that in fact are the same. The probabilities of making errors of the two kinds depends on the quality of the technique and the data, on the objective skill of the examiner, and on the subjective expectations and consequences of any given decision as judged by the examiner.

In addition, the committee has recognized that in the practice of voice identification the alternative of rendering *no opinion* after examination of speech samples decreases the rate of error as compared with the rate of error yielded by laboratory experiments, where the examiner is not allowed this alternative.

The report of the National Academy of Sciences has clarified in many ways the situation of voice identification by aural and spectrographic examination of speech samples, providing recommendations which might enhance the possibility of its complete acceptance by the scientific community.

Any lawyer who desires to find expert witnesses in this field of evidence may contact the International Association of Voice Identification which can provide names and addresses of available professionals to be consulted by defense or prosecution. The Association was founded and incorporated in Michigan as a nonprofit corporation in May 1971. Founding members were Lawrence Kersta, Ernest Nash, and the author. The purposes of the Association are to set quality standards, develop a code of ethics for the field, and encourage research in all methods of voice identification. To become a professional examiner, the Association requires a candidate to possess an academic background in audiology and speech sciences and to work on practical field cases of voice identification during a minimum of 2 years as a trainee of the Association. After this traineeship is completed, the candidate takes theoretical and practical examinations on voice identification and acoustic phonetics. After successfully passing these examinations, the candidate is granted membership as a professional examiner.

Among the standards set by the Association are the following:

1. A minimum of 10 good similarities or matchings between the unknown and known samples must be available to allow the examiner to produce a positive identification.
2. The examiner must be allowed as many samples and as much time as he feels he needs in order to produce a positive opinion in each examination.
3. According to the particular conditions encountered by the examiner in each case, the following alternative opinions should be adhered to:
   a. Positive identification;
   b. Probability of identification;
   c. Positive elimination;
   d. Probability of elimination;
   e. No opinion one way or the other.

FIELD PROCEDURES

Outline of Procedures

In the actual practice of voice identification and elimination by aural and visual examination of spectrograms, there are several steps to be completed from the moment the alleged criminal has used his or her voice in the commission of the delict until a suspected person is tried in a court of law, presenting the voice as evidence either for identification or for elimination.

The first step consists of recording the criminal or unknown voice. The next step is discovering the suspected persons and obtaining samples of their voices using the same text as the questioned call. All these materials should be sent to a professional examiner on voice identification who will prepare suitable examplars for aural and visual comparisons of the unknown and known voices. After the examination is completed and a decision is reached by such an examiner, the prosecution itself must determine whether or not this evidence will be offered in court. Defense lawyers may also request independently an examination of the voices of their clients for purposes of elimination. In both situations the technical procedures will be the same. A description of these procedures is presented in the next sections.

Recordings of the Questioned Voice

The questioned voice (criminal call) recording is obtained in different manners, according to circumstances:

1. The unknown person calls a police headquarters, a plant, a business office, etc., producing a bomb threat, a false alarm, information connected with a crime, etc. Many police headquarters possess a 24-hour tape recorder that registers all incoming calls. The portion of the 24-hour tape is then transcribed to a cassette or an open-reel tape recorder. Usually the quality of the 24-hour tape is poor, but if the machine is properly maintained, this evidence is usable for purposes of identification. Transcription of the unknown call should be properly done through patching wires. Some actual cases in which this manner of recording the unknown caller was used are given below.

    Call to a police headquarters:

    Minnesota v. Constance Trimble, Ramsey Co. District Ct., St. Paul, No. 24,049.
    Michigan v. Frederick Lemon, 61st District Ct., Grand Rapids.
    Michigan v. Chaisson, District 54-1, City of Lansing.
    Call to a plant:
    U.S. v. Betty Phoenix, So. District Indiana, No. 70-Cr-428.

2. An unknown caller telephones a private person or a home with the purpose of extortion, to request ransom money, or to produce an obscene call. In this case the victim may request the assistance of the police. Usually, police, properly instructed by a crime laboratory, will attach a tape recorder to the victim's telephone. They will instruct the victim to turn on the tape recorder any time the telephone rings, prior to answering. Then if it is a normal call, the recorder can be turned off or the tape can be erased. In case the call is made by the criminal, the entire conversation is recorded. The tape recorder can be connected directly to the telephone line or through a pickup (i.e, a magnetic toroidal pickup adjusted to the receiver). The tape recorder must be plugged into the power line to avoid failures of low-voltage batteries. A clean tape or cassette should always be available in the tape recorder, and the system should be tested frequently to avoid electrical or mechanical problems. Some actual cases in which questioned voice calls were obtained in this manner include:

    U.S. v. Moses Brown, Superior Ct., District of Columbia.
    Commonwealth vs. Edward Lykus, Superior Ct., New Bedford, Mass.
    U.S. v. Earl F. Brown, Jr., U.S. District Ct., Eastern District of Tennessee, No. 13130.
    Michigan v. Larry Nelson, Circuit Ct., County of Oakland.

3. Recordings from an alleged criminal can be obtained by an agent or

informer using a body-attached and concealed tape recorder or a transmitter. Usually this type of recording is noisy and of a poor quality. Bars and public places are the usual environments where the agent or informer goes to meet the alleged criminal to talk. This manner of recording was used in the case of *U.S. v. Lucas* (Supreme Ct., New York, 1974).

Recording Exemplars of Known Suspects and Defendants

To produce recording exemplars, an accurate transcript of the questioned voice text should first be made. The interrogator who obtains the recordings should become familiar with the transcript, rate, and aural characteristics of the questioned voice. Then a system including a telephone line should be set up, if the questioned recording was obtained through the telephone. The line should be as similar as possible to the line used by the criminal, if some knowledge of this particular item is available. At the end of the line where the interrogator sits, a tape recorder should be connected to that telephone. The telephone at the other end of the line is used by the person. The system should be tested prior to the actual recording of exemplars. When all the people involved are ready and communication is established between the two ends of the line, and interrogator should state the date, time, place, his name, and the name of the defendant, who is listening at the other end of the line. Then the interrogator requests the suspect or defendant to utter the first sentence of the questioned transcript, saying, for example: "Please, Mr. X, repeat after me: I will plant a bomb." The person repeats this sentence. If the interrogator is not satisfied for any reason, due to errors or marked deviations from the natural rate, pitch, or articulation of the defendant's speech, he should have the defendant repeat the sentence as many times as necessary. The recording now continues with the second sentence, in the same manner as with the first, until the whole content of the transcript is completed.

The complete procedure can be repeated several times. In addition, a direct tape recorder registration can be obtained at the end where the defendant sits. Sometimes a direct recording can help the examiner. Placement, type of microphone, and a reasonably quiet environment are required for recordings of known voices. The microphone should be unidirectional and place about 30 cm from the mouth of the defendant at an approximate angle of 70 degrees. The recording system should ensure a frequency response the same as, or better than, the telephone line. If particular areas of resonance due to environment or system are known or detected, they should be corrected, if possible, or information on this problem should be provided to the voice identification examiner.

Recordings should be played back before the suspect or defendant leaves the scene in order to allow time to correct any detected deficiency. Cooperation of the defendant is crucial to obtain these exemplars and should be ensured by court order if necessary.

All these materials might be properly dubbed through patch wires, using recorders well maintained and checked, connected to power plugs. Open-reel or cassette tape used should be of a good quality and clean. Bias voltage of the tape recorders utilized should be properly adjusted to the tape used. Tapes should be properly labeled regarding content and mailed or delivered to the examiner, thus ensuring the chain of custody. The examiner should also be careful to protect the chain of custody as required by law, to initial all materials received, and to keep a record with dates and events concerning the case.

Preparation of Spectrograms and Aural Materials

Prior to preparing aural elements and spectrograms for analysis, the examiner should listen carefully to the recordings and check the transcripts to detect any discrepancy with the text spoken. If the examiner did not receive a transcript of the unknown and known voices text, he should prepare one.

The recordings received by the examiner should first be dubbed into one-track, 1.2 mil open-reel tapes at 7.5 inches per second. These tapes are set in the spectrograph, and the first 2.4 second text segment from the unknown call is selected. Settings of the spectrograph for voice identification purposes usually include broad-band filtering, lineal expanded scale 60 to 4,000 Hz, and high shaping (12 dB per octave amplification). A spectrogam of this segment of speech is produced and examined. Frequency marks of this spectrogram are checked. If noise in particular bands is observed, attempts to filter it should be made without losing speech information. Furthermore, particular bands may need to be amplified. A spectrogram using a "flat shaping" should be produced and compared with the previous one. The experience of the examiner will help him to find the best compromising settings to obtain the optimum information. A spectrogram with a scale of frequencies up to 7,000 Hz should be obtained in case fricative information of high bands is included in the recording.

All spectrograms from the unknown caller are obtained in this fashion. Immediately after each spectrogram is taken out of the machine, it should be labeled "unknown," and the name of the case, the date, and the correlative number of the spectrogram should be stated at the superior edge, using a pen or pencil of a selected color, usually red. At the bottom of the spectrogram the text should be written, targeting properly to the corresponding spectrographic patterns. A phonetic writing or the normal spelling or both, one above the other, may be used for this purpose. Correct targeting is crucial, and a professional examiner is expected to do a proper job concerning this matter. An electronic gate, suggested by the author to the producers of the spectrograph some years ago, may help in some instances to difficult targeting.

The known voices text should be processed in the same manner, and the corresponding spectrograms should be labeled with the name of the speaker, the case, the date, and the correlative number of the spectrogram, using a pen or pencil of a different color than the one used for the "unknown" spectrograms. In addition, the text should be written at the bottom of the spectrogram, following the same directions as in the unknown spectrograms.

Preparation of Aural Materials

A convenient way of arranging the unknown and known voices text for comparison of perceptual features by using the short-term memory process is to dub the segments of these texts into continuous loop cartridges of 1.5 minutes duration. Four tracks can be used in each cartridge. In each track a segment of about 2 seconds should be recorded as many times as the duration of the loop allows. The segment should correspond to a sentence or a grammatical unit to avoid cutting the melodic speech pattern of the speaker. Output from the spectrograph or a Cannon loopcorder tape recorder may be used to simplify these recordings. Playing back each track allows the examiner to listen continuously to each segment.

As many cartridges as necessary should be used to record in this manner the complete text from the unknown and known voices. Cartridges must be properly labeled and numbered correlatively in such a manner that track n of cartridge m from the unknown speakers contains the sentence similar to that on track n and cartridge m of the known speakers. Two cartridge tape recorders should be connected to an amplifier and loudspeaker or earphones with a system of switches to select alternatively and quickly any of the unknown and known recordings to be compared aurally. Recording levels of all these loops should be adjusted to the same overall volume.

The examiner should fit the 90-second loop cartridges containing the same sentences from the unknown and known voices in two tape recorders connected to a common stereo amplifier. He can then play back and listen successively to both voices, as often and as long as he deems necessary. The examiner can compare perceptual features from the two voices, such as melody pattern, pitch, quality, respiratory group, and any peculiar, observable common feature. For instance, in a particular case, both the questioned speaker and the defendant produced a peculiar whistling at the end of some sentences which served as a clue for identification. In many cases a difference in pitch is observed between the questioned voice and the known voice. Often the questioned recording presents a higher pitch than the known recording exemplars. In this situation, a good practice is to alter the pitches from both recordings by matching them, using the Varimax tape recorder. In most cases a more precise articulation and a slower rhythm are observed in the known voice than in the unknown one. A trained examiner expects to find these differences and could recognize the usual range of intraspeaker variation through the examination of a considerable number of cases.

If there is more than one known voice, the procedure is repeated, comparing each of these suspected voices with the unknown one. Sometimes comparisons are done among several unknown voices to determine whether or not they belong to the same person.

The examiner may reach a tentative decision after this aural examination. Eventually a panel of listeners also may be utilized to judge on similarities or dissimilarities of the compared voices.

Visual Examination of Spectrograms

The examiner can compare visually the same phonetic elements from the unknown and known spectrograms by matching mean frequencies and bandwidths of formants, slopes and transient patterns, interformant densities, type and distance of vertical striations, distribution of acoustic energy of fricatives and plosives, gaps of plosives, and onset time of vibration of vowels following an invoiced plosive. Important clues for identification can be found in acoustic density distribution patterns if located in the same frequency-time coordinates of the unknown and known spectrograms. For instance, in a recent case, a characteristic isolated spike was found in both the unknown and the known spectrograms of the word "damn" below the second formant and midway of the duration of this word. This type of similarity gives substantial weight to a positive identification. Indeed, the chance that such a particular spike of energy at these coordinates of a word was produced by different persons is very remote (Fig. 51-8).

An examiner never expects to find two spectrograms so similar that they can be overlapped. This is also the case in most systems of identification, including handwriting, fingerprinting, and ballistics.

Dissimilarities found in both sets of spectrograms can be attributed to intraspeaker or interspeaker differences. For instance, some difference in pitch or coarticulation due to slight phonetic variations may alter the mean frequencies of formants in spectrograms of similar sentences produced by the same person. The experience and judgment of a professional examiner can determine whether these differences are due to intra- or interspeaker variability, producing identification or elimination respectively. Only in cases beyond doubt—subjectively speaking—can the examiner honestly produce positive identification. In all other instances he should give probability of identification or elimination, or offer no opinion one way or the other.

It is the author's opinion that reliable evaluations for the courts can be given only be experienced, professional forensic examiners of spectrograms who have spent a number of years performing such evaluations. A general speech scientist with no special training in voice identification cannot offer an expert opinion on this subject, no matter how thorough his knowledge of speech sciences.

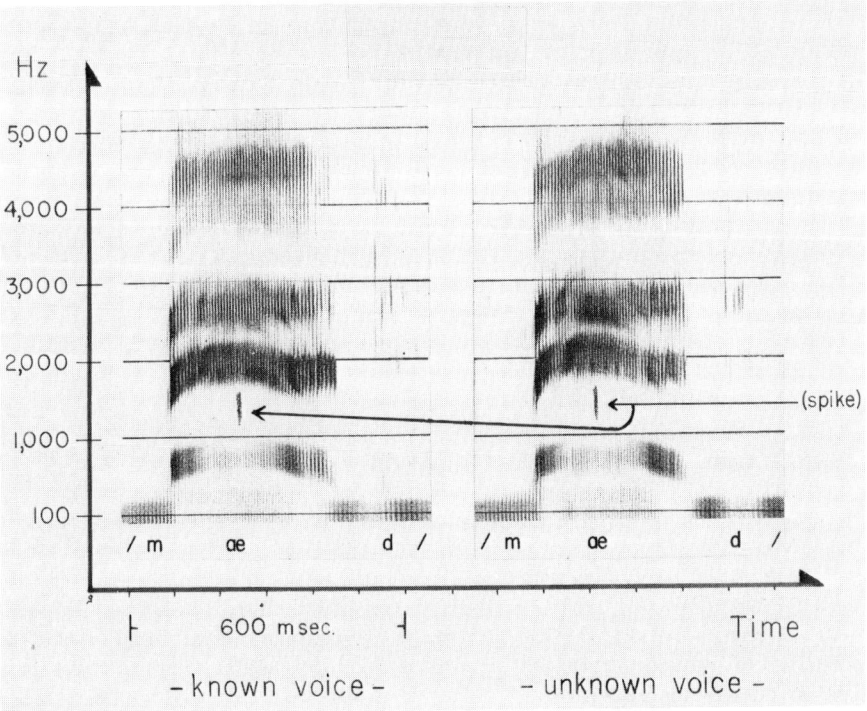

FIGURE 51-8. Spectrograms of the word "mad" corresponding to an unknown and to a known voice respectively. The spike between the second and the third formants is a strong indication that these two spectrograms correspond to the same person.

COURT APPEARANCES

Through all the cases involving voice identification, a typical pattern of courtroom examination of expert witnesses in voice identification has developed. Its description may help prosecuting attorneys and defense counselors alike in preparing their own trial strategy in the event that they should deal with this type of evidence. In this description it is assumed that the voice of the defendant has been positively identified by a professional examiner. Therefore, the prosecutor takes the direct examination, and the defense counselor the cross-examination, of the expert witness for the prosecution. It is assumed that there are rebuttal expert witnesses for the defense.

In direct examination, after the usual questions to qualify the examiner, an attempt is generally made to restrict the field of voice identification to those who practice this specialty on a professional and continuous basis. The reason is that the expert witness for the defense usually is a general speech scientist rather than a professional voiceprint examiner.

At this point in the examination, the defense attorney usually objects to the admission of voiceprint evidence on the basis of the Frye rule; that is, that the technology is not accepted as reliable by the scientific community. Upon this objection, the judge must make a ruling before the witness can go any further in his substantive-opinion testimony. If a jury is present, the judge may exclude the jury while this issue is being presented by both sides.

The criteria for application of the Frye rule vary in different jurisdictions. Some require acceptance of reliability in the entire community of speech scientists, while others limit the test to acceptance among scientists in the field of voice identification.

Normally the prosecutor then proceeds to ask his expert to describe voice identification methods generally and voiceprint spectrography in particular. The various experimental projects described earlier in this chapter are usually presented, especially the Tosi project because of its size and scope. The opinion is offered that the technology is accepted as reliable in the scientific community.

After this presentation, the defense usually offers rebuttal by its witness, a general speech scientist, who states his opinion that the method is unreliable and scientifically unsound and that voiceprint technology is not accepted in the scientific community of which he, the witness, is a part.

As a part of the rebuttal, the defense counsel often tries to dismiss conclusions from favorable laboratory experiments to real-life cases of voice identification, arguing that the many different factors encountered in real life, as opposed to laboratory experiments, render such conclusions not applicable to actual legal cases. In re-direct examination of the prosecution witness this argument is countered by stating that all conditions that may produce differences in the spectrograms from the unknown and known voices can lead to only a probability of identification, or, at the worst, to a false elimination rather than to a false positive identification. Only when the examiner is convinced beyond doubt that the unknown and the defendant's samples belong to the same person does he produce a positive identification. In any other situation he abstains from giving an opinion one way or the other or states only probabilities.

After these presentations, the trial court judge makes his ruling. If it is favorable to admission of the evidence, the voiceprint examiner is allowed to continue with his testimony in the presence of the jury, if it is a jury trial.

Later in the trial, during the submission of evidence for the defense, the defense attorney will place his rebuttal witness on the stand and attempt to qualify him as an expert in the voice-identification field. In the cross-examination by the prosecutor, questions are asked concerning the experience of the witness specifically in voice identification, rather than in speech and hearing sciences in general. Many well-recognized scientists, brought to the court by subpoena or by their own will, have failed to qualify as experts on voice identification, some of them by their own admission. This point should be considered by the defense counselors. Rather than to attack the voiceprint method as unacceptable, they may consider the option of securing a professional examiner who can testify in behalf of the defendant if such an examiner has found only a probability of identification or elimination, or no opinion one way or the other, after examination of the tapes. When voiceprint evidence is admitted, the court often allows submission of spectrographs and tape recordings as court exhibits. These exhibits consists of spectrograms from the unknown and the defendant's voice uttering the same sentences. Very often a tape recording containing sequences of unknown and defendant sentences is also introduced and played back to the jury.

Similarities from both sets of spectrograms are shown and explained to the court and the jury if the defense insists on this procedure. It is preferable not to do so because in these situations each member of the jury tends to feel that he or she can become an instant expert in matching spectrographic similarity. If this situation does occur, the attorney should ask an instruction against the practice, which is often highly detrimental to the prosecution's effort to support the expertness of the evaluation.

The defense, on the other hand, could have prepared spectrograms and tapes of the same questioned text produced by a person with a voice with the same general characteristics as the defendant's voice. These materials could eventually convince a jury about the difficulty of identifying a person through his or her voice.

Another rebuttal that the defense may offer is to demand the disclosure of the receiver-operating characteristic of the prosecutor's expert witness or to request that this examiner be given an "open" test, including the voice of the defendant among the voices of other people, identified by a number rather than by a name. These rebuttals would need to be conducted in open court, an unlikely practice in most jurisdictions.

TRAINING OF VOICE IDENTIFICATION EXAMINERS

There are several institutions that offer training for voice identification examiners using oral and visual examination of speech spectrograms. One of these is the Michigan State University Institute of Voice Identification, which offers periodic workshops that are held for eight hours a day, five days a week, for one month, in cooperation with the crime laboratory of the Michigan Department of State Police. The workshops include both theoretical and practical training in voice identification by aural and visual examination of spectrograms. The theoretical training consists of lectures on acoustic phonetics, theory of voice production, and speech spectrography. Practical training consists of aural examination of voices and visual examination of spectrograms of voices from laboratory experiments and from real-life cases.

The theoretical aspects of acoustic phonetics and voice production are presented at an elementary level, including instruction on the general characteristics of sound, simple harmonic motion, representation of waves in the temporal and in the frequency domain, complex waves, Fourier analysis, resonances, production of speech, acoustic characteristics of speech sounds, formants, areas of higher acoustical density, and coarticulation phenomena. Also provided are a comprehensive discussion of phonetics and a practicum on the usage of the international phonetic alphabet.

The practical training of students in the workshop starts with very simple cases of identification using closed trials and contemporary spectrograms. Explanations are given of the kinds of similarity patterns that should be detected in order to identify properly an unknown voice from several known voices. Training continues with more complicated cases involving noncontemporary spectrograms and open trials until the students achieve an accuracy of at least 90 percent. Then more complicated cases are offered, including noise interference and closely similar voices. Aural examination is also discussed. Aural trials are presented to the students in graduated degrees of difficulty, from very simple cases, closed trials, and contemporary recordings, to more complicated cases involving noncontemporary recordings, open trials, and, later, recordings with noise.

Once the students have reached at least a 90 percent success rate in identifications and eliminations and have shown proficiency in handling combined aural and visual examinations, they are ready to consider actual field cases from the Voice Identification Unit of the Michigan Department of State Police. They are left on their own to prepare the whole process from original recordings to final results.

A final examination is given to the students, covering both the theoretical aspects and the practical tasks, including a field case. In addition, the students, are trained to obtain samples from known voices in an actual setting that imitates a field situation. Instruction is given in preparing a transcript and in presenting the questions to a suspected person for recording a satisfactory voice exemplar.

The workshop on voice identification and elimination is offered to both scientists and crime laboratory technicians with good scientific background. It should be pointed out that the Michigan State University Institute of Voice Identification does not provide a certificate of professional competency, but only a certificate of attendance at the workshop. Another institution that provides training in spectrography as applied to voice identification is Voiceprint, Inc.

THE FUTURE OF VOICE IDENTIFICATION

No method or combination of methods can presently produce absolutely positive identifications or eliminations in all cases submitted. It could be stated reasonably that the better the quality and extension of available samples, the better the qualifications of the examiner, and the more comprehensive the cluster of methods used, the better the chance of obtaining valid results in a large percentage of cases. Continued research in this area, using both subjective and objective methods, is needed.

Practical forensic experience will dictate whether aural and visual examinations should be complemented with semiautomatic or automatic methods when these techniques become available and are proved reliable.

Better practices also can be developed to assure the qualifications of voiceprint examiners, including a continuing test of competency through periodic review of the examiner's receiver-operating characteristic.

REFERENCES

1. Wolf, J.: Efficient Acoustic Parameters for Speaker Recognition. *J. Acoustical Soc. Am.* 51:2044–2056, 1972.
2. Atal, B.: Automatic Speaker Recognition Based on Pitch Contour. *J. Acoustical Soc. Am.* 52:1687–1697, 1972.
3. Tosi, O., et al.: Experiment on Voice Identification. *J. Acoustical Soc. Am.* 51:2030–2043, 1972.
3. Holmgren, G.: Physical and Psychological Correlates of Speaker Recognition. *J. Speech Hearing Res.* 10:57–66, 1967.
5. Tosi, et al., op. cit.
6. McGehee, F.: The Reliability of the Identification of the Human Voice. *J. Gen. Psychol.* 17:249–271, 1937.
7. Pollack, I., Pickett, J., and Sumby, W.: On the Identification of Speakers by Voice. *J. Acoustical Soc. Am.* 26:403–406, 1954.
8. Bricker, P., and Pruzansky, S.: Effect of Stimulus Content and Duration on Talker Identification. *J. Acoustical Soc. Am.* 40:1441–1449, 1966.
9. Stevens, K. N., Williams, C. E., Carbonell, J. R., and Woods, B.: Speaker Authentication and Identification: A Comparison of Spectrographic and Auditory Presentation of Speech Material. *J. Acoustical Soc. Am.* 44:1596–1607, 1968.
10. Holmgren, op. cit.
11. Black, J. W.: The Quality of a Spoken Vowel. *Arch. Speech* 2:7–27, 1937.
12. Potter, R., Kopp, G., and Green, H.: *Visible Speech*. Van Nostrand, New York, 1947 (reprinted by Dover, New York, 1966).
13. Presti, A. J.: High-Speed Sound Spectrograph. *J. Acoustical Soc. Am.* 40:628–634, 1966.
14. Gray, C. H., and Kopp, G. A.: Voiceprint Identification. Bell Laboratories Report, 1944, pp. 1, 3, 13, 14.
15. Kersta, L. G.: Voiceprint Identification. *Nature* 196:1253–1257, 1962.
16. Ladefoged, P., and Vanderslice, R.: The Voiceprint Mystique. *Working Papers in Phonetics*, Vol. 7. University of California, Los Angeles, 1967.
17. Young, M., and Campbell, R.: Effects of Contexts on Talker Identification. *J. Acoustical Soc. Am.* 42:1250–1254, 1967.
18. Stevens, et al., op. cit.
19. Hazen, B.: Effects of Different Phonetic Contexts on Spectrographic Speaker Identification. *J. Acoustical Soc. Am.* 54:650–660, 1973.
20. Tosi, et al., op. cit.
21. Bolt, R., et al.: Speaker Identification by Speech Spectrograms: Some Further Observations. *J. Acoustical Soc. Am.* 54:531–534, 1973.
22. Wolf, op. cit.
23. Hair, G., and Rekieta, T.: Speaker Identification Final Report. Stanford Research Institute Report No. 1363, Stanford, Cal., 1972.
24. Atal, op. cit.
25. Wolf, op. cit.
26. Su, L., and Fu, K.: Automatic Speaker Identification Using Nasal Spectra and Nasal Coarticulation as Acoustic Clues. Air Force Office of Scientific Research Grant 69-1776. Report TR-EE 73-33, Purdue University School of Electrical Engineering, Lafayette, Indiana, 1973.
27. Bordone, C., et al.: Invariances of Talkers' Choral Spectra. Paper presented at the 87th meeting of the Acoustical Society of America, New York, April 23–26, 1974.
28. Tosi, O.: *Voice Identification: Theory and Legal Applications*. University Park Press, Baltimore, 1979.

CHAPTER 52

Joseph P. Buckley is Director of the John E. Reid and Associates Laboratory in Chicago, and is a lecturer in polygraph technology at Northwestern University School of Law. A graduate of Loyola University and Reid College of Detection of Deception, Mr. Buckley is Vice President of the American Polygraph Association and is Chairman of the Legal Information Committee of the Illinois Polygraph Society. He has contributed to the second edition of *Truth and Deception: The Polygraph ("Lie Detector") Technique,* by J. E. Reid and F. E. Inbau.

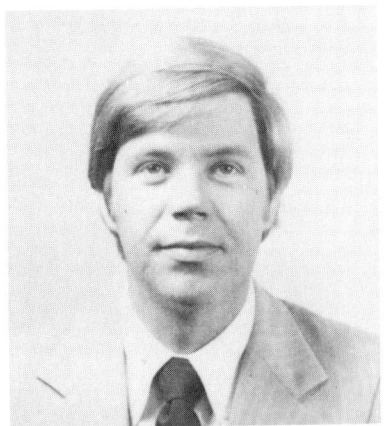

POLYGRAPH TECHNOLOGY

Joseph P. Buckley, M.S.

The primary purpose of this chapter is to provide the reader with a general description of the theory and principles of the polygraph technique. It would be impossible in a single chapter to attempt a discussion and explanation of all of the details and intricacies involved in the scientific detection of deception. Therefore, the following material is designed to provide only a general overview of the procedural aspects of the polygraph technique.[1]

A DIAGNOSTIC PROCEDURE

To the general public the polygraph is more commonly referred to as the "lie-detector" and is often perceived to be a mechanical device that provides a sensory signal (such as a ringing bell or flashing light) when a subject lies to a test question. On the other hand there are some individuals who believe the opposite to be true; that is, they consider it impossible for any type of mechanical device to be used to determine whether or not a person is truthfully answering a question. Both of these views, however, are unfounded.

Although there is no instrument that mechanically signals whether a person is lying or telling the truth, it is a demonstrable fact that there are available instruments (polygraphs) which are capable of producing recordings of physiologic data that may be used as the basis for the application of a reliable technique for diagnosing deception.

HISTORICAL DEVELOPMENT

The first attempt to use a scientific instrument in an effort to determine truth or deception occurred about 1895. At that time Cesare Lombroso published an account of his experiments in which he attempted to detect deception on actual criminal suspects by recording their blood pressure-pulse changes by means of a device called a "hydrosphygmograph." Since this instrument was already in existence at the time of Lombroso's experiments, he cannot be considered a "lie-detector" inventor but certainly should be accorded the distinction of being the first individual to utilize a scientific instrument for the purpose of detecting lies.

Subsequent to Lombroso's work, numerous other individuals experimented with various scientific instruments in an effort to determine their applicability in the detection of deception.[2] These efforts culminated in the development of the "Reid polygraph," by John E. Reid in 1945, which recorded blood pressure, pulse, respiration, the galvanic skin reflex or electrodermal response (generally referred to as the GSR), and muscular activity. This instrument, which will be subsequently described in greater detail, is presently considered to be the most practical and effective scientific instrument available for the detection of deception.

CONTROL QUESTION TECHNIQUE

At the present time there are basically two types of testing techniques used by polygraph examiners: the relevant/irrelevant question technique, and the control question technique. Due to severe limitations in the relevant-irrelevant question technique, the material in this chapter is confined to the control question technique, which has proved to be the far more reliable of the two.

THE INSTRUMENT

The instrument that is used in the proper application of the polygraph technique is essentially a pneumatically operated mechanical recorder of changes in respiration, blood pressure, and pulse. These basic features may be supplemented by a unit for recording the galvanic skin reflex or electrodermal response, which is presumably based upon the change of electrical conductivity of the skin, and a unit for recording muscular movements and pressures.

Any instrument that does not record, as a minimum, respiration and blood pressure-pulse changes is totally inadequate for polygraph testing in actual case situations.

The polygraph is attached in the following manner to the person being tested. One pneumograph tube, with the aid of a beaded chain, is fastened around the chest and another one around the abdomen of the subject to measure the respiration patterns. A blood pressure cuff, of the type used by physicians, is fastened around the subject's upper right arm. Electrodes are then attached to the subject's left hand or fingers. No attachment is necessary to record body movements or pressures; they are obtainable by means of a rubber bladder affixed to the backrest of the chair occupied by the subject. These attachments, as well as the entire polygraph instrument itself, are shown in Figure 52-1.

THE EXAMINATION ROOM

Polygraph examinations should be conducted in a quiet, private, semi-soundproof room. Extraneous noises, such as the ringing of a telephone or the conversation of persons outside the examination room, or the pres-

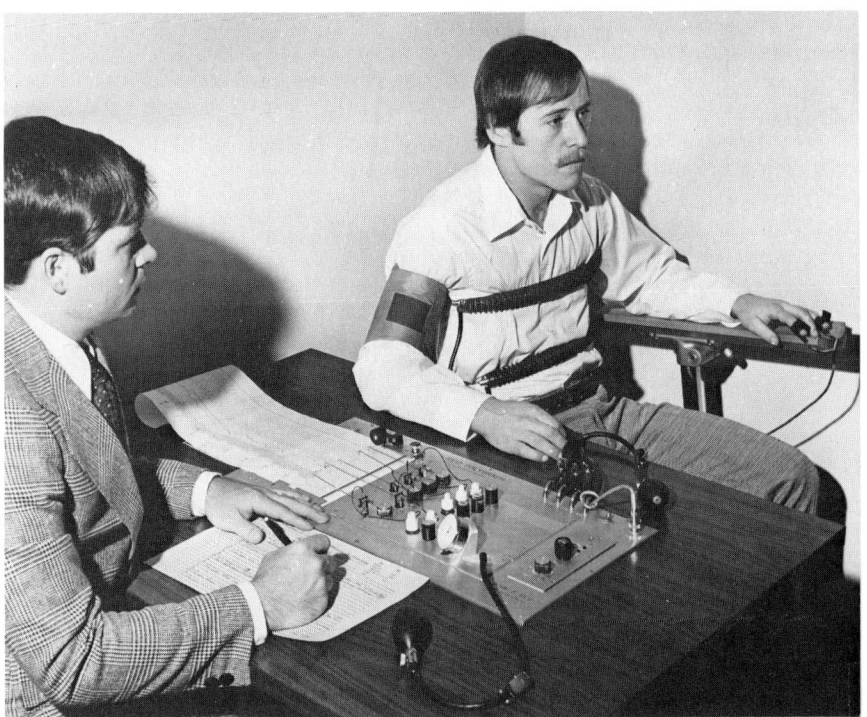

FIGURE 52-1. This photograph illustrates the Reid polygraph in operation. Observe the pneumograph tubes around the subject's chest and abdomen, the blood pressure cuff around the upper right arm, and the electrodes attached to two fingers on the left hand. The back of the chair is equipped with an inflatable rubber bladder for the purpose of recording muscular contractions and pressures. The subject is placed in a position so that he or she looks straight ahead, with the instrument to the right side and rear. The examiner is portrayed by Stanley M. Slowik, Director of the John E. Reid and Associates Laboratory in Denver. The subject is portrayed by Michael T. Reid, a licensed Illinois examiner, presently an attorney at law in Chicago.

ence of investigators or other spectators in the room itself, would induce disturbances and distractions that in turn would distort the various physiologic recordings and seriously interfere with a satisfactory polygraph diagnosis.

EXAMINER QUALIFICATIONS AND TRAINING

Although the type of instrument and technique used in any given polygraph examination are important, the critical factors involved in any examination are the ability, experience, education, and integrity of the examiner himself. An examiner must be an intelligent person with a reasonably good educational background, preferably a college degree. Since the examiner will be dealing with people in sensitive situations, he must also possess the ability to "get along" well with others and to be sincere in his dealings with them. He must be able to view each examination objectively and must always guard against allowing his personal views, prejudices, or biases to distort his performance. It is critical that the training of a polygraph examiner has included an internship under the guidance of a competent, experienced examiner with a sufficient volume of actual cases to permit the trainee to make frequent observations of polygraph examinations and to conduct tests himself under the instructor's personal supervision. Too often the training of a polygraph examiner merely consists of sitting in a lecture room for 6 weeks, never being afforded the opportunity to learn from the experience of actual case examinations under the supervision of an expert.

The trainee should also have read and received instruction in the relevant phases of psychology and physiology, and particularly in the examination and interpretation of a considerable number of polygraph test records in verified cases, where the status of the respective case has been positively established as definite by some independent evidence. The required period of this individualized training should be a minimum of 6 months.

TEST PROCEDURE

Pretest Interview

Before administering a polygraph examination, it is imperative that the examiner conduct a pretest interview, usually lasting 30 to 40 minutes. During this interview the instrument should be explained to the subject, as well as the purpose and nature of the examination itself. It is at this time that the actual test questions are developed and reviewed with the subject, particularly those which will serve as the control questions. In addition, the pretest interview involves the casual asking of a series of questions which are predesigned to elicit verbal and nonverbal responses that may give the examiner an indication of the subject's truthful or deceptive status.

The pretest interview allows the examiner an opportunity to relieve the apprehensions of the truthful subject, as well as to satisfy the deceptive subject as to the efficacy of the technique.

The interview must not be accusatory; its main purpose is to permit examiner observations and to formulate test questions. At no time during the pretest interview should the examiner indulge in any interrogation aimed at determining the subject's deception or truthfulness, or at obtaining a confession. To do so would place the accuracy of any subsequent testing in total jeopardy.

TEST QUESTIONS

Irrelevant Questions

For the purpose of ascertaining the subject's normal pattern of responsiveness, he is asked several questions that have no bearing on the case investigation. These are known as "irrelevant" questions—questions which the examiner knows the subject is answering truthfully. An example of such a question is one regarding the subject's age, as, for instance, "Are you over 21 years of age?" Reference might be made to some other age unquestionably but reasonably, and not ridiculously, below that of the subject. Usually four irrelevant questions are asked during a polygraph test.

Control Questions

For a polygraph examination to be both fair to the subject and accurate in its indications of truthfulness or deception, it is a necessity that the examiner use control questions. A control question is one which is unrelated to the matter under investigation but of a similar, though less serious, nature, and one to which the subject will, in all probability, lie; or at least his answer will give him some concern with respect to either its truthfulness or its accuracy. For instance, in a theft-motivated case, the control question might be: "Did you ever steal anything in your life?" or "Since the age of 18, did you ever steal anything?" If the subject were to make any admissions to the proposed control question during the pretest interview, it would be rephrased to include them (e.g., "Except for what you've told me, did you steal anything else in your life?"). Usually two control questions are utilized during a polygraph test.*

Relevant Questions

Questions pertaining to the particular issue under investigation are known as "relevant" questions. There usually are three or four relevant questions in a polygraph test, and each must be unambiguous, unequivocal, and thoroughly understandable to the subject.†

The relevant test questions should all be related to one issue or to one particular criminal act. If, in a single polygraph examination, the examiner were to inquire about the subject's possible participation in several

---

*The admissions made by a subject on the control question should be kept in confidence by the examiner, and in many instances the examiner will make such a promise of confidentiality to the subject. The purpose of the control question is to insure the accuracy of the technique, not to develop incriminating admissions against the person being tested.

†The relevant-irrelevant question technique was originally developed by John Larson and Leonarde Keller in the 1920s, and is still used by many polygraph examiners today. This questioning technique contains two types of test questions, those pertaining to the issue under investigation (relevant questions) and other questions which are irrelevant, such as those dealing with the subject's name, age, and residence. The responses on the relevant and irrelevant questions are compared, and if the subject responded more to the relevant questions, he is considered as not telling the truth, but if no significant responses occur to either the relevant or irrelevant questions, the subject is reported as truthful. The limitations of this technique are: (1) a lying subject who is naturally unresponsive would be erroneously reported as truthful since they would show no response to either the relevant or irrelevant questions; (2) some truthful subjects may initially show a response to the relevant questions as a result of nervousness or apprehension, and without something more substantial with which to compare their responses than an irrelevant question, they stand a greater chance of being reported as deceptive with this technique than with the control question technique, and (3) using the relevant-irrelevant question technique there was found to be an inconclusive rate of over 20 percent, as compared to a rate of about 5 percent inconclusive findings with the control question technique. The limitations of the relevant-irrelevant question technique were overcome with the development and introduction of the control question technique in 1947 by John E. Reid. The control question technique is considered by all polygraph authorities in this country to be the most reliable and effective questioning technique in the scientific detection of deception.

unrelated offenses, the accuracy of the test results may be severely limited. For example, if during the polygraph examination of a lying subject, he were to be asked four relevant questions, each dealing with a separate and distinct rape offense, there would be a strong possibility that he may only show deceptive responses to the particular rape which was, to him, the most devastating or emotionally weighted one. Let us assume that in one offense the victim died as a result of injuries suffered during the rape; in the second case the victim was beaten up but recovered; in the third the rape took place without the victim's suffering any physical injury; and in the fourth the rape was attempted, but the perpetrator fled before accomplishing the act. If the subject who committed all four offenses were to be questioned simultaneously during one polygraph examination about all of the offenses, in all probability he would only show deceptive responses to the one or two most serious ones, namely the one in which the victim died or the one in which the victim was seriously injured. It is highly probable that no deceptive responses would appear to the relevant questions dealing with the third or fourth offenses, because they would be less meaningful and less weighted in the mind of the subject. Consequently, an examiner could mistakenly interpret the lack of responses to the latter offenses as indicative of truthfulness as to them.

In addition to confining the relevant test questions to one issue, it is important to limit the number of relevant questions in a given examination. If the examiner were to ask more than four or five relevant questions, in addition to the two control questions and the four irrelevant questions, the danger exists that responses occurring on the additional relevant questions may be the result solely of the discomfort the subject may be feeling from the inflated blood pressure cuff. Also, it would be more difficult for a deceptive subject to maintain an emotional tension to each relevant question if it were disseminated over 10 or 15 questions, rather than if there were only three or four relevant questions.

Finally, the relevant test questons should go to the very heart of the issue and be very specific in nature to obtain the most accurate results. The relevant questions should be phrased in similar terms, as illustrated by the following examples with respect to four different polygraph case situations:

> Last Monday did you kill John Jones?
> Last Monday did you steal that missing $50,000 from the First National Bank?
> Did you force Mary Smith to have sexual intercourse with you?
> On June 4, 1977, did you force a man at gunpoint to give you money?

At the conclusion of the pretest interview, and prior to the first test, the subject is told precisely what all the test questions will be, and he is also assured that no questions will be asked about any other offense or matter than that which has been discussed with him by the examiner. Surprise has no part in a properly conducted polygraph examination. If the examiner were to ask a question that he did not review with the subject, any subsequent response could be due to the "surprise" aspect of the question or even to the subject's uncertainty as to the meaning of the question.

CONSTRUCTION AND NUMBER OF TESTS

The following is a list of the types and arrangement of questions asked during a typical polygraph test. Questions 1, 2, 4, and 7 are irrelevant.

Questions 3, 5, 8, and 9 are relevant. Questions 6 and 10 are the control questions. During each test the subject is required to answer only "yes" or "no" to each question. These questions are based on a hypothetical arson case in which the subject's place of business was totally destroyed by the fire. (Since the suspected motive for the fire was to fraudulently obtain the insurance money covering the property, whether or not the subject ever cheated anyone in his life is deemed the appropriate primary control question.)

1. Do they call you James? (The pretest interview has disclosed that he is generally called James.)
2. Are you over 40 years of age? (Alternatively, reference is made to some other age unquestionably but reasonably below that of the subject.)
3. Last Saturday night, did you set fire to the White Department Store at First and Main Streets?
4. Are you in Chicago [or another city] now?
5. Did you start the fire in your store?
6. Besides what you told about, did you ever cheat in any other way in your life?
7. Did you ever go to school?
8. Did you plan or arrange with anyone to set fire to your store?
9. Do you know who started the fire in your store?
10. Did you ever do anything that was against the law?

The time interval between each question is 15 to 20 seconds.

The asking of the foregoing questions in one test *does not constitute a polygraph examination;* there must be at least three, and usually more, tests of a similar design before a diagnosis can be attempted, because even the truthful subject may show a response to a relevant question on one of the tests, for a variety of reasons. Therefore, it is necessary that a full series of tests be given to establish the degree, and most importantly, the consistency of responses. The entire examination usually takes approximately 60 minutes.

THE DIAGNOSIS

At the conclusion of the testing, the examiner studies and evaluates the polygraph records. At the risk of oversimplification, it may be said that a lie reaction is ordinarily indicated in the tracings by a suppression or distortion in respiration and by a change in blood pressure-pulse, or in the galvanic skin reflex, immediately after the subject has answered the questions asked by the examiner. If the subject responds or reacts to a greater degree, and consistently so, to the control questions than to the relevant questions, he is considered truthful. If, on the other hand, a greater degree and consistency of reaction or response occur on the relevant questions in comparison to no response, or only a slight response, to the control questions, that is suggestive of deception.

The following reproductions of actual polygraph recordings are illustrative of the type of responses that are considered indicative of truthfulness (Figs. 52-2, 52-3, and 52-4) and of deception (Figs. 52-5, 52-6, and 52-7), using only the respiration blood pressure-pulse criteria.

In many instances the person being tested will attempt to distort the polygraph tracings or, as it is sometimes said, to "beat the test." These

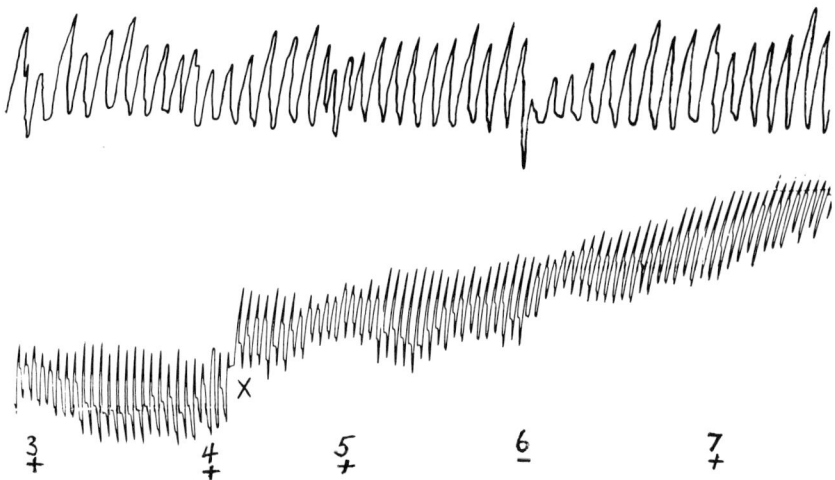

FIGURE 52-2. Record of a truthful 15-year-old subject who claimed that he and a friend were the victims of excessive physical force by the police. Questions 4 and 7 were irrelevant. At questions 3 and 5, the subject was asked whether the police threatened and struck his friend, as alleged by the subject. His "yes" answers did not produce any significant responses, whereas his "no" answer at question 6, the control question, did. At question 6, he was asked whether he had ever done anything that he would not want his parents to know about. His response in respiration and blood pressure at that point clearly indicated that his "no" answer was a lie. Based on the lack of any comparable response at questions 3 and 5, the examiner concluded that the accusations of excessive force were truthful. The X marked above question 4 indicated an adjustment of the blood pressure recording by the examiner at that point.

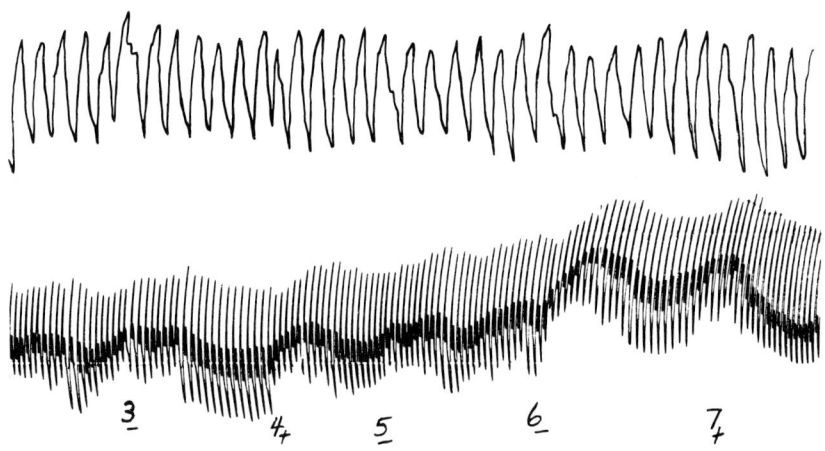

FIGURE 52-3. Record of a truthful theft suspect. Questions 4 and 7 were irrelevant. At questions 3 and 5, the subject was asked whether he had stolen any merchandise (medical instruments) from his employer. Question 6 was the control question, "Did you ever steal anything?" The only significant response appeared in the blood pressure tracing at control question 6. In view of the response at 6, and the lack of response at relevant questions 3 and 5, the proper interpretation was one of truthfulness regarding the subject's theft of merchandise from his employer.

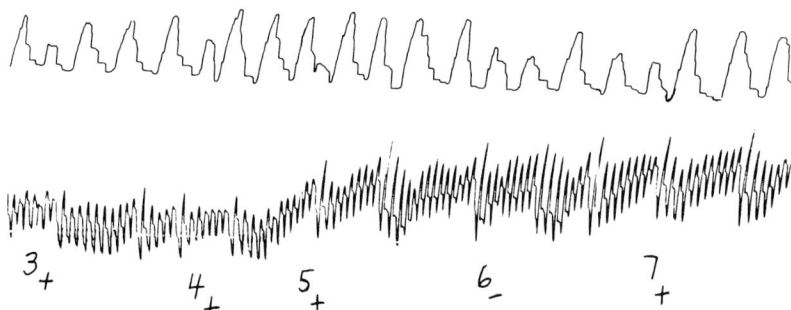

FIGURE 52-4. Record of a truthful subject who claimed that one of his male coworkers had made sexual advances toward him. Questions 3 and 5 pertained to the allegations, the former being, "Did Williams tell you that John D. said he wanted to have sex with you?" and the latter being, "Did John D. ever tell you that he wanted to make love to you?" Questions 4 and 7 were irrelevant. Observe the suppression in respiration at control question 6, when the subject was asked: "Did you ever cheat anyone in your life?" The respiration response at control question 6, compared to the lack of response on relevant questions 3 and 5, indicated that this subject was telling the truth. This conclusion was later verified as accurate.

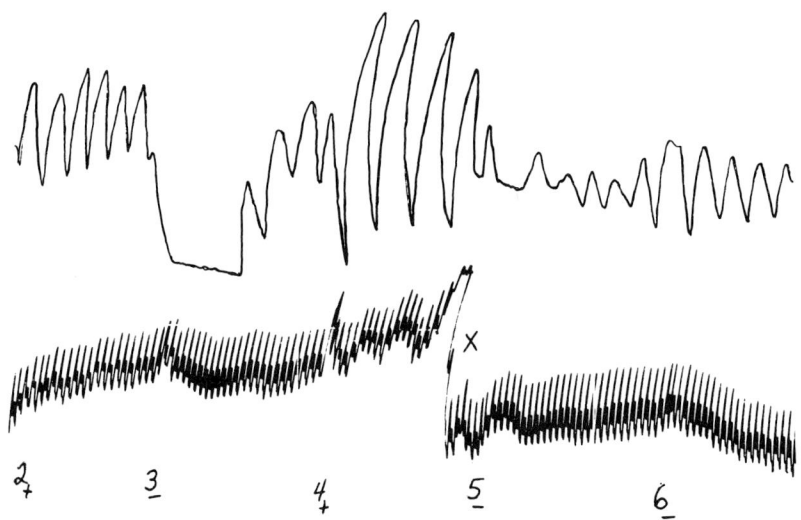

FIGURE 52-5. Record of a lying law enforcement official alleged to have made derogatory racial comments to a fellow official. Questions 3 and 5 pertained to the alleged racial statements; question 4 was irrelevant, and question 6 was the control question: "Did you ever break any department rules or regulations?" Significant deceptive responses appear in the respiration tracing at questions 3 and 5, whereas no response occurred at question 6. The subject's lies to the relevant questions (3 and 5) dealing with the accusations were of greater concern to him than lying to the general control question. This is the reverse of the situation of a person who is telling the truth regarding the main issue; his principal concern on the test is the control question lie. The X above question 5 indicates an adjustment of the blood pressure tracing by the examiner at that point.

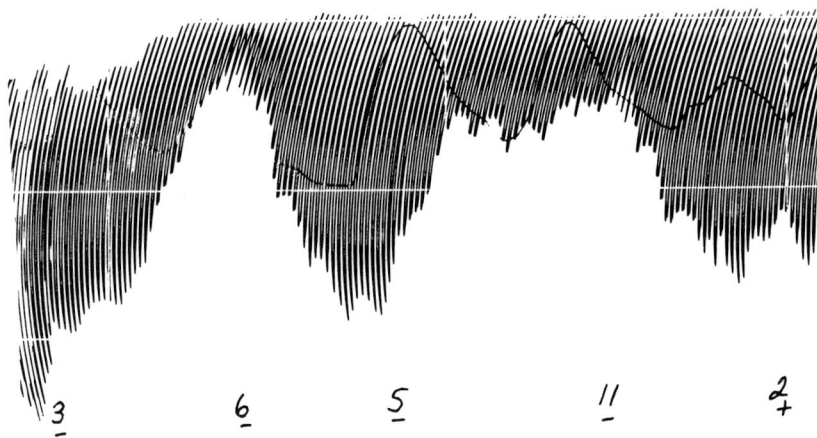

FIGURE 52-6. Record of a lying theft suspect. Question 2 was irrelevant; questions 3 and 5 referred to the theft of a diamond; questions 6 and 11 were control questions. The dramatic rise in the blood pressure level at relevant questions 3 and 5 followed by the return of the blood pressure to its normal level at control questions 6 and 11 are clear indications of the subject's deception about the diamond theft. This record is a portion of the subject's mixed question test. On the mixed question test the questions are read to the subject in sequence such that each relevant question is paired with a control question.

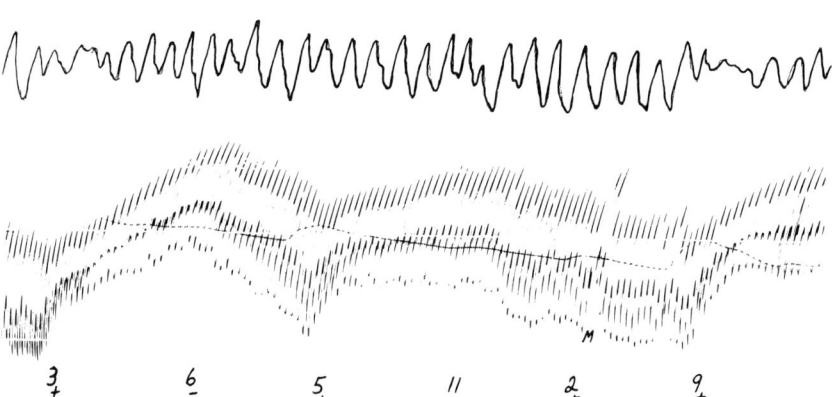

FIGURE 52-7. Record of a lying subject. Questions 3, 5, and 9 referred to whether the subject complied with the provisions of his sentence; question 2 was irrelevant; questions 6 and 11 were control questions. Observe at questions 3, 5, and 9, the rise in the blood pressure level, and at questions 3 and 9, the respiration responses. These specific responses at the relevant questions, and the lack of comparable responses at control questions 6 and 11, are indicative of deception. The M above question 2 indicates a movement by the subject at that point.

evasive efforts can, in themselves, be reliable indicators of deception, as illustrated in Figures 52-8, and 52-9.

There are several extraneous factors which can influence the outcome of the polygraph test results. One such factor would be lack of concern about the test on the part of the person being tested. If the subject is not concerned and has little or no fear about having his deception detected, his test results would probably be inconclusive (i.e., no decision could be rendered as to his truthfulness or deception on the relevant questions).

In order for the polygraph examiner to render a definite diagnosis as to truth or deception there must be a consistency of response or reaction to either the relevant questions or the control questions.

The basic psychological factor underlying the polygraph technique is fear of detection. Unless the person being tested is concerned about, or even fearful of, the instrumental technique indicating his deception, the test would be ineffective. There must be an emotional involvement on the part of the subject; he must feel motivated to lie, either on the relevant questions or the control questions, in order to obtain significant responses. It is the fear of detection or motivation to lie, due to a feeling that something is at stake, which stimulates the subject's sympathetic nervous system, thereby causing the physiologic changes recorded by the polygraph instrument.

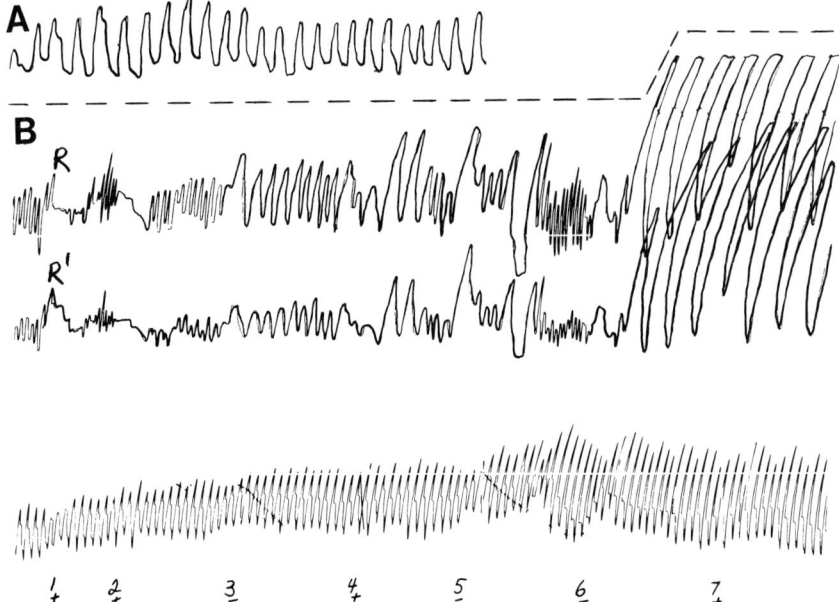

FIGURE 52-8. Record of a lying embezzlement suspect. A is an example of the subject's normal respiration pattern obtained before the actual testing began. B is a portion of the subject's test in which he was asked about the embezzlement at questions 3 and 5. Questions 1,2,4, and 7 were irrelevant, and question 6 was the control question: "Did you ever steal anything?" Observe the subject's attempt to distort his respiration pattern by engaging initially in very fast, rapid breathing and then very deep, heavy breathing at questions 6 and 7. These distortion efforts can be seen in both the abdominal respiration tracing (R) and the thoracic respiration tracing (R'). The lying subject engages in this type of deliberate distortion in the hope that he may be able to mislead the examiner or render the test inconclusive. However, distortion efforts of this magnitude are clear indications of deception in themselves.

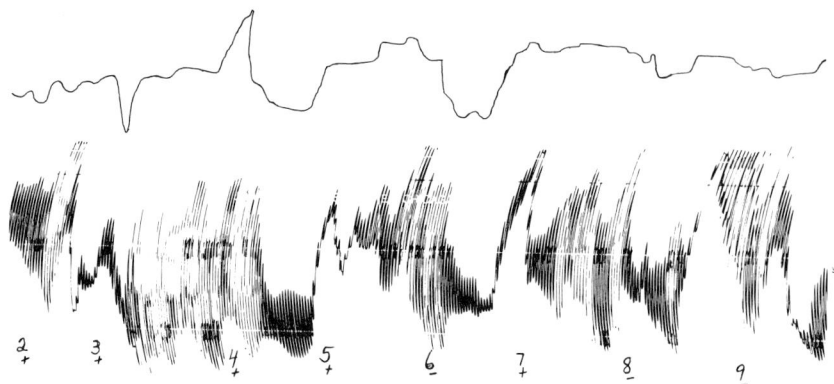

FIGURE 52-9. Record of a lying subject suspected of stealing $60,000. During the examination of this subject, he attempted to distort his test records by flexing his biceps muscle (as reflected by the erratic nature of the blood pressure recording) and also tried to hold his breath throughout most of the test. These deliberate distortion efforts were clear indications of deception.

A second factor to be considered is that the polygraph test results will only reflect a person's beliefs, not necessarily what in fact took place. For example, if a witness to a crime fully believed, and in his mind was positive, that he saw the man now identified as Joe Jones shoot John Smith last Saturday night, his polygraph examination would indicate that his statements were the truth, even though, in fact, he was mistaken as to the actual identity of the perpetrator.

A third factor, and one which is often thought by the general public to adversely affect the polygraph test results, is extreme nervousness. The control question technique, however, has various built-in protections against such an eventuality. First of all, the pretest interview usually serves to decrease the apprehension of a truthful, tense, or nervous subject, particularly when the areas to be covered on the test are fully described to the subject. Secondly, with a subject whose nervousness persists throughout the testing, that factor will be revealed by the uniformly irregular nature of the polygraph tracings. In other words, physiologic changes or disturbances induced only by nervousness usually appear on the polygraph record without relationship to any particular question or questions; they are usually of no greater magnitude or significance when relevant questions are asked than when irrelevant or control questions are asked.

One additional factor to be considered which could affect the results of the polygraph examination would be the taking of several polygraph tests on the same issue by one subject. If a deceptive subject were to take several polygraph tests on the same issue at different laboratories, he might eventually reach a stage where he becomes so emotionally drained that he no longer shows deceptive responses on the relevant questions, possibly leading the examiner to conclude that he is in fact telling the truth. This phenomenon may result from the fact that at the time of his initial polygraph examination the subject was identified as lying about the matter under investigation. Subsequently he may "give up," feeling that he has already been "caught," but goes to a second or possibly third laboratory for another polygraph test in "search" of a favorable report. If he is doing so, for example on behalf of his attorney, the combined factors of his possibly "giving up" as a result of failing a prior test and the knowledge that the results of this test will never be known to anyone but his attorney if it again indicates his deception, may cause him to be unresponsive to the relevant questions.

There are other factors which could affect the test results, but the ones already discussed are probably the most troublesome to the polygraph examiner.

SUPPLEMENTARY TESTS

In addition to the previously described test consisting of relevant, irrelevant, and control questions, there are several other and different types of tests that may be used. One of these is called the "peak of tension" test. This test can only be used in those instances where the subject has not been informed by the investigators (or the media) of all the important details of the offense in question. The "peak of tension" test consists essentially of the asking of a series of questions in which only one has any bearing upon the matter under investigation. This one pertinent question refers to some detail of the incident or occurrence (e.g., the kind of object stolen, the kind of implement used in a crime, etc.) which could not have been known by an innocent person or by anyone who had not been informed previously of such a detail. For instance, if a suspected murderer has not been told about the identity of the murder weapon, he may be asked a series of questions which refer to various weapons, one of which will be the actual one used. The theory behind the peak of tension test is that if the person tested is the one who killed the victim, for instance, he will be apprehensive about the question referring to the exact weapon used, whereas an innocent person would not have such a particularized concern.

Before conducting a peak of tension test, the examiner prepares a list of about seven questions, among which, near the middle, is the question pertaining to the actual detail. The list is then read off to the subject, and he is informed that during the test those questions, and no others, will be asked, in that precise order. A truthful subject, unaware of the accuracy of any one question, will not ordinarily be concerned about that one any more than the others. On the other hand, a lying subject will have that question in mind as the test is being conducted and, in anticipation of it, he is apt to experience a buildup of tension that will climax at the crucial question; in other words, at that point he will reach a "peak of tension."

Another supplementary type of test which can be used in those instances when the subject is overly responsive is called the "guilt complex" test. In those instances when the examiner is unable to determine whether or not the subject is telling the truth about the issue under investigation because of the similarity in both degree and consistency between the responses to the relevant and control questions, a guilt complex test could be administered.

The guilt complex test contains, in addition to the irrelevant and control questions, a new series of relevant questions dealing with a real incident that the subject *could not* possibly have committed; in other words, a totally fictitious incident. The subject is advised by the examiner that at the request of the agency submitting the subject for the test, he is to be questioned about a second offense. The examiner then reviews with him the relevant questions dealing with this new issue and briefly interviews the subject as to his possible participation in, or knowledge of, the offense. Then two or three tests are conducted with these relevant questions. If the subject responds to the guilt-complex questions in a manner similar to those responses on the real-issue questions, then the examiner would be unable to draw any definite conclusion as to the subject's status on the real offense in question. However, if the subject does not respond to these guilt-complex questions in the same fashion as he did to the real-issue questions, this would indicate that the subject was being deceptive as to the primary or real issue under investigation.

A third supplementary test, which may be advisable in certain situations, is commonly referred to as the "silent answer" test. This test consists of the same irrelevant, relevant, and control questions as those used during the standard test. However, on the silent answer test, the subject is instructed to answer the questions silently, to himself, without making any verbal response. This type of test is particularly effective in those instances when the subject's verbal responses cause a distortion in the tracings such as a sniff or clearing of the throat.

Figures 52-10 annd 52-11 illustrate the appearance in a polygraph record of this peak of tension in the blood pressure tracing, as well as the value of the galvanic skin reflex tracing in peak of tension testing.

THE ACCURACY OF EXAMINATION RESULTS

Percentage of Definite Decisions

In about 25 percent of the polygraph examinations conducted by a competent examiner, truth or deception may be so clearly disclosed by the

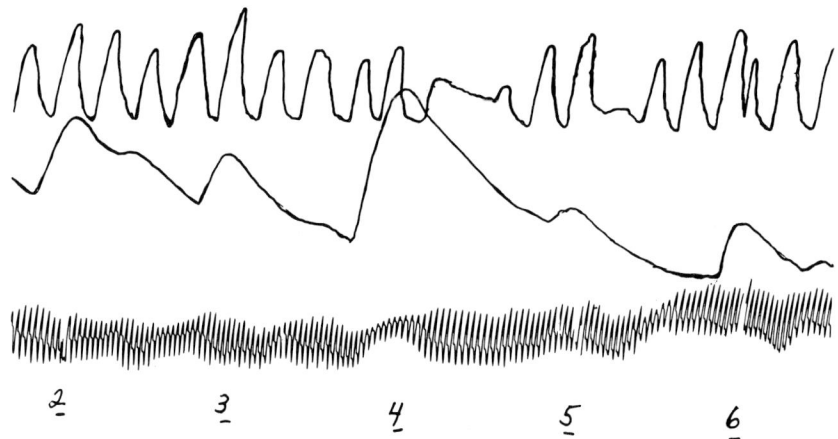

FIGURE 52-10. The "peak of tension" test record of a bank thief. In this case approximately $50,000 had been stolen from a bank. Due to the nature of the circumstances of the theft, it appeared as though there was collusion between a bank employee and the outside perpetrator who had successfully arranged for the fraudulent transfer of $50,000 from a large corporation account at the bank into his own personal account. The subject of this examination, a female employee of the bank, claimed that she had no knowledge of the theft or the name of the account to which the money had been fraudulently transferred. On this "peak of tension" test, the subject was asked whether the account which falsely received the money was opened in the name of _____. The blank was filled in with seven different names. Observe at question 4 (which referred to the actual name used to open the account) the pronounced peak of tension in the GSR tracing (the middle one) and the significant respiration response. This test confirmed the subject's involvement in that only the guilty suspect could have known this name.

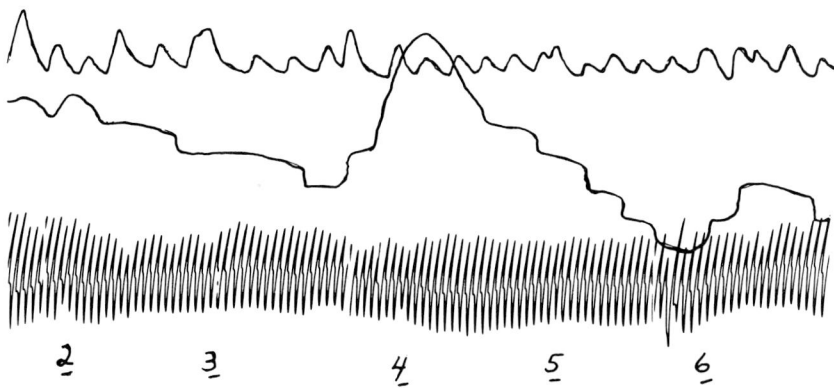

FIGURE 52-11. The "peak of tension" test of a subject suspected of stealing money from his employer. During this test the subject was asked the question: "Did you steal _____ in money from the XYZ Corporation?" The blank was filled in with seven different amounts ranging from $300 to $2,000. Observe at question 4 ($800) the pronounced peak of tension in the GSR tracing (the middle one). When confronted with an actual display of this record, the subject indicated that he had in fact stolen $800 from the company and agreed to make full restitution.

nature of the reactions to relevant or control questions that the examiner will be able to point them out to any nonexpert and satisfy him of their significance. In about 65 percent of the cases, however, the indications are not that clear; they are sufficiently subtle in appearance and significance to require expert interpretation of their significance. In roughly 10 percent of the examinations, the examiner may be unable to make any diagnosis at all.

Degree of Accuracy

The accuracy of the polygraph technique is difficult to estimate.* In many cases the truth as to who committed an offense may never be ascertained by confession or subsequently developed factual evidence. Proof is often lacking, therefore, as to whether the examiner in any given case was right or wrong. It has been demonstrated, however, that the technique, when properly applied by a trained and competent examiner, is very accurate in its indications,[3] and the relatively few errors that do occur favor the innocent, since the known mistakes in diagnosis almost always involve a failure to detect lies of deceptive subjects rather than a finding of lying on the part of a truthful person.

The polygraph technique does, of course, have its detractors. These views are often strongly held and have resulted in statutory and court-imposed limitations on the use of polygraph technology and on its judicial admissibility. These views are discussed below and will be found expressed in the additional readings presented at the end of this chapter.

---

*Four recent validity studies have indicated that when properly applied by a competent, trained and experienced examiner, the polygraph technique is over 85 percent accurate when decisions were based solely on the interpretation of the polygraph records. This accuracy increased to over 90 percent when the examiner had available for consideration, in addition to the polygraph records themselves, such auxiliary information as the test questions, the case history, and the behavior symptoms exhibited by the subject during the course of the polygraph examination.

THE LEGAL STATUS OF THE POLYGRAPH TECHNIQUE

At the present time the judicial status of the polygraph technique is generally one of inadmissibility, except in some jurisdictions as discussed below. (See also Chapter 56.)

The primary reason for this exclusionary policy as expressed by the courts has been the failure of the polygraph technique to gain "general acceptance" in the particular field in which it belongs. The "general acceptance" rule for the admissibility of polygraph evidence was established in 1923 by a federal court in *Frye v. United States*,[4] the first appellate court decision addressed to the admissibility issue. In the Frye case, the results of a systolic blood pressure test were excluded as evidence because the court felt that the test was still in the experimental state and had not as yet gained acceptance by psychologists and physiologists as an accurate and reliable means of determining whether or not a person is telling the truth.*

Numerous attempts have been made to introduce the results of a polygraph examination in the wake of the Frye decision, but for the most part the status of the test results as probative evidence remains the same. One notable exception, however, is the 1975 case of *State v. Dorsey*.[5] The trial court excluded evidence concerning the results of a polygraph examination offered in behalf of the defendant, who was on trial for murder, upon objection by the prosecutor. On appeal the New Mexico Supreme Court ruled that it was in error for the polygraph test results to be excluded. The court held that once the competency of the examiner had been established, to deprive the defendant of the use of the favorable evidence would violate his constitutional right to "due process."

Another court decision favorable to the defense usage of test results is *Commonwealth v. a Juvenile* (No. 1),[6] in which the Massachusetts Supreme Court held by a 5 to 1 decision that if a defendant offered to submit to an examination by a competent examiner and agreed to have the results admitted, he was to be accorded that privilege.

In several jurisdictions polygraph test results have been ruled admissible pursuant to a stipulated agreement *between the opposing parties*. The 1962 case of *People v. Valdez*[7] has served in many instances as the model stipulation case. In this case, the trial court, over the objection of defense counsel, honored the prior stipulation agreement signed by the defendant, his counsel, and the prosecutor, and allowed the polygraph examiner to testify. Upon appeal the Arizona Supreme Court upheld this ruling and stated that "although much remains to be done to perfect the lie-detector as a means of determining credibility, we think it has been developed to a state in which its results are probative enough to warrant admissibility upon stipulation." The court then set forth the following procedures for stipulation cases:

1. That the prosecuting attorney, the defendant, and his counsel all sign a written stipulation providing for defendant's submission to the test and for the subsequent admission at trial of the graphs and the examiner's opinion thereon on behalf of either the defendant or the state.

---

*It is interesting to note that another person subsequently confessed to the murder for which Frye was convicted.

2. That notwithstanding the stipulation, the admissibility of the test results is subject to the discretion of the trial judge (i.e., if the trial judge is not convinced that the examiner is qualified or that the test was conducted under proper conditions, he may refuse to accept such evidence).
3. That if the graphs and examiner's opinion are offered in evidence, the opposing party shall have a right to cross-examine the examiner respecting (a) the examiner's qualifications and training; (b) the conditions under which the test was administered; (c) the limitations of, and the possibilities for error in the polygraph technique; and (d) at the discretion of the trial judge, any other matter deemed pertinent to the inquiry.
4. That if such evidence is admitted, the trial judge should instruct the jury that the examiner's testimony does not tend to prove or disprove any element of the crime with which a defendant is charged but at most tends only to indicate that at the time of the examination, the defendant was or was not telling the truth. Further, the jury members should be instructed that it is for them to determine what corroborative weight and effect such testimony should be given.

FUTURE LEGAL STATUS

According to John E. Reid and Fred E. Inbau in their publication *Truth and Deception: The Polygraph ("Lie-Detector") Technique* (second edition, 1977), polygraph test results are ready for judicial acceptance, provided that the following conditions are met: (1) that the examiner possess a reasonably good educational background, preferably a college degree; (2) that he has received at least 6 months of internship training under an experienced, competent examiner with a sufficient volume of case work to afford frequent, supervised testing in actual case situations; (3) that the examiner witness have at least 3 years' experience as a specialist in the field of polygraph examinations; and (4) that the examiner's testimony must be based upon polygraph records which he must produce in court in explanation of his opinion and for purposes of cross-examination.

A very important development with respect to the legal status of the polygraph technique occurred in 1973. At that time the New Jersey Supreme Court appointed a "committee on criminal procedure dealing with polygraph tests." This committee, upon a comprehensive review of the literature and the law regarding polygraph tests, issued a report at the New Jersey Judicial Conference in which the majority of the committee concluded that in the absence of a stipulation between the prosecution and the defense, the test results should not be admitted in evidence. However, a minority report of the committee expressed the view that where a test has been administered by a competent examiner, even without prior stipulation between the opposing parties, the results should be admissible. This report is reproduced in the *New Jersey Law Journal* of May 10, 1973 (volume 96, page 525).

THE TESTIMONY OF THE POLYGRAPH EXAMINER

The important areas that may affect the accuracy of the reported test results, and therefore the areas about which to question the polygraph examiner witness, would be (1) his polygraph training, (2) the extent of his experience with respect to the years and number of tests he has conducted, (3) the operation of the polygraph instrument itself, (4) the type of questioning technique used by the examiner, and (5) the accuracy of the polygraph technique. In addition, special consideration should be given to the number of tests and the number of questions asked during the tests. If a person is overtested or asked an excessive number of test questions (four relevant questions are usually considered to be the maximum number that would yield reliable results), the subject may have a tendency to become emotionally unresponsive. The examiner should also be questioned as to the type of pretest interview he conducted. If the interview was accusatory in nature, the subsequent test results could very well be unreliable.

There are several other factors which can affect the test results and which should be developed during the examination of the examiner witness, but if the examiner is well trained, using a reliable technique, and has been actively engaged in the testing of criminal suspects for a minimum of 3 years, he should be able to adequately explain the polygraph technique and the specific test results in question.

REFERENCES

1. Reid, J. E., and Inbau, F. E.: *Truth and Deception: The Polygraph ("Lie-Detector") Technique.* ed. 2. Williams & Wilkins, Baltimore, 1977.
2. Trovillo, P. V.: A History of Lie Detection. *J. Crim. Law Criminol.* 29(6):848–881, 1939; 30(1):104–119, 1939.
3. Horvath, F. S., and Reid, J. E.: The Reliability of Polygraph Examiner Diagnosis of Truth and Deception. *J. Crim. Law Criminol. Police Sci.* 62:276–284, 1971; Hunter, F. L., and Ash, P.: The Accuracy and Consistency of Polygraph Examiners' Diagnosis. *J. Police Sci. Adm.* 1:370–375, 1973; Slowik, S. M., and Buckley, J. P.: Relative Accuracy of Polygraph Examiner Diagnosis of Respiration, Blood Pressure and GSR Recordings. *J. Police Sci. Adm.* 3:305–309, 1975; Wicklander, D. E., and Hunter, F. L.: The Influence of Auxiliary Sources of Information in Polygraph Diagnosis. *J. Police Sci. Adm.* 3:405–409, 1975.
4. 54 U.S., App. D.C. 46, 293 Fed. 1013 (1923).
5. 88 N.M. 184, 539 P. 2d 204 (1975).
6. 365 Mass. 421, 313 N.E. 2d 120 (1974).
7. 91 Ariz. 274, 371 P. 2d 894 (1962).

ADDITIONAL READINGS

1. Over 20 states have adopted licensing statutes for polygraph examiners. For a typical statute, see Oklahoma Stats. Ann. Title 59, §§ 1451–1476. Illinois Rev. Stat. ch. 111, § 2401–2432, 1977.
2. Sixteen states have statutorily limited the use of polygraph tests. Statutes of this type have withstood constitutional attack. See State v. Community Distributors, 64 N.J. 479, 317 A.2d 697 (1975).
3. For a detailed examination of the appellate court cases in the United States on admission of polygraph evidence, see Note, "Physiological and Psychological Truth and Deception Tests," American Law Reports, 2d, pp. 1306–1410, 1972. Also see cases collected and discussed in People v. Barbara, 400 Mich. 352, 255 N.W.2d 171, 1977. The use of polygraph evidence is not exclusively a prosecution tool as was pointed out in this chapter. For a review of the use of polygraph evidence to aid in proving innocence, see Axelrod, R.M.: The Use of Lie Detectors by Criminal Defense Attorneys, 3 National J. of Criminal Defense 107, 1977.
4. For further commentary on the legal issues concerning polygraph evidence, including articles critical of admissibility of such evidence even under stipu-

lation, see Note, Emergence of the Polygraph at Trial, 73 Columbia L.Rev. 1120, 1973; Wilner, R. C.: Polygraph: Short Circuit for Truth?, 29 U. of Florida L.Rev.286, 1977; Abbell, M.: Polygraph Evidence: The Case Against Admissibility in Federal Criminal Trials, 15 American Criminal L.Rev. 29, 1977; Radek, L. J.: The Admissibility of Polygraph Results in Criminal Trials: A Case for the Status Quo, 3 Loyola U.L.J. 289, 1972; Kaplan, A. G.: The Lie Detector: An Analysis of Its Place in the Law of Evidence, 10 Wayne L. Rev. 381, 1964; Skolnick, J. H.: Scientific Theory and Scientific Evidence: An Analysis of Lie Detection, 70 Yale L.J. 694, 1961. For the latest comprehensive review of admissibility issues, see Admissiblity of Polygraph Evidence in Criminal and Civil Cases, edited by Ansely, N., American Polygraph Association, Linthicum Heights, Md., 1979.

CHAPTER 53

Charles S. Petty is Director of the Southwestern Institute of Forensic Sciences at Dallas, Chief Medical Examiner of Dallas County, Director of the Dallas County Criminal Investigation Laboratory, and Professor of Pathology and Forensic Sciences at the University of Texas Southwestern Medical School at Dallas. Dr. Petty holds degrees in pharmacy and physiology from the University of Washington and received his medical education at Harvard Medical School. He is a diplomate of the American Board of Pathology in pathologic anatomy, clinical pathology, and forensic pathology. Dr. Petty is former President of the American Academy of Forensic Sciences and is a Fellow of the American Association for the Advancement of Science, the American College of Physicians, the American Society of Clinical Pathologists, and the British Academy of Forensic Sciences.

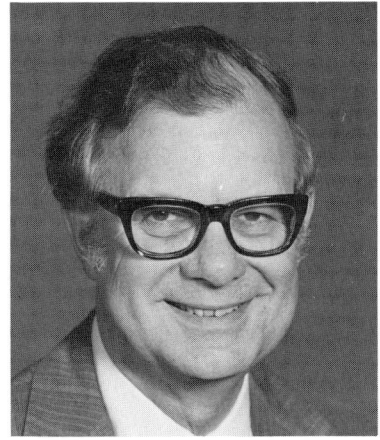

IDENTIFICATION PROCEDURES IN DEATH INVESTIGATION

Charles S. Petty, M.D.

The ultimate, positive identification of the dead body presented in an unidentified state is a major goal of the medicolegal official. This goal is illusive and sometimes remains beyond the reach of the involved official. There are many pragmatic reasons for effecting positive identification. Among them are the following:

1. To resolve the anxiety of the next of kin of a person missing and presumed dead. Great effort has been expended to accomplish the goal of identification for this single reason: witness the expenditure of large sums of money and much time to effect positive identification of Americans who died in the Korean and Vietnam conflicts and in recent airliner crashes.
2. To settle the estate of the person missing and presumed dead. Proof of death depends upon the identification of the dead individual. In our modern age of documentation, a certificate of death is required by insurance companies, the Social Security agency, the Veterans Administration, and retirement systems, among others, for the payment of a variety of benefits. In the absence of proof of death, estate settlement may be delayed for long periods of time (perhaps until the "presumed dead" statutes are applicable, which may be 5 years or more, depending upon the jurisdiction).
3. To establish the *corpus delicti* (the body or proof of the crime) to permit prosecution for homicide.
4. To allow the medicolegal official to release the body to the next of kin for burial. This practical problem faces all medicolegal officials who do not have satisfactory long-term holding facilities for bodies. Identification is also sought by public officials who must, without identification, eventually dispose of the body at public expense.

There are, no doubt, other reasons for desiring the positive, final identification of the dead body. All of them, however, call for positive identification to be effected by the easiest, most practical means. There are methods available by which to establish positive, undeniable identification. These are listed below:

1. Fingerprints, footprints, or handprints;
2. Dental patterns or restorations;
3. Frontal sinus patterns;
4. Skull suture patterns and vascular grooves;
5. Normal and abnormal bone comparisons;
6. Other fortuitous comparisons.

In each of the techniques listed above there must be premortem, specifically comparable material available with which to match the material collected in the postmortem state. Note also that each of the techniques provides for documentation of the comparison so that the match between the premortem and postmortem materials can be preserved and subjected to retest whenever desired.

FINGERPRINTS

Since the turn of the century, fingerprints have been used as a very efficient means of establishing the identity of individuals. Indeed, the popularity of this method of identification has led to the establishment of large fingerprint card files, and many plans for "universal fingerprinting" have been advanced. For a variety of reasons, such a seemingly useful system has never been adopted in the United States or in other countries. The idea of fingerprinting every citizen seems to engender fears of totalitarianism. The largest central file of fingerprints in the world is maintained by the Federal Bureau of Investigation. Each of the states maintains some central fingerprint file capability, utilizing the Department of Public Safety or state police jurisdiction. Large and small municipalities also maintain fingerprint files. Any or all such files may be referred to when attempting to effect identification of unknown dead individuals.

The use of fingerprints as a method of identification, like all comparison methods, is easier to accomplish if the dead individual has another potential means of identification. This allows the fingerprint file to be searched by name; if there are fingerprints on file for such an individual, comparison of that set with those taken after death is an easy task. Positive identification can be effected quickly and with a minimum of time expenditure. However, if the fingerprint file is to be searched by the method of classifying the fingerprint set obtained after death and matching by the classification formula, a much more time-consuming process is involved, and certain obstacles are apt to be interposed. A complete set of fingerprints is necessary in order to classify the fingerprint pattern. Fingerprints for classification must be clear, complete, and comparable. Each of the 10 fingerprints must be available. The procurement of such a set from the body is not always easy and may be impossible. The act of fingerprinting the body and the procurement of a set of prints do not always make it possible to classify the fingerprint set and to search the files by means of the classification technique.

There are many reasons why it may be difficult, if not impossible, to obtain good fingerprints from a dead body. The most important of these include foreign material such as blood or grease on the fingers; rigor mortis making it difficult to open the hands to spread and manipulate the fingers; postmortem drying of the fingerpads; decomposition, burning, and other injury to the fingers; and immersion in water or other fluid for a prolonged time.

The usual technique employed to make fingerprints is to ink the print area and to press the inked area against heavyweight paper or cardboard. The manipulation of the fingers against the paper to produce a clear print is not easily accomplished, particularly in view of the inflexibility of the fingers due to rigor mortis. Despite this, in the majority of instances, clear, utilizable prints can be obtained where these problems do not exist or where they can be corrected or avoided. There are many variations of the technique. Rather than using the standard FBI fingerprint card some officials prefer to use strips of paper with each strip designed to accommodate in premarked spaces each of the five prints from a single hand. Others prefer to use small squares of paper with a separate square for the print from each finger. Still others use curved card holders and claim that adequate prints are more easily obtained in such a manner.

At the Southwestern Institute of Forensic Sciences in Dallas, the standard FBI cards are folded in such a manner as to make a strip of five boxes for the prints for one hand and are then refolded to permit the other hand to be printed. This has proven to be quite satisfactory for most situations (Fig. 53-1). Two sets of fingerprints are obtained from each body. One set is sent to the law enforcement agency with jurisdiction over the place where death occurred; the other set is sent to the Federal Bureau of Investigation. In this way, both the local law enforcement agencies and the FBI can purge their active files of those known to be dead. It is of interest to realize that over 40 percent of the sets of fingerprints sent to the Federal Bureau of Investigation are matchable with those on file (Table 53-1). It should be emphasized that the files against which the postmortem prints are matched are not merely those collected from persons involved in crime, but include other fingerprints as well. The latter file includes those fingerprinted incident to entry into the armed forces, those who have applied for federal civil service positions, and other groups.

As indicated above, there are many factors which may make satisfactory printing of the fingers of the dead body difficult and at times impossible. To help cope with the wrinkled skin of the fingerpads resulting from immersion of the body in water, injection of air or various liquids into the

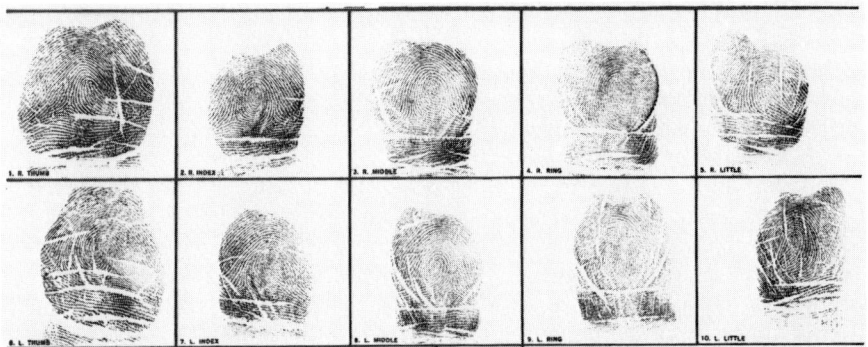

FIGURE 53-1. Fingerprints obtained from a dead body by inking the fingerbulbs and by rolling a folded standard FBI fingerprint card over the bulbs. (FBI form FD-249 [Rev. 3-13-72].)

TABLE 53-1. FINGERPRINTING OF BODIES*

Number of medical examiner cases	1523
Not printed	252
Infants, young children	
Decomposed bodies, burned bodies	
Cases certified without viewing	
Printed	1271
Fingerprints lost, misplaced, etc.	26
Number of cases with fingerprints	1245
Number of cases with no FBI fingerprint record, or postmortem fingerprints not satisfactory for comparison	717
Number of cases with FBI retrievable fingerprints: identified by prints	528

*Results of 6 months of body fingerprinting at Southwestern Institute of Forensic Sciences (January 1 to June 30, 1978); 42 percent of all bodies fingerprinted (and where fingerprints were submitted to the Federal Bureau of Investigation) were identifiable by postmortem fingerprints.

fingerpads has been advocated.[1,2] This may be accomplished by injecting the fluid through a very fine 28 to 30 gauge needle. In some instances this is a considerable aid in obliterating the wrinkles of the skin. If immersion is prolonged or decomposition is advanced, or in some instances of radiant heat burns, the skin of the hands and fingers can be peeled away from the underlying tissue. Satisfactory fingerprints can sometimes be made by inserting the technician's finger into the "skin glove," inking the area to be printed, and rolling the inked surface against a fingerprint card. It must also be realized that in instances where the epidermis is absent as a result of decomposition, immersion, scalding, or other causes, the printing of the remaining, not external, skin can be productive of useful fingerprints. In such instances, the detail will not be as great, and because the ridges are less well defined, much care and a "light touch" of the fingerprinter are essential.

In some cases of contractures, and with decomposing tissues, removal of the fingers from the hands may permit more satisfactory printing by allowing easier and more gentle access to the fingerpad area. Occasionally when rigor mortis is well developed and the need for fingerprints is urgent, incision into the palmer surface of the fingers at the proximal interphalangeal joint will enable the fingers to be straightened, and printing can be carried out. Such an approach will make it unnecessary to remove the fingers in their entirety. One of the unconsidered problems of totally removing the fingers is that of increased potential for mix-up of the separated members.

Other techniques have been utilized to help make available usable prints from fingers that are less than ideal for printing. A substance which will fill in the furrows between the ridges, such as liquid latex, can be helpful. If the latex, with a hardener added, is painted on the fingers, or if the fingers are dipped into the liquid, hardening of the thick layer of latex will result in a mirror image of the pattern of the ridges of the fingerpad. This can then be inked and the ink then transferred to paper, or the pattern photographed.[3] A somewhat similar technique employs cellophane tape.[4] Black fingerprint powder is dusted onto the finger, and the opaque film is then applied to the bulb of the finger. When the tape is pulled away from the finger, the black powder adheres to the finger ridges. Then the tape can be applied to transparent vinyl so that the fingerprint is both preserved and accessible.

FOOTPRINTS

Footprints as a means of identification have been used in some countries where bare feet are apt to be encountered. In Hawaii an active criminal footprint file is maintained. In this tropical area, such a file is of practical importance. Throughout the United States, many newborn infants are footprinted so as to have a ready means of positive identification in the event of a nursery mix-up. Such footprints are ordinarily made part of the hospital record and can be used for comparison purposes should the need arise. In the author's experience, the prints are frequently smudged and unsatisfactory for comparison purposes. This appears to be due to a failure to use good technique, since the pattern is clear if the print is properly taken.[5] The potential of footprint comparison remains little used but should be kept in mind by the forensic scientist for use in those instances where the fingers and hands have been destroyed or where fingerprints have never been taken prior to death. This applies particularly in the case of children. Footprints of U.S. Air Force pilots are on the file since the feet, encased in shoes or boots, may survive an aircraft crash in better condition than would the hands.

PALM PRINTS

Palm prints have very rarely been used in identification but are occasionally useful in establishing the presence of an individual at the crime scene. Palm prints may be obtained quite easily by inking the palm of the dead individual and then rolling over the inked area, the paper wrapped about a pasteboard roller 4 to 8 cm in diameter.

FINGERPRINTS ON SKIN

Fingerprints on the skin of bodies are not the subject of this discussion. These have been found, and the principle of their deposition is the same as that for so-called latent fingerprints. The print is left on suitable surfaces because of the fatty substances contained in the sweat which exudes from the fingerpads as well as from most skin surfaces. The greasy impression of the fingerprint can be left on skin as well as on other surfaces. Nevertheless, fingerprints are rarely found on skin. Various techniques have been developed to search for such latent prints and to develop these prints so that they may be transferred or photographed.[6,7] The preservation of the body in such a manner as to prevent the smudging of such prints is an additional burden to those who must transport the body from the scene of death to the place where it can be adequately examined. This new requirement for physical evidence preservation has not yet been studied in detail, and the problems associated with it have not been resolved.

DENTAL PATTERNS AND RESTORATIONS

Teeth and dental alterations have been used for many years in successful attempts to establish identity. The teeth are highly individualistic. It is possible to make comparisons so as to effect identification by using:

1. Comparisons of the teeth and dental charts;
2. Comparisons of x-rays of the teeth and dental x-rays;

3. Comparisons of the teeth with dental casts of the teeth;
4. Comparisons of protheses with dental charts, casts, etc.

The extent of usefulness of dental patterns and restorations is indicated by the growth of the discipline of forensic dentistry or odontology. A section of the American Academy of Forensic Sciences is devoted to this highly specialized activity. Several textbooks in forensic dentistry dealing with identification have been published in very recent years.[8-11] Most large medicolegal investigative systems have one or more dentists interested in the forensic aspects of dentistry available as consultants (see Chapter 50).

The type of comparison possible between pre- and postmortem dental x-ray films is illustrated in Figure 53-2. This illustrates one method of comparison. The mandible and the maxilla are bisected in the midline after removal and are then subjected to x-ray with the two halves of each bone (and, of course, the included teeth) lying flat on the ordinary x-ray cassette. This is a quick and easy way to produce usable x-ray films for comparison purposes. L. E. Norton[12] was probably the first forensic pathologist to use this technique. Perhaps more precisely comparable films may be made by using a dental x-ray machine and the usual dental film packs, but in the absence of such equipment, the Norton technique is quite satisfactory. The angle at which the jaws, including teeth and dental restorations, are viewed is critical for fine matching of the shape of the restorations. The jaws may be easily repositioned at a slightly different angle by inserting a 2 to 3 mm radiotransparent wedge under one edge of each of the bisected jaws and remaking the x-ray exposure.

In addition to dental restoration (filling) outlines, root canal fillings, the results of apicoectomy, crowns, posts used to hold inlays in place, and bone structure are visible by x-ray examination. In the instance of multiple reconstructions, many points of coincidence can be found.

The usefulness of prostheses and casts for identification purposes has often been emphasized. However, no comparison is possible without the

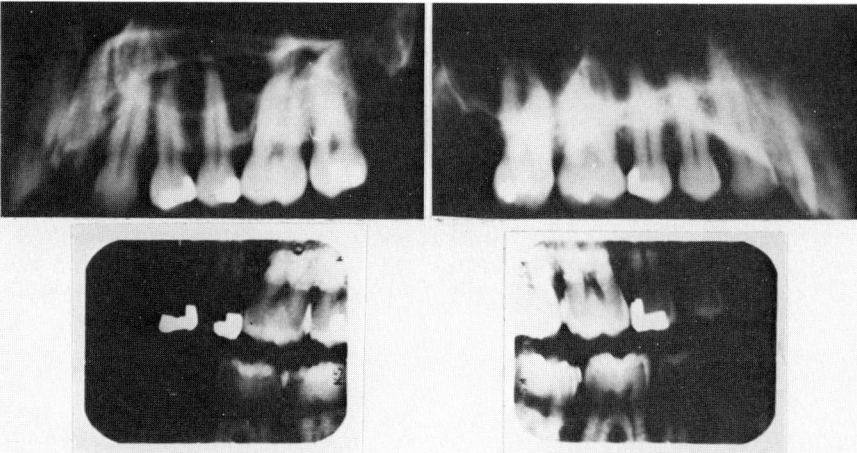

FIGURE 53-2. Comparison of pre- and postmortem x-ray films of the teeth and jaws. The postmortem demonstration of the jaws is accomplished by dividing the maxilla and the mandible in the midline and placing the bisected jaws on the cassette. Films at upper right and left were made after death. Those at lower right and left are dental films made before death.

procurement of the jaws with the included teeth. The removal of both the maxilla and mandible is a simple procedure, and retention in a plastic bag filled with a formalin solution is readily accomplished. Jaw specimens can be stored indefinitely.

FRONTAL SINUS PATTERN

In recent years, the individuality of the x-ray pattern of the frontal sinuses has become recognized. No two patterns appear to be the same. Comparison of premortem x-ray films with those taken after the death are most useful in enabling comparison for identification purposes. An investigative lead, a suspicion of the identity of the unidentified dead, the location of the premortem x-ray films, and the comparison of such films with those taken after death combine to form a quick, easy, and documentable system. Some special expertise may be necessary to help position the head for the proper angle of projection; a radiologist or perhaps an x-ray technologist can supply the needed aid. Figure 53-3 shows several frontal sinus patterns selected at random. Note how they are all quite different. It has been suggested that the sella turcica (hypophyseal fossa) can be used for identification purposes in a manner similar to the frontal sinuses.[13]

SKULL SUTURE PATTERN AND VASCULAR GROOVES

The suture patterns of the skull appear to be quite individualistic. The sagittal and lambdoid sutures are especially complicated and quite different from one person to another. Two major factors most often prevent the use of these suture patterns for comparison: (1) the sutures close, and the patterns are more or less obliterated; and (2) the suture patterns are not well demonstrated in those premortem x-ray films most commonly available.

The vascular grooves, such as those related to the middle meningeal vessels, are much more apt to be visible in x-ray films than are the suture lines. They are, therefore, more useful for purposes of comparison to establish identity (Fig. 53-4).

NORMAL AND ABNORMAL BONE COMPARISONS

Abnormal bones such as cervical and lumbar ribs, wormian bones (small bones in the skull caused by abnormal suture patterns leaving islands of bone surrounded by sutures, sometimes referred to as "sutural" or "intrasutural bones"), and sesamoid bones (bones included in tendons, frequently seen in the hands and feet) may provide definite points for comparison and positive identification. It should be noted that some sesamoid bones are of rather constant occurrence; five are usually present in the hand, and several are rather constantly present in the foot. Others are inconstant, and the pattern may be quite variable from one person to another. Abnormally formed bones such as the bicepital rib may present such a bizarre appearance that a comparison for identification purposes may be effected. The trabecular fine structure of all bones (excluding the bones of the skull) may be defined with enough precision to permit comparisons. The usefulness of xeroradiography for this purpose has been demonstrated. The usefulness of comparison of fracture or orthopedic intervention sites and of trephine or other operative defects of the skull has stood the test of time. The use of x-ray films of bones as the field of

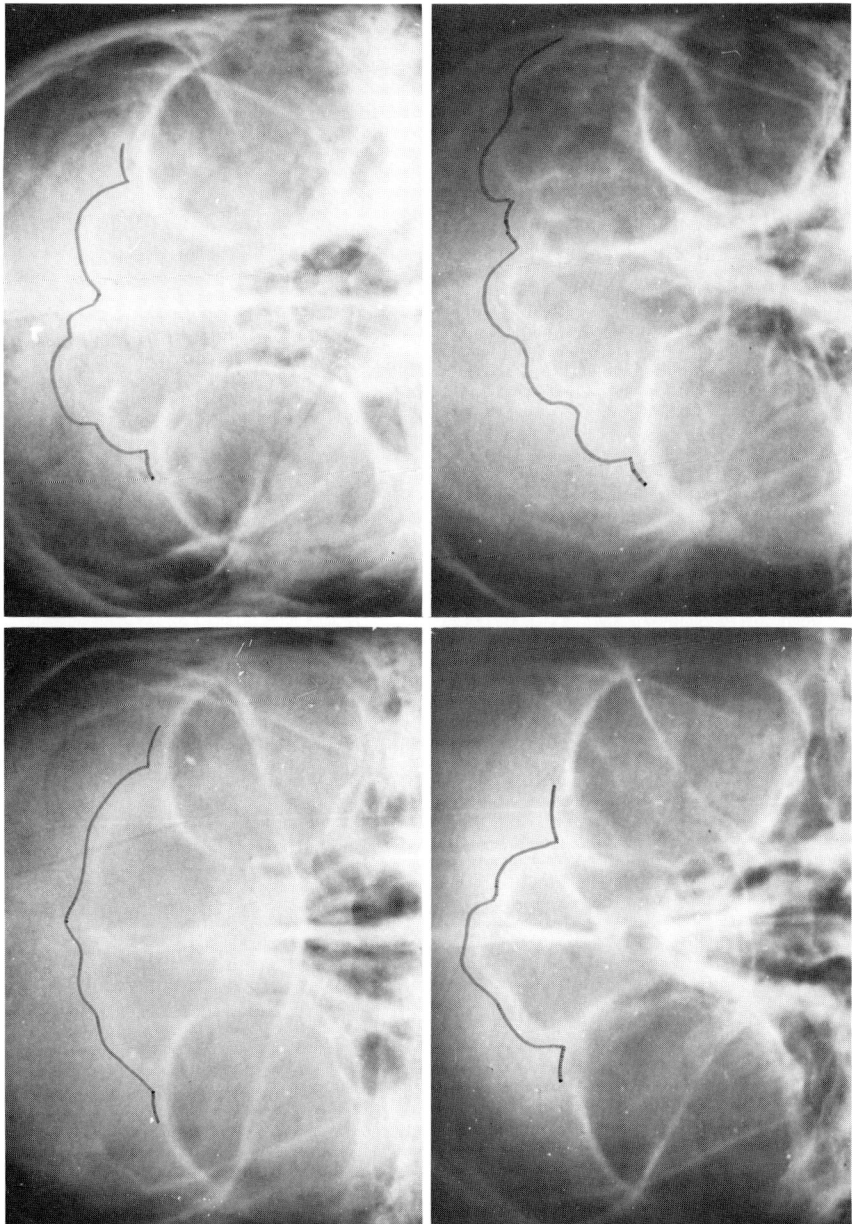

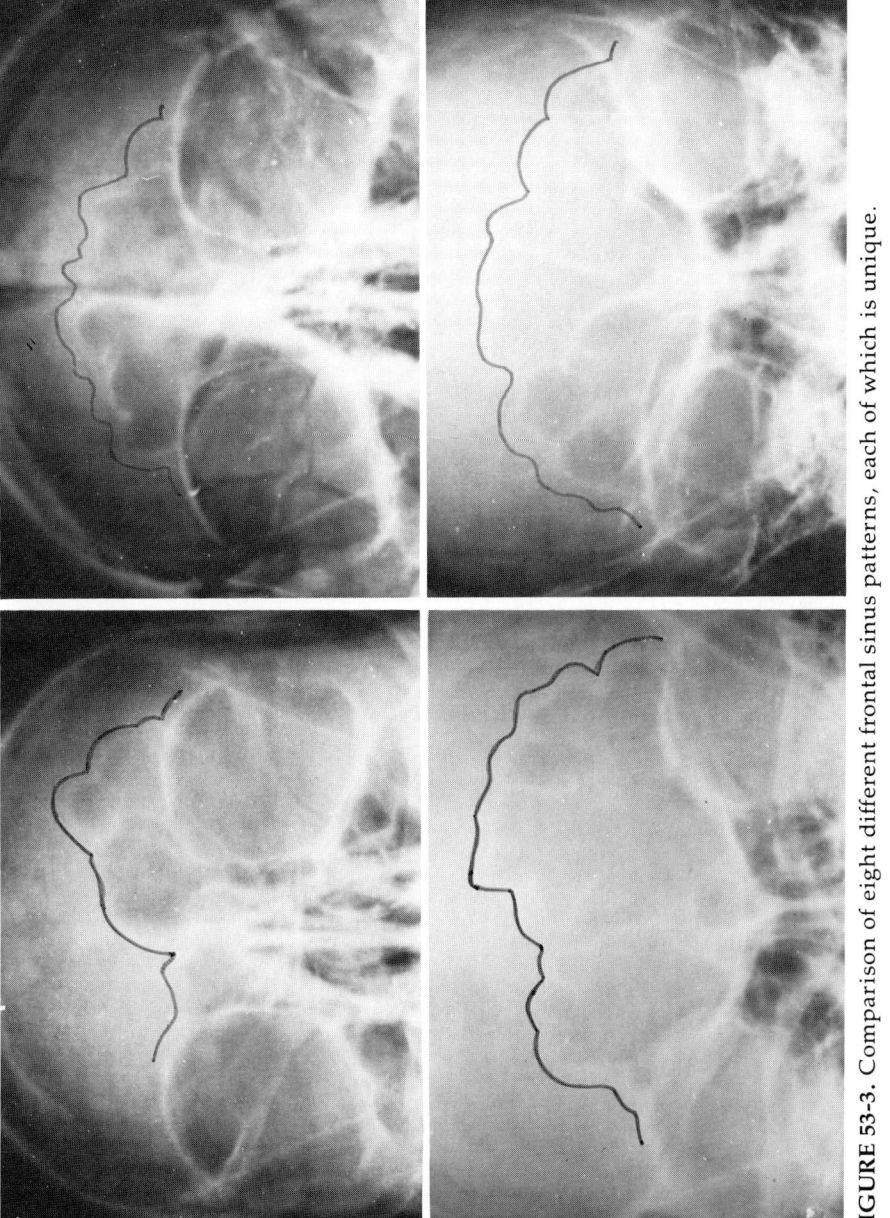

FIGURE 53-3. Comparison of eight different frontal sinus patterns, each of which is unique.

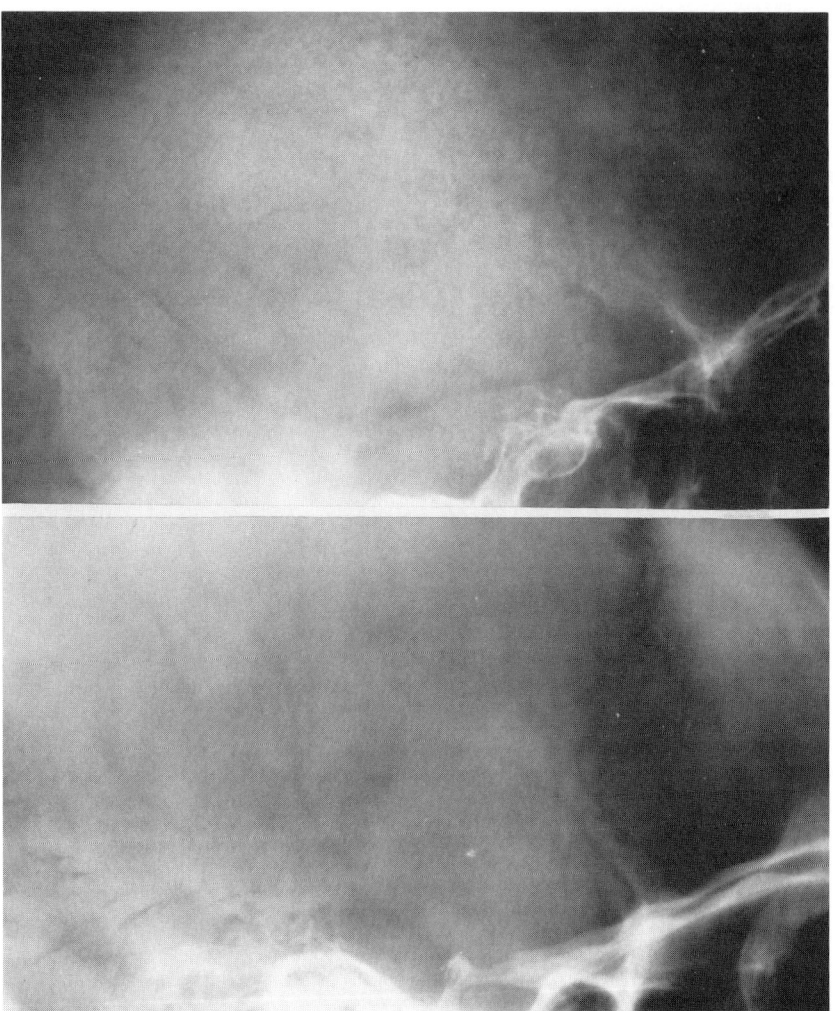

FIGURE 53-4. Comparison of the vascular patterns of two different skulls in lateral x-ray examinations. The two patterns are obviously different.

comparison of pre- and postmortem views is limited only by the imagination and ingenuity of the forensic pathologist and the radiologist working together to effect identification of the body. Here, as with other comparison techniques, the starting point must be the names of those whom the body *may* represent.

OTHER FORTUITOUS COMPARISONS

TATTOOS. Some tattoos are undoubtedly unique. The author has seen tattoos of the individual's name, his armed forces serial number, his social security number, and even his complete name and home address. The more combinations of tattoos an individual has, the greater the chance for a positive identification by tattoos alone. Some tattoos are so common as to make them useless when attempting identification. Such markings as "Born to lose," "Mother," and the fouled anchor are repeated over and over again by tattoo artists. Tattoos tend to fade somewhat and to become less distinct with the passage of time. Infrared photography is sometimes quite useful to clarify these older tattoos. Subjecting the tattooed area to heat furnished by a photographer's tungsten lamp (ordinarily used to provide illumination for taking photographs) will cause local heating. The epidermis can then be easily separated from the dermis (true skin), and the details of the tattoo will be quickly and easily revealed.

WIRE SUTURES. Wire sutures, frequently used by surgeons in repairing sternum-splitting and abdominal laparotomy incisions, are completely individual in size, number, and form. Comparison can be effected by x-ray examination so as to facilitate identification.

PACEMAKERS. The implantation of pacemakers has become a frequently employed method of providing for proper heart rhythm and rate. Each pacemaker bears not only the manufacturer's name, but also a model and serial number. Thus the recovery of a pacemaker from a body is very like recovering the individual's calling card. A query addressed to the manufacturer will reveal the name and address of the person who wore the device in life.

BULLETS. The author can recall a badly decomposed body which was recovered from an open field. No dental restorations were present. Decomposition of the body was so advanced that fingerprinting was impossible; and the soft structures of the face were so decomposed that virtually only the skull remained. However, a bullet was recovered from the chest. By comparison this was shown to have been fired from the service revolver of a state trooper who, it was known, had fired at a man who had been stopped for a driver's license check. When the man fled, the trooper called upon him to stop. He then shot in the general direction of the fleeing man. A search of the area failed to reveal the man, and no evidence of wounding (in the form of blood spots) was found. It was after nearly 2 weeks that the body was found in a field adjacent to the woods into which the man had fled. Since the trooper had retained the driver's license following the incident, identification was effected by this unusual manner. A remarkable case to be sure, but such do exist and such "backhanded" identification is sometimes possible.

PROTHESES. Implanted artificial heart valves; hip, knee, and elbow joints; plates in the skull; and other devices may be used as a means of effecting identification. Some of these implants are so individual as to offer a means of positive identification. Others are much less personalized but may be used at least to eliminate certain possible misidentifications. Some dentures may even carry an identifying number, and in rare instances the owner's name may be found on a piece of paper imbedded in the plastic matrix of the dentures. No doubt there are other prosthetic devices that serve to make either imperfect or precise identification possible.

LESS POSITIVE METHODS OF IDENTIFICATION

Identification by other means than those discussed above may be much less positive. For many years identification of the dead has been effected by visual examination of the face. To be sure, faces are all quite individual, but the recognition of a person depends upon many subtle things about the person and not merely the facial features. Voice, gait, mannerisms, facial expression, and gestures are all used to effect recognition. With a dead body, however, these aids to recognition no longer exist. The face is still, the eyes are closed, and the tissues are relaxed or stiff due to rigor mortis. Moreover, the face may be compressed because the body has been resting on it when lying in the prone position, or it may be distorted by the presence of endotracheal tubes, airways, or wounds, and the whole face rendered less than easy to recognize. Add to this the terror experienced by many people who have never before seen a dead person, as well as the emotion brought about by the fear of recognizing a close relative or friend lying dead in the morgue, and there is small wonder that sight recognition is not always reliable. In some of the newer morgue facilities another barrier is interposed: that of protective windows through which the identifying person is expected to view the body. In other morgues the ultimate, modern, all-seeing technical aid is present: a closed-circuit television system. There are many good reasons for employing this device, but another layer of impersonality is interposed, and sometimes identification by sight is precluded.

It is the experience of many investigators, trained in the scientific method, that sight identification is more than occasionally affected by items associated with the body but of little use in effecting true identification. Clothing is frequently included as a conscious or unconscious addition to the identification process, even by intelligent individuals anxious to effect identification. Consider the insidious effect upon the viewer of the body if it is clad in blue jeans. How many million people in the United States are wearing blue jeans at any given time? Yet the identification by sight of the body is skewed by the presence of blue jeans known to have been worn by that person whom the viewer is attempting to recognize. Jewelry is also used to bolster the positivity of the identification. How many plain, uninitialed yellow metal bands are worn on the left fourth finger at any time?

Items found in pockets do not establish positive identification and furnish at best only a lead to identification. Frequently encountered is the loaning of a driver's license or other card for various reasons. Death comes to the borrower, and the wrong person is thought to be dead. False identification can also be planted.

Identification by photograph, that is, comparing a photograph of the face of the body with predeath photographs, is even more apt to be in error than identification effected by sight. One point of most useful comparison is the ear. Ears of one person are very different from those of another. The ear does not relax or change its shape as a result of death or rigor mortis. The ear is a prominent individual characteristic, as was noted in the late nineteenth century by Bertillon.[14] An entire system of identification based upon the individuality of the ear has been published by Iannarelli.[15] Ears can be compared, in shape at least, from photograph to body. Frequently, however, good photographs of the ears are not available because hair obscures them, and many portraits are taken of the person in a more or less full-face alignment showing little of the ear detail.

IDENTIFICATION BY CIRCUMSTANCE

Occasionally the circumstances under which the body is found are such that identification is not positive but circumstantial. Most frequently this situation occurs in relation to fires, as in the following example:

> A fire occurs in a residence; the only known inhabitant is an old woman. A body is discovered in the bedroom. Charring of the body has obliterated all possibility of sight identification, fingerprints, and even stature estimation (see below). There is no question but that the body is that of an elderly woman. No teeth are present, but it is known that the single resident of the dwelling has no teeth. Dentures are found in another part of the residence, but the fire destruction of the jaw structures is so great that it is impossible to match the dentures with the jaw contours.

In such a situation, identification is circumstantial. The expected body was found after the fire. Perhaps it is known that the resident of the house was a smoker, and nicotine was found in the urine or in the liver; she was known to take diazepam, and this drug was found in the tissues. All evidence points to this body as being that of the expected householder. Furthermore, the old woman is missing after the fire, and her pension check remains uncashed. Who could doubt but that the body is that of the woman who lived there? Yet something is missing: positive identification has not been established. The body is identified only by circumstance — strong circumstance, of course, but still only circumstance. It is unlikely that the charred body represents the remains of someone else, but such situations have occurred. The author is aware of instances of body substitution for reasons of insurance fraud or concealment of homicide.

How then is such a death to be certified by the medicolegal official? One way to resolve the situation described is to indicate on the death certificate in the space provided for the name of the deceased, "Circumstantially identified as [name]." It is certainly better to so state than to indicate with apparent complete confidence the name of the deceased individual with no modifying phrase or indication of lack of positive identification.

ANTHROPOLOGIC IDENTIFICATION

The discovery of a skeleton is often the exposure of an enigma. The anthropologist can estimate with considerable accuracy the sex, race, age, and stature. However, in the absence of dental material with which to work, or without specific bony abnormality, positive identification remains an illusive goal. The physical anthropologist can be of great help to the medicolegal official; no medicolegal investigative office should fail to count among its consultants an interested and well-qualified physical anthropologist. The value of the services of such a technically competent person is considerable. Nevertheless, positive identification of skeletal remains will not usually be effected by such a consultant, and he should not be expected to do so.

"POSITIVE" IDENTIFICATION

There is no question but that positive identification of a body sometimes results from the overconfident application of techniques that actually afford less than positive identification. Sight identification, with all of the associated shortcomings, is not infrequently utilized as a positive identification technique. There is no question that positive recognition will obtain in a high percentage of instances when the body is viewed by a relative or friend who knew the deceased person and who has had continued and recent contact with him. Sight identification of a less than ideally preserved body by a casual acquaintance who has not had recent association with the person now presumed dead is an unsatisfactory exercise that may well yield misleading results.

As the examination into the identity of the dead person continues, an aggregation of nonpositive identification features may appear. The size and nature of clothing, laundry marks, general habitus, color of hair, nonspecific tattoos, and other factors may comprise this aggregation. Positive identification features may remain undiscovered despite intensive search. At some point the aggregation of nonspecific features becomes an aggravation to those attempting to effect identification. The goal seems so close at hand, yet remains so far away. It is at this point that the unwary may succumb and assign positivity to a nonpositive analysis. The legal phrase *caveat emptor* (let the buyer beware) should be kept in mind in such situations, and it should be realized that only presumptive identification has been realized in such situations, no matter how much they are labeled as positive.

REFERENCES

1. *The Science of Fingerprints: Classification and Uses.* Federal Bureau of Investigation, Washington, D.C., 1977, pp. 138–141.
2. Moenssens, A. A.: *Fingerprint Techniques.* Chilton, Philadelphia, 1971, pp. 146–147.
3. Soule, R. L.: Personal communication, 1971.
4. Principe, A. H., and Verbeke, D. J.: Fingerprinting of the Deceased by the Dusting-Tape Method. *J. Crim. Law Criminol. Police Sci.* 63:439–443, 1972.
5. Shepard, K. S., Erickson, T., and Fromm, H.: Limitations of Footprinting as a Means of Infant Identification. *Pediatrics* 37:107, 1966.
6. Adcock, J. M.: The Development of Latent Fingerprints on Human Skin: The Iodine-Silver Plate Transfer Method. *J. Forensic Sci.* 22:599–605, 1977.
7. Reichardt, G. J., Carr, J. C., and Stone, E. G.: A Conventional Method for Lifting Latent Fingerprints from Human Skin Surfaces. *J. Forensic Sci.* 23:135–141, 1978.
8. Gustafson, G.: *Forensic Odontology.* Staples Press, London, 1966.
9. Sopher, I. M.: *Forensic Dentistry.* Charles C Thomas, Springfield, Ill., 1976.
10. Cameron, J. M., and Sims, B. G.: *Forensic Dentistry.* Churchill Press, London, 1974.
11. Luntz, L. L., and Luntz, P.: *Handbook for Dental Identification.* J. B. Lippincott, Philadelphia, 1973.
12. Norton, L. E.: Personal communication, 1977.
13. Reynolds, J.: Personal communication, 1973.
14. Bertillon, A.: Identification of the Living, in Peterson, F., Haines, W. S., and Webster, R. W. (eds.): *Legal Medicine and Toxicology.* W. B. Saunders, Philadelphia, 1923, pp. 63-131.
15. Iannarelli, A. V.: *The Iannarelli System of Ear Identification.* Foundation Press, Brooklyn, 1964.

CHAPTER 54

Maureen Casey is Chief Document Examiner in the Criminalistics Division of the Chicago Police Department. She is a Fellow and Past Chairman of the Questioned Documents Section of the American Academy of Forensic Sciences, and is a member of the American Society of Questioned Documents Examiners. Ms. Casey, who has published a number of papers and articles on various aspects of documents examination, is a diplomate of the American Board of Questioned Document Examiners, Inc.

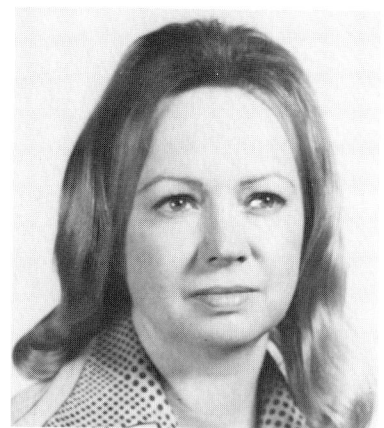

QUESTIONED DOCUMENT EXAMINATION

Maureen Casey, B.A.

SCOPE OF THE FIELD

The field of document examination covers a wide variety of types of evidence, and, in almost all cases, these will involve the contents of a piece of paper or the paper itself. Documents are, in many cases, the foundation of legal, financial, and business proceedings and also play an important role in social intercourse today. Out of the millions of documents that come into existence daily, only a small number will become suspect at some point in their existence. These documents may become suspect as to their authenticity or may provide a link between a person and a situation. In either case, an individual's integrity, monetary situation, or even freedom may be dependent upon the correct interpretation of such evidence as the document has to offer. It therefore becomes incumbent upon the investigator to recognize those situations where document evidence will play a positive role and then to secure the best expertise available in the evaluation of such material.

Documents may prove important in both criminal and civil cases. In too many instances they are associated only with certain types of financial crime (e.g., bogus checks, credit card fraud, and embezzlement). While this type of crime is abundant, it by no means exhausts document evidence possibilities. The astute criminal investigator will recognize the importance of document evidence in many types of investigations, including death investigations (suicide notes, hotel registration cards, letters of explanation); burglaries (pawn tickets, burglary notes, negotiated checks and credit cards); robberies (pawn tickets, robbery notes); auto thefts (titles, bills of sale, altered or fraudulent vehicle license plates); gambling (burnt papers, water-soluble papers, carbon papers, indented writing); confidence games (receipts, wrappings, notes of information);

arsons and bombings (pieces of paper or tape which may provide valuable information in tracing material to an origin); and so on. In civil work, the nature of the cases may often be different than that of criminal cases; however, the types of document examinations are quite similar. Civil cases may involve land rights, patent rights, internal frauds or deception, contested wills, contract and financial disputes, and malpractice suits.

THE FORENSIC DOCUMENT EXAMINER

At present, there is no formal, university-type schooling in document examination which would lead to a degree in this field. Whether this will happen in the near future is uncertain as the field of document examination is a relatively small and specialized one. A college education provides an excellent background for work in the field of document examination, and most document examiners do hold a baccalaureate degree. Trainees entering the profession today must have a bachelor's degree to qualify for membership in two of the professional organizations.

Document examiners receive their training in recognized questioned document laboratories on an appreticeship basis. Normally, such training will encompass a period of 2 to 3 years and be under the direct supervision of a well-qualified and experienced document examiner. Training will cover all areas of document examination (i.e., handwriting, mechanical impressions, alterations, photography, papers, and inks), and experience will be gained by working on actual cases submitted to the laboratory. Document examination is not learned by correspondence courses, 2-week seminars, 2-hour lectures, or attendance at scientific meetings. Such programs can only serve the purpose of expanding one's knowledge or keeping abreast of new techniques and advances in the field.

The profession of questioned document examination includes examiners in government service (federal, state, and municipal laboratories) and examiners in private practice; those in government service comprise approximately 90 percent of the profession in the United States. Document examiners in private practice maintain an office and a well-equipped laboratory and devote their full time to this work.

Most qualified document examiners are members of at least one of the professional organizations in the field of questioned documents. These are the American Society of Questioned Document Examiners and the Questioned Documents Section of the American Academy of Forensic Sciences. Both of these organizations have definite minimum requirements of education, training, and experience to qualify for associate or provisional membership and additional requirements to meet the criteria for full membership. The ASQDE was formally founded in 1942 by Albert S. Osborn and is an outgrowth of the yearly "get togethers," since 1913, of a small but steadily expanding group of document examiners who met to discuss mutual problems. The Questioned Documents Section of the AAFS, founded in 1948, is one of nine forensic disciplines in that organization.

In 1977, document examiners took the initial steps toward certification with formation of the American Board of Forensic Document Examiners, Inc., sponsored by the ASQDE and the AAFS. Certification began in 1978, and is open to all document examiners who meet the published minimum requirements and successfully pass a series of testing procedures designed to assess their knowledge and capabilities in all areas of document work.

Successful applicants are known as diplomates of the ABFDE. One of the primary reasons for certification in the field of questioned documents is to provide the user of forensic science services with some means of evaluating the qualifications of individuals who purport to be document examiners.

THE COMPARISON OF HANDWRITING

Individuality and Bases of Identification

The comparison of handwriting, including hand printing* (or lettering) and numerals, comprises a majority of the document examiner's day to day practice. It is the most difficult and time-consuming area of document examination to master, for here we are dealing with a product of the human individual and all of the physical, emotional, and surrounding conditions in which writing may be prepared. It is the area in which the examiner must be fully trained and experienced in order to properly evaluate these conditions, for identification is not predicated on a pen but on a person.

Handwriting is accomplished by a complex interaction of nerves, memory, and muscular movement. An individual's writing is a composite of many factors but most importantly includes the system of writing learned, a person's ability to imitate characteristics of the system, the modification of system characteristics through use, and the incorporation of designs to suit one's personal taste. Handwriting does not remain static but changes gradually over a period of time, much as one's physical appearance changes over the years. Handwriting is as individual to a person as is the combination of physical characteristics which serves to distinguish one person from another. Although the act of writing is a conscious one, through repeated use it becomes a habitual, almost automatic exercise so that thought is concentrated on the subject matter of the writing rather than on the individual letter forms which make up the writing.

Identification of handwriting, hand printing, and numerals is based on a significant combination of class and individual characteristics common to both the known and questioned writings and on a lack of any fundamental divergent characteristics. In this regard, the presence of one fundamental divergent characteristic between the known and questioned writings would serve to indicate that the writings are by different authors. A fundamental divergent characteristic is one that is repeated consistently throughout a writing, indicating it to be a personal habit of the author and, significantly, not found in the comparison writing. Essentially, in an identification, all of the characteristics of the questioned writing will fall within the range of the known writing and be capable of explanation through the known writing (Figs. 54-1 and 54-2).

Obviously, then, an identification is not based on the similarity of one or two letter forms. It takes into account all of the features of the writing, including letter forms, proportions, size, spacing, slant, beginning and ending strokes, shading, pressure, pen lifts, quality, and movement. While two or more people may be found to have writing pictorially simi-

---

*Although certain aspects of hand-printing identification could well be the subject of a separate discussion, for purposes of the present work, it is included here with the discussion of handwriting.

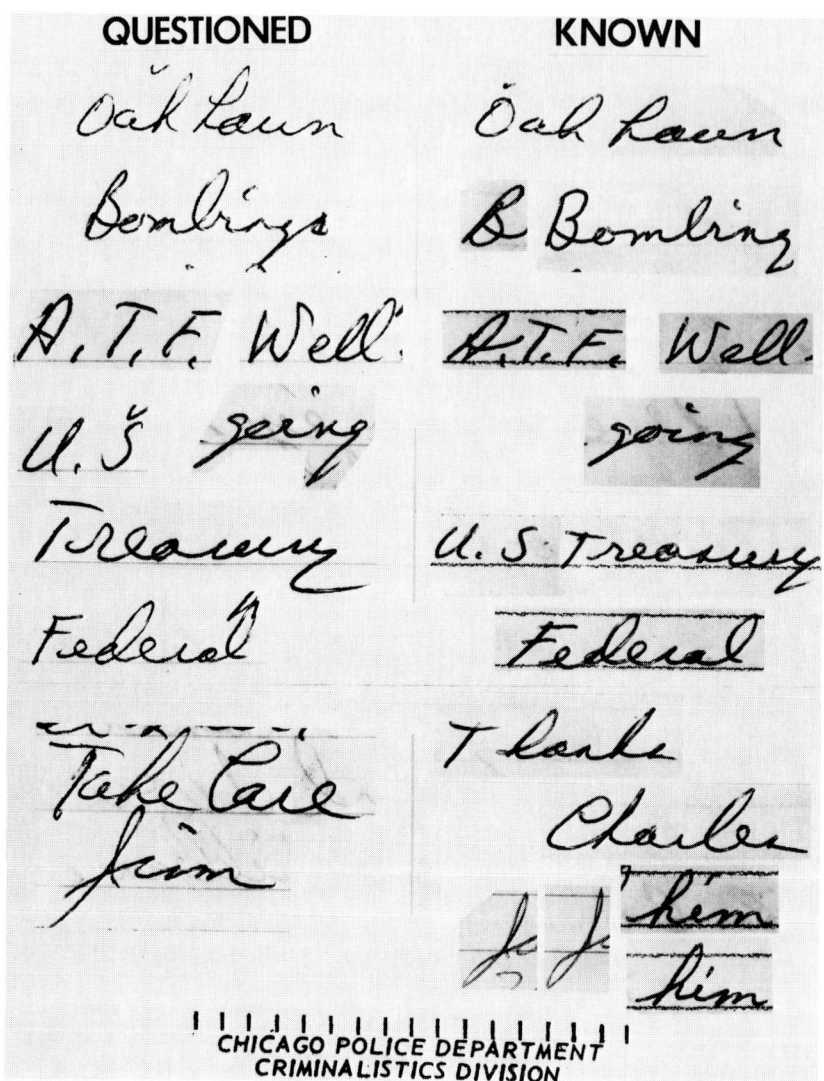

FIGURE 54-1. Comparison chart used to demonstrate identification of the writer of a handwritten anonymous letter. Note the one-trough "w" in the word Lawn, the formation of letter "g" and the dot on the "i" in the word Bombing, the formation of letter "W" in Well, the ending of letter "y" in Treasury, the printed "F" in Federal, and the proportions of the upper loops in Take, Thanks, and Charles.

lar to one another, when all of the features of the writing are detected and properly evaluated, the writers can be distinguished. It is, then, the unique combination of writing features which serves to distinguish between two writings as well as to indicate the identity of authorship of two writings.

Writing contains another characteristic which is of vital consideration in the total picture of identification and which must be properly understood and evaluated. This characteristic is natural variation, which may be defined as slight modifications of the basic form throughout successive specimens of writing. Natural variation, an inherent quality of writing,

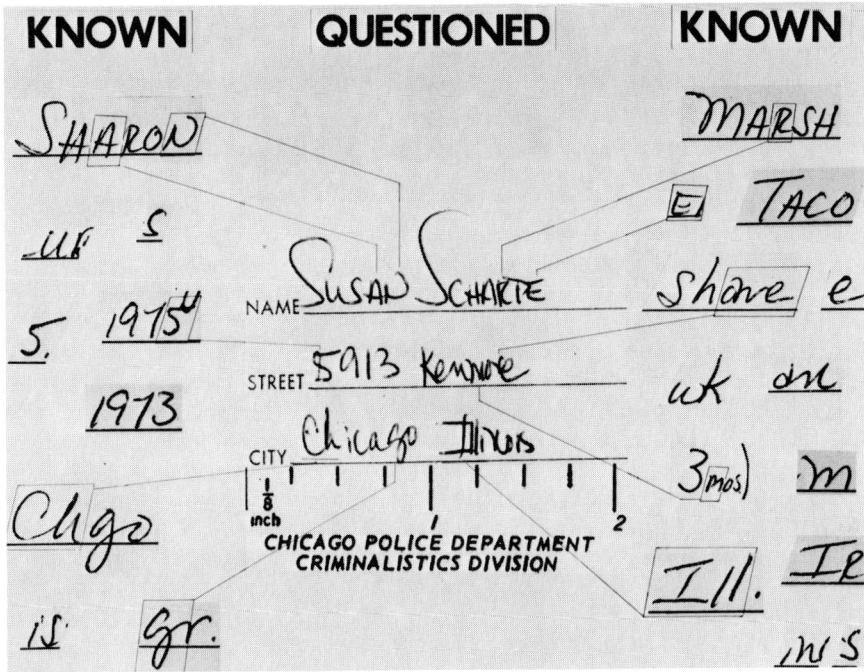

FIGURE 54-2. Comparison chart used to demonstrate identification of the writer of a hand-printed motel registration card in a homicide case. Note the connecting of certain letter forms.

occurs because no two writing specimens of one person are ever written exactly alike. The extent of natural variation will vary among writers and can be assessed from a sufficient quantity of an individual's writing.

Standards of Comparison

Obtaining proper or suitable handwriting standards for comparison with the questioned writings is crucial not only for a correct evaluation of the material, but also to provide the basis for determining the degree of definiteness of the findings or opinion. In general, proper handwriting standards should consist of (1) a sufficient amount of writing, and (2) writing which is suitable for comparison with the questioned material. These conditions are interdependent, and one cannot be considered without the other in obtaining suitable standards.

A sufficient amount of writing is undefinable in the strictest sense. What would prove to be sufficient in one case may be clearly unacceptable in another. Basically, the amount of known writing needed will depend upon the variation in a person's hand, the suitability of the standards for comparison with the questioned writing, and the amount of questioned writing that is to be compared. Normally, the greater the variation in a person's hand, the greater the amount of writing required to encompass the full range of writing characteristics. Also, if the writing in question consists of a limited amount of material (e.g., one sentence or less), more known material will be required for comparison than would be needed if the questioned document were an extended piece of writing, such as a letter. This is because extended writing exhibits a more extensive picture of the individual's writing habits

To be suitable for comparison with the questioned material, known writing should approximate the type of matter and conditions under which the questioned document was prepared. For example, it is necessary to compare disputed signatures with genuine signatures; general handwritten material with general handwritten material; hand-printed material, whether upper case, lower case, or block style, with hand printing of a similar nature; and numerals with numerals (Fig. 54-3). However, not just any known standards containing signatures, handwriting, hand printing, or numerals will be suitable in every instance. It may be necessary that the type of known standards conform generally to the type of disputed material under investigation in order to provide a basis of comparability, as will be explained later. In addition, certain conditions of writing will also affect the type of standards to be secured. Questioned writings prepared in a hurried manner, in ill health, in an unusual writing position, on an unusual writing surface, in an effort to disguise, or in other similar circumstances would have to be considered on an individual basis.

Each handwriting case is different because of the many variables involved, and each must be considered on its own merits. A general guide can be given to the type of handwriting standards which should be obtained, and in the majority of cases these will suffice. There should also be communication between the person handling a case and the document examiner so that the facts and special circumstances surrounding a particular case are clearly understood.

DICTATED STANDARDS

Dictated standards are those obtained directly from an individual for the purpose of comparison with a particular disputed or questioned writing. Most document examiners make use of a handwriting standard form in obtaining a portion of the dictated material.[1] Figure 54-4 is the handwriting standard form used by the Chicago Police Department. It is produced here to explain the value of such a form in obtaining a good quantity of

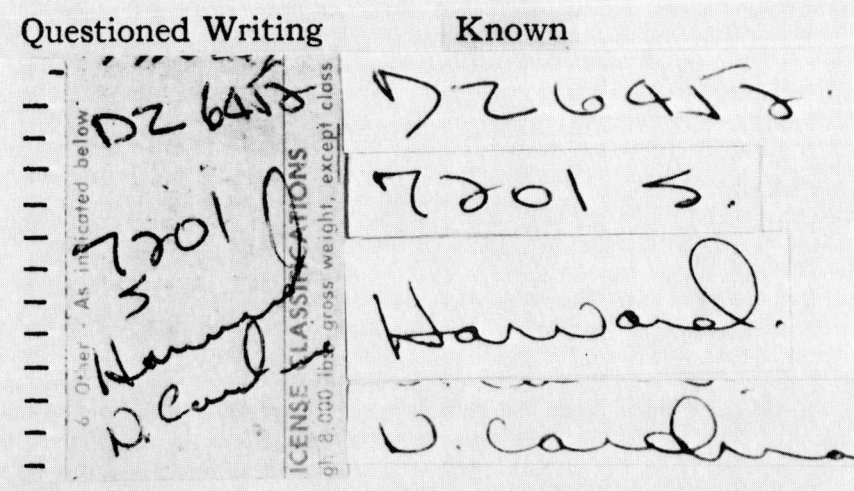

FIGURE 54-3. Identification of notations—numerals, hand printing, and handwriting—on the back side of a driver's license. Only a small portion of the original comparison material is shown.

the initial dictated writing. The top portion of the face is laid out much like an application form, providing an initial ease and familiarity with the subject matter. The lower half of the face is a list of some of the more common names in the Chicago area and includes almost all of the upper and lower case letters of the alphabet in addition to common combinations of letters used to form other names or words, such as "son," "ert," "ard," and "man." Similarly, the top back portion of the form is a listing of common names, abbreviations, and numerals. The center back portion includes words most commonly found in anonymous letters of any variety, and the space for dictated material accommodates dictated contents from the questioned material. Taken as a whole, the handwriting standard form is an initial attempt to obtain suitable and sufficient standards of comparison. No handwriting standard form, however, could be devised which would provide sufficient and suitable material for comparison in each and every case; thus it should be expected that the handwriting form will fall short of the examiner's needs in a number of instances.

It is wise for the investigator to supplement the handwriting form with additional dictated specimens (Figs. 54-5 and 54-6) whenever possible. These may take the form of plain white sheets of paper or simulated copies (hand-drawn or machine copies from a blank form) of the questioned documents and are used for the purpose of dictating the contents of the questioned writings. Each of the questioned writings should be dictated several times. These supplements to the standard form provide the examiner not only with additional specimens of writing, but also with material more comparable to that in question. It is also suggested that the handwriting standard form or initial writing be completed with a ballpoint pen, while the supplemental material should be completed with the same type of writing instrument used to prepare the questioned document. The reason for doing so is that ballpoint pens usually provide a clearer indication of the fine points of the writing, while pencils and fiber-tipped pens may tend to hide some of these.

When obtaining dictated handwriting standards, certain rules should be observed in order to secure the best possible comparable material. The subject should be seated in a quiet room or in an area apart from any conditions which would tend to distract him. The person witnessing the standard should remain in the presence of the subject and watch the execution of all specimens. The subject should be allowed or required to rest at intervals. If it is observed that the subject is attempting to disguise the specimens, additional writing should be taken, for disguise usually becomes less effective with more lengthy material.

COURT-ORDERED STANDARDS

Where an arrested person refuses to give handwriting standards voluntarily, he may be compelled to do so by the court of jurisdiction. Likewise, a person presumed to have knowledge or a part in certain events may be subpoenaed before a grand jury investigating the matter and ordered to provide handwriting exemplars. In either case, a refusal to comply with the order can result in a contempt of court citation. Handwriting evidence has been held by the U.S. Supreme Court to be nontestimonial or noncommunicative evidence and therefore not protected by the self-incrimination clause of the Fifth Amendment.[2]

Court-ordered handwriting standards are not necessarily a panacea for successfully resolving the disputed handwriting problem under investi-

A

NAME	William M. Riordan
DATE	March 17, 1977
ADDRESS	3550 Lake Shore Drive
CITY & STATE	Chicago, Ill
PHONE	338-1793
MARRIED OR SINGLE	Married
NAME OF SPOUSE	Elizabeth
CITY & STATE OF BIRTH	Chicago, Ill
DATE OF BIRTH	12-25-49
NAME OF PERSON LIVING WITH	Elizabeth
RELATIONSHIP	Wife
OCCUPATION (IF STUDENT LIST SCHOOL)	Plumber
SOCIAL SECURITY NUMBER	306-17-5261
NAME OF EMPLOYER OR FORMER EMPLOYER	Metropolitan Construction Co.
SALARY	23,000
ADDRESS OF EMPLOYER	3640 Garland Court
PHONE	893-7676
NAME OF NEAREST RELATIVE	Mary Anne McKay
RELATIONSHIP	Sister
ADDRESS OF NEAREST RELATIVE	1209 State Parkway
CITY & STATE	Chicago, Ill

WRITE THE FOLLOWING

Printed	Written
DONALD O'CONNOR	Donald O'Connor
ALBERT JOHNSON	Albert Johnson
ROBERT OLSEN	Robert Olsen
EDWARD YOUNGBERG	Edward Youngberg
PETER FISHER	Peter Fisher
MICHAEL SMITH	Michael Smith
JACK KOWALSKI	Jack Kowalski
CHARLES QUINN	Charles Quinn
U. X. ZIMMERMAN	U. X. Zimmerman
GEORGE KELLY	George Kelly
ELIZABETH VAUGHN	Elizabeth Vaughn
DAVIES McINTYRE	Davies McIntyre
FRANKLIN PATRICK	Franklin Patrick
WILLIAM BROWN	William Brown
LAWRENCE HARRISON	Lawrence Harrison
RAYMOND TAYLOR	Raymond Taylor
THOMAS NOVAK	Thomas Novak

YOUR SIGNATURE: William M. Riordan

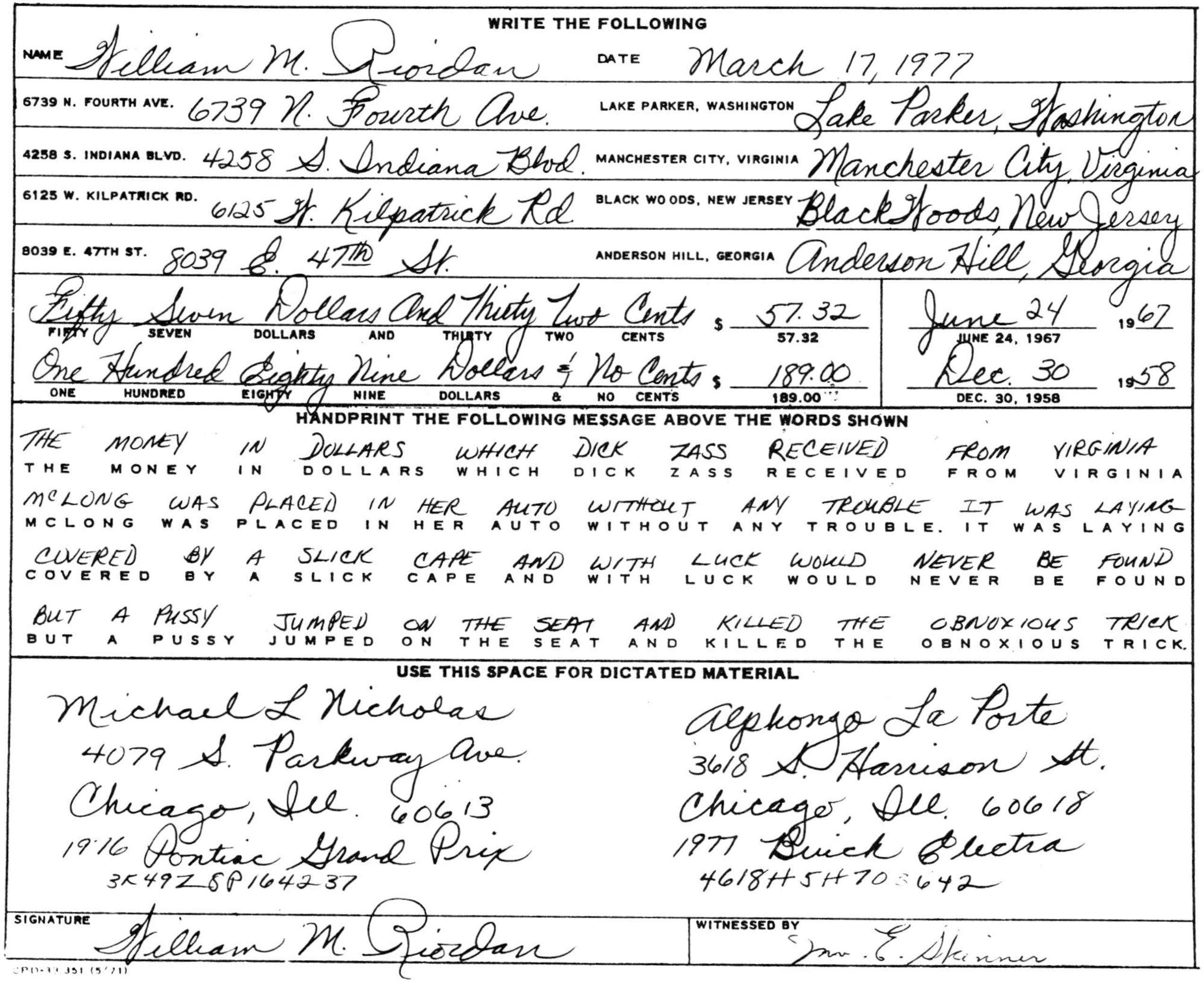

WRITE THE FOLLOWING

NAME William M. Giordan DATE March 17, 1977

6739 N. FOURTH AVE. 6739 N. Fourth Ave. LAKE PARKER, WASHINGTON Lake Parker, Washington

4258 S. INDIANA BLVD. 4258 S. Indiana Blvd. MANCHESTER CITY, VIRGINIA Manchester City, Virginia

6125 W. KILPATRICK RD. 6125 W. Kilpatrick Rd. BLACK WOODS, NEW JERSEY Blackwoods, New Jersey

8039 E. 47TH ST. 8039 E. 47th St. ANDERSON HILL, GEORGIA Anderson Hill, Georgia

Fifty Seven Dollars and Thirty Two Cents $ 57.32 June 24, 1967
FIFTY SEVEN DOLLARS AND THIRTY TWO CENTS 57.32 JUNE 24, 1967 19 67

One Hundred Eighty Nine Dollars & No Cents $ 189.00 Dec. 30, 1958
ONE HUNDRED EIGHTY NINE DOLLARS & NO CENTS 189.00 DEC. 30, 1958 19 58

HANDPRINT THE FOLLOWING MESSAGE ABOVE THE WORDS SHOWN

THE MONEY IN DOLLARS WHICH DICK ZASS RECEIVED FROM VIRGINIA
THE MONEY IN DOLLARS WHICH DICK ZASS RECEIVED FROM VIRGINIA

MCLONG WAS PLACED IN HER AUTO WITHOUT ANY TROUBLE IT WAS LAYING
MCLONG WAS PLACED IN HER AUTO WITHOUT ANY TROUBLE. IT WAS LAYING

COVERED BY A SLICK CAPE AND WITH LUCK WOULD NEVER BE FOUND
COVERED BY A SLICK CAPE AND WITH LUCK WOULD NEVER BE FOUND

BUT A PUSSY JUMPED ON THE SEAT AND KILLED THE OBNOXIOUS TRICK
BUT A PUSSY JUMPED ON THE SEAT AND KILLED THE OBNOXIOUS TRICK.

USE THIS SPACE FOR DICTATED MATERIAL

Michael L. Nicholas   Alphonzo La Porte
4079 S. Parkway Ave.   3618 S. Harrison St.
Chicago, Ill. 60613   Chicago, Ill. 60618
1976 Pontiac Grand Prix   1977 Buick Electra
3K49Z6P164037   4618H5H703642

SIGNATURE William M. Giordan   WITNESSED BY Jane E. Skinner

FIGURE 54-4. Handwriting standard form: (A) face, (B) back.

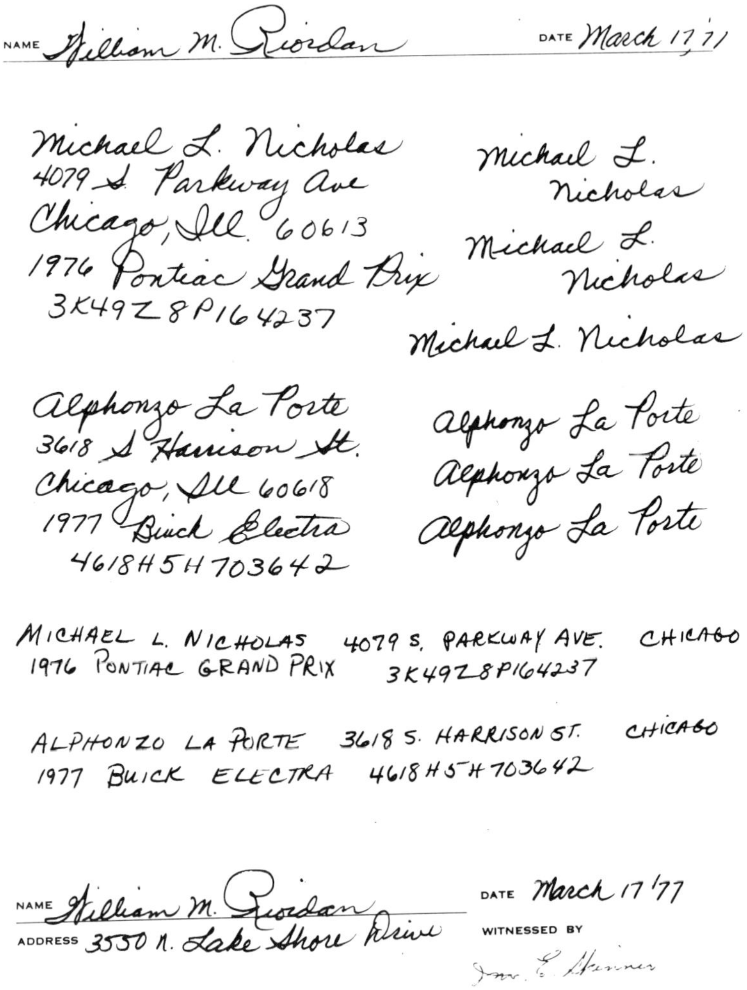
NAME William M. Riordan DATE March 17 '77

Michael L. Nicholas
4079 S. Parkway Ave
Chicago, Ill. 60613
1976 Pontiac Grand Prix
3K49Z8P164237

Michael L. Nicholas
Michael L. Nicholas
Michael L. Nicholas

Alphonzo La Porte
3618 S Harrison St.
Chicago, Ill 60618
1977 Buick Electra
4618H5H703642

Alphonzo La Porte
Alphonzo La Porte
Alphonzo La Porte

MICHAEL L. NICHOLAS 4079 S. PARKWAY AVE. CHICAGO
1976 PONTIAC GRAND PRIX 3K49Z8P164237

ALPHONZO LA PORTE 3618 S. HARRISON ST. CHICAGO
1977 BUICK ELECTRA 4618H5H703642

NAME William M. Riordan DATE March 17 '77
ADDRESS 3550 N. Lake Shore Drive WITNESSED BY

FIGURE 54-5. Format for obtaining dictated writing wherein plain white paper is used by the subject for writing the questioned material as it is dictated to him.

gation. Court-ordered standards are not voluntarily produced, and the problem of disguise becomes a major consideration in many of these cases. The investigator should be aware of this fact and make every effort to obtain sufficient and suitable standards of comparison. Where the material is disguised to the extent that the document examiner can make no adequate comparison with the disputed writing, such fact should be reported to the court in the examiner's written report. An attempt to disguise court-ordered handwriting standards is, in many cases, regarded as evidence of contempt of the order.

COLLECTED STANDARDS

Collected standards are writings prepared at a time and for a purpose other than the present investigation. As a rule, such specimens contain undisputedly normal writing of an individual, since there would usually have been no reason to disguise it. For this reason, collected standards can be an excellent source of comparison material and should be strongly

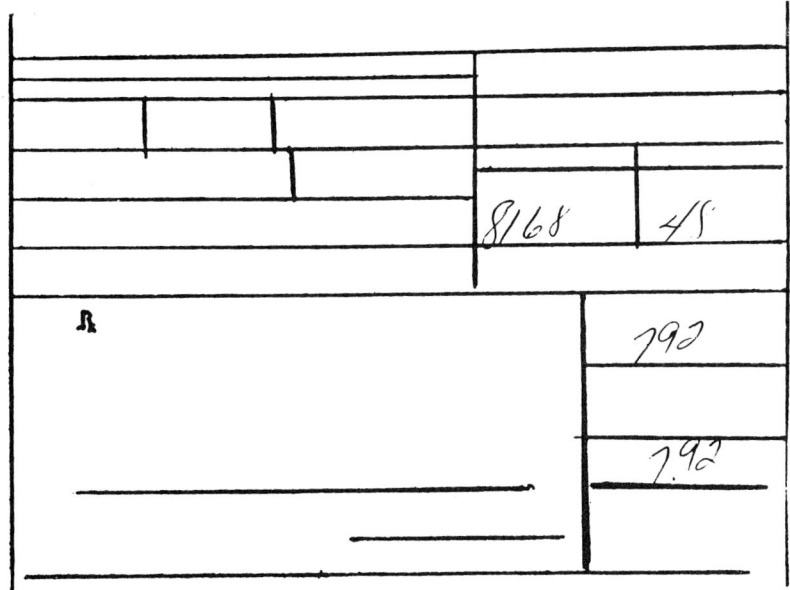

FIGURE 54-6. This is a simulation of the format of a prescription form which constituted the questioned evidence in a case. It was prepared by hand-drawing the lines on a piece of paper the approximate size of the questioned document and reproducing this form to obtain numerous standards for dictated material. Since the pricing portion of the prescription form was in question, these dictated standards provided comparable material with regard not only to the specific combinations of numerals, but also to the arrangement of the material.

considered by the investigator when obtaining standards. Sources of collected writings include application forms, W-4 forms, cancelled business and personal checks, writings prepared in the course of business transactions, and social correspondence. To be useful, collected standards must be comparable with the material in question and must also contain the quality of provability in court.

Disguised Writings

It is not uncommon to examine a case wherein disguise is a factor. Disguise is a deliberate attempt on the part of the writer to alter his natural habits of writing in order to make identification of the writing impossible. The problem in dealing with disguise is the extent to which the writer has achieved his goal.

Disguise is observed more often in standards of comparison than in questioned writings. When the questioned material has been effectively disguised, no amount of known writing will be useful in identifying it. If the questioned material is not disguised, or not effectively disguised, there will always be a possibility of identifying it. The problem in most cases is to obtain suitable, undisguised standards of comparison.

It is well for the investigator to be aware of some of the more common tactics used in attempting to disguise dictated handwriting specimens. In this way, he can recognize gross disguise in the writing and request additional specimens from the subject until a more normal writing is produced. The more common methods of disguise include (1) writing with extreme rapidity so that the material resembles a series of strokes rather than a legible script; (2) writing with extreme slowness and forming each letter with inordinate care; (3) writing with a heavy pressure; (4) writing with an opposite slant; (5) writing extremely small and crowded so that the material is barely readable; and (6) writing extremely large and out of proportion (Fig. 54-7). In some cases, a writer may combine handwriting and hand printing, or a combination of the above methods, which is easily recognizable because of the inconsistency of the overall material. Writing with the unaccustomed hand, a method less often used in disguise, can be recognized because of the poor quality and inconsistency of the writing.

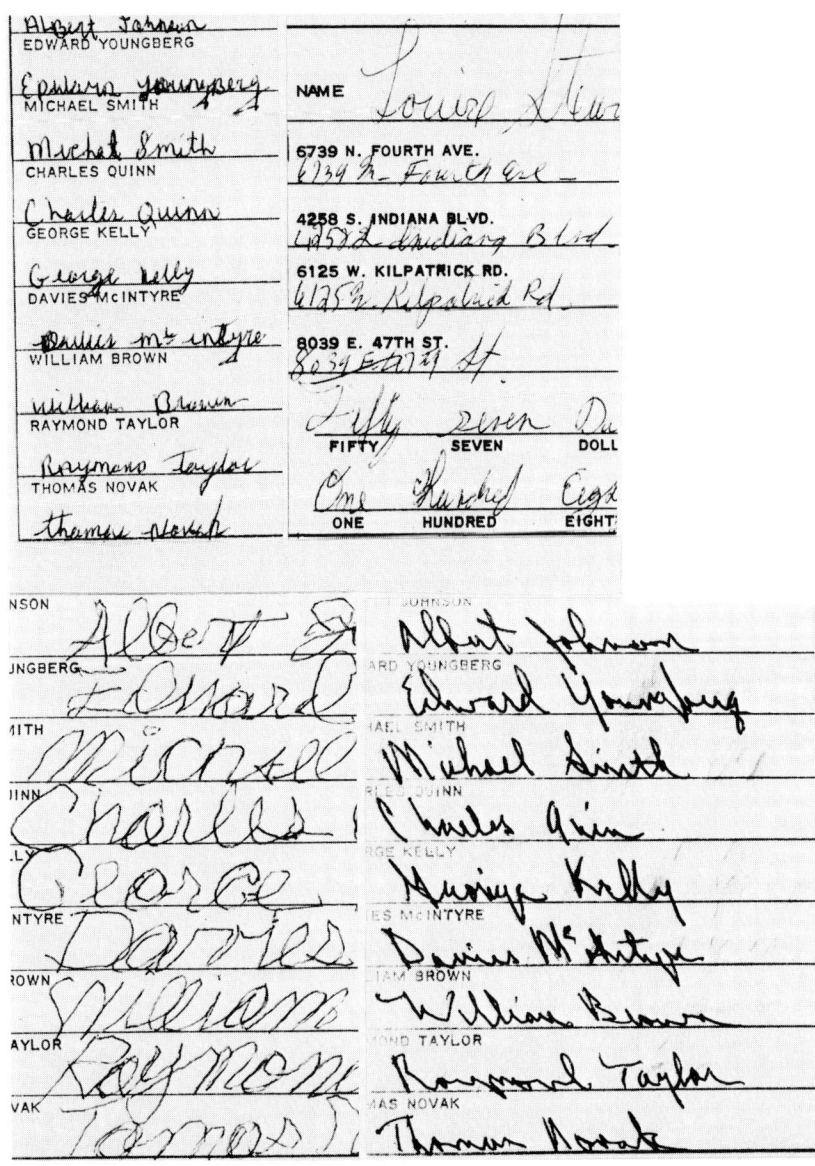

FIGURE 54-7. Examples of disguised writings. The last example was photographed with side light to show the embossing effect from heavy writing pressure used throughout the form.

SIGNATURE COMPARISON

Genuineness and Forgery

The comparison of signatures or detection of forgery may be regarded as a specialized area of handwriting identification. Signatures, through repeated use and the incorporation of characteristics designed to suit the writer, may become highly individualized and reflect features not found in the general handwriting of an individual. For this reason, when a comparison is requested to determine genuineness or forgery of a signature, the standards must consist of signatures of that individual. Generally, these standards of comparison should encompass a sufficient number of known signatures to incorporate the extent of variability in the writing, signatures prepared as close in time to the date of the questioned signature as possible, and signatures of the same general class (e.g., formal, informal, and hastily prepared specimens). Much will depend upon the individual circumstances of the signature writing as to the most appropriate material for comparison (Fig. 54-8).

The identification of a signature as genuine is based upon the principles of handwriting identification discussed previously; however, certain aspects of the writing will assume greater importance in signature comparison than would be the case with general handwriting. The writing movement used to produce a signature is an important consideration in determining whether a signature is genuine or forged (Fig. 54-9). Genuine signatures will exhibit a certain degree of speed, skill, freedom, continuity, and pen motion, all of which contribute to the individual writing movement. These elements are among the most difficult to imitate and constitute the area in which forgeries are usually deficient.

Signature forgery generally may be grouped into three classes: traced, simulated, and what may be termed spurious forgery. A traced forgery is the outlining of a genuine signature from one document onto another document upon which the forger wishes it to appear. Basically, two methods are used to achieve this result. One method utilizes transmitted light wherein the area of the document upon which the signature is to be copied is placed directly over the document containing the genuine signature, both having been placed over a strong background light and the forged signature traced from the genuine either directly or by lightly penciling the outline and then overwriting the penciled outline. The second method involves placing the document which is to receive the signature underneath the document bearing the genuine signature and, by tracing the genuine signature with a writing instrument, produce an indented outline on the underneath page or, as an alternative, interleaving the documents with carbon paper to produce a carbon outline on the forged document. In both cases, the outline is overwritten to produce the final signature (Fig. 54-10).

A simulated forgery is an attempt to copy in a freehand manner the characteristics of a genuine signature either from memory of the signature or from a model. It is accomplished without the aid of an outline. A spurious forgery is one prepared primarily in the author's own handwriting wherein little or no attempt has been made to copy the characteristics of the genuine writing.

Traced signatures are basically drawings and, as a result, lack much of the free, natural movement inherent in a person's normal writing. Simu-

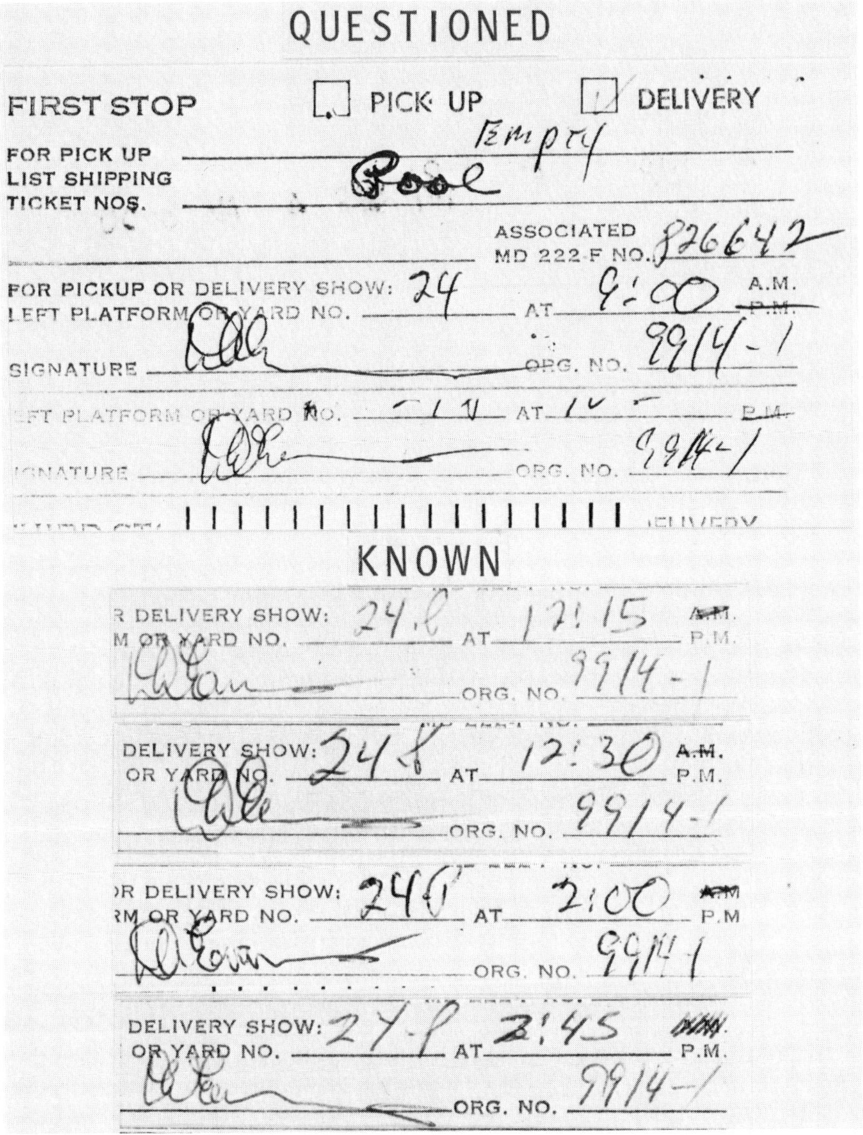

QUESTIONED

FIRST STOP ☐ PICK UP ☑ DELIVERY

FOR PICK UP LIST SHIPPING TICKET NOS. Empty Pool

ASSOCIATED MD 222-F NO. 826642

FOR PICKUP OR DELIVERY SHOW: 24 LEFT PLATFORM OR YARD NO. AT 9:00 A.M.

SIGNATURE ORG. NO. 9914-1

LEFT PLATFORM OR YARD NO. AT P.M.

SIGNATURE ORG. NO. 9914-1

KNOWN

DELIVERY SHOW: 24 AT 12:15 P.M. ORG. NO. 9914-1

DELIVERY SHOW: 24 AT 12:30 A.M. P.M. ORG. NO. 9914-1

DELIVERY SHOW: 24 AT 2:00 P.M ORG. NO. 9914-1

DELIVERY SHOW: 24 AT 2:45 P.M. ORG. NO. 9914-1

FIGURE 54-8. The questioned signatures "D.W. Evans" on shipping forms are prepared in an informal, careless, and hurried manner. Dictated handwriting standards, prepared in a formal and unhurried manner, were unsuitable for comparison. When collected signatures were obtained which were prepared under circumstances similar to those involving the questioned signatures, identification was possible.

lated signatures, on the other hand, will vary in quality according to a number of factors, including the writer's skill as a penman; the difficulty of the signature being imitated; the writer's ability to recognize and incorporate detail; practice of the signature to be imitated; the writer's ability to concentrate on the important features of the signature; and throughout all of the writing, his ability to simultaneously discard all of his own natural habits of handwriting. In addition, the forger must choose a signature in the relevant time period and pay close attention to

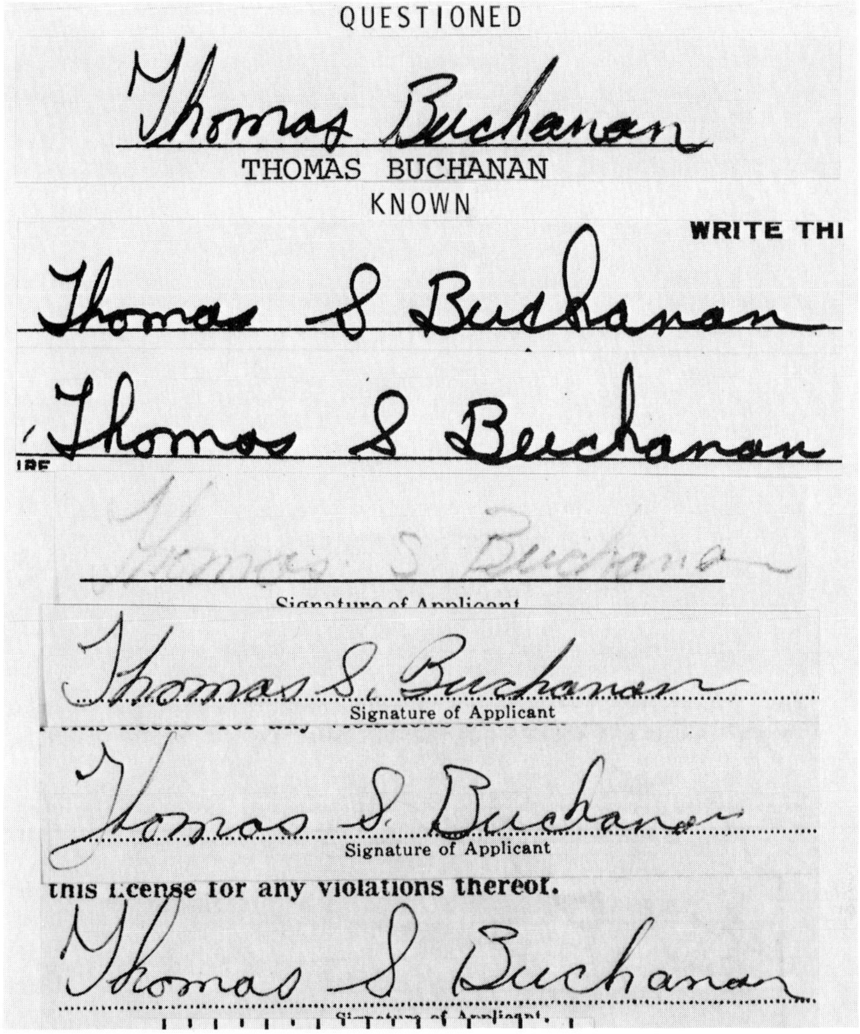

FIGURE 54-9. The questioned signature, appearing on an affidavit, was denied by the subject. The top two known signatures are from the dictated specimens, and the remaining known signatures are representative of the collected standards. It is seen that the collected standards encompass more of the variation in the individual's hand and are helpful in proving the genuineness of the denied signature. Examination reveals the questioned signature to be prepared freely, in a continuous writing motion, and with a speed and skill comparable to that shown in the known signatures.

natural variation in the writing, particularly when more than one forgery must be prepared. The difficulty of executing the so-called perfect forgery becomes apparent, and although simulated signatures are generally the better of the above two classes of forgery, they will usually not go undetected under close scrutiny (Fig. 54-11).

Traced and simulated forgeries are sometimes recognizable in themselves, traced forgeries showing evidence of an outline, and both types showing evidence of a drawn appearance (i.e., slow and uncertain pen movement). Upon comparison with genuine signatures of the individual,

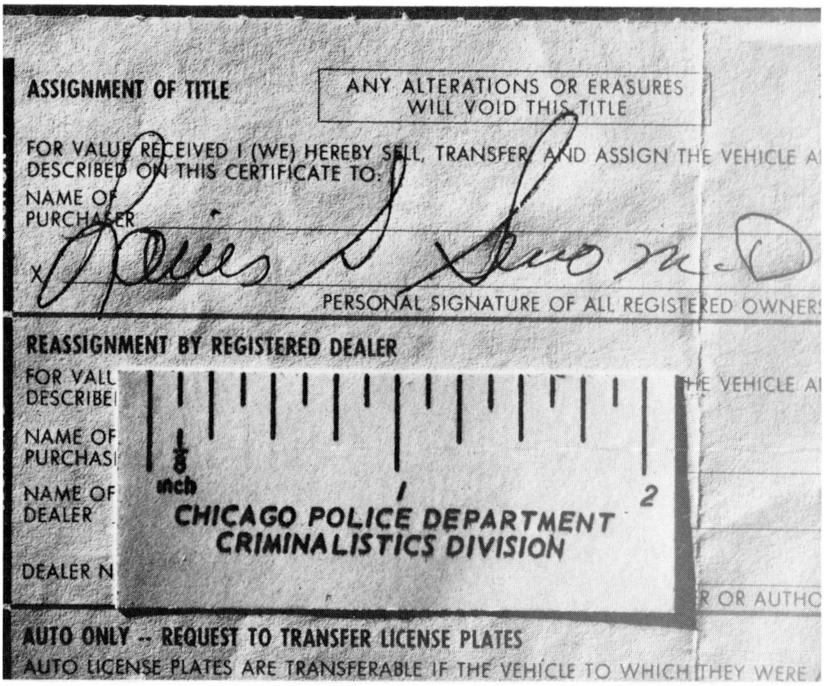

FIGURE 54-10. A traced forgery prepared by inking over an indented outline of a genuine signature. The indentations are seen when viewed with side light.

specific defects become more apparent. Among these defects are hesitation points in the writing, liftings of the pen in unusual places, patchings, incorrect manner of forming some letters, incorrect shading or lack of shading, tremorous movements, abrupt beginning and ending strokes, and a lack of inconspicuous details (Fig. 54-12).

Because of the nature of traced and simulated signatures (i.e., the attempt to copy another's handwriting characteristics), the authors of these types of forgeries are seldom identified. Only if the author of such a forgery were to do a particularly unskillful imitation or to imitate only a portion of the genuine signatures (e.g., only the capital letters, thereby leaving the greater portion of the writing to contain his own natural habits) would the possibility of identification exist. Spurious forgeries, on the other hand, because they are prepared without benefit of a model signature, always possess the possibility of identification.

Special Signature Cases

Signature problems wherein the writing is directly affected by a physical condition of the writer will occasionally come to the document examiner's attention. Such cases may involve writing of the aged, the infirm, the handicapped, the blind, or writing prepared under the influence of alcohol or drugs. The purported guided-hand signature (i.e., where one person claims to have helped guide the hand of another in preparing the latter's signature) also falls into this category. These signature problems differ from those described previously in that the writing may be badly deteriorated, executed with great difficulty, contain irregular or confused movements, or appear erratic in portions.

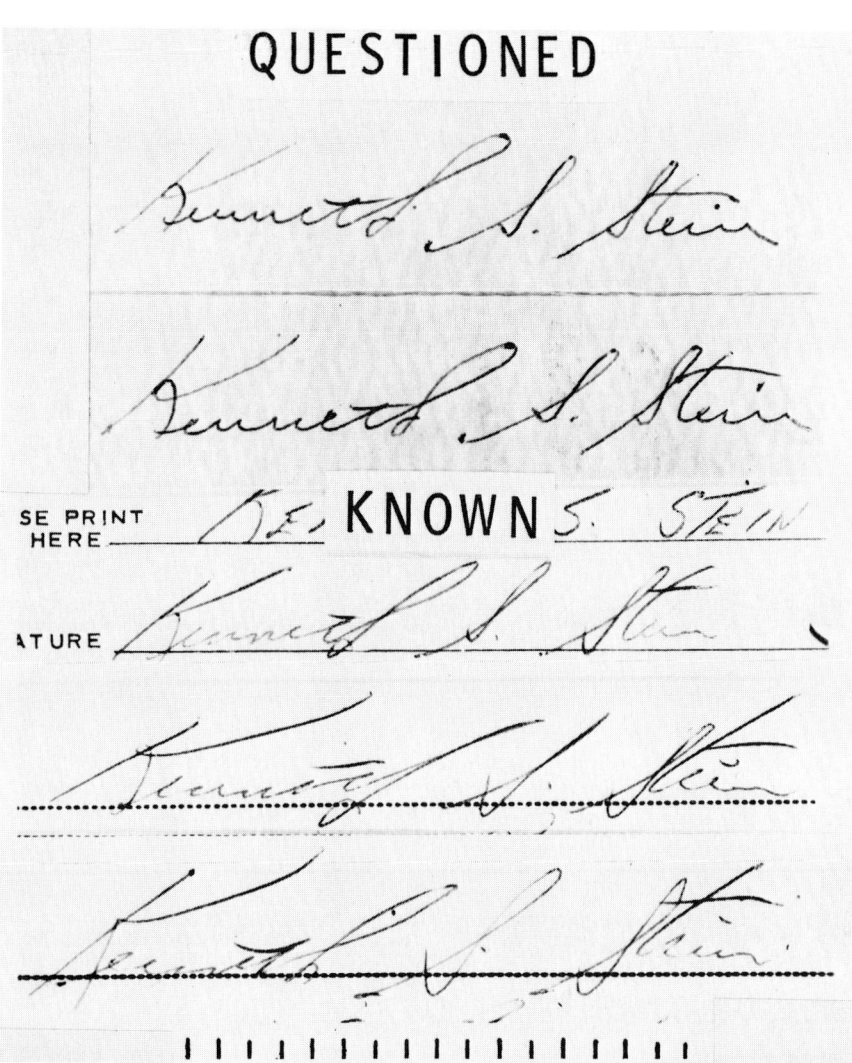

FIGURE 54-11. The questioned signatures are simulated forgeries of a genuine signature of Kenneth S. Stein. Note the lack of variation between the two questioned signatures, indicating that they were probably copied from the same model signature. Observe also the tremorous movements, particularly in letters "K," "h," "S," and "t," indicating a slow, drawn effect, and the definite beginning and ending strokes in the questioned signatures as opposed to the tapered strokes in the known.

Cases of this type must be considered in light of the individual circumstances of the writing. Standards must be available which reveal the previous and present writing habits of the person. Such signatures, even those of the poorest quality, may be distinguished from forgeries, but only by very careful and experienced observation and evaluation of the written material.

The comparison of initials may also be included as special signature cases because normally these involve only two or three letter forms. Even so, if initials are used regularly by a person in signing certain types of documents, they become as individual to the person as his signature (Fig.

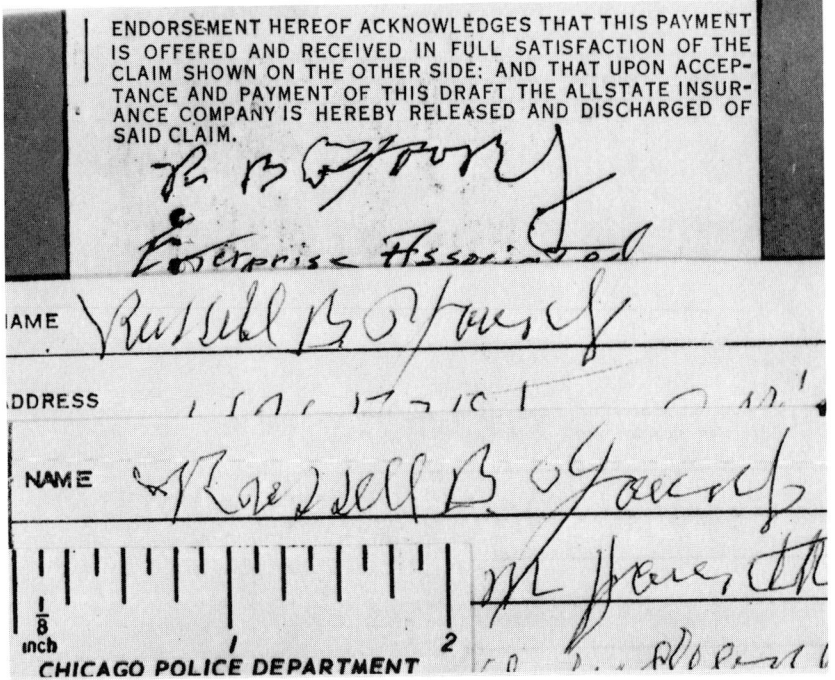

FIGURE 54-12. The questioned signature "R.B. Young" is a poorly executed, simulated forgery. The genuine signatures are those of an aged person whose quality of writing has deteriorated to some degree. However, there are many fine movements in the known signatures which the forger has disregarded completely, concentrating more on the quavery movements of the writing.

54-13). Great care must be exercised in examining such limited material, and good standards of comparison are a must.

THE COMPARISON OF MECHANICAL IMPRESSIONS

Typewriting

Typewriting identification is a most important aspect of questioned document work as it involves a good portion of those communications which are not handwritten and a good bulk of legal and business documents in existence today. Typewriting problems are often thought of only in terms of identifying a typewritten communication with a specific machine, the more common typewriting problem, when in fact other possibilities exist. The addition of typewritten matter to an existing typewritten document after it has been signed or legalized in some manner may serve to alter the contents or the context of the document. The addition may be in the form of characters, words, phrases, or even paragraphs prepared on the same machine or on one having a typeface closely resembling that used to prepare the original document. In many cases, additions to an existing document can readily be recognized by a close inspection of the size and design of type and measurement of the vertical and horizontal alignments of the material, using specially designed typewriter test plates (Fig. 54-14), or by differences in the ink intensity of the typewriting.

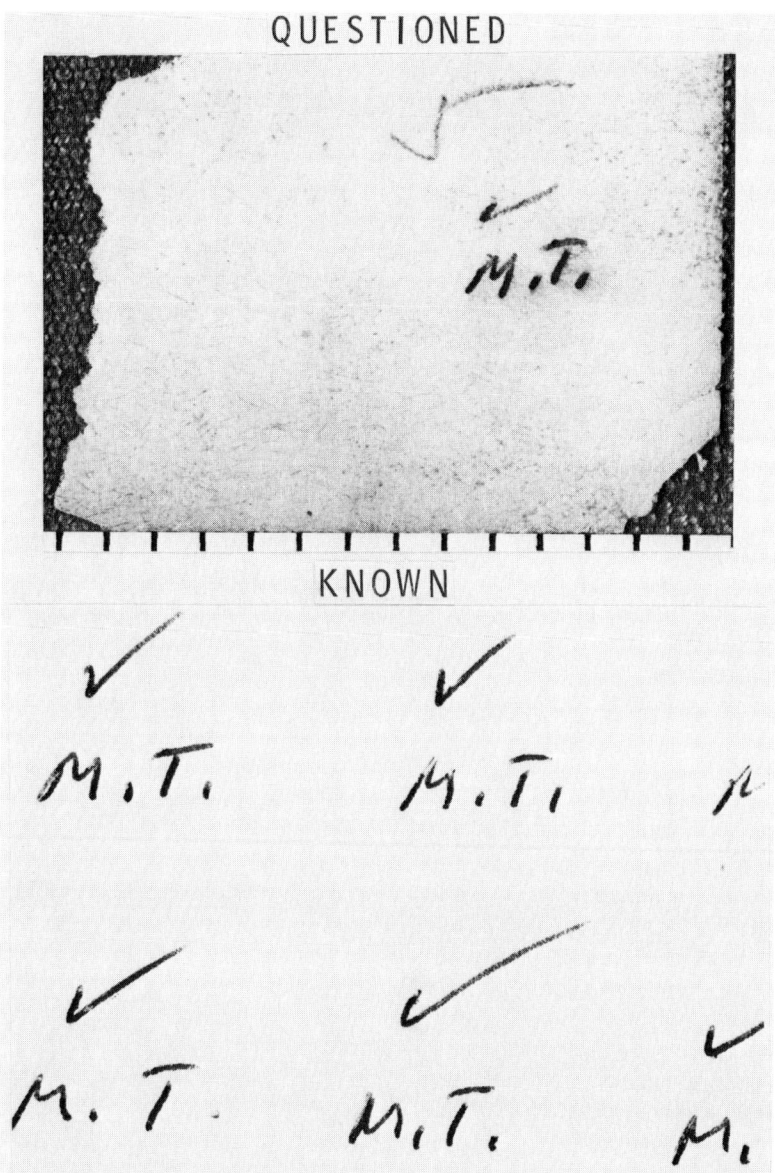

FIGURE 54-13. Initials and check mark on a small piece of paper attached to a stack of currency notes were an important factor in determining the owner of the money. Note the form of the letters, the starting point of letter "M," the length and angularity of the center of the "M," the relative lengths of the downstroke and crossbar of the "T," the curvature of the crossbar and distance above the downstroke, the size and spacing of the letters, and the manner of forming the periods. Note also the placement and proportions of the check mark.

Substitution is another manner of tampering with a typewritten document. The original material is removed via an appropriate physical method, and the new material inserted in its place. Substitutions can usually be recognized by the evidence of tampering (i.e., the physical indicators of the method used) when examined microscopically or under various light

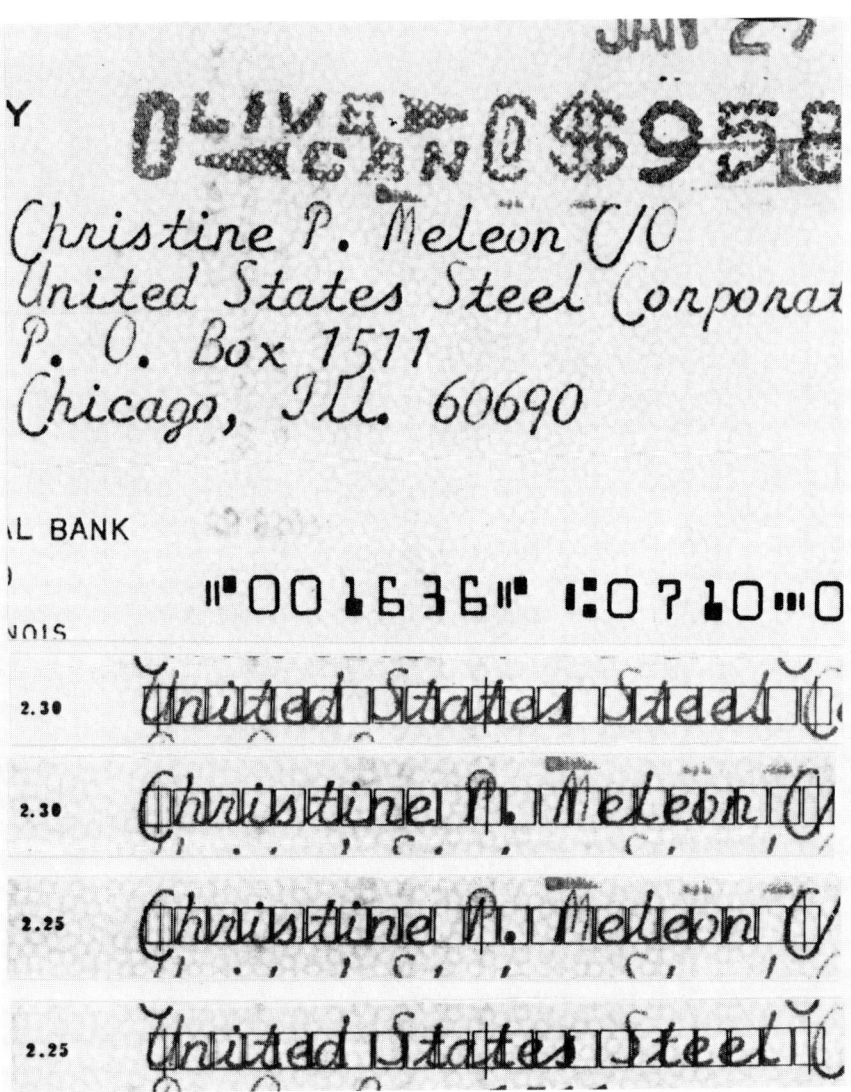

FIGURE 54-14. The line "Christine P. Meleon C/O" was added to the payee area of a check after it had been stolen from the mail. The addition was made with a similar design but different size of type (i.e., a pitch of 2.25 mm as opposed to 2.30 mm). Vertical and horizontal misalignment is also apparent.

sources, and also by a close inspection of the typeface and measurement of the vertical and horizontal alignments. Establishing the relative time period in which a typewritten document was prepared through the typewriting itself is another possibility. This may be accomplished through dating of the typeface or deterioration of the typewriter used to prepare the document. In some instances, it can be demonstrated that a particular typewriter ribbon was used in preparing a specific typewritten document. This is true where the characters on the typewriter ribbon can be deciphered to read the same material, in the same order, as it appears on the disputed document, and where, of course, the type style is the same. This evidence is even more convincing when the same errors, in the same order, are present (Fig. 54-15).

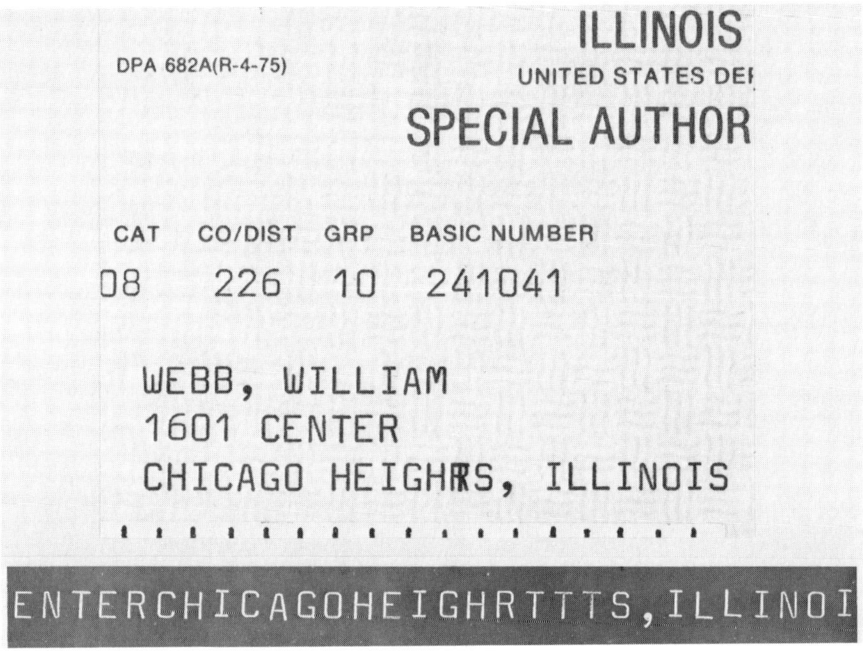

```
                          ILLINOIS
   DPA 682A(R-4-75)       UNITED STATES DE
                       SPECIAL AUTHOR

      CAT   CO/DIST  GRP   BASIC NUMBER
      08     226     10     241041


         WEBB, WILLIAM
         1601 CENTER
         CHICAGO HEIGHRS, ILLINOIS

    ENTERCHICAGOHEIGHRTTTS,ILLINOI
```

FIGURE 54-15. Identification of the typewriter ribbon used in preparing the faces of a series of checks. The letter "R" in HEIGHTS was typed in error and overtyped several times with the letter "T."

TYPEWRITER STANDARDS

The most common typewriting problem is that of identifying a questioned typewritten document with the typewriter used in preparing the document. The first step to an identification is the classification of the type style in an effort to determine the make of machine in question and thereby eliminate numerous other brand-name machines.* Once a suspect machine has been located, standards may be obtained and a comparison with the questioned document initiated. Whenever possible, the suspect typewriter should be submitted to the document examiner. When this is not possible, suitable typewriter standards may be provided following a format similar to that shown in Figure 54-16.

The format for obtaining typewriting standards should include all pertinent data of the machine including make, model, serial number, and any additional features such as the capability to accommodate a two-ribbon system. The entire keyboard should be typed at least two times, and the questioned material, depending upon its extensiveness and repetition, should be typed two times, adhering as closely as possible to the arrangement and spelling of the questioned text. The pressure used in typing the standards should vary, on a manual machine, from light to medium to heavy in an attempt to simulate the conditions of the original typing. A carbon impression, duplicating the above, is obtained by plac-

---

*For this and other typewriting problems, document examiners maintain an extensive typewriter reference file covering domestic and foreign styles of type, dates of introduction of type styles, dates of changes in type styles and design modifications of typewriters.

FORMAT FOR TYPEWRITING STANDARDS

INSTRUCTIONS

TYPEWRITER IDENTIFICATION	IBM Electric Typewriter, Serial Number 11-95342, located at 1111 South Michigan, 5th floor, Room 599, owned by the Neverready Company and assigned to Mr. J. Jones.
ENTIRE KEYBOARD --TWICE	ABCDEFGHIJKLMNOPQRSTUVWXYZ abcdefghijklmnopqrstuvwxyz 1234567890-=½;',./ !@#$%¢&*()_+¼:",.? ABCDEFGHIJKLMNOPQRSTUVWXYZ abcdefghijklmnopqrstuvwxyz 1234567890-=½;',./ !@#$%¢&*()_+¼:",.?
MESSAGE	This is a warning to you and your family. We know where you live. If you don't put $10,000 in a brown envelope and place it under the rock near the second pillar North of the "L" station on Ashland Ave. we will kill your son. We mean business. This is a warning to you and your family. We know where you live. If you don't put $10,000 in a brown envelope and place it under the rock near the second pillar North of the "L" station on Ashland Ave. we will kill your son. We mean business.
CARBON PAPER IMPRESSION	
ENTIRE KEYBOARD	ABCDEFGHIJKLMNOPQRSTUVWXYZ abcdefghijklmnopqrstuvwxyz 1234567890-=½;',./ !@#$%¢&*()_+¼:",.? ABCDEFGHIJKLMNOPQRSTUVWXYZ abcdefghijklmnopqrstuvwxyz 1234567890-=½;',./ !@#$%¢&*()_+¼:",.?
MESSAGE	This is a warning to you and your family. We know where you live. If you don't put $10,000 in a brown envelope and place it under the rock near the second pillar North of the "L" station on Ashland Ave. we will kill your son. We mean business.
TYPIST, IDENTIFICATION	This material was typed by Det. Earl E. Morn, #1961, 45th Dist., on 31 January 1971 at the above listed location.

TO OBTAIN CARBON PAPER IMPRESSION--SET MACHINE FOR STENCIL AND PLACE CARBON PAPER IN FRONT OF TYPING PAPER

WHEN TYPING, VARY DEGREE OF TOUCH--HEAVY, MEDIUM AND LIGHT

FIGURE 54-16. Format for obtaining typewriting standards.

ing the machine on stencil and typing directly through a fresh piece of carbon paper placed in front of the paper. The carbon impression is taken for the purpose of obtaining a clear picture of the condition of the typeface.

TYPEWRITER IDENTIFICATION

TYPE-BAR MACHINE. The identification of a type-bar machine with its product is based upon a consideration of the class and individual characteristics of the machine. Once it has been established that the class characteristics, size and design of type, and line spacing are in agreement, the actual identification is based upon the machine's individual characteristics (i.e., those peculiarities which serve to distinguish it from any other machine bearing similar class characteristics). Generally, individual characteristics fall into two classes: defects in the typeface and defects in alignment. Such defects are most often caused through wear or misuse of the machine, although manufacturing defects are a possibility. Occasionally, machine defects, such as skipping of a space, irregular margin stops, improper letter spacing, improper ribbon actions, or improper platen alignment which cuts off tops or bottoms of letters, can add to the identification formula.

A standard type-bar machine contains 44 keys or type bars (88 characters), operating independently of one another, each of which is liable to potential damage. Damage can result from a variety of occurrences and affect either the metal typeface or the alignment of the type bar. This damage is observed in the typewritten impression as typeface and alignment defects. Typeface defects include broken or missing serifs and dented or otherwise defective characters. Alignment defects include characters which print above or below the base line of typing, to the right or left of the center line of typing, canted from the perpendicular, or more heavily in one area than another.

The actual identification of a typewriter with its product or of two typewritten documents having been prepared on the same machine is based primarily upon a unique combination of typeface and alignment defects in common plus the same combination of nondefective characters. This is not simply a matter of counting up defective and nondefective characters, however, since not all typeface and alignment defects bear equal weight or consideration in an identification. The manner in which characters are defective, possible causes of the defects, and incidence of letter usage all contribute to the final evaluation. The end result of this combination of defects must be such that the possibility of another machine of the same size and design of type having exactly the same defects is virtually nonexistent (Fig. 54-17).

SINGLE-ELEMENT MACHINE. The IBM Selectric typewriter, introduced onto the market in 1961, represented a significant departure in typewriter design. Instead of having type bars, it contained a single, interchangeable typewriting element and a stationary platen. The typewriting element was mounted on a carrier unit which acted to move the element across the paper and to control its movements of rotation, tilt, and forward motion in the typing process. Because the operation of this machine was entirely different than that of a type-bar machine, the usual criteria for establishing identification was no longer entirely valid. The identification problem had to be reanalyzed in light of the basic principles of operation of the Selectric typewriter.

The Selectric typewriter contains two basic components, the removable typing element and the machine itself, both interacting to form a system. It is this system, the combination of a particular typing element used on a particular machine, that is identified when comparison is made with a questioned document. If the typing element were to be destroyed after the questioned document had been typed, that particular system, would no longer exist. Similarly, each new typing element used on a machine creates a new system. This thought should be kept in mind when obtaining standards for comparison. All elements having the same size and

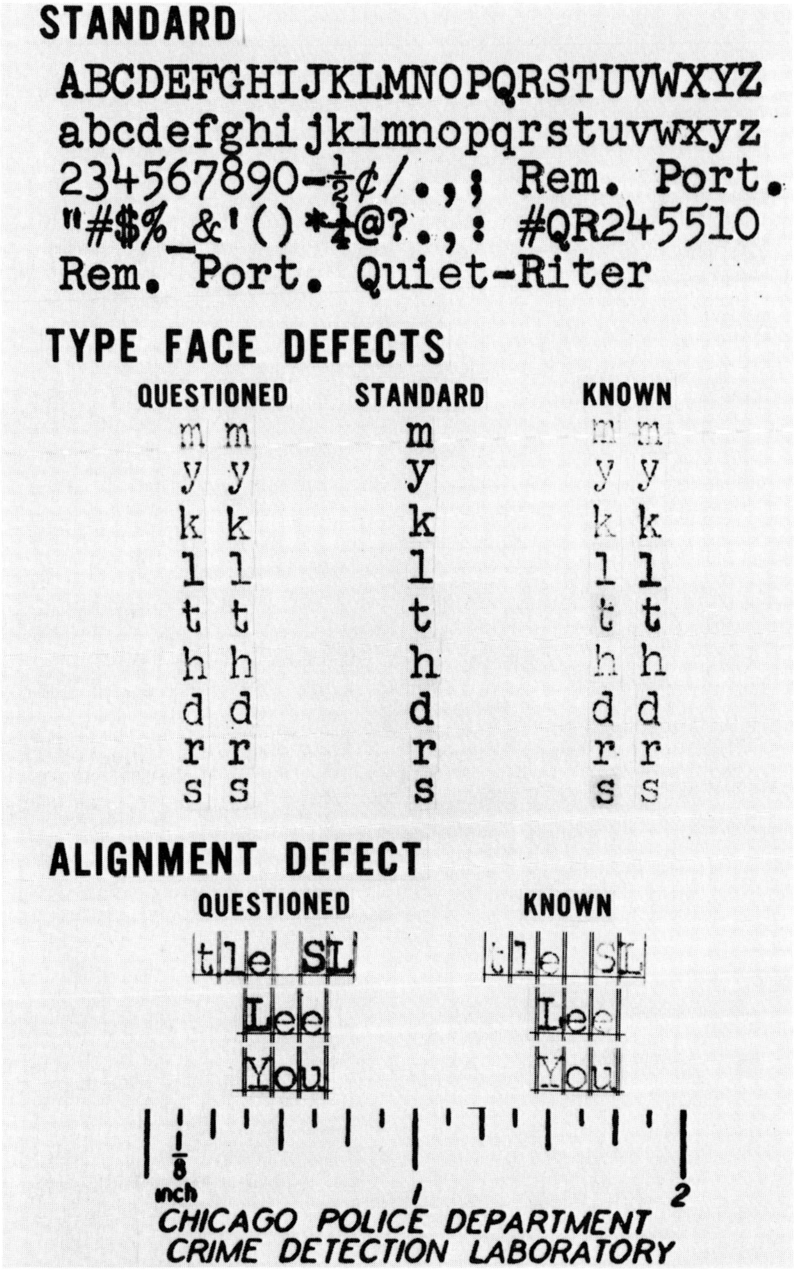

STANDARD

ABCDEFGHIJKLMNOPQRSTUVWXYZ
abcdefghijklmnopqrstuvwxyz
234567890-½¢/.,; Rem. Port.
"#$%_&'()*¼@?.,: #QR245510
Rem. Port. Quiet-Riter

TYPE FACE DEFECTS

QUESTIONED	STANDARD	KNOWN
m m	m	m m
y y	y	y y
k k	k	k k
l l	l	l l
t t	t	t t
h h	h	h h
d d	d	d d
r r	r	r r
s s	s	s s

ALIGNMENT DEFECT

QUESTIONED   KNOWN

CHICAGO POLICE DEPARTMENT
CRIME DETECTION LABORATORY

FIGURE 54-17. Chart used for demonstration of a typewriter identification. Typeface defects include the broken serifs on letters "m," "y," "k," "h," and "d"; the short left foot of "l"; the dented "t," "r," and "s"; and the bent right arch of "m." An alignment defect resulting from a maladjusted shift-stop causes all capital letters to print above the base line of typing

design of type as that used in preparing the questioned document should be used on all suspect machines to obtain typewriting standards. Obviously, elements and machines must be carefully marked to identify the various systems.

Identification of a system is primarily dependent upon a unique combination of typing-element defects and machine defects in common and a similar combination of nondefective characters. With the Selectric machine, however, individual typeface defects do not occur as commonly as with the type-bar machine and, in most cases, will play a minor role in the final identification. Alignment defects, arising from irregularities in both the operation of the typing element and the operation of its controlling mechanism, will constitute the primary basis for identification. Occasionally, type-element defects, occurring as a result of the manufacturing process, will be a contributing factor in the identification. Extreme care must be used in evaluating defects from a Selectric machine as they are significantly more subtle than will be found with a type-bar machine. One must also be fully aware of how a Selectric machine works, which mechanisms control the various operations, and which operations affect the various letters in order to avoid the possibility of error.[3]

In the years since 1961, modifications of the basic Selectric machine have been developed and introduced as the Selectric II, commonly called the dual-pitch machine, and the Correcting Selectric. The Selectric II is basically the same machine except that it contains a dual-escapement mechanism, rendering it capable of accepting and typing both 10-pitch(pica) and 12-pitch(elite) elements. This could further complicate a problem if one is not aware of this feature. The Correcting Selectric typewriter utilizes a correctable film ribbon in conjunction with a lift-off tape to effect removal of a typed image from the paper. While the ink is removed from the paper, an indentation still remains from the striking force of the typing element, and the possibility of detection and decipherment of the original character exists.

The single-element mechanism is no longer exclusive to IBM. In the last several years, other typewriter companies, including Royal, Remington, Adler, Facit, Hermes, and Olivetti, have introduced their own single-element models. With increased volume and usage of this machine, single-element typewriter problems will become more prevalent in the years to come.

Word Processors

A brief mention of word processors should be made here since typewriters are involved in many of these systems. IBM was the first company to introduce such a system utilizing the Selectric typewriter as the input/output (I/O) unit. In its simplest form, a word-processing system consists of a typewriter and a magnetic card or magnetic-tape control unit. The typewriter is adapted with an interface to the electronic control unit. Text is entered at the typewriter keyboard at the fastest draft speed and automatically recorded, via the electronics, on a magnetic card or magnetic tape. Control or code keys, located on either the keyboard or control unit, instruct the system to perform various operations of editing and formating. The completed text, in its revised form, is then automatically played out on the typewriter.

Since IBM's introduction of these systems in the late 1960s, many other companies have introduced word-processing systems using the IBM Selectric typewriter as the I/O unit, adapting the machine to be compatible with their control units. More sophisticated systems which do not use typewriters, but rather keyboard and offline or high-speed printers, may also be found on the market. The systems utilizing the typewriter, however, were geared to small or medium-sized office needs and are the more likely to be encountered by the document examiner.

The relatively new Xerox 800 word-processing system, introduced in 1974, deserves special mention because of its unique single-element printer, formerly the Diablo printer. The print mechanism is a simple plastic or metal disk, termed a Daisy wheel, consisting of 96 petals each of which carries a print character. The unit is capable of printing in either direction, left to right and right to left, making it a faster typing system than that used by IBM.

Checkwriters

Checkwriter problems encountered by the document examiner most commonly involve checks stolen in a burglary, where the checkwriter may also be taken as part of the proceeds, or internal company problems, where an office employee uses the company checkwriter to imprint stolen company checks. When a suspect machine is located and a comparison required with checkwriter impressions on questioned checks, the machine along with the checks should be submitted to the document examiner.

In those cases where it is impossible to submit the checkwriter because of daily use in an office, standards obtained by the investigator should follow a certain format. Standards should be obtained to include all of the characters on the suspect checkwriter. This procedure will facilitate a comparison with any numerical amount of checks not yet in hand. It may be accomplished by setting all dials at the zero position and impressing this amount, carrying the procedure through to the number nine position. Standards duplicating the amount on each questioned check available should also be secured. It is preferable to secure specimens on separate pieces of paper cut to the approximate size of a business check or on blank checks if available. The reason for submitting the suspect checkwriter to the laboratory whenever possible is that the document examiner is better able to simulate the conditions under which the questioned impressions were made. Differences in inking and pressure between the questioned and known specimens can be important considerations in the examination process. Then, too, the examiner is able to evaluate peculiarities of the machine on a first-hand basis.

Basically, the printing mechanism of a checkwriter consists of cast typefaces bonded to a number segment shaped in the form of a half circle and attached to an operating arm. The typefaces are milled to form either grooves or pin holes, depending upon the manufacturer, and these in turn mesh with a platen which has been grooved or contains pin points, to form the perforated impressions. The inking mechanism is either an inked roll, which passes over the typefaces prior to each printing, or an inked ribbon through which the characters impress directly. It should be noted that some checkwriters bear a removable slug which may contain a prefix such as "The Sum of" or the company name, but all other parts of the machine are permanently affixed.

Identification of a checkwriter is possible because of imperfections which may be developed in the manufacturing process—casting of the type characters, milling of the grooves, assembly of the machine parts—and defects which occur through wear and use of the machine. Because there are relatively few checkwriter manufacturers, class characteristics are easily defined on the basis of the design of the characters.

Hand Stamps

There are many varieties of hand stamps, manufactured for many different purposes, which range from the specially made, single-purpose stamp to the mass-produced, common-use stamps. Rubber is the most versatile material for hand stamps, although occasionally plastic, metal, linoleum, or wood stamps will be encountered. Hand stamps will be recognized in forms such as the facsimile signature stamp, the name and/or title stamp, the word or phrase stamp (e.g., "Registered," "Do not handle"), date stamps, and marking stamps.

Basically, rubber stamps are made by assembling metal type in a chase, impressing the type through heat and pressure into a hardened piece of material to form the mat or matrix, and then contacting the mat with a sheet of gum, again through heat and pressure, to form the raised rubber dies. The dies are then cut from the sheet, in many cases by hand, and glued to mounts or, in the case of moveable stamps, affixed to a frame. Some rubber type is sold in kits, usually consisting of a font, to be assembled into a holder by the user.

Class characteristics of rubber stamps include not only the size and design of letters, but also the spacing and arrangement of material. Individual characteristics are most often acquired through wear, age, use, or misuse of the stamp, although it is quite possible for imperfections to occur through any of the steps in the manufacturing process, even backtracking to imperfections in the metal typefaces (Fig. 54-18).

When it becomes apparent that a comparison will be required between a particular hand stamp and impressions on certain questioned documents, the hand stamp should be taken out of use and packaged to protect the surface from alteration. It should be submitted to the document examiner along with the questioned impressions.

Machine Stamps

Machine stamp cases involve machines which have mechanical printing units and print onto paper. Evidence includes adding machine tapes, meter print-outs, cash register receipts, accounting machine print-outs, computer print-outs, and time cards (Fig. 54-19). In a broader sense, machine stamps also include those which have a mechanical printing unit and print into a metal surface, such as an automobile identification tag (VIN), or a plastic surface, such as a credit card or addressing plate. Although paper is the primary domain of the document examiner, his familiarity with number and letter design and causes of defective characters may contribute to the latter investigations.

Printed Matter

Some of the reasons for examining printed matter are to determine whether or not a document is counterfeit; the makeup of a document such as a business form, certificate, or handbill; or whether two or more documents have been printed from the same plate, indicating a common source. An examination of printed matter entails not only a consideration of the printing method, but also of the paper, the manner of cutting or perforating edges, the design of the font, arrangement or format of the material, registration or alignment of the printing, or any other evidence which may aid in individualizing the document.

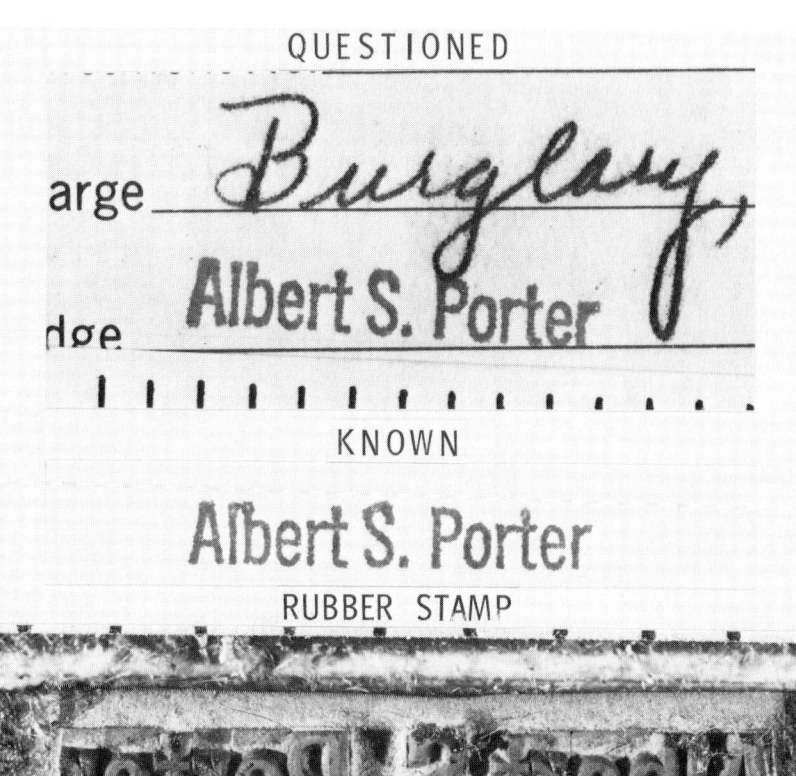

FIGURE 54-18. The size, design, spacing, and arrangement of letters in the questioned and known impressions are similar. The rubber stamp also contains an accumulation of foreign material—ink, paper fibers, and dirt—firmly adhering to portions of letters. This foreign material is inked with the stamp and causes it to print irregularly in those letter portions.

When examining a suspect counterfeit document, comparison must always be made with a genuine document (Fig. 54-20). Usually, documents are counterfeited by the offset method, which means that a genuine document has been photographed to prepare the plates for the counterfeit. In some cases, unwanted material from the genuine document is not properly eliminated in the photographic process, and remnants remain visible in the counterfeits (Fig. 54-21). Identification of the model document used in the preparation of the counterfeits is therefore sometimes possible from an examination of these traces.

The document examiner is sometimes asked to examine the makeup of a document for the purpose of providing investigative leads to the author or printer of the material. While such specificity is usually not possible, the examiner can aid in determining such things as type of materials and equipment used in preparing the original layout of the work; the availability of, and knowledge required to use, such materials and equipment;

FIGURE 54-19. The questioned cash register receipt was found in a garbage can. Upon decipherment of the store's name and address, investigation disclosed that the receipt was for the purchase of a gun. Receipts to be used as standards were obtained from the store's cash register and compared with the questioned document. Proof was offered that the questioned receipt was prepared on the cash register used to prepare the standards.

the methods of printing; and the overall quality of the printing job. Armed with this knowledge, the investigator is in a better position to recognize evidence pertinent to the case should the print shop be located.

Some knowledge of printing materials and methods is helpful to the investigator when conducting a search of a print shop. Items to look for

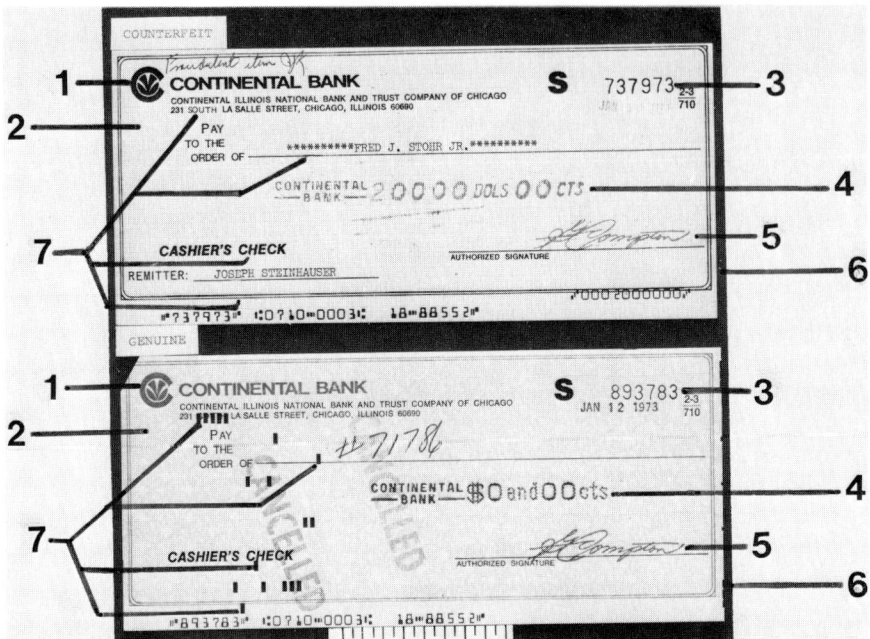

FIGURE 54-20. Examination and comparison of an alleged counterfeit document with a genuine specimen show differences in (1) color of ink, (2) background safety design, (3) method of printing numerals, (4) printed vs. original checkwriter impression, (5) offset-printed vs. machine-printed signature, and (6) perforations on the edge of the check. Where punch holes in the genuine document interfered with printed material (7), these areas were touched up when preparing the counterfeit.

are the setup of the type chase, if it has not yet been torn down; the proof or inked impression of the type setup; the negative of the job; and the printing plate. In many cases, the proof, the negative, and the printing plate remain in the files of the shop for a certain period of time. The rubber printing blanket, used on the offset press, should be examined for an impression of the questioned document. Even though the blanket has been wiped clean of ink from a previous job and a new job begun, previous impressions are retained (Fig. 54-22). A cleaner or wipe-off sheet, similar to blotting paper and sometimes used to clean ink off the blanket, may contain an impression of the material under investigation. Finally, the trash can is a source of waste material from the initial stage of the run or problems which may develop during the run.

ALTERATIONS AND METHODS OF DECIPHERMENT

Documents are altered for a variety of reasons, many of which involve some type of fraud or an attempt to protect one's interests. Some of the more common types of alterations to be found are the raising of the amount on a check or other negotiable instrument; altering of the date on a letter, contract, will, or other legal document; changing of the contents of a ledger, log, or record book; and altering of vital information on papers of ownership, certificates, and forms of identification. Alterations usually take the form of additions to a document, deletion of material from a document, substitution of material (a combination of deletion and addi-

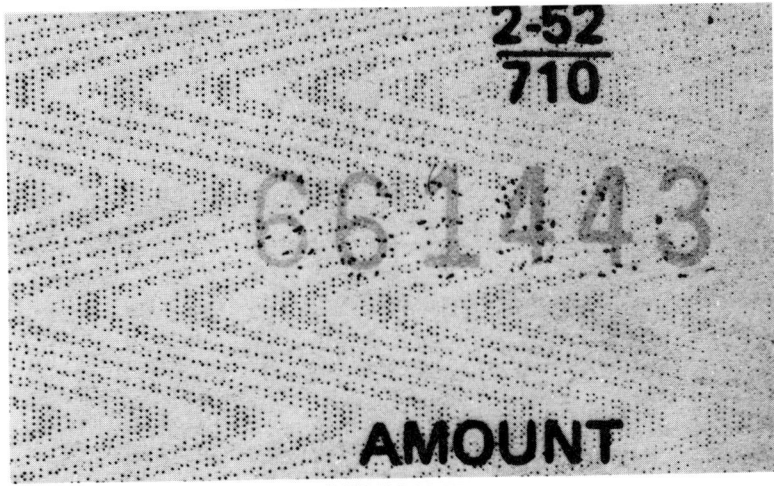
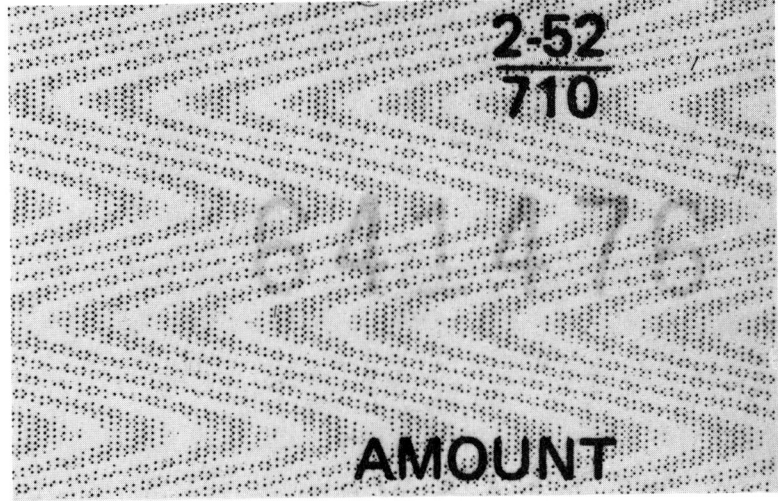

FIGURE 54-21. In photographing a genuine check to produce the negative for the printing plate, the number was not properly filtered out. Remnants of the original number were visible on the counterfeit checks, and an attempt was made to decipher these based upon the size and design of the numerals and the disturbance to the background pattern on the checks.

tion), and obliteration of the original matter. The quality of any alteration is primarily dependent upon a knowledge of the paper and writing materials used in preparation of the genuine document, the availability of materials needed to accomplish alteration of the specific item, and the skill necessary to use these materials effectively. Few alterations are of such high quality that they should go unnoticed by a normally observant person. The most probable reason that altered documents exchange hands without being questioned is that people simply do not take the time to look closely at the instrument.

Additions may take the form of added strokes to an existing character, to "raise" a check, for example, or they may be letters, words, or sentences

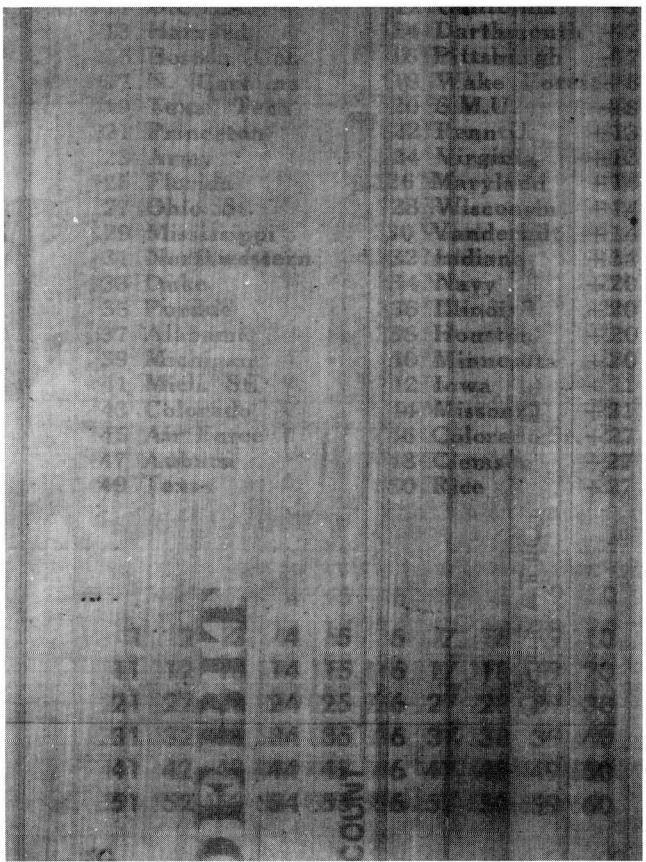

FIGURE 54-22. The rubber printing blanket was found in the print shop and photographed to show the run of a football parley card. It can be seen that the blanket was also used to print an accounting job.

included to change the essential meaning of a document. Additions to a handwritten document are potentially discoverable because of differences in the writing instrument or inks (Fig. 54-23), crowding of the inserted material (Fig. 54-24), overwriting to make other parts of the document appear uniform with the insertion, modifications to the arrangement of material, or differences in the handwriting. Similarly, some factors indicating additions to typewritten documents are differences in the size or design of type, differences in alignment, ribbon variation, or crowding of the material (Fig. 54-25).

When matter is deleted from a document, the purpose is usually to substitute new material. Deletions are most commonly made by means of mechanical erasure (i.e., rubber, emery paper, or a sharp blade used to scrape the ink off the paper). Chemicals are not widely used as they do not effectively penetrate ballpoint pen writing inks; water-based inks used in many fiber-tipped pens, however, are amenable to a certain type of chemical erasure, but the results are not necessarily satisfactory. Safety papers, such as those used for checks, will immediately expose a chemical erasure.

Erasure is most effective with pencil writing, particularly if a hard-surfaced paper is used. Some pencil erasures can be made with little

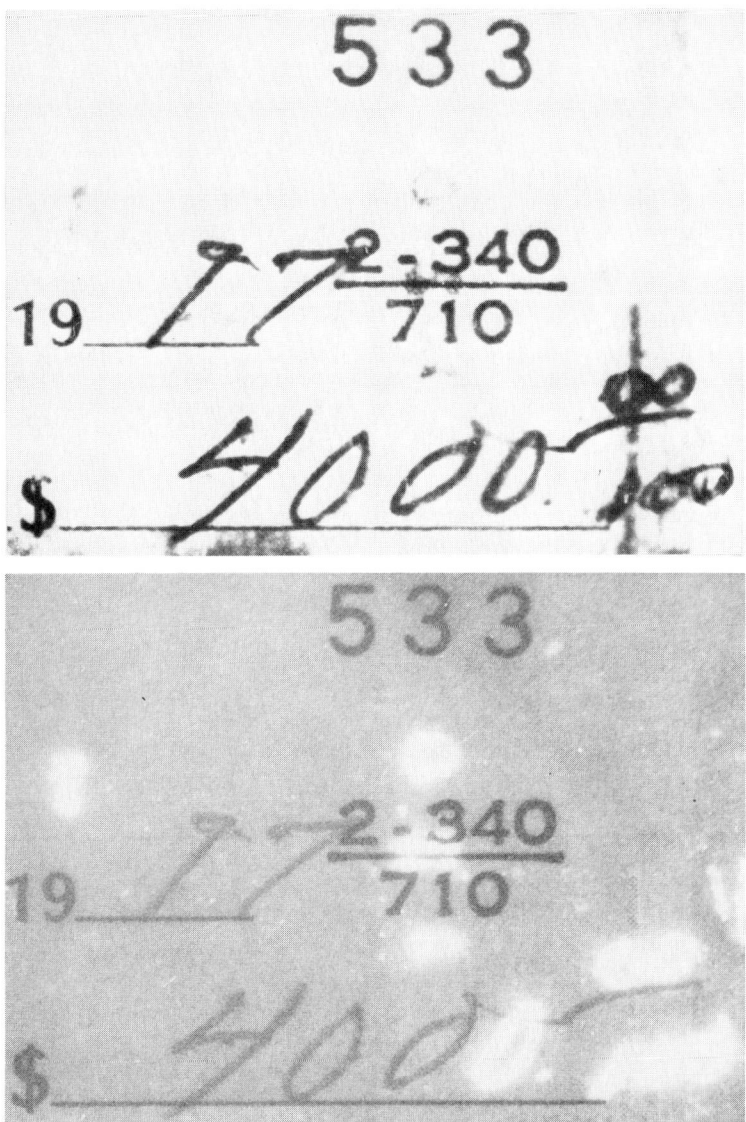

FIGURE 54-23. The check was raised from $400.00 to $4000.00 by the addition of a zero with a ballpoint pen ink similar in color to the original ink. An infrared luminescence photograph clearly demonstrates the different inks.

disturbance to the paper fibers, while others are so poor that not only are the fibers disturbed, but graphite particles remain imbedded in the paper. Decipherment of the former may be possible from indentations left in the paper from the original writing, and the latter from indentations plus the remaining graphite particles (Fig. 54-26).

Erasures of ballpoint pen writing and typewriting are often apparent because of the effort needed to remove the image from the paper.[4] Such erasures usually exhibit a considerable disturbance of paper fibers and a thinning of the paper in the area of the erasure. If an attempt is made to remove the image completely, there is a good possibility of tearing the paper; as a result, ink particles often remain imbedded in the paper due

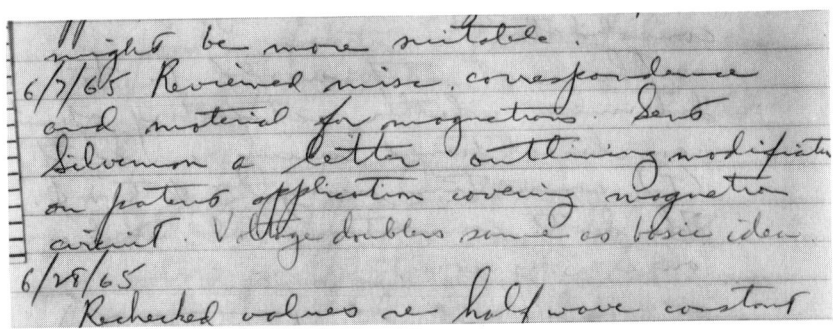

FIGURE 54-24. A device was marketed by Company B, allegedly copying the patent of Company A, which had introduced the device some years earlier. The notebook of the research engineer of Company B became important, in particular, one dated entry which was a key factor in the patent. Examination of the notes revealed that the one sentence "Voltage doubles same as basic idea" was prepared in a different ink than that used to prepare the prior portion of the entry and the subsequent entry. More importantly, the handwriting of this line is restricted when compared with the handwriting of the remainder of the entry which is more spread out. The spacing between letters and words has been reduced to fit the sentence into the only available space. (Courtesy of David J. Purtell, Private Consultant, Chicago.)

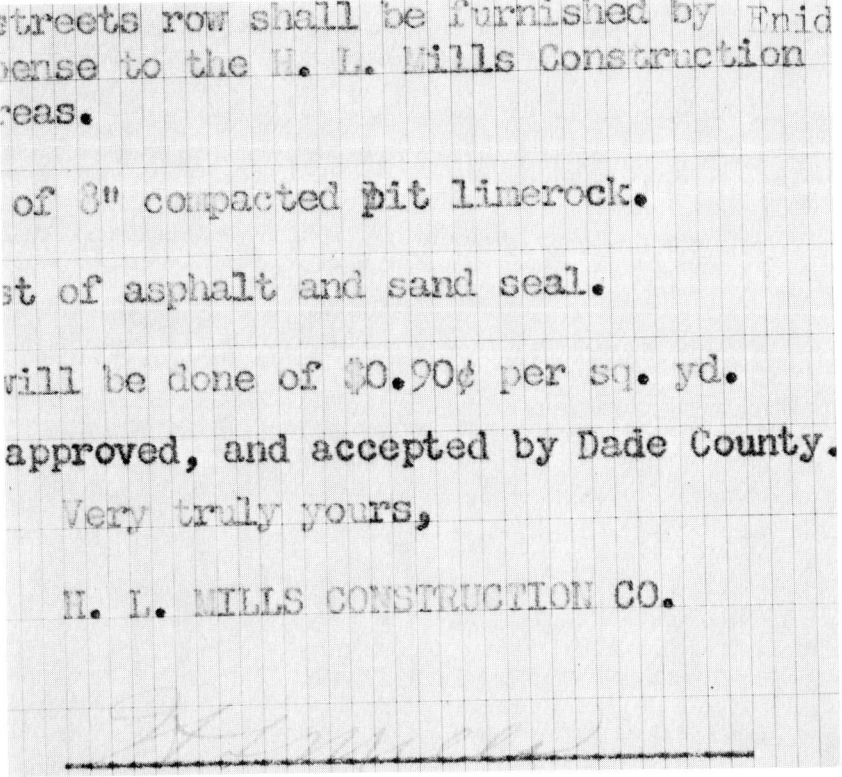

FIGURE 54-25. The last line above the closing was inserted after the contract was completed and signed. Note the horizontal misalignment under a test plate and the difference in ribbon intensity. (Courtesy of Ordway Hilton, Private Consultant, New York.)

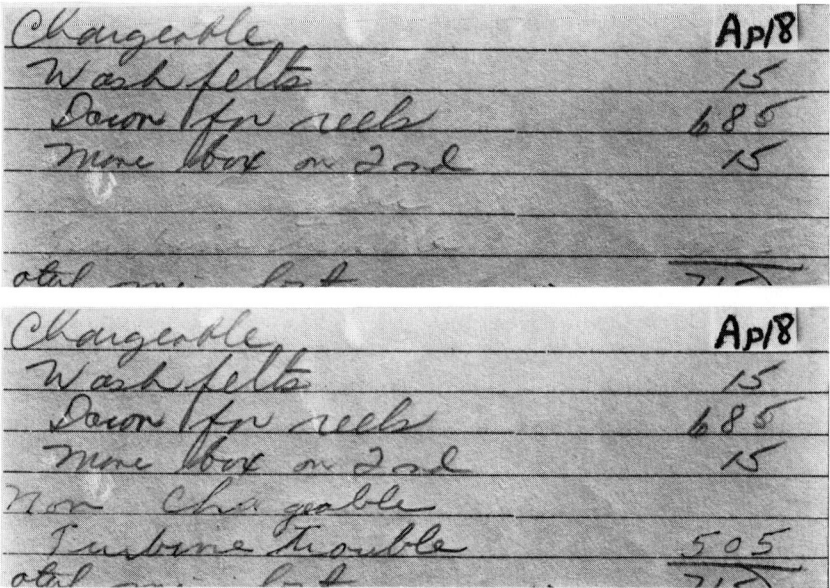

FIGURE 54-26. This document was one of a series of essential records in a suit and countersuit between a paper mill and the manufacturer of a device for winding paper as it came off the machines. The numbers represent minutes of chargeable and nonchargeable time. The erased pencil notations were deciphered from the indentations remaining in the paper. (Courtesy of Ordway Hilton, Private Consultant, New York.)

to incomplete erasure. A decipherment of the original material is dependent upon the ink traces which remain as well as the indentations resulting from the writing instrument. If new material has been inserted in the erased area, decipherment may become more difficult.

Obliteration problems occur when one writing medium is rendered imperceptible by covering with the same or another writing medium. Any type of hand or machine writing instrument may be involved—pencil, ball point pen, fiber-tipped pen, fluid-ink pen, typewriter, checkwriter, rubber stamp, or printing matter. If the original and covering materials consist of different writing mediums or the same writing medium but different inks, there will exist a possibility of differentiating between the two inks so that the original matter is essentially restored and can be read. Differentiation between two inks is possible because of color differences or constituents in the inks susceptible to intensification or deletion in the different ranges of the visible and invisible spectrum. In cases where the obliterated and obliterating instrument is the same, no such ink differences exist, but decipherment may still be possible through microscopic examination.

The document examiner may employ one or more of a number of methods useful in the discovery, decipherment, or restoration of alterations. The first method is usually a visual and microscopic examination to determine the specific problem and the best means of attacking it. Aids to a visual examination will include various types of light sources such as infrared, infrared luminescence, ultraviolet, reflected, point-source, and transmitted light; various colored filters; and ruled plates. Photography is also used as an examination tool, and each of the visual aids may be employed with special films to record the alteration. Chemical means, where the removal of an ink is indicated, are used only if all other methods fail to solve the problem and then only if there is sufficient reason to believe that these will be effective.

RESTORATION OF BURNT, CHARRED, AND WATER-SOLUBLE PAPERS

Burnt, charred, and water-soluble papers are the most delicate types of document evidence to handle. Most often they constitute evidence in gambling cases. This material should always be submitted to the laboratory with the utmost care and at the earliest opportunity. If at all possible, burnt and charred papers should be submitted in the container in which they are found. If this is not possible, for example, if burnt papers are found lying on the floor, they can be picked up with a sheet of paper and placed, not dumped, into a sturdy, boxlike container. The most important thing to remember is to keep the burnt pieces as intact as possible so that if written or printed material is present, it can be deciphered with some meaning. When the evidence is brought into the laboratory, it is processed to provide better handling capabilities, placed between glass plates for preservation, and photographed in an attempt to intensify and decipher the contents (Fig. 54-27).

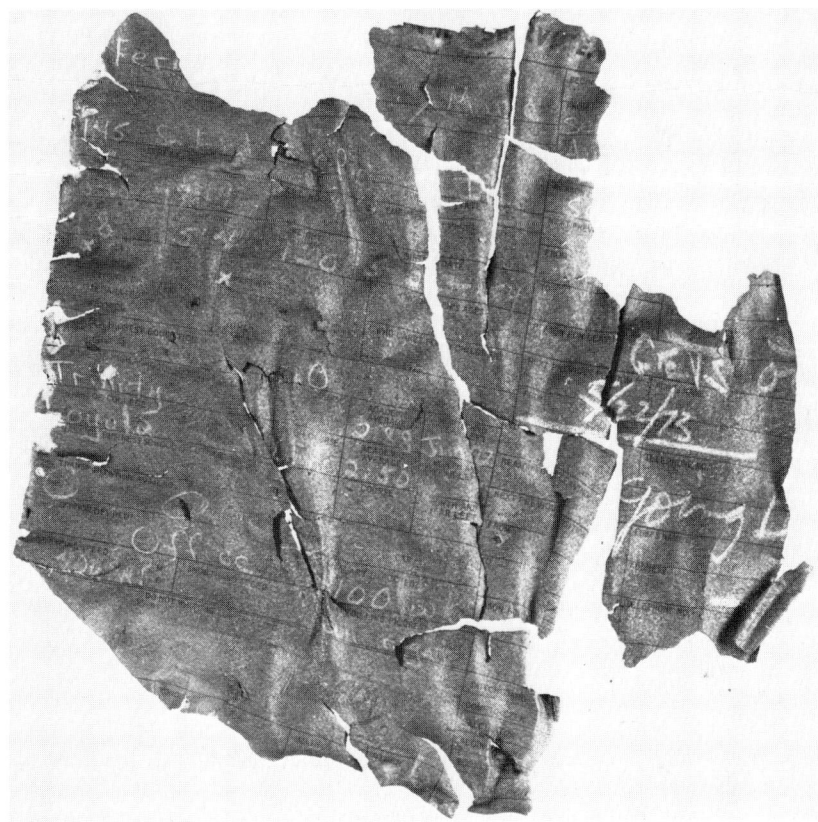

FIGURE 54-27. These burnt papers have been photographed under glass to show one side of an application form filled out by the victim prior to an attempted rape. The application form was burned by the defendant to destroy the evidence.

Water-soluble papers should be taken from the liquid and placed on a material to which they will not adhere. Newspaper and cardboard should be avoided. In the laboratory, the papers will be dried to a certain point so that they can be handled, separated if necessary, and photographed to render a decipherment. The success of the operation will, of course, depend upon the condition of the papers when they are found and submitted.

DECIPHERMENT OF INDENTED WRITING

Indented writing occurs when two or more pieces of paper are in contact; writing on the top sheet of paper will produce indentations on the second sheet. Decipherment of a readable message will depend upon the depth of the indentations. The depth of the indentations will in turn depend upon the types of paper used, the type of writing instrument used, the pressure exerted in writing, and the nature of the surface upon which the writing was executed.

Indented writing is generally deciphered by means of oblique lighting, sometimes with the aid of a finely ruled plate. These sources act to create a series of highlight and shadow areas, rendering definition to the latent writing. The writing is photographed in the same manner (Fig. 54-28). In

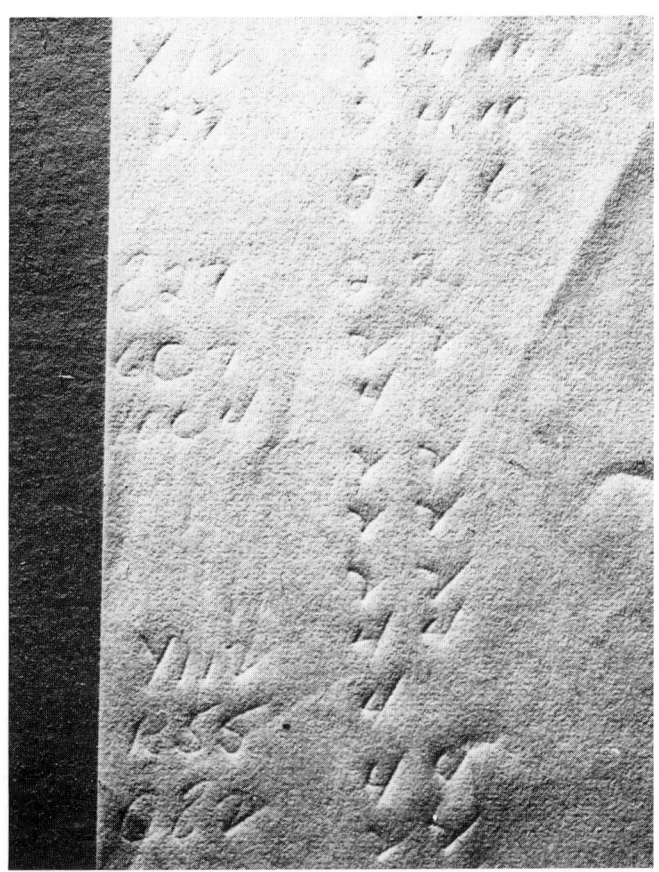

FIGURE 54-28. The decipherment of indented writing in a gambling case.

some cases, it may be possible to make a comparison of indented writing with known standards, but only if the indented impressions are of an extremely good quality.

PAPER EXAMINATIONS AND COMPARISONS

Paper constitutes the basis of almost all documents and certainly is an important consideration in the examination of any document case. Occasionally, however, the question arises as to the comparison of two or more papers and whether they are similar to, or different from, one another. A preliminary examination and comparison of all of the physical characteristics of the papers, including color, size, thickness, texture, and finish, may provide a sufficient basis to distinguish between the papers. If all physical characteristics prove to be similar, it may be requested, depending upon the criticalness of the issue, that a comparison of the chemical composition be made. This is normally not within the purview of the document examiner, and outside specialists in paper analysis will be recommended or consulted. In most instances, however, unless the issue is critical (i.e., the whole case revolves about the paper and no other evidence can support a finding), the need for a chemical breakdown of the paper is superfluous.

Questions also arise as to the source of a piece of paper or the use for which it is intended. Watermarks in some papers provide information as to the manufacturer of the paper, and a study of the physical characteristics may disclose its most likely uses.

Paper comparisons also involve the matching of torn or fractured edges to determine whether two pieces of paper were originally one document (Fig. 54-29). Perforated edges may be similarly matched (Fig. 54-30).

DATING OF A DOCUMENT

Frequently, the question is raised, "Can you date the ink of the writing or the ink of the signature on this document?" In reality, the question is most often one of determining whether the document was prepared at the time it is alleged to have been prepared. In past years, the dating of writing inks was a difficult problem and at best could usually only be determined within considerable time periods. This is because determinations usually rested upon the introduction of new writing instruments or basic changes in the formulations of writing inks. It is only in recent years that the dating of some writing inks, particularly ball-point pen inks, in more specific time periods has become feasible.

In the mid-1960s, the Laboratory of the Bureau of Alcohol, Tobacco and Firearms (ATF) recognized the need for dating ball-point pen inks, which resulted in the establishment of a ball-point pen ink library and the refinement of procedures to analyze such inks. The laboratory has in its ink library the formulations of all known U.S. ball-point pen ink manufacturers since 1968, a good assortment of domestic ink formulations manufactured prior to 1968, and a representative sampling of foreign ball-point pen inks. At present, limitations to dating ball-point pen inks exist because the library has an incomplete collection of foreign inks and of domestic inks prior to 1968. As the library increases its data on these inks, such limitations as now exist will be minimized.[5]

The ATF Laboratory has also been instrumental in implementing a program of "tagging" inks. Most U.S. manufacturers of ball-point pen

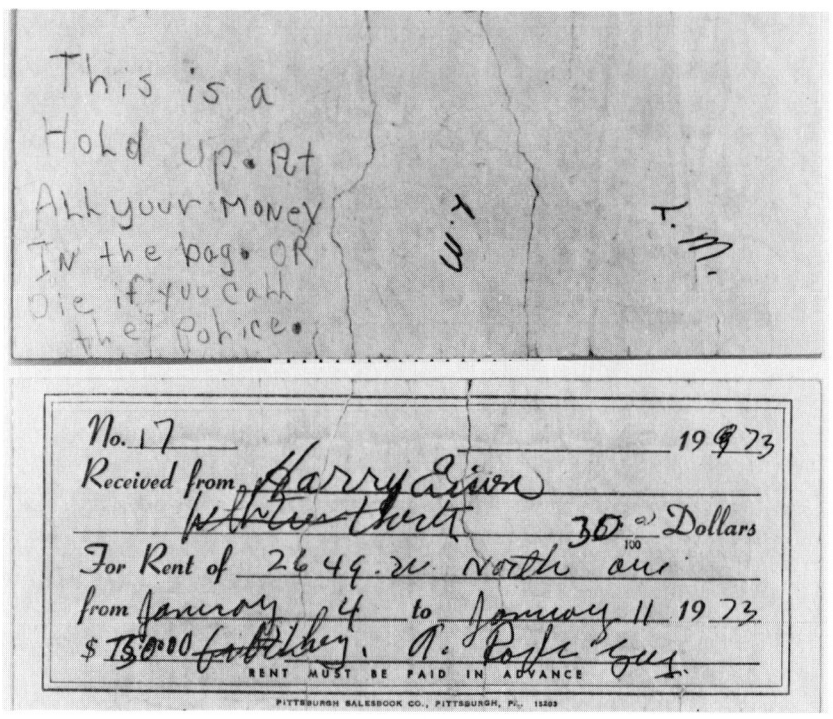

FIGURE 54-29. Matching of torn edges of paper. The holdup note was left at the scene of the crime. The other two portions of paper were found on a table in the suspect's home.

inks now "tag" inks on a yearly basis for dating purposes. Such tagging is eventually intended to include fluid and fiber-pen inks.

Ink, however, is not the only means by which a document may be dated, and, in fact, other methods may provide dating within a narrower time frame. Paper may contain watermarks which are coded as to the year of manufacture; design changes in watermarks also can indicate a date. The paper itself represents a possibility if it contains materials which could not have been available on the alleged date; however, paper dating can usually be stated only in general terms. Typewriting may be placed in a specific time period by the date of introduction of the type design or by deterioration of the typewriter itself. Concerning the latter, if dated work from a typewriter covers a period of time about the alleged date of the disputed document, a study of the changes in identifying characteristics may confirm or disprove when the document was prepared (Fig. 54-31). Printed matter on a document, such as letterheads or printed forms, may be dated where design changes have been made or additional runs cause slight changes in the printing (Fig. 54-32). Handwriting, and in particular a signature, can sometimes be placed within a certain time period because of changes which may occur in the writing due to a particular condition. For example, where writing has deteriorated rapidly because of ill health, a time sequence may be developed. When examining a document to determine whether or not it was prepared at the time alleged, all materials used in the preparation of the document are considered on the basis of their relevancy to the time period under investigation.

QUESTIONED DOCUMENT EXAMINATION

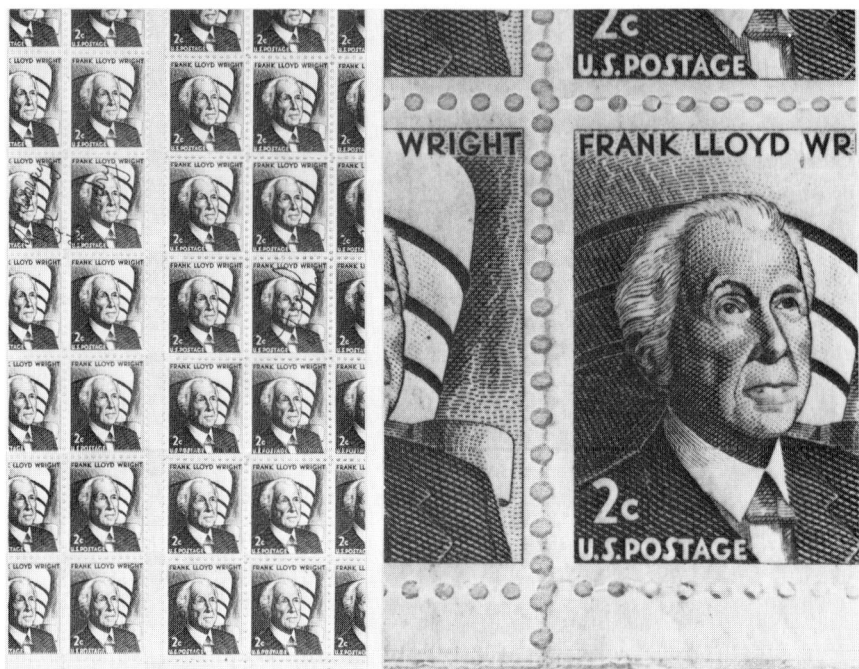

FIGURE 54-30. As part of the proceeds of a burglary, 80 stamps were torn from a 100-stamp sheet in the owner's collection. When found, the suspect had the 80-stamp portion folded up in his breast pocket. The perforations of the two portions were matched and identified as having originally been one sheet of 100 stamps.

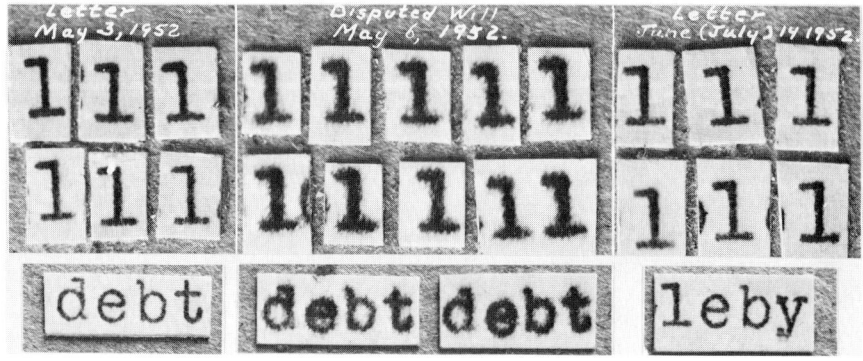

FIGURE 54-31. A disputed, typewritten will (a carbon copy the original of which was never found) bore the date May 6, 1952. Letters which had been prepared on the same typewriter were obtained prior to and after the date of the disputed document. Examination disclosed that the disputed typewriting contained two character defects not found in the comparison typewritten letters: the left foot of the letter "l" had been broken off, and the letter "e" was typing low. These defects were not present in the machine on the alleged date of the will, and therefore it could not have been prepared at that time. In many cases, disproving the alleged date on a document may be more firmly established than substantiating its date. (Courtesy of Ordway Hilton, Private Consultant, New York.)

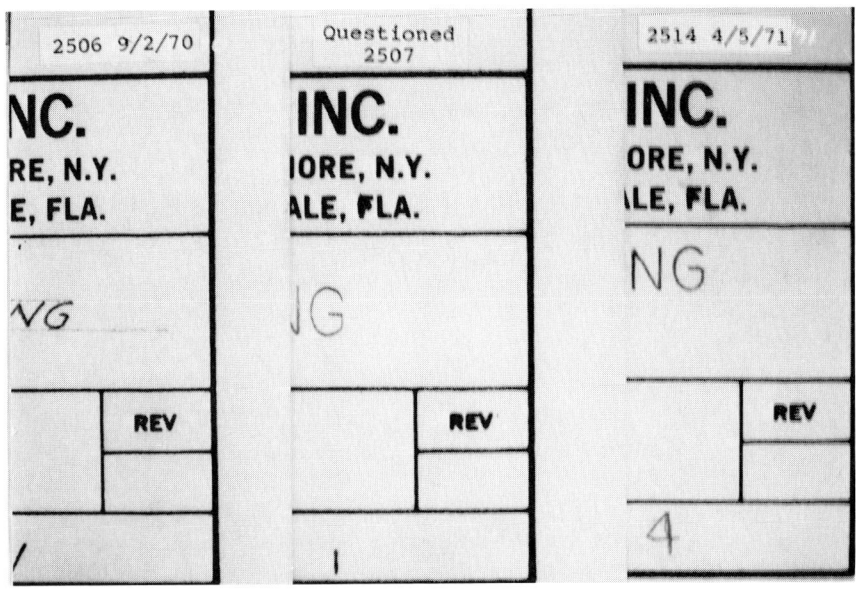

FIGURE 54-32. The questioned document is a drawing of a cargo net alleged to have been prepared in September 1970, and subsequently patented. Another firm challenged the validity of the patent, stating that it was copied from a device developed by a European and could not have been seen by the defendant until well after the alleged date on his drawing. Forms 2506, dated September 2, 1970, and 2514, dated April 5, 1971, are from the files of the defendant. These forms show a sharper printing than the questioned form and do not contain the flawed "F" and the filled-in "R." The questioned form, which is a second printing, appears to have been made by using a sheet from the first printing to produce a new offset plate. (Courtesy of Ordway Hilton, Private Consultant, New York.)

THE EXAMINATION OF MACHINE COPIES

Machine copies have become so much a part of the business world's operations today that almost every office, large or small, has its own copying machine or ready access to one. In fact, copies have become so integrated in the paper maze that, in some cases, they substitute as original documents. It is the occasional machine copy, out of the thousands and thousands produced daily, that will be used for a fraudulent purpose or come under scrutiny for some other reason.

Most copiers in use today are electrostatic machines which use either plain or coated paper. The plain-paper copiers prove more versatile in copier forgery than do the coated-paper copiers. Among the problems encountered in copier forgery are the fitting together of selected areas from original documents to form a "new" document; changing selected areas on a copy, such as a date or amount, and recopying to form another document; and, if all of the materials used in the preparation of the original document are available, creating a new original containing the desired changes and then copying this new document. Questions to be resolved in such cases include, "Can it be shown that parts of documents have been fitted together to form a new original?" (Fig. 54-33); "Is this a first or subsequent generation copy?" and "Was this copy made from this original?"

It is sometimes desirable to prove that a particular copy was made on a

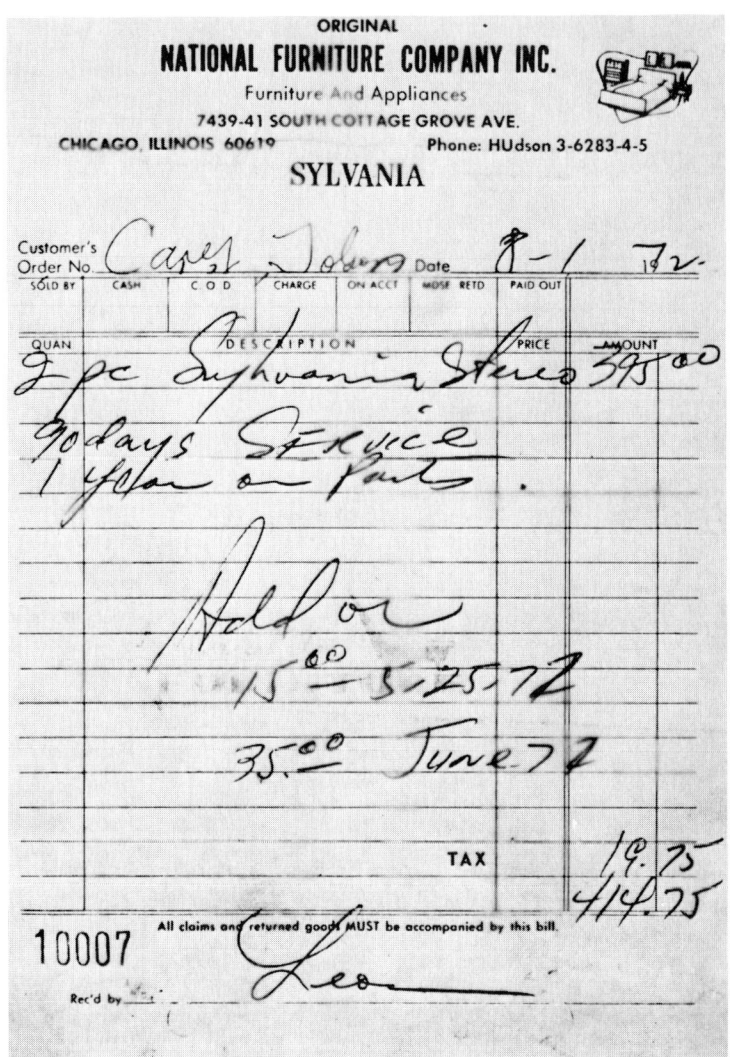

FIGURE 54-33. The top portion (to include the name) of one receipt and the remaining portion of a second and similar receipt have been fitted together and machine-copied to form a new document. It was submitted, along with other copies, to an insurance company for payment for items stolen in a burglary. Note that the bottom portions of the letters "y," "T," and "o" in the name and the numeral "8" in the date have been cut off. The extraneous markings above the boxes labeled "C.O.D." and "ON ACCT." are from other writings on the document comprising the top segment. Similarly, the extraneous markings in the boxes labeled "SOLD BY" and "CHARGE" are from other writings on the document comprising the bottom segment. The date on the bottom segment was altered from "71" to "72" to agree with the top portion.

particular machine. Because copy machines vary as to the type of paper used, the manner in which copy paper is accepted into the machine, the process by which a copy is made, and the method of "photographing" the original document, and because copy machines develop their own peculiar defects, the identification of a copy with a particular machine is possible.

SEQUENCE OF WRITINGS

When two written lines intersect in one or more places, and it can be determined which ink is on top, positive proof is offered of which writing was prepared first and which writing last, or the sequence of writings. Such a determination may assume importance where writings are "fitted in" to an existing document (Fig. 54-34) or where a document is not prepared in the usual or fixed order. Written lines in this instance also include inked impressions prepared by machine or rubber stamp. Sequence of writing problems may be broadened to include the intersection of writing and folds, writing and punch holes, or writing and other disturbances to the paper.

The most effective method of examining the sequence of written lines is microscopically with controlled lighting. It is a difficult problem, and, in many cases, no solution is possible. When findings are rendered, they should be capable of being clearly demonstrated and logically explained.

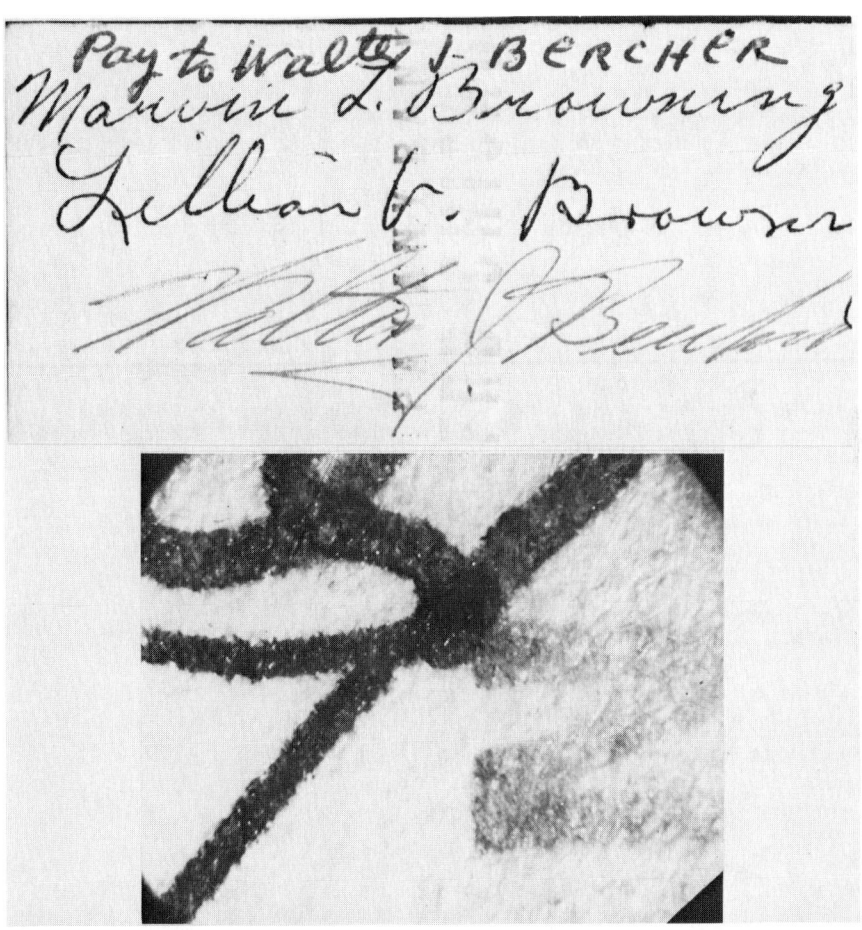

FIGURE 54-34. The writing "Pay to Walter J. Bercher" has been fitted into the limited space above the first endorsement on the check, and the writer has signed his name below the second endorsement. Note the attempt made to write the "ter" of Walter around the initial "L" and the hand printing of the middle initial and last name. The letter "r" of Walter intersects the initial "L" of the first endorsement, and under microscopic examination the sequence of writings can be established.

LATENT FINGERPRINTS ON PAPER

The document examiner should be consulted whenever there is a need to process paper evidence for latent fingerprints. Where the possibility of a handwriting, typewriting, or other comparison is evident, it is advisable to submit such evidence for chemical development, rather than to process this material in the field. In this way, the evidence will not be disturbed by powders, and it may be examined and photographed prior to latent processing.

The primary chemical methods used by the document examiner are ninhydrin, silver nitrate, and iodine fuming. Ninhydrin is one of the best methods developed since it works well on both fresh and old prints, does not generally disturb the written or printed matter on the document if handled properly, and leaves a relatively permanent print. Prints developed on paper are photographed and submitted to a fingerprint examiner for evaluation and comparison.

PRESERVATION OF DOCUMENT EVIDENCE

The reason for placing the discussion of document preservation near the end of the chapter is that at this point the reader should have a better understanding of document evidence possibilities and should appreciate the reasons why this evidence should be kept in the best possible condition. Paper can easily be mutilated, particularly the evidential portions of the document, by excessive handling, stapling, clipping, punch holes, folding and unfolding, and writing on the document. When paper evidence is to be submitted to the document examiner, it should be protected in some manner, such as by placing in a folder, a cellophane envelope, or between two sheets of paper. The document may be marked by the investigator, in a corner away from any written or printed matter, but should contain no other writings. Any notes or instructions should be placed on a separate piece of paper. If it is desired that the document be processed for latent fingerprints, this should be clearly indicated so that the evidence is treated properly. Standards of comparison should be treated in a similar manner. Such precautions will help to insure the best possible evaluation of all evidence possibilities the document has to offer.

The investigator should always make every effort to submit the original questioned document. Copies, no matter how good the quality, impose limitations on an examination, and, in many instances, these limitations will be reflected in inconclusive reports or restricted findings. Copies simply do not exhibit the fine detail in writing and are essentially lifeless when viewed under a microscope. They are particularly hazardous where questions of genuineness or forgery of signatures are concerned.* Similarly, when submitting collected standards, every effort should be made to obtain the original of these.

---

*There will be situations where the original document has been destroyed or cannot be located and an examination of a copy is the only alternative. It is not implied that copies of all documents are entirely useless for comparison; on the contrary, definite opinions as to authorship are possible under certain conditions.

THE DOCUMENT EXAMINER AS AN EXPERT WITNESS

After a case has been examined and findings rendered in a written report, the document examiner may be subpoenaed to testify in the forthcoming trial or proceedings. In most cases, the examiner will prepare demonstrational material for the court, usually charts containing enlarged photographic representations of the evidence, or 35 mm slides. These are employed to help demonstrate to the court the reasoning used in arriving at the stated opinion.

The testimony of the document examiner, like that of many other expert witnesses, is opinion testimony. Credence is based upon the person's qualifications—his or her education, training, knowledge, experience, and research—in the area of the testimony. The document examiner will usually provide the attorney with a list of questions designed to elicit his particular qualifications. A pretrial conference between the examiner and attorney is an absolute necessity to the proper presentation of the document evidence. It is also helpful if the attorney is informed on legal precedents germane to the document matter at hand.

Throughout this discussion, importance has been placed upon the role of the investigator/attorney in a document case, as it is he who submits the evidence upon which an opinion must be based. Not every document problem will possess a solution, and sometimes the findings will necessarily be less than conclusive. However, the quality of the evidence submitted, particularly the standards of comparison, is of paramount importance in the solution of many document problems.

REFERENCES

1. Purtell, D. J.: Handwriting Standard Forms. *J. Crim. Law Criminol. Police Sci.* 54(4):522–528, 1963.
2. *Gilbert v. California,* 388 U.S. 263, 87 S. Ct. 1951 (1967); *Schmerber v. California,* 384 U.S. 757, 86 S. Ct. 1826 (1966).
3. Hilton, O.: Identification of the Work from an IBM Selectric Typewriter. *J. Forensic Sci.* 7(3):286–302, 1962.
4. Casey, M. A., and Purtell, D. J.: IBM Correcting Selectric Typewriter: An Analysis of the Use of the Correctable Film Ribbon in Altering Typewritten Documents. *J. Forensic Sci.* 21(1):208–212, 1976.
5. Crown, D. A., Brunelle, R. L., and Cantu, A. A.: The Parameters of Ballpen Ink Examination. *J. Forensic Sci.* 21(4):917–922, 1976.

ADDITIONAL READING

Books

Conway, J. V. P.: *Evidential Documents.* Charles C Thomas, Springfield, Ill., 1959.
Harrison, W. R.: *Suspect Documents, Their Scientific Examination.* Frederick A. Praeger, New York, 1958.
Harrison, W. R.: *Forgery Detection.* Frederick A. Praeger, New York, 1964.
Hilton, O.: *Scientific Examination of Documents.* Callaghan, Chicago, 1956.
Osborn, A. S.: *Questioned Documents.* ed. 2. Boyd Printing Company, Albany, 1929.
Quirke, A. J.: *Forged, Anonymous and Suspect Documents.* George Routledge, London, 1930.
Scott, C. C.: *Photographic Evidence.* Vernon Law Book Company, Kansas City, 1942; 3-volume ed., 1969.

Articles

Alford, E. F.: Disguised Handwriting. *J. Forensic Sci.* 15(4):476–488, 1970.
Anderson, G.: Systematic Thefts of Food Stamps Involving Erasures and Alterations. *J. Police Sci. Adm.* 3(1):15–18, 1975.
Bartha, A.: Restoration and Preservation of Typewriting and Printing on Charred Documents. *Can. Soc. Forensic Sci. J.* 6(3):111–114, 1973.
Bartha, A., and Duxbury, N. W.: Restoration and Preservation of Charred Documents. *Can. Soc. Forensic Sci. J.* 1:1–2, 1968.
Beacom, M. S.: Handwriting by the Blind. *J. Forensic Sci.* 12(1):37–59, 1967.
Beck, J.: Printed Matter as Questioned Documents. *J. Forensic Sci.* 12(1):82–101, 1967.
Black, D.A.: Forgery Above a Genuine Signature. *J. Crim. Law Criminol. Police Sci.* 50(6):585-590, 1960.
Casey, M.A.: The Alteration of Pari-Mutuel Tickets. *J. Crim. Law Criminol. Police Sci.* 62(2):282-285, 1971.
Casey, M.A., and Paholke, A. R.: A Dual View to Identifying Metal Stamped Impressions. *J. Police Sci. Adm.* 3(2):177-182, 1975.
Caywood, D.: Decipherment of Indented Writings—A New Technique. *J. Police Sci. Adm.* 1(1):50-55, 1973.
Conway, J.V.P.: The Identification of Hand Printing. *J. Crim. Law Criminol. Police Sci.* 45(5):605–612, 1955.
Costain, J., and Lewis, G.: A Practical Guide to Infrared Luminescence Applied to Questioned Document Problems. *J. Police Sci. Adm.* 1(2):209–218, 1973.
Crown, D. A.: Class Characteristics of Foreign Typewriters and Typefaces. *J. Crim. Law Criminol. Police Sci.* 59(2):298–323, 1968.
Dick, R. M.: A Comparative Analysis of Dichroic Filter Viewing, Reflected Infrared and Infrared Luminescence Applied to Ink Differentiation Problems. *J. Forensic Sci.* 15(3):357–363, 1970.
Doud, D: Charred Documents, Their Handling and Decipherment. *J. Crim. Law Criminol. Police Sci.* 43(6):812–826, 1953.
Evett, I. W.: The Decipherment of Impressions in Paper—Some Methods Old and New. *J. Forensic Sci. Soc.* 13(2):83–90, 1973.
Godown, L.: Forgeries Over Genuine Signatures. *J. Forensic Sci.* 14(4):463–468, 1969.
Godown, L.: New Nondestructive Document Testing Methods. *J. Crim. Law Criminol. Police Sci.* 55(2):284–285, 1964.
Godown, L.: Sequence of Writings. *J. Crim. Law Criminol. Police Sci.* 54(1):101–109, 1963.
Grant, J.: The Role of Paper in Questioned Document Work. *J. Forensic Sci. Soc.* 13(2):91–95, 1973.
Harris, J. J.: Disguised Handwriting. *J. Crim. Law Criminol. Police Sci.* 43(5):685–689, 1953.
Harris, J. J.: Preparation for Trial from a Document Examiner's Viewpoint. *J. Forensic Sci.* 7(3):351–356, 1962.
Hilton, O.: A Study of the Influence of Alcohol on Handwriting. *J. Forensic Sci.* 14(3):309–316, 1969.
Hilton, O: Consideration of the Writer's Health in Identifying Signatures and Detecting Forgeries. *J. Forensic Sci.* 14(2): 157–166, 1969.
Hilton, O.: Dating Typewriting by an Analysis of Variable Defects. *J. Crim. Law Criminol. Police Sci.* 51(3):373–377, 1950.
Hilton, O.: Identification of Typewriting. *J. Crim. Law Criminol. Police Sci.* 48(2):219–223, 1957.
Hilton, O.: Identification of Work from a Selectric II Typewriter. *J. Forensic Sci.* 18(3):246–253, 1973.
Hilton, O.: Influence of Age and Illness on Handwriting: Identification Problems. *Forensic Sci.* 9:161–172, 1977.
Hilton, O.: The Care and Preservation of Documents in Criminal Investigation. *J. Crim. Law Criminol. Police Sci.* 31(1):103–110, 1940.

Hilton, O.: The Complexities of Identifying the Modern Typewriter. *J. Forensic Sci.* 17(4):579—585, 1972.

Kelly, J. H.: Effects of Artificial Aids and Prostheses on Signatures. *J. Police Sci. Adm.* 3(4):394–399, 1975.

Kelly, J. H.: Spectrofluorometric Analysis of Ball Point Ink. *J. Police Sci. Adm.* 1(2):175–181, 1973.

Kelly, J. H.: Identifying the Copying Machine Used in Preparation of Simulated Forgeries. *J. Forensic Sci.* 18(4):410–413, 1973.

Kessell, T. R.: Mechanical Addressing Methods. *J. Forensic Sci.* 21(2):422–426, 1976.

Kreuger, W. C.: Paper Analysis in Forensic Sciences. *Identification News* 22(11):3–6, 15, 1972.

Lacy, L. P.: Modern Printing Processes. *J. Crim. Law Criminol. Police Sci.* 47(6):730–736, 1957.

Lile, J. E., and Blair, A. R.: Classification and Identification of Photocopies: A Progress Report. *J. Forensic Sci.* 21(4):923–931, 1976.

Mathyer, J., Veillon, P., and Rothenbuehler, O.: Some Remarks on the Optical Examination of Inks. *Int. Crim. Police Rev.* No. 262, 1972.

Mathyer, J.: The Expert Examination of Signatures. *J. Crim. Law Criminol. Police Sci.* 52(1):122–133, 1961.

McCarthy, J. F.: On Playing the Game of Expert Witness in a Two-Value Logic System. *J. Forensic Sci.* 19(1):131–135, 1974.

McNally, J. P.: The Adversary System: Role of the Document Examiner. *J. Forensic Sci.* 18(3):188–192, 1973.

Miller, F. M.: The Approximate Age of a Document. *FBI Law Enforcement Bull.* 35(2):1966.

Miller, J. T.: Professionalization of Document Examiners: Problems of Certification and Training. *J. Forensic Sci.* 18(4):460–468, 1973.

Miller, J. T.: Role of Check Protector Identification in Law Enforcement Exemplar and Comparison Problems. *J. Police Sci. Adm.* 3(3):259–266, 1975.

Mortimer, J. H.: Court Ordered Handwriting Exemplars—How Effective? *J. Forensic Sci.* 15(4):448–454, 1973.

Nemecek, J.: A Deep Look into Typewriter Alignment. *J. Forensic Sci.* 10(1):23–33, 1965.

Osborn, P. A.: The Trial of a Document Case. *J. Forensic Sci.* 10(4):422–432, 1965.

Purtell, D. J.: Effects of Drugs on Handwriting. *J. Forensic Sci.* 10(3):335–346, 1965.

Purtell, D. J.: The Identification of Checkwriters. *J. Crim. Law Criminol. Police Sci.* 54(2):229–235, 1954.

Purtell, D. J.: The Identification of Rubber Stamps. Crime Detection Laboratories Seminar No. 4, Royal Canadian Mounted Police, May 10–11, 1956.

Sellers, C.: Assisted and Guided Signatures. *J. Crim. Law Criminol. Police Sci.* 53(2):245–248, 1962.

Shaneyfelt, L. L.: Obliteration, Alteration and Related Document Problems. *J. Forensic Sci.* 16(3):331–342, 1971.

CHAPTER 55

Irving C. Stone, Jr. is Chief of the Physical Evidence Analysis Section of the Southwestern Institute of Forensic Sciences at Dallas and is Assistant Professor of Forensic Sciences (Pathology) at the Southwestern Medical School of the University of Texas. Dr. Stone holds degrees in geology and geochemistry from Iowa State University and The George Washington University. He has served as a Special Agent in the Physics and Chemistry Section of the FBI Laboratory in Washington, D.C. Dr. Stone was Vice President of Geochemical Surveys, Inc., of Dallas prior to joining the staff of the Southwestern Institute.

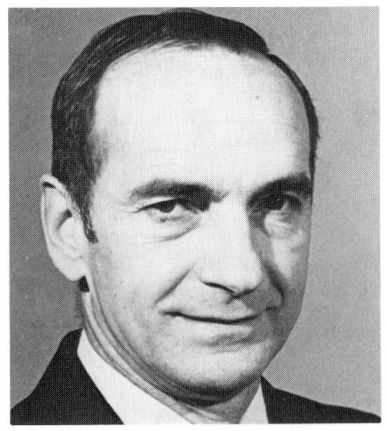

STATISTICAL ASPECTS OF FORENSIC SCIENTIFIC EVIDENCE

Irving C. Stone, Jr., Ph.D.

The scientist working in a forensic laboratory has a responsibility to consumers of his product or service which is different from that of most professions. The consumer is one or another phase of the justice system, whether it be a police department, a federal investigative agency, or a criminal or civil court. The responsibility under our adversary system is to justify the analytical or comparative technique used, and to present the findings in a useful and accurate manner.

PREPARATION AND ORGANIZATION OF DATA

It is important to perform analyses of evidence in a sequence so that the least destructive technique is employed first with progression to methods which may consume part or all of the material. In the same logical manner, the forensic scientist needs to organize his findings or results in reports to the investigative body. These results must be supported by work sheets, photographs, and various graphic data such as instrument charts. In court, the forensic scientist must be prepared to explain to the jury and judge how and why he treated the evidence submitted as described in the work notes. This can range from simple explanation of a certain piece of analytical instrumentation to a relatively detailed description of how a particular drug can be identified positively in the presence of a number of other similar compounds.

In certain disciplines, such as the examination of questioned documents and fingerprints, exhibits are prepared for the information of the court. Most often, though, the forensic scientist is faced with justification of the employed technique based on references in the literature and peer acceptance. Beginning with the acceptance by the court of a scientist's credentials, based on education and experience, through the foundation laid by explanation of methods and instruments, the scientist proceeds to a stated conclusion. This conclusion may be a positive, conclusive opinion that a metal piece found at a burglary scene was at one time attached to a screwdriver found in the defendant's possession. On the other hand, the expert may state that he does not know, or cannot state with reasonable certainty, that the metallic elements found on the hands of the deceased were due to gunshot residue. This leads to the discussion of some of the mistakes frequently made by forensic scientific experts in arriving at conclusions.

COMMON PITFALLS

LACK OF PROFESSIONALISM. The forensic scientist must separate personal from professional opinion; he or she must rely only on the data obtained, or facts discovered, in arriving at conclusions. The forensic scientist must expect that his findings and conclusions will be challenged and be prepared to have the same evidence examined or analyzed by another bona fide expert. If this simple concept is followed, most pitfalls can be avoided.

DEMEANOR. The demeanor of the forensic scientist on the witness stand should be natural and unaffected. One should not try to emulate a scientist whom one respects or admires as this almost always projects an unnatural manner. Each person has his own voice tone, modulation, and language style. It is much more understandable to the court if the expert presents his methods, findings, and conclusions in terms of his own personality, not one borrowed or copied from another.

OUTSIDE INFLUENCE. Outside influence is to be guarded against; by this is meant the apparently helpful suggestions of the attorney, whether the prosecutor or defense counsel, on how to "emphasize" the findings. It is acceptable to receive advice on the sequence of testimony, but the findings and conclusions, including the lack of a conclusion, must be those of the witness. It is the forensic scientist who places his reputation on the line during each court appearance, and there is a great responsibility to the accused and the court to state neither more nor less than can be reproduced and proven.

DIRECT ANSWERS TO DIRECT QUESTIONS. There is a natural tendency in testifying to assist the attorney posing questions by anticipating the direction of his line of inquiry or to answer swiftly before formulating a responsive, intelligent reply. It is better to listen intently, wait momentarily to assure understanding, ask for clarification or restatement if necessary, and then to respond in as simple and brief a manner as possible. Certainly, some answers must be lengthy because of the very nature of the subject or the questions, but a consistent partner of poor expert testimony is verbose answers to simple questions.

UNDERSTANDING THE QUESTION. Experienced witnesses learn to recognize and anticipate lines of inquiry. It is true that this knowledge aids in avoiding "traps" or virtually unanswerable questions. It is important, however, even for these persons, to be certain that they understand the question. A measured pause, rather than an immediate reply to a question posed, serves to avoid this pitfall.

STATISTICS IN TESTIMONY

A number of excellent references are available to the scientist regarding statistical manipulation of data. One of the best, most readable statistical method texts, written primarily for chemists, is by Youden.[1] Several useful chapters dealing with probability in the forensic sciences are contained in a book edited by Peterson.[2] Legal authorities and important cases are discussed in Chapter 56.

In considering the use of statistical principles, we should define our boundaries. On the one hand, qualified expert witnesses can testify with great certainty in some instances (e.g., the positive association of a particular person with a fingerprint taken from the crime scene). The forensic scientist can also state with reasonable certainty that a fragment of headlamp lens came from a particular headlamp when the random fracture edges match like pieces from a jigsaw puzzle. What is often overlooked is that the scientist can state with equal positiveness a negative finding (e.g., that a blood stain found at a crime scene did not originate from the suspect). This could be termed a "positive-negative" conclusion.

From these two types of conclusive findings, we pass into a gray area when something from the crime scene is similar to something having relation to the person suspected of committing the crime but is not singular and conclusive. It is in this type of situation that statistical principles and techniques may provide the court with useful information pertaining to the relative uniqueness of the finding.

Finally, the other boundary would seem to be the enigmatic, frustrating area where findings are inconclusive. It seems to the author that this type of conclusion can be a perfectly valid finding. However, it may sometimes cloak the incompetence of an examiner. It is only a valid finding when experience and meticulous care in analysis or examination fail to produce a more conclusive result.

In the forensic laboratory there are obvious uses for the statistical handling of analytical data. The forensic serologist, for example, must be prepared to justify the techniques used and the results obtained. The courts are showing increasing interest in methods that give weight to these results. Every newly developed technique, newly discovered blood group, or enzyme system increases the possibility of reducing the population from which a given blood stain could have originated. Many data are available, based upon blood bank determinations of the blood group and type of blood donors and recipients. This analysis has been used as the basis for determining how unusual a particular blood group system is when compared with the general population.[3,4] There are variations in the distribution of blood groups, types, and other genetic markers based upon the racial origin of the individual in question.[5]

Law of Probability

The simplest, most used statistical relationship in the forensic sciences is the law of probability. It states that probabilities combine according to the multiplication rule. The probability of A and B occurring together when A and B are two independent events is the product of A and B. Assume that a laboratory performs blood determinations in the ABO, Rh, and MNSs systems. For the blood stain examined, the following are obtained with probabilities shown for a Caucasian subject:[4]

O	45%
Rh [R¹r(CDe/cde)]	32%
MN	50%
Ss	45%

The frequency of the blood group system follows P(A,B,C,D) = P(A) + P(B) + P(C) + P(D), or P = 0.45 × 0.32 × 0.50 × 0.45 = 0.032, or 3.2 percent of the population. Thus the serologist can testify as to the relative uniqueness of the blood stain (occurring in 3.2 percent of the Caucasian population), explaining it in terms a layman may understand. The number of persons from whom the blood stain could have originated is further reduced as more blood group, enzyme, and protein systems are determined.

In a recent case in Texas, a suspect was apprehended and charged with the murder of a woman. The only actual physical evidence associating him with the murder was blood found on his clothing. The data obtained from this analysis, in addition to the fact that the suspect was blood group O, were as follows:

Blood Group System	Victim's Blood Groups	Blood on Suspect's Coat	Frequency
ABO	B	B	0.11
Rh	rr (cde/cde)	rr (cde/cde)	0.12
MN	MM	MM	0.28
Ss	SS	SS	0.11
EAP	BB	BB	0.32
Es-D	2-1	2-1	0.18
PGM	1-1	1-1	0.57

The frequency of this combination of blood groups yields 0.000013 (0.0013 percent), or 13 in each one million persons. Thus a degree of uniqueness is developed with respect to the findings; the court is supplied with another view as to the weight of the evidence.

There are less well known but nonetheless important forensic uses for statistics. New procedures for analysis and comparison of glass evidence are now providing a data base for determining the relative uniqueness of glass.[6,7] A caution should be sounded here because the probability law described above holds only for functions that are independent of one another. In the analysis of glass, refractive index and density are the two properties most often measured. These two physical properties of glass are related to each other; thus there is a high degree of correlation between them, as reported by Dabbs and Pearson.[8] If one calculates probability on the basis of these two physical properties, it will be in error if the assumption is made that the refractive index and density are independent variables.

In the author's laboratory, a rather painstaking effort is under way to assess the relative uniqueness of window glass, or flat glass as it is referred to in the industry. Data for known glass specimens (i.e., glass collected from crime scenes) are being obtained and stored in a computer. Both refractive indices and density are measured, as well as the quantitative levels of five trace elements. The data base being established will be representative not so much of flat glass now being manufactured, but will be a collation of flat glass involved in crimes. Much is said about the relatively narrow range for quality control in the manufacture of flat glass. Often overlooked, however, is the fact that it is not necessarily new glass, such as window panes, that is broken in the commission of crimes. Thus the data base reflects more accurately the existing glass in the Dallas area with respect to relative uniqueness. For example, in a burglary which occurred in a suburb of Dallas, glass was submitted from the broken window at the scene (K1), as well as a fragment of glass (Q1) found on the floorboard of the suspect's vehicle. Refractive indices were determined at three wavelengths of light to obtain the physical property called dispersion. The analytical data are shown for 656 nm (nC), 589 nm (nD), and 486 nm (nF) wavelengths.

	K-1	Q-1
nC	1.5200	1.5199
nD	1.5229	1.5227
nF	1.5294	1.5295
Density, gm/cc	2.509	2.509

Previous work in the author's laboratory had shown that the variation expected within a single window pane for the techniques was ±0.0003 for refractive index and ±0.001 gm/cc for density. X-ray fluorescence techniques for analysis of arsenic, strontium, rubidium, iron, and zirconium revealed, within experimental error, identical values. At the time the data were needed for courtroom presentation, the data base consisted of 140 crime-scene glass samples. No probability calculation or other statistical manipulation was performed, as the base was considered to be too limited. It was possible, however, to testify that the glass samples in question, Q-1 and K-1, were the same within experimental limits and were unique in the population of 140 glasses. Given below are the data for all glass samples in the population with similar properties according to the nD computer sort (76P1362 is the K-1 crime scene glass):

	nC	nD	nF	Density
G 59	1.5179	1.5220	1.5324	2.494
G 16	1.5194	1.5221	1.5288	2.503
76P1362	1.5200	1.5229	1.5294	2.509
G 60	1.5205	1.5231	1.5300	2.503
G 87	1.5205	1.5233	1.5301	2.507

Below is shown the same data base sorted by density:

	nC	nD	nF	Density
G 87	1.5205	1.5233	1.5301	2.507
G 39	1.5182	1.5210	1.5278	2.508
76P1362	1.5200	1.5229	1.5311	2.509
G 109	1.5214	1.5242	1.5311	2.510
G 12	1.4212	1.5240	1.5309	2.510

As the base expands to 1000 or more, it is believed that calculations may be in order to assess the probability that the two glasses, Q-1 and K-1, came from other than the same window.

The first papers have appeared on applying statistics to hair comparisons by microscopy.[9,10] Neutron activation analysis has utilized such data handling in analysis of a diverse range of forensic applications, including hair and gunshot residues.[11]

The purpose here has not been to explain statistical techniques, but to call attention to areas where the forensic scientists can utilize the power of statistics. Analytical procedures in the forensic laboratory need not be developed independently, as the scientific literature is replete with new and advanced analytical techniques. As these methods are adapted to forensic analysis, however, they must be evaluated, using acceptable standards or reference materials.

The use of statistics, not just as a laboratory tool but in explaining analytical results to the jury, is not of recent origin. However, the employment of statistics by the forensic scientist who is making reports or testifying as an expert witness has not been widespread. Perhaps the reluctance to introduce elementary statistical principles is due to the unfamiliarity of the attorneys with the concepts involved or the suspicion that the jury will not understand the calculations, or perhaps because the forensic scientist himself does not have a sufficient grasp of statistical methods to utilize them adequately and to explain them to the attorneys, the courts, and the juries concerned with the administration of justice in this country.

REFERENCES

1. Youden, W. J.: *Statistical Methods for Chemists.* John Wiley & Sons, New York, 1951.
2. Peterson, J. L.: *Forensic Science and Scientific Investigation in Criminal Justice.* AMS Press, New York, 1975.
3. Culliford, B. J.: *The Examination and Typing of Bloodstains in the Crime Laboratory.* Report PR 71-7. U.S. Department of Justice, Law Enforcement Assistance Administration, Washington, D.C., 1971.
4. *Technical Methods and Procedures.* ed. 6. American Association of Blood Banks, Washington, D.C., 1974.
5. Race, R. R., and Sanger, R.: *Blood Groups in Man.* ed. 4. Blackwell Scientific Publications, Oxford, 1962.
6. Reeve, V., Mathiesen, J., and Fong, W.: Elemental Analysis by Energy Dispersive X-ray: A Significant Factor in the Forensic Analysis of Glass. *J. Forensic Sci.* 21:291–309, 1976.
7. Stone, I. C., and Fletcher, L.: Variations in Window Glass—Refractive Indices, Density and Trace Elements. Paper presented at the 28th Annual Meeting of the American Academy of Forensic Sciences, Washington, D.C., February 1976.
8. Dabbs, M. D. G., and Pearson, E. F.: Some Physical Properties of a Large Number of Window Glass Specimens. *J. Forensic Sci.* 17:70–78, 1972.
9. Gaudette, B. D., and Keeping, E. S.: An Attempt at Determining Probabilities in Human Scalp Hair Comparison. *J. Forensic Sci.* 19:599–606, 1974.
10. Gaudette, B. D.: Probabilities and Human Pubic Hair Comparisons. *J. Forensic Sci.* 21:514–517, 1976.
11. Lyon, W. S., and Miller, F. J.: Forensic Application of Neutron Activation Analysis. *Isotopes and Radiation Technology* 4(4), Summer 1967.

CHAPTER 56

William J. Curran is Frances Glessner Lee Professor of Legal Medicine at Harvard University and Chairman of the State Medicolegal Investigation Committee of Massachusetts. Professor Curran writes regularly for the *New England Journal of Medicine* and teaches at the Medical School, Law School, and School of Public Health at Harvard. He was formerly Robert R. Utley Professor of Legal Medicine and Director of the Law-Medicine Institute of Boston University. He also served as Assistant Professor of Law and Government and Assistant Director of the Institute of Government at the University of North Carolina. Professor Curran is the author of several books in the medicolegal field including *Law, Medicine and Forensic Science* (with E. D. Shapiro); *Trauma and the Automobile; The Doctor as a Witness;* and *Medicolegal Proof in Litigation.* He is an Associate Editor of the *American Journal of Law and Medicine* and was formerly Medicolegal Editor of the *Massachusetts Law Quarterly.*

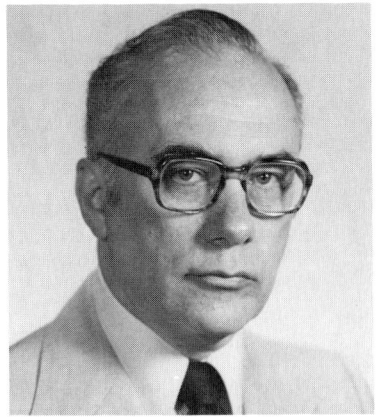

COURTROOM PRESENTATION OF FORENSIC SCIENTIFIC EVIDENCE

William J. Curran, J.D., LL.M., S.M.Hyg.

FORENSIC SCIENTISTS AND THE COURTS

The literature of judicial administration and courtroom presentation of expert testimony seems largely to ignore the overall field of forensic science while concentrating attention upon its separate parts: from forensic pathology to forensic psychiatry, from toxicology to criminalistics, from polygraph technology to questioned documents examination. Like the Cheshire Cat of Lewis Carroll, it often seems composed of unconnected parts, but with no whole body.

There are some fine commentaries on the general issues of scientific proof in the judicial system.[1] Many of these concern medical evidence, but most of the articles and books provide a wider scope in both basic science and technological fields.

As was pointed out earlier, the term "forensic," as used in this text, means "of the court." Actually, any kind of scientific data presented in court is being used in a forensic sense. Thus a geneticist, a physicist, or a pharmacologist called as a witness to give an expert opinion about his field is, on that occasion, a forensic scientist. However, he or she is not a specialist in the field of forensic science. The specialist deals with a scientific subject which is either exclusively or very frequently utilized in law enforcement and judicial systems. Such a specialist may actually appear in court only infrequently, but his or her evaluations and reports are regularly used in legal controversies, police investigations, and court proceedings.

EXPERT OPINION IN THE COMMON LAW SYSTEM

The common law system requires that most opinion evidence be presented by the parties as adversaries rather than be gathered by the courts in an impartial manner. Moreover, the courts are quite minimal in their interpretation of the standard for "expertness." The expert is merely a person who has knowledge beyond that of the ordinary jury member. Thus the American courts have never encouraged the development of forensic medical and scientific experts. If anything, the common law system has worked against the concentration of court advice or consultation in any small group or groups. Only in recent years have the various forensic specialty organizations, on their own, begun to move effectively toward certification.

SCIENTIFIC EVIDENCE: RULES OF ADMISSIBILITY

The liberal and open acceptance of "expert" testimony and opinion is in direct contrast to a very strict attitude toward accepting scientific proof based on tests and technical procedures. This firmly entrenched attitude results from a deep distrust in the Anglo-American common law of non-testimonial evidence. It is said that "machines can't be cross-examined" in the traditional way, and therefore their credibility cannot be challenged by the lawyers and the judges who rule over the contest grounds. It is feared that the simple, unsophisticated jurors will be unduly impressed by scientific techniques and may allow these machines to replace them in their assigned functions of weighing the evidence and judging the credibility of the testimonial witnesses. The most feared technical tests of all have been those which deal directly with human credibility: the polygraph and "truth serum."

Two issues are presented whenever scientific proof is submitted to the courts. The first is the issue of admissibility. The second is the issue of the relative weight to be given the evidence once it is admitted.

The initial issue of admissibility is put to the trial judge, not to the jury. The judge must decide whether the scientific test or procedure has received adequate general acceptability or endorsement within the scientific community to be considered reliable.[2] The most famous case setting forth this principle was decided in 1923 in a Federal court. In *Frye v. United States*,[3] the court held:

> Just when a scientific principle crosses the line between the experimental and the demonstrable stages is difficult to define. Somewhere in this twilight zone the evidential force of the principle must be recognized, and while the courts will go a long way in admitting expert testimony deduced from a well-recognized scientific principle or discovery, the thing from which the deduction is made must be sufficiently established to have gained general acceptance in the particular field to which it belongs.[4]

This single case has had a widespread and chilling effect on scientific proof in the decades since it was decided. Some scientific-technical advances, such as photography, have been admitted relatively quickly and have been utilized effectively, except where the characterization of the pictures as gruesome or indecent has prevented admissibility.[5] Radiology was also accepted fairly rapidly, and x-ray pictures,[6] along with photographs, are still the most heavily utilized scientific products in the American court system.

Some technological advances are admitted into court as a part of expert opinion, particularly medical opinion, which might not otherwise have met the Frye case standard if they had been forced to stand alone. Various laboratory tests have been relied upon by physicians, chemists, hematologists, and toxicologists without perhaps even being mentioned by name in the reports or oral opinions presented in court. In other situations, the results of a clinical test may be accepted without question because of the high standing and prestige of the medical expert. He or she is trusted to have screened out "unreliable" techniques and to have come to court with an opinion strengthened by his or her overall experience and judgment. Justice Oliver Wendell Holmes thus characterized expert testimony in the late nineteenth century. A physician was testifying on whether a person found dead in a fire had suffered consciously before death. The physician had no personal experience with such cases, but had read the literature of the field and formed his opinion in part on his reading. Justice Holmes ruled the opinion admissible, concluding,

> . . . his general competence as an expert seems not to have been questioned . . . when one who is competent on the general subject accepts from his experience as probably true a matter of detail which he has not verified, the fact gains an authority it would not have had from the printed page alone, and, subject perhaps to the exercise of some discretion, may be admitted.[7]

This is a common attitude of the courts, and it covers many situations. The liberality of the expert-opinion rule escorts much scientific data into court on the coattails of the highly respected authority. I wrote of a case[8] where the California Supreme Court admitted a psychiatric evaluation based in part on the technique of narcoanalysis, even though the use of the technique alone as "truth serum" to gain admission of the actual statements of the patient probably would have been strongly resisted and excluded from evidence.[9]

Many of the techniques of forensic science cannot ride this protective cloak of the medical or other high-prestige expert. (Persons with doctoral degrees are particularly esteemed in court, along with full professors from well-known local or national universities.) The weaker presentations tend to contain some or all of the following elements:

1. The presenter of the results is a technician with little or no advanced scientific training.
2. The presenter is not legally licensed and rarely has even a certificate of competence from a generally well-respected professional group or educational institution.
3. The presenter does not understand the underlying scientific principles upon which his machine is supposed to be based.
4. The witness who is available to testify concerning the scientific acceptance and reliability of the technique is often its inventor or a close collaborator with the inventor, or has a financial interest in the method, or runs the only school for training technicians in the field.
5. Proof of the scientific acceptance of the technique is severely limited by one or both of the following factors:
   a. the technique is used only in forensic science applications for law-enforcement agencies, investigations, and courts;
   b. the witness is the inventor and only user of the technique.

Any experienced forensic scientist will recognize some or all of the foregoing points; they usually have the deep scars to prove it. Technicians have been abused in court, accused of bias, ridiculed concerning their training, and accused of out and out fraud and chicanery, all by implication from the elements given above.

The most frequently attacked specialized technique in this class has been the polygraph. It is not surprising that the evidence offered in the Frye case was based upon the polygraph. The defendant in a murder case offered his own polygraph results in his own defense. The polygraph was rejected in 1923, and has suffered a similar fate in most courts ever since. Ironically, in a later review of the Frye case by an author interested in issues of scientific proof and the polygraph, it was found that the defendant Frye was released some years after his conviction when another person confessed to the murder.[10]

The first three points above are being dealt with more effectively in recent years as technicians are being selected and trained better and as programs for the licensing of technicians are being instituted. Numbers are still too small to move toward public licensing at the state level; the move is more toward national accreditation by special boards composed of the leaders of the groups. Recent court cases on the polygraph have endorsed these moves in the field.

The last two points in the list above are particularly difficult for techniques exclusively designed for use in the law-enforcement and judicial systems. How are these discoveries to gain "general acceptance" in the outside scientific community where they are not used and where suspicion and prejudice are often attached to "cops and robbers" technology? The more liberal political groups, often very well represented in scientific and academic circles, tend to react negatively to procedures which may help the police and the prosecuting arms of the state. It is not realized that these techniques are also extremely useful to provide objective proof of innocence.

The most difficult situation of all under the last two points above is the use of still experimental techniques of a forensic scientific nature, or the conduct of an experiment in the courtroom. Under the Frye rule, the first type of technique is generally excluded. On the other hand, the courts do allow many courtroom-performed experiments.[12] Care must be taken to make the experiments representative of what is at issue in the case. Moreover, the party presenting the experiment runs the risk that the test, always perfectly executed out of court, will "go wrong" in court. There seems to be a pernicious tendency in court to prove the everlasting validity of "Murphy's law"—what can go wrong will go wrong. Judges rarely, if ever, give the experimenter a second chance in court.

There are exceptions to the rule on use of still experimental techniques where no other method of proof is available. The most recent application was in the famous Coppolino murder trial in New Jersey, during which a toxicologist was allowed to offer evidence based upon a new test developed by him for the purposes of the case to detect the existence of succinylcholine chloride in the corpse of the alleged murder victim. The toxicologist testified that, based on his own new test, he found abnormal amounts of a breakdown product of succinylcholine in the body. The defense fought vigorously against admission of the testimony. The upper court found that the trial judge had not abused his discretion in admitting the test results and the expert opinion of the forensic toxicologist.[13]

If readers are interested in earlier history of admission of evidence of experimental techniques in poison cases, there is a rich literature of European cases in the field, particularly from the nineteenth century.[14]

PRELIMINARY MATTERS ON ADMISSION

In addition to the substantive issue of scientific acceptability and reliability, there are other preliminary steps to the submission of the results of scientific tests or exhibits in court. These are generally called "laying the foundation" for admission. Usually, the issue is the matching up of the data presented with the party or parties involved, or with the scene which is depicted in a photograph. A witness is usually required to provide this "connecting" evidence or identification. The best witness is usually the technician who performed the test, or the photographer who took the pictures. He or she can testify that the test was done or that the photograph was taken of the party in the litigation. When the picture is of an accident or crime scene, any persons who were actually present at the scene can give an opinion as to whether the picture is a "true representation" of the scene as they saw it. This opinion makes it unnecessary to call the photographer. Thus a forensic pathologist can lay the foundation for photographs taken during an autopsy, even though a photographer actually operated the equipment.

On many tests, the procedure is more complex. The witness must describe the procedure used to mark the particular specimen, or plate, or graph, and then identify that mark with the party in question. This is necessary when the exhibit itself cannot be identified on its face with the person involved.

Closely related to the above is the issue of offering evidence on the chain of custody of a specimen or piece of evidence where there is any danger of its contamination, alteration, or misidentification. In the criminal system, with crime laboratories and medicolegal laboratories as well as police, coroners, and medical consultants all involved, the chain of evidence issues are often pressed very closely and observed to the letter in trial courts. The time of laboratory technicians is often taken up with courtroom appearances of a brief nature which should either be handled by out of court dispositions or not raised at all. Nevertheless, in serious criminal cases where every minor point is heatedly contested, these matters still seem to occupy the time of the adversaries. Methods of marking evidence and maintaining the chain and escort of evidence are discussed in other chapters of this text.

THE WEIGHT OF THE EVIDENCE

The second point mentioned earlier concerning scientific proof was the relative weight to be given the data once received by the fact finder. There is a belief that scientific data generally has greater weight than testimonial evidence for several reasons: (1) it is considered more objective; (2) it is considered less biased than interested witnesses called by the parties; and (3) it is considered less fallible or subject to honest error than eyewitness observations or human memory of the same events. These points overlap in the minds of most people and result in a general feeling of greater reliability for scientific proof over testimonial statements by lay people, or even expert opinions of witnesses who seem to offer only subjective evaluations—"my experience" or "my clinical judgment"—as the basis for their testimony.

Judges and lawyers are aware of these tendencies, and they generally resent them. Legally trained minds value testimonial evidence and trust vigorous cross-examination to expose its weaknesses. They feel that the richer parties in litigation can purchase "science" and prostitute it in the courtroom with no jurors the wiser. In instructing juries, judges often try (by using a disparaging manner or tone of voice) to bring the scientific evidence into parity (or less) with the testimonial evidence. Great injustices have resulted. Perhaps the most famous case was the paternity suit against Charles Chaplin, the late actor and film artist extraordinary, in which the undisputed blood-test evidence excluded Chaplin as the father. The trial judge allowed the case to go to the jury on the basis of the "equally persuasive" testimony of the plaintiff that Chaplin was the only man who had had sexual intercourse with her at the relevant times. Incredibly enough, the appellate court upheld the judges's instructions and the verdict that Chaplin was the father.[15] Just in case readers should assume this case an anomaly, a peculiarity of the California courts in dealing with rich movie stars, the same result was reached and upheld 6 years later in New Jersey.[16] For blood-test evidence in paternity and other identification cases, it took legislative action and the Uniform Act on Blood Tests to curb this tendency of the trial-court judges and their juries. Under the statutes, when the results of the test indicate that the man is not the father, the test results are now conclusive. Where the results indicate compatibility, they must be interpreted as such and cannot alone support a finding that the accused man is the father. Similar problems were presented concerning the weight to be given alcohol-blood levels and breath tests for alcohol. Statutes now create presumptions of alcoholic "influence" at certain levels and binding inferences or evidentiary support for a "drunkenness" finding, based upon the test results alone. No amount of testimonial "denial" is allowed to offset the test results. In effect, the defendant is convicted of the objective fact of having had such an alcohol level in his blood stream, rather than of the more subjective effect the alcohol may or may not have had on his driving.

POSSIBILITIES, PROBABILITIES, AND PROOF

Science deals with mathematical probabilities. Some tests can *exclude* even possibilities (as in the blood-test identification cases above) of an event or a connection. It is much more difficult to prove a positive finding scientifically. Moreover, many tests cannot produce *any* reliable results on certain people or under certain circumstances. The polygraph is an example of the latter at its present stage of development. Some individuals are not susceptible to reliable testing at the time of the demonstration.[17] Such people do not "fool" the machine; they merely do not respond to pretest material in such a way as to enable the trained technician to measure their reactions to stressful questions later in the examination.

Like other experts, the witness offering scientific test results is interpreting against a norm, and the score of the subject is given in relation to the norm. Further interpretation can be offered, and different experts may question the reliability of the test, its applicability to the particular subject, and its scoring criteria. Current controversies over scores on IQ tests are examples discussed in Chapter 31 of this book.

The courts have not developed mathematical standards of reasonable certainty. In fact, the less susceptible the matter is to being placed in a probability table, the more the courts seem willing to admit it on the basis of the willingness of the expert witness, to characterize it by adjectives and adverbs such as "most likely," "more likely than not," and "reasonably certain, based on current standards in the field." Thus most medical testimony on diagnosis and prognosis and most forensic pathology testimony on the cause, mechanism, and manner of death are devoid, quite intentionally, of mathematical formulas. Ironically, the application of tables is found in estimates of time of death, an area notoriously considered to be riddled with uncertainty (see Chapter 7). The same disenchantment is now found in clinical psychiatric evaluations of "dangerousness" (see Chapter 32).

Efforts to apply the calculus of probabilities to courtroom estimates of events have generally been a failure. Appellate courts become surprisingly sophisticated when reviewing the efforts of mathematical experts on the witness stand and usually find the experts to have failed to take into account the actual realities of the case at hand which should have had a bearing on their calculations. In addition, they have applied very strict rules of admissibility of the qualifications of these experts and the reliability of their calculus formulas. The most notorious case in this field has been *People v. Collins*,[18] decided in California. The use of the calculus of the witness was rejected. In addition to its attack on the actual calculation, the appellate court found that the jury was unable to cope with "the mystique of the mathematical demonstration." There have been many commentaries on these cases and on other similar ones, the best being by Tribe[19] and Ball.[20] A sociologist questioned trial judges about instructions to juries based upon mathematical formulations of probabilites and found them *almost unanimously opposed*.[21] There are writers who take a more positive view toward the use of probabilities in the courtroom.[22]

COURTROOM APPEARANCES

Other chapters in this text have provided suggestions on the style of courtroom testimony. The primary recommendations would seem to be (1) that the witness have a pretrial conference with the direct questioner to assure a complete, understandable, and truthful presentation, and (2) that the witness testify as impartially as possible, avoiding all appearances of bias or advocacy for any side in the litigation. All other suggestions seem secondary to these two key points.

On cross-examination, the forensic science witness should continue to maintain an appearance of impartiality and should avoid sparring or debating with the cross-questioning lawyer. Nevertheless, the technician or scientist should not abandon his or her position too quickly, merely to seem impartial. The position taken on direct testimony should be defended where it can be, and should be explained in lay terms where possible. The cross-examiner often tries to use other terms to characterize what the expert witness or technician has said on direct examination. For example, the following are contrasting characterizations commonly heard in court:

Direct Examination	*Cross-Examination*
reasonable certainty	inexact science
probability	possibility
hypothesis	theory
finding	opinion
test	experiment
apparatus	bag of tricks
polygraph	truth box
calculation	conjure up
consultant	paid employee

estimate of probability   speculation, guesswork
opinion   guesswork,
evaluation   and more guesswork!

Similar contrasting characterizations in regard to medical witnesses can be found in my earlier text[23] and in Simpson's[24] excellent handbook for the British courts. The cross-examiner's practices differ very little; they are highly adaptable to time and place. The appellate courts usually frown on mere word-games with the witnesses, unless the cross-examiners are able to secure substantively damaging admissions which they back up with independent evidence of their own.

REFERENCES

1. Boyd, A.: Judicial Recognition of Scientific Evidence in Criminal Cases. *Utah Law Rev.* 8:313–330, 1964; Kirk, E.: The Interrelationship of Science and the Law. *Buffalo Law Rev.* 13:393–415, 1964; Korn, J.: Law, Fact, and Science in the Courts. *Columbia Law Rev.* 66:1080–1111, 1966; Ormrod, R.: Scientific Evidence in Court. *Crim. Law Rev.* 1968 ed., pp. 240–250; Moenssens, A., and Inbau, F. E.: *Scientific Evidence in Criminal Cases.* ed. 2. Mineola Press, New York, 1978.
2. Strong, W. J.: Questions Affecting the Admissibility of Scientific Evidence. *U. Illinois Law Forum* 1–21, 1970.
3. *Frye v. U.S.,* 54 U.S. App. D.C. 46, 293 Fed. 1013, 1923.
4. *Ibid.,* p. 1014.
5. Scott, C. C.: *Photographic Evidence.* ed. 2. West Publishing Company, St. Paul, 1969.
6. Donaldson, S. W.: *Roentgenologist in Court.* Charles C Thomas, Springfield, Ill., 1954.
7. *Finnegan v. Fall River Gas Works,* 159 Mass. 311, 34 N.E. 523, 1893.
8. Curran, W. J.: Expert Psychiatric Evidence of Personality Traits. *U. Pa. Law Rev.* 103:999–1014, 1955.
9. Polen, J.: Admissibility of Truth Serum Tests in Court. *Temple Law Rev.* 35:401–420, 1962.
10. Wicker, D. H.: The Polygraphic Truth Test and the Law of Evidence. *Tenn. Law Rev.* 22:711–725, 1953.
11. *U.S. v. Redding,* 350 F. Supp. 90 (Mich. 1972); How Some Courts Have Learned to Stop Worrying and Love the Polygraph. *N.C. Law Rev.* 51:900-914, 1973; The Emergence of the Polygraph at Trial. *Columbia Law Rev.* 73:1120–1226, 1973; Reid, J. E., and Inbau, F. E.: *Truth and Deception.* ed. 2. Williams & Wilkins, Baltimore 1977.
12. Cleary, E. W. (ed).: *McCormick's Handbook of the Law of Evidence.* ed. 2. West Publishing Company, St. Paul, 1972, pp. 524–542.
13. *Coppolino v. State,* 223 So. 2d 68 (Fla. App. 1969); appeal dismissed, 234 So. 2d 120 (Fla. 1969); cert. denied, 399 U.S. 927 (1970); see also Bailey, F. L.: *The Defense Never Rests.* Stein & Day, Briarcliff Manor, N.Y., 1971.
14. Borowitz, A.: *Innocence and Arsenic.* Harper & Row, New York, 1977; Thorwald, J.: *The Century of the Detective.* Harcourt, Brace & World, New York, 1965; Saunders E.: *The Mystery of Marie LaFarge,* Crerke & Cockeran, London, 1951.
15. *Berry v. Chaplin,* 74 Cal. App. 2d 652, 169 P.2d 442, 1946.
16. *Ross v. Marx,* 24 N.J. Super. 25, 93 A. 2d 597, 1952.
17. Reid and Inbau, op. cit.
18. *People v. Collins,* 68 Cal. 2d 319, 438 P.2d 33, 66 Cal. Rptr. 497, 36 A.L.R. 3d 1176.
19. Tribe, L.: Trial by Mathematics. *Harvard Law Rev.* 84:329–340, 1971.
20. Ball, S.T.: The Moment of Truth: Probability Theory and Standards of Truth. *Vanderbilt Law Rev.* 14:807–820, 1961. See also Conrad, R.: The Expert and

Legal Certainty, *J. Forensic Sci.* 9:445–452, 1964; Ennis, B. J., and Litwack, T. R.: Psychiatry and the Presumption of Expertness: Flipping Coins in the Courtroom, *Cal. Law Rev.* 62:693–752, 1974.
21. Simon, R.: Judges' Translations of Burdens of Proof into Statements of Probability. *Trial Lawyers' Guide* 13:29–35, 1965.
22. Finkelstein, J.E., and Fairley, F.J.: A Bayesian Approach to Identity Evidence. *Harvard Law Rev.* 83:489–520, 1970; Kingston, J.: Probability and Legal Proceedings. *J. Crim. Law Police Sci.* 57:93–102, 1966; Liddle., J.: Mathematical and Statistical Probability as a Test of Circumstantial Evidence. *Case Western Reserve Law Rev.* 19:254–265, 1968.
23. Curran, W.J.: *Tracy's The Doctor as a Witness.* ed. 2. W. B. Saunders, Philadelphia, 1965.
24. Simpson, K.: *A Doctor's Guide to Court.* ed.2. Butterworth, London, 1967.

INDEX

ABDOMEN, autopsy opening of, 114–116
Abortion, 219–220
Abrasion
  blunt-force trauma and, 346–367
  medicolegal significance of, 367
Abuse
  alcohol. See Alcohol abuse.
  child, 236–240. See also Pediatric death.
  controlled substances and, 915–921
  drug. See Drug(s).
Academic programs in forensic toxicology, 1043–1044
Accident vs. suicide, 845–846
Accidental multiple death, 631–633
Addiction, 879–880
Additives, food, 1000–1101
Adipocere, 164
Adipose tissue and drug concentration, 1059
Administrative issues in criminal cases, 1005–1006
Admissibility
  preliminary matters of, 1283
  rules of, 1280–1282
Adversary system of justice, 930–931, 993–995
Advertising, unethical, 45
Advocacy and truth, 36–37
Aerial applicator aircraft, 348–349
Age determination, 1134–1137
Agent or impartial expert, 749–750
Aggression, sexualization of, 538
Aircraft
  aerial applicator, 348–349
  air transport, 351–352
  fighter-type, 349–350
  light, 347–348
  rotary wing, 350–351
Aircraft death
  aerial applicator aircraft in, 348–349
  air transport aircraft in, 351–352
  autopsy in, 352–353, 358
  crash site investigation and, 344–346
    civil aircraft accidents in, 344–346
    military aircraft accidents in, 346
  crop dusters in, 348–349
  death certification in, 358–359
  documentation in, 353–355
    photographs in, 353–354
    roentgenograms in, 354–355
  fighter-type aircraft in, 349–350
  general considerations in, 352–353
  investigation of, 338–361
    authority in, 343–344
    developing principles in, 339–342
    ejection seats in, 341
    human factors concept in, 341–342
    pilot error in, 340
  light aircraft in, 347–348
  magnitude of problem of, 342–343
  National Transportation Safety Board and, 343–344
  natural disease in, 357–358
  pathology in, 346–359
  patterns of injury in, 346–352
  rotary wing aircraft and, 350–351
  toxicology in, 355–357
    carbon monoxide in, 355

Aircraft death—*continued*
  drugs in, 355–356
  ethanol in, 355
  sample collection and processing in, 356–357
  vitreous humor in, 357
Akathisia, 898
Alcohol abuse, alcoholism and, 864–876, 882
  beverage control legislation and, 871–872
  civil commitment procedures in, 868–869
  client's bill of rights and grievance procedure in, 874
  criminal law and intoxication in, 866–868
  driving while intoxicated and, 870
  drunk-driving laws and, 870–871
  education in public schools and, 872–873
  funding treatment programs and, 874
  historical perspective in, 865–866
  industrial alcoholism programs and, 874
  insurance and, 873
  medical assistance and, 873
  supplementary security income and, 874
  treatment in, 888–889
Alcohol impairment
  automobile death and, 314–316
  blood level in, 121, 1011
  Widmark's formula in, 316
Alcohol testing, laboratory space for, 1027–1029
Alcohol in treatment of dangerousness, 793–794
Alcoholic Beverage Control Agency, 872
Alcoholics, legal rights of, 868
Algor mortis, 154–156
Allergy, drug, 597–598
Allopathic definition of health, 911
Ambivalences and suicide, 183
American Academy of Forensic Sciences, 104, 1002
  Code of Ethics of, 34–36
American Board of Forensic Psychiatry, 648
American Journal of Criminology and Police Science, 22
American Jury, The, 931
Amicus curiae of Roman law, 2
Ammunition types, 433–435
Amnesia, 759
Amotivational syndrome, 885, 890
Amphetamines
  abuse of, 882–883
  history of prescription of, 917–918
Amputations, 731
Anaphylaxis, 597–598
Ancient origins, 1–2
Ancillary services in drug abuse, 891–892
Anesthesia deaths, 600–601
Animal toxins, 1112–1113
Anoxia, 249

Antabuse, 889
Antagonist, narcotic, 887–888
Anthropologic identification of dead body, 1219
Anthropology
  forensic, 993
  forensic dentistry and, 1134
Antianxiety drugs, 899–900
Antidepressant drugs, 899
  abuse of, 885–886
Antipsychiatry attitude, 965
Antipsychotic drugs, 897–898
Antisocial disorders, 900–902
Antisocial personality, 798–813
  biological substrates of, 808–810
  dangerous, 703–704
  defective role-taking in, 804–808
  early formulations of, 800–804
  etiologic perspectives in, 804–808
  heterogeneity of, 810–811
  sociological and psychiatric variables in, 805–808
Arachnoid, 390–392
Arsenic, 1059
Arson
  concealed homicide and, 296–298
  fraud and, 298–300
Artifactual fractures, 282
Artifactual hematoma, 282
Asphyxia
  autoerotic, 584–587
  in children, 226–228
Asphyxial deaths, 248–266
  autopsy findings in, 253–258
  death certification in, 261–262
  drowning in, 262–264
  foreign body inhalation in, 254–255
  hanging and strangulation, 255–258
  investigation and reporting of, 258–261
    autopsy report in, 261
    gathering evidence in, 260
    interpretation of autopsy reports in, 259–260
    key clinical findings in, 260
    laboratory tests in, 260–261
    scene investigation in, 258–259
  mechanical, 249–252, 254
  scuba death in, 264–266
  smothering and gagging in, 254
  sudden death mechanisms, 252–253
  traumatic, 258
Aural examination of voices, 1160–1163
Aural material preparation, 1178–1179
Autoerotic asphyxia, 584–587
Automatism, drug, 846–847
Automobile death
  cause of crash in 309–310
  crash phase investigation in, 320–323
    impact decelerative forces formula in, 320
    skid mark formula in, 320–321
  history of, 307–308
  homicide by motor vehicle in, 330–331
  intentional crashes in, 330
  investigation and preventive programs in, 306–337

Automobile death—*continued*
  post-crash fire hazard in, 329–330
  post-crash medical care in, 331–333
  pre-crash factors in, 310–319
    alcohol impairment in, 314–316
    carbon monoxide in, 317
    driver skill in, 310–311
    drug impairment in, 316–317
    human factor in, 310–314
    natural disease in, 318–319
    postmortem series on, 319
    sudden death in, 318–319
    vehicular interior in, 310
  prevention of, 334–335
  problems in, 308–309
  tort liability in, 333–334
Autopsy
  aircraft death and, 352–353, 358
  asphyxial death and, 253–258, 261
  clothing in, 111–112
  crime laboratory examination and, 120
  diagnosis and, 119
  disposition of evidence and, 118
  drowning and, 263–264
  drug abuse and, 1125–1130
  external evidence of injury and, 112–113
  external evidence of therapy and, 113–114
  external examination in, 112
  firearms injury and, 465–467
  head in, 116
  heart disease, trauma, death and, 187–195
  histopathology in, 122–123
  hospital vs. medicolegal, 129–130
  internal evidence of injury and, 117
  internal evidence of therapy and, 117
  internal examination in, 116
  medical vs. medicolegal, 480–481
    clinical correlation in, 482
    clothing examination in, 481
    external examination elements in, 481–482
    external and internal evidence of injury in, 482
    provisional anatomic diagnoses in, 482
    toxicologic examination in, 482
  medicolegal
    blunt force injury and, 484–488
    common mistakes during, 124–125
    examples in, 482–488
    fundamental procedures of, 110–126
    practical perspectives of, 128–138
    special problems in, 123–124
    stab wound and, 483
  medicolegal vs. hospital, 129–130
  medicolegal photography in, 125–126
  neck in, 115
  opening thorax and abdomen in, 114–116
  organ system description in, 117–118
  pattern of injuries and, 113
  parenteral drug abuse and, 1123–1124
  photographs and, 119
  pneumothorax and, 114
  pregnancy and, 114
  preservation of evidence in, 130–138
  protocol summary in, 119
  psychological, 845
  serologic or biologic examination in, 120–121
  specimens and samples to be recovered in, 118–123
  step by step procedure in, 115–116
  strangulation and, 115
  toxicologic examination in, 121–122
  trauma and, 479–488
Aviation accidents
  natural disease in, 357–358
  pathology in, 346–359
  toxicology in, 355–357

Barium enema, 603–604
Battered baby syndrome, 236
Baxstrom patients, 783–784
Beck, Theodoric R., 13
Bender-Gestalt test, 771
Bile, drug concentration in, 1058
Bill of rights, client's, 874
Binet tests, 767
Bioavailability and drug interaction, 595–597
Biochemical reactions in time of death, 157–160
Biological substrates of sociopathy, 808–810
Bite marks, 1146–1147
Black lung disease, 64
Bleeding by trauma, 390
Blood alcohol determination, 121, 1011
Blood loss determination, 389
Blood test evidence, 1284
Blunt force injury
  autopsy in, 484–488
  pediatric death and, 228–233
Board certification in forensic toxicology, 1045–1047
Body, exhumed, toxicologic examination of, 1071–1072
Body-cavity searches, 40
Body processing in fire death, 272–285
Body removal, 84–86
Brain
  contusion of, 373, 399–403
  coverings of, head injury and, 390–392
  drug concentrations and, 1059
Brain death, 143–149
  development of concept of, 143–145
  laws about, constitutionality of, 147–148
  medicolegal aspects of, 145–147
  time of death and, 148–149
  transplantation and, 146
Bullets
  death identification and, 1217
  types of, 433–435
Bumper fractures, 325–326
Burden of proof, 974–975
Burking, 579
Burn. *See also* Fire death.
  first-degree, 277
  flash, 278
  full-thickness, 278

Burn—*continued*
  partial thickness, 278
  psychiatric-legal problems and, 731
  second-degree, 277–278
  third-degree, 278

CADAVER organ donation, 624
Cadaveric spasm, 152
Cafe coronary, 254
Caliber determination by x-ray examination, 445–446
California Achievement tests, 768
California Association of Criminalists, 36
Cancer deaths and medical care, 605–607. *See also* Neoplastic disease.
  complications of therapy in, 607
  diagnosis delay in, 606–607
Capital punishment, 661
Carbon dioxide death, 632–633
Carbon monoxide deaths, 631–633
  aircraft, 355
  automobile, 317
  fire, 273–276, 301–303
  pediatric, 233–234
Cardiac arrest, 601–602
Cardiac conduction system, 195
Cardiomegaly, 189–192
Cardiomyopathy, hypertrophic, 192
Cardiovascular causes of sudden death, 196
Cardiovascular disease, 188
Causality in psychiatric-legal problems, 732
Central nervous system hemorrhage, 391
Cerebral fat embolism, 385
Cerebrospinal fluid and time of death, 157
Chain of custody, 558
Charge to jury, 946–948
Checkwriter identification, 1248
Chemical-involved death
  incidence of agents in, 1063
  pathologist in, 1118–1131
Chemline, 1044
Children
  abuse of, 236–240. *See also* Pediatric death.
    forensic dentistry and, 1145–1146
  drugs and, 900
  molestation of, 581-582
  psychiatric-legal problems and, 731
  sexual arousal to, 817–818
Children's Apperception Test, 776
Chlorpromazine, 897–898
Chopping wounds, 412–415
Christison, Sir Robert, 10
Chromatography
  gas, 1054
  thin-layer, 1053
Clean Air Act Amendments of 1970, 1101–1102
City, county, state government, medicolegal investigative system and, 70–71
Civil aircraft accidents, 344–346
Civil law and psychiatry, 720–736

Civil trial proceedings, 928–930
Clinical medicine and forensic pathology, 105–106
Clinical Use of Psychotherapeutic Drugs, 897
Clothing
  autopsy and, 111–112, 481
  firearms victims and, 446–451
  sharp instrument injury and, 413 414
Cocaine abuse, 883
Code of Bamberg, 6
Code of Hammurabi, 2
Code of Nuremberg, 41
Cold exposure death, 291–295
  ancillary studies in, 294–295
  body processing in, 292-294
  data correlation in, 295
  gathering information in, 292
Commitment procedures in alcoholism, 868–869
Common grave discovery, 639
Common knowledge, 964–965
Common law system and expert opinion, 1279–1280
Commonwealth of Massachusetts v. a Juvenile, 1202
Commonwealth of Massachusetts v. Lykus, 1173
Competency to manage one's affairs, 734
Competency screening test, 779
Competency to stand trial, 741, 750–758
Comprehensive Drug Abuse Prevention and Control Act of 1970, 1107–1109
Compression, 386, 389
Compurgation, 10
Conditional release, 792–793
Confessions, improperly obtained, 41–42
Confidentiality
  drug-abuse treatment and, 892–893
  medicolegal records and, 76–78
Congenital malformations, 598–599
Contact-range firearms wounds, 418–422
  mechanism of, 419
  muzzle imprint in, 421
  types of, 419–421
  varying factors in, 419
Contracts, 734
Controlled substances. *See also* Drugs.
  conflicting schools of medical thought about, 916–917
  cure-all psychoactive drugs and, 917–918
  drug abuse concepts and, 919–921
  FDA schedules of, 911–913
  freedom to prescribe, 906–915
  Harrison Act prosecutions and, 907–909
  legal context of, 906–915
    allopathic definition of health and, 911
    benefits to medical profession of, 910–911
    medical community's response to legal regulation of, 909–911
    medical/legal cooperation and consequences in, 911–915
  medical use, abuse, recreational use of, 915–921

Controlled substances—*continued*
  methadone maintenance and, 913–915
  postwar attitudes concerning, 909–910
  prescribing, physician's rights and responsibilities in, 904–925
Contusion
  brain, 399–403
  contracoup, 400
  deep tissue and organ, 373–375
  medicolegal significance of, 376
  superficial, blunt-force trauma and, 367–373
Conversion reaction, 724
Cooling, postmortem body, 154–156
Coordination in criminal cases, 1001–1002
Coronary artery in autopsy, 188–189
Corneal transplantation, 623
Coroner. *See also* Medical examiner.
  legal liability problems of, 59–61
  medical examiners and, 16–17
Correctional psychiatry, 676–719
Corrosive substance, 1094
Cost of crime laboratory, 1037
Cost-benefits for criminal justice system, 670–671
Cot death, 224–226
Counterfeiting, 1249–1252
Courtroom appearances, 1285–1286
Courtroom presentation of evidence, 490–506. *See also* Evidence.
  correcting examiner in, 500–501
  cross-examination and, 502–504
  demonstrative evidence in, 498–499
  direct examination and, 497–498
  direct interrogation and, 500
  distinguishing characteristics of death cases and, 491–492
  forensic pathologists as expert witnesses and, 495–496
  forensic scientific evidence and, 1278–1287
  general situations of, 496–497
  "gruesome" photography and, 499–500
  judicial proceeding types and, 504
  medical certainty and, 501–502
  medicolegal investigative system and, 68–69
  nonpartisanship in, 500
  preparation for trial and, 492–493
  pretrial consultation and, 494–495
  psychiatric and psycholegal, 962–987
  story to be told in, 493–494
  testimonial style and, 501
  voice identification and, 1181–1182
Covert sensitization, 791
Crash site investigation, aircraft, 344–346
Crib death, 224–226
Crime laboratory
  accessibility of, 1013
  administration of, 1020–1021
  air conditioning and heating in, 1018–1019
  alcohol level evaluation by, 1011
  asphyxial death and, 260–261
  case records of, 1033–1034
  communications system of, 1018
  cost and, 1037
  crime scene evaluation by, 1010–1011
  definitions and misconceptions of, 1009–1010
  director of, 1015
  document examination by, 1011, 1026
  drug identification by, 1011, 1024–1025
  emergency equipment in, 1020
  emergency power system of, 1018
  evidence handling procedures in, 1031–1033
  evidence receipt by, 1000
  evidence rooms in, 1019–1020
  fire death and, 285–286
  firearms and toolmarks and, 1011
  furnishings of, 1019
  gas and volatiles in, 1020
  hierarchy of, 1012–1013
  implied consent alcohol and drug testing in, 1027–1029
  integration of, 1014
  laboratory systems in, 1017–1020
  latent prints and, 1011–1012, 1029
  location of, 1016–1017
  need for, 1010
  operating procedures in, 1034–1036
  organization of, 1008–1038
  parent organization of, 1014
  parking facilities of, 1018
  personnel in, 1029–1031
  photography by, 1012, 1027
  physical facility of, 1015–1031
  plumbing in, 1019
  police sophistication and, 1013–1014
  procedures in, 1031–1036
  quality control measures for, 1047
  rape and, 557, 558–559
  records of, 1033–1034
  resources allocation and, 1001
  scene evaluation by, 1010–1011
  scientific classifications in, 1030–1031
  security in, 1017–1018
  serology and, 1012, 1025–1026
  service features of, 1010–1012
  size and sophistication of, 1014–1015
  special sectional needs in, 1020–1029
  specimens and samples for, 120
  teamwork in, 1000
  toxicology and, 1012, 1053–1065
  trace evidence and, 1012
  trace evidence and firearms and, 1021–1024
  transportation and, 1036
  utility of, 1013
  work records of, 1034
Criminal cases
  administrative and financial issues in, 1005–1006
  communicating results to users in, 1002–1003
  coordination with examiners in, 1001–1002
  defense attorney in, 1004
  evidence receipt by laboratory in, 1000

Criminal cases—*continued*
  evidence and testimony in, 1005
  forensic science and, 995–1006
  initial police response in, 995–996
  investigation in, 996–999
  laboratory resources allocation in, 1001
  laboratory teamwork in, 1000
  preparing case for court in, 1003–1004
  pretrial conferences in, 1004–1005
  routing evidence for analysis in, 999
  scientific investigation of, 17
  severity of, 934–935
  special outside expertise in, 1002
Criminal justice system
  cost benefits for, 670–671
  intoxication and, 866–868
  mental retardation and, 861–862
  rape and, 562–564
Criminal responsibility
  drugs and, 902–903
  psycholegal examinations and reports in, 758–759
Criminal trial proceedings, 928–930
Criminalist, 997
Criminalistics, identification and, 11–15, 992
Crop dusters, 348–349
Cross-examination, 502–504
  illustrative case of, 977–982
  techniques in, 972–973
Custodial institutions, 609
Cytotoxic reactions in drug allergy, 598

DANGEROUSNESS
  mental retardation and, 862
  predictive accuracy in, 783–786
    approaches toward increasing, 786–790
    base-rate information in case-specific decisions and, 788–789
    implications for treatment and, 782–797
    parole board prediction system and, 789–790
    social-environmental factors in, 787–788
  treatment implications in, 790–794
    alcohol and, 793–794
    conditional release in, 792–793
    desensitization techniques in, 791–792
Dates of historical significance, 19–24
De praestigiis daemonum, 4–5
De relationibus medicorum, 3–4
Death
  brain. *See* Brain death.
  definition and time of, 140–169
  mores for, 51–54
  pronouncement and certification of, 142
  sudden. *See* Sudden death.
  time of
    algor mortis and, 154–156
    biochemical reactions and, 157–160
    brain death and, 148–149
    early postmortem period and, 151–160
    estimation of, 150–151
    eye in, 156
    late postmortem changes and, 160–164
    livor mortis and, 153–154
    practical problems in, 80–82, 164–167
    rigor mortis and, 151–153
    serum and cerebrospinal fluid in, 157
    stomach contents and, 156–157
    supravital reactions and, 156
    vitreous humor and, 158–160
  unified concept of, 142–143
Death certificate, 78–80
Death certification
  aircraft death in, 358–359
  asphyxial death and, 261–262
Death investigation
  basic steps in, 270
  identification procedures in, 1206–1220
    anthropologic, 1219
    circumstance and, 1218–1219
    dental patterns and restorations in, 1211–1213
    fingerprints in, 1208–1210
    fingerprints on skin and, 1211
    footprints in, 1211
    frontal sinus pattern in, 1213
    less positive methods in, 1217–1218
    normal and abnormal bone comparisons in, 1213–1216
    pacemakers and, 1217
    palm prints and, 1211
    positive identification and, 1219–1220
    prostheses in, 1217
    reasons for, 1207
    skull suture and vascular grooves in, 1213
    tattoos and, 1216–1217
    wire sutures in, 1217
  medicolegal, 490–506
Decipherment, 1252–1258
Declaration of Tokyo, 41
Defendant characteristics, 935–937
Defense attorney
  criminal cases and, 1004
  medicolegal investigative system and, 70
Defense wound, 415
Delaney clause, 1101
Deliberations in trial process, 945–946
Delinquents, defective, 702
Denial and suicide, 182
Dentistry, forensic, 993, 1132–1149
  age determination and, 1134–1137
  anthropology and, 1134
  bite mark examination and, 1146–1147
  child abuse and, 1145–1146
  death investigation and, 1211–1213
  personal habits and, 1138–1139
  race determination and, 1137–1138
  radiologic evaluation and, 1141–1144
  sex determination and, 1140–1141
  sinus examination and, 1144–1145
  skeletal identification and, 1148–1149
Dependence, psychological, 880
Dependency reaction, 725–727
Dermal irritation, 1093–1094
Desensitization techniques, 791–792

Detective and criminal investigation, 996
Detoxification, 887
Diagnosis and autopsy, 119
Disability in psychiatric-legal problems, 732–733
District attorneys, 69–70
Document(s), questioned
    alterations and decipherment in, 1252–1258
    burnt, charred, water-soluble paper restoration in, 1258–1259
    crime laboratory examination by, 1011
    dating of, 1260–1261
    examination of, 993, 1222–1269
    forensic examiner of, 1224–1225
    handwriting comparison in, 1225–1234
    indented writing decipherment in, 1259–1260
    laboratory space for, 1026
    latent fingerprints on paper in, 1266
    machine copy examination in, 1263–1264
    mechanical impression comparison in, 1240–1252
    paper examinations and comparisons in, 1260
    preservation of evidence in, 1266
    scope of field of, 1223–1224
    sequence of writings in, 1265
    signature comparison in, 1235–1240
Document examiner as expert witness, 1267
Documentation in aircraft death, 353–355
Donation, cadaver organ, 624
Draw-A-Person test, 778
Driving and intoxication, 314–316, 870
Drowning, 262–264
    autopsy findings in, 263–264
    childhood, 241
    pathophysiology of, 263
    victim and environment in, 262–263
Drug(s). *See also* Controlled substances; Toxicology, forensic.
    abuse of. *See* Drug abuse.
    aircraft death and, 355–356
    antianxiety, 899–900
    antidepressant, 899
    antipsychotic, 897–898
    children and, 900
    criminal responsibility and, 902–903
    deaths due to, 1122–1131
    identification of
        crime laboratory in, 1011
        laboratory space for, 1024–1025
    impulse or antisocial disorders and, 900–902
    ingestion and inhalation of, 1125
    inherent toxicity of, 1067
    mainlining, 1123
    nonscheduled, prescription of, 1110–1111
    psychoactive, 896–903
    regulation of, 1107–1111
        commercial offenses and, 1110
        Comprehensive Drug Abuse Prevention and Control Act of 1970, 1107–1109
        fraudulant offenses and, 1110
        prescription of nonscheduled drugs and, 1110–1111
        scheduling in, 1108–1109
    skin-popping, 1122–1123
    stimulant, 900
    suicide and, 173–174
    testing of, laboratory space for, 1027–1029
    therapeutic and toxic concentrations of, 1067
    tolerance, to 1065–1066
    toxic and lethal levels of, 1130–1131
    types of fatalities and, 1122
Drug abuse
    ancillary services in, 891–892
    automobile death and, 316–317
    controlled substances and, 919–921
    fatal
        autopsy and sample collection in, 1125–1130
        ingestion in, 1127–1128
        pulmonary findings in, 1126–1127
        skin-popping and mainlining in, 1128–1130
    parenteral, 1122–1123
        autopsy findings in, 1123–1124
        skin in, 1123–1124
        visceral changes in, 1124–1125
    patterns of, 880–886
        alcohol and, 882
        amphetamines and, 882–883
        antidepressants and, 885–886
        cocaine and, 883
        hallucinogens and, 884–885
        lithium and, 886
        major tranquilizers and, 885
        marijuana and, 885
        minor tranquilizers and, 881–882
        opiates and, 883–884
        sedatives and, 880–882
        sleeping pills and, 881
        stimulants and, 882–883
        tobacco and, 886
    psychological dependence and, 880
    treatment in, 886–891
        confidentiality in, 892–893
        hallucinogen and, 890
        inhalant abuse and, 890–891
        marijuana and, 890
        narcotic addiction and, 887–888
        programs for, 878–894
        sedatives, minor tranquilizers, alcohol and, 888–889
        stimulant and, 889–890
    trends in, 893
Drug allergy, 597–598
    anaphylaxis in, 597–598
    cytotoxic reactions in, 598
    serum sickness in, 598
Drug automatism, 846–847
Drug interaction and bioavailability, 595–597
    absorption in, 596
    displacement from albumin carrier sites and, 596
    liver enzyme induction and, 596–597

Drunk-driving laws
  enforcement of, 870–871
Dura mater, 390
Dyskinesia
  tardive, 898
Dyslexia
  tests for, 769
Drug reactions and drug related deaths, 593–599
  analysis of problem of, 594–595
  congenital malformations in, 598–599
  drug allergy in, 597–598
  drug interaction and bioavailability in, 595–597
  magnitude of problem of, 593–594

ECOLOGICAL toxicology, 1084
Education in forensic pathology, 98–99
Educational achievement tests, 768–770
Ejection seats, 341
Elderly patient deaths, 609–610
Embalming, 52
  arterial, 52
  trochar, 52
Embolism
  fat, 385
  pulmonary, 608
Emergency medical technicians, 63
Emotional release in suicide, 182
Endocardial fibroelastosis, 221
Enema, barium, 603–604
Environmental regulations, 1101–1107
  Clean Air Act Amendments of 1970, 1101–1102
  Federal Insecticide, Fungicide, and Rodenticide Act, 1106
  Federal Water Pollution Control Act of 1972, 1104
  National Water Quality Standards Program, 1104
  Occupational Safety and Health Act of 1970, 1102–1103
  Resource Conservation and Recovery Act, 1106
  Solid Waste Utilization Act of 1976, 1106
  Toxic Substances Control Act, 1103–1104
  toxicity and, 1080–1081
Environmental toxicology, 1084
Epidemic death, 630
Epidural space, 390
Epilepsy, 1120–1121
Esquirol, Jean, 8
Ethanol and aircraft death, 355
Ethical inquiry, 29
Ethical standards, 28–48
  enforcement of, 45–46
  excessive publicity and, 38–39
  forensic pathology and, 43–45
  forensic science and, 31–36
  general, 34–36
  general interprofessional, 32–33
  impartiality in public agencies and, 37–38
  improperly obtained confessions, 41–42
  investigational procedures and, 39–41
  monopoly and legal enforcement, 31
  professional, 30–31
  psychiatric and psychological issues in, 42–43
  specific, 33–34
  truth and advocacy in, 36–37
  unethical advertising and publicity in, 45
Ethyl alcohol
  blood concentration of, 1072
  childhood poisoning and, 233
  forensic toxicology and, 1072–1074
  postmortem concentrations of, 1073
  urine concentration of, 1072
  vitreous humor concentration of, 1072
Evidence
  autopsy disposition of, 118
  autopsy preservation of, 130–138
    photography in, 130–131
  blood test, 1284
  common pitfalls of, 1272–1273
  courtroom presentation of, 490–506. *See also* Courtroom presentation of evidence.
  forensic toxicologist and, 1082
  handling procedures for, 1031–1033
  laboratory receipt of, 1000
  manner and style of giving, 970–971
  possibilities, probabilities, and proof in, 1284–1285
  preparation and organization of, 1271–1272
  presentation of, 1005
  psychiatric, 669–670
  rooms for, 1019–1020
  routing for analysis of, 999
  search for, 998–999
  scientific, rules of admissibility of, 1280–1282
  "show it to me cold," 132–134
  statistical aspects of, 1270–1276
  technician for, 997
  testimony statistics and, 1273–1276
  "the best case," 137–138
  trace, 1012
  weight of, 1283–1284
  "what's it all about?" 134–137
Evidentiary chains, 131–132
Examination
  external, autopsy and, 112
  psycholegal, 738–760
Examiner as agent or impartial expert, 749–750
Exhibitionism, 826–838
  case studies in, 830–836
  classification in, 835–836
  common law definition of, 827–828
  history of, 828–829
  patient management in, 829–830
  patient population characteristics in, 830–831
  psycholegal aspects of, 830
  therapy in, 832–834
    masturbation and, 832–833
    pain inducement and, 833
  treatment in, 829–830
    anticipation in, 834
    follow-up in, 835

Exit wounds. *See* Outshoot or exit wounds.
Expert witness
    common law system and, 1279–1280
    document examiner as, 1267
    forensic pathologists as, 495–496
    forensic toxicology and, 1048–1049
    impartial, 749–750
    outside, 1002
External evidence of injury, 112–113
External evidence of therapy, 113–114
Extraalveolar air syndrome, 265
Extradural space, 390
Eye. *See also* Vitreous humor.
    irritants to, 1096–1097
    time of death and, 156
    transplantation of, 623

FAMILY and suicide, 181–184
FDA drug schedules, 911–913
Federal Insecticide, Fungicide, and Rodenticide Act, 1106
Federal Water Pollution Control Act of 1972, 1104
Female, sex-related death of, 578–580
Fighter-type aircraft, 349–350
Figure drawing test, 778
Financial issues in criminal cases, 1005–1006
Fingerprints
    death identification and, 1208–1210
    finger removel in, 1210
    laboratory space for, 1029
    latent, 1011–1012
    on paper, 1266
    postmortem difficulties with, 1208–1209
    on skin, 1211
    technique in, 1209
Fire death, 271–286
    body processing in, 272–285
        artifactual fractures in, 282
        artifactual hematoma in, 282
        carbon monoxide saturation in, 273–276
        cause of death in, 282–285
        concealed homicide and, 272–273
        cutaneous reaction to heat and flame in, 276
        injury and disease in, 276–282
        percentage total body surface and, 276–277
        pugilistic attitude in, 279–280
        was victim alive or dead? 273–276
        who is burned victim? 273
        why didn't victim escape? 285
    carbon monoxide level in, 301–303
    concealed homicide in, 296–298
    delayed, 285
    gathering information concerning, 271–272
    identification problems in, 298–300
    incomplete investigation in, 295–296
    laboratory and x-ray studies in, 285–286
    scene investigation in, 272
Fire department, 63
Firearms
    blunt and sharp instruments and, 362–489

crime laboratory and, 1011
examination room and, 1023
trace evidence and, 1021–1024
Firearms injury, 415–472
    alteration of gunshot wounds in, 452–454
    ammunition types in, 433–435
    autopsy facilities for, 465–467
        equipment in, 466
        personnel in, 466–467
        place in , 465–466
        x-ray equipment in, 466
    clothing of victims in, 446–451
        examination techniques in, 451
        medicolegal importance of, 450–451
    contact-range wounds in, 418–422
    description of, 462–465
        medicolegal, 464–465
        physician's, 462–464
    long-range wounds in, 425–428
    medium-range wounds in, 423–425
    misconceptions in, 467–472
    missile velocity in, 431–433
    nonwounding area telltales in 451–452
    outshoot or exit wounds and, 428–430
    range of fire determination in, 416–418
    residue in, 454–459
    residue on hands of suspect in, 459–461
        flameless atomic absorption for, 460
        neutron activation for, 460
        paraffin test for, 460
    residue on victim and wound of entrance in, 461–462
    short-range wounds in, 423
    shotgun wounds in, 435–443
    substances discharged in, 415–416
    x-ray examination of, 444–446
        caliber determination in, 445–446
        reasons for, 444–445
        surprise missiles in, 445
Flameless atomic absorption and firearms residue, 460
Floppy mitral valve disease, 192
Florida accident, 328–329
Florida v. Otero, 1172
Fluid overload death, 608
Fluorocarbon toxicity, 1093
Fluoroalkanes, 1093
Foam cone, 403
Food additives, 1100–1101
Food Additive Amendment, 1100–1101
Food poisoning death, 630
Foodborne disease, 1113
Footprints, 1211
Foreign body inhalation, 254–255
Forensic anthropology, 993
Forensic dentistry. 993
Forensic medical expert pool concept, 75–76
Forensic pathology. *See* Pathology, forensic.
Forensic science
    American beginnings of, 13–17
        medical examiners and coroners in, 16–17
        medicolegal decline in, 14
        twentieth century, 14–16

Forensic science—*continued*
  criminal cases and, 995–1006
  emergence of, 9–17
    American beginnings of, 13–17
    forensic toxicology in, 10
    identification and criminalistics in, 11–13
  ethical codes in, 31–36
  specialty areas in, 992–993
    criminalistics, 992
    forensic anthropology, 993
    forensic dentistry, 993
    forensic pathology, 992–993
    forensic toxicology, 993
    questioned documents examination, 993
  team approach in, 990–1006
Forensic Sciences Foundation, 105
Forensic scientists and courts and, 1279
Forgery, signature, 1235–1238
Fouling, 423
Fracture, 381–386
  artifactual, 282
  bumper, 404
  compound or open, 381–382
  fat embolism in, 385
  forensic importance of, 383
  healing of, 383–384
  medicolegal significance of, 383
  pathophysiologic effects of, 384–385
  propensity to, 382
  simple, 381
  skull, 385–386
  x-ray demonstration of, 382–383
Frontal sinus pattern, 1213
Frostbite, 293
Frye v. United States, 1202
Funeral directors
  medicolegal investigative system and, 71–72
  objectives of, 52

GAGGING, 254
Gastrointestinal tract disorders, 223
Gates-McKillop Reading Diagnostic Tests, 769
Genitals, trauma and mutilation of, 577–578
Gilmore Oral Reading Test, 769
Glass specimens, 1274–1275
Goddard, Calvin, 21–22
Goodenough Draw-A-Person Test, 766
Grievance procedure and alcoholism, 874
Gross, Hans, 17
Guardianship
  mental retardation and, 860–861
  psycholegal examinations and reports in, 745–749
Guilt complex test, 1199–1200
Gunshot wound. *See* Firearms injury.

HABILITATION and mental retardation, 857–858
Hallucinogen abuse, 884–885
  treatment for, 890
Halothane, 600

Halstead-Reitan Neuropsychological Test, 771
Hand stamp identification, 1249
Handbook of Psychiatry Therapy, The, 897
Handwriting
  comparison of, 1225–1234
  disguised, 1233–1234
  fundamental divergent characteristic in, 1225
  individuality and bases of identification, 1225–1227
  natural variation in, 1226–1227
  standards of comparison in, 1227–1233
    collected, 1232–1233
    court-ordered, 1229–1232
    dictated, 1228–1228
Hanging, 255–258
Harmonic motion, 1155–1156
Harrison Narcotic Act, 906–909
Hazard ratings in toxicity, 1080
Head and autopsy, 116
Head injury, 390–405
  brain contusion in, 399–403
  coverings of brain and, 390–392
  epidural hemorrhage in, 392
  hyperextension in, 397–399
  patterns of injury in, 404–405
  subarachnoid hemorrhage in, 396–399
  subdural hemorrhage in, 392–395
Health, allopathic definition of, 911
Health departments
  death investigation and, 616
  location of, 617–618
Heart
  contusion of, 375
  weight of, 189–192
Heart disease, trauma, death and, 186–206
  autopsy procedures in, 187–195
    cardiac conduction system examination in, 195
    cardiomegaly and, 189–192
    coronary artery and, 188–189
    myocardial examination in, 192–195
  cardiovascular disease classification in, 188
  diagnosis of, 196
  scene investigation, historical data in, 195–203
Heat exhaustion, 290–291
Heat and flame, cutaneous reaction to, 276
Heat stroke
  death in, 290–291
  in nursing home, 300–301
Helicopters, 350–351
Helmet regulations, 323–325
Hematoma
  artifactual, 282
  epidural, 392
  subdural, 392–395
Hemorrhages
  ball, 402
  blunt-force trauma in, 387–389
  central nervous system, 391
  epidural, 392
  estimation of blood loss in, 389
  hypertension and, 389

Hemorrhages—*continued*
  predisposing conditions in, 390
  subarachnoid, 396–399
  subdural, 392–395
Hepatitis, serum, 604–605
Hesitation marks, 174, 415
Heterogeneity of sociopathy, 810–811
Highway design, 334–335
Hippocratic Oath, 30
Histopathology, 122–123
Historical review of correctional psychiatry, 678–681
History and development, 1–26
  amicus curiae of Roman law, 2
  ancient origins, 1–2
  contemporary conditions in, 18–19
  emergence of forensic science, 9–17
  medicolegal specialization, 6–9
  methods of proof, 5–6
  Middle Ages, 2–5
  scientific criminal investigation in, 17–18
  seventeenth and eighteenth centuries, 5
  significant dates in, 19–24
Hittite Code, 2
Homicide
  childhood, 242–245
  concealed
    fire in, 272–273
    fire death and, 296–298
  detection of, 56
  motor vehicular, 330–331
  multiple, 633–636
    scene investigation in, 633–634
    suicide and, 634–636
  sex-related, 580–581
Homicide-suicide pacts, 184
Homosexuality, pedophilia and, 821
Homosexually related deaths, 582–584
Hospitals and medicolegal investigative system, 72–74
Hospital death. *See also* Medical care death.
  nosocomial infections and, 607–609
  nursing home and, 616–617
Hot liquid death, 286–289
Hot objects death, 286–289
Household products, pediatric death from, 235–236
Human factors concept in aircraft death, 341–342
Human rights and mental retardation, 858–860
Humanistic aspect of law as justice, 666–668
Hypertension and hemorrhage, 389
Hyperthermia
  malignant, 601
  systemic, 290–291
Hypostasis, postmortem, 153–154
Hypothermic death, 291–295

Iatrogenic injuries, suspicious, 590
Identification and criminalistics, 11–13
Identification procedures in death investigation, 1206–1220
Imhotep, 1
Immunity law for medical examiners, 58
Impact decelerative forces formula, 320
Impartiality in public agencies, 37–38
Impulse disorders, 900–902
Incarceration, 685–687
Incised wounds, 406
Income, supplementary security, 874
Incompetency to stand trial, 699–700
Incomplete sentences test, 778–779
Index Medicus, 593
Individualization in law as justice, 664–666
Industrial alcoholism programs, 874
Industrial illnesses, 727
Industrial toxicology, 1085–1087
Information access in product labeling, 1097–1098
Ingestion of drugs, 1125, 1127–1128
Inhalant abuse, 890–891
Inhalation
  drug, 1125
  food, 608
  testing, 1092–1093
Injury
  internal evidence of, 117
  pattern of, 113
  previous, suicide and, 850
Inmate experience, 683–687
  jail experience and, 683–684
  prison experience and, 684–687
Insanity, not guilty by reason of, 700
Insects, late postmortem and, 164
Insect toxins, 1112–1113
Institutionalization of retarded, 857–858
Institutionalized and elderly patients, 609–610
Instruments and firearms, 362–489
Insurance
  alcoholism and alcohol abuse and, 873
  medicolegal investigative system and, 64–66
  suicide and, 847–849
Intelligence
  evaluation of, 765–766
  quotient, 767
  testing of, 766–768
    Binet tests in, 767
    Goodenough Draw-A-Person Test in, 766
    Raven Progressive Matrices Test in, 766
    Wechsler tests in, 767–768
Intensive care unit incidents, 602–603
Interchange, theory of, 12
Intercousre, anal and oral, 559
Internal evidence of injury, 117
Internal evidence of therapy, 117
International Association of Coroners and Medical Examiners, 104
Interspeaker variability, 1160
Interview data in psychological testing, 770
Intestinal contents of drug concentrations, 1059
Intoxication
  criminal law and, 866–868

Intoxication—*continued*
  driving and, 870
  pathological, 882
Intraspeaker variability, 1160
Investigation of criminal cases
  criminalist in, 997
  detective in, 996
  evidence search in, 998–999
  evidence technician in, 997
  health departments and, 616
  medical examiner in, 997–998
  preservation in, 998
Investigational procedures, 39–41
Iowa Tests of Basic Skills, 768
Irritants, 1094
  eye, 1096–1097
  neoplastic disease and, 213–214
  primary, 1095–1096

JAIL
  experience in, 683–684
  medicolegal investigative system and, 68
  psychoses, 690–691
  suicide in, 695–697
  why work in one? 711
Jesness Inventory, 774–775
Journal of the Water Pollution Control Federation, 1106
Judge in trial process, 946–948
Judge trial vs. jury trial, 931–934
Jury and trial process
  adversary process in, 930–931
  alternative approaches to organizing research in, 928
  charge to jury and, 946–948
  civil and criminal trial proceedings and, 928–930
  defendant characteristics and, 935–937
    physical attractiveness in, 936–937
    psychological attractiveness in, 935–936
  deliberations in, 945–946
  future research in, 938–941
  judge in, 946–948
  jury in, 931–935
    Kalven and Zeisel study and, 931–934
    severity of punishment and crime and, 934–935
  jury size and decision rules in, 937–941
  lawyers in, 948–950
  psycholegal research and, 954–955
  psychological perspectives of, 926–961
  review of research findings in, 930–953
  sequestration in, 944–945
  six vs. twelve member juries in, 937–938
  unanimous vs. nonunanimous verdicts in, 938
  voir dire in, 941–944
  witness in, 950–953
Jury trial vs. judge trial, 931–934
Justice
  administration of, 654–674
  adversary system of, 993–995
  cause of, psychiatry and, 664
  law as

humanistic aspect of, 666–668
individualization in, 664–666

KALVEN and Zeisel study, 931–934
Kinetic energy formula, 432–433

LABELING, product, 1091–1098
Laboratory. *See* Crime laboratory.
Laceration, 375–381
Langer's lines, 408
Law
  civil, psychiatry and, 720–736
  conflict with forensic psychiatry and, 671–673
  humanistic aspect of, 666–668
  individualization in, 664–666
  medicolegal investigative system and, 62–63
  mental retardation and, 854–863
  objective and subjective theory of, 664–666
  rape and, 525
Law Enforcement Assistance Administration, 1037
Lawyers in trial process, 948–950
Lead intoxication, 236
Legal considerations in rape, 513–516
Legal enforcement, monopoly and, 31
Legionnaire's disease, 61
Lethality scale, 178–179
Liability, product, 1098–1100
Liability insurance, 16
Life stage, rape and, 519–520
Light aircraft, 347–348
Lithium, 886, 899
Litigation, 973–974
Liver
  drug concentration and, 1058
  drug interaction and, 596–597
  hemangioendothelioma of, 605
Livor mortis, 153–154
Locard, Edmond, 12
Lombroso, Cesare, 9
Long-range firearms wounds, 425–428
Lucid interval, 392
Lung lesions, 222

MACHINE copy examination, 1263–1264
Machine stamp identification, 1249
Mainlining drugs, 1128–1130
Make-A-Picture Story test, 777
Malingering, 730
  psycholegal examinations and reports in, 759
Malpractice suits, 734–735
  suicide and, 850–852
Manie sans delire, 801
Manslaughter, vehicular, 330–331
Marijuana abuse, 885
  treatment of, 890
Maryland Post Mortem Examiners Law, 87–90
Mastery needs, 537
Masturbation
  death during, 576–577
  exhibitionism and, 832–833

Mechanical impression comparison, 1240–1252
  checkwriters in, 1248
  hand stamps in, 1249
  machine stamps in, 1249
  printed matter in, 1249–1252
  typewriting in, 1240–1247
  word processors in, 1247–1248
Mechanical violence, 1121–1122
Medical care deaths, 588–613
  adverse drug reactions and drug-related deaths in, 593–599
  anesthesia and, 600–601
  approach and analysis of, 589–592
  cancer and, 605–607
  cardiac arrest in, 601–602
  drug involvement in, 591
  institutionalized and elderly patients and, 609–610
  intensive care unit incidents and, 602–603
  medical and hospital personnel in, 591
  physician involvement in, 591
  researching medical literature and, 592–593
  surgical care and, 599–600
  suspicious iatrogenic injuries and, 590
  transfusion reactions and serum hepatitis in, 604–605
  x-ray procedures and, 603–604
Medical certainty, 501–502
Medical examination in rape, 555–557
Medical examiner, 20, 997–998. *See also* Coroner.
  coroners and, 16
  establishment of, 54–55
  immunity law for, 58
  legal liability problems of, 59–61
Medical Jurisprudence of Insanity, The, 14
Medical literature, researching, 592–593
Medical report form for rape, 565–569
Medical schools, 66–68
Medical societies, 63–64
Medico-Legal Society of New York, 16
Medicolegal death investigation, 490–506
  city, county, state government and, 70–71
  courts and, 68–69
  defense counsel and, 70
  district attorneys and, 69–70
  emergency medical technicians and, 63
  fire department and, 63
  funeral directors and, 71–72
  government support and protection of, 56–59
  hospitals and, 72–74
  insurance companies and, 64–66
  jails and prisons and, 68
  law enforcement groups and individuals and, 62–63
  legal provisions of, 58
  legal source for, 54–56
  medical schools and, 66–68
  operational aspects of public, 51–94
  operational goals of, 53
  operational interfaces of, 61–75
  practitioners of medicine and, 64
  professional medical societies and, 63–64
  relatives and friends of deceased and, 74–75
  service and civic organizations and, 71
Medicolegal officer, 55
Medicolegal records, 76–78
Medicolegal specialization, 6–9
Medium-range firearms wound, 423–425
Medline, 593, 1044
Menard 18, 784
Mental age, 767
Mental retardation and law, 854–863
  categories of, 855–856
  criminal justice system in, 861–862
  dangerousness and, 862
  definitional concepts in, 855–856
  guardianship and, 860–861
  human rights and, 858–860
  institutionalization in, 857–858
  legal issues in, 856–857
  prisoners and, 692–693
  right to treatment or habilitation in, 857–858
  sterilization and, 859–860
Mental status examination, 645
Mentally ill offender, 682–683
Metastases, 210
Methadone maintenance, 887, 913–915
Methane death, 632–633
Metropolitan Achievement Tests, 768
Michigan Picture Story Test, 776–777
Middle Ages, 2–5
Military aircraft accidents, 346
Minnesota Multiphasic Personality Inventory, 774
Minnesota v. Trimble, 1172
Missile velocity, 431–433
  kinetic energy formula and, 432–433
  tissue and organ damage in, 432
  wounding and, 432–433
Mississippi v. Winton, 1173
MMPI, 774
Monopoly and legal enforcement, 31
Mores of death, 51–54
Motorcycle deaths, 323–325
Multiple death investigations, 628–639
  accidental, 631–633
  common grave discovery and, 639
  homicide in, 633–636
  medicolegal, 637–638
  natural death in, 629–631
  police and, 636–637
Mummification, 162–164
Muzzle imprint, 421
Myocardial examination, 192–195
Mycotoxins, 1113–1114
Myxomatous mitral valve degeneration, 192

NARCISSISM and rape assailant, 537
Narcotic(s). *See also* Controlled substances.
  addiction to, 887–888
  forensic toxicology and, 1074–1075
  pediatric death and, 235
Narcotic antagonist, 887–888

National Association of Medical Examiners, 104
National Interprofessional Code for Physicians and Attorneys, 32–33
National Transportation Safety Board, 343–344
National Water Quality Standards Program, 1104
Natural death, 1120–1121
  multiple, 629–631
Natural disease
  aircraft death and, 357–358
  automobile death and, 318–319
Neck autopsy, 115
Neoplastic disease
  medicolegal investigator in, 214
  relationship of trauma to tumors in, 210–211
  repeated minor trauma and chronic irritation in, 213–214
  significance of trauma in, 209–210
  trauma to abnormal tissue in, 213
  trauma and death related to, 208–216
  trauma to normal tissue in, 211–213
Neuropsychological tests, 771
Neurosis
  anxiety, 722–724
  hysterical (conversion type), 724
  traumatic, 722
Neutron activation and firearms residue, 460
Nonwounding area telltales in gunshot cases, 451–452
Nosocomial infections and hospital death, 607–609
Nursing home death, 609, 616–617. *See also* Medical care death.

OCCUPATIONAL Safety and Health Act, 1089–1091, 1102–1103
Offenders
  mentally abnormal, 698–699
  normal, correctional psychiatry and, 682
  sex, 700–701. *See also* Rape assailants.
Operational aspects of forensic psychiatry, 642–653
Opiate abuse, 883–884
Orfila, J.M.B., 10
Organ contusion, 373–375
Organic deficiency evaluation, 770–771
Organ disease in pediatric death, 222–223
Organ system in autopsy, 117–118
Organ transplant programs, 82
Outshoot or exit wounds, 428–430
  lack of, 430
  misconceptions about, 467
  shored, 429–430
  shotgun wounds and, 438
  variation in shape of, 428

PACEMAKERS, 1217
Pain, prolonged, 731
Palm prints, 1211
Paper
  burnt, charred, water-soluble restoration of, 1258–1259
  examinations and comparisons of, 1260
Paraffin test, 460
Parole board prediction system, 789–790
Paternity suits, 1284
Pathologists, forensic
  as expert witness, 495–496
  qualifications for, 1042–1043
Pathology
  anatomic, 97
  clinical, 97
  forensic, 98–108, 992–993
    certification in, 99–105
    clinical medicine and, 105–106
    crime-laboratory related areas and, 106–108
    ethical standards in, 43–45
    issues of, 150–151
    personal characteristics in, 108
    professional education in, 98–99
    qualifications for examination in, 100–102
    qualifications and training for, 97–108
    special areas of trauma and, 106
  subspecialities of, 98
Peak of tension test, 1199
Pedestrian fatalities, 325–328
Pediatric deaths, 218–246
  abortion in, 219–220
  asphyxia in, 226–228
  blunt force trauma in, 228–233
  carbon monoxide poisoning and, 233–234
  child abuse in, 236–240
  childhood drowning in, 241
  childhood suicide and homicide, 242–245
  endocardial fibroelastosis in, 221
  ethyl alcohol intoxication and, 233
  gastrointestinal tract disorders in, 223
  household products in, 235–236
  lead intoxication in, 236
  lung lesions in, 222
  narcotic abuse and, 235
  organ disease in, 222–223
  poisoning in, 233–236
  respiratory infections in, 222
  stillbirths in, 220
  sudden infant death syndrome in, 224–226
  sudden natural, 220–224
Pedophiles, 815
  classification of, 816
  heterosexual, 816
  homosexual, 816
Pedophilia, 814–824
  heterosexual, 818–820
  homosexual, 821
  preventive factors in, 816–817
  sexual arousal to children in, 817–818
  treatment in, 821–823
    behavioral approaches and, 821
    physiologic techniques and, 821
    traditional psychotherapy and, 821
Penis, trauma and mutilation of, 577–578
Pennsylvania v. Toppa, 1173
People v. Valdez, 1202
Personal injury, suits involving, 721–722

Personal injury—*continued*
  survivor syndrome in, 722
  traumatic neuroses in, 722
Personality functioning evaluation, 771–780
  objective approaches to, 774–775
    Jesness Inventory in, 774–775
    Minnesota Multiphasic Personality Inventory in, 774
  projective approaches to, 775–780
    competency screening test in, 779
    figure drawing in, 778
    incomplete sentences test in, 778–779
    Rorschach test in, 779–780
    Thematic Apperception Test in, 776–777
Personnel, crime laboratory, 1029–1031
Pharmacological Calvinism, 913
Phonetic code, 1158
Photography
  aircraft death and, 353–354
  autopsy and, 119
  crime laboratory and, 1012
  "gruesome," 499–500
  laboratory space for, 1027
  medicolegal, 125–126
  preservation of evidence and, 130–131
Physical attractiveness of defendant, 936–937
Pia mater, 390
Pilot error, 340
Pinel, Philippe, 7–8
Plant toxins, 1111–1112
Pneumothorax, 114
Poisons
  blood concentrations of, 1067
  childhood, 233–236
  food, 630
Police
  multiple death investigation and, 636–637
  response in criminal case of, 995–996
  sophistication of, 1013–1014
Polygraph technology, 1186–1204
  accuracy of, 1200–1201
    degree of, 1201
    percentage of definite decisions and, 1200–1201
  construction and number of tests and, 1192–1193
  control question technique in, 1188
  diagnosis in, 1193–1199
  diagnostic procedure and, 1187
  examination room in, 1188–1189
  examiner qualifications and training in, 1189–1190
  examiner testimony and, 1203–1204
  future legal status of, 1203
  guilt complex test in, 1199–1200
  historical development of, 1187–1188
  instrument in, 1188
  legal status of, 1202–1203
    Commonwealth of Massachusetts v. a Juvenile, 1202
    Frye v. United States, 1202
    People v. Valdez, 1202
    State v. Dorsey, 1202
  peak of tension test in, 1199

pretest interview in, 1190
rules of admissibility and, 1282
supplementary tests in, 1199–1200
test procedure in, 1190
test questions in, 1190–1192
  control, 1191
  irrelevant, 1190–1191
  relevant, 1191–1192
Postimmersion syndrome, 265–266
Postmortem examination
  crime laboratory examination and, 120
  definition of, 51
  histopathology in, 122–123
  late
    adipocere in, 164
    biology in, 164
    insects and, 164
    mummification in, 162–164
    putrefaction in, 160–162
    time of death and, 160–164
  serologic or biologic examination in, 120–121
  specimens and samples to be recovered in, 119–123
  time of death and, 151–164
  toxicologic examination in, 121–122
Postmortem purge, 160
Powder tattooing, 423–425
Pregnancy
  air embolus during, 578
  autopsy in, 114
Press and media, 82–83
Prescription of nonscheduled drugs, 1110–1111
Preservation in criminal cases, 998
Pretrial conferences, 1004–1005
Pretrial preparation, 967–968
Printed matter identification, 1249–1252
Prison experience, 684–687. *See also* Jail.
  authority and control in, 685
  temporal profile of incarceration in, 685–687
Prison psychoses, 691–692
Prison violence, 693–695
Prisoners
  classification of, 707–708
  difficult characters and, 697–698
  incompetency to stand trial and, 699–700
  jail psychoses and, 690–691
  mental retardation and, 692–693
  mentally abnormal offenders and, 698–699
  mentally ill, 688–689, 701–702
  not guilty by reason of insanity and, 700
  prison psychoses and, 690–691
  prison violence and, 693–695
  psychiatric problems of, 687–704
  psychiatric and psychological profiles of, 689–690
  sex offenders and, 700–701
  suicides and, 695–697
Probability in testimony statistics, 1273–1276
Probative value of forensic psychiatry, 645–646
Product labeling, 1091–1098

Product labeling—*continued*
  acute dermal toxicity and, 1094–1095
  corrosive substance and, 1094
  dermal irritation and, 1093–1094
  eye irritants and, 1096–1097
  highly toxic substance and, 1091–1092
  information access and, 1097–1098
  inhalation testing and, 1092–1093
  irritants and, 1094
  primary irritant substances and, 1095–1096
  product use and, 1098
  toxic substance and, 1092
Product liability, 1098–1100
Product use, 1098
Proof, historical methods of, 5
Prosecution
  rape and, 526
  sexual assault suspect and, 560–561
Prostheses, 1217
Protocol, autopsy, 119
Provisional anatomic diagnoses, 482
Psychiatric fact-finding, 658–659
  ethical issues of, 42–43, 659–664
Psychiatric involvement in legal settings, 643–644
Psychiatric profiles of prisoners, 689–690
Psychiatric and psychological evidence
  courtroom presentation of, 962–987
  criticisms of, 669–670
  general and special evaluations in, 966
  illustrative testimony in, 975–986
  judicial and legal practices in, 964–965
    common knowledge and, 964–965
    legal hostility and, 965
    weak standards for testimony and, 965
  state of art problems in, 963–964
  testimonial presentation in, 966–975
Psychiatric report to court, 976–977
Psychiatric-legal problems, 730–735
  amputations and, 731
  burns and, 731
  causality in, 732
  children and, 731
  competency to manage one's affairs and, 734
  contracts and, 734
  legal competency and, 733
  medical malpractice cases and, 734–735
  percentage of diability and, 732–733
  prediction and, 733
  prolonged pain and, 713
  scars and, 731
  sexual molestation and rape and, 732
  wills and, 733–734
Psychiatry
  administration of justice and, 654–674
  antisocial personality and, 805–808
  civil law and, 720–736
  correctional, 676–719
    as agent of change, 704
    classification of prisoner and, 707–708
    dangerous psychopaths and, 703–704
    defective delinquents and, 702
    definition of field, 678–683
    difficult characters and, 697–698
    future directions of, 682–683
    historical review of, 678–681
    incompetency to stand trial and, 699–700
    inmate experience and, 683–687
    jail psychoses and, 690–691
    mental retardation and, 692–693
    mentally abnormal offenders and, 698–699
    mentally ill offender and, 682–683
    mentally ill prisoner and, 688–689, 701–702
    normal offender and, 682
    not guilty by reason of insanity and, 700
    present scene in, 681–682
    preservation of therapeutic identity and, 709–711
    prison psychoses and, 691–692
    prison violence and, 693–695
    prisoner problems and, 687–704
    rehabilitation and, 705–709
    role of, 704–711
    sex offenders and, 700–701
    suicides in prisons and jails and, 695–697
    why work in prison? 711
  forensic
    capital punishment and, 661
    cause of justice and, 664
    clearer questions and more relevant answers in, 644–645
    conflict with law and, 671–673
    cost-benefits for criminal justice system and, 670–671
    ethical issues of fact finding in, 659–664
    fact-finding for legal purposes and, 658–659
    history and development of, 7–8
    mental status examination in, 645
    operational aspects, training, and qualifications in, 642–653
    probative value and, 645–646
    psychiatric involvement in legal settings and, 643–644
    qualifications and training for, 648–649
    security facilities and, 647–648
    toward standard for, 650–651
    statutory attempts to establish, 649–650
    structure and operation of, 646–647
Psychoactive drugs, 896–903
  classification of, 880
  cure-all, 917–918
Psychodiagnosis, 763–765
Psycholegal examinations and reports, 738–760
  amnesia and, 759
  competency to stand trial and, 750–758
  criminal responsibility and, 758–759
  examiner as agent or impartial expert and, 749–750
  ethical standards and, 42–43
  guardianship and, 745–749
  important elements of, 739–740

Psycholegal examinations and reports—*continued*
  malingering and, 759
  testamentary capacity and, 740–745
  ultimate questions and, 968–970
Psychological attractiveness of defendant, 935–936
Psychological autopsies, 845
Psychological dependence, 880
Psychological profiles of prisoners, 689–690
Psychological tests
  definition of, 764
  dyslexia and, 769
  educational achievement tests in, 768–770
  evaluation of intelligence and, 765–766
  intelligence testing in, 766–768
  interview data in, 770
  in legal settings, 762–781
  major areas of, 765–780
  neuropsychological tests in, 771
  organic deficiency evaluation in, 770–771
  personality functioning evaluation and, 771–780
  psychodiagnosis and, 764–765
  scores on, 764
Psychology of rape assailant, 532–551
Psychopathy. *See* Antisocial personality.
Psychophysiologic reaction, 725
Psychoses
  jail, 690–691
  prison, 691–692
Public agencies, impartiality of, 37–38
Public health aspects of medicolegal death investigation, 614–618
Public health deaths, 615–616
Public schools and alcohol education, 872–873
Publicity
  excessive, 38–39
  unethical, 45
Pugilistic attitude, 279–280
Pulmonary fat embolism, 385
Pulmonary findings in drug abuse, 1126–1127
Punishment, severity of, 934–935
Purge, postmortem, 160
Putrefaction, 160–162

QUALIFICATIONS
  in forensic pathology, 96–108
  in forensic psychiatry, 642–653
Quality control measures, 1047
Questioned documents. *See* Document(s), questioned.
Questiones medico-legales, 4

RACE determination, 1137–1138
Radiologic evaluation, 1141–1144
Range of fire, 416–418
Rape, 508–531
  aftermath of, 524
  agency investigation of, 554
  aggressive aim, 543–544
  anal and oral intercourse in, 559
  assessment of criminal justice system in, 562–564
  chain of custody and, 558
  community investigation of, 553–572
  counseling issues and, 521–527
    assault in, 525
    law enforcement in, 525
    medical concerns in, 525
    physical safety in, 526
    preparation for victim responses in, 526–527
    prosecution in, 526
    social support system in, 526
  crisis centers for, 522–523, 561–562
  definition of, 509
  divorced or separated woman and, 520
  dynamics of, 540–548
    classification in, 540
    theme of motivation in, 540–543
  examination in
    instruction sheet for, 564–565
    male, 570–571
  fantasies of, 510
  group, 511
  impulsive, 548
  incidence of, 509
  instruction sheet for (male), 569–570
  kit for medical examination in, 556–557
  laboratory analysis in, 558–559
  laboratory examination in, 557
  legal considerations in, 513–516
    consent in, 514–515
    corroboration in, 513
    defense and, 514
    judge vs. jury trial in, 515
  life stage considerations in, 519–520
  long-term consequences of, 520–521
  medical examination in, 555–557
  medical report form for, 565–569
  medicolegal considerations in, 527–529
  middle-aged woman and, 520
  mythology of, 510–512
  physical force in, 511
  psychiatric-legal problems and, 732
  race and, 511
  recommendations and considerations about, 527–529
  reported incidence of, 512
  serologic or biologic examination in, 120–121
  sex-aggression diffusion in, 546–548
  sexual aim, 544–546
  single young woman and, 519–520
  stress and, 516–519
    phases in, 517
    responses to, 518
  uncontrollable urge theory of, 510–511
  victim behavior in, 511
  victim's experience of, 510
  victims other than adult females and, 560
  victimhood and, 512
  violence and, 511–512
  woman with children and, 520
Rape assailant
  basic assumptions about, 534

INDEX

1305

Rape assailant—*continued*
  clinical evaluation of, 548-549
  developmental history of, 538–539
  examination of, 560
  outpatient management of, 549
  prognosis and treatment of, 548-551
  prosecution of, 560–561
  psychological functioning of, 532–551
    evaluation of, 534–535
    feelings about women and, 535–536
    impairment in healthy narcissism and, 537
    level of sexual development in, 536
    mastery needs and, 537
    reality testing in, 535
    sexualization of aggression in, 538
    sublimation defects in, 536–537
  residential treatment of, 549–551
Rapist. *See* Rape assailant.
Raven Progressive Matrices Test, 766
Ray, Isaac, 18
Reality testing, 535
Receiver-operating characteristics in voice identification, 1154
Records, medicolegal, 76–78
Recreational use of controlled substances, 915–921
Rehabilitation, 705–709
Reinsch test, 1063
Reiss, R.A., 12
Relatives and friends of deceased, 74–75
Release, conditional, 792–793
Reports, psycholegal, 738–760
Residue, firearm, 454–462
Resource Conservation and Recovery Act, 1106
Respirator lung, 603
Respiratory infections, 222
Rigor mortis
  cadaveric spasm and, 152
  time of death and, 151–153
Roentgenograms in aircraft death, 354–355
Role-taking, defective, 804–808
Rorschach test, 779–780
Rotary wing aircraft, 350–351
Routing, analysis of evidence and, 999

Sample collection in drug abuse, 1125–1130
Scars, 731
Scene alteration, 175–176
Scene examination, 84–86
  asphyxial death and, 258–259
  fire death and, 272
  heart disease, trauma, death and, 195–203
Scientific criminal investigation, 17–18
Scientific evidence
  courtroom presentation of, 1278–1287
  rules of admissibility of, 1280–1282
Scuba death, 264–266
Secondary gain, 729–730
Security in crime laboratory, 1017–1018
Security facilities and forensic psychiatry, 647–648
Sedative abuse, 880–882, 888–889
Semantic disorder, 804

Sensitization, covert, 791
Sequential Tests of Educational Progress, 768–769
Sequestration, 944–945
Serology, 1012
  laboratory space for, 1025–1026
  specimens and samples in, 120–121
Service and civic organizations, 71
Serum, time of death and, 157
Serum sickness, 598
Seventeenth and eighteenth centuries, 5
Sex determination, 1140–1141
Sex hanging, 584–587
Sex offenders, 700–701. *See also* Rape assailants.
Sex-aggression diffusion, 546–548
Sex-related deaths, 574–587
  autoerotic asphyxia, 584–587
  child molestation, 581–582
  female death during, 578–580
    burking in, 579
    suffocation in, 579
  homicide in, 580–581
  homosexual, 582–584
  sexual activity and, 576–577
  simultaneous, 580
  trauma and mutilation of genitals in, 577–578
Sexual arousal to children, 817–818
Sexual molestation, 732. *See also* Rape.
Sexualization of aggression, 538
Sharp instrument injury, 405–415
  chopping wounds in, 412–415
  clothing defects in, 413–414
  defense wound in, 415
  hesitation marks in, 415
  incised wounds in, 406
  stab wounds in, 408–412
  various weapons in, 413
Short-range firearms wounds, 423
  fouling in, 423
  shotgun in, 423
Shotgun wounds, 435–443
  barrel diameter in, 442–443
  exit wounds in, 438
  range in, 436
  rifled slugs in, 437–438
  short-range firearms wounds and, 423
  types of shot in, 436–437
  wad mark in, 438–441
Signature comparison, 1235–1240
  genuineness and forgery in, 1235–1238
  special signature cases in, 1238–1240
Sinus examination, 1144–1145
Skeletal identification, 1148–1149
Skid mark formula, 320–321
Skin in parenteral drug abuse, 1123–1124
Skin-popping drugs, 1128–1130
Skin transplantation, 623
Skull
  death identification and, 1213
  fracture of, 385–386
Sleeping pills, 881
Smothering, 254
Social-environmental factors in dangerousness, 787–788

Social support systems, 526
Sociology, antisocial personality and, 805–808
Sociopathy. See Antisocial personality.
Solid lung system, 603
Solid Waste Utilization Act of 1976
Soot tattooing, 1128
Sound spectra, 1155–1159
　complex, 1157
　frequency range in, 1159
　phonetic code in, 1158
　simple harmonic motion and, 1155–1156
Soundness of mind, 974–975
Speaker recognition
　objective methods of, 1168–1172
　　automatic systems of identification in, 1169–1172
　　semiautomatic systems of identification in, 1169
　subjective methods of, 1160–1168
　　aural examination of voices in, 1160–1163
　　visual examination of spectrograms in, 1163–1168
Speaker variability, 1159–1160
Specialty areas in forensic science, 992–993
Specimens
　autopsy, 118
　handling and storage of, 1061
　histopathology and, 122–123
　obtaining, 1056–1061
　postmortem examination and, 119–123
　serologic or biologic examination of, 121–122
　toxicologic examination of, 121–122
Spectrograph room, 1023
Spectrography, speech, 1163–1164
Spectrogram
　preparation of, 1178
　visual examination of, 1163–1168, 1179–1180
　　Kersta's studies and, 1164–1165
　　Tosi and associates studies in, 1166–1168
　　voiceprint identification in, 1164
　　Young and Campbell, Stevens and associates and Hazen in, 1165–1166
Spectrometer, mass, 1056
Spectrophotometry, ultraviolet, 1053
Speech
　acoustic parameters of, 1159–1160
　production of, 1154–1160
　　sound spectra and, 1155–1159
　　speech acoustic parameters and speaker variability in, 1159–1160
SRA Achievement Series, 769
Stab wounds, 408–412
　autopsy in, 483
　contusion with, 411
　external appearance of, 408–409
　wound patterns in, 409–411
Stanford Achievement Test, 769
Stanford Diagnostic Reading Tests, 769
START program, 703
State v. Dorsey, 1202

Steam death, 286–289
Sterilization in mental retardation, 859–860
Stillbirths, 220
Stimulant abuse, 882–883, 900
　treatment for, 889–890
Stomach contents
　drugs and, 1058
　time of death and, 156–157
Strangulation, 255–258
　autopsy in, 115
Stress, rape and, 516–519
Stress inoculation, 791
Stringham, James S., 13
Subdural space, 392
Sublimation defects, 536–537
Sudden death
　asphyxial, 252–253
　automobile death and, 318–319
　cardiovascular causes of, 196
Sudden infant death syndrome, 224–226
Suicide
　accident vs, 845–846
　assessment in, 852–853
　automobile drivers as, 330
　case studies in, 843–844
　certification of, 841–844
　childhood, 242–245
　common characteristics in, 177
　common law and, 841–842
　concealment of, 842
　crisis of, 180–181
　degrees of, 842–843
　drugs in, 173–174
　drug automatism and, 846–847
　family and, 181–184
　　ambivalences in, 183
　　assessment of, 183–184
　　denial in, 182
　　emotional release phase in, 182
　　general guidelines for, 181–182
　hesitation marks in, 174
　homicide-suicide pacts and, 184
　insurance and, 847–849
　investigation of, 170–185
　lethality scale in, 178–179
　long-range firearms wounds and, 426
　medical malpractice and, 850–852
　multiple homicide and, 634–636
　physical signs of, 172–176
　previous injury and, 850
　in prisons and jails, 695–697
　psycholegal aspects of, 840–853
　psychological autopsies in, 845
　psychological signs of, 176–180
　scene alteration in, 175–176
　self-immolation, 279
　suspicions of, 174–175
　worker's compensation and, 849–850
Supervisory qualifications in forensic toxicology, 1044–1045
Support facilities, 83–84
Supravital reactions, 156
Surgical care deaths, 599–600
Surprise missiles, 445
Survival syndrome, 722

Synergism, 1066

TATTOOS, 1216–1217
  powder, 423–425
Technicians in forensic toxicology, 1043
Testamentary capacity, 740–745
Testimonial issues in forensic toxicology, 1048–1049
Testimonial presentation, 966–975, 1005
  cross-examination techniques in, 972–973
  examinations for litigation and, 973–974
  manner and style of giving evidence in, 970–971
  practical suggestions in, 966–967
  pretrial preparation in, 967–968
  psycholegal issues and ultimate questions in, 968–970
  reasonable certainty of conclusions in, 968
  soundness of mind and burden of proof in, 974–975
  vulnerability of professional narcissist and, 971–972
Testimonial statistics, 1273–1276
Testimonial style, 501
Texas Medical Examiner Law, 90–94
Thematic Apperception Test, 776–777
Theory of interchange, 112
Theory and Practice of Voice Identification, 1174
Therapeutic community, 888
Therapeutic identity, 709–711
Therapy
  external evidence of, 113–114
  internal evidence of, 117
Thermal death, 268–304
  cold exposure in, 291–295
  fire in, 271–286
  heat exhaustion and heat stroke in, 290–291
  hot liquid, steam, hot objects in, 286–289
  scope of investigation in, 269–271
Thorax in autopsy, 114–116
Thorium dioxide, 605
Time of death. *See* Death, time of.
Tobacco abuse, 886
Tolerance
  drug, 1065–1066
  WHO definition of, 920
Toolmarks, 1011
Tort liability, 333–334
Toxic substances, 1079–1080, 1092. *See also* Drugs; Poisons.
  acute dermal, 1094–1095
  animal, 1112–1113
  environmental factors in, 1080–1081
  fluorocarbon, 1093
  hazard ratings and, 1080
  highly, 1091–1092
  insect, 1112–1113
  microbiological, 1113
  plant, 1111–1112
  stability of, 1067–1071
Toxic Substances Control Act, 1090, 1103–1104
Toxicologist, evidentiary responsibility and, 1082

Toxicology, 1012
  aircraft death and, 355–357
  analytic, 1119
  autopsy and, 482
  clinical, 1083–1084
  ecological, 1084
  environmental, 1084
  forensic, 10–11, 993
    academic programs in, 1043–1044
    board certification in, 1045–1047
    expert qualifications and testimonial issues in, 1048–1049
    general considerations about, 1050–1077
    general qualifications for, 1041–1042
    interpretation of results in, 1065–1075
      ethyl alcohol and, 1072–1074
      exhumed body and, 1071–1072
      individual condition in, 1066–1067
      inherent toxicity of drug and, 1067
      narcotics and, 1074–1075
      synergism in, 1066
      therapeutic and toxic blood concentrations in, 1067
      tolerance in, 1065–1066
      toxic substance stability and, 1067–1071
    laboratory considerations in, 1053–1065
      conventional equipment and methodology in, 1053–1056
      handling and storage of specimens in, 1061
      incidence of agents in chemical-involved deaths and, 1063
      limitations of, 1063–1065
      specimens in, 1056–1061
    laboratory quality control measures in, 1047
    pathologists and, 1042–1043
    qualifications and training for, 1041–1049
    screening in, 1061–1063
    specialty areas of, 1078–1117
    specimens and samples in, 121–122
    supervisory qualifications in, 1044–1045
    technicians in, 1043
  industrial, 1085–1087
  interpretative, 1119
  veterinary, 1087–1088
  wildlife, 1084
Toxline, 1044
Trace evidence, 1012
  firearms and, 1021–1024
Traffic fatalities, 334–335
Tranquilizer abuse, 881–882, 885
  treatment in, 888–889
Transfusion reactions, 604–605
Transplantation programs and medicolegal investigation, 620–627
  brain death and, 146
  donor types and, 621
  legal consent for cadaver organ donation in, 624
Transportation, 1036
Trauma

Trauma—*continued*
  abnormal tissue and, 213
  autopsy records in, 479–488
  blunt-force, 364–390
    abrasion in, 364–367
    combined abrasion, contusion, laceration in, 381
    compression in, 386
    deep tissue and organ contusion in, 373–375
    fracture in, 381–386
    hemorrhage in, 387–389
    laceration in, 375–381
    patterns of injury in, 404–405
    superficial contusions in, 367–373
  death by, 362–489
    firearms injury in, 415–472
    sharp instrument injury in, 405–415
  delayed death after, 474–476
  genitals and, sex-related death and, 577–578
  heart disease, death and, 186–206
  lethal, no external indication of, 474
  multiple weapon, 479
  natural disease and, 478
  neoplastic disease and, 208–216
  normal tissue and, 211–213
    postmortem vs. predeath, 472
  purposeful acts after, 476–477
  quantitation of, 477
  questions and answers on, 472–479
  repeated minor, 213–214
  resuscitation and, 474
  survival with medical assistance and, 478–479
  tumor and, 210–211
  wound alteration in, 479
  incompetency to stand, 699–700
  preparation for, 492–493
  psychological perspectives of, 926–961
Trial by ordeal, 15
Truth and advocacy, 36–37
Tumors and trauma, 210–211. *See also* Neoplastic disease.
Typewriting identification, 1240–1247
  single-element machine in, 1245–1247
  type-bar machine in, 1244–1245
  typewriter standards in, 1243–1244

ULTIMATE questions, 968–970
Uniform Alcoholism and Intoxication Treatment Act, 868–869
Uniform Anatomical Gift Act, 146
Uniform Brain Death Act, 146
Uniform Commercial Code, 1099
University instruction in medicolegal specialization, 6–9
Urine and drug concentration, 1059–1060

VERDICTS, 938
Veterinary toxicology, 1087–1088
Victimhood and rape, 512
Violence, prison, 693–695
Visceral changes in parenteral drug abuse, 1124–1125
Vitreous humor
  aircraft death and, 357
  drug concentrations and, 1060
  time of death and, 158–160
Voice identification
  closed tests in, 1154
  court appearances and, 1181–1182
  discrimination tests in, 1153
  field procedures in, 1175–1180
    recording exemplars of known suspects and defendants, 1177–1178
    recordings of questioned voice and, 1176–1177
    spectrogram and aural material preparation in, 1178–1179
    visual spectrogram examination in, 1179–1180
  fundamentals of, 1150–1184
  future of, 1183–1184
  history of, 1151–1152
  legal acceptance of, 1172–1175
    Commonwealth of Massachusetts v. Lykus, 1173
    Florida v. Otero, 1172
    Minnesota v. Trimble, 1172
    Mississippi v. Winton, 1173
    Pennsylvania v. Toppa, 1173
  methods of, 1153–1154
  model of voice communication in, 1152–1153
  open tests in, 1153–1154
  receiver-operating characteristic in, 1154
  speech production and, 1154–1160
  subject methods of speaker recognition in, 1160–1168
  training examiners for, 1182–1183
Voice communication, cybernetic model of, 1152–1153
Voiceprint identification, 1164
Voir dire, 929, 941–944
  conducting of, 942–943
  kinds of challenges in, 941–942
  what to look for during, 943–944
    demography in, 944
    nonverbal cues and, 944
    personality and, 943

WATER quality, 1105
Wechsler Tests, 767–768
Wad-cutter bullet, 433
Wad mark, 438–441
Weight of body, 112
Weyer, Johann, 4–5
Widmark's formula, 316
Wildlife toxicology, 1084
Wills, 733–734
Wire sutures, 1217
Witness in trial process, 950–953
  articulation and, 953
  expert. See Expert witness.
  external factors in, 952–953
  internal factors in, 950–951
Women, rape assailant feelings about, 535–536
Word processor identification, 1247–1248
Worker's compensation, 1088–1089
  claims of, 727–729
  laws of, 16
  suicide and, 849–850

Writing, indented, 1259–1260

X-RAY examination
   in firearms injury, 444–446, 466
   in fire death, 285–286

X-ray related death, 603–604

ZACCHIAS, Paulo, 4
Zootoxins, 1113

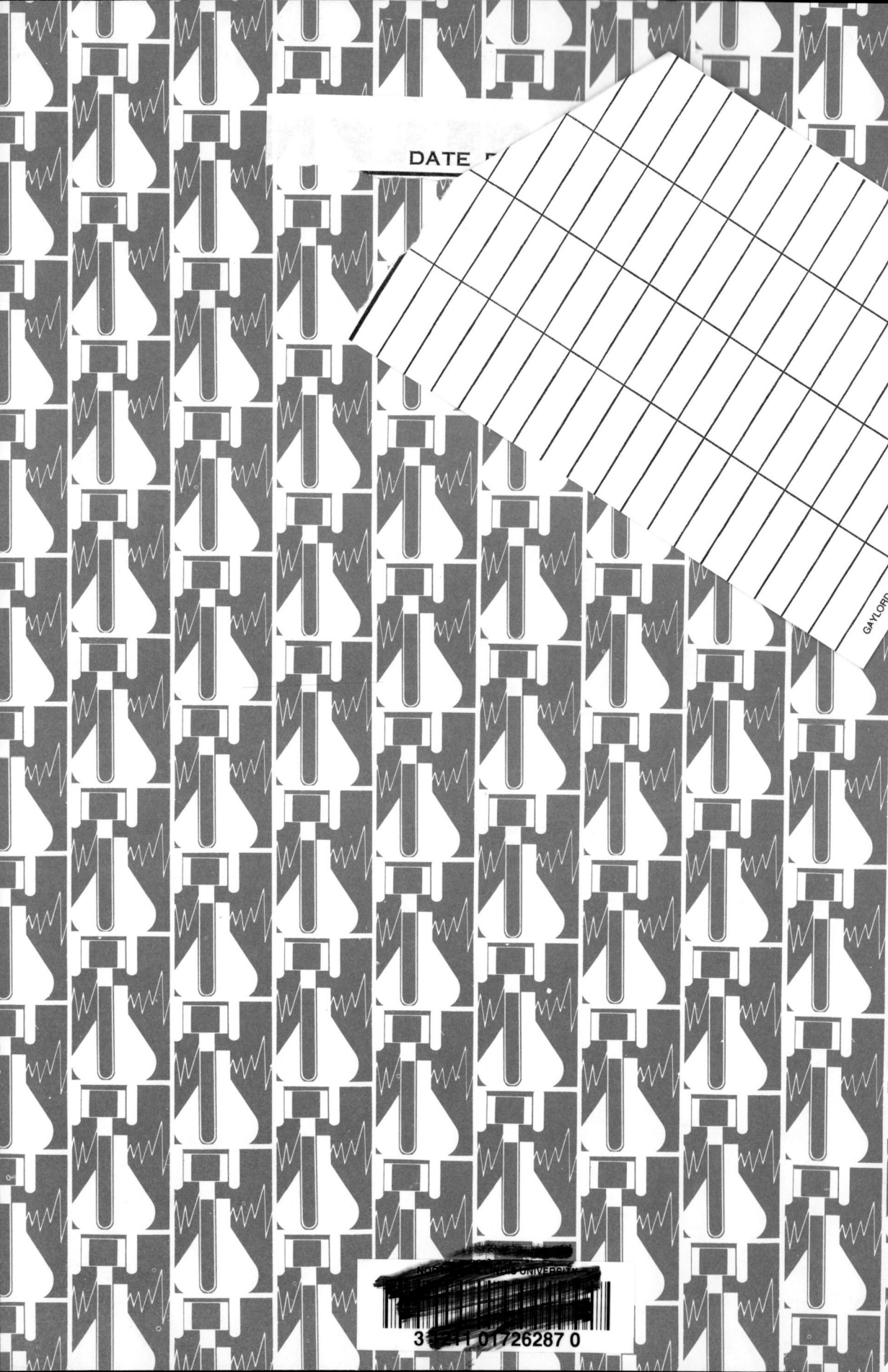